Praise for the
American Dietetic Association Complete Food and Nutrition Guide

"The gold standard, go-to guide for reliable, practical nutrition information."

—Ellie Krieger, MS, RD, bestselling author and host
of Cooking Channel's *Healthy Appetite*

"Jam-packed with practical eating and food safety tips."

—*USA Today*

"This book will appeal to those who want to know a little bit about everything in nutrition but don't have a science background."

—Chris Rosenbloom, PhD, RD, *The Atlanta Journal-Constitution*

"Of the five books closest to my keyboard, this guide is one of the most frequently used. A dynamite resource!"

—Antonia Allegra, CCP, executive director, Symposium for
Professional Food Writers; food, wine, travel author

"Bottom line, this is the best consumer nutrition book out. It's user-friendly, and it's complete. From a tidbit to a chapter, if it matters in nutrition, Roberta Duyff has included it. This book is worth its weight in gold."

—Keith Ayoob, EdD, RD, Associate Professor of Pediatrics,
Albert Einstein College of Medicine, New York City

"This nutrition bible is a good bet. This reputable resource separates fads from facts and answers questions from apples to zucchini, allergies to vegetarian diets."

—Nancy Clark, MS, RD, *Running Network* and *Sweat* magazine

"Turns a complicated subject into everyday practical information . . . a fun read."

—Claire Lewis, *Today's Health* and *Wellness* magazine

"Sorting out the constantly changing world of nutrition information, diets, and weight loss fads can be tricky, but this book provides all the facts in an easy-to-read format."

—Connie Diekman, MEd, RD, Director of University Nutrition, Washington University

"A remarkable reference."

—Graham Kerr, author, culinary expert, TV personality

eat right. Academy of Nutrition and Dietetics

AMERICAN DIETETIC ASSOCIATION

Complete Food and Nutrition Guide

4TH EDITION

Roberta Larson Duyff
MS, RD, FADA, CFCS

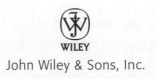

WILEY

John Wiley & Sons, Inc.

About the Academy of Nutrition and Dietetics

The Academy of Nutrition and Dietetics is the largest group of food and nutrition professionals in the world. As the advocate of the profession, the Academy's vision is to optimize the nation's health through food and nutrition.

For more information . . .

Visit the Academy's Web site at www.eatright.org, where you'll find nutrition news, tips, and information. Click on the "Find a Registered Dietitian" button to locate a dietetics professional in your area.

This book is printed on acid-free paper. ∞

Copyright © 2012 by the Academy of Nutrition and Dietetics. All rights reserved

Illustrations on part and chapter openers and on pages 345, 424, and 426 copyright © 2002 by Jackie Aher.

Published by John Wiley & Sons, Inc., Hoboken, New Jersey
Published simultaneously in Canada

Design and Production by Forty-Five Degree Design LLC.

No part of this publication may be reproduced, stored in a retrieval system, or transmitted in any form or by any means, electronic, mechanical, photocopying, recording, scanning, or otherwise, except as permitted under Section 107 or 108 of the 1976 United States Copyright Act, without either the prior written permission of the Publisher, or authorization through payment of the appropriate per-copy fee to the Copyright Clearance Center, 222 Rosewood Drive, Danvers, MA 01923, (978) 750-8400, fax (978) 646-8600, or on the web at www.copyright.com. Requests to the Publisher for permission should be addressed to the Permissions Department, John Wiley & Sons, Inc., 111 River Street, Hoboken, NJ 07030, (201) 748-6011, fax (201) 748-6008, or online at http://www.wiley.com/go/permissions.

The information contained in this book is not intended to serve as a replacement for professional medical advice. Any use of the information in this book is at the reader's discretion. The author and the publisher specifically disclaim any and all liability arising directly or indirectly from the use or application of any information contained in this book. A health care professional should be consulted regarding your specific situation.

For general information about our other products and services, please contact our Customer Care Department within the United States at (800) 762-2974, outside the United States at (317) 572-3993 or fax (317) 572-4002.

Wiley also publishes its books in a variety of electronic formats and by print-on-demand. Some content that appears in standard print versions of this book may not be available in other formats. For more information about Wiley products, visit us at www.wiley.com.

ISBN 978-0-470-91207-2 (paper); ISBN 978-1-118-17401-2 (ebk);
ISBN 978-1-118-17402-9 (ebk); ISBN 978-1-118-17403-6 (ebk)

Printed in the United States of America

10 9 8 7 6 5 4 3 2

Contents

PART VI   Resources: More about Healthful Eating

Foreword

Wellness, a goal that we all have, can be achieved. It takes awareness, planning, and a passionate belief in ourselves. A can-do attitude will steer our progress. When we know *what* to do, *how* to do it, and *why* we want to do it, we can do great things for our health and well-being. Making good food choices is one of the most important actions we can take on that road to wellness.

That is what this book is about. It is a tool designed to answer the whats, hows, and whys about food and nutrition as you make this journey.

It's no secret that good food choices are the cornerstone of wellness. Every day, new messages about food and nutrition show up in the media or in advertising. What does it all mean, and how can a well-intentioned consumer make sense of it all? The members of the Academy of Nutrition and Dietetics, the world's largest organization of food and nutrition experts, are committed to gathering the research and evidence and translating it into sound advice for the public. In fact, our vision statement is "Optimizing the nation's health through food and nutrition."

Since the first edition, this book has earned a permanent place on the bookshelves of individuals, families, and healthcare professionals alike. It's no surprise why. Backed by the latest science and published under the Academy moniker, the information in this book has earned the respect and trust of hundreds of thousands of readers. But beyond that, it's a good read. Roberta Duyff presents a wealth of information in an entertaining, easy-to-read style.

What's changed since the last edition? As public attention has turned increasingly to the obesity epidemic in children and adults, you'll find more solid information and advice about weight management. Also, there's a greater focus on food. While the right mix of nutrients keeps us going, the idea of food—its smells, tastes, and textures—*gets* us going. There is plenty of advice, ideas, and kitchen tips to satisfy the foodie in us all. More than ever, this book is about you and the personal choices you make. Regardless of your life stage and health status, you'll find plenty of information that suits you, from grocery shopping to planning meals to managing diet-related health conditions to food safety and more.

Armed with this information, we can influence our family and friends. As parents, we can model a healthy lifestyle for our children. As a spouse, we can guide our partner's food choices at mealtimes. If we care for aging parents, we can plan meals and activities to help them maintain independence and to manage any chronic conditions they may have. In short, we will be empowered by this guide to make needed changes and to support the good habits we already have. Indeed, we all can eat well to live well.

Happy reading, happy eating . . . a toast to your health!!

Sylvia Escott-Stump, MA, RD, LDN
President, Academy of Nutrition and Dietetics
2011–2012

Acknowledgments

For every edition of the *American Dietetic Association Complete Food and Nutrition Guide*, I am grateful and indebted to the many professionals, colleagues, and friends—in the fields of nutrition and dietetics, health, family and consumer sciences, food sciences, culinary arts, education, communications, and public policy—who have shared their insights, knowledge, and experience, as well as their time throughout my career, and certainly during the development of this book. I'm especially grateful to:

The Academy of Nutrition and Dietetics, for the honor and opportunity to write this comprehensive food and nutrition resource on behalf of the association's more than 70,000 members.

Academy staff for their editorial and marketing support: Diana Faulhaber, Publisher and Director of Academy Books and Resources, and Laura Pelehach, Manager, Acquisitions and Development, who provided their editorial support for the opportunity that the academy provided me to write this consumer-focused, healthy-eating book; Sharon Denny, Wendy Marcason, and Eleese Cunningham in the Academy Knowledge Center, for their quick, enthusiastic help in answering today's nutrition questions; Georgia Gofis, Academy Director of Marketing, for the book's many promotional efforts; the Academy staff who previously worked with me on the first, second, and third editions; and all those who have supported these Academy staff members.

Academy members, registered dietitians, nutrition experts, and all reviewers who volunteered countless hours to review manuscripts for this fourth edition, for content accuracy, clarity, and comprehensiveness:

● Jennifer Autodore, Keith-Thomas Ayoob, Christina K. Biesemeier, Mary Anne Burkman, Nancy Clark, Nancy Copperman, Connie Diekman, Diana Cullum-Dugan, Joy Dubost, Marianne Smith Edge, Nancy Patin Falini, Susan Finn, Anthony Flood, Ruth Frechman, Barbara L. Grant, Alice Henneman, Betsy Hornick, A. Christine Hummell, Julie Miller Jones, Wendy Reinhardt Kapsak, Ellen Karlin, Lisa Katic, Sarah B. Krieger, Cynthia Kupper, Lindsey Loving, Jacqueline B. Marcus, Martha Marino, Melissa Ventura Marra, Laura E. Matarese, Mildred Mattfeldt-Beman, Holly L. McClung, Linda McDonald, Rita Mitchell, Farida Mohamedshah, Susan Nitzke, Beth Ogata, Christine M. Palumbo, Antigoni Pappas, Kerry Phillips, Catharine Powers, Elizabeth Rahavi, Susan Randall, Valentina M. Remig, Paula Ritter-Gooder, Christine Rosenbloom, Tami A. Ross, S. Marlene Schmidt, Mary K. Sharrett, Madeleine Sigman-Grant, Denise Sofka, Kris Sollid, Cathie Squatrito, Tricia Thompson, and Suzanne Vieira.

Those who helped with previous editions, especially Betsy Hornick, editor and registered dietitian, on behalf of ADA Publications (now Academy Books and Resources), for her nutrition expertise, editorial guidance, and commitment to excellence; Sherri

Hoyt, colleague and registered dietitian, for her contributions on food sensitivity, infant feeding, and nutrition during pregnancy and breast-feeding; the many registered dietitians and dietetic technicians, registered, who served as reviewers; and dietetic interns for their careful fact checking of nutrient data.

Registered dietitians and other food, nutrition, and health professionals in government agencies, the food industry, and educational institutions throughout the country, who served as ongoing resources and insightful experts.

Organizations who granted permission for the use of supporting illustrations and graphics.

The excellent team of editors, designers, and staff at John Wiley & Sons, especially Tom Miller, Executive Editor; Jorge Amaral, Assistant Editor; and John Simko, Senior Production Editor, who expertly handled the editing and production; the design team; Laura Cusack, Senior Marketing Manager; Senior Publicist Matthew Smollon; as well as the John Wiley & Sons publishing teams responsible for the second and third editions and the Chronimed Publishing team responsible for its first edition.

Other friends and family who reviewed this book in earlier editions from their unique consumer and professional perspectives: Linda Carpenter, Julie Duyff, Phil Duyff, Patty Fletcher, Ann Hagan Brickman, Karen Marshall, Patricia McKissack, and Linda Valiga.

Edith Syrjala Eash, Dr. Diva Sanjur, and Dr. Hazel Spitze, my mentors and academic advisors, who encouraged me in my early career as a registered dietitian and as a food and nutrition educator and professional.

Anne Piatek and Nancy Schwartz—the colleagues and registered dietitians who first encouraged me to write this healthful-eating, science-based book for consumers and professionals.

The many readers, media representatives, university students, and colleagues who've called this book their "bible" of nutrition from its very first edition, who've shared their insights for subsequent editions, and who've helped to make this book a best-seller from the start!

My family, especially my mother, Jeane Larson, and my friends, who shared their support, understanding, and encouragement—and others in my family, who always encouraged my pursuit of life-long learning, my commitment to the public well-being, and my ability to communicate with accuracy, and informed, balanced viewpoint—and with a joy for empowering others.

My husband, Phil, who has read every word in all four editions to ensure clarity of the content and the positive voice of the message . . . and offered the loving support I needed to write and continually update this book

To your health!

Roberta Larson Duyff, MS, RD, FADA, CFCS
Author/Food, Nutrition, and Culinary Consultant
Duyff Associates, St. Louis, Mo.

About the Author . . . an award-winning author, national speaker, media spokesperson, and food industry/government consultant, Roberta Larson Duyff, MS, RD, FADA, CFCS, promotes "the power of positive nutrition" to consumers of all ages with practical, science-based, great-tasting ways to eat and stay active for health.

Among her books, Roberta has authored three other titles for the Academy, including *365 Days of Healthy Eating from the American Dietetic Association* and *Food, Nutrition and Wellness* (a high school textbook), and several children's healthy-eating books. She was the guiding force behind and contributor to the *American Dietetic Association Cooking Healthy Across America* cookbook as Chair of the American Dietetic Association's Food & Culinary Professionals Dietetic Practice Group. Among her awards, she has been recognized with the American Dietetic Association's (now the Academy of Nutrition and Dietetics) prestigious Medallion Award for professional excellence, as an ADA Fellow, and with ADA's First Annual President's Lecture.

Unless otherwise noted, the nutrient and calorie data in this book were derived from the U.S. Department of Agriculture, Agricultural Research Service, 2011. *USDA National Nutrient Database for Standard Reference,* Release 24. Nutrient Data Laboratory Home Page, http://www.ars.usda.gov/ba/bhnrc/ndl.

Introduction

The *American Dietetic Association Complete Food and Nutrition Guide* has been created for you—as your practical, up-to-date resource on healthful eating and active living for your personal wellness. It reflects the 2010 Dietary Guidelines for Americans; the interactive, individualized healthy eating advice represented by MyPlate; the latest food and nutrition research; and today's food, culinary, and lifestyle trends. But it's much more. It goes beyond guidelines with clear, easy-to understand advice and practical ideas to eat healthier and be more physically active, one step at a time.

Making healthy choices isn't always easy. Full of solutions for your everyday eating dilemmas, this book's practical, science-based advice is flexible enough for your lifestyle or needs. From weight control and portion control to heart-healthy eating, savvy food shopping to safe food handling, the basics of home cooking and kitchen nutrition, eating out wisely, vegetarian food styles to sports nutrition, helping kids eat right to smart eating for aging, food sensitivities (e.g., gluten intolerance, allergies), and eating for diabetes to other food-related health issues, in this book you'll find sensible solutions that are easy, effective, and great tasting. Skim the pages for many other "hot" food and health issues, too, including making calories count, eating healthy as a cost-effective healthcare strategy, being green with food, getting the most nutri-

tion for your food dollar, using dietary supplements wisely, today's food agriculture, and much more.

As your complete resource on healthy eating, you can refer to this book again and again at every age and stage of your life—from choosing the healthiest baby food or feeding a child or teen to dealing with unique nutrition needs at different points in a woman's life or with the special challenges of aging. It's also filled with advice for preventing, slowing, and dealing with heart disease, cancer, diabetes, and other common health problems. This book is meant for you and for all those you care about—perhaps a child, a spouse, a companion, an aging parent, or a friend.

For your personal nutrition check-up, you'll find opportunities to assess your own everyday food choices. Start in chapter 1 with "Looking for Healthy Solutions?" to identify your personal eating challenges. For more information, each question refers you to in-depth answers throughout the book. In fact, in almost every chapter, "Your Nutrition Check-Up" gives you a close-up look at your own food decisions. Use the websites within each chapter to delve more into topics of concern or interest to you.

Whenever nutrition makes the news (print, television, radio, online), this book can help you judge the headlines and separate facts from perceptions and fads. It reflects current science-based advice, as presented in the position papers of the Academy of Nutrition and Dietetics (formerly the American Dietetic

Association), the authority America turns to for food and nutrition guidance, with nearly one hundred years of nutrition expertise and research. As a registered dietitian and author, I've compiled this comprehensive resource with ways to make healthful eating, quality food, and great flavor go hand in hand at your family table.

With questions posed to nutrition experts—in part through the Academy's Knowledge Center—thousands of consumers have helped me shape the focus and content of the *American Dietetic Association Complete Food and Nutrition Guide* from its success-

ful first edition to this fully updated fourth edition. I hope the answers to their food and nutrition questions will also answer many of your own, and help you find practical, positive ways to take simple steps for your own and your family's good health!

From my table to yours, read, enjoy, be active, and eat healthy . . . for life!

Roberta Larson Duyff, MS, RD, FADA, CFCS
Author/Food, Nutrition, and Culinary Consultant
Duyff Associates, St. Louis, Mo.

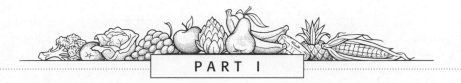

PART I

Wellness
Eat Smart, Get Active, Live Well

CHAPTER 1

Food and Lifestyle Choices

A Healthy You!

Your life is filled with choices! Every day you make thousands of choices, many related to food. Some seem trivial. Others are important. A few may even set the course of your life. But as insignificant as a single choice may seem, when made over and over, it can have a major impact on your health—and your life!

This book is about choices—those you, your family, and your friends make every day about food, nutrition, physical activity, and health. Within its pages, you'll find reliable nutrition information and sound and positive advice based on current scientific evidence. You'll find useful "how-tos" for making healthful food choices in almost any situation and at every stage of life. You'll learn about preparing healthful food at home and ordering carefully when you eat out—and to enjoy the pleasures and flavors of mealtime. After all, taste is the number one reason most people choose one food over another.

Most important, the practical tips, flexible guidelines, and simple tools in these pages help you choose nutritious, flavorful foods to match your personal needs, preferences, and lifestyle—even as your life and family situation change. Eating for health is one of the wisest decisions you'll ever make!

Wellness: Your Overall Health

What does wellness mean to you? Perhaps being free of disease and other health problems? Or having plenty of energy, a trim or muscular body, or the ability to finish a 10K run or fitness walk? Actually, wellness is far broader and more personal. It refers to your own optimal health and overall well-being. Wellness, or fitness, is your good health at its very best. Being nutritionally fit is a wellness essential!

Wellness defines every aspect of health—not only your physical health but also your emotional and mental well-being. In fact, they're interconnected. And smart eating and active living are fundamental to all three. When you're fit, you have:

- energy to do what's important to you and to be more productive;

- stamina and a positive outlook to handle the mental challenges and emotional ups and downs of everyday life, and to deal with stress;

- reduced risk for many health problems, including serious, often life-changing diseases such as heart disease, cancer, type 2 diabetes, and osteoporosis;

- the chance to look and feel your best;

- physical strength and endurance to protect yourself in case of an emergency;

- a better chance for a higher quality of life, and perhaps a longer one, too!

The benefits of overall wellness are ageless! Well-nourished, physically active children and teens grow, develop, and learn better. Good nutrition helps ensure a healthy pregnancy and successful breast-feeding. Healthful eating and active living help people at every age and stage of life feel their best, work productively, and lower their risks for some diseases—and may even slow aging. The sooner healthful eating and regular physical activity become priorities, the better your overall health will be.

The Health Equation

Healthful eating and active living are among your best personal investments. Your genes, age, surroundings, lifestyle, health care, and culture strongly influence your health. What and how much you eat and how much you move profoundly impact your health and weight, too.

For wellness you don't need special or costly foods, or fancy exercise equipment or a health club mem-

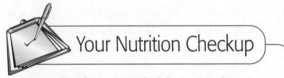

Your Nutrition Checkup

Ready for Healthier Eating?

Where do you fit on this healthy eating readiness test?

☐ *"My food choices are okay as they are."* Okay, that's your decision. But read on to find out why you might consider a few steps in the future to eat for better health (and perhaps to move more, too).

☐ *"I'll change my eating habits sometime, but I can't make myself do it now."* Good initial thought. Consider the pros and the cons as you decide. Check here for sensible, realistic ways to eat smarter (and get active)—but now rather than later. The sooner you start, the greater the benefits.

☐ *"I'm ready to eat smarter, starting now."* Good—you can do it! Check the tips throughout the book for small steps to healthful eating that work for you. As you achieve them, try a few more. Be active, too.

☐ *"I'm already a 'healthy eater.'"* Great, keep it up! Flip through this book for more practical ways to eat smart. In fact, get adventuresome with your eating. And take time for active living.

☐ *"Healthy eating and active living are second nature to me."* Excellent! Share the practical advice here and your own success with someone else. The health benefits are your rewards. If you stray from time to time, identify why, address the reason or reasons, and get back on board.

bership. You don't need to give up your favorite foods, or set up a tedious system of eating rules or calorie counting. And you don't need to hit a specific weight on the bathroom scale. You do need a sensible way to eat smart and be active, with an approach that's right for you. You're in control. You can do that, one simple step at a time.

Nutrition: You've heard the term all your life. In a nutshell, nutrition is how food nourishes your body. Being well nourished depends on getting enough of the nutrients and calories your body needs—-but not too many calories-—and on keeping your weight within a healthy range.

Being active? It's not being busy. It doesn't mean being an athlete. Instead it's making physical activity a regular part of your daily routine, even with every-day tasks of living such as using the stairs, doing yard work, and walking the dog.

These two priorities certainly aren't the only ones that promote fitness. Other lifestyle choices throughout your life are important, too: get enough sleep, avoid smoking, manage stress, drink alcoholic beverages only in moderation (if you drink and are of legal age), wear your seat belt, observe good hygiene, get regular medical checkups, obtain adequate health care—to name a few.

Smart Eating Matters!

Our understanding of nutrition is based on years of scientific study. Yet interest in food and health actually dates back at least to the ancient Greeks. Hippocrates, the "Father of Medicine" born about twenty-five hundred years ago, is quoted as saying, "If every individual could have the right amount of nourishment and exercise, not too little and not too much, we should have found the safest way to health."

Not until the nineteenth century, however, did the mysteries of nutrition begin to unravel. Today, although scientists have answered many nutrition questions, new ones arise as knowledge evolves. Research continues as scientists explore emerging issues related to food, nutrients, and phytonutrients, and the many roles they play in promoting health and protecting against disease. New knowledge is evolutionary, not revolutionary!

Today we know that healthful eating and active living can lower your risks for overweight and obesity, high blood pressure, high blood cholesterol, high blood glucose, and low bone density. All are risk factors for serious diseases such as heart disease, certain cancers, type 2 diabetes, stroke, and osteoporosis, which are among the main causes of disability and death in the United States.

Today's nutrition guidance is supported by scientific evidence. So unlike the ancients, you have a well-founded basis for making wise food choices for health and your own well-being.

Smart Eating: Right for You, Too!

Why do you choose one food over another? Your food choices reflect you and what's important to you: your culture, your surroundings, the people around you, your view of yourself, the foods available to you and those foods you like, your emotions, and likely what you know about food and nutrition.

Besides the nutrition benefits, food is also a source of pleasure, adventure, and great taste. It's no surprise that people entertain and celebrate with food, or look forward to a special dish.

Good nutrition can go hand in hand with pleasurable meals. Throughout this book, you'll find many easy ways to make your "plate" more appealing—and at the same time, more nourishing. You'll not only learn the "whys" of healthful eating and being active, you'll also learn how to be successful at managing your weight—and how to keep your family healthy. In addition, you'll gain insights and get tips about buying, preparing, serving, and eating foods you like in the right portion size—and about trying new foods—to promote health.

For a quick visual cue to healthful eating, see "MyPlate" in this chapter and chapter 10.

Smart Eating, Active Living: Guidelines for Americans

What's the secret to health? There's no secret, just solid advice. Most Americans need to make wiser food choices, to reach and keep a healthy weight, and to get active. To set the stage and promote healthful eating and physical activity, guidelines have been established by the federal government to help: Dietary Guidelines for Americans and Physical Activity Guidelines for Americans.

Eat Smart: Dietary Guidelines for Americans

The Dietary Guidelines for Americans (DGA) provides advice for making informed food choices, consuming the right amount of calories for you, and being physically active. The goals: to promote overall health and a healthy weight, and to reduce the chance of disease. Issued jointly by the U.S. Department of Agriculture (USDA) and the U.S. Department of Health and Human Services (USHHS), the DGA 2010 presents authoritative guidance for Americans ages two and over, including people who are at higher risk for chronic disease. The advice reflects current scientific evidence. To form that advice, experts completed a rigorous, systematic review of the evidence in a process that was transparent and open to the public.

Reviewed and updated as necessary, the Dietary Guidelines are published every five years to reflect the evolving body of scientific evidence about nutrition and health. Nutrition is, after all, a dynamic science that continues to expand our knowledge over time. The latest guidance also takes into account the many factors that affect food and physical activity choices.

You may wonder why this advice doesn't apply to toddlers and infants. There are two main reasons: First, their nutritional needs and eating patterns vary and depend on their developmental stage, and second, their needs differ a lot from those of older children, teens, and adults.

Although the DGA is meant to set policy, its messages are applied in many places where you can access food. These guidelines provide the scientific basis underlying many nutrition initiatives such as setting nutrition policies; designing nutrition programs for children and mothers, school food service providers, those receiving food assistance, older adults, and more; teaching children and teens about nutrition; and communicating with consumers about sound nutrition and active living.

The Dietary Guidelines for Americans, 2010, fit into four key areas, with twenty-three general recommendations and six more for special groups such as pregnant and breast-feeding women and older adults. The guidelines overlap in many ways, making it easier to

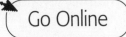

Track Your Food Choices, Make Your Eat Smart Plan!

Want a snapshot view of what you eat and how much you move in a day, several days, or even over weeks? There's an easy, personalized way to plan, track, and assess your overall eating pattern and physical activity level.

Whether from a cell phone or a home computer, use the SuperTracker at www.ChooseMyPlate.gov to compare your food choices to the 2010 Dietary Guidelines for Americans to find out about foods in the marketplace and to see steps you can take to improve. Online and interactive, the SuperTracker can be your coach, journal, and source of social media support.

fit the advice into your total diet. *See the appendices for all recommendations.* The guidelines are summed up in two overarching concepts with an important premise: most nutrients should come from food.

- Maintain calorie balance over time to achieve and sustain a healthy weight.

- Focus on consuming nutrient-dense foods and beverages.

Let's start with an overview of the four key areas of the Dietary Guidelines' advice. Then, armed with information and practical strategies throughout this book, apply the advice to your food and lifestyle choices—and do it your way, as long is as you stay within your calorie needs! *To start, refer to "Ready, Set, Take Action" in this chapter.*

Healthy Weight, Healthy Life

Balance Calories to Manage Weight

The incidence of overweight and obesity is much higher in the United States today than just a few decades ago. The risks are significant. At every age, a healthy weight is fundamental to a long, healthy, and productive life. For children and adults, even a few excess pounds may be riskier than you think. Research shows that being overweight or obese increases the risk for high blood pressure, unhealthy blood lipid

(fats) levels, and prediabetes. But obesity also is linked to type 2 diabetes, heart disease, certain cancers, and even premature death. *Chapter 2 addresses reasons for the rise in overweight and obesity, including scientific evidence that links food choices to weight.*

Calorie balance is key to a healthy weight. Calorie balance is achieved when the calories consumed from food and drinks equal the calories used for physical activity and metabolic processes. On the flip side, calorie *imbalance*, or consuming more calories than the body uses, is the reason for the growing national and global epidemic of overweight and obesity, and not just among adults. Overweight among children and teens has risen dramatically within recent decades.

No matter what your age, pay attention to your weight. Set your goal on achieving or keeping a weight that's healthy for you. Your calorie needs will likely decrease gradually over adulthood. Strive to keep your healthy weight over the years; children and teens who keep their healthy weight as they grow have less chance of becoming overweight or obese as adults.

Reaching and keeping a healthy weight isn't always easy. Lifestyle, your food environment, and social pressure are among the many barriers that enable overeating and inactivity.

To achieve and maintain a healthy weight, improve your eating habits and be physically active. That means controlling the calories you consume from all your food and beverage choices and cutting back on your intake if you need to lose weight. Also, fit more physical activity into your day and spend less time in sedentary activities such as TV watching and computer time.

What's your measure of health? *Check chapter 2 to learn how to be successful at weight management.*

Click Here! Websites to Know . . .

- Dietary Guidelines for Americans, 2010, www.dietaryguidelines.gov
- 2008 Physical Activity Guidelines for Americans, www.health.gov/paguidelines
- MyPlate (visual cue for healthful eating), www.ChooseMyPlate.gov
- Let's Move, www.letsmove.gov

For specific advice on healthy weight for children, pregnant and breast-feeding women, and those with chronic disease, see chapters 17, 18, and 22.

Eat Less of These!

Foods and Food Components to Reduce

Whether you're at a healthy weight or not, you may need to limit certain foods and food components.

Regardless of body weight, many people (children and teens included) consume too much of these: sodium; solid fats (major sources of saturated fats and *trans* fats); cholesterol (by most men); added sugars; refined grains; and by some Americans, alcoholic drinks. Too much of these may increase the risks of certain chronic diseases. When too much of them replaces nutrient-dense foods, it's harder to meet nutrient recommendations and control calories.

Evidence shows that most people can cut back and so reduce their health risks while getting the nutrients they need. What should you cut back on?

Sodium. Sodium is an essential nutrient, and besides adding flavor, it has many important uses as a food ingredient. So why eat less?

Most Americans consume much more sodium than they need, on average 3,400 milligrams (mg) a day. Generally speaking, evidence shows that the higher the sodium intake, the higher the blood pressure. Conversely, when sodium intake goes down, so may blood pressure. Keeping blood pressure in a normal range decreases the risk for heart disease, congestive heart failure, and kidney disease.

Recommendation: Reduce sodium intake to less than 2,300 milligrams of sodium daily, or 1,500 milligrams if you are age fifty-one years or older, or if, for any age, you are African American or have high blood pressure, diabetes, or chronic kidney disease. The 1,500-milligram daily recommendation applies to about half the U.S. population, including children and most adults.

The main source of sodium in the U.S. diet is processed food, not the salt shaker. Use the Nutrition Facts on food labels to find and buy foods with less sodium; remember, it all adds up. Consume more fresh foods and fewer processed foods that are high in sodium. Eat more foods prepared at home, where you control the amount of sodium, and use little or no salt or salt-

Have You Ever Wondered ?

. . . what "nutrient-dense" and "nutrient-rich" mean? Nutrient-dense foods and beverages provide vitamins, minerals, and other substances that may have positive health effects with relatively few calories. All vegetables, fruits, whole-grain foods, seafood, eggs, beans and peas, unsalted nuts and seeds, fat-free and low-fat milk and milk products, and lean meats and poultry—when prepared without solid fats or added sugars—are nutrient-dense. You'll also see the term "nutrient-rich," commonly used to mean "nutrient-dense." For food labeling, the term "rich" has a regulated definition, however, meaning that one label serving of the food has 20 percent of more Daily Value for the nutrient.

. . . if your exercise level is of moderate intensity? Take the "talk-sing" test to find out. If you can talk comfortably as you move, that's moderate activity. If you're too breathless to talk, that activity may be vigorous. If your goal is moderate activity, you might need to slow down, but remember that vigorous activity has added benefits. If you can sing, that's light-intensity activity; step up your pace! *For another way to target your workout intensity, refer to "Your Physical Activity: How Intense?" in chapter 20. Also see "Moderate Activity: What Is It?" in this chapter.*

containing seasonings. When you eat out, order lower-sodium items if you can, or ask that salt be left out.

Sodium is found in a wide range of foods, so the more foods and drinks consumed, the greater potential for more sodium intake.Cutting back on food portions to cut calories also may help to reduce sodium.

For more about sodium, refer to chapters 6 and 7. Chapter 10 describes the DASH Eating Plan, which targets sodium at 2,300 mg daily or less. For more ways to manage blood pressure, see chapter 22.

Fats. Fat is another nutrient that's essential for health—and for children's growth. Besides supplying energy, it contains essential fatty acids and carries fat-soluble vitamins (A, D, E, and K) and carotenoids (phytonutrients) into your bloodstream. Fat has other roles in health as well. The Institute of Medicine recommends 20 to 35 percent of calories from total fat intake for adults. This range is linked to a lower risk of chronic disease, yet allows for an eating plan with enough essential nutrients. *The appendices and chapter 5 list ranges for other age groups.*

Scientific evidence shows that the type of fat consumed affects heart disease risk more than the amount. Too much solid fats (saturated fats and *trans* fats) and cholesterol are linked to a higher risk for unhealthy levels of blood cholesterol and for heart disease. The effect of dietary cholesterol is small compared to the effect of solid fats. High-fat diets tend to be high in solid fats and excess calories.

Recommendations: Strive to eat less than 10 percent of calories from saturated fats; replace saturated fats with monounsaturated and polyunsaturated fats, and consume fewer than 300 milligrams of cholesterol per day. Keep *trans* fatty acids as low as possible by limiting foods that contain *trans* fats, such as partially hydrogenated oils; limiting other solid fats; and reducing calories from solid fats.

As your sources of fat, choose foods such as oily fish, nuts, and vegetable oils, which contain mostly heart-healthy oils (high in polyunsaturated and monounsaturated fatty acids). Limit saturated fats and replace them with heart-healthy oils. Limit solid fats in your cooking and food choices, too. For example, trim fat from meat, remove poultry skin, use less butter and stick margarine, and choose low-fat and fat-free foods such as milk and milk products. Eat smaller portions of foods that contain solid fats, such as regular cheese, sausage, bacon, pizza, and grain-based desserts. When you limit saturated fats, you often lower cholesterol in your food choices, too.

For more about fats, solid fats, and cholesterol, refer to chapter 5, "Fat Facts."

Added Sugars. Added sugars supply calories, but certain foods with added sugars deliver little else nutritionally. Then why are they added? To sweeten foods and drinks, to add flavor, to help preserve food, and to provide other qualities, such as improved texture, that add appeal.

While sugars are naturally present in food, most sugars in the typical U.S. diet are added during food processing, preparation, or at the table. Added sugars contribute 16 percent of the total calories in the U.S. diet; cutting back on foods and drinks with added sugars can lower calories without compromising nutrition adequacy. That said, a little sweetener has a role in

---

Eat Better Today, Stay Healthy for Tomorrow

The Dietary Guidelines describes a healthy eating plan as one that limits the intake of sodium, solid fats, added sugars, and refined grains, and emphasizes nutrient-dense foods and beverages, vegetables, fruits, whole grains, fat-free or low-fat milk and milk products, seafood, lean meats and poultry, eggs, beans and peas, and nuts and seeds.

A healthy eating pattern with careful food handling does more than promote health and help to decrease the risk of chronic disease. It also helps to prevent food-borne illness.

MyPlate, as well as the USDA Food Patterns and the DASH Eating Plan (*see chapter 10*), can help you use the Dietary Guidelines to:

- find your balance between food and physical activity to manage your weight;
- reduce food and food components linked to increased health risks;
- increase food and nutrients that promote health while staying within your calorie needs;
- build a healthful eating pattern.

Source: Based on the Dietary Guidelines for Americans, 2010.

---

healthy eating. For example, a little sweetener added to some yogurts and breakfast cereals may encourage people to consume them and get the vitamin D, calcium, and/or fiber they provide.

Recommendation: Reduce calories from added sugars and caloric sweeteners, such as those in sugar-sweetened drinks. Simply replacing sweetened drinks with water or with unsweetened options or using less table sugar makes a difference.

What about tooth decay? Both added sugars and naturally occurring sugars contribute to decay, as do starches, another form of carbohydrate.

For more about carbohydrates refer to chapter 3.

Solid Fats and Added Sugars. The 2010 Dietary Guidelines expresses concern about calories from excessive amounts of both solid fats (saturated fats and *trans* fats) and added sugars. Together they provide about 35 percent of calories, or nearly 800 calories a day on average for Americans who eat 2,000 calories daily. Foods that contain them may not contribute much nutrition.

For weight management, the source of calories isn't really the issue; eating too many calories is. Foods with solid fats and added sugars won't promote weight gain any more than other calorie sources do—if calorie intake balances with calorie need (calories used).

For most people, no more than 5 to 15 percent of calories, or 100 to 300 calories in a 2,000-calorie eating plan, should come from solid fats and added sugars. A higher percentage makes it difficult to get enough vitamins, minerals, and fiber and still stay within calorie limits.

How do you limit foods and drinks with added sugars and solid fats? Eat more nutrient-dense foods such as an apple rather than a slice of apple pie, or lean ham instead of bacon. Read food labels and be aware—Nutrition Facts list only amounts of total carbohydrates and total sugars, not added sugars; you'll need to read the ingredient list, too. Solid fats are shown as saturated fats and *trans* fats in the Nutrition Facts. *Chapter 12 gives label reading tips.* When you do choose to consume soda, cake, or other foods or drinks with solid fats or added sugars, take smaller portions and eat these foods less frequently.

Refined Grains. Switch your grains. Eat more whole grains and fewer refined grain products. Here's why: When grains are refined, vitamins, minerals, and fiber are lost. Although refined grains are enriched to add some nutrients back, all the nutrients and fiber found in whole grains aren't routinely restored to refined grain products. That said, refined grain products are typically enriched with B vitamins and iron and fortified with folic acid. Limit those high in solid fats and added sugars. This includes cookies and cakes.

Recommendation: Make at least half of all grain choices whole grains. Choose enriched, refined grain products with less solid fat and added sugars.

Alcohol. Alcoholic beverages should be consumed only in moderation—up to one drink a day for women and two for men—and only by adults of legal drinking age. A drink is 12 ounces of regular beer (5 percent alcohol), 5 ounces of wine (12 percent alcohol), or 1.5 fluid ounces of 80-proof (40 percent alcohol) distilled spirits.

Moderate drinking may have some health benefits,

perhaps lowering the risk for heart disease. It also may help people retain their cognitive function as they age. Yet, these possibilities are no reason to start drinking or to drink an extra glass or two. In fact, even moderate drinking can be a health issue. As little as one drink a day may increase slightly a woman's risk for breast cancer. Drinking is also linked to a higher risk for violence, drowning, and injuries from falls and motor vehicle accidents.

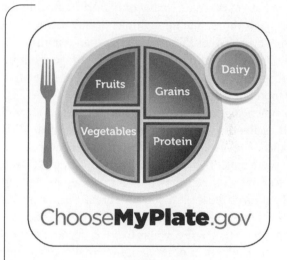

Ready, Set, Take Action!

Make food choices for a healthier lifestyle. Choose steps like these—and start today!

Balancing Calories
- Enjoy your food, but eat less.
- Avoid oversized portions.

Foods to Increase
- Make half your plate fruits and vegetables.
- Make at least half your grains whole grains.
- Switch to fat-free or low-fat (1 percent) milk.

Foods to Reduce
- Compare sodium in foods like soup, bread, and frozen meals—and choose the foods with lower numbers.
- Drink water instead of sugary drinks.

Throughout this book, you'll find many more easy steps like these. *See chapters 10 and 11 to learn how to set your table with MyPlate website advice.*

Source: www.ChooseMyPlate.gov.

Excessive drinking is risky and has no benefits. In fact, it's linked to higher chances of liver disease (cirrhosis), high blood pressure, stroke, type 2 diabetes, certain cancers, injury, and violence. Over time, excessive drinking is linked to weight gain and can impair both short- and long-term mental function. It also leads to about seventy-nine thousand deaths in the United States annually. Binge drinking is linked indirectly to more risks, including sexually transmitted diseases, unintended pregnancy, and violent crime.

What's excessive? Heavy or high-risk drinking for women is more than three drinks on any day or more than seven a week; for men, more than four drinks a day or more than fourteen per week. Binge drinking is four or more drinks in two hours for women, and five or more for men.

When should you avoid drinking? Whenever you put yourself and others at risk! Don't drink at all if you can't restrict your drinking to moderate amounts; if you're under the legal drinking age; if you're taking prescription or over-the-counter medications that can interact with alcohol; if you have certain medical conditions (such as liver disease, hypertriglyceridemia, or pancreatitis); or if you plan to drive, operate machinery, or take part in other activities that require your attention, skill, and coordination, or in situations where impaired judgment could cause injury or death. Also, don't drink if you're pregnant or think you may be pregnant, as drinking, especially in the first few months, is linked to behavioral and nervous system problems for the offspring.

For more about alcoholic beverages, advice and risks, refer to "Alcoholic Beverages: In Moderation" in chapter 8. For guidance related to breast-feeding, see chapter 18.

Eat More of These!

Foods and Nutrients to Increase

Eating a variety of nutrient-dense foods every day is basic to good nutrition, health, and weight management. Nutrient-dense foods provide relatively few calories for the nutrients they contain.

Today we know much more about the health-promoting nutrients in vegetables; fruits; whole grains; fat-free and low-fat milk and milk products; protein foods, including seafood, lean meat and poultry, eggs,

beans and peas, soy products, and unsalted nuts and seeds; and oils. Together, these foods also provide nutrients such as potassium, calcium, vitamin D, and fiber, which many people don't consume enough of. Their lack is a public health concern.

Vegetables and Fruits. Despite their health benefits, most people don't consume enough vegetables and fruits. Whether they're fresh, frozen, canned, or dried, fruits and vegetables are major sources of often under-consumed nutrients, including folate, magnesium, potassium, fiber, and vitamins A, C, and K. Evidence shows that consuming enough fruits and vegetables is also linked to a lower risk of many chronic diseases and may help protect against certain types of cancer. If prepared without adding fats or sugars, fruits and vegetables are relatively low in calories. As a result, eating more of them may help you achieve and keep your healthy weight.

Recommendation: Eat more vegetables and fruits. Include a variety of colorful vegetables, especially dark-green, red, and orange vegetables, and beans and peas.

Many children and young adults consume more than half of their fruit as juice. Instead, for the fiber benefits, choose mostly whole fruit rather than juice. When choosing juice, make sure it is 100 percent juice. Also, choose fruit canned in juice rather than syrup to limit added sugars.

Whole Grains. While most people eat enough grain products, very few consume enough whole grains.

Recommendation: Make at least half the grains you eat whole, replacing refined grains with whole grains. Whole-grain foods are made from the entire grain kernel: the fiber-rich bran and germ, and the endosperm. Refined grains contain mostly the endosperm.

Why emphasize whole grains? They're important sources of iron, magnesium, selenium, B vitamins, and fiber. Eating whole grains may help reduce the risk of heart disease and may be linked to a lower body weight. Although evidence is limited, eating whole grains also may be associated with less risk of type 2 diabetes.

The fiber in whole grains varies. So choose those with more fiber (at least 3 grams or more per label serving) for more health benefits.

If at least half of your grains are whole, what about the other half? Make them enriched or whole grain, too. Enriched grain products are fortified with certain B vitamins and iron to replace those lost when grains are refined. They're also fortified with folic acid, whereas whole grains may not be.

Making at least half your grains whole can be tricky. *See chapter 10 to learn how.*

Low-Fat/Fat-Free Dairy Foods. These foods deliver many important nutrients, including some that people often lack enough of: calcium, vitamin D (if vitamin D–fortified), and potassium. Beyond that, consuming dairy foods appears to be linked to better bone health, a reduced risk of heart disease and type 2 diabetes, and lower blood pressure in adults.

Despite the benefits of milk, milk products, and fortified soy beverages, most people from ages four and up, and even many two- and three-year-olds, don't consume enough. Females consume less than males, and intake tends to decline with age. Of the dairy foods consumed in the United States, a relatively small percentage are low-fat or fat-free. Nearly half is in the form of cheese, little of which is low-fat.

Recommendation: Consume more low-fat and fat-free milk and milk products, and replace whole and full-fat products with low-fat and fat-free choices as a way to eat less solid fats. Low-fat and fat-free milk and yogurt also have more potassium and vitamins A and D and less sodium, cholesterol, and saturated fat than cheese.

If you don't or can't drink milk, try low-lactose and lactose-free milk products and/or soy beverages fortified with calcium and vitamins A and D.

Lean Protein Foods. Whether from seafood, meat, poultry, eggs, beans, peas, soy products, nuts, or seeds, these foods provide more than protein. They're all good sources of B vitamins, vitamin E, iron, zinc, and magnesium. Seafood, nuts, and seeds deliver more unsaturated fats than meat does.

Recommendations: Replace meat and poultry that have solid fats with those lean protein foods that are lower in solid fats and calories; some are good sources of oils, too. Eating a variety of protein foods delivers a host of benefits. For example, moderate evidence indicates that eating peanuts and tree nuts reduces risk factors for cardiovascular disease. Consume them in small amounts and in place of other protein foods; their oils may play a role in heart health. Fiber and other nutri-

ents in beans and peas have many health benefits; *see chapter 3.*

More variety means eating more seafood in place of some meat and poultry, too. Among seafood's unique benefits are its omega-3 fatty acids; *see chapter 5.* How much seafood should you eat? Eight ounces or more a week (less for young children), or about 20 percent of your protein foods, is linked to lower cardiac deaths for those with and without preexisting cardiovascular disease. *For guidelines on eating seafood during pregnancy and breast-feeding, see chapters 13 and 18.*

Oils. Why have advice about oils? First, they contribute essential fatty acids and vitamin E. Second, oils that are high in unsaturated fats are heart healthier than solid fats, which are more saturated. Most Americans consume more solid fats—and less oil—than advised.

Recommendation: Because oils are a concentrated calorie source, switch from solid fats to oils rather than consume more oil. Small amounts are enough! Among the sources are vegetable oils such as canola, corn, olive, and soybean oils, as well as avocados, nuts, olives, and seafood. *See chapter 5 to learn more.*

For more about all these nutrient-dense foods, the amounts you need, and fitting them into your daily meals and snacks, refer to chapters 10 and 11. Check chapter 17 for specific advice for children and teens.

Nutrients of Concern. Potassium, calcium, vitamin D, and fiber come up short in the eating patterns of most Americans. Some groups of people also are short on iron, folate, and/or vitamin B_{12}. *Refer to chapter 6 to learn about these vitamins and minerals, and chapter 3 to learn about fiber. Check the appendices for nutrient amounts recommended for you.*

Plan Your Meals and Snacks
Building Healthy Eating Patterns

How can you apply the advice just described to your day's food choices? How can you choose meals and snacks to stay within your calorie limit, to deliver the nutrients you need, and to reduce your risk for chronic disease? How can you plan healthy meals and snacks for your family?

Several flexible food guides—the USDA Food Patterns, with lacto-ovo-vegetarian and vegan versions, and the DASH (Dietary Approaches to Stop

Hypertension) Eating Plan—can help you. They all take cultural, ethnic, traditional, and personal preferences, as well as food costs and food availability, into account. They give you a range of options and respect your personal preferences. Each of these guides categorizes foods into food groups based on nutrient content, and each recommends food group amounts for several calorie levels. They also take into account building a healthful eating pattern with a variety of foods over time. *To learn about the food guides, see chapter 10.*

As you build your own healthy eating pattern:

● Focus on nutrient-dense foods: vegetables, fruits, whole grains, fat-free and low-fat milk and milk products, lean meats and poultry, seafood, eggs, beans and peas, nuts, and seeds. In preparing them, add little or no solid fats, sugars, or sodium. Limit foods and beverages with solid fats, sodium, and added sugars. *To fit them into healthful, everyday meals and snacks, refer to chapters 10 and 11.*

● Remember that beverages count! You may be surprised that American adults (ages nineteen or over) *drink* about 400 calories a day, many from regular soda, energy and sports drinks, and alcoholic beverages. Consider drinking milk and juice instead, which provide essential nutrients. Make your milk choices fat-free or low-fat, and choose 100 percent fruit juice. To limit excess calories and maintain a healthy weight, drink water and other beverages with few if any calories. *Refer to chapter 8 for more about beverages.*

● Be food safe. Foodborne illness strikes more than forty-eight million individuals each year, according to 2011 statistics from the Centers for Disease Control and Prevention, causing mild to severe and even life-threatening symptoms. A substantial number of outbreaks likely come from unsafe food practices at home. A healthful eating pattern is both nourishing and safe.

Keeping food safe is up to you, not just farmers, food manufacturers, retailers, and restaurant workers. Many cases of foodborne illness could be avoided if consumers handled food carefully. Clean your hands, food contact surfaces, and vegetables and fruits. Cook foods to safe internal temperatures. Separate raw, cooked, and ready-to-eat foods while shopping for, storing, and preparing them. And chill (refrigerate) perishable foods promptly.

Some foods pose a high risk for foodborne illness. *Refer to chapter 13 for tips on keeping food safe.*

● Be savvy with supplements and fortified foods. *Remember:* foods first for good nutrition. Besides their essential vitamins and nutrients, nutrient-dense foods provide fiber and other health-promoting components. For some people or in certain situations, supplements and fortified foods are advised, such as vitamin D, folic acid, vitamin B_{12}, or iron supplements. *See chapter 23 for appropriate supplement use.*

Move It! Physical Activity Guidelines for Americans

Wellness takes more than healthful eating. Regular physical activity promotes health, a sense of well-being, and a healthy weight. Yet most Americans don't get enough.

The 2008 Physical Activity Guidelines for Americans (PAG), issued by the U.S. Department of Health and Human Services (USHHS), provides science-based guidance on physical activity and health. Meant for Americans ages six and older, these guidelines can help you improve your health through appropriate physical activity—and have fun, too! This advice complements Dietary Guidelines' advice.

Why be physically active? Evidence shows that regular physical activity reduces the risks for many health problems; some activity is better than none. Most health benefits come from at least 150 minutes (2 hours and 30 minutes) a week of moderately intense physical activity. If you move longer or with more vigor, you get even more benefits. Endurance (aerobic) and muscle-strengthening (resistance) activities are beneficial, too. *Refer to "Ten Reasons to Make the 'Right Moves'" in this chapter.*

Being physically active is important at every age, including for those with physical disabilities. Just choose activities that work for you. *The bottom line:* Benefits of appropriate physical activity far outweigh possible injury or other health risks for almost everyone.

Unless you have a health concern, you probably can start moving more now. Talk to your healthcare provider first if you have an ongoing health problem—including heart disease, high blood pressure, diabetes, osteoporosis, arthritis, or obesity—or if you're at high risk for heart disease, if you have a disability, or for women, if you are pregnant. Together determine the amount and type of activities that are right for your abilities or condition.

For the 2008 Physical Activity Guidelines for Americans, refer to the appendices.

Get Active, Stay Active, Be More Active

Spread out your physical activity, or do it all at once. Either way you get benefits. If you have been inactive, start gradually. Work up to longer, more intense activities. The 2008 Physical Activity Guidelines and the 2010 Dietary Guidelines provide consistent messages:

● Limit screen time—especially important for kids! That's the amount of time spent watching TV or using other media, such as video and computer games. When you do watch TV, try to move around and "multitask" as you watch or listen; perhaps do some sit-ups, stepping in place, or other exercises.

● Do it your way. Choose activities that fit your lifestyle. For kids, make them fun and appropriate for their physical ability. *See "Twenty Everyday Ways to Get Moving" in chapter 2.*

● Build up slowly. For your physical activity of choice, do a little more, a little longer, each time. Then do it more often! Move enough to keep fit without overdoing. Keep track with a journal.

● Choose activities with moderate or vigorous intensity. *See "Moderate Activity: What Is It?" below.* You might gradually replace some moderate activity with vigorous activity for similar health benefits in half the time.

● Vary your activities. Different activities use different muscles: for example, gardening for your arm muscles, power walking or bicycling for your heart and leg muscles, and sit-ups for abdominal muscles. For overall fitness, choose activities that build cardiovascular

---

MODERATE ACTIVITY: WHAT IS IT?

If some activities use more energy than others, you may wonder what moderate physical activity really means. It equates to the energy you need to walk 2 miles in 30 minutes.

Moderate physical activity uses about 3½ to 7 calories a minute, 150 calories a day, or about 1,000 calories a week. For that amount of energy expenditure, you might spend more time on less vigorous activities such as brisk walking, or spend less time on more vigorous activities, such as running.*

COMMON CHORES	DURATION	*Less Vigorous, More Time** ↑↓ *More Vigorous, Less Time*	SPORTING ACTIVITIES	DURATION
Washing and waxing a car	45–60 min.		Playing volleyball	45–60 min.
Washing windows or floors	45–60 min.		Playing touch football	45 min.
Gardening	30–45 min.		Walking 2 miles	30 min
Wheeling self in wheelchair	30–40 min.		Basketball (shooting baskets)	30 min.
Pushing a stroller 1½ miles	30 min.		Dancing fast (social)	30 min.
Raking leaves	30 min.		Water aerobics	30 min.
Shoveling snow	15 min.		Swimming laps	20 min.
Stairwalking	15 min.		Basketball (playing a game)	15–20 min.
			Jumping rope	15 min.
			Running 1½ miles	15 min.
			1 mile	10 min

* Some activities can be performed at various intensities. The suggested durations correspond to the expected intensity of effort.

Source: Your Guide to Lowering Blood Pressure, NHLBI, www.nhlbi.nih.gov/hbp/prevent/p_active/m_l_phys.htm. Accessed January 1, 2012.

endurance (walking, running, distance biking), muscle strength (heavy gardening, working with resistance bands), bone strength (walking, tennis), and flexibility (stretching, yoga, dancing).

● Get a partner. Being active with family and friends can make it easy and fun!

● *Remember:* Some physical activity is better than none. So avoid too much sitting. Start with ten-minute chunks, three times a day, three days a week. Perhaps walk; then gradually walk longer, more often, and at a faster pace.

Your Food Choices: The Inside Story

While you enjoy the sensual qualities of food—the mouth-watering appearance, aroma, texture, and flavor—your body relies on the life-sustaining functions that nutrients in food perform. Other food substances, including phytonutrients (or plant substances), appear to offer health benefits beyond basic nourishment. *See chapter 6 to learn about phytonutrients.*

Ten Reasons to Make the "Right Moves"

Whether you're involved in sports or live an active lifestyle, physical activity pays big dividends. The more you do, the greater the health. Physical activity is the right move for fitness for almost everyone. Consider a few reasons why:

1. *Trimmer body.* If you're physically active, you'll have an easier time maintaining a healthy weight, or losing weight and keeping it off if you're overweight. *For more about physical activity for weight management, refer to chapter 2, "Your Healthy Weight."*

2. *Less risk for health problems.* An active lifestyle—or a sports regimen—can help protect you from many ongoing health problems.

   Studies show that regular physical activity helps lower risk factors. For example, physical activity helps to lower total and LDL ("bad") cholesterol and triglyceride levels while boosting the HDL ("good") cholesterol level, control blood pressure, and improve blood glucose levels. Your risks for heart disease, high blood pressure, type 2 diabetes, and certain cancers go down when you fit physical activity into your daily life.

   Active living also may reduce or eliminate the need for medication to lower blood lipids, lower blood pressure, or manage diabetes.

3. *Stronger bones.* Regular, weight-bearing activities—such as walking, running, weight lifting, and cross-country skiing—help make your bones stronger. Even in adulthood, weight-bearing exercise helps maintain bone strength and reduce your chance of fractures and osteoporosis.

4. *Stronger muscles.* Strength-training activities, such as lifting weights, at least two times a week keep your body strong for sports and everyday living. When you're strong, it's easier to move, carry, and lift things. When you exercise your muscles, you also give your heart a workout. It's a muscle, too. A strong heart pumps blood and nutrients more easily through your sixty thousand miles of blood vessels.

5. *More endurance.* You won't tire as easily when you're physically active. And you may have more stamina during the rest of the day, too.

6. *Better mental outlook.* Active people describe feelings of psychological well-being and self-esteem when they make active living a habit. It's a great way to reinforce an empowered attitude and a positive outlook.

7. *Stress relief and better sleep.* Research shows that physical activity helps your body relax and release emotional tension. That promotes longer, better-quality sleep, and you may fall asleep faster.

8. *Better coordination and flexibility.* Your body moves with greater ease and range of motion when you stay physically active.

9. *Injury protection.* When you're in shape, you more easily can catch yourself if you slip or trip, and can move away from impending danger more quickly.

10. *Feel better and perhaps younger longer.* Research suggests that physical activity slows some effects of aging. Active people have more strength and mobility and fewer limitations.

One more reason: physical activities can be fun!

Exercise Your Options

For more about the benefits of physical activity—and ways to be more physically active—check here:

- For most healthy people, including those managing their body weight, refer to "Get Physical!" and "Twenty Everyday Ways to Get Moving" in chapter 2.
- For children, refer to "Active Play for Toddlers and Preschoolers" and "Get Up and Move!" in chapter 17.
- For teens, refer to "Move It!'" in chapter 17.
- For older adults, refer to "Never Too Late for Exercise" in chapter 19.
- For travelers, refer to "When You're on the Road" in chapter 20.
- For athletes, refer to chapter 20, "Athlete's Guide: Winning Nutrition."

Nutrients: Classified Information

Your body can't make most substances it needs to function normally, repair itself, produce energy, or grow. You need the varied and adequate nutrient supply that food delivers for nourishment—and for life itself.

To access these nutrients your food choices are digested, or broken down. Then the nutrients are absorbed into your bloodstream and carried to every cell in your body. Most of your body's work takes place in your cells. Food's nutrients are essential. More than forty nutrients in food, classified into six groups, have specific and unique functions. Their work is linked, as they work together in your body's many metabolic processes.

Carbohydrates. As your body's main source of energy, or calories, carbohydrates are both starches (complex carbohydrates) and sugars. Fiber, another form of complex carbohydrate, aids digestion, promotes health, and helps protect against some diseases. Despite its role in health, fiber isn't a nutrient; it isn't digested and then absorbed into the body. *See chapter 3, "Carbs: Sugars, Starches, Fiber."*

Fats. Fats supply energy. They support other functions, too, such as nutrient transport, growth, and being part of many body cells. Fats are made of varying combinations of fatty acids. Fatty acids aren't all the same. Some are highly saturated (solid at room temperature), while others are more unsaturated. Essential fatty acids are required for your health, although your body can't make them. *You'll learn about fat and cholesterol (a fatlike substance) in chapter 5, "Fat Facts: Cholesterol, Too."*

Proteins. Proteins are sequenced combinations of amino acids, which build, repair, and maintain body tissues. Your body makes nonessential amino acids; others, from food, are considered "essential" because your body can't make them. Proteins provide energy, especially when carbohydrates and fats are in short supply. If they're broken down and used for energy, amino acids can't be used to maintain body tissue. *For more about protein, see chapter 4, "Protein Power."*

Vitamins. Vitamins work like spark plugs, triggering chemical reactions in body cells. Each vitamin regulates different body processes. Because their roles are so specific, one cannot replace another. *Refer to chapter 6, "Vitamins, Minerals, Phytonutrients: Variety on Your Plate."*

Minerals. Somewhat like the actions of vitamins, minerals spark body processes. They, too, have unique job descriptions. *Refer to chapter 6.*

Water. Water makes up 45 to 75 percent of your body weight—and it's a nutrient, too. It regulates body processes, helps regulate your body temperature, carries nutrients and other body chemicals to your cells, and carries waste products away. *See chapter 8, "Fluids: Water and More!"*

Nutrients: How Much?

Everyone needs the same nutrients—just in different amounts. For healthy people, age, gender, and body size make a difference. Children and teenagers, for example, need more of some nutrients for growth. Pregnancy and breast-feeding increase the need for some nutrients and for calories. Because their bodies are typically larger, men often need more of most nutrients than women do.

How much of each nutrient do you need? Dietary Reference Intakes (DRIs) established by the Food and

Nutrition Board of the Institute of Medicine, National Academy of Sciences, make daily nutrient recommendations for healthy people in the United States and Canada based on age and gender. The DRIs include four types of recommendations:

● *Recommended Dietary Allowances (RDAs)* are recommended nutrient levels that meet the needs of almost all healthy individuals in specific age and gender groups. Consider these recommendations as your goal for getting enough nutrients.

● *Adequate Intakes (AIs)* are similar in meaning to RDAs. They're used as guidelines for some nutrients that don't have enough scientific evidence to set firm RDAs.

● *Tolerable Upper Intake Levels (ULs)* aren't recommended amounts. In fact, there's no scientific consensus for recommending nutrient levels higher than the RDAs for most healthy people. Instead, ULs represent the maximum intake that probably won't pose health risks for most healthy people in a specific age and gender group.

● *Estimated Average Requirements (EARs)* are used to assess groups of people, not individuals.

For carbohydrates, fats, and proteins (all macronutrients), which supply calories (energy), there's also an Acceptable Macronutrient Distribution Range (AMDR). That range not only reflects what's enough, it's also the amount linked to reduced chronic disease risk.

Groups of scientific experts regularly review and update the DRIs to reflect the most current research evidence. *The DRIs appear in the appendices.*

How do you use the DRIs? For the most part, you don't need to add up the numbers; it takes considerable effort to calculate the nutrients in all your food choices and then to make an assessment with DRIs. The Dietary Guidelines for Americans—and the USDA Food Patterns and the DASH Eating Plan—take the DRIs into account.

If you choose to calculate your nutrient intake, remember that the recommendations—RDAs and AIs—apply to your average nutrient intake over several days, not just one day and certainly not one meal. *For ease, follow a food guide discussed in chapter 10 instead.* A registered dietitian can help you; *see chapter 24 to find expert help.*

More Than Nutrients: Food's Functional Components

Food contains much more than nutrients. Science is uncovering the benefits of other components in food, such as phytonutrients (including fiber), omega-3 and -6 fatty acids, plant stanols and sterols, and pre- and probiotics, to name a few. Described as "functional," these substances do more than nourish you. They appear to promote your health and protect you from health risks related to many major health problems, including heart disease, some cancers, diabetes, and macular degeneration, among others.

At least for now, no DRIs exist for functional components in food, except for fiber. And scientists don't yet fully understand their roles in health. However, within this book, you'll get a glimpse of emerging knowledge about some functional components in food. You're bound to hear more as new studies unfold.

Healthful Eating, Active Living: One Step at a Time!

Are you ready to eat healthier or get active? (*See "Your Nutrition Checkup" earlier in this chapter*.) Even if it takes effort, it's worth it. To reach your goals, take one easy step at a time. The sooner you invest in your health, the greater the benefits!

Audit your food choices and lifestyle. Start by keeping track of what you eat or drink, along with how much, when, and why. For example, do you snack when you feel stressed or bored? Use a food journal to pinpoint eating behaviors you want to change and a physical activity log to track how active you are. *Refer to "Dear Journal . . ." in chapter 2 for tips on keeping a log, or use the SuperTracker, noted in "Go Online," in this chapter. Take the personal assessments in "Your Nutrition Checkup" throughout the book.*

Set personal goals. Know what you want—perhaps a healthier weight or lower cholesterol levels. Be realistic. Change doesn't mean giving up a food you like. Smaller portions, different ways of cooking, or being more physically active give you "wiggle room" to occasionally enjoy foods with more calories.

Make a plan for change. Divide big goals, such as "I will eat better," into smaller, more specific goals, such as "I will eat more vegetables" or "I will eat more whole-grain foods." List practical steps to achieve your goals. For example:

Goal: Consume at least half of all your grains as whole grains.

Steps: Make sandwiches and French toast with whole-grain bread. Switch to brown rice. Eat oatmeal for breakfast. Snack on plain popcorn. Add whole barley when you make vegetable soup.

Be patient. Make gradual changes. Long-term change takes time, commitment, and encouragement. Most health goals take a lifelong commitment. Stick with your plan. Remember that small steps toward a goal add up over time.

Monitor your progress. If you get off track, pick up where you left off, and start again. You're in control!

Seek help from a qualified health professional. A registered dietitian can help you on your fitness journey; *see chapter 24.*

Reward yourself. Change is effort that deserves recognition. "Pat yourself on the back" with a bike ride, a walk with a friend, a new phone app, or a bouquet of flowers. Feeling good is the best reward!

Reevaluate your plan every month or two. See how changes you made—the simple steps you took—fit with your goals. Plan a few more simple steps; even tackle a new goal!

Looking for "Healthy Solutions"?

Looking for a practical approach to sound nutrition? Check here for sensible, easy solutions to eat for fitness. It's within your power to make changes!

DO YOU . . .	YES OR NO?	FOR "HEALTHY SOLUTIONS," CHECK HERE . . .
Feel confused by conflicting nutrition headlines and emerging research?	☐ Yes ☐ No	*Chapter 24, "Well Informed?,"* to decipher today's and tomorrow's news about food and health. Refer to this whole book to learn what's known about nutrients, phytonutrients, and health and how that translates into smart eating.
Find it hard to lose weight and keep it off?	☐ Yes ☐ No	*Chapter 2, "Your Healthy Weight: Key to Wellness,"* to find ways to reach and keep your healthy weight that work—and sort through diets that don't.
Want to make the right beverage choices—with so much to choose from?	☐ Yes ☐ No	*Chapter 8, "Fluids: Water and More!"* to decide what to drink and how much.
Think you need to give up your favorite foods to eat healthy?	☐ Yes ☐ No	*Chapter 10, "Planning to Eat Smart,"* to see how you can enjoy all kinds of foods and eat for good health.
Feel life's just too hectic to eat healthy?	☐ Yes ☐ No	*Chapter 11, "Meals and Snacks: Healthy Solutions!"* to find quick, healthful, easy meals and snacks when you're tight on time and low on energy.
Want to devise a personal, customized plan for healthful eating—a plan that's right for you or your family?	☐ Yes ☐ No	*Chapter 10, "Planning to Eat Smart,"* for tips on creating an eating plan that's right for you, your calorie needs, and your food "style."
Want to know more about the array of foods in supermarkets and farmers' markets?	☐ Yes ☐ No	*Chapter 9, "What's on Today's Table?"* to keep updated on today's "new" foods (functional, health-positioned, organic, ethnic, others), food regulations, and more.

(continued)

Looking for "Healthy Solutions"? *(continued)*

Do you . . .	Yes or No?	For "Healthy Solutions," check here . . .
Want to get the most nutrition—and the best value—for your food dollar?	☐ Yes ☐ No	*Chapter 12, "Savvy Shopping,"* to shop for taste, convenience, price—and good health.
Wonder if the "bug" you caught might be foodborne illness?	☐ Yes ☐ No	*Chapter 13, "The Safe Kitchen,"* for essential ways to keep your food safe to eat.
Have limited cooking skills, or think healthful home-prepared meals take too much effort?	☐ Yes ☐ No	*Chapter 14, "Kitchen Nutrition: Cooking Matters,"* for simple ways to prepare healthful and flavorful meals in your kitchen.
Want to make smarter choices when you eat out at a restaurant?	☐ Yes ☐ No	*Chapter 15, "Your Food Away from Home,"* for ways to make eating out healthful, adventuresome, and enjoyable—without overdoing on calories!
Need assurance that you're feeding your baby right?	☐ Yes ☐ No	*Chapter 16, "Off to a Healthy Start: Feeding Baby,"* for infant-feeding basics, from breast- and/or bottle-feeding to solids.
Want stress-free tactics to feed growing kids, whether they're picky eaters or busy teens?	☐ Yes ☐ No	*Chapter 17, "Food to Grow On: Toddlers to Teens,"* for strategies that help your child or teen learn to eat for health and a healthy weight now and in the long run.
Wonder what food and nutrition strategies can help address women's unique health issues?	☐ Yes ☐ No	*Chapter 18, "For Women Only,"* for sound eating advice for pregnancy, breast-feeding, menopause, and more.
Want to eat smart as you age, and even slow the aging process?	☐ Yes ☐ No	*Chapter 19, "For Adults: Age Fifty Plus!,"* for smart eating if you're fifty years or over or if you're caring for someone that age.
Want to maximize your athletic performance?	☐ Yes ☐ No	*Chapter 20, "Athlete's Guide: Winning Nutrition,"* for ways to eat for your physical best before, during, and after a workout or competition.
Wonder if your (or your teen's) vegetarian eating is healthful enough?	☐ Yes ☐ No	*Chapter 10, "Planning to Eat Smart,"* for practical advice no matter what your approach to vegetarian eating.
Think you have a food allergy or need to eat gluten- or lactose-free food?	☐ Yes ☐ No	*Chapter 21, "Sensitive to Food,"* to deal with lactose intolerance, gluten intolerance, a food allergy, or other food sensitivities.
Want to reduce your risks for—or deal with—certain food-related health problems?	☐ Yes ☐ No	*Chapter 22, "Smart Eating to Prevent and Manage Disease,"* to know how to eat for health to reduce the risks for or manage common health problems—heart disease, diabetes, cancer, osteoporosis, GI problems, and anemia, among others. (This book also is filled with tips!)
Think you need a nutrient or herbal supplement, but you're still cautious?	☐ Yes ☐ No	*Chapter 23, "Dietary Supplements: Use and Misuse,"* to sort smart advice from misinformation about dietary supplements.

Every "yes" is one more reason to use this book as your guide to healthful eating and active living!

Your Healthy Weight
Key to Wellness

We often take it for granted, but good health is one of the most precious gifts of life. A healthy weight—maintained throughout life—helps you achieve good health in many ways: look your best, feel your best, and reduce your risk for many serious and ongoing diseases.

Yet today's high rates of overweight and obesity are causes for concern. Among all ages—children, teens, and adults—in the United States, obesity has become epidemic, with the incidence doubling and in some cases tripling over the past four decades. *See "Weighing the Risks" later in this chapter.* Health risks related to underweight are of concern, too, *as addressed later in this chapter in "Underweight: Hazards to Health."*

What is a healthy weight? It's the weight that's best for you—not necessarily the lowest weight you think you can be. A healthy weight actually is a range that's statistically related to good health. Being above or below that range increases the risk of health problems, or decreases the likelihood of good health.

The smart approach to your best weight is really no secret—only common sense. A healthful lifestyle, with regular physical activity and an eating pattern chosen to meet your nutrient needs within your calorie limits, makes all the difference. Everyone has a personal calorie limit. Achieving and sustaining your healthy weight throughout life is healthier than trying to lose weight after gaining too much.

Calorie balance matters! The key to your healthy weight is simple—balance calories consumed with calories used for physical activity and many body processes. *See "Calories in Balance!" in this chapter.* From food shopping to cooking to eating out, this book provides practical and positive ways to reach and keep your healthy weight.

What's Your Healthy Weight?

The answer isn't as simple as stepping onto a bathroom scale, then comparing your weight to a chart. Your healthy weight likely differs from someone else's weight, even if you are the same height, gender, and age.

Why a difference? Your genetic makeup plays a role because it determines your height and the size and shape of your body frame. A genetic link to body fat also may exist. Of course, genetics isn't the only reason why weight differs. Your metabolic rate, the rate at which your body burns energy, depends in large part on your body composition. Muscle burns more calories than body fat does. Your overall health is a factor that defines your healthy weight range, too.

To determine your right weight, your healthcare provider takes several things into account: (1) your body mass index, or your weight in relation to your height; (2) the location and amount of body fat you have; and (3) your overall health and risks for weight-related problems such as diabetes or high blood pressure.

Body Mass Index: Indicator of Health Risk

Body mass index (BMI) is a measure of body weight in relation to height, which is considered a reasonably reliable indicator of total body fat. That in turn suggests the risk of disease and death. BMI doesn't directly measure body fat. For adults, there's no difference in BMI weight ranges for age. For those under age 65, health risks related to a higher BMI appear to be the same, regardless of age.

BMI ranges of healthy weights allow for individual differences. Higher weights within a healthy range typically apply to people with more muscle and a larger frame. After all, muscle and bone weigh more than fat. Gaining or losing weight within these ranges isn't necessarily healthful for you.

People with a higher percentage of body fat tend to have a higher BMI. Carrying excess body fat puts them at greater risk for health problems such as heart disease, diabetes, certain cancers, and high blood pressure. The higher the BMI, the greater the risk. Although rare, some people who are obese are metabolically normal.

What's Your BMI?

You don't need to do calculations. For your adult BMI (both men and women), *check the BMI chart in this chapter*, or use the website www.nhlbisupport.com/bmi. Growth charts with BMI for children and teens differ, taking individual growth patterns for their gender and age into account. For kids, *use the growth charts in the appendices* or on www.cdc.gov/growthcharts, or use the calculator at apps.nccd.cdc.gov/dnpabmi.

If you fit within the healthy range—BMI 18.5 to 24.9—that's good. Take steps to keep it there, especially if your BMI starts to creep up. *Be aware:* Some people fit within the healthy range but still have excess body fat and little muscle.

What if your BMI is above 25? For most people, that's less healthy—unless the extra weight is muscle, not fat. For adults, a BMI of 25 to 29.9 is considered overweight; 30 or above is considered obese. These describe weight ranges that are greater than what is considered healthy for a given height. The higher your weight is above the healthy range, the greater your risk for weight-related problems. Take steps to lower your BMI and to achieve and maintain your healthy weight.

What if your BMI falls below "healthy"? That may be okay for you, but also may suggest a health problem. A BMI under 18.5 may indicate increased risk for menstrual irregularity, infertility, or osteoporosis. It also may be an early symptom of another health problem or an eating disorder. Check with your health professional if you lose weight suddenly or unexpectedly.

Use the BMI *only* as a guideline. Age, gender, and ethnicity impact how BMI relates to body fat. For people who have lost muscle mass, including some elderly people, even a BMI within the "healthy" range may not be healthy. Healthy muscular people may have a BMI above the healthy range since muscle weighs more than fat. Your BMI alone doesn't determine whether your weight is healthy. The location and amount of body fat you carry, and your weight-related risk factors, including your family history of health problems, count, too.

Fit at Any Size

Healthy people come in many sizes and shapes: tall or short, stocky or lanky, muscular or not. These differences are a unique part of being human. For this reason, there's no such thing as a "perfect body," or an ideal body weight, shape, or size, that everyone should strive for. The most important thing is being healthy, so you can enjoy life with the body you have.

Likewise, losing weight, or maintaining a healthy weight, is easier for some than others—in spite of their commitment to healthful eating and physical activity. After physical activity, genetics play a role.

Regardless of your size and shape, you can choose a healthful lifestyle—and so live a fuller, more productive life and reduce your risk for health problems.

● Assess your own health habits. Make choices with health in mind.

● Be active—no matter what your body size. Start by doing what you can do, anything that gets you moving, even for a few minutes.

● Eat for health with a sensible approach. *See chapter 10.*

● Get regular physical checkups.

● Monitor your "numbers" (blood cholesterol, triglycerides, blood pressure, fasting blood glucose levels). Keep them within a healthy range. *See chapter 22 for normal levels.*

● Make your goal your personal healthy weight, not some unattainable goal!

Body Weight, Body Fat?

Your body composition (how much of your weight is body fat versus bone or muscle), not necessarily where you fit on any chart, is important for evaluating your weight. The location and amount of body fat counts, too. Even though the BMI is useful for most men and women, it has some limits:

● It may overestimate body fat in athletes and others with a muscular build.

● It may underestimate body fat in older adults and others who have lost muscle.

How can you determine how much of your weight is body fat (often referred to as percent body fat)? Short of expensive tests such as underwater weighing, getting an exact measure isn't easy, and it's especially hard to figure it out on your own. A health or fitness professional might use a skinfold caliper to measure the fat layer on several parts of your body, such as your arm, midriff, and thigh. Today's electronic scales and other devices also can measure body fat percentages.

Remember: Your weight on a scale by itself can't tell you if you're carrying too much fat and how your weight is distributed. Most importantly, body weight shouldn't dictate how you feel about yourself.

Here are some other ways to judge how you are doing in terms of body fat and health.

Of Apples and Pears

Stand in front of a full-length mirror, preferably nude. How do you look? Be your own judge. Are you shaped like an apple or a pear? For health, being an "apple" can be riskier than being a "pear."

Where your body stores fat is a clue to your healthy weight. Abdominal or upper body fat (applelike shape) increases the risk for some health problems such as diabetes, high cholesterol levels, early heart disease, and high blood pressure, even when BMI falls

DOES YOUR BMI PUT YOU IN A RISKY ZONE?*

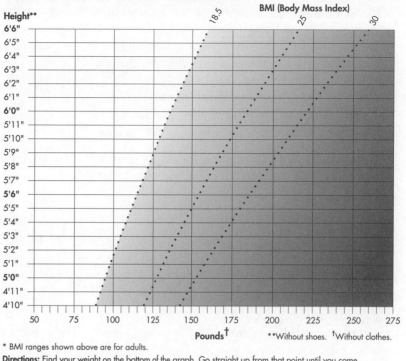

Pounds†   **Without shoes. †Without clothes.

* BMI ranges shown above are for adults.

Directions: Find your weight on the bottom of the graph. Go straight up from that point until you come to the line that matches your height. Then look to find your weight group.

■ BMI 18.5 to 24.9: not a risk factor for weight-related health problems

■ BMI 25 to 29.9: some increased risk for weight-related health problems

■ BMI 30 or higher: significant increased risk for weight-related health problems

Source: Adapted from Report of the Dietary Guidelines Advisory Committee, Dietary Guidelines for Americans, 2000.

within a healthy range. In contrast, excess weight carried in the hips, buttocks, and thighs (pearlike shape) doesn't appear to be as risky for most health problems. However, it may increase your risk for varicose veins and orthopedic problems.

For the most part, being an "apple" or a "pear" is an inherited tendency for those who carry extra weight. In other words, fat distribution is partially influenced by genes. However, smoking and drinking too many alcoholic beverages also seem to increase fat carried in the stomach area; as a result, they increase the risk of weight-related health problems. Conversely, vigorous exercise can help to reduce fat everywhere, helping to decrease these health risks.

After menopause many women tend to add weight around the midriff.

Waist Whys. Health risks go up as waist size increases. That's especially true if your waist measures more than

35 inches for a woman or more than 40 inches for a man. So a simple tape measure is a tool for assessing abdominal fat. Stand, and measure your waist around your bare abdomen just above your hipbone. (*Hint:* Relax, breathe out, measure. Don't cinch in the tape measure or pull in your stomach!)

The higher your BMI and waist measurement and the more weight-related risk factors you have, the more likely you'll benefit from losing a few pounds.

For more about the risks from and the causes of overweight and obesity, refer to "Weighing the Risks" later in this chapter.

Calorie Balance Basics

You can't touch them or see them. Food supplies them. Your body burns them to keep you alive—and moving. What are they? They're calories! To understand how to achieve and maintain a healthy weight, start with calorie basics.

A Measure of Energy

Calories are units of energy. Back in science class, you probably learned the technical definition: One calorie is the amount of energy needed to raise the temperature of 1 gram of water by 1 degree Celsius. In the world of nutrition and health, the term "calorie" refers to energy in food and the energy the body uses.

Click Here! Websites to Know . . .

- Academy of Nutrition and Dietetics, http://www.eatright.org/Public/content .aspx?id=6843
- International Food Information Council Foundation, www.foodinsight.org/Resources/ Weight-Management
- Steps to a Healthier Weight, USDA, www.ChooseMyPlate.gov
- My Food-a-pedia, USDA, www.myfoodapedia.gov
- Weight-control Information Network, win.niddk.nih.gov/index.htm

In food, calories are energy locked inside three groups of nutrients: carbohydrates, fats, and proteins. These nutrients are released from food during digestion, then absorbed into the bloodstream and at some point converted to blood glucose, or blood sugar. Alcohol delivers calories, too.

In your body, the food energy in glucose finally gets released into trillions of body cells, where it's used to power all your body's work—from your heartbeat, to push-ups, to the smile that spreads across your face. Calories from food you don't need can be stored as body fat for later use or perhaps as glycogen, a storage form of carbohydrate.

Calories in Food and Beverages

Read food labels or check a calorie-counting book, website, or phone app. You'll see that nearly all foods and drinks supply calories—some more than others. What accounts for the differences?

Three nutrient groups—carbohydrates, proteins, and fats—and alcohol supply calories, in food and beverages. Gram for gram, fat and alcohol supply more than either carbohydrate or protein. Fats provide 9 calories per gram; alcohol, 7 calories per gram; and carbohydrates and proteins, 4 calories per gram. Most foods provide a combination of these nutrients. Vitamins, minerals, and water don't provide calories; neither do cholesterol and fiber.

Foods that are watery, watery-crisp (rather than

Balancing Calories to Manage Weight

Dietary Guidelines' Key Recommendations

- Prevent and/or reduce overweight and obesity through improved eating and physical activity behaviors.
- Control total calorie intake to manage body weight. For people who are overweight or obese, this will mean consuming fewer calories from food and beverages.
- Increase physical activity and reduce time spent in sedentary behaviors.
- Maintain appropriate calorie balance during each stage of life—childhood, adolescence, pregnancy and breast-feeding, and older age.

Source: Dietary Guidelines for Americans, 2010.

greasy-crisp) such as lettuce and greens, or fibrous tend to have fewer calories and more volume than foods that are more fatty or greasy. (Water and fiber are calorie-free.) For example, celery, which has more water and fiber than French fries, also has fewer calories. To turn up the volume on your plate, choose bulky foods with more water or fiber that may fill you up with fewer calories. *Check "Eat More Food, Fewer Calories!" in chapter 10.*

To find the calories in a food or to compare two foods, click here: www.myfoodapedia.gov.

How Many Calories for You?

Your body's need for energy, or fuel, never stops. Every minute of every day, your body needs a constant supply of energy to stay alive and to function well.

Powering your body with energy can be compared to fueling your car. Both your car and your body need an energy source just to keep idling. When you move, your body (and your car) burns more fuel to go faster and farther. Some bodies—and some cars—are more fuel efficient than others. That is, they use less energy to do the same amount of work.

How many calories do you need? Most people don't know. Calorie needs vary from person to person. Everyone has a personal limit. Even your own energy needs change from day to day and at different ages and stages of life. Your age, basal metabolic rate, body size and composition, physical health, and activity level contribute to your caloric needs. What's more, wanting to lose, gain, or maintain your weight affects how many calories you need to consume.

The Institute of Medicine advises Acceptable Macronutrient Distribution Ranges (AMDR): for adults, calories from carbohydrate (45 to 65 percent), from fat (20 to 35 percent), and from protein (10 to 35 percent).

To lose, gain, or maintain your weight, the proportion of each of these nutrients makes little difference. It's your total calories—in and out—that count! However, the fewer calories you consume overall, the greater percent of calories you need from protein (within the AMDR range) to also meet your protein need.

Check "Estimated Calorie Needs per Day by Age, Gender, and Physical Activity Level" in the appendices to estimate your calorie needs, or use the online SuperTracker tool at www.ChooseMyPlate.gov.

Calories in Balance!

There's nothing magical about controlling weight!

To maintain weight: balance calories you consume from foods and beverages with calories expended. In other words, let calories in equal calories out.

The amount of calories you can consume to match your body's energy (calorie) expenditure is your energy allowance. Think of it as a calorie budget. How do you want to "spend" those calories? If you need to lose or gain, tip the calorie balance:

● *For weight loss:* Consume fewer calories than you burn each day. Either cut back on calories in, or move more. Better yet, do both!

● *For weight gain:* Tip calorie balance the other way. Take in more calories than your body uses. Still keep moving!

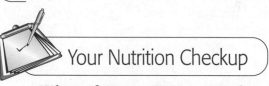

Your Nutrition Checkup

What If Your BMI or Waist Size Is High?

If your BMI is between 25 and 30 and you are otherwise healthy, you may need to look into healthy ways to improve your eating and physical activity habits.

Talk to your healthcare provider about losing weight if:

● Your BMI is 30 or above, *or*

● Your BMI is between 25 and 30, you are under age 65 years, *and* you have two or more of these health problems: type 2 diabetes, high blood pressure, heart disease and stroke, some types of cancer, sleep apnea, osteoarthritis, gallbladder disease, liver disease, irregular menstrual periods *or*

● A family history of heart disease or diabetes, *or*

● Your waist measures over 35 inches (women) or 40 inches (men)—even if your BMI is less than *25—and* you have:

   ● Two or more of the health problems listed above *or*

   ● A family history of heart disease or diabetes.

Source: Weight-control Information Network, NIH Publication No. 04-5283, 2008.

For more about these health risks, see chapter 22, "Smart Eating to Prevent and Manage Disease."

Metabolism: Energy for Body Basics

Energy for basal metabolism (basic needs) is energy your body burns on "idle" or what you need to stay alive. In scientific terms, basal metabolic rate (BMR) is the energy level that keeps involuntary body processes going: pumping your heart, breathing, generating body heat, perspiring, transmitting brain messages, and producing thousands of body chemicals. For most people, basal metabolism represents about 60 percent of their energy needs!

Why can one person consume more calories day after day and never gain a pound? For another person of the same age, height, and activity level, weight control is a constant challenge. Age, gender, genetics, and body composition and size, among other factors, affect basic energy needs. Although you don't need to know your BMR to achieve and maintain a healthy weight, that may be useful information for some people, perhaps athletes in training. Health or fitness professionals, especially a registered dietitian, can determine that for you. *Worth noting:* A handheld palm device is available that individuals can use to measure their metabolic rate at rest.

Age Factor. Young people—from infancy through adolescence—need more calories per pound than adults do for growing bone, muscle, and other tissues. During infancy, energy needs are higher per pound of body weight than at any other time in life. And just watch a growing teenager eat; you know that energy needs are high during adolescence!

By adulthood, food energy (calorie) needs—and BMR—start to decline: 2 percent for each decade. For example, a woman who needs about 2,200 calories per day for her total energy needs at age twenty-five might need 2 percent less, or 2,156 calories per day, at age thirty-five. She may need another 2 percent less by age forty-five, and so on.

Why the decline in BMR? Body composition and hormones change with age. And with less physical activity, muscle mass decreases; body fat takes its place. Because body fat burns less energy than muscle, fewer calories are needed to maintain body weight, and the basal metabolic rate goes down. (As an aside, regular physical activity can help keep your metabolic rate up.)

If you continue to follow your teenage eating habits—and live a less active lifestyle—the extra pounds that creep on with age should come as no surprise! Unused calories get stored as body fat.

Family Matters. Genetic makeup and inherited body build account for some differences in basal metabolic rate—differences you can't change! (Families tend to pass on food habits to one another, too, which also may account for similarities in body weight.)

Body Size, Shape, and Composition. Consider their impact on BMR and energy needs:

● A heavy, full-size car usually burns more fuel per mile than a small, sleek sports car. Likewise, the more you weigh, the more calories you burn. It takes somewhat more effort to move if you weigh 170 pounds compared to 120. That's one reason why men, who often weigh more, use more calories than women.

● A lean, muscular body has a higher metabolic rate than a softly rounded body with more fat tissue. Why? Ounce for ounce, muscle burns more energy than body fat does. So the higher your proportion of muscle to fat, the more calories you need to maintain your weight. A softly rounded body type has a greater tendency to store body fat then a lean, muscular body. *Tip:* Stay physically active to maintain your muscle mass—and give your BMR a boost.

● A tall, thin body also has more surface area than a short body, and as a result, more heat loss; the net result—more calories burned (higher BMR) to maintain normal body temperature.

Gender Gap. The ratio of muscle to fat differs with gender, accounting for differences in BMR. Up to age ten or so, energy needs for boys and girls are

---

How Does Your Body Use Energy?

If you're like most people, here's how your body uses the energy it "burns" each day:

Basic energy needs (basal metabolism)	60%
Physical activity (all movements)	30%
Digestion of food and absorption of nutrients	10%
Total energy use for the day	*100%*

about the same, but then puberty triggers change. When boys start developing more muscle, they need more calories; their added height and size demand more energy, too.

By adulthood, men usually have less body fat and 10 to 20 percent more muscle than women of the same age and weight. That's one reason why men's basic energy needs are higher. In contrast, women's bodies naturally keep body fat stores in reserve for pregnancy and breast-feeding, when a woman's energy needs go up. *Refer to chapter 18.*

Hot . . . or Cold? Outside temperature affects internal energy production. On chilly days, your BMR "burns" a little higher to keep you warm during prolonged exposure to cold. Shivering and moving to keep warm use energy, too. And in hot temperatures, your body's air conditioning system burns a bit more energy—for example, as you perspire to cool down.

Diet Factor. Do you think that skipping meals or following a very-low-calorie eating plan offers a weight-loss edge? Think again. Severe calorie restriction can make your body more energy efficient and cause the rate at which your body burns energy to slow down! Your body then requires slightly fewer calories to perform the same processes. This slow-down in metabolic rate is your body's survival strategy.

Physical Activity: An Energy Burner

Movement of any kind—a blink of your eye, a wave of your hand, or a jog around the block—uses energy. In fact, about 30 percent of your body's energy intake is used to power physical activity of all kinds, not just

BURNING CALORIES WITH ACTIVITY

CALORIES BURNED PER HOUR, BY BODY WEIGHT			CALORIES BURNED PER HOUR, BY BODY WEIGHT		
ACTIVITY	**120 LBS.**	**170 LBS.**	**ACTIVITY**	**120 LBS.**	**170 LBS.**
Aerobic dance	335	500	Racquetball	380	540
Archery	190	270	Reading	70	100
Basketball	330	460	Rowing, stationary	380	540
Bicycling (<10 mph)	220	310	Running, 10 mph	870	1,235
Bowling	165	230	Sitting (watching TV)	55	75
Calisthenics	190	270	Sitting (writing, typing)	100	140
Driving a car	110	155	Skating, roller	380	540
Eating	80	115	Skiing, cross-country	435	615
Food preparation	120	175	Skiing, downhill	325	460
Gardening	220	310	Sleeping	50	70
Golf (walking)	245	345	Soccer	380	540
Hiking	325	460	Swimming, leisure	380	540
Horseback riding	220	310	Tennis	380	540
Housework	135	190	Walking, brisk	205	295
Jogging	380	540	Weight training	165	230
Mowing lawn	245	345			

Calculated from: Ainsworth, BE. *The Compendium of Physical Activities Tracking Guide. Prevention Research Center,* Norman J. Arnold School of Public Health, University of South Carolina, 2002.

the time spent in a gym! At best, that estimate is imprecise because activity levels differ so much. Very active people need more calories, about 40 percent of their total energy for physical activity.

The amount of energy used to power physical activity actually depends on three things, nicknamed F.I.T.: frequency, intensity, and time (how long you do it). Walking up stairs takes more calories than using an escalator. Or suppose you walk with a friend of the same age and body size. The one who pumps his or her arms and takes an extra lap around the block burns more energy for that activity. *The chart "Burning Calories with Activity" in this chapter shows the energy (calories) used for common, nonstop activities.*

The Food Connection

Eating itself actually burns calories. Digesting food and absorbing nutrients use about 10 percent of your day's energy expenditure—about 200 calories if you consume 2,000 calories daily. But don't count on these processes to burn up all the energy in anything you eat!

Calorie Myths

Do these unfounded notions sound familiar?

Myth: A rich, fudgy brownie, before bedtime, is more fattening than the same brownie eaten at lunchtime.

Fact: What you eat, not when, makes the difference. No matter when they're eaten, calories seem to have the same effect in the body. Too many can add up to extra body fat. Timing has no direct effect on how your

body uses the calories. However, evidence does suggest that eating regular meals, especially breakfast, helps promote weight loss by reducing fat intake and minimizing impulsive snacking later.

Weight gain from late-night snacking may come from eating out of habit, boredom, or stress—not hunger—and from eating more calories than planned. Listen to your body's hunger cues and avoid impulsive and mindless eating. To avoid late-night snacking eat dinner later, save dessert for later, or go to bed earlier.

Myth: Potatoes and bread are fattening.

Fact: By themselves, they're not high in calories— 88 calories for a medium (4-ounce) potato and 70 calories for an average-size slice of bread. However, high-fat toppings or spreads can add up to excess calories. Consider the calories in one tablespoon: sour cream (about 30 calories), butter or margarine (about 100 calories), and regular mayonnaise (about 100 calories).

Myth: Skip nuts for weight loss.

Fact: A small portion (an ounce or two) of nuts can be okay—and may take the edge off hunger. Enjoy these nutrient-rich foods in small amounts for their healthy oils, protein, fiber, and magnesium. Be prudent: a half ounce, or a small handful, of mixed nuts has about 84 calories.

Myth: Going vegetarian is a sure way to lose weight.

Fact: Not necessarily. Although a vegetarian eating plan is often lower in calories, cutting out meat, poultry, and dairy foods won't automatically mean fewer calories. Even vegetarians can overeat—with excessive portions and with too many high-calorie foods with more added sugars and fat.

Myth: Carbs cause weight gain.

Fact: Excess carbohydrates are no more fattening than excess calories from any source: fats, carbohydrates, and proteins. When it comes to weight gain, a calorie is a calorie, regardless of its source.

Limited research notes that carbohydrate-rich food may cause weight gain in "insulin-resistant" people. For these individuals, it's speculated that the body reacts to sugars and starches by overproducing insulin—and so causes too much carbohydrate to be stored as fat. However, most of us don't gain weight on

Have You Ever Wondered

. . . if stress promotes weight gain? The role of chronic stress and weight is an area of research. Among the questions: Do hormones released with stress increase appetite, and do these hormones promote fat production and deposits, especially in the abdomen? That said, for many people, stress triggers emotional overeating.

. . . what to do when your weight seems to plateau? Be patient. Plateaus are normal with weight loss. Your body requires fewer calories to function as you lose weight. Allow time to readjust. Gradually adding more activity may help nudge you off the weight plateau.

a high-carbohydrate diet unless it provides excess calories. *See "Metabolic Syndrome" in chapter 22.*

Weighing the Risks

Overweight, obesity, or underweight: all pose health risks!

Overweight and obesity are epidemic—and on the rise—in the United States and in many other parts of the world. According to the Centers for Disease Control and Prevention, 34 percent of U.S. adults were obese in 2008, compared to about 15 percent of adults in the late 1970s; in 2008 72 percent of men and 64 percent of women were overweight or obese in the United States. For youth in the United States, an estimated 20 percent of children ages six to eleven years are considered obese today, compared to 4 percent in the early 1970s. Among children ages two to five years, obesity has jumped from 5 to 10 percent over these decades, and from 6 percent to 18 percent among adolescents.

Weight Problems: The Causes

What Causes Overweight and Obesity?

The simple answer is calorie imbalance, in this case meaning more calories are consumed than used. However, the underlying reasons are far more complex: environmental, lifestyle, social, psychological, and physical. Consider the world we live in: temptation from food that's easily available, limited options for nutrient-rich foods and beverages in some places, and communities that are designed for driving, not walking or bicycling. Lifestyles are often overscheduled, leaving less time for physical activity. And the list goes on.

Today's technology means people expend fewer calories for daily tasks. Think of the impact of the computer. In past decades a typist on a manual typewriter burned 15 more calories more per hour than someone doing the same work on a computer today. For four hours of work, that's 60 calories a day, or 300 calories over a workweek. Add up the impact from escalators and moving sidewalks, cars and motorbikes, work-saving appliances and electric car door openers, and more! The amount of screen time—TV, video games, computers—is also linked to inactivity and the rise in obesity. Inactivity has become a way

> ## Have You Ever Wondered **?**
>
> *. . . if my weight problem is really a thyroid problem?* Maybe—but before you blame your thyroid, check with your doctor, who may order a test to find out. Hypothyroidism, when the thyroid doesn't produce enough thyroid hormone, is the most common form of thyroid disease; one symptom is weight gain. On the flip side, an overactive thyroid causes hyperthyroidism; one symptom is weight loss. *See chapter 22, for more about thyroid disease and high blood cholesterol.*

of life, and weight control has become an everyday challenge. The more you sit, the less energy you need, and the more likely you are to gain weight if your food intake stays the same!

The food supply has changed, too. Compared to the 1970s, people today have, on average, 600 more calories a day available to consume! That comes from bigger portions and choosing more higher-calorie foods with added sugars and fats such as sugary drinks, grain-based desserts, and vending machine snacks. Studies show: Portion size is linked to body weight.

Because it runs in families, genetics may play a role in being overweight or obese—especially if the conditions are right. For example, people who inherit a "sluggish" metabolism are more likely to have a weight problem. A child's surroundings and upbringing are factors. Families pass on their diet and lifestyle habits. With one obese parent, the chances of being overweight are 40 percent; that doubles when both parents are obese.

Other factors also are linked to weight gain, obesity, or problems with weight loss. Those include certain diseases, such hypothyroidism, polycystic ovary syndrome, and Cushing's syndrome. Some medications may stimulate appetite, may cause water retention, or may affect basal metabolic rate; check with your doctor. Lack of sleep also may contribute to weight problems.

What about Being Too Thin?

The reasons for being underweight are as complex and unique as being overweight. Genetics may be a factor. As with obesity, thinness tends to run in families. Some people may inherit a speedy metabolism. For many reasons, the brain's appetite center may not signal hunger, so people may feel full even when they're not. Other psychological, physical, economic, social, and lifestyle factors also may get in the way of eating well.

Overweight and Obesity: Hazards to Health

Sometime spend an hour or so carrying around a 5-pound bag of flour, a 10-pound bag of potatoes, or a heavy phone book. Tiring? That's the extra burden on your body and heart when you carry extra pounds of body fat. The more excess body fat you have, the greater that burden. Every body system—including the lungs, the heart, and the skeleton—has to work harder as you move.

Have you ever finished a physical exam feeling that your weight was within a healthy range, only to have your doctor advise losing a few pounds? For some physical conditions, such as high blood pressure, diabetes, high blood cholesterol, or arthritis,

---

Your "Weigh": Figuring Your Energy Needs

How much energy does your body need in a day? For a rough guesstimate, do the following "energy math."

1. *Figure your basic energy needs (BMR).* Multiply your healthy weight (in pounds) by 10 for women and by 11 for men. If you see from your BMI that you're overweight, use the average weight within the healthy weight range for your height in "Does Your BMI Put You in a Risky Zone?" on page 23.

   weight × ____ (either 10 or 11) = ____ calories for basic needs

2. *Figure your energy needs for physical activity.* Check the activity level that matches your lifestyle for most days of the week:

   ____ Sedentary: mainly sitting, driving a car, lying down, sleeping, standing, reading, typing, or other low-intensity activities

   ____ Light activity (for no more than 2 hours daily): light exercise such as light housework, grocery shopping, walking leisurely

   ____ Moderate activity: moderate exercise such as heavy housework, gardening, dancing, or brisk walking (and very little sitting)

   ____ Very active: active physical sports, or in a labor-intensive job such as construction work

   Multiply your basic energy needs by the percent that matches your activity level: sedentary, 20%; light activity, 30%; moderate activity, 40%; or very active, 50%.

   ____ calories for basic needs
   × ____% for activity level
   = ____ calories for physical activity

3. *Figure energy for digestion and absorbing nutrients.* Add your calories for basic needs and calories for physical activity, then multiply the total by 10%.

   (____ calories for basic needs + ____ calories for physical activity) × 10% =

   ____ calories for digestion and absorbing nutrients

4. Add up your total energy needs by adding calories for each purpose.

   + calories for basic needs

   + calories for physical activity

   + calories for digestion and absorbing nutrients

   = ____ calories for your total energy needs

   As an example, consider this 40-year-old female, who works at a desk and walks during her lunch hour. She weighs 125 pounds, which is healthy for her height.

   Basic energy needs: 125 pounds × 10 = 1,250 calories

   Energy for moderate physical activity: 1,250 calories × 0.30 = 375 calories

   Energy for digestion and absorbing nutrients: (1,250 + 375 calories) × 0.10 = 162.5 calories

   Total energy needs: 1,250 calories + 375 calories + 162.5 calories = *1,787.5 calories*

Check the appendices for the Dietary Reference Intake's Estimated Energy Requirements, as well as the "Estimated Calorie Needs per Day by Age, Gender, and Physical Activity Level."

RISKY BUSINESS

**OVERWEIGHT AND OBESITY:
KNOWN RISK FACTORS FOR . . .**

- Type 2 diabetes
- Heart disease and stroke
- High blood pressure
- Gallbladder disease
- Osteoarthritis (degeneration of the cartilage and bone in joints)
- Sleep apnea and other breathing problems
- Some forms of cancer (uterine, breast, colorectal, prostate, perhaps others)

OBESITY: ASSOCIATED WITH . . .

- High blood pressure
- High blood cholesterol
- Complications of pregnancy
- Menstrual irregularities
- Excess body and facial hair
- Stress incontinence (urine leakage cause by weak muscles in the pelvic area)
- Psychological disorders such as depression
- Increased surgical risk

Source: National Institute of Diabetes and Digestive and Kidney Diseases/National Institutes of Health.

your doctor may offer that advice, even if your weight appears to be in a healthy range.

Many health problems and premature death are linked to overweight and obesity. *See the chart "Risky Business" above. See chapter 22 to learn about links between excess body weight and heart disease, diabetes, and some cancers.*

Obesity can lead to a cycle of inactivity. Often extra body weight makes physical activity more tiring—even for everyday activities such as walking up stairs or through a mall. Inactivity can lead to more weight gain, more muscle loss, and other health problems. Obesity can have an emotional price tag, too, if a negative body image leads to poor self-esteem and social isolation.

Now consider the upside: The health benefits of trimming down. If you need to lose, dropping 5 to 10 percent of your body weight may improve your health and quality of life, and prevent these health problems. For someone who weighs 200 pounds, that's a loss of 10 to 20 pounds. Even this small weight shift can help lower the risk factors for many chronic diseases: lower blood pressure, total and LDL blood cholesterol levels, triglyceride level, and blood glucose level. In addition, HDL cholesterol levels may go up. *See the "'Fat' Dictionary" in chapter 5. For women, see "Every Age and*

Stage of Life: Why a Healthy Weight?" in chapter 18.

Your weight is healthy? Smart eating and active living help you prevent weight gain and stay healthy as you age. In fact, keeping your healthy weight over time is better than trying to lose weight after you gain. Once someone becomes obese, it takes more effort—and more time—to get to a healthy weight.

Obesity and Kids: A Heavy Burden

America's youth are getting fatter. They're less active physically. And health risks—such as high blood cholesterol, high blood pressure, and type 2 diabetes—related to excess body fat are more common today among kids. In the past these conditions were primarily found among adults. Effects of childhood overweight and obesity can last a lifetime.

Although obese children don't automatically become obese adults, there's reason for concern. Eating and activity patterns for life often are established during childhood. For these children, the risk for being overweight as teens and adults is higher. Research says those who are overweight as teens have a significantly greater chance for ongoing health concerns such as diabetes as adults. And weight problems affect self-image and, as a result, self-esteem. How children feel about themselves can affect almost every aspect of their lives now—and into adulthood.

Prevent obesity at an early age! Often increased physical activity, rather than cutting calories, is enough to help overweight children achieve a healthful weight. For them, the goal is to reduce the rate of weight gain as they grow and develop. Young people need enough calories and nutrients for their growth and development. Before devising a plan to help your child or teenager lose weight, talk to your doctor or registered dietitian (RD). Weight-loss programs for adults are not meant for children or teens.

For more about healthful food choices and lifestyles

Weight Cycling

Have you gained and lost the same 10, 20, or even 30 pounds over and over again? The cycle of repeatedly losing and regaining weight sometimes happens to those who go on weight-loss diets. Weight cycling may lead to feelings of frustration, failure, and poor self-esteem. According to some studies, weight cycling may even increase the risk for ongoing health problems such as high blood pressure, high cholesterol, and gallbladder disease.

Weight cycling is often an outcome of quick-fix diets, weight-loss gimmicks, and other risky strategies and may be linked to binge eating, *described later in this chapter*. If repeated "ups and downs" of dieting describe your weight problem, shift your approach to one of lifetime weight management. Break the cycle with long-term approaches rather than short-term results. Make gradual and permanent changes in the way you eat, your physical activity level, and your lifestyle. It's the only way to be healthy—for life.

If you have weight-cycling history, here's some insight. Most research indicates that weight cycling itself doesn't affect, or lower, your metabolic rate, according to the National Institutes of Health, Weight-Control Information Network. Most people return to their original weight, with the same percentage of lean muscle and fat as before—if their activity level and calorie intake return to the original levels, too. Weight cycling doesn't increase abdominal fat, either. If you adopt a healthier approach to weight loss or maintenance, your past history won't get in the way.

for children and teens, see chapter 17, "Food to Grow On." There you'll also find guidelines for helping young people reach and maintain a healthy weight.

Underweight: Hazards to Health

Is being too thin a problem? Maybe. Being too thin can be a health risk, especially if underweight results from undereating. An eating pattern with too few calories may not supply enough nutrients to keep the body running normally. Children who undereat may not get enough nutrients or energy for growth and development either. A lack of food energy may cause fatigue, irritability, and lack of concentration. And those with a poor diet may have trouble warding off infections.

For normal-weight people, a layer of body fat just under the skin helps protect the body from cold. But very thin people have only a very thin fat layer, so they lack enough insulation to keep them warm. That is even more of a health concern for the thin, frail elderly, especially without adequate heating in their homes.

If you lose weight suddenly and don't know the cause, talk to your doctor. This may be an early symptom of other health problems.

A doctor may advise some weight gain, perhaps to replace weight loss and aid recovery after a prolonged illness or surgery, or to help withstand some medical treatments, perhaps cancer treatment.

Weight Management: Strategies That Work!

The key to managing your weight throughout your life? A positive "can do" attitude and the right kind of motivation! If you're trying to lose weight to fit into a bathing suit before vacation, or to look good for your school reunion, or because your spouse is nagging you to drop a belt size, your commitment and efforts are likely to fizzle out over time. Internal motivators—health, increased energy, self-esteem, feeling in control—increase your chances for lifelong success.

If you're at your healthy weight, these strategies for weight management are meant for you, too.

Caution: If your weight problem is excessive—too much or too little—or if you have health problems, talk to your doctor before starting a weight-loss plan. Children, pregnant women, those with chronic diseases, and people over age sixty-five shouldn't attempt weight loss without advice from their health professional.

Look for more ways to manage your weight in other chapters in this book.

Ready? Set . . . Go with the Right Mind Set!

Whether your objective is weight loss, weight gain, or weight maintenance, lifelong success may mean new ways of thinking. And while you can't control the way your body uses calories for its metabolic processes, you can control what you eat and drink and how many calories you use in physical activity.

● Make health your weight-management priority. Strive for your best weight for health, not necessarily the lowest weight you could be—or what you consider your "ideal" number. *A potential bonus:* Positive changes in your appearance!

● For weight loss or gain, follow these tactics: (1) healthful eating, (2) regular physical activity, and (3) acceptance of the weight you can achieve through healthful eating and a healthful lifestyle.

● Set realistic, attainable goals—for you! Start with your current weight or lifestyle, not where you want to be. The challenge of trimming 5 pounds at a time may seem more doable than losing 25 or more pounds.

● Focus on a healthful lifestyle—for a lifetime—not on "dieting." Dieting alone is often a short-term tactic without long-term results. The concept of "dieting" carries negative baggage: guilt, "shoulds," and "can't haves." For most people, "dieting" results in failure.

● Focus your strategies: action-oriented, doable, specific, and one step at a time. Perhaps you'll walk for 15 minutes each day during your break, or you'll drink low-fat or fat-free milk rather than a milk shake with your fast-food lunch.

● Tailor your strategies to you: your schedule, budget, family situation, and personal needs, to name a few. Experts have found that two out of three people who were successful at weight control personalized their efforts to fit their lifestyles.

● Think long-term; act gradually. Fasting and starvation-type diets can peel off pounds, but most weight that's lost quickly is water loss, which will come back as fast as it's lost. Grueling exercise regimens may tone the body, but for most people, these tactics aren't realistic ways to live—nor healthful, either.

Instead of trying quick fixes, plan for a gradual weight shift of $1/2$ to 1 pound a week. That's safe and healthy. With any more weight loss, you may be exercising too much or eating too little.

If you need to lose weight, losing about 10 percent of your weight over 6 months likely is safe; that's 20 pounds in 6 months (26 weeks) for someone who weighs 200 pounds. Your extra pounds didn't appear overnight. They don't disappear that way, either!

● Be realistic with your self-talk. Skip the absolutes—"always," "never," and "must" in your tactics. "I'll never eat another French fry." "I must swim twenty laps every other day." Get rid of "shoulds," too. "I should get up early and walk."

● Cut yourself some slack. Nobody's perfect. Allow for occasional slipups in your eating strategies, without feeling guilty.

● Plan to indulge sensibly. Plan for occasional "treats" and "splurges." You may be more successful in the long run.

● Expect success. Reaching life's goals is often a self-fulfilling prophecy. Positive self-talk and an enthusiastic approach to weight management can set you up for success!

Get Physical!

Move it to lose it! Physical activity is a powerful tool for weight management. A physically active lifestyle offers many other rewards—from heart health to strong bones to stress relief and more. *See "Moderate Activity: What Is It?" in chapter 1.*

For Your Health, for Calorie Balance . . .

● Consume foods and drinks to meet, not exceed, calorie need.
● Plan ahead to make better food choices.
● Track food and calorie intake.
● Limit calorie intake from solid fats and added sugars.
● Reduce portions, especially of high-calorie foods.
● Cook and eat more meals at home, instead of eating out.
● Think about choosing healthy options when eating out.
● Limit screen time.
● Increase physical activity.
● Choose moderate- and vigorous-intensity physical activity.
● Avoid inactivity. Some activity is better than none.
● Slowly build up the amount of physical activity you choose.

Source: Dietary Guidelines for Americans, 2010 .

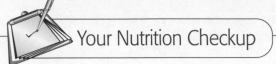

Weight-Loss Readiness Test

Your attitude affects your ability to succeed at weight loss. Take this readiness quiz to see if you're mentally ready before you begin.

Mark each statement as "true" or "false." Be honest with yourself! The answers should reflect the way you really think—not how you'd like to be!

1. I have thought a lot about my eating habits and physical activities. I know what I might change.

2. I know that I need to make permanent, not temporary, changes in my eating and activity patterns.

3. I will feel successful only if I lose a lot of weight.

4. I know that it's best if I lose weight slowly.

5. I'm thinking about losing weight now because I want to, not because someone else thinks so.

6. I think losing weight would solve other problems in my life.

7. I am willing and able to increase my regular physical activity.

8. I can lose weight successfully if I have no slipups.

9. I am willing to commit time and effort each week to organize and plan my food and activity choices.

10. Once I lose a few pounds but reach a plateau (I can't seem to lose more), I usually lose the motivation to keep going toward my weight goal.

11. I want to start a weight loss program, even though my life is unusually stressful right now.

Now Score Yourself

Look at your answers for items 1, 2, 4, 5, 7, and 9. Score "1" if you answered "true" and "0" if you answered "false." For items 3, 6, 8, 10, and 11, score "0" for each "true" answer and "1" for each false answer.

No one score indicates if you're ready to start losing weight. But the higher your total score, the more likely you'll be successful.

If you scored 8 or higher, you probably have good reasons to lose weight now. And you know some of the steps that can help you succeed.

If you scored 5 to 7 points, reevaluate your reasons for losing weight and the strategies you'd follow.

If you scored 4 or less, now may not be the right time to start. You may be successful initially, but you may not be able to sustain the effort to reach or maintain your weight goal. Reconsider your reasons and approach.

Interpret Your Score

Your answer gives clues to stumbling blocks to your weight management success. Any item you scored as "0" suggests a misconception about weight loss, or a problem area for you. Look at each item more closely.

1. You can't change what you don't understand, and that includes your eating habits and activity pattern. Keep records for a week to pinpoint when, what, why, and how much you eat—as well as patterns and obstacles to regular physical activity.

2. You may be able to lose weight in the short run with drastic or highly restrictive changes in your eating habits or activity pattern. But they may be hard to live with permanently. Your food and activity plans should be healthful ones you can enjoy and sustain.

3. Many people fantasize about reaching a weight goal that's unrealistically low. If that sounds like you, rethink your meaning of success. A reasonable goal takes body type into consideration—and sets smaller, achievable "mile markers" along the way.

4. If you equate success with fast weight loss, you'll likely have problems keeping weight off. "Quick-fix" approaches often backfire when you face the challenges of weight maintenance. The best and healthiest approach is slow weight loss while learning ways to keep it off permanently.

5. The desire for and commitment to weight loss must come from you—not others. People who lose weight, then keep it off, take responsibility for their weight goals and choose their own approach.

6. Being overweight may contribute to some social problems, but it's rarely the single cause. While body image and self-esteem are strongly linked, thinking you can solve all your problems by losing weight isn't realistic. And it may set you up for disappointment.

7. A habit of regular, moderate physical activity is key to successfully losing weight—and keeping it off. For weight control, physical activity doesn't need to be strenuous. Any moderate physical activity that you enjoy and do regularly counts.

8. Most people don't expect perfection in their daily lives, yet they often feel they must stick to a weight-loss program perfectly. Perfection at weight loss isn't realistic. Rather than viewing lapses as catastrophes, see them as opportunities to find what triggers your problems and develop strategies for the future.

9. To successfully lose weight, take time to assess your challenges, then develop an approach that's best for you. Success requires planning, commitment, and time.

10. A plateau in an ongoing weight-loss program is perfectly normal, so don't give up too soon! Before you lose your motivation, think about past efforts that failed, then identify strategies to help overcome hurdles.

11. Weight loss itself can be a source of stress, so if you're already under stress, you may find a weight-loss program somewhat difficult to implement right now. Try to resolve other life stressors before starting to lose weight.

Source: Academy of Nutrition and Dietetics.

Study after study shows that people who keep physically active are more successful at losing—and keeping off—extra pounds of body fat. These are some reasons why physical activity promotes a healthy weight:

- *Burns calories.* The longer, more frequently, and more vigorously you move, the more calories you burn. When you burn more than you consume, your body uses its energy stores, and you lose weight. Just adding thirty minutes of brisk walking to your day makes a difference!

- *Helps you keep and build muscle and lose body fat.* Without physical activity, you tend to lose lean body tissue.

- *Helps relieve stress.* Stress may lead to nibbling on more food and consuming more calories than your body needs.

- *Creates a "trimmer" mind-set.* As people get more physically active, they often opt for foods with fewer calories, less fat, and less added sugars. The reason? It just seems to "feel good."

- *"Looks good" on you.* A firm, lean body from physical activity looks trimmer than one that's flabby with more body fat, even at the same weight. Think of your body as a "package" of lean tissue and body fat; muscles take less space than body fat. Although looks aren't the only reason for being physically active, they're a great side effect!

What if you need to *gain* weight? Because the benefits go beyond weight control, everyone needs to move! To gain weight, there's no need to cut back on physical activity unless a person's physical activity pattern is excessive—or if a physician advises a slower pace.

Weight control is just one reason to keep physically active. *For other benefits, see "Ten Reasons to Make the 'Right Moves'" in chapter 1.*

Live an Active Lifestyle

An active lifestyle is key to calorie balance, weight management, and many more health benefits. You don't need to be an exercise fanatic with strenuous daily workouts. Step aerobics, kickboxing, or thirty minutes on an exercise bike every day may not be right for you. That's okay; any kind of moderate, consistent physical activity can do the job. In fact, any activity you enjoy and stay with can be the right one for you. If it's enjoyable, you're more likely to stick with it.

What's the daily goal for physical activity? That depends on your calorie intake—and it varies depending on your age. For a healthy body weight, the 2008 Physical Activity Guidelines for Americans advises 150 minutes of aerobic moderate-intensity physical activity each week for most adults. *See "Moderate Activity: What Is It?" in chapter 1.* You may need to boost your level of physical activity to reach and keep your healthy weight, perhaps to 300 minutes or more a week. Do activities that build muscle, too, at least twice weekly: legs, hips, back, chest, stomach, shoulders, and arms; for kids, three times weekly for these activities is advised. *Refer to the appendices for Physical Activity Guidelines for children, teens, and older adults.*

Do it all at once, or spread it out: for example, ten minutes of brisk walking during your lunch hour, fifteen minutes of leisure bike riding, and five minutes of sidewalk sweeping at home. If you haven't been physically active, then build up gradually. Get a pedometer to count your steps; work up to 10,000 steps a day. Even a little more physical activity—and a little less TV and computer time—can make a difference.

Remember: The energy expenditure of physical activity goes up in three ways. The longer, the more frequent, and the more intense your activity, the more energy you burn.

Even though some weight-loss regimens make "spot-reducing" promises, your body can't get rid of fat in just the problem places. Abdominal crunches alone won't help you lose weight around your stomach. As you exercise and burn more calories than you

---

Twenty Everyday Ways to Get Moving

Fitting physical activity into your life may be easier than you think—even with a busy lifestyle. These everyday activities count toward your day's total if they're done with moderate intensity. Most take only a little extra time. Fit activity in 10 minutes at a time.

1. Wake up 30 minutes earlier, and take a brisk walk to start your day. Need someone to get you going? Schedule your walk with your spouse or a neighbor.

2. Forget the drive-through car wash. Wash the car yourself. *Bonus:* You'll save money at the same time.

3. Take stairs instead of the elevator or escalator. Walking up stairs is a great heart exerciser, calorie burner, and muscle builder!

4. Park at the far end of the parking lot for a longer walk. Get off the bus a stop ahead, then walk the rest of the way to your destination. Walk your kids to and from school.

5. Give yourself at least 5 minutes off for every hour or two of computer time: walk to the water fountain, or go up and down a few flights of stairs.

6. Walk around your building—outside or inside—during your lunch or coffee break. You'll burn energy rather than being tempted to nibble on a snack.

7. Get a dog, and walk together. Your dog needs the exercise, too! No dog? Then borrow a neighbor's dog or push a baby stroller.

8. Play actively with your kids, grandkids, or pets. Some dogs like to play with a Frisbee as much as kids do!

9. Before and after dinner, walk—and talk—with your family. To burn more energy if you have an infant, use a baby carrier on your back rather than pushing a stroller.

10. Do backyard gardening. (*Bonus:* Grow fresh vegetables and herbs if you can.) In the fall, rake leaves.

11. Ride your bike (the kind you pedal) to work or to a friend's home—if it's safe to do. Walk to do nearby errands, such as grocery shopping for small things or going to the post office.

12. While you watch television, do household chores or projects: mop the floor or refinish a piece of furniture. Avoid "couch potato" syndrome.

13. Catch up with your around-the-house work: wash the windows, vacuum or shampoo the carpet, clean the garage or basement, sweep the sidewalk.

14. Use the exercise equipment you already own. Do two things at one time: ride your stationary bicycle while you read the morning paper or a newsmagazine. Watch the morning news while you work out on your rowing machine.

15. Push your lawn mower instead of using the power-assisted drive. Skip the snow blower; shovel the snow by hand if you're fit.

16. Make homemade bread. Knead the dough by hand, not with a bread machine or a food processor.

17. Use a rest room at the other end of the building so you get an opportunity to walk.

18. Plan an active family vacation or a weekend outing. Rather than sit on a beach, go canoeing, hiking, or snow skiing.

19. "Walk your talk!" Move your body while you talk on the phone. (Use hand weights while talking on the phone.)

20. Rent an exercise video or DVD rather than a movie. And work out as a leisure-time activity.

consume, your body draws energy from all its fat stores, including the problem spots. If you keep on moving, fat will eventually disappear in all the right places.

Eat Smart for Weight Loss

The good news: Eating for weight control and for good health are one and the same. A simple food plan with regular physical activity, based on guidelines from the USDA Food Patterns or the DASH Eating Plan, can accomplish both goals. Use it to tip your calorie balance toward weight loss; at the same time, make the calories in your food choices count for good nutrition! *Refer to chapter 10 for a healthful eating plan, created at a calorie level to lose or maintain your weight.*

What's slow, steady weight loss? It's a safe rate of about ½ to 1 pound per week. Experts say that striving for a 250- to 500-calorie deficit per day can help you achieve that. *Remember:* One pound of body fat contains 3,500 calories worth of stored energy. For weight loss, you need to create a 3,500-calorie deficit for each pound you want to lose: cut back on what you eat, be more physically active—or better yet, do both!

Be Calorie Savvy

To trim your calorie intake, should you count calories? Perhaps—monitoring food intake is an effective strategy. Counting calories does take time and effort. Eating smarter can also help. Cut back to smaller portions. Make calories count by choosing mostly nutrient-rich foods and fewer high-calorie foods.

Being calorie aware is the first step toward weight loss and keeping your healthy weight.

● Know your calorie needs. Set your calorie limits to shed pounds or avoid weight gain. And try to hit that target. *See "How Many Calories for You?" earlier in this chapter.* Weigh yourself and see how your clothes fit. Then, if needed, adjust what and how much you eat and perhaps adjust your physical activity level, too. For children and teens, remember that they need enough calories and nutrients for growth, as well as normal body function and physical activity.

● Know the calories in food and beverages. Get a calorie counter in print, on a hand-held device, or online, perhaps with a phone app. Check www.my foodapedia.gov for calorie amounts. Use Nutrition Facts on food labels to check and compare calories per label serving, the serving size, and servings per package. Remember that a serving isn't necessarily the whole package! *Check "Label Lingo: Calories" in this chapter for the meaning of nutrient content claims on labels, too.*

● *Remember:* A single food isn't "fattening." To manage your weight, it's your total diet that counts.

Trim Calories Wisely

Your total calorie intake, over several days, counts in a healthful eating pattern for weight loss.

● Follow the advice of the USDA Food Patterns, at a calorie level targeted for your weight loss. For a ½- to 1-pound a week drop, pick the plan to help you consume up to 250 to 500 calories a day less—without going below 1,600 calories a day (USDA Food Patterns are set at twelve calorie levels; *refer to chapter 10 and the appendices*.) If you use an extra 150 calories a day with physical activity, you need to trim only 100 to 150 calories from your day's food choices to lose about ½ pound in a week!

● Watch your portion sizes, and the amount you serve to others. Excess calories from any foods can tip your calorie balance toward weight gain when portions are bigger than you need. *See "Get Portion Savvy" in this chapter.*

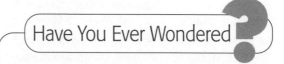

Have You Ever Wondered

. . . why some people gain weight when they stop smoking? First, when smokers quit, they may feel hungrier, but generally only for the first few weeks. Second, they may snack or consume more alcoholic drinks after they stop. Third, as nonsmokers, they may burn slightly less calories during the day; smoking makes the body temporarily burn calories faster. For those who do gain weight, the average gain is about 10 pounds. To help keep those 10 pounds off, take a walk instead of a cigarette.

. . . if drinking water can help you lose weight? Maybe, but it's not a magic weight-loss beverage. That said, foods with a high water content such as fruits, vegetables, and soups can increase short-term satiety and, as a result, may lead to a reduction in total caloric intake—if it means you still take in fewer calories than your body burns.

● Reduce the amount of foods and drinks that often are overconsumed. That includes sugar-sweetened beverages and alcoholic beverages, which supply calories but few nutrients. Strong evidence shows that young people who consume more sugar-sweetened beverages also have higher body weights; it's also an issue for adults. Monitor the amount of 100 percent

Get Portion Savvy

"It's not too big. It's not too small. It's just right!" Keep tabs on portion sizes to manage the number of calories you consume. Even lower-calorie foods can add up to a hefty calorie count when portions get big.

How portion savvy are you? Without using a measuring cup, try pouring one cup of dry cereal—or scooping a half cup of ice cream—into a bowl. Now check the size with a measuring cup. Chances are, you've overestimated. Most people do. That's why many people quite innocently overdo their calorie intake.

● Eat from plates, not packages. When you nibble chips or crackers from a package or snack on ice cream from the carton, you may not know how much you've eaten. It may be more, much more, than you think!

● Plate food in the kitchen—no serving bowls at the table. Control the amount of food by serving on dinner plates, not in serving bowls. Use smaller bowls and dinner plates so small portions look like more.

● Replace large portions of higher-calorie foods, such as sugary desserts, with lower-calorie foods, such as fruit.

The USDA Food Patterns give guidelines for healthful amounts in household measures. Use measuring cups and spoons, and perhaps a kitchen scale to compare your helpings with food group recommendations or the serving sizes listed on the Nutrition Facts of food labels.

Need specific strategies to be more portion savvy? Check here for "how-tos":

● Size up your servings—see chapter 10.

● Be aware of portion size—see chapter 11.

● Control restaurant portions—see chapter 15.

fruit juice, too, especially for youth who are overweight or obese.

● Eat enough fruits, vegetables, and whole-grain foods. Being high in fiber and usually low in calories, they can help satisfy you faster. *Bonus:* They may take more time to chew—which may help you eat less.

● Limit the calories you take in from solid fats (saturated and *trans* fats) and from added sugars. It's an effective weight loss strategy *if* total calories are reduced, too. For foods high in added sugars and/or solid fats, eat just small amounts, less often. *Refer to chapters 3 and 5 to learn about them.*

● After eating enough nutrient-rich foods, spend any extra calories with discretion, perhaps small amounts of foods with more fat and added sugars. If you're physically active, you have more calories to spend!

● Learn how to eat what you like! You're more likely to stick with an eating plan if you don't deprive yourself. Just eat small amounts of higher-calorie food. No one food can make you fat.

● Go easy on wine, beer, spirits, and other alcoholic drinks: no more than one drink a day for women and two for men. Alcohol supplies calories—7 calories per gram. A 12-ounce 5 percent beer contains about 150 calories, a 5-ounce glass of white wine has about 120 calories, and 1½ ounces of 80-proof spirits have about 100 calories. Alcoholic drinks are top calorie contributors for many adults. Downing a six-pack of beer on a hot summer day can add up to a whopping 900 calories, and splitting a 1-liter bottle of wine can supply 360 calories or more; excessive amounts aren't healthful, either. Drinking alcoholic beverages also can stimulate your appetite so you may eat more.

● Ask a registered dietitian for more guidance on choosing healthful foods for weight loss.

Eat Mindfully: Slimming Habits

Look at your eating habits. Do you snack at work because everyone else does? Do you eat fast so you can get on quickly with your day? Do you eat standing up?

● Know your personal daily calorie limit. Use the SuperTracker on www.ChooseMyPlate.gov to find out. Keep that number in mind as you make your food choices.

● Rethink your ways of eating. Do any habits promote weight gain? Consider what, when, why, where, and how you eat. If you need to, make some changes.

● Plan meals and snacks ahead to make better choices. Haphazard eating often becomes high-calorie eating. Pack low-calorie snacks, such as raw vegetables, to eat at work or school.

● Think before you eat. Ask yourself: Is it worth the calories?

● Keep healthful, nutrient-rich snacks available at home. Or carry them with you, perhaps as a snack at work. It's easy to think about meals, yet forget about snacks.

● Shop on a full stomach to help avoid the temptation to buy extra goodies or to nibble on free samples. Write your shopping list when you're not hungry.

● Stick to a regular eating schedule. (There's no hard-and-fast rule about eating three meals a day.) Studies show that missed meals can lead to impulsive snacking and overeating and may lower the rate at which your body burns energy. Eat breakfast!

Check It Out!

Ready to start a healthful and effective weight control plan? Ask yourself a few questions before you begin. Does the program include:

● A variety of foods from all the food groups and in the right amount (enough, not too much)? (*See chapter 10.*)

● Appealing foods you will enjoy eating for the rest of your life, not just a few weeks or months?

● Foods that are available where you usually shop for food?

● The chance to eat your favorite foods—in fact, any foods?

● Eating strategies that fit your lifestyle and budget?

● Enough regular physical activity?

If you *cannot* answer "yes" to all these questions, chances are this weight-loss program won't bring long-term success because you may not stick to it. Success is possible only when you make healthful, permanent changes in your eating and physical activity habits.

● Cook and eat at home more often. Then you're in control of the calories. Meals you prepare can include foods with fewer calories and more nutrients: vegetables, fruits, whole-grain foods, fat-free and low-fat dairy foods, and soy products, seafood, or lean meat or poultry. Experiment! *See chapter 14 for cooking skills and kitchen nutrition tips.*

● When you eat out, consider the calories. And choose healthful options. *For tips on eating smart when eating out, see chapter 15.*

● Eat slowly. Savor the flavor of each bite. After all, it takes about twenty minutes for your stomach to signal your brain that you're full—which curbs your urge for a second helping. Slow down by putting down your fork between bites. Eat with chopsticks if they slow you down. Sip, rather than gulp, beverages. Swallow before refilling your fork.

● Eat when you're hungry; stop when you're satisfied, not full. Learn body signals for fullness and real hunger. Forget the "clean-plate club." You don't need to eat everything on your plate if you're satisfied.

● Sit down to eat, rather than nibble while you do other things. Focus on your food. That way you know that you've eaten.

● Make eating the only event—and enjoy it. Eating unconsciously or when distracted while you watch television, read, talk on the phone, or drive may lead to eating more than you think. If you do eat as you watch TV, portion out just a small serving.

Need specific calorie-cutting strategies that deliver good nutrition, too? Check here for "how-tos":

● Take control of calories in alcoholic drinks—see chapter 8.

● Snack smart for fewer calories—see chapter 10.

● Get "calorie-wise" as you shop—see chapter 12.

● Cut calories by trimming fat and added sugars in food "prep"—see chapter 14.

● Eat out with calorie savvy—see chapter 15.

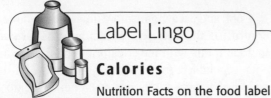

Label Lingo

Calories

Nutrition Facts on the food label list the calories in a single serving. In addition, "calorie lingo" on the package can alert you to lower-calorie food products as you search supermarket displays.

LABEL TERM	MEANS
Calorie-free	Less than 5 calories
Low-calorie	40 calories or less
Reduced or fewer calories	At least 25% fewer calories*
Light or lite	One-third fewer calories or 50% less fat*; if more than half the calories are from fat, fat content must be reduced by 50% or more
Low-calorie meals	120 calories or less per 100 grams
Light meal	"Low-fat" or "low-calorie" meal

*As compared with a standard serving size of the traditional food

● Choose foods that take more time to eat. For example, peeling and eating an orange takes longer than drinking a glass of orange juice.

● Stop eating when you leave the table. Avoid the urge to nibble on leftovers as you clean up.

● When you get the urge to nibble (especially if you're not hungry), do something else. Jog, call a friend, walk the dog, or step out into your garden.

● Be aware of the influence of others. You don't need to eat cake, muffins, or bagels in the break room just because your officemate brought them!

● Limit beverage calories, especially from sugary drinks and alcoholic beverages. Their calories add up.

Eating Triggers

You have the best intentions. Then something triggers your desire to eat—even though you're not hungry. Get in touch with the emotions and situations that trigger your eating. Learn to differentiate between physical hunger and emotionally driven hunger instead of looking inside the refrigerator or diving into a bowl of snacks. Find an appropriate diversion. Limit temptations when possible. Avoid mindless eating!

● Do you eat when you're bored or stressed? Find other options: Enjoy your garden, play with the dog, go shopping, call a friend, or play with your kids. *See "Emotional Overeating: Take Control!" later in this chapter.*

● Be aware of social situations where there's food: parties, entertaining, dating, talking around the coffeepot at work, and happy-hour meetings. Create your ways to avoid overeating.

LOW-"CAL" AND LOW-FAT: NOT THE SAME!

Read the label! Compare the calories. Being fat-free doesn't make a food calorie-free. A fat-free or reduced-fat product may have as many (even more) calories per serving than full-fat products—sometimes even more. Fat may be replaced with ingredients that add calories, such as sugar, flour, or starch thickeners that add flavor and texture. Many people eat larger quantities of fat-free or low-fat foods, believing they are healthier and lower in calories.

Fig cookie (1)	
Fat-free	48 calories
Regular	56 calories
Vanilla frozen yogurt (½ cup)	
Nonfat	110 calories
Regular	117 calories
Caramel topping (2 tablespoons)	
Fat-free	105 calories
Regular	103 calories
Peanut butter (2 tablespoons)	
Reduced-fat	166 calories
Regular	188 calories
Cereal bar (1.3 ounce)	
Low-fat	133 calories
Regular	140 calories

Source: U.S. Department of Agriculture, Agricultural Research Service, 2005; U.S. Department of Agriculture, National Nutrient Database for Standard Reference, Release 24, 2011; and food industry websites, as appropriate.

● *Remember:* Out of sight, out of mind. If the sight of candy, chips, and other high-calorie foods lures you, store them in an inconvenient place. Better yet, don't keep them around. Instead stock up on fruit, raw vegetables, and other foods with fewer calories.

● Accomplished something special? Reward yourself, but not with food. Treat yourself to a massage. Buy something new to wear or read. Or go to a play, concert, or sports event.

● Watch out for seasonal triggers: perhaps nibbling while watching fall and winter sports on television, "cooling off" in hot weather with a few beers or an extra-large soft drink, or eating and entertaining during the holidays. Or eat smaller portions or different foods if only eating will do. If you're not sure what triggers your eating, keep a food journal for a week or two. *See "Dear Journal . . ." below.*

Dear Journal . . .

Help yourself to weight control by keeping tabs on what you eat. Research shows that people who keep a food and activity journal or log are often more successful at weight management than those who don't.

There's nothing complicated about keeping a record. Use a notebook to keep a hand-written food and activity journal. Or use a diary on a phone app or online Website.

Keep track of the amounts and kinds of foods and beverages you eat. To get a handle on any eating "triggers," write your mood and rate your hunger level each time you eat. Put down the time and place, too. List the amount of time you spend in physical activity, along with what you do. Keep your food and activity record for at least a week or two. Then review it for a close look at your eating and physical activity habits. You don't need to count every calorie.

Most people can spot problem areas easily. Keeping records offers one way to identify areas you might need to change. It also can help you focus on your weight and physical activity goals—and think twice before indulging in a high-calorie snack when you're not hungry or sitting too much.

For an online food and physical activity tracker, check the SuperTracker at www.ChooseMyPlate.gov. Or to track physical activity, use www.presidents challenge.org, or use a log like the one on www.health .gov/paguidelines.

Emotional Overeating: Take Control!

To relax, quell anger, or overcome depression or loneliness, mood-triggered eating may feel good—at first. But eating to cope with emotions can lead to more negative feelings (guilt, lack of personal control, and poor self-esteem) and perhaps to a cycle of mood-triggered eating and excessive calorie intake. As important, using food to satisfy emotions may distract you from handling serious life issues.

On the plus side, learning to control mood-triggered eating promotes feelings of personal power and self-esteem!

Learn to deal with emotions in a positive, appropriate way. Address the real problems. Resolve your moods with positive self-talk or a brief change of scenery. Compared with nibbling, physical activity—perhaps a brisk walk, a bike ride, or a tennis game—often does the trick. Regular physical activity is a great stress buster!

Party "Tid-bites"

Sharing and enjoying a traditional holiday meal and party foods with family and friends doesn't need to destroy healthful food habits nurtured all year. Any foods—even traditional holiday fare—can fit into a healthful calorie-conscious eating plan. These party tips can help you hold the line:

● Be realistic. Trying to lose weight during the holidays may be a self-defeating goal. Instead strive to maintain your weight.

● Think ahead. Balance party eating with other meals. Eat small, lower-calorie meals during the day so you can enjoy celebration foods, too—without overdoing your calorie intake for the day.

● Take the edge off your hunger before a party. Eat a small, low-calorie snack such as fruit or whole-grain toast. Hunger can sabotage strong willpower!

● When you arrive at a party, avoid rushing to the food. Greet people—conversation is calorie-free! Get a beverage, and settle into the festivities before eating. You may eat less.

● Ask for sparkling water and a lime twist rather than wine, champagne, or a mixed drink. Sparkling water doesn't supply calories.

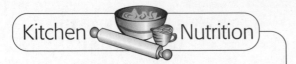

Celebration Meals Go Lean!

Celebration menus—or almost any meal—may be modified to lower the calories and the added sugars and fat content. Often the differences go almost unnoticed. Compare this traditional menu with its lower-calorie version. *Then see chapter 14 for tips on trimming calories in food preparation.*

ORIGINAL MENU	LOWER-CALORIE MENU
3½ oz. roasted turkey with skin	3½ oz. skinless, roasted turkey
½ cup stuffing	½ cup wild rice pilaf
½ cup broccoli with 2 tbsp. hollandaise sauce	½ cup broccoli with lemon juice
½ cup cranberry relish	¼ cup cranberry relish
1 medium crescent roll	1 whole-grain roll
1 slice pecan pie	1 slice pumpkin pie
Total calories: 1,140	*Total calories:* 735

● Move your socializing away from the buffet to avoid unconscious nibbling.

● Make just one trip to the party buffet. And be selective. Only choose the foods you really want to eat; keep portions small. Often just a taste satisfies a craving or curiosity.

● Opt for lower-calorie party foods. Enjoy raw vegetables with a small dollop of dip, just enough to coat the end of the vegetable. Try boiled shrimp or scallops with cocktail sauce or lemon. Go easy on fried appetizers and cheese cubes.

● If you're bringing a dish, make it healthfully delicious—and low-calorie. That way, you'll know there's something with fewer calories. Bring raw vegetables with a yogurt or cottage cheese dip, or bring a platter of fresh fruit.

● Enjoying a sit-down dinner party? Make your first helping small—especially if your host or hostess expects you to take seconds.

● Forget the all-or-nothing mind-set. Depriving yourself of special holiday foods, or feeling guilty when you do enjoy them, is neither a healthful eating strategy nor part of the holiday spirit!

● Balance "party calories" with more physical activity.

Motivation Boosters for Weight Loss

With weight control as part of your lifestyle, healthful eating and physical activity become second nature. When you need a boost to stay on track, try this!

● Make lifestyle changes with a friend or a family member! A partner increases the enjoyment factor of physical activity and healthful eating.

● Enlist support. Family and friends can help you keep on track. Those who have the support of family members, particularly a spouse, more likely manage their weight successfully. Watch out for those who attempt to sabotage your efforts. If it's right for you, join a support group.

● Track your weight-loss progress—daily or weekly, whichever way helps keep you on track. Be aware that weight fluctuates from day to day due to fluid loss and retention. If daily weighing is confusing or discouraging, know that once a week is enough.

● Track your steps to help you keep your body moving. Get a pedometer. Aim for 10,000 steps a day.

● Give it time. For women, weight gain from water retention may be a normal part of a monthly menstrual cycle. Usually that passes in a few days.

● Celebrate any success. If you carry around excess pounds, even small changes can make a difference in your health and reduce your disease risk.

● Enjoy how good your healthy weight feels. Reward yourself with a new garment, a bouquet of flowers, a new CD, or a special outing. Still, there's no greater motivation or reward than knowing you're in control and caring for yourself and improving your health!

Eat Smart for Weight Gain

There's plenty written about weight loss. However, some people need to gain weight. Weight gain can be as hard as weight loss!

The obvious approach for weight gain is this—consume more energy than your body burns. For every pound of body weight you gain, you need to consume 3,500 calories more than your body burns. As with weight loss, do so in a healthful way. *Note:* The suggestions indicated here are not meant for people with eating disorders, whose weight problems are complex and often life-threatening, or for people with chronic disease.

● Eat more nutrient-rich foods. The USDA Food Patterns have twelve plans for healthy eating, each at a different calorie level. To make your calories count for good nutrition, pick a plan with more calories than you eat now. You may have room for "extra" calories from foods with more fat or added sugars. *Refer to chapter 10.*

● Even though higher-fat foods deliver more calories, be fat savvy. Keep your overall eating plan low in solid fats. Replace solid fats with oils. *See chapter 3.*

● Choose some foods with concentrated calories. Try dried fruits and peanut butter. Fortify soups, casseroles, and fluid milk with dry milk powder. Garnish with olives, avocados, nuts, and cheese, which have more calories.

● Eat more frequently. Try five to six small meals a day if your appetite is small. Eating two or three large meals during the day may be too much to handle at one time.

● Drink fluids thirty minutes before and after meals—not with meals. By limiting beverages at mealtime, you'll have more room for food.

● Focus on nutrient-rich foods and beverages. Don't fill up on low- and no-calorie foods or drinks, such as diet sodas or diet candies. Rather than coffee, tea, and water, drink juice, milk, and shakes. Sweet foods that also provide nutrients are better choices than calorie-rich candy and cake; try a yogurt parfait or trail mix bars.

● Enjoy a snack before bedtime.

● Stimulate your appetite if you don't feel like eating. *See "No Appetite?" on this page.*

● Use the Nutrition Facts on food labels to choose nutrient-rich foods, which also supply more calories. *See chapter 12 for more on label reading.*

● Try adding a commercial liquid meal replacement.

Make a shake or smoothie if you can't get enough calories from regular meals and snacks.

● Get more guidance from a registered dietitian. *See chapter 24, "Well-Informed?" for tips on finding a qualified nutrition expert in your area.*

● Stay physically active—good for muscle building, adding bulk to your body, and feeling energetic.

Source: Adapted from Gail Farmer, American Dietetic Association.

No Appetite?

People lose their appetite for all kinds of reasons: illness, pain, fatigue, depression, stress, medication, disease, or a combination of these.

If that happens, the appetite control center of your brain might be affected, signaling that you're not hungry even when you should be. You may lose your appetite and tolerance for food when you're sick—even though you need nourishment to get well. Or emotional stress may affect your desire for and ability to handle food.

Cope with a loss of appetite. Eat by the clock rather than by hunger. It may be easier to consume all the calories you need. Take advantage of the "up" times. When you feel well and your appetite is good, eat and enjoy! To stimulate your appetite:

● Add some pizzazz to your foods! Colorful foods, appealing texture, and an appetizing aroma are helpful aids to increasing food intake.

● Drink a glass of beer or wine before meals. This often gives your appetite a jump start. But check with your doctor about any medication interactions first.

● Eat meals with friends. The pleasure of being with others may be an appetite booster.

● Fill the house with enticing food aromas such as freshly baked bread, cake, or cookies.

● Keep favorite foods on hand. You may eat more when food is readily available.

● Make mealtimes pleasant. A relaxed and attractive setting with soft music or flowers on the table may perk up your appetite.

● Try eating your meal away from the dining room table, such as picnic style in the living room or at a candlelit table in front of the fireplace. Sometimes a change of place helps.

● Plan for longer mealtimes. Don't schedule activities close to meals.

● Walk before meals. A short walk often helps stimulate an appetite.

● Stay away from unpleasant or unsettling topics of conversation at mealtimes, especially if stress is a problem for you.

Source: Adapted from Gail Farmer, American Dietetic Association.

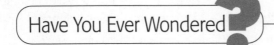

Have You Ever Wondered

. . . why it seemed easy to lose weight in your teens and twenties . . . and why it's so hard now? There could be several reasons why it seems harder as an adult—a less active lifestyle, different eating habits, or changes in your body. Metabolism slows during each decade of your adult years.

Being inactive complicates the picture if you lose muscle mass and put on extra body fat, too. Fat tissue requires fewer calories to maintain than muscle does. The remedy? Get more active. Physical activity burns fat and can build muscle, making weight loss easier. Increased physical activity can boost the rate at which your body uses energy for your basic energy needs.

. . . what it takes to lose weight and keep it off? Maintaining weight loss isn't easy! Success stories and research shared through the National Weight Control Registry offer insight (www.nwcr.ws/default.htm). In their studies nearly all participants changed their food intake in some way and increased their physical activity, most often by walking to lose weight. To keep it off, most continued to maintain a low-calorie, low-fat diet and to do high levels of activity. About three-quarters ate breakfast daily and weighed themselves once a week. About 90 percent fit in about an hour a day, on average, of physical activity, and 62 percent said they watched less than ten hours of TV weekly.

. . . if your stomach shrinks when you eat less? No, your body doesn't work that way. Although your stomach can expand to accommodate a large intake of food, it doesn't stretch out indefinitely. As stomach contents pass into your intestines, the stomach goes back to its normal size. When you cut back on calories, your stomach keeps its normal size, even if your appetite isn't as big.

. . . if every person's body has a unique set point, or a preset weight, that it tries to return to? That's a theory with no conclusive evidence. Even if a set point exists, it's probably a range that can be set a little lower with more physical activity and food choices with fewer calories for someone who's too thin, eating a few extra calories may help adjust the set point a bit higher.

Disordered Eating: Problems, Signs, and Help

Up to 24 million Americans suffer from disordered eating, according to the National Association of Anorexia Nervosa and Associated Disorders (ANAD). Eating disorders—anorexia nervosa, bulimia, and binge eating disorder—are actually distorted eating habits often related to emotional problems. Those with eating disorders have the highest death rate of any mental illness.

Anorexia typically results in low body weight; it's linked to menstrual irregularity, osteoporosis in women, and greater risk of early death in women and men. Bulimia may or may not be linked to low body weight. And binge eating disorder, probably the most common eating disorder, typically results in overweight and often in repeated weight gain and loss. All require qualified medical attention. Yet despite the potential health risks, only 10 percent of those with eating disorders get treatment.

Anorexia and Bulimia: What Are They?

Anorexia nervosa is sometimes called the "starvation sickness." Obsessed with food, weight, and thinness, people suffering from anorexia typically see themselves as overweight and deny their hunger and refuse to eat—even after extreme weight loss. As they consume too few calories for their basic needs, their bodies slowly waste away. By starving themselves, people with anorexia don't get the nutrients they need for normal bodily functions. They may also lose weight with excessive exercise, self-induced vomiting, or misuse of laxatives, diuretics, or enemas.

Bulimia nervosa is marked by binge eating and purging (self-induced vomiting). The person gorges, usually on high-calorie foods, and then intentionally vomits or uses laxatives or diuretics. The consequences are serious: dehydration, organ damage, internal bleeding from the stress of vomiting, tooth decay from stomach acids in vomit, and in some cases, death. Many people with these eating disorders alternate between anorexia and bulimia. Reports indicate that 25 percent of college-age women resort to bingeing, then purging to keep weight off. Unlike anorexia, people with bulimia may have a healthy weight for their age and height.

Disordered eating is more than the "big three." Also getting attention: night eating syndrome (not just eating at night) and orthorexia nervosa, a popular name for obsessive, compulsive attitudes and behavior about healthful eating. Compulsive exercising is a related concern. Another growing concern that's not an eating disorder but has similar causes and serious health risks is the growing trend among some young women with diabetes to manipulate insulin as a way to lose weight.

When does an eating disorder start? Generally it begins with an ordinary weight-loss diet, begun just before or after a major life change or trauma. However, there's no clear understanding of the exact causes.

We do know, however, that eating disorders are more than food problems. The person's whole life—schoolwork or career, family life, overall health—gets wrapped up in the eating issues.

Who's at Risk for Anorexia and Bulimia?

People of almost any age and either gender may develop an eating disorder, with incidence increasing among adults and even children as young as eight, nine, and ten years old! However, some groups of people are more at risk than others.

- Females: They're clearly more susceptible. About 90 to 95 percent of people with anorexia are women. It's estimated that as many as 1 in every 100 teenage girls in the United States will develop ANAD.

- Adolescents: Anorexia is the third most common chronic illness among teens.

- Athletes: Dancers, gymnasts, wrestlers, and jockeys, who must control their weight, are susceptible.

- Males: Eating disorders are increasingly identified in males. An estimated 5 to 15 percent of those with anorexia or bulimia are male.

Anorexia and Bulimia: The Warning Signs

Eating disorders produce warning signs. If you or someone you know shows any combination of these symptoms, be concerned!

People with anorexia may:

- Eat tiny portions, refuse to eat, deny hunger, and diet continuously.

- Show abnormal weight loss—15 percent or more of body weight—or a large weight loss in a short time, and refuse to maintain a normal weight.

- Act hyperactive, depressed, moody, or insecure.

- Have an intense, persistent fear of being fat.

- See themselves as fat, wanting to lose more weight, even when they are very thin.

- Exercise excessively and compulsively.

- For females, have irregular or missing (at least three in a row) menstrual periods.

Body Image: Dissatisfied, Distorted—or Not?

In a society that values thinness as the ideal, body weight and shape too often impact body image and inappropriately define self-worth—especially among teens and young women. Body shapes considered "acceptable" are limited. The "ideal body" is portrayed culturally, typically originating in media; in addition, family and peer expectations and reactions from others influence a person's body image and, ultimately, self-worth.

When a poor body image leads to loss of self esteem, many aspects of life suffer: the way people socialize, build relationships, participate in physical activities, and function psychologically at school, work, and daily life. Being dissatisfied with one's body image is both a symptom and a risk factor for body distortion, but also for anorexia nervosa and bulimia nervosa, among other health risks.

To help build a positive body image for ourselves and others, reflect on your own ideas of body size and image. Recognize that healthy people come in many sizes and shapes. Skip comments that reinforce body size stereotypes, such as "I feel fat today." Talk about other personal qualities, and make them positive.

● Develop fine, downy hair on their arms and face because of inadequate protein intake.

● Experience hair loss and sensitivity to cold.

● May binge-eat, then purge, perhaps by vomiting or using laxatives or diuretics.

People with bulimia may:

● Binge-eat mainly in private.

● Disappear after eating—often to the bathroom.

● Show great fluctuations in weight, and may be of normal weight or be overweight.

● Be preoccupied with food.

● Feel out of control when eating.

● Eat enormous meals but not gain weight.

● Feel ashamed and depressed after gorging.

● Binge-eat, then purge or vomit.

● Abuse laxatives, diuretics, emetics, or diet pills to lose weight. Emetics such as syrup of ipecac induce vomiting.

● Develop dental problems caused by stomach acids from vomiting. Acids eat away at tooth enamel.

● Have swollen parotid glands. The parotid glands, near the ears, are one type of salivary glands.

● Have broken blood vessels in the eyes.

Binge Eating Disorder: A More Common Problem

Binge eating disorder (BED), different from occasional overindulging, is the uncontrollable eating of large amounts of food in a short time. Unlike bulimia, a person with BED usually doesn't purge, fast, abuse diuretics or laxatives, or overexercise. Estimates suggest that 2 percent of Americans have this disorder—many are obese or overweight.

The concerns are physical, psychological, and social. Large amounts of food eaten by binge eaters are typically high in fats and added sugars, and may lack sufficient vitamins and minerals. With the likelihood of overweight and obesity comes an increased risk for serious health problems, including diabetes, heart disease, high blood pressure, gallbladder disease, and some cancers. Binge eating often results in

Three Things to Know about Disordered Eating

Experts aren't certain about the exact causes of disordered eating. But they do agree on these key points:

1. Food itself is not the primary problem. Instead, eating patterns are symptoms of serious psychological distress.

2. Early detection is crucial. The sooner the person gets help, the better the chance for permanent recovery.

3. Help is available. Team treatment, including medical and dental care, psychotherapy, nutrition education, and family counseling, provides the best results.

depression, embarrassment, and social isolation; those with the disorder are often upset by both the problem and their inability to control their eating.

Although the cause of BED isn't clear, there's a link to depression and other negative emotions. Among the areas of research: the effect of brain chemicals and metabolism, and whether depression is a cause or a result of binge eating disorder.

Who's at Risk for Binge Eating Disorder?

Many people with BED are overweight or obese (often severely obese); even normal-weight people have this disorder. More women than men deal with BED, but it's the most common eating disorder among men.

BED: The Warning Signs

Being overstuffed after an exceptional meal isn't necessarily a warning sign. Instead, people with binge eating disorder typically have several characteristics:

● Feel out of control when eating.

● Eat unusually large amounts of food.

● Eat very fast.

● Eat until they feel uncomfortable.

● Eat a lot, even when they aren't hungry.

● Feel embarrassed about the amount of food they eat, so eat alone.

● Feel disgusted, depressed, or guilty about overeating.

What to Do

If you suspect a friend or a family member has anorexia, bulimia, or binge eating disorder, don't wait until a severe weight problem or a serious medical problem proves you are right. There's plenty you can do before that happens:

● *Act to get help.* Speak to the person about your concern. Enlist assistance from family and friends. Talk to medical professionals, a social worker, or the school nurse or counselor if the person is a student. Call your local mental health association. A registered dietitian also can give you an expert perspective on eating disorders. *See chapter 24 to locate a registered dietitian in your area.*

People with disordered eating may encourage disordered eating among others; today that problem has spread and been encouraged through websites with private chat rooms and through other social media.

For people with BED, a weight-loss diet alone may not be successful. Losing weight and keeping it off may be harder (for physical and emotional reasons) than for people without an eating disorder. Normal-weight people with binge eating disorder shouldn't be on a weight-loss diet.

The best treatment for disordered eating combines medical, psychological, and nutrition counseling. Participation in self-help groups for the patient, as well as group counseling for family members, are important parts of treatment.

● *Expect resistance.* Someone with anorexia usually doesn't believe that he or she needs help or is in any danger. Someone with bulimia or BED may acknowledge the problem but refuse to seek help. The faster he or she gets help, the greater the chances for recovery.

● *Prepare for long-term treatment.* Recovery may take several months to several years. Symptoms and attitudes related to eating disorders rarely disappear quickly. Treatment includes helping people achieve an appropriate weight. Family support groups are particularly effective in helping relatives of people with disordered eating survive the long ordeal.

For more guidance, see "Weighty Issues for Children—Teens, Too!" and "Pressure to Be Thin" in chapter 17.

"Diets" That Don't Work!

Every year Americans spend billions of dollars on the weight-loss industry—often for diet plans, diet books, services, and gimmicks that don't work! The lure of quick, easy weight loss is hard to resist, especially for those unwilling to make a commitment to lifelong behavioral change. Although the diets are ineffective in the long run, weight-loss hopefuls willingly give the next craze a chance. The result? Perhaps temporary results. But overall, wasted money, weight regained, a feeling of failure, and perhaps damage to health. *The bottom line:* If a diet or product sounds too good to be true, it probably is. And any diet that's taken to the extreme can add up to trouble.

The next dieting craze is often a past craze that's simply resurfaced with a new name, a new twist, yet still no sound science to back up the claims. Fad diets typically rely on nonscientific, unproved claims, personal stories, testimonials, or poorly controlled studies. Not surprisingly, many people feel confusion and diet fatigue as they sort through contradictory popular approaches to weight loss. Sound familiar? For those who try one fad diet after another, weight cycling becomes a common, frustrating problem. *See "Weight Cycling" earlier in this chapter.*

Fad Diets: Be Cautious!

Popular diets may not work—at least not in the long run—if they promote:

● Rapid weight loss. *The facts are . . .* Quick weight loss is often muscle and water loss, too—not just body fat. Losing weight slowly and steadily—½ to 2 pounds per week—is more likely to last than a dramatic weight change.

● No need to exercise. *The facts are . . .* The best way to keep a healthy weight, to lose body fat, and to build muscle is to eat smart and move more! Find physical activities that you enjoy, then aim for 30 to 60 minutes of activity on most days of the week.

● Rigid meal and snack plans. *The facts are . . .* Rigid plans can take a lot of effort and may not match your own food preferences or lifestyle. If you can't follow the plan for the rest of your life, it's not right for you.

● Specific food combinations. *The facts are . . .* No

scientific evidence suggests that combining certain foods or eating them in careful sequence, perhaps at specific times of day, aids weight loss or causes food to turn to body fat or produce toxins in your intestines.

● Unlimited amounts of some foods; severe restrictions of others. *The facts are* . . . Diets that allow unlimited amounts of a single food (such as rice, grapefruit, or cabbage soup), that eliminate a food group (such as dairy foods), or try to eliminate a nutrient (such as carbohydrate) or food substance (such as gluten) have no unique ability to melt body fat and lose weight. Because they lack food variety, they likely won't provide all the nutrients needed for health, especially if some foods are off-limits. That can have unintended health consequences such as bone loss if dairy is eliminated to save calories. Even by taking a multivitamin supplement, you'd miss some essentials. And a diet plan that requires you to eat the same foods all the time is monotonous and hard to stick to.

The bottom line: No super food or food combination can reverse weight gain resulting from inactivity and overeating. Eliminating a food or food category doesn't work, either. Also, because these diets don't teach new eating habits, people usually don't stick with them!

Very-Low-Calorie Liquid Diets

Very-low-calorie liquid formulas have been developed for short-term use under a doctor's supervision. To help some obese people, they may aid short-term weight loss—if there's also a commitment to new eating and active living habits. Used as a liquid diet without other foods, they're very low in calories, providing just 400 to 800 calories a day.

These formulas were changed after deaths were attributed to their use. Newer formulas have more vitamins, minerals, and high-quality protein.

The facts are . . . Without medical supervision and nutrition education, liquid diets don't teach new ways of eating. They don't provide adequate nutrition. Since people usually don't stay with them, there's

Have You Ever Wondered

. . . if a high-protein/low-carb diet has any weight-loss advantage? The truth is, it's the overall calories that count! If your total calorie intake is lower than your calorie expenditure, you'll lose weight, no matter where your calories come from.

The best approach is a healthful eating pattern that's also right for you—within the recommended ranges for energy nutrients (carbohydrate, fat, and protein); *see "How Many Calories for You?" earlier in this chapter* to learn recommended intake ranges for each. Low- to moderate-carbohydrate diets for weight loss may be appropriate for some people, perhaps those with insulin resistance; *see "Metabolic Syndrome" in chapter 22.*

A moderate-carbohydrate diet with more protein may help some people lose body fat while maintaining muscle as they lose weight. If you choose a diet higher in protein, make sure your choices are mostly lean protein foods (lean meat, skinless chicken, seafood, and beans).

A high-protein diet may be risky for those with some chronic diseases, such as kidney disease; talk to your doctor.

. . . if you can lose weight if you go gluten free? Gluten free is neither no-carb nor low-calorie. Instead it's an eating plan for those with celiac disease, who can't tolerate gluten-protein in foods made with wheat, barley, or rye. Other grain products replace these foods, but not their calories. In fact, gluten-free foods may have more calories if fats or sugars replace some of the wheat products. There also are risks related to avoiding wheat products such as bread that are fortified with folic acid, a nutrient that protects against birth defects.

. . . if skipping meals can help with weight loss? No, in fact research indicates that meal-skipping is often linked to weighing more. That may happen when people eat more than normal to satisfy hunger when they do eat. The best advice is to eat meals that are smaller, lower-calorie, and nutrient-rich, as well as satisfying enough to manage your hunger.

usually no long-term weight loss. They also may result in fatigue, constipation, nausea, diarrhea, hair loss, or heart arrhythmia. For people with some health problems, such as insulin-dependent diabetes or kidney disease, a very-low-calorie liquid diet can be harmful.

Fasting

As a tactic, does fasting jump start weight loss?

The facts are . . . As with very-low-calorie diets, fasting deprives the body of energy and nutrients needed for normal functions. Any rapid weight loss is mostly water and muscle loss. Fasting also may cause fatigue and dizziness, with less energy for physical activity. And it feeds the cycle of "yo-yo" dieting.

As an aside, there's a misconception that fasting "cleans out" the system, removing toxic wastes. If you're healthy, your body does that naturally as part of its metabolic processes, whether you fast or not.

Recognize that fasting is an important part of some religious observances, such as Ramadan for Muslims and some Hindu practices. Like other food patterns, both fasting and breaking the fast later in the day can be done in a healthful way. If you're breaking a fast, drink enough fluids to avoid dehydration and choose nutrient-rich foods, perhaps with more protein and fiber, with sustaining power to help feel full longer.

Gimmicks, Gadgets, and Other "Miracles"

Promoters advertise "easy ways to weight loss"—weight-loss patches, electric muscle stimulators, spirulina (a species of blue-green algae), starch and fat blockers, creams that melt fat away, and many others. *Chapter 23 addresses some weight-loss supplements.*

The facts are . . . No super foods can alter your genetic code. No products can magically melt fat while you watch TV, sleep, or sweat. All these products have been offered for sale and purport to promote weight loss. Yet none proves effective. Some ingredients in supplements and herbal products can be dangerous—even deadly for some people. And they divert money away from buying nutrient-rich foods.

The popular press often advertises massages and other therapies for losing "cellulite," dimpled fat

Have You Ever Wondered

. . . if over-the-counter diet pills help with weight loss? Over-the-counter diet pills, or appetite suppressants, work by curbing appetite, but usually just for a few weeks. Some have unpleasant side effects, and some can be addictive, with potential damage to the heart and the nervous system. They may be prescribed to help a person start a lifelong program for weight management, but they're not a substitute for healthful eating habits over the long term. They should never be taken for very long—and only under a doctor's supervision.

. . . if high-fiber bulk fillers can reduce hunger? Probably, but they aren't advised. First they absorb liquid, then swell in the stomach. These products can be harmful when they obstruct the digestive tract. *See "Supplement Watch: Fiber Pills and Powders" in chapter 3 to learn more.* Eating enough fiber-rich food, as part of a healthful weight-loss plan, is a smarter idea!

. . . if obesity can be controlled with medication? For some people, medication may be prescribed—under a doctor's care—as part of an obesity treatment program. Such medication isn't effective for everyone, and can have potential side effects. The U.S. Food and Drug Administration (FDA) has approved orlistat for long-term use. Over-the-counter orlistat reduces the absorption of dietary fat; however, it may reduce the absorption of some fat-soluble vitamins, too. The U.S. FDA warns that in rare cases orlistat can cause severe liver injury. The FDA has approved two others for short-term use: phentermine and diethylpropion, which both work as appetite suppressants. Each has possible side effects and should be taken under a doctor's supervision Research continues on medications to manage obesity.

on thighs and hips. Cellulite is simply normal body fat under the skin that looks lumpy when the fat layer gets thick, allowing connective, fibrous-looking tissue that holds fat in place to show. The lumpy look can lessen or disappear with normal weight loss.

You've probably seen weight-loss programs that sweat off extra weight. Sweating in a sauna—or wearing a rubber belt or nylon clothes that make you perspire during exercise—may cause weight loss. However, the pounds that disappear are water loss, not body fat. When you drink or eat, weight returns.

Instead of helping to achieve a healthful weight

goal, "sweating off" pounds may damage health through dehydration. *See chapter 8 for more about the need for water. See chapter 24 to learn how to detect health fraud.*

Healthy Weight: Your Support Team

If you have weight problems of any kind or more questions about controlling your own weight, it's okay to seek outside advice and help. But be wary. Not every weight-loss "professional" is qualified to give the help you need.

First and foremost, choose a program that suits your personality and lifestyle. In addition, find a program with a maintenance plan that includes physical activity, and counseling that focuses on realistic behavioral changes. Your workplace might have a wellness program that can help you be more physically active and manage your weight; find out! In the end, you supply your own motivation, but the plan must promote your good health. Choose a sound plan you can live with.

If you need help finding a weight-control program, talk with a registered dietitian, who is trained to help you figure out what kind of weight-management system will fit your lifestyle. *For more help in finding a qualified nutrition professional and for reliable information about nutrition and health, see chapter 24.*

If you become ill after using a weight-loss product or service, contact the U.S. Food and Drug Administration at 1-800-332-1088.

Have You Ever Wondered

. . . if meal replacements are effective for weight loss? Research has shown that meal replacements (liquid drinks, meal bars, and portion-controlled meals) can be an effective weight management aid for some. They can offer convenience, ease, and portion and calorie control, and perhaps reduce sensory stimulation from food itself. Like any food, they should be nutrient rich.

Have You Ever Wondered

. . . if the glycemic index is a useful tool for a weight-loss diet? The glycemic index (GI) measures how individual foods affect blood glucose levels. But it's not easily applied to real-world eating. Choosing carbohydrate foods and drinks with a low GI isn't effective for weight loss, according to strong research evidence. *For more about GI, refer to chapter 3.*

. . . if getting more sleep helps with weight loss? Maybe. Scientists are investigating if sleep affects hormones that regulate hunger, feeling full, or metabolic rate. Research also is looking at the links between sleep and heart disease, diabetes, and immunity. Snooze enough, and stay tuned!

. . . why clothes look different on a mannequin than on you? Most store mannequins don't represent average women in the United States. Mannequins are typically 6 feet tall, with a 34-inch bust, 23-inch waist, and 34-inch hips! And the body type you generally see in advertising or on a runway? Only about five percent of American females have that shape naturally!

Questions to Ask . . . about Weight Loss Programs

Millions of Americans participate in organized weight-loss programs each year. Today the Internet also provides this service. Many of these programs are run by qualified medical and nutrition experts who can effectively help their clients lose weight and keep it off permanently. However, others make overblown claims and tout products that are ineffective and costly, and their staff may not have appropriate credentials. Before you sign on the dotted line, ask:

● What is the approach? What are the program goals?

● Does the program have any health risks?

● How will you assess my health status before recommending the program? Many programs recommend a medical checkup before starting.

● Will the program include instruction, guidance, and skill building to help me learn to eat in a positive, healthful way for the long term? How?

● Will the program include guidance on physical activity for a lifetime? How?

● Does the program address challenges like eating at social gatherings or on the road?

● What data can you share that shows your program works? What has been written about the program's success besides individual testimonials?

● Do customers keep off the weight after they

Eat What You Crave!

If the sight of certain foods puts your mind into a tailspin, you may need to readjust your approach to eating. An overly restrictive diet may "feed" a food craving—and set you up to overindulge!

The jury is still out on the true cause of food cravings. It may be physiological, psychological, or both. We don't yet know if food cravings are linked to a need to resupply the body with nutrients it lacks, or if cravings are reinforced by positive emotional and social links to certain foods.

Studies suggest that avoiding certain foods altogether often makes them irresistible. The result? Giving in to a food craving, and perhaps overeating. Then guilt creeps in, and people try to resist those foods once again, only to overindulge and feel guilty again.

What's a better approach? Eat a small portion of any food you enjoy—even if it's higher in fat or calories. Even when you're trying to shed pounds, you can enjoy some high-calorie foods as long as your eating plan is healthful, and you eat fewer calories overall than your body uses. As another option, try to satisfy your palate with a low-fat, low-calorie version.

Need more strategies for sensible, effective weight management? Check here for "how tos":

● Help your child or teen keep a healthy weight—see chapter 17.

● Encourage your kids to move more and sit less—see chapter 17.

● Stay physically active in your later years—see chapter 19.

● Gain, maintain, or lose weight as an older adult—see chapter 19.

Have You Ever Wondered

... if surgery and liposuction are options for weight loss? Not for most people. Gastric bypass surgery, done by shortening the small intestine or by making the stomach smaller, does promote weight loss. However, because the side effects can be harmful with lifelong implications, doctors generally advise surgery only as a final resort for people who are at least 100 pounds overweight when other approaches haven't worked. Another approach, called adjustable gastric banding, can alter stomach capacity and emptying time. Liposuction, the surgical removal of fat tissue from various body areas, is often only a short-term solution. If eating and exercise habits remain the same, it's likely that weight will be regained.

... if you should join a support group to lose weight? Perhaps, but that's an individual matter. Weight-loss organizations and support groups often educate participants as they offer psychological support. And many, but not all, are coordinated by qualified nutrition experts. The section *"Questions to Ask ... about Weight Loss Programs"* can help you judge. For some people, peer support offers motivation, especially if they pay to attend the program. There's a downside, however. Without a weight maintenance program, many people gain weight again when they're no longer in the group.

leave the diet program? Ask for results over two to five years. The Federal Trade Commission requires weight-loss companies to back up their claims.

● What are the costs for membership, weekly fees, food, supplements, maintenance, and counseling? What's the payment schedule? Are any costs covered under health insurance? Do you give refunds if I drop out?

● Will you monitor my success at three- to six-month intervals, then modify the program if needed? How?

● Do you have a maintenance program? Is it part of the package, or does it cost extra?

● What kind of professional support is provided? What are the credentials and experiences of these professionals? (Detailed information should be available on request.)

● What are the program's requirements? Are there special menus or foods, counseling visits, or exercise plans? Can I make changes based on my food preferences or food allergies?

Logging on to the Internet may offer support for weight loss. Some people like the anonymity; others like personalized help with feedback at home. Some research suggests that well-designed, interactive programs are effective—at least in the short term. The challenge is finding a site that offers sound guidance and privacy of personal data, rather than one that's mostly in business to sell products. There's another potential problem. Face-to-face weight-loss counseling with a registered dietitian addresses other issues—related health problems, personal lifestyles, and food preferences, among others—that may affect your weight-loss success; cyberdieting may not. *See "Nutrition in Cyberspace" in chapter 24.*

For more guidance on evaluating a weight-control plan, see "Check It Out!" earlier in this chapter.

Once you choose a weight-loss program, go prepared to talk with the healthcare professional. *See chapter 24, "When You Consult an Expert . . ."*

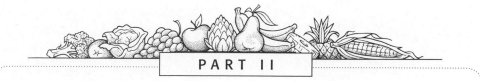

PART II

Well Nourished
The Basics

CHAPTER 3

Carbs
Sugars, Starches, Fiber

When you think of carbohydrates, what comes to mind: hearty whole-grain bread, piping hot oatmeal, tender fettuccini, freshly popped popcorn, naturally sweet potatoes, crunchy celery, summer-fresh corn on the cob, juicy peaches or sweet mangoes, a fresh banana, savory baked beans, or fruit yogurt?

All these nourishing foods put carbohydrates, in one form or another, on your plate, along with other essential nutrients. For your health and your healthy weight, make your carbohydrate foods count for good nutrition!

Carbs: The Basics

Sugars, starches, and fiber: they all belong to a nutrient category called carbohydrates. As energy nutrients, sugars and starches (complex carbohydrates) are your body's main fuel sources. Fiber, another complex carb, has other unique health benefits. For the record, "carbs" is the nickname for a nutrient category, not for bread, pasta, rice, and other carbohydrate-containing foods.

All carbohydrates are made of the same three elements: carbon, hydrogen, and oxygen. Their name comes from their chemical makeup. The first part, "carbo-," means carbon; "-hydrate" means water, or H_2O. To make different types of carbohydrates, these elements first are arranged as single units. Sugars contain one or just a few of these units; that's why sugars are considered simple carbohydrates. Made of many sugar units, starches and fiber are complex carbohydrates.

Sugars: Carbohydrate's Short Form

Table sugar may come to mind when you hear the word "sugar." Yet that's just one of several sugars, or simple carbohydrates.

In scientific language, sugars are monosaccharides with one sugar unit, disaccharides with two linked sugar units, and oligosaccharides with three to ten sugar units. ("Mono-" means one, "di-" means two, "oligo-" means few, and "-saccharide" means sugar.) Monosaccharides are fructose, galactose, and glucose.

When two monosaccharides join chemically, they become disaccharides:

- sucrose = glucose + fructose
- lactose = glucose + galactose
- maltose = glucose + glucose

Some sugars occur naturally in foods. Others are added. Regardless, both provide calories, or food energy. Fructose is the naturally occurring sugar in fruit, root vegetables, and honey. When fructose occurs naturally, it's always in food with other sugars, such as glucose. Lactose is the naturally occurring sugar in milk. Maltose is formed when starch breaks down to simple sugars. Sucrose is another name for table sugar; this same sugar is found naturally in many fruits, some vegetables, and some grains.

Were you born with a "sweet tooth"? Probably yes.

Studies show that newborns respond to the sweet tastes of sugars quicker than to the other four tastes: bitter, sour, salty, and umami (meaty or savory). At any age, sweetness adds pleasure to eating!

Complex Carbohydrates: Made of Many Sugars

Starches and fiber have something in common. Called complex carbohydrates, or polysaccharides, they're longer chains of many sugar units. "Poly-" means many.

You may wonder—if starch is made of sugars, why doesn't it taste sweet? Molecule size makes the difference. Starch molecules are bigger. Unlike sugars, which are smaller, starch molecules are too big to fit on receptors of your taste buds, so they don't taste sweet. But keep a starchy cracker in your mouth for a while. Once digestive enzymes in saliva break down its starch into sugars, the cracker starts to taste sweet.

Starch comes from plant-based foods such as rice, pasta, potatoes, beans (legumes), and other vegetables and grain products. Whole-grain foods, as well as beans, other vegetables, and fruit, deliver fiber.

Glycogen, another polysaccharide, comes from animal sources. It's the form of carbohydrate that's stored in your body. During endurance sports glycogen is an important energy source. *For more about energy for sports, refer to "Energy to Burn" in chapter 20.*

Fiber: Not All Alike

We talk about fiber as a single food component, but it's not that simple. Actually, fiber is a general term, referring to different polysaccharides and lignin. All contribute to healthful eating.

Like starch, fiber is a complex carbohydrate, made of many linked sugar units. Unlike starch, fiber can't be digested, or broken down, into simple sugars for absorption into the bloodstream. As a result, it can't provide energy as other carbohydrates can. Instead, fiber passes through to the large intestine undigested.

Various types of fiber often are grouped in two categories: soluble and insoluble. Soluble fibers dissolve in water; insoluble fibers don't. Known as "roughage," insoluble fibers give structure to plant cell walls. These differing qualities also allow them to keep you healthy in different ways, as you'll learn later in this chapter. Some major health benefits are attributed to both types

Have You Ever Wondered?

. . . if honey, brown sugar, or other so-called natural sweeteners are more nutritious than white sugar? That's a common misperception. While promoted as healthier options, sweeteners such as agave nectar, honey, grape juice concentrate, date sugar, and molasses don't differ significantly in calories and nutrients from table sugar. For those with diabetes, they affect blood glucose levels in a similar way. If you like the flavor, enjoy, but only in limited amounts, as you would any added sugars.

Honey, formed from nectar by bees, is composed of several sugars (fructose, glucose, sucrose, and others). Ounce for ounce, the nutrients in honey and white (or table) sugar are nearly the same. A teaspoon of honey has slightly more calories and carbohydrates. That's because honey weighs slightly more. One teaspoon of white (table) sugar has about 16 calories and 4.5 grams of carbohydrates; a teaspoon of honey, about 21 calories and 6 grams of carbohydrates. Both are broken down into glucose and fructose in your body. Honey is sweeter than white sugar, so you need less honey to sweeten foods.

Brown sugar is merely sugar crystals flavored with molasses. Nutritionwise it too has about 17 calories and 4 grams of carbohydrate per teaspoon—about the same amounts as white sugar.

. . . if molasses, which is a natural sugar, is more nutritious than other sweeteners? Molasses does have measureable amounts of some nutrients. Because the flavor is strong, the amount generally consumed isn't likely enough to provide an appreciable nutrient contribution—and it does supply calories. A tablespoon of molasses has about 40 mg of calcium, 1 mg of iron, and 60 calories.

of fiber. With the mixture of foods most people eat, about two-thirds to three-quarters of their fiber intake is likely soluble.

More recently, soluble fibers also have been categorized by their viscosity. Viscous fibers are soluble fibers that gel or thicken in water.

Digestion: From Complex to Simple

Both sugars and starches break down to single sugars during digestion. From a calorie standpoint, the body doesn't distinguish their food source.

In a nutshell, going from a complex carbohydrate to a simple sugar happens when starches are digested. Before they can be absorbed from your digestive tract into your bloodstream, starches are broken down by human enzymes to the simplest sugars: glucose, galactose, and fructose. Then, in the bloodstream, single sugars move into body cells where they're converted to energy.

Monosaccharides such as the fructose in fruits can be absorbed as they are. That's not true for disaccharides: sucrose, lactose, and maltose. Digestive enzymes break them down. That said, some people don't produce enough of a digestive enzyme called lactase; as a result, they may feel discomfort digesting lactose, or milk sugar. *Refer to "Lactose Intolerance: A Matter of Degree" in chapter 21.*

Only fiber remains relatively intact through the body's small intestine. Digestive enzymes in the intestine can't break down fiber to sugar units. That's why fiber isn't a significant source of energy, or calories. In the large intestine, fiber can bind to water and add bulk to waste, or it can be fermented by friendly bacteria to form gases and short-chain fatty acids, which have unique health benefits. Short-chain fatty acids are absorbed and provide a small amount of calories and other health benefits.

Have You Ever Wondered

. . . what refined sugar is? Refined sugar is described most simply as sugar separated either from the stalk of sugarcane or from the root of a sugar beet. The sugar-containing juice of the plant is extracted, then processed into dried sugar crystals. It's sold as granulated or white sugar. Molasses is the thick syrup that's left after sugar beet or sugarcane is processed for table sugar.

. . . what raw sugar is? Raw sugar comes from processing sugarcane. Raw sugar is a coarse, granulated solid sugar left when clarified sugarcane juice evaporates. Because of its impurities, you can't buy 100 percent raw sugar. But you can buy turbinado sugar. Light-tan turbinado sugar is raw sugar refined in a centrifuge under sanitary conditions. Nutritionally speaking, its caloric and carbohydrate contents are the same as in refined, or table sugar. So-called natural sugars (raw sugar, date sugar, honey, maple syrup) aren't nutritionally better than other sugars.

For your health, when eating carbohydrate-containing foods:

- Reduce the intake of calories from added sugars.
- Cut back on foods and drinks with added sugars (sugar-sweetened beverages).
- Limit the consumption of foods that contain refined grains, especially refined grain foods that contain solid fats, added sugars, and sodium.
- Consume at least half of all grains as whole grains. Increase whole-grain intake by replacing refined grains with whole grains.*
- Increase vegetable and fruit intake.

*When choosing a refined grain product, check the ingredient list to make sure it's made with enriched flour.
Source: Dietary Guidelines for Americans, 2010.

Carbohydrates: For Energy and Health

Carbohydrates are one of six nutrient categories—and they're your body's preferred and major energy source!

Your Body's Power Source

Carbohydrates power everything from jogging to breathing to thinking and even to digesting food. Actually, glucose is the main form of carbohydrate used for energy—and the only energy source your brain normally can use. Because glucose circulates in your bloodstream, it's often called blood glucose. It's carried to all body cells; each cell has its own power-house that uses glucose to produce energy.

When carbohydrates are absorbed, blood glucose levels rise. Insulin helps glucose enter cells, where it's used for energy.

Your body doesn't turn all blood glucose to energy at once. As blood glucose levels rise above normal, insulin (a pancreatic hormone) signals your liver, muscles, and other cells to store the extra. Some gets stored in the muscles and liver as glycogen, a storage form of carbohydrate. Some glucose may be converted to body fat—if you consume more calories than your body uses, or burns.

When blood glucose levels drop below normal, another hormone, called glucagon, triggers the conversion of glycogen to glucose. That's how blood glucose levels stay within normal range between meals. Once glucose is back in your bloodstream, it's again ready to fuel body cells.

Your body also derives energy from fat and protein, but carbohydrates should be your main energy source. As such, they can spare, or save, protein for what only protein can do: build and repair body cells and tissues. (*See chapter 4 for more about protein.*) If your calorie intake is less than what your body needs and if your limited glycogen stores are spent, body proteins are broken down for energy. In a low-carb, high-fat eating plan, fat becomes an energy source. In the process, ketones from incomplete fat breakdown may build up in the bloodstream, which has been linked to health problems such as kidney damage and gout.

Just a Spoonful of Sugar . . .

1 teaspoon honey	21 calories
1 teaspoon jelly	16 calories
1 teaspoon brown sugar	17 calories
1 teaspoon table sugar	16 calories
1 teaspoon maple syrup	17 calories
1 teaspoon corn syrup, light or dark	19 calories

Have You Ever Wondered ?

. . . what resistant starch is? It's a complex carbohydrate that resists digestion in the small intestine. Instead it passes into the large intestine, where it's fermented and may promote the growth of healthy bacteria. Resistant starch performs like fiber and so contributes fewer calories than other complex carbohydrates. Naturally occurring resistant starch is found in beans (legumes); underripe and slightly green bananas; cold, cooked potatoes; and unprocessed whole grains. It also may be produced through food processing.

. . . what inulin is? Inulin—not to be confused with insulin—is considered to be a soluble fiber and is found naturally in many vegetables and fruits, including Jerusalem artichokes, asparagus, leeks, onions, bananas, and raisins. It's also added to many foods in the marketplace, such as some breads and pasta, without affecting the taste and texture.

Because it isn't digested or absorbed in the stomach or small intestine, inulin—when replacing other carbohydrates—doesn't affect blood glucose levels, offering possible benefits for those with diabetes. Instead it passes into the large intestine, where it has other health benefits as a fermentable fiber.

As a soluble fiber, inulin may play a role in reducing levels of blood cholesterol and promoting regularity.

As a prebiotic, inulin is food for good bacteria such as *bifidobacteria* and *lactobacilli*, the same bacteria in yogurt with active cultures and fermented dairy foods.

As a source of short-chain fatty acids, it may promote gut health and help keep the large intestine functioning normally, may help support the immune system, and may help to improve calcium absorption, among other functions; *see chapter 6 for more about pre- and probiotics.*

Too much inulin can result in gas *(see "Fiber's Health Benefits" in this chapter)* and diarrhea. Try to eat a variety of fiber sources, not just inulin.

. . . what fructo-oligosaccharides (FOS) are, and what they do? FOS, which are polymers of fructose, are found naturally in some foods. Like inulin, FOS are only partially digested by humans and may help improve gastrointestinal health. Providing fewer calories than sugars or starches, they're often used as an alternative sweetener. They too work as a prebiotic. Not enough evidence suggests if they're effective as supplements or prebiotics for preventing traveler's diarrhea, constipation, high blood cholesterol levels, or other conditions.

. . . what the difference is between lignin and lignan? The terms often get confused. Classified as an insoluble fiber, lignin actually isn't a carbohydrate but a complex molecule that's a woody part of the stems and seeds of fruits and vegetables and the bran in cereals. Its properties may help prevent cancers. Lignans are phytonutrients in whole grains and flaxseeds; research is examining their roles as phytoestrogens and anticancer agents.

From sugar or starch, 1 gram of carbohydrate fuels your body with the same amount of energy, 4 calories per gram. By comparison, protein supplies 4 calories per gram and fat supplies 9 calories per gram.

The bottom line: For your health's sake, make nutrient-rich carbohydrate foods your body's main energy source.

Dispelling Carbohydrate Confusion

Over the decades, many misconceptions have been associated with carbohydrates. The following facts dispel some common myths.

Do Carbs Make You Fat?

No. Eating too many calories from any source—carbohydrates, fats, proteins, or alcohol—causes your body to produce extra body fat. Actually, when you eat a variety of food with enough carbohydrates, excess calories from fats turn into body fat first before extra calories from carbohydrates do.

Contrary to some popular beliefs, sugar won't cause your body to make or store fat. It's true that insulin levels rise when carbohydrates are absorbed. That's normal. Insulin regulates energy storage, allowing your body to move blood glucose elsewhere, perhaps to your cells for energy or to your muscles or liver for storage. Once accomplished, insulin and glucose levels drop to normal if you're healthy. Glucose is converted to body fat only if you consume more calories than your body needs.

Neither sugar itself nor a carbohydrate-rich diet causes an insulin reaction that will result in weight gain. And consuming carbohydrate-rich foods doesn't cause insulin resistance. People who are overweight and sedentary may have symptoms of insulin resistance, a condition often diminished with moderate physical activity and weight loss.

To maintain a healthy weight, control calories from all your food choices, and stay physically active.

Are Carbs Linked to Hyperactivity?

Following an afternoon of sweet snacks, friends, and active play, kids may be wired up. But don't blame the candy, cupcakes, or sweet drinks for a sugar high. Sugar has been wrongly accused as a cause of hyperactivity or attention deficit-hyperactive disorder (ADHD). Even though scientific evidence doesn't support a link between the intake of sugars and hyperactivity, many parents and other caregivers seem reluctant to put this notion aside.

Causes of nervous, aggressive, and impulsive behavior and a short attention span aren't understood completely. But experts advise adults to take stock of a child's overall environment. The excitement of a party or a special event, such as trick-or-treating or a visit to Santa—not the sweet snacks that go with the fun—may account for unruly behavior. To the contrary, some studies suggest that sugars may have a calming effect. There's not enough research yet, but a body chemical called serotonin produced in and released from the brain may be a factor.

Do Carbs Cause Diabetes?

Again, the answer is no. Sugars—and other carbohydrates—don't cause diabetes. Although the scientific community debunked this myth decades ago, the misperception persists.

With diabetes, the body can't handle blood glucose (blood sugar) normally, which affects your body's ability to produce energy from the food you eat. The causes are complex. Genetics certainly play a role, but illness, being overweight or obese, or simply getting older also may trigger diabetes. Being overweight seems to be a key factor in the growing diabetes epidemic, including type 2 diabetes among kids.

While food choices don't cause diabetes, diet along with physical activity and perhaps medication is part of managing diabetes. To control blood glucose levels, people with diabetes need to manage the overall carbohydrates, as well as proteins, fats, and alcoholic drinks, in their meals and snacks.

In the past, people with diabetes were warned to avoid or strictly limit sugar in their food choices. Today, experts recognize that all sugars and starches affect blood glucose levels. According to current advice from the American Diabetes Association, moderate amounts of sugar—in fact, all carbohydrates—can be part of a well-balanced diet for managing diabetes. A registered dietitian or certified diabetes educator can help plan and monitor their diet. *For more on diabetes, as well as insulin resistance, refer to chapter 22, "Diabetes: A Growing Concern."*

Do Carbs Trigger Hypoglycemia?

It's highly unlikely. Yet many people explain away anxiety, headaches, and chronic fatigue as hypoglycemia caused by eating foods with sugar. Often self-diagnosed, hypoglycemic disorders are actually quite rare.

Hypoglycemia, or low blood glucose, is a condition, not a disease. Between meals, glucose levels

---

Hot Topic: Glycemic Index

Glycemic index (GI) and glycemic load (GL) are receiving attention as people seek ways to manage their weight, blood glucose levels, or other health conditions. Yet, notes the *Dietary Guidelines Advisory Report, 2010,* GI and/or GL aren't associated with body weight; using them as tools doesn't lead to more weight loss or better weight maintenance. There may be a link between GI and type 2 diabetes, although the evidence isn't conclusive.

Just what is glycemic index? It's a way of rating carbohydrate-containing foods on how they affect the body's blood glucose levels after eating them. How high it rises, and for how long, depend on the quality of the carbohydrates. Some are digested faster; others, more slowly. A food's GI is ranked against a glucose solution on a scale of 1 to 100: 55 or under is low; 56 to 69 is medium; and 70 or above is high. Foods with a higher glycemic index produce a greater increase in blood glucose levels (blood glucose response) than low GI foods.

What's glycemic load then? It takes both the quality and the quantity of carbohydrates into account. The rise and the fall of blood glucose levels after eating depend on both. The GL equals the GI times the amount of carbohydrates in grams divided by 100; for example, an apple has a GI of 40 x 15 grams of carbohydrate ÷ 100 = a GL of 6 grams. In contrast, a small baked potato with a GI of 60 would have a GL of 12 grams, or twice the metabolic impact. For GL, less than 10 is low, 11 to 20 is medium, and 21 or over is high.

That said, figuring the body's response sounds simpler than it really is. Glycemic index is calculated for a specific amount of food, usually 50 grams of total carbohydrate minus the fiber. Many factors affect glycemic index for a single food, including its ripeness, its variety, how it's prepared or processed, the type of sugar and starch, how much fat and fiber it contains, and how long it takes to digest. Portion size varies, too, for providing the standard 50 grams of carbohydrate; both 7 carrots and 640 grams (about 4 cups cubed) of watermelon supply that amount.

In general, nonstarchy vegetables, most fruits, beans (legumes), and milk tend to have a low glycemic index. For example, ½ cup of kidney beans has a glycemic index of 52; a medium apple, 38. White bread (from refined flour), crackers, and cornflakes are high-GI foods. The glycemic index of a medium baked potato (no skin) is 85, considered high. Yet this rule of thumb doesn't always hold true. Watermelon and carrots—a vegetable and a fruit—also have a high glycemic index.

The glycemic index of a single food isn't reliable for helping most healthy consumers make food choices. Why? First, the food is usually eaten with other foods; glycemic index doesn't measure what happens with mixed foods. A high-GI food eaten with a low-GI food may give a moderate GI response. Second, the amount eaten may be more or less than the amount for calculating glycemic response; to address that issue, glycemic loads for standard portions have been determined. And third, the GI response to a food can vary from one person to another. A person's individual response may vary from day to day, too.

That said, glycemic index is being used in research related to type 2 diabetes, heart disease, and obesity—with potential for more use in the future. Currently, however, no evidence shows that eliminating foods with a higher glycemic index, such as baked potatoes or cornflakes, promotes weight loss or helps with appetite control. And these foods may offer nutrient and phytonutrient benefits.

Research does imply that when choosing carbohydrate foods, heed their calories, caloric density, and fiber content, without concern for their glycemic index or glycemic load. If you choose to use the GI, choose lower-GI foods more often.

For people with diabetes, glycemic index may be useful as one tool to manage blood glucose levels, along with blood glucose monitoring and monitoring total grams of carbohydrate. Its use should be guided by a registered dietitian or other health professional. *Refer to "Diabetes: A Growing Concern" in chapter 22.* Sometimes endurance athletes use high-GI foods to resynthesize muscle glycogen.

naturally drop but they remain fairly constant, between 60 and 110 milligrams per deciliter (mg/dL). A signal for hypoglycemia is when levels drop below about 40 mg/dL. When blood glucose falls below normal levels, there's not enough glucose immediately available for cells to produce energy. That can cause several symptoms, including sweating, rapid heartbeat, trembling, and hunger.

Among people with diabetes, hypoglycemia is caused by taking too much insulin, by exercising too much, or by not eating enough. In most other cases, low blood glucose is linked to other serious medical problems, such as liver disease or a pancreatic tumor.

In rare cases, a disorder called reactive hypoglycemia occurs. As a rebound effect, the body secretes too much insulin after eating a large meal. The result is a drop in blood glucose well below normal, and symptoms such as shakiness, sweating, rapid heartbeat, and trembling may occur—but not until about two to four hours after eating. These symptoms shouldn't be confused with extreme hunger, with symptoms of gradually increased stomach rumbling, headache, and feelings of weakness, usually occurring six to eight hours after a meal.

If you think you're among the few with symptoms of reactive hypoglycemia, pay attention to how you feel two to four hours after eating. Then talk to your physician about testing your blood glucose level while you're experiencing symptoms.

Also, be cautious of so-called health clinics that diagnose sugar-induced hypoglycemia and offer treatment with costly remedies.

Your Smile: Carbohydrates and Oral Health

Imagine the wide smile that comes with those popular words "Look, Mom, no cavities!" Good oral hygiene and dental care, along with the widespread presence of fluoride toothpaste, fluoride rinses, sealants, and fluoridated water, can make smiles healthier than ever.

What causes cavities, and how can you protect your teeth? Whether you get cavities depends on many things, including your food choices. Heredity, as well as the makeup and flow of saliva, are factors, as are your nutritional status, oral hygiene, fluoride exposure, use of medications, and general health. Although part of the nutrition equation, sugars—both naturally occurring and added—aren't the only carbohydrates

---

Keep Teeth and Gums Healthy

- Eat healthy! An adequate supply of nutrient-rich foods from all five food groups promotes healthy teeth and gums. *See chapter 10 to learn more.*

- Go easy on between-meal snacks. When you do snack, try to eat the snack at one time rather than over a longer period.

- Brush twice a day, in the morning and before bed; brush your tongue, too. Be aware that brushing too often may be abrasive to your tooth enamel.

- Use a fluoride toothpaste with the American Dental Association Seal of Acceptance. The optimal amount of fluoride from toothpaste comes from brushing twice a day, not any more often.

- Teach children over age two years to brush with just a pea-size amount of fluoride toothpaste and to spit out, not swallow, toothpaste to reduce the chances of mottled teeth (dark spots) from too much fluoride. For kids under age two, talk to your doctor about fluoride toothpaste.

- Floss daily to help remove food particles and plaque between teeth. Or use an interdental cleaner; ask your dentist if it's right for you.

- Use a fluoride mouth rinse with your dentist's advice; don't swallow it. A fluoride rinse for those under age six years isn't advised.

- Have regular dental checkups, which include a thorough cleaning.

- Talk to your dentist about sealants, which protect against decay in the pits and fissures of your teeth (they're not just for kids).

- For infants, avoid the urge to pacify your baby with a bottle of juice, formula, or milk. If you choose to use a bottle as a pacifier, fill it with water only.

- For children, talk to your dentist, doctor, or pediatric nurse about what amount of fluoride your child should have. If you live in a community that doesn't have an optimal amount of fluoride in the water, supplements may be recommended.

linked to cavity formation. Starches, or fermentable carbohydrates, contribute to cavities (also called caries), too.

Plaque Attack!

Tooth decay starts when bacteria in your mouth mix with carbohydrates—both sugars and starches—to make acids. Bacteria are found in dental plaque, an invisible film that forms in your mouth and clings to the surfaces of your teeth and along your gumline.

Acids, produced by oral bacteria, can eat away tooth enamel, causing tooth decay, also known as dental caries. Every time you eat sugars and starches, acids begin to bathe your teeth. The cavity-producing action continues for 20 minutes or more after you eat something starchy or sugary.

These two equations offer a quick summary of action that takes place in your mouth when bacteria in plaque mix with carbohydrates in food:

plaque + carbohydrates = acid

acid + tooth enamel = potential tooth decay

A Sticky Issue

Hard candy offers no more threat to your teeth than pasta does. Surprised? Any food that contains carbohydrates—pasta, bread, rice, chips, fruit, even milk, as well as cake, cookies, and candy—can "feed" bacteria in plaque.

Likewise, table sugar, or sucrose, isn't the only sugar that affects oral health. Any sugar—whether it's added or naturally occurring—can promote cavities. Fructose in fruit and lactose in milk also cause bacteria to produce plaque acids. Cookies sweetened with juice have the same cavity-promoting potential as cookies made with table sugar.

Among young children, baby-bottle tooth decay happens when teeth or gums are exposed for extended periods of time to milk, breast milk, formula, fruit juice, or another sweet drink. When babies fall asleep sucking on a bottle or fall asleep frequently while breast-feeding, the chances go up. (*For more on baby-bottle tooth decay, refer to "Caring for Baby Teeth" in chapter 16.*)

Do some foods promote cavities more than others? No definitive list ranks the cavity-forming potential of food. However, some factors make a difference: how often you eat (or how often carbohydrate comes

---

Snack for a Healthy Smile

Keep your smile healthy! For everyone, especially children, smart snacking can lead to good oral health.

- Overcome the urge to snack frequently. Bacteria in plaque produce acids that can damage teeth for 20 minutes or more after each exposure to carbohydrates.

- Choose snacks wisely for a well-balanced eating plan. Eat raw vegetables, fruits (such as apples), plain yogurt, cheese, milk, and popcorn.

- Even though sugars from hard candy, cough drops, and lollipops may leave your mouth faster than snacks that stick between your teeth, go easy on sugary snacks that dissolve slowly in your mouth. Sucking on foods prolongs the time when sugar bathes your teeth. Slowly sipping a sugar-sweetened beverage or soft drink has the same effect.

- Brush as soon as you can after snacking. This removes plaque and so stops the cavity-producing action of bacteria. Or at least rinse your mouth with water to get rid of food particles.

---

in contact with your teeth) and how long carbohydrate stays on your teeth. In fact, a food's form (liquid, solid, or stick and how slowly it dissolves), the frequency of consuming its sugar or starch, other nutrients, its potential to stimulate saliva, foods it's eaten with, and the order of food intake all make a difference.

Frequency. The more often you eat carbohydrate foods, especially between meals, the more likely acid attacks teeth. Sucking hard candy or cough drops, nibbling chips, or slowly sipping a sugar-sweetened drink nourishes bacteria and bathes teeth with plaque acids for a while. The action continues for 20 minutes or longer after you finish each candy, nibble on chips, or drink each sip of regular soft drink or juice.

Type of Food. Because some foods stick to your teeth, plaque acids continue their action long after you stop eating or drinking. The word "sticky" may conjure up thoughts of caramels. Yet caramels dissolve and leave your mouth faster than bread or chips that stick between your teeth or in the pits of your molars. It may take hours for the food particles to finally leave your mouth. The faster food dissolves and leaves your mouth, the less chance it has to produce plaque acid. For example, sticky dried fruit, granola bars, and raisins may stay on your teeth longer than a soft drink or a hot fudge sundae.

Will a box of raisins or a bunch of grapes be more cavity-promoting than a single raisin or a single grape? Eaten at one time, portion size makes no difference. Any amount of carbohydrate gets the decay process going. It's the frequency of snacking that seems to have a bigger impact on cavity formation than snack size.

Brushing after eating and flossing remove the decay duo of plaque and food particles. Swishing water around your mouth after meals and snacks may help rinse away food particles and sugars but won't remove plaque bacteria.

Oral Health: Beyond Carbohydrates

Carbohydrates aren't the only nutrition factor linked to oral health. Some nutrients make teeth stronger. And some are described as anticavity foods.

For children, overall healthful eating promotes healthy teeth, making them stronger and more resistant to cavities. Several nutrients are especially important, including calcium, phosphorus, and vitamin D. These nutrients also build the jawbone, which helps keep teeth in place. For adults, calcium and vitamin D intake have little effect on keeping teeth healthy. But these same nutrients help keep the jawbone strong.

Tooth loss, common among the elderly, may be linked to periodontal, or gum, disease. Constant infection causes the bone structure of the jaw to gradually deteriorate. (*Refer to "Keep Smiling: Prevent Gum Disease" in chapter 22 for more information.*)

Before fluoridation of water was common, tooth decay was much more prevalent. Now, adding fluoride to drinking water, toothpaste, and mouth rinses is one of the most effective ways to prevent cavities. Fluoride makes the structure of teeth stronger by helping to add minerals back to microscopic cavities on the surface of tooth enamel. Bottled water generally isn't fluoridated. With more fluoride sources today, municipalities may adjust the fluoride level in their water supply to lower the chance of fluorosis, when teeth can become discolored or spotty from too much fluoride. (*Refer to "The Fluoride Connection" in chapter 8.*)

Saliva itself is beneficial. Your body produces up

Have You Ever Wondered

. . . if presweetened cereals are more cavity-promoting than unsweetened cereals? There's really no difference. Carbohydrates in both starches and sugars nourish bacteria that promote decay. The cavity factor depends on how long any cereal sticks between teeth or in the crevices in molars. Cavity-causing potential doesn't depend on the amount of sugars or starches.

Although not a dental health issue, presweetened cereals are sources of added sugars, but perhaps adding no more sugar than the amount in a spoonful of sugar sprinkled on unsweetened cereal. There is a trend among some cereal manufacturers to lower the sugar content of cereals marketed to children. Check the ingredient list on the food label to compare; choose those that help you reduce added sugars.

Something else to consider: Whether presweetened or not, ready-to-eat cereals offer a quick, convenient way to fit breakfast in and to get significant nutrient intake. Many cereals are nutrient-fortified; many are whole-grain or high-fiber. Topped with milk or yogurt, cereal also provides a way to consume calcium and vitamin D. Interestingly, breakfast eaters, including those who eat cereal, tend to have lower BMIs than those who don't.

to one quart of saliva a day, especially if you drink enough fluids. That's good news, because saliva helps protect your teeth from decay. By clearing carbohydrates from your mouth faster, saliva helps to reduce the time during which plaque acids can form. Minerals in saliva—calcium, phosphorus, and fluoride—may have a protective effect, too.

Some aged cheeses, such as sharp Cheddar, Monterey Jack, and Swiss, also may offer modest cavity protection. By increasing saliva flow, they lower acid levels. Both milk and cheese contain nutrients, including calcium, phosphorus, and protein, that may help protect tooth enamel.

Fiber's Health Benefits

Life doesn't depend on fiber, but your overall health may. Fiber promotes health, including optimal digestive and gut health. A high-fiber eating pattern also may help reduce the risks for obesity, heart disease, diabetes, and other chronic diseases. The 2010 Dietary

Guidelines advise choosing foods that provide more dietary fiber in the form of fiber-rich fruits, vegetables, and whole grains. Here's why.

Soluble and Insoluble: Different Missions

Most foods contain both soluble and insoluble fibers; each is unique. Soluble fiber dissolves in water while insoluble fiber doesn't. These different qualities provide different health benefits. Just as different vitamins are needed for optimum nutrition, different types and sources of fibers are needed, too.

● Insoluble fibers, such as cellulose, hemicellulose, and lignin, aid digestion. Although they don't dissolve, insoluble fibers do hold on to water. And they move waste through the intestinal tract without being broken down, earning fiber its title as "nature's broom." By adding bulk and softness to stools, insoluble fibers promote regularity and help prevent constipation. By moving wastes through the colon, insoluble fibers increase the rate at which wastes are removed. Wheat bran, for example, is high in insoluble fiber.

● Soluble fibers such as gums, mucilages, pectin, and some hemicelluloses offer different protective benefits. Instead of giving a coarse texture to food, some soluble fibers, such as those in oat bran, dissolve to become gummy or viscous. Viscous fibers help reduce cholesterol absorption and help control the amount of glucose in the bloodstream. They're often used in low-fat and fat-free foods to add texture and consistency. Soft, liquid foods may have fiber, but usually this soluble fiber isn't viscous.

Defining Fiber

If you read about fiber, you'll likely see a slew of terms: dietary fiber, functional fiber, total fiber, and a few more. What's the difference? What we understand about fiber is in flux. There's much more to learn about measuring food's fiber content and its many physiological effects. This includes fiber's ability to bind cholesterol, how it speeds intestinal transit time to protect against cancer and constipation, and how its fermentation benefits intestinal (gut) health. These issues impact how we talk about fiber.

The IOM's Dietary Reference Intakes use "total fiber," defined as dietary fiber plus functional fiber. In this book, dietary fiber is the fiber that's naturally present in plant-based foods. Also with health benefits, functional fiber is manufactured from plant or animal products. For example, inulin and FOS (fructooligosaccharides or frucan) work as prebiotics; methylcellulose is a bulking agent.

For labeling, dietary fiber is used, yet the definition differs around the world. As more is learned, fiber's definitions will be clarified. Nutrition truly is an evolving science!

FUNCTIONAL NUTRITION: A QUICK LOOK AT DIETARY FIBER

DIETARY (FUNCTIONAL AND TOTAL) FIBER	POTENTIAL BENEFIT	SOME FOOD SOURCES
Insoluble fiber	● supports maintenance of digestive system; may reduce the risk of some types of cancer	● wheat bran, corn bran, fruit skins
Beta glucan*	● may reduce the risk of coronary heart disease (CHD)	● oat bran, oatmeal, oat flour, barley, rye
Soluble fiber*	● may reduce risk of CHD and some types of cancer	● psyllium seed husk, peas, beans, apples, citrus fruit
Whole grains*	● may reduce the risk of CHD and some types of cancer; supports maintenance of healthy blood glucose levels	● cereal grains, whole-wheat bread, oatmeal, brown rice

* The U.S. Food and Drug Administration has approved a health claim for this food component.
Source: International Food Information Council Foundation, 2011.

If you've ever made jam or jelly, you're probably familiar with pectin. Pectin provides their thick, gel-like consistency. In your body, pectin plays a different role, binding to fatty substances and promoting their excretion as waste. This quality seems to help lower blood cholesterol levels. Viscous fibers also may help regulate the body's use of sugars.

Fiber, Healthy Weight, and Satiety

A fiber-rich diet may help you reach and keep your healthy weight. In fact, research shows that a fiber-rich diet is linked to lower body weight. Why?

● Fiber-rich foods are often lower in calories than the same volume of high-fat foods, and may displace other sources of food energy.

● Fiber itself isn't digested, so it provides few calories. The few calories come from short-chain fatty acids, produced when fiber ferments in the large intestine.

● Fiber-rich foods tend to be more satiating than low-fiber foods, meaning they help you feel full on fewer calories. Because fiber-rich foods often take longer to chew, you may eat more slowly, giving your body time to register that you're full.

● Fiber adds bulk to food and slows the time it takes to pass through your gastrointestinal tract. So a meal or a snack may seem bigger as it fills you up and it may stay with you longer. As a result, you may be less likely to overeat.

● And as fiber ferments in the intestine, that too may affect satiety.

As an aside, different types of fiber added to food and drinks aren't equally satiating; some have little or no effect.

To make a fiber-rich diet work for your waistline, avoid excess calorie intake, too, and stay physically active. *To learn more about healthy weight, see chapter 2.*

Fiber and Type 2 Diabetes

For people with diabetes, a fiber-rich diet (especially with viscous fiber) may help to control the rise of blood glucose levels after eating. The reason why soluble fiber may help lower blood glucose levels isn't fully understood. Perhaps it's because fiber makes the stomach contents more viscous (more sticky

What Is a Whole Grain?

A whole grain is the entire edible part of any grain, such as wheat, corn, oats, and rice, among others. In the life cycle of plants, it's the seed from which other plants grow. Nutrients in these seeds supply the first nourishment for the plant before the roots are formed. The whole grain, or seed, contains three parts: endosperm, bran, and germ.

The bran makes up the outer layers of the grain. It supplies antioxidants, B vitamins, trace minerals, and dietary fiber.

The endosperm, which is the inner part of the grain, has most of the proteins and carbohydrates, and just small amounts of vitamins and minerals. White flour is ground from the endosperm.

The germ is small but very important. It sprouts, generating a new plant. It has B vitamins, vitamin E, trace minerals, antioxidants, and essential fats.

While whole grains have more fiber than their refined forms, some grains have much more fiber than others. While very nutritious, brown rice isn't a huge fiber source.

The bran and the germ of a whole grain supply most of the fiber. When milled to produce white flour, only the endosperm remains. Most of the fibrous bran and the germ are removed—along with important nutrients and phytonutrients, including fiber. Since they contain nutrients, fiber, and other phytonutrients found naturally in grains, whole-grain foods are usually a healthful choice!

and gummy) and so prolongs its emptying. Because carbohydrates break down more slowly, sugar is released and absorbed more slowly, too. That in turn may slow the rise of blood glucose levels.

The reasons why fiber benefits weight control also apply to those managing diabetes; fiber-rich foods tend to be less energy-dense, bulkier, and take longer to eat. They provide satiety and help prevent overeating.

In an overall healthful eating plan to manage diabetes, a fiber-rich diet that includes foods with viscous fiber such as beans (legumes) and oats is wise. For some with diabetes, fiber's role in blood glucose control may help reduce the need for insulin, or medication.

If you have diabetes and want to consume more fiber to help control blood glucose, talk to a registered dietitian or certified diabetes educator.

To learn more about blood glucose and its role in diabetes, see "What Is Diabetes?" in chapter 22.

Fiber and GI Health

You already read about the benefits of insoluble fiber, the kind in wheat bran. And you read that fiber holds onto water, helping to soften and add bulk to waste. This action promotes gastrointestinal (GI) health. It helps stools pass through the intestinal tract more quickly with normal frequency and ease. As a result, fiber helps prevent constipation and the discomfort that goes with it. It also may help solidify loose, watery stools.

When soft stools easily pass out of the body, there's no need for strained bowel movements. As a result, hemorrhoids—a painful swelling of the vein near the anus—are less likely to form. Softer, bulkier stools put less pressure on the colon walls and so reduce the chance of hemorrhoids, too. *To learn about diverticulosis and diverticulitis, see "Gastrointestinal Conditions" and "Achieve Optimal Digestive Health" in chapter 22.*

Potential fiber benefits to gut health come from many health-promoting bacteria. Fermentable fibers help create an environment for healthy bacteria, which

Have You Ever Wondered?

. . . if carbohydrates affect your mood? Maybe, but the evidence isn't conclusive. Studies have investigated the link between stress and serotonin, a body chemical synthesized as more tryptophan (a nonessential amino acid) enters the brain. Serotonin, a mood regulator, breaks down to help relieve stress. Although carbohydrates may help replenish the body's serotonin, no conclusive research suggests a calming effect. Does a bowl of ice cream or a mug of hot chocolate give you a feeling of comfort or calm? Perhaps it's really a link to pleasant memories.

. . . if whole grains are always a healthier choice than refined grains? Not necessarily. Most whole-grain foods provide significantly more fiber, vitamin E, potassium, selenium, zinc, and phytonutrients than refined or enriched grain products. However, enriched grain products generally provide more folate, certain B vitamins, and iron. So the best advice: enjoy both, and make half your choices whole. For a young woman who may become pregnant, enriched grain products are important sources of folic acid. *See chapter 18 to learn more.*

Over the Years: A Grain of Truth

Your ancestors consumed much more fiber than you do!

Before advanced milling technology, gristmills were used to grind wheat, corn, and other grains into meal or flour. Using the water power of a river, grain was milled between two coarse stones. Then it was sifted to remove the inedible chaff, or husk, leaving all the edible parts of the grain. The bran and the germ that contain fiber and many essential nutrients remained. Whole grains were the foods of the masses. In some parts of the world, that continues to be true. In fact, some people still pound their grain by hand to make flour.

As technology improved, the bran and the germ were separated and removed, leaving refined white flour. With this new process came new status. White bread, with its softer texture and high-class appeal, became more desirable than coarser, darker bread. But white bread was more expensive and available only to

those who could afford it—as far back as Roman times. For the same reasons, white rice became more desirable than brown rice. Simply put, refined was in!

With the switch to refined grains, however, people became shortchanged on many nutrients and fiber without knowing it. In the 1940s, recognizing the health consequences, manufacturers began enriching many grain products with some nutrients lost during processing—thiamin, riboflavin, niacin, and iron. In some, fiber was added back, too. Since the late 1990s, enriched grain products also have been fortified with folic acid.

Only within the past thirty-five or so years have health experts recognized that fiber offers more than bulk to food. It's loaded with health benefits. Today whole-grain products, along with other fiber-rich foods—vegetables, fruits, and beans—are in again. And today's experts advise that you make at least half your grains whole grains!

may help promote immunity, may help the body eliminate waste, and may help reduce discomfort from some food intolerances. Short-chain fatty acids (SCFAs) produced from fermentable fiber also help the body absorb some key nutrients and may help suppress harmful bacteria that create inflammation, and so may lower the chance of infections and colon cancer. SCFAs also may help reduce risk factors for other health concerns. It may help lower blood cholesterol and triglyceride levels, improve HDL:LDL cholesterol ratio, and lower blood glucose response.

Which Bread Is Whole Grain?

Being brown doesn't make bread whole wheat. Being white may not mean that bread is made with just refined white flour, either. Here's why you need to read the label!

- Whole-grain breads usually are browner than breads made with refined white flour. However, a rich brown color may come from coloring, often listed on the label as caramel coloring.

- Today, some whole-wheat bread looks white. The whole-wheat flour is made from a different grain variety, white wheat, with a lighter color and a milder flavor. Refined white flour is made traditionally with a red wheat, with its darker color and slightly bitter taste. If you don't eat traditional whole-wheat bread, white whole-wheat bread is a way to fit whole grains in!

Terms such as "seven-grain" or "multigrain" are no assurance that bread is whole grain. Those two terms simply mean that the bread is made with flour from more than one grain.

Finding whole-grain bread takes label-reading skills. Any bread labeled "whole wheat" must be made with 100 percent whole-wheat flour. "Wheat bread" may contain both white refined and whole-wheat flours; proportions vary. The ingredient list gives a general idea; the flour listed first is in the greater amount. Find loaves made mostly with whole-wheat or other whole-grain flour.

Other whole-grain label clues: (1) a whole-grain health claim, which requires the product to contain 51 percent or more whole-grain ingredients by weight (it doesn't mean 100 percent whole grain) and (2) the Whole Grains Council's voluntary Whole Grain Stamp. *Refer to chapter 13 on labeling.* Whole-grain breads may or may not be high in fiber.

Fiber: Heart Healthy, Too!

Another potential benefit: Fiber (from food or supplements) may help reduce the risk of cardiovascular disease by improving blood cholesterol levels, lowering blood pressure, and reducing inflammation in the body. Research suggests that 12 to 33 grams of fiber a day from food, or up to 42.5 grams of fiber per day from supplements with viscous fiber, such as psyllium and beta glucan, may provide these benefits. Studies indicate that whole grains also protect against heart disease and that bran is likely protective.

Some soluble fibers (mostly beta glucan) may help lower the level of total blood cholesterol, mainly by lowering LDL, or "bad," cholesterol. How? In the small intestine, soluble fiber acts like a sponge, binding cholesterol-rich bile acids. As a result, they can't be reabsorbed, but instead pass through the intestine as waste. Thus the body absorbs less dietary cholesterol, and the liver pulls more cholesterol from the blood to replace the lost bile acids. That may make blood cholesterol levels drop. Fermentation of soluble fiber in the large intestine to short-chain fatty acids also helps inhibit cholesterol synthesis in the liver.

Years of research show that soluble fiber in beans, psyllium, oats, flaxseed, and oat bran help lower blood cholesterol levels in some people. And the insoluble fiber in flaxseed and other foods may have a different cholesterol-lowering effect.

As you can see, the benefits of fiber-rich foods for heart health are truly complex. That said, there's enough sound research for the U.S. Food and Drug Administration to allow foods to carry health claims linking oats, psyllium, and whole grains to heart health. (*See "Health Claims on the Label" in chapter 12 for more about health claims.*) Those same high-fiber foods may be lower in fat, too, and may have other substances besides fiber that affect the way the body uses lipids (fats), such as omega-3 fatty acids in flaxseed. Yet another benefit is that fiber-rich foods may displace fattier foods in meals and snacks. Research also suggests a potential link between higher fiber intake and reduced blood pressure.

As more is learned about fiber and heart health, consume fiber-rich foods of all kinds—and follow other advice for heart health. *See "If You Need to Improve Your Lipid Levels" in chapter 22.*

Cancer Protection

The link between a high-fiber diet and a lowered risk for some cancers, such as colorectal cancer or polyps, hasn't been clearly established, although they seem associated. Despite the inconsistency in studies, most scientific research shows there are benefits to consuming a fiber-rich diet.

A high-fiber diet may help reduce cancer risk in several ways: (1) by speeding the time it takes for waste to pass through the digestive tract; (2) by forming a bulkier, heavier stool; and (3) by controlling the intestinal pH balance (the level of acidity or alkalinity). Slow movement of food waste through the digestive tract allows more time for potentially harmful substances to come in contact with intestinal walls. Bulkier stools help dilute the concentration of potential carcinogens. And insoluble fibers help keep the pH at a level that reduces the ability of intestinal microbes to produce carcinogens.

Is fiber the potential protector, or is it something else? It's difficult to know. Many fiber-rich foods supply plenty of nutrients, including antioxidants and phytonutrients, too. Any anticancer power of fiber-rich foods may come from the complex interaction or the additive benefits of their many components.

Other Fiber Benefits

Ongoing research suggests that fiber has other roles in health. Some, such as inulin, may work as prebiotics. (*See "Functional Nutrition: Prebiotics and Probiotics—What Are They?" in chapter 6.*) Others may affect the absorption of minerals such as calcium and, as a result, bone health, perhaps in a positive way.

Intestinal Gas: Part of Fiber's Action

People complain and sometimes joke about beans and vegetables in the cabbage family, saying they cause gas. Intestinal gas is a common complaint, and a normal side effect, of moving to a high-fiber diet.

Gas forms in the intestines because humans lack the right enzymes to digest certain carbohydrates, leaving people feeling gassy and bloated. Other foods or ingredients reported to cause gas for some include milk, wheat germ, onions, carrots, celery, bananas, raisins, dried apricots, prune juice, and sorbitol. Sorbitol, which is slowly digested, is actually a sugar

alcohol, not a sugar. (Any discomfort from milk likely results from lactose intolerance, *which you can learn about in chapter 21.*)

Intestinal gas results from undigested carbohydrates that are fermented by intestinal bacteria. Beans in particular have these carbohydrates. Interestingly, this fermentation may have health benefits. For example, fermentable fiber may improve absorption of minerals, especially calcium, iron, and magnesium. Also, the production of short-chain fatty acids during fermentation may reduce the risk of colorectal cancer among other health benefits.

If your typical eating plan is low in fiber, minimize the discomfort that comes with bulking up your fiber intake. Increase slowly over several months. Drink

Supplement Watch: Fiber Pills and Powders

Taking a fiber pill or powder may not offer the extra health benefits you may think—although it may help soften stools and relieve constipation, depending on the type of fiber. Some fiber supplements offer only small amounts of fiber, so even if they have a laxative effect, it would take many fiber pills to meet the recommended amount.

If you do choose to take a fiber supplement for regularity, your body eventually may rely on them if your overall diet lacks fiber. Fiber supplements also can inhibit the absorption of some minerals, as well as some medications such as aspirin and warfarin. If you take insulin to manage blood glucose levels, you also may need to adjust your insulin dosage.

Fiber-rich foods—vegetables, fruits, whole grains, and beans—are better options. They supply vitamins, minerals, and phytonutrients along with other benefits associated with a high-fiber diet. Moreover, these foods can provide more pleasure than a fiber pill!

Can fiber supplements help you lose weight and keep it off? No scientific evidence supports this claim. Research doesn't show a link between fiber supplements and reduced cancer risk, either.

While fiber supplements are generally safe, talk to your healthcare professional or pharmacist before taking them, especially if you have intestinal problems. With some digestive disorders, a doctor may recommend taking a fiber supplement. If you take a fiber supplement, also drink plenty of fluids.

enough water, too, to help reduce the effects of intestinal gas and prevent impacted stools.

To help tame the gas caused by beans, try these tips:

● When preparing dry beans, soak them overnight, then discard the soaking water, since it will contain some gas-producing carbohydrates. Cook the beans in fresh water.

● Allow enough time to cook dry beans thoroughly. That makes them easier to digest.

● If bean dishes or other foods cause gas, take smaller helpings.

● De-gas canned beans by draining, then rinsing the beans. That also reduces the sodium significantly.

If you need more relief from intestinal gas, several nonprescription products may help. Products containing charcoal taken at the end of a meal help absorb gas in the intestines. However, they can interfere with the absorption of medications and aren't recommended for children. Products such as Beano with a food enzyme called alpha-galactosidase help convert gas-producing carbohydrates to more easily digestible sugars. They're sold as tablets or drops, taken before a meal. Products with simethicone help relieve gas symptoms but don't prevent them. This substance works by breaking large pockets of gas in the intestines into smaller bubbles.

Other gas-reducing or gas-preventing products are sold, some with questionable claims. Check with your doctor before using any gas-reduction products.

Carbohydrates: How Much Is Enough for You?

Sugars and Starches: How Much?

For your optimal health, how many grams of carbohydrates are right for you? That exact amount is unknown. However, the Institute of Medicine (IOM) recommends carbohydrate (starch and sugars) intake in two ways: as an Adequate Intake (AI) level and as Acceptable Macronutrient Distribution Range (AMDR), set for energy nutrients.

The AI is based on the minimum level of sugars and starches needed to provide enough glucose (blood glu-

Have You Ever Wondered

. . . if a "sugar-free" food is also "calorie-free"? Not necessarily, so don't let the term confuse you. A sugar-free food may not contain sugar, but it may contain calories from other carbohydrates, fats, and proteins. To find the calories and total sugars in one label serving of any packaged food, read the Nutrition Facts. Total sugars listed on the label are the combination of added and naturally occurring sugars.

. . . what "no sucrose" or "no refined sugar" means? Perhaps not what you think. Instead of using an added sugar, such as high-fructose corn syrup (HFCS), the food may be sweetened with ingredients such as agave syrup, juice concentrates, or date sugar. Check the Nutrition Facts; their calories may be no different.

. . . if "low-carb" is "low-calorie"? No again. If protein or fat replaces carbohydrates, the calories per label serving may not change. If you're out to manage your weight, you can't count carbs and ignore the calories. Read the Nutrition Facts!

. . . what goes in when food manufacturers take carbohydrates out? Traditional products may use higher-protein ingredients in place of some carbohydrates—for example, soy flour, soy protein, or wheat protein in place of wheat flour. Or, as in candy, ice cream, and other sweets, sugar alcohols may replace some sugars. High-fiber fillers also may replace whole grains in products promoted as high-fiber; however, by replacing whole grains, the product misses out on their nutrient and phytonutrient benefits.

cose) daily for normal brain function. For people ages one year or over, that's a minimum of 130 grams of carbohydrate, which equals 520 calories, or 25 percent of the calories in a 2,000-calorie daily diet. That's more than the amount recommended in the early stages of some weight loss regimens! The AI for pregnancy is 175 grams; for breast-feeding, 210 grams.

An eating plan that simply meets the AI for carbohydrates is likely inadequate for providing other nutrients and fiber, and it may be high in fat or protein. For that reason, the IOM also established an AMDR. For carbohydrates, that's a range of 45 to 65 percent of total daily calories, adding up to 225 to 325 grams of carbohydrates daily in a 2,000-calorie-a-day eating plan. The amount for young children is different, since they need a somewhat higher proportion of fat; *see chapters 16 and 17.*

The actual amount you need depends on your total calorie need. If you're physically active, consume on the high end of the AMDR range (65 percent). If you're on a low-calorie eating plan, consume at the low end (45 percent). At the lowest end of this range, it is difficult to meet daily recommendations for fiber. Usually protein replaces carbohydrate as an energy source if you're eating low-calorie. (*See chapter 2 to learn more.*)

There is no Tolerable Upper Intake Level (UL) for carbohydrates.

How Much Added Sugars?

Added sugars are those sugars, syrups, and other caloric sweeteners added for sweetness, preservation, and other functional qualities, such as browning or texture. They may be added during food processing or preparation, or at the table. Or they may be consumed separately, perhaps in candy, sugary desserts, or soft drinks.

No ideal intake level for added sugars has been set by the IOM. However, it has advised limiting added sugars intake to a maximum of 25 percent of total calories, or 125 grams or less, based on a 2,000-calorie diet. Why limit added sugars?

● Added sugars just contribute calories. Many foods high in added sugars supply energy but few other nutrients or fiber. And they may replace more nutritious foods that contain important vitamins and minerals.

● People who consume more than 25 percent of added sugars are more likely to have poor intakes of some essential vitamins and minerals according to the IOM.

However, just cutting back on added sugars may not be enough to improve nutrition. You still may need to eat more fruits, vegetables, whole grains, and low-fat and fat-free dairy products. In fact, added sugars in some nutrient-rich foods may help increase the intake of nutrients that come up short, such as fiber from whole-grain muffins, and calcium and vitamin D from flavored milk.

Hot Topic: High-Fructose Corn Syrup

Fructose is a natural sugar in fruit. It's also part of a sweetener used in processed foods and beverages. Crystalline fructose, which is pure fructose, can be manufactured from any source of glucose and looks and tastes much like sucrose, although slightly sweeter. High-fructose corn syrup (HFCS) comes from cornstarch and has virtually the same composition and taste as sucrose. Currently HFCS is one of the most common sweeteners in the United States, commonly used because it blends well with other ingredients and it costs less than sugar. Like any sugar, HFCS and crystalline fructose supply 4 calories per gram.

Does HFCS contribute to obesity? Calorie for calorie, HFCS contributes no more than other sugars may when consumed to excess. It's the amount, not the type, of sugar that can lead to weight gain. Like sucrose (table sugar), HFCS delivers 4 calories per gram. And like sucrose, HCFS has about equal parts of fructose and glucose. As absorbed into the bloodstream, the metabolites of these sugars are indistinguishable. Flavorwise, HFCS is no sweeter than sucrose.

Despite the recent controversy, no convincing scientific evidence indicates that HFCS is processed by the body differently than sucrose, that it increases body fat in a unique way, or that it boosts appetite or causes sugar cravings. In fact, the American Medical Association recently concluded that HFCS doesn't appear to contribute to obesity any more than other caloric sweeteners.

As an added sugar, high-fructose corn syrup does provide calories. The more calories consumed from any source, the greater their influence on weight gain. To help trim your calorie intake, ease up on added sugars of all kinds, including HFCS. If you consume regular soft drinks, fruit drinks, sports drinks, and other sugary drinks, consider moderation and portion size. And go easy on all kinds of foods with added sugars, such as salad dressings, baked goods, syrup, candies, sugary desserts, jams, yogurts, condiments, canned and packaged foods, and other sweetened foods. *The bottom line:* Rather than trying to just avoid HFCS, limit your intake of *all* added sugars.

● As with starches and naturally occurring sugars, added sugars can promote tooth decay, especially with frequent snacking. Poor oral hygiene and sticky foods enhance sugars' ability to promote decay, too.

Energy Carbs: Too Much

Any calorie source—carbohydrates, fats, proteins— can contribute to weight gain when calorie intake

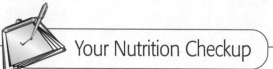 Your Nutrition Checkup

Sweet and Nutrient-Rich, Too?

Here's your chance to check your sweet choices. Are they packed with nutrients, too? Or do they provide mostly calories, added sugars, and few nutrients? Check the space that describes what choices you make!

Do You . . . ?	ALWAYS	MOSTLY	SOMETIMES	NEVER
☐ Drink 100 percent juice—or milk—with lunch or dinner, rather than soft drinks?	____	____	____	____
☐ Reach for fruit as a snack, rather than candy or cookies?	____	____	____	____
☐ Top your cereal with fruit instead of sugar?	____	____	____	____
☐ Sweeten waffles, pancakes, or French toast with fruit or fruit puree, rather than syrup?	____	____	____	____
☐ Top ice cream with fruit, not just chocolate or caramel syrup?	____	____	____	____
☐ Choose water or milk as a snack beverage instead of sweetened fruit drinks?	____	____	____	____
☐ Choose fruit for dessert, not a sugary, high-calorie dessert?	____	____	____	____
☐ Go for a small rather than a big slice of pie or cake?	____	____	____	____
☐ Snack on two or three cookies with milk, rather than simply down five or six cookies, or the whole package?	____	____	____	____
☐ Limit sodas: 8 or 12 ounces rather than a 20-ounce (or larger) serving?	____	____	____	____

Now rate your choices.

Total the points in each column. For each answer, give yourself:

    4 points for always

    3 points for mostly

    2 points for sometimes

    1 point for never

If you scored . . .

30 or above. Your sweet choices are mostly high in nutrients, too. In fact, enjoy a bit of sugar now and then to add pleasure to eating.

20 to 29. If your overall diet is balanced and you're not overspending your calorie budget, your preference for sweets is probably okay.

10 to 19. Your sweet tooth may be crowding out nutritious foods. Check them out and consider some sweet options such as fruit, with few or no added sugars. You'll find great ideas for nutrient-rich options in this chapter!

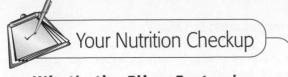

Your Nutrition Checkup

What's the Fiber Factor in Your Food Choices?

That's up to you—and what you choose to eat. If you had a choice, which would you pick for your meals or snacks?

1 medium unpeeled apple	or	½ cup applesauce
1 slice whole-wheat bread	or	1 slice white bread toast (from refined flour)
3½-oz. cooked meat patty	or	½ cup baked beans
⅓ cup bran flakes	or	⅓ cup corn flakes
1 carrot stick	or	1 bread stick
½ cup white rice	or	½ cup brown rice
½ cup strawberries	or	½ cup grapes
½ cup spinach	or	½ cup peas
½ cup peanuts	or	1 oz. cheese
2 figs	or	2 dried plums (prunes)
2 tbsp. bean dip (hummus)	or	2 tbsp. sour cream
¾ cup orange juice	or	1 orange
1 baked potato with skin	or	½ cup mashed potatoes (no skin)
1 tbsp. wheat germ	or	1 tbsp. wheat bran

Now check your answers . . .

For each pair, these foods contain more fiber: unpeeled apple, whole-wheat bread, baked beans, bran flakes, carrot stick, brown rice, strawberries, peas, peanuts, figs, bean dip (hummus), orange, baked potato with skin, and wheat germ.

To compare the specific amounts of fiber in these food pairs, see the table *"How Much Total Carbohydrate and Fiber?" later in this chapter.* Give yourself 5 points each time you picked the higher-fiber choice; 70 points is the highest score you can get. The higher your score, the more fiber in your diet—if these foods truly would be your "picks" for the day!

exceeds calorie output. The same goes for any type of sugar (added or naturally occurring) or starch; all have calories and share equally in the potential for weight gain when calorie balance tips toward excess calorie intake.

That said, added sugars provide about 16 percent of total calories in the United States. By reducing added sugars you also limit calorie intake, which can help you reach and keep a healthy weight without compromising the nutrient adequacy of your eating plan.

How Much Fiber?

If you're like most Americans, your day's meals and snacks come up seriously short on fiber, supplying only about half (about 15 grams) of the amount your body needs per day.

Fiber recommendations depend on age and gender. For men to age fifty, the IOM advises an AI of 38 grams daily; for women in that age range the recommendation is 25 grams daily. During pregnancy and breast-feeding, the recommendation is slightly higher. If you're age fifty-one or more, the AI is less: 30 grams of total fiber daily for men, 21 grams for women. *Chapter 17 gives fiber recommendations for children and teens.*

To meet your fiber goal, follow the advice of the USDA Food Patterns (*see chapter 10*).

● Eat 4½ cups of fruit and vegetables daily if you eat 2,000 calories daily, and slightly more if you need more calories.

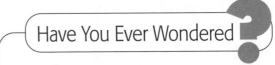

Have You Ever Wondered

. . . if cornmeal is a whole grain? Yes—but only if it's made with the whole corn kernel. Cornmeal that's labeled degerminated or degermed has been refined and is not whole grain.

. . . what grains are whole grain? Buckwheat, brown rice, bulgur, whole kernel corn (hominy), millet, popcorn, quinoa, sorghum, triticale, whole oats and oatmeal, wheat berries, whole barley (not pearl barley), whole farro (emmer), whole rye, and whole wheat are more common whole grains in the United States. Cracked wheat is whole berry wheat, too—it's just broken into coarse, medium, or fine particles.

● Make at least half your grain choices whole: equal to 3 ounces of whole-grain foods or more each day.

● Consume beans (legumes) often (about 1½ cups a week on a 2,000 calorie-a-day eating plan).

If you boost your fiber intake, do so gradually over several weeks. Give the friendly bacteria in your intestines time to adjust. If you boost your fiber intake too quickly or consume too much regularly, you may end up with gas, diarrhea, cramps, and bloating.

When you eat more fiber, drink plenty of water and other fluids, too. Fiber acts like a large sponge in your GI tract. It holds water as it keeps waste moving along. That's how it helps prevent constipation and related intestinal problems. For fiber to do its job, you need to consume enough fluids. How much fluid a day? *Refer to chapter 8 to see how much fluid you need.*

Older adults (age sixty-five or over) and those who have had gastrointestinal (stomach, intestines, or rectum) surgery may feel the effects of added fiber more than others and should take caution and check with their doctor before adding fiber to meals and snacks.

Fiber: Too Much

Although uncommon, you can overdo a good thing and consume too much fiber, more likely from abuse of high-fiber supplements than from food. By consuming more than 50 to 60 grams of fiber a day, your body's absorption of vitamins and minerals, among them zinc, iron, magnesium, and calcium, may go down. An excessive amount of fiber may cause gas, diarrhea, and bloating.

Although rare, you can get too much fiber from food by eating a lot of bran or very-high-fiber cereals, or using a fiber supplement in an eating plan that already has plenty of vegetables, fruits, and whole grains.

Carbohydrates in Food

We casually refer to a vast array of foods as carbs when we really mean carbohydrate-containing foods. Good carbs and bad carbs are also misnomers that typically refer to nutrient-rich and energy-dense foods with carbohydrates. So, what foods contain carbohydrates? And are some better choices than others?

Most carbohydrates come from plant-based foods. Through photosynthesis, plants transform the sun's

Have You Ever Wondered

. . . which one to buy: wheat germ or wheat bran? They're two different parts of the grain, so their benefits differ. The germ is the nutrient-rich inner part, and the bran is the outer coating. From a nutritional standpoint, 1 ounce (⅓ cup) of wheat bran has a lot more fiber, about 13 grams, than the 4.4 grams of fiber in 1 ounce (¼ cup) of wheat germ. Wheat germ has more protein, and more of some vitamins and minerals.

. . . what psyllium is? (When you pronounce it, the "p" is silent.) Psyllium—high in soluble fiber—is a seed husk used in some bulk-forming natural laxatives; it also has potential cholesterol-lowering qualities. Some supplements have it. Its source is plantago, a plant that grows in India and the Mediterranean. Although some people may be allergic to psyllium, in moderate amounts it's safe for most people.

. . . if "whole grain" is "high fiber"? And if "high fiber" is "whole grain"? In either case, not necessarily. First, the amount of fiber differs naturally in different types of grain, depending on their proportion of bran, germ, and endosperm. Other ingredients and moisture in whole-grain foods also affect fiber content. Second, high-fiber foods, such as bran cereals, may have more fiber even though they aren't whole grain. For fiber content, read the label's Nutrition Facts; if a label serving has 20 percent or more Daily Value, it's high fiber. *As another clue, check for a whole-grain labeling claim, described in chapter 12.*

energy into carbohydrates as food for their own growth. As a result, carbohydrates—sugars and starches—naturally form in fruits and vegetables, including beans and peas, grain products, nuts, and seeds. All these foods are good sources of other nutrients, too.

Carbohydrates change as plants mature. As fruit matures, its carbohydrate shifts from starch to sugars, making fruit sweeter and more appealing. By contrast, many vegetables—among them peas, carrots, and corn—are sweetest when young. As they mature, their sugars change to starches. What's the chef's lesson? If you're buying fresh produce, look for young vegetables and serve them at their peak. Don't store them too long. Serve fruits when they're ripe; you may need to allow ripening time after you buy them.

Plants and foods of plant origin count on fiber for their shape. It's fiber that gives celery its rigid stalk and gives spinach the strong stems that hold up its leaves. That same structure bulks up the contents inside your GI tract.

Carbs in Foods: Choose by the Company They Keep

Many carbohydrate-containing foods are nutrient-rich. Others qualify as empty-calorie foods. The best choices deliver a nutrient bundle without excess calories.

Vegetables, fruits, beans and peas, and whole-grain products are nutrient-rich. From a nutrition standpoint, they're a calorie bargain. As a group, they're packaged with vitamins A and C, folic acid, iron, and fiber, which are nutrients that typically come up short in the eating patterns of most Americans.

Low-fat and fat-free dairy foods contain another carbohydrate: the naturally occurring sugar called lactose. Lactose in milk and some other dairy foods is packaged with high-quality protein, calcium, vitamin D, and more.

Fiber isn't a lonely component in food, and its benefits can't be easily separated from the contributions of other nutrients and plant substances. Most fiber-rich foods, such as beans and peas, whole-wheat bread, berries, and broccoli, are packed with carbohydrates (complex and simple), other essential nutrients, and some phytonutrients with different health-promoting benefits. Consider these examples:

● Many fruits and vegetables contribute potassium and folate, as well as antioxidant vitamins such as beta carotene and vitamin C, which may help protect against some cancers.

● Whole grains contain vitamin E and selenium as well as iron, magnesium, zinc, and B vitamins. Some whole-grain foods supply lignan, which may block estrogen activity in cells and perhaps reduce the risk of some cancers. Whole grains also supply phytic acid, which may prevent free radicals from forming and perhaps reduce cancer risk by binding to minerals.

● Beans supply protein as well as B vitamins and iron.

● Foods with more fiber often have less fat, too.

To visualize healthy proportions of nutrient-rich, carbohydrate-containing foods in a meal *see chapters 10 and 11. For more about the vitamins, minerals, and phytonutrients in these foods, see chapter 6.*

In contrast, some carbohydrate-containing foods have a limited nutrient package yet deliver significant calories. That includes sugary drinks such as soda and fruit-flavored drinks, candy, and grain-based desserts that are high in added sugars and/or solid fats. Choose them less often. Food patterns with a lot of added sugars are often low in some essential nutrients.

Sugars: In Healthful Eating

Whether naturally occurring or added, sugars make many foods more appealing. They contribute to the

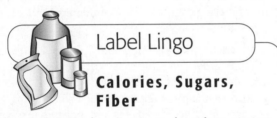

Label Lingo

Calories, Sugars, Fiber

Although the FDA hasn't approved nutrient content claims for total carbohydrates, you may find claims related to calories, sugar, or fiber. Look for these terms as you walk the supermarket aisles:

LABEL TERM ...	MEANS ...
Calorie free	less than 5 calories per serving
Sugar-free	less than 0.5 gram sugars per serving
Reduced sugar or less sugar	at least 25 percent less* sugar or sugars per serving
No added sugars, without added sugar, no sugar	no sugars added during processing or packing, including ingredients that contain sugar such as juice or dry fruit
High-fiber	5 g or more per serving
Good source	2.5 to 4.9 g per serving
More or added fiber	at least 2.5 g more* per serving

*As compared with a standard serving size of the traditional food.

taste, aroma, texture, color, and body of the foods we all enjoy. For overall good health, a smart goal is to enjoy most of their appeal from naturally occurring sugars in fruit, milk, and some other foods, and to consume foods with added sugars judiciously, in limited amounts.

Naturally Sweet Choices

Packaged with many nutrients essential to health, enjoy the sweet flavors of foods with naturally occurring sugars—and get their bundle of health benefits, too:

- Enjoy fruit—in salads, salsas, sauces, toppings, and more. For fruits that are sour or bitter, such as cranberries and limes, a little added sugar may make these nutritious fruits or their juices more enjoyable.

- Snack on fruit instead of candy, cookies, and pastries. Tuck an apple, peach, pear, banana, grapes, or dried fruit in your carry bag.

- Make a switch. Eat whole or sliced fruit for dessert rather than cake, cookies, ice cream, or other sugary desserts.

Fruit Snacks: Sweet and Nutritious

Next time you crave a sweet snack, reach for fruit! Besides satisfying a taste for sweets, fruit is packed with nutrients, phytonutrients—and delivers fiber, too.

Fruit pops. For a nutritious fruit pop, freeze pureed fruit (mango, papaya, or apricot) or juice in ice cube trays or paper cups with wooden sticks.

Frozen bananas. Push a wooden stick into half of a peeled banana. Roll in yogurt or a light coating of chocolate syrup, then in crunchy cornflakes. Wrap; freeze.

Fruit mix. Mix a zipper-top bag of dried fruits of your choice: apple slices, apricots, blueberries, cherries, cranberries, pear slices, and raisins, among others. (*Hint:* Brush your teeth—or rinse your mouth with water—after nibbling. Dried fruit sticks to teeth!)

Frozen chips. Slice bananas into thin rounds. Spread them flat on a baking pan; cover. Freeze and serve frozen as a fun snack. (The same technique works for seedless grapes or berries.)

Frugurt. Top a rainbow of cut-up fruit with low-fat yogurt.

Have You Ever Wondered

… if chocolate milk is okay for kids? Like unflavored milk, chocolate and other flavored milks are an excellent source of calcium and vitamin D, important for growing strong, healthy bones. Flavored milk offers children who don't like plain milk a way to still get the calcium and vitamin D they need. And the sugars in flavored milk are no more cavity-promoting than other carbohydrates. When available, choose fat-free or low-fat flavored milks.

- Drink milk. It derives some of its pleasing flavor from lactose, its own naturally occurring sugar. If you prefer a sweeter taste, choose flavored low-fat or fat-free milk. The benefits of its calcium and vitamin D outweigh the calories from added sugars in flavored milk. Many dairies are also reducing added sugars in flavored milk; check the label to compare.

- Choose 100 percent fruit juice.

Foods with Added Sugars: Some, Not Much

For the many foods with added sugars, be prudent!

- Use a light touch with the sugar spoon. Sweeten coffee or tea with just a bit of sugar, use low-calorie sweeteners, or add a hint of sweetness with a sprinkle of cinnamon. Use the same tip on cereal or French toast. Better yet, sweeten them with sliced or pureed fruit instead.

- Limit or skip regular soft drinks and other sugary beverages. There are about 10 packets of sugar in a 12-ounce can of soda! Quench your thirst with water (with a citrus slice) or unsweetened beverages instead.

- Choose 100 percent fruit juice instead of fruit-flavored drinks.

- Go 50/50 to cut calories in half. Share a sugary dessert or snack with a friend; eat it slowly for the most enjoyment.

- Eat just small, infrequent portions of sugary snacks. Choose a miniature instead of a large candy bar, or a 6-ounce can of soda instead of a 20-ounce bottle.

● Read food labels to compare packaged foods. Choose mostly those with little or no added sugars on the ingredient list. Look for "no sugar added" on canned and frozen fruit as a nutrient content claim. Some such as candy, beverages, yogurt, and baked foods may be sweetened with a sugar alternative with fewer or no calories.

For more ways to sweeten with fruit and reduce added sugars in your food prep, see chapter 14.

Added Sugars in Food: What They Do. Eighty-five years ago, homemakers baked with white and brown sugar and honey; prepared jellies, jams, and syrup with sugar; and flavored homemade baked beans with molasses or sorghum molasses. As a home cook, you likely prepare food with some type of sugar, too, especially if you bake.

Today sugars are added during commercial food processing as more and more households depend on the convenience of store-bought foods and drinks. Soft drinks, candy, other sweet snacks, desserts, and sweet baked goods are obvious sources of added sugars. However, they're added to many other processed and prepared foods. *See "Added Sugars: Top Sources" on this page.*

Sweetness is the attribute that gets attention. Yet sugars contribute far more to food. For kitchen chemistry, sugars work as multipurpose ingredients, fulfilling functions that you may not even think about:

● In all kinds of food: sugar adds to the flavor, aroma, texture, color, and body of food. Sometimes just a small amount of added sugar can bring out the flavors of other ingredients, such as in tomato-based sauce or salad dressing.

● In yeast breads: sugars are "food" for yeast, allowing dough to rise. Yeast doesn't consume all the sugar, however. The rest adds flavor and contributes to the aroma and delicate-brown color of the crust.

● In cakes: sugars contribute to the bulk, tenderness, smooth crumb texture, and lightly browned surface. In cakes that have air whipped in, such as angel food cake and sponge cake, sugars help hold the form.

● In cookies: as sugars and shortening are creamed together, sugars help bring air into the dough. Sugars also contribute to the light-brown color, crisp texture,

Added Sugars: Top Sources

	PERCENT* OF ADDED SUGARS INTAKE
● Soft drinks, energy drinks, sports drinks	35.7
● Grain-based desserts (such as cakes, pies)	12.9
● Fruit drinks	10.5
● Dairy-based desserts (such as ice cream)	6.5
● Candy	6.1
● Ready-to-eat cereals	3.8
● Sugars and honey	3.5
● Tea (sweetened)	3.5
● Yeast breads	2.1
● All other food categories	15.4

*For the amount of added sugars in common foods, check the USDA Database for Added Sugars Content of Selected Foods, 2006: www.nal.usda.gov/fnic/foodcomp/Data/add_sug/addsug01.pdf.

Source: Dietary Guidance for Americans, 2010.

and even to the cracked surface of sugar cookies and gingersnaps.

● In canned jams, jellies, and preserves: sugars help inhibit the growth of molds and yeast by tying up the water that these microorganisms need to multiply. For this reason, sugars act as preservatives.

● In candy: sugar contributes to the texture—for example, the smoothness of hard candy and the creaminess of fudge. And as it cooks, turning from white to yellow to brown, sugar develops a unique, tasty flavor.

Can you cut back on sugar in recipes? That depends. For some recipes, the results wouldn't be much different—except for taste. In others, the volume, texture, color, and aroma may not be the same. And in jams, jellies, and preserves, mold grows quickly without added sugar, even if refrigerated. *See chapter 14 for tips on preparing food with less added sugar.*

Starchy Foods: Complex, Healthful, and Easy!

Many starchy foods deliver more nutrients than complex carbohydrates. Choose nutrient-rich options such as these:

● Prepare or order starchy vegetables and beans in soups, salads, casseroles, and sides: for example, sweet potatoes, squash, peas, pumpkin, kidney beans, chickpeas, lima beans.

● Substitute whole-grain products—whole-wheat bread and pasta, brown rice, oat muffins, for example—for some of those made with refined flour. Make at least half of your grain choices whole grain.

● Partner grain foods with other nutrient-rich foods. For example, serve brown rice with vegetable stir-fry, whole-wheat pita stuffed with a garden salad, or baked potato (skin on) topped with chili beans.

● Choose grain products with fewer fats and added sugars—for example, bagels in place of doughnuts, *trans*-fat free crackers rather than chips, and baked potatoes for fries.

● Be sensible about portions. It's all too easy to serve 3 cups of pasta when half that amount may be enough!

● For refined grains, choose those that are enriched and fortified with folic acid.

Food's Fiber Factor

Do you like to nibble on popcorn? This whole-grain snack is a fiber booster, with 3.5 grams of fiber and just 95 calories in 3 cups of plain popcorn.

Most fruits, vegetables, and whole grains provide about 1 to 3 grams of fiber per standard serving. Some are better sources than others. A heaping bowl of fresh greens may seem loaded with fiber, but greens are mostly water. One cup of lettuce contains about 1 gram of fiber. In contrast, $\frac{1}{2}$ cup of a three-bean salad (mainly beans) supplies more than 3 fiber grams. Beans are an excellent fiber source, and nuts are good sources.

Food provides two types of fiber:

● *Insoluble fibers:* whole-wheat products; wheat, oat, and corn bran; wheat germ; flaxseeds; nuts; and many vegetables (such as cauliflower, green beans, and potatoes), including the skins of fruits and root vegetables, and beans. In fact, their tough, chewy texture comes from insoluble fibers.

● *Soluble fibers:* dried beans and peas, oats, barley, flaxseeds, seeds, and many fruits and vegetables (such as apples, oranges, and carrots). When cooked, their soft, mushy texture comes from their soluble fibers. Psyllium seed husks also supply soluble fiber.

Plant-based foods actually contain a mixed bag of these fibers. Fruits and vegetables have both pectin (soluble) and cellulose (insoluble). Fruit, however, usually has more pectin, and vegetables have more cellulose. Oatmeal and beans have both soluble and insoluble fiber. Beta glucan is the soluble fiber in oats and barley. The bran in wheat, rice, corn, oats, and other grains isn't alike, either. Wheat bran has a higher concentration of fiber than most other bran, and its bran is mainly insoluble. Oat bran contains mainly soluble fiber.

Grain products made from refined flour supply fiber, too, but not much compared to whole grains. If foods such as white bread, traditional pasta, and potatoes are your main source of fiber, you may fall short of your daily fiber needs. They may not be as fiber-rich as other options. To increase your fiber intake choose foods with more dietary fiber such as brown rice instead of those with less, such as white rice. Still consume the appropriate amount of calories to manage your weight. For the benefits of different types of fiber, enjoy a variety of plant-based foods such as vegetables (including beans), fruits, whole-grain foods, and nuts.

Food preparation or processing can affect some of fiber's functions. Just as the ability of a sponge to hold water changes when it's chopped into very fine pieces, so do properties of fiber change when food processing or preparation alter its structure. In some cases, by grinding fiber, viscous complexes may form more

Have You Ever Wondered

... what graham flour is? It's whole-wheat flour that's a little coarser than regular whole-wheat flour. Try it!

... if soybeans or tofu are good fiber sources? Half a cup of soybeans has more than 5 grams of fiber. That's great! But when soybeans are processed to make tofu, fibrous substances are strained out. What's left is high in soy protein. One-half cup of tofu has less than 1 gram of fiber.

readily. Minimally processed foods are generally better fiber sources; fiber content drops when the fiber-rich part of a food, such as the bran or the peel on fruit, is removed. (*See "Which Apple for Fiber?" on this page to compare the fiber in different forms of an apple, including juice.*)

"Fiber Up" Your Food Choices

Ready to eat more fiber? Use these tips to help put your fiber intake within the recommended range. All these options are nutrient-rich, too!

● Start with breakfast. Choose a fiber-rich breakfast cereal, perhaps bran; check food labels to find one with 5 or more grams of fiber per serving. Top cereal with fruit or wheat bran for a little more fiber. Other options include oatmeal, whole-bran muffins, whole-wheat waffles, or fiber-rich breakfast/cereal bars.

● Switch to whole grains. Make more of your grain choices fiber-rich whole grains rather than eating more grains. Choose breads, buns, and bagels with whole-grain flour as the first ingredients on the label—for example, whole-wheat flour, oat flour, rye flour, whole ground cornmeal. Five grams or more (or 20 percent or more Daily Value) of dietary fiber per label serving is an excellent fiber source; 2.5 to 4.9 grams (or 10 to 19 percent Daily Value) per serving is a good source. Eat breads made with bran, too, such as bran muffins. Try whole-wheat tortillas and pasta, too.

● Experiment with other whole grains. Give brown or wild rice a try, or mix half brown and half white rice. *Refer to "Cooking Grain by Grain" in chapter 14.*

● Eat beans, peas, and lentils. They're among the best fiber sources around. And they add flavor and texture to salads, soups, casseroles, salsas, and more.

● Fit fruits and veggies into your meals and snacks: about 4½ cups total a day if you eat 2,000 calories a day. Perhaps plan cooked vegetables and a salad for dinner, and whole fruit and carrot sticks for lunch. How about a fruit or veggie snack? And make them varied!

● Speaking of snacks, go fiber-rich with raw veggies, fruit (including dried fruit), whole-grain pretzels or crackers, plain popcorn, or a small handful of nuts.

● Enjoy fruits and vegetables with the skin on. With the skin, a medium potato has 3.8 grams of fiber. Skinless, it has less: 2.3 grams. Also enjoy the flavor,

---

Which Apple for Fiber?

Apple juice, applesauce, a whole apple—which has the most fiber? An apple of any variety with the peel on has more fiber than an apple without the peel. And as food changes form, its fiber content may change, too.

1 whole medium apple with peel	3.3 grams fiber
1 whole medium apple without peel	1.7 grams fiber
½ cup applesauce	1.5 grams fiber
¾ cup apple juice	0.2 gram fiber

---

crunch, and fiber benefits of edible seeds in berries, kiwifruit, and figs.

● Choose whole fruit more often than juice. Fiber comes mainly from the peel and pulp; usually both are removed when fruit is juiced. Juice usually has almost no fiber. *See "Which Apple for Fiber?" above.*

● Keep fiber-rich foods on hand so they're easy to add to dishes, for example, frozen and canned vegetables, and whole-grain crackers.

● Fiberize your cooking style. Substitute higher-fiber ingredients in recipes, such as using part whole-wheat flour in baked food. Fortify mixed dishes with high-fiber ingredients, perhaps bran, crushed bran cereal, or oatmeal added to meat loaf or ground flaxseeds added to baked goods. Add veggies of all kinds to soups, stews, pizzas, and pasta sauces.

For more ways to boost the fiber in food preparation, see chapter 14.

Carbohydrates on Food Labels

Hunting for the carbohydrate content of food? Check the food label. Clues come in three places: nutrient content claims, the Nutrition Facts, and the ingredient list.

Check the Claims

Nutrient content claims such as "sugar-free" or "no added sugar" appear on some food containers, such as on flavored yogurt, canned fruit, and breakfast cereal. You may see a "high fiber" or "added fiber" claim on packages of bread, breakfast bars, or cereal. These claims are regulated by the U.S. Food and Drug

Administration (FDA). If they catch your attention, check the Nutrition Facts for specific amounts. *Refer to "Label Lingo: Calories, Sugars, Fiber" in this chapter to know their meaning.*

What do terms such as "net carbs," "low carb," or "net impact carbs" on labels mean—and not mean? Often they're defined as consumer confusion! Although currently allowed, these terms aren't regulated by the FDA, at least not now. Their meaning is unclear, varying among food manufacturers and weight-loss plans. "Net carbs" on a label may be total carbohydrates minus fiber, or minus fiber and sugar alcohols. The idea behind them is this: Because fiber isn't digested and absorbed and sugar alcohols aren't completely absorbed, their carbohydrates don't count; however, this issue is under scientific debate. Until regulated, the FDA recommends that labels explain the term and its calculation. For diabetes management, talk to your registered dietitian or certified diabetes educator about how foods labeled with these terms fit in your food plan.

Check the Facts

Almost all food labels carry Nutrition Facts with the amount of calories, total carbohydrates, sugars, and fiber in a standard label serving. As defined by FDA for the Nutrition Facts panel:

● *Total carbohydrates* include starches, naturally occurring and added sugars, sugar alcohols, and fiber as well as organic acids and preservatives (which don't weigh much).

● *Sugars* are the sum of all naturally occurring and added sugars. All contribute to the total carbohydrate amount. You'll find sugars in all kinds of foods, including those with no added sugars—such as milk, fruit, and grain products. On the label, added sugars are included in sugars; they're not listed separately in the Nutrition Facts. You need to check the ingredient list to identify relative amounts of added sugars.

● *Dietary fiber*, also part of total carbohydrates, is listed. By checking the label, you'll see that whole-grain foods usually have more fiber than those made from refined grains.

● *Sugar alcohols, discussed later in this chapter*, might appear on a separate line in the Nutrition Facts.

Check the Ingredients

Added Sugars. To identify added sugars in processed foods, check the ingredient list (naturally occurring sugars aren't listed). If a sugar appears as the first or second ingredient, or if several sugars are listed, the food likely has a lot of added sugars.

Even if you don't see the word "sugar" in the ingredient list, it may have added sugars. Terms ending in "-ose" mean sugars. Words such as maltose, dextrin, and corn syrup are sugars, too, often made of several types of sugars. Among the many sugars that

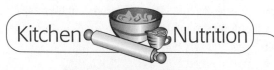

Kitchen Nutrition

Sweet Seasons

Bring out the flavors of foods with seasonings that offer the perception of sweetness: allspice, cardamom, cinnamon, ginger, mace, nutmeg, and citrus juices.

● Add ginger to a fruit glaze. Blend frozen raspberries with a pinch of ginger and a small amount of fruit juice concentrate or sweetener. Toss the glaze with fresh berries or sliced fruit.

● Add a sweet spice of your choice to dry coffee grounds before brewing.

● Add zest and sweet flavor to oatmeal and other cooked breakfast cereals with allspice, mace, or nutmeg. In place of water, cook it in fruit juice (or milk for more calcium and phosphorus). Toss with dried fruits such as cranberries or apricots, or top with fresh fruit.

● For a hint of sweet flavor in rice, cook with cardamom, cinnamon, or ginger. You might substitute juice for part of the cooking liquid. Perhaps toss in raisins or other dried fruits, too!

● Add a touch of sweetness to cooked vegetables. For example, add ginger to carrots, cinnamon to mashed sweet potatoes, and a sprinkle of nutmeg to spinach.

● Squeeze citrus juice—lemon, lime, or orange—over fresh fruit to enhance the flavor. *Calorie-saving tip:* You save about 45 calories with a squeeze of juice rather than 1 tablespoon of sugar.

● Make your own syrup for pancakes or waffles. In a blender, puree sliced peaches, berries, or apples with a little fruit juice, honey, and a pinch of cinnamon.

may appear, besides those ending in "–ose," are the following:

brown sugar	high-fructose corn
cane sugar	syrup (HFCS)
confectioner's sugar	invert sugar
corn sweeteners	malt syrup
corn syrup	maple syrup
crystallized cane sugar	molasses
dextrin	raw sugar
evaporated cane juice	syrup
fruit juice concentrate	turbinado sugar
honey	

Evaporated fruit juices and jams are mostly just sugars, too.

Fiber. To spot fiber-rich grains, learn which ones are whole grain. Look for terms such as "bran," "whole-grain," or "whole-wheat flour." *See "Which Bread Is Whole Grain?" in this chapter and "Is It Really Whole Grain? Check the Label!" in chapter 12.*

Alternatives to Sugar

"Low in calories" and "sugar-free"! As a way to minimize added sugars and calories, these are sweet messages, especially for people who want options to manage their weight, control their blood glucose levels, or limit their exposure to tooth-decay-promoting sugary foods. Two types of sugar alternatives can help achieve those goals: sugar replacers (a category of nutritive sweetener) and low-calorie sweeteners. *Stevia, further addressed in "Have You Ever Wondered?" on page 82, is another option.*

Sugar Replacers (aka Sugar Alcohols)

Sugar alcohols, or polyols, are a category of nutritive sweeteners. Why nutritive? Like sugars, they provide energy, or calories. Usually they replace sugar on an equal basis by weight. Why the term "sugar alcohol"? To clarify, the words "sugar" and "alcohol" in this context refer only to their chemical structure. Sugar alcohols don't contain ethanol, as alcoholic beverages do. They also may be referred to as sugar replacers or reduced-calorie sweeteners.

Sugar alcohols are carbohydrates naturally present in many foods you already enjoy, including berries, other fruits, and vegetables. They usually aren't used in home cooking. Derived from sucrose, glucose, and starch, sugar alcohols also can be manufactured—for example, erythritol, isomalt, lacititol, maltitol, mannitol, sorbitol, xylitol, and hydrogenated starch hydrolysates.

Their sweetness varies, from 25 percent to 100 percent as sweet as sugar. Sorbitol and mannitol, for example, may be half as sweet as table sugar; however, xylitol is just as sweet. They're often combined with low-calorie, or intense, sweeteners such as aspartame or saccharin, for a sweeter flavor. *See "Sweet Comparisons" in this chapter.*

Sweet Benefits

"Sugar-free" doesn't mean "calorie-free"! Sugar alcohols do supply energy, but fewer calories per gram than sugar does: from 1.5 to 3 calories per gram. Sugars provide 4 calories per gram. To compare, sorbitol has 2.6 calories per gram; mannitol, 1.6 calories per gram. Since they're lower in calories than sugars, sugar alcohols have potential advantages for people managing their weight.

For those with diabetes, sugar alcohols offer another benefit. As an energy source, they're absorbed more slowly than sugars and incompletely, and they require little or no insulin for metabolism. Their glycemic response is low. That said, for diabetes management, sugar alcohols aren't "free foods." In other words, they aren't calorie-free; instead, 2 grams of sugar alcohols are generally counted for 1 gram of carbohydrate. If you're managing diabetes, have a registered dietitian or certified diabetes educator help you fit foods with sugar alcohols into a healthful eating plan.

Another benefit is that sugar alcohols don't promote cavities. Why? They aren't converted to acids by oral bacteria that produce cavities. In fact, the FDA has approved a health claim for gum, candies, beverages, and snack foods with sugar alcohols, noting that sugar alcohols in these foods do not promote tooth decay.

For some people, sorbitol and mannitol may produce abdominal gas or discomfort or may have a laxative effect when consumed in excess. You might see this statement on a label: "Excess consumption may have a laxative effect. Eat foods with these sweeteners in moderation or perhaps with other foods if your tolerance is lower."

What about their safety? The FDA regulates their use. The following sugar alcohols are on the GRAS ("generally recognized as safe") list or are approved as additives: erythritol, hydrogenated starch hydrolysates (HSH), isomalt, lactitol, maltitol, mannitol, sorbitol, and xylitol.

Sugar Replacers in Foods

Besides adding sweetness to some sugar-free foods, sugar replacers add texture and bulk to a wide range of foods such as baked goods, fruit spreads, ice cream, frozen desserts, and candies. They also help food stay moist, prevent browning when heated, and add a cooling sensation. Baked foods made with sugar alcohols won't have a crisp brown surface unless the color comes from another ingredient. Sugar alcohols also are used in chewing gum, toothpaste, and mouthwash.

Pairing Sugars and Chocolate

A love for chocolate can be traced through the centuries. Known as a food of the gods, chocolate was highly prized in the Americas in pre-Columbian times. Native Americans from what is now Mexico served chocolate to European explorers as early as the 1500s.

By itself, chocolate has a bitter taste. But sugar, transported from plantations in the American and Caribbean colonies, made chocolate tasty to the European palate. By the mid-1600s, the popularity of chocolate, sweetened with sugar, had spread throughout Europe. In 1847, milk chocolate was created, and it quickly became popular around the world.

As an ingredient with a distinctive flavor, chocolate and its main ingredient, cocoa, can fit within a healthful eating plan. They may add a flavor spark that makes nutritious foods, such as milk, more appealing. Chocolate, a plant-based ingredient, also contains a category of phytonutrients potentially beneficial to health called flavanols, which may offer some health benefits, as well as stearic acid, a saturated fat that may have a neutral effect on blood cholesterol levels. *For more on flavanols refer to chapter 6 on phytonutrients.* Research is exploring links to heart health. Chocolate appears to have significant antioxidant potential; dark chocolate has more flavanols than milk chocolate does.

The chocolate challenge? Sugary, chocolate-flavored foods are typically high in calories, added sugars, and fat, and often low in other nutrients. And they may crowd out more nutritious foods—for example, if a chocolate bar replaces fruit in your lunch bag—or when you can't control a chocolate urge. Much of the chocolate we consume is in confectionery and baked products that are fat-laden, too. *The bottom line:* Go easy on chocolate!

Now let's melt away a few chocolate myths:

- *Myth: Chocolate causes acne.* That misconception has captured the attention of teens for years. However, hormonal changes during adolescence are the usual cause of acne, not chocolate.

- *Myth: Carob bars are more healthful than chocolate bars.* Actually, a carob bar has the same amount of calories and fat as a similar-size chocolate bar. Carob, a common substitute for chocolate, comes from the seeds of the carob tree, which are different from cocoa beans.

- *Myth: Chocolate has a lot of caffeine.* Chocolate supplies caffeine, but the amount is quite small. Eight ounces of chocolate milk have about 5 milligrams of caffeine, compared with 3 milligrams in 5 ounces of decaffeinated coffee. In contrast, 5 ounces of regular-brew coffee contains 115 milligrams of caffeine.

- *Myth: Some people are "chocoholics."* Not true—although some people do have a stronger preference for chocolate than others, perhaps because of its taste, aroma, and texture. While popping chocolate candies may become a high-calorie habit with a pleasurable sensation, eating chocolate itself can't become truly addictive. Research is exploring any potential role of chocolate to brain neurotransmitters that regulate serotonin and dopamine, often referred to as feel-good body substances.

How can you spot foods with sugar alcohols? The ingredient list on a food label may give the specific name, perhaps sorbitol. If a nutrition content claim is made, such as "sugar-free," the sugar alcohol content must appear with the Nutrition Facts separately, under carbohydrates. Look for grams of sugar alcohols or of the specific sugar replacer. The label also may say that the food has fewer calories per gram than other similar foods with nutritive sweeteners, such as honey, corn syrup, or sucrose.

Low-Calorie Sweeteners: Flavor without Calories

When it comes to sweetness, sugar is at the top of one's mind. Yet low-calorie, also called very-low-calorie, sweeteners deliver sweet taste while providing virtually no calories. Being many times sweeter than the same amount of sugar, they're also aptly named intense sweeteners. Just a very small amount delivers a lot of sweetness. *Refer to "Sweet Comparisons" in this chapter to learn more.* In comparison, nutritive sweeteners such as sugars and sugar alcohols supply calories.

Just about anyone can safely consume low-calorie sweeteners. Alone or blended with other sweeteners, they sweeten foods such as yogurt and pudding, and beverages without adding calories or promoting tooth decay. If foods or drinks with low-calorie sweeteners substitute for higher-calorie foods and drinks, they may help tip the calorie balance toward weight loss.

Sweet Options

Perhaps no ingredient has been scrutinized by researchers as much as low-calorie sweeteners. Before being used in food—or as a tabletop sweetener—they're first tested extensively to meet the guidelines and safety standards of the FDA. That includes assigning Acceptable Daily Intakes (ADIs).

Currently in the United States, six intense sweeteners have been approved: acesulfame potassium, aspartame, neotame, saccharin, sucralose, and tagalose. But watch for news about others. Approval from the FDA has been sought for alitame and cyclamate. Both are approved in some other countries, including cyclamate in Canada. If you travel abroad, you may hear of stevioside or thaumatin, too.

Have You Ever Wondered ?

. . . what stevia is? It's an herb with a substance much sweeter than sugar, yet virtually calorie-free. From a bush native to South America, stevia has been used there as a sweetener for hundreds of years; it's also used for medicinal purposes. Until recently in the United States, stevia was available only as a supplement. In 2008 the FDA granted GRAS ("generally recognized as safe") status to Rebaudioside A, a highly purified compound in stevia. It's sold under brand names such as Pure Via and Truvia. This very refined stevia product can be used as a replacement for calorie-containing sweeteners—with a reminder that it's not a magic bullet for weight loss or blood glucose control and that it may cause nausea, bloating, or other mild side effects. GRAS status has not been given to whole-leaf stevia or its crude extracts due to concerns about potential unhealthy side effects. The best advice is to talk to a health professional before using it. Sometimes stevia is marketed as "natural," but remember that this term has no legal FDA definition. While safe as a tabletop sweetener and as an ingredient, no data show that stevia has benefits over other low-calorie sweeteners.

Acesulfame Potassium. Acesulfame potassium (or acesulfame K) entered the food world in 1967. Approved for use in the United States in 1988, acesulfame potassium is marketed under the brand names Sunette, Sweet 'n' Safe, and Sweet One.

A white, odorless, crystalline sweetener, it provides no calories. Like saccharin, acesulfame potassium can't be broken down by the body, and it's eliminated in the urine unchanged. Again, no calories and a potential benefit for people with diabetes.

Acesulfame potassium is 200 times sweeter than table sugar, adding its sweet taste to candies, baked goods, desserts, noncarbonated drinks, dairy products, sauces, alcoholic drinks, and tabletop sweeteners such as Sweet One and Swiss Sweet. By itself in some foods, a high concentration of acesulfame potassium may leave a slight aftertaste, so it's often combined with other sweeteners, both traditional and intense.

Cooking tip: Because acesulfame potassium is heat-stable, you can use it in cooked and baked foods. Like saccharin, it gives no bulk, or volume, as sugar does, so it may not work in some recipes. *Refer to "Cooking with Low-Calorie Sweeteners" later in this chapter.*

Aspartame. Aspartame is also about 200 times sweeter than table sugar. Developed in 1965 and approved by the FDA in 1981, aspartame was first marketed as NutraSweet and sold as the tabletop sweeteners: Equal, NutraSweet, and NutraTaste. Aspartame is now available in a variety of tabletop sweeteners.

Aspartame isn't sugar. Instead it's a combination of two amino acids—aspartic acid and the methyl ester of phenylalanine. While amino acids are the building blocks of protein, aspartic acid and phenylalanine are joined in a way that's perceived as sweet to your taste buds. These same two amino acids are also found naturally in common foods such as meat, fat-free milk, fruit, and vegetables. When digested, your body treats them like any other amino acid in food.

Like other protein, aspartame has 4 calories per gram. Because so little is used, the calorie impact is negligible.

Have You Ever Wondered

... whether the FDA has guidelines for sugar replacers? The FDA has set Acceptable Daily Intakes (ADIs) for sugar replacers (sugar alcohols and low-calorie sweeteners) used as food additives. The ADI for each one, set at a very conservative level, is how much can be consumed daily over a lifetime without posing a risk.

... why low-calorie sweeteners don't promote tooth decay? As sweeteners, they won't promote cavities because they aren't broken down by bacteria in plaque. Since they don't feed bacteria, no acids form. Sugarless gum, flavored with a low-calorie sweetener, may actually promote dental health. Not only does it not have carbohydrates, but also chewing sugarless gum increases saliva flow, which helps neutralize plaque acids.

... if foods with low-calorie sweeteners increase your appetite and potentially promote weight gain? Although inconclusive, research evidence doesn't show that these sweeteners stimulate appetite. That said, they can aid weight management by adding flavor to food and beverages while limiting calories.

Because aspartame contains phenylalanine, people with the rare genetic disorder called phenylketonuria (PKU) need to be cautious about consuming foods and beverages that contain it. The ingredient list on food labels must list "aspartame"; these labels display this statement: "Phenylketonurics: Contains Phenylalanine." PKU doesn't allow the body to handle phenylalanine properly. PKU afflicts about one in fifteen thousand people in the United States, where all infants are screened for PKU at birth. *Refer to chapter 21, "Sensitive to Food."* If you don't have PKU, you can drink diet soda without this concern.

Contrary to rumors spread by unidentified online sources, aspartame has been intensely studied for its safety. No scientific evidence shows links between aspartame and health problems, including attention deficit disorder and seizures among children. It is approved as safe by the FDA.

Because it's not heat-stable, aspartame is used mostly in foods that don't require cooking or baking. Most aspartame consumed in the United States is in soft drinks. Among other commercial uses are in puddings, gelatins, frozen desserts, yogurt, hot cocoa mix, powdered soft drinks, teas, breath mints, chewing gum, and tabletop sweeteners such as Equal and SweetMate.

Cooking tip: When aspartame is heated for a long time, it may lose its sweetness. When you prepare food with a tabletop sweetener containing aspartame, add it toward the end of cooking. Or sprinkle it on a cooked or baked product after removing it from the heat.

Neotame. Neotame was approved by the FDA in 2002. Neotame is a noncaloric sweetener that's 8,000 times sweeter than table sugar and is used in food and beverages. Although it contains aspartic acid and phenylalanine as aspartame does, the chemical structure differs. Because it isn't digested as aspartame is, neotame isn't absorbed. As a result it doesn't need to carry a warning label for PKU.

Saccharin. Developed in 1879, saccharin has been used as a noncaloric sweetener for about a hundred years. It's produced from a naturally occurring substance in grapes. Today saccharin is used in soft drinks and in tabletop sweeteners such as Sweet'n Low and Sweet 10. The benefits? Calorie-free, not cavity-promoting, not metabolized by humans, and safe.

Being 300 to 500 times sweeter than table sugar, a small amount of saccharin adds a lot of flavor without adding calories. Just 20 milligrams of saccharin gives the same sweetness as one teaspoon (4,000 milligrams, or 4 grams) of table sugar. Because the body can't break it down, saccharin doesn't provide energy. Instead it's eliminated in urine.

What about its bitter aftertaste? It's usually blended with other sweeteners to make the flavor pleasing.

After decades of research, saccharin was removed from the government's list of potential carcinogens and, since the 1970s, has had interim approval. Scientific consensus in the government's *2000 Report on Carcinogens* deemed that cancer data on rats was not relevant to human physiology. In the past, a few studies hinted that saccharin—in very large amounts (equivalent to 750 cans of soft drinks or 10,000 saccharin tablets daily)—may cause cancer in laboratory rats. No human studies have ever confirmed the findings. As of 2000, a warning label isn't required for products that contain saccharin. As with any food or food substance, keep moderation in mind.

Cooking tip: Saccharin keeps its sweet flavor when heated, so it can be used in cooked and baked foods. Because it doesn't have the bulk that sugar has, it may not work in some recipes. *Refer to "Cooking with Low-Calorie Sweeteners" in this chapter.*

Sucralose. Of the low-calorie sweeteners, sucralose is the only one that's made from sugar. It's actually 600 times sweeter. Developed in 1976 and approved in 1998 for U.S. use, sucralose is marketed as Splenda, among other brands.

Unlike sugar, the body doesn't recognize sucralose as a carbohydrate. As a result, it doesn't promote tooth decay and supplies no calories. Sucralose can't be digested, absorbed, or metabolized for energy, so it doesn't affect blood glucose levels or insulin production, either. Instead it passes through the body unchanged—a benefit for people with diabetes. As a low-calorie powder, it's used in beverages, processed foods, chewing gum, and tabletop sweeteners.

Cooking tip: Sucralose offers the sweet sugar flavor, without the calories, and performs like sugar in cooking and baking. However, it doesn't give bulk to baked goods. It's highly heat-stable, even for a prolonged time. And it keeps its flavor in foods even when

Sweet Comparisons

Many ingredients have a sweet flavor. Some, much more than others. Most sugar alcohols aren't as sweet as sucrose. For *low-calorie* sweeteners such as saccharin, a little bit goes a long way!

SWEETENER	COMPARING THE SWEETNESS TO SUCROSE (WHITE OR TABLE SUGAR)
Hydrogenated starch hydrolysates	0.25–0.5
Lacititol	0.3–0.4
Isomalt	0.45–0.65
Sorbitol	0.5–0.7
Mannitol	0.5–0.7
Erythritol	0.7
Maltitol	0.9
Tagatose	0.92
Sucrose (table sugar)	1.0
Xylitol	1.0
High-fructose corn syrup (HFCS)	1.5
Fructose (crystalline)	1.5
Cyclamate*	30
Aspartame	200
Acesulfame K	200
Saccharin	300–500
Sucralose	600
Alitame*	2,000
Neotame	8,000

*Not yet approved for use in food or beverages in the United States.

stored for a long time. Like sugar, it dissolves easily in water. Use sucralose as a sweetener in food preparation and beverages.

Tagatose. Considered by the U.S. FDA as "generally recognized as safe," tagatose is a low-calorie sweetener (1.5 calories per gram) derived from lactose, which is found in some dairy foods. Tagatose is 92 percent as sweet as table sugar. Unlike lactose, tagatose passes through the stomach and small intestine without being digested or absorbed. Instead, it's fermented in the large intestine, providing about 1.5 calories per gram; there it also works as a prebiotic. Sold as Nutralose, it may be used as a food and beverage ingredient; check the ingredient list to find out. Because it doesn't promote tooth decay, as other sugars do, it can carry a health claim about dental health.

Low-Calorie Sweeteners: For Whom?

The 1970s brought a focus on slimness, the 1980s on fitness, and from the 1990s until today, diabetes and obesity have become bigger issues. The growing use of low-calorie sweeteners paralleled these health interests and concerns. From a health perspective, almost anyone can consume foods and beverages flavored with low-calorie sweeteners. It's a matter of personal choice.

Low-calorie sweeteners can be part of a weight management strategy. However, just consuming foods or drinks with these sweeteners won't result in weight loss or keep you from gaining weight! You must limit calories from other sources, too, and avoid replacing the calories saved with higher-calorie foods later.

For people with diabetes, foods and drinks with low-calorie sweeteners can satisfy a taste for sweetness without affecting insulin or blood glucose levels. And they can help with weight control, which is important for managing diabetes.

Need more carb-smart strategies for healthful eating? Check here for how-tos:

● Shop to make carb foods count for good nutrition—chapter 12.

● Sweeten food and boost the fiber as you cook for health—chapter 14.

● Enjoy sweet flavors in restaurant foods—and eat smart, too—chapter 15.

● Manage carbs if you're an athlete—chapter 20.

● Handle carbohydrates on a diabetic eating plan—chapter 22.

Low-calorie sweeteners are safe but are not intended in foods for infants and young children. Kids need ample calories for rapid growth and active play. Foods and beverages sweetened with low-calorie sweeteners are okay occasionally if children eat enough from a variety of nutrient-rich foods.

Cooking with Low-Calorie Sweeteners

With their sugarlike flavor, low-calorie sweeteners can replace sugars and so reduce calories in many recipes. For example, sweetening an apple cobbler with saccharin rather than brown sugar might save 67 calories per serving (if a recipe to serve four calls for ½ cup of brown sugar).

If you use low-calorie sweeteners, remember that their unique cooking qualities differ from those of sugar. You likely need to adjust your recipe or food preparation technique. As ingredients in baked goods, low-calorie sweeteners have limitations.

● Check label directions for food preparation tips. Or check the manufacturer's website. You'll likely see the sugar equivalents. Since some low-calorie sweeteners have ingredients added for bulk, the substitution equivalents vary among products.

● Experiment. Add just a little sweetener until you get the sweetness you want. Adding too much can ruin the flavor.

● Use any low-calorie sweetener in recipes that don't require heat, such as cold beverages, salads, chilled soups, frozen desserts, or fruit sauces.

● Use saccharin, acesulfame potassium, and sucralose-based sweeteners in all kinds of recipes—uncooked, cooked, and baked—according to package directions. They are heat-stable and retain their sweetness when heated. Even then, you may get better results if you substitute only some of the sugar with a low-calorie sweetener.

● Add aspartame-based sweeteners, if used, near the end of the cooking or baking. Aspartame isn't heat-stable. Prolonged and high heat breaks down aspartame; that causes a loss of sweetness. If heated, aspartame is still safe to consume.

Know that recipes prepared with low-calorie sweeteners may not turn out the same as recipes made

How Much Total Carbohydrate and Fiber?

Selected Foods	Serving Size	Calories	Total Carbohydrates (g)	Dietary Fiber (g)
Legumes, Lentils				
Kidney beans, canned	½ cup	105	19	6.8
Lentils, cooked	½ cup	113	19	7.8
Navy beans, cooked	½ cup	127	24	9.6
Soybeans, cooked, mature	½ cup	149	8	5.2
Split peas, cooked	½ cup	114	20	8.1
Vegetables				
Artichoke, globe, cooked	½ cup hearts	43	10	7.2
Broccoli, cooked, chopped	½ cup	27	6	2.6
Collard greens, cooked	½ cup	25	5	2.7
Green peas, cooked	½ cup	67	12	4.4
Mixed vegetables, canned	½ cup	40	8	2.4
Okra, cooked	½ cup	18	4	2.0
Potato, baked, with skin	1 medium	130	29	2.9
Parsnips, cooked	½ cup	55	13	3.1
Pumpkin, canned	½ cup	42	10	3.6
Spinach, canned	½ cup	25	4	2.6
Sweet potato, baked with skin	1 medium	105	24	3.8
Tomato paste	¼ cup	54	12	2.7
Turnips, cooked	½ cup	17	4	1.6
Winter squash, acorn, cooked	½ cup	57	15	4.5
Fruits				
Apple with skin	1 small	77	21	3.6
Asian pear	1 small	51	13	4.4
Banana	1 medium	105	27	3.1
Blackberries	½ cup	31	7	3.8
Dates, chopped	¼ cup	104	28	2.9
Figs, dried	¼ cup	93	24	3.7
Orange	1 medium	62	15	3.1
Plums, dried (prunes), stewed	¼ cup	104	28	3.1
Pear	1 medium	103	28	5.5
Raspberries	½ cup	32	7	4.0

SELECTED FOODS	SERVING SIZE	CALORIES	TOTAL CARBOHYDRATES (G)	DIETARY FIBER (G)
Breads, Pasta, Other Grains				
Bulgur, cooked	½ cup	76	17	4.1
Bran flakes ready-to-eat cereal	¾ cup	96	24	5.3
Bread, white	1 slice	66	12	0.7
Bread, whole-wheat	1 slice	69	12	1.9
English muffin, whole-wheat	½ muffin	67	13	2.2
Oat bran muffin	1 small	178	32	3.0
Pearled barley, cooked	½ cup	97	22	3.0
Rice, brown, cooked	½ cup	108	22	1.8
Rice, white, cooked	½ cup	103	22	0.3
Rye wafer crackers, plain	2 wafers	73	18	5.0
Shredded wheat ready-to-eat, spoon size	1 cup	172	40	6.1
Spaghetti, enriched, cooked	½ cup	110	21	1.3
Spaghetti, whole-wheat, cooked	½ cup	87	19	3.1
Nuts				
Almonds	1 ounce	163	6	3.5

Source: U.S. Department of Agriculture, National Nutrient Database for Standard Reference, Release 24, 2011.

with sugar, especially baked products such as cookies, cakes, muffins, and quick breads. Sugar does more than add flavor. With a low-calorie sweetener, expect:

- Lower volume and different texture. Sugar adds bulk, but low-calorie sweeteners may not unless they have a bulking agent to help bring up the volume. Another option: go 50/50 by substituting saccharin- or acesulfame potassium-based sweeteners for half the sugar, according to package directions. The volume still won't be as high as with 100 percent sugar. Crispy cookies may not have the same texture.

- Lighter color. Sugar caramelizes and has a browning effect. Intense sweeteners don't.

- Different baking time.

- Somewhat different flavor—an issue if you're sensitive to the sweetener's aftertaste.

- Shorter keeping time. Sugar holds moisture. With low-calorie sweeteners, baked foods may dry out faster.

For baking buy a blend—part sugar, part low-calorie sweetener. Blends have fewer calories and carbohydrates than sugar, but they aren't calorie- or carbohydrate-free.

CHAPTER 4

Protein Power

The word "protein" may conjure up thoughts of steak, soy, or the latest high-protein, weight-loss diet. Yet protein is a nutrient, not a food. With the recent interest in fat and carbohydrates, health issues surrounding protein have been overlooked. And since protein-rich foods are so readily available in the United States and other developed countries, this essential nutrient is typically taken for granted. Now protein is getting the attention it deserves!

Why is there growing interest in protein? Among the reasons: High-protein diets are being used for weight loss, and many people are choosing vegetarian eating patterns with plant-based sources of protein. Beyond that, and for the first time, protein received significant attention in the 2010 Dietary Guidelines Advisory Committee Report.

Protein Basics, Protein Foods

We often think of protein as a single nutrient. Yet, proteins in both foods and body cells are made of amino acids. Although many more appear in nature, the body uses about twenty amino acids as raw materials to make at least ten thousand unique body proteins, each with a somewhat different structure. In food it's the unique composition and arrangement of amino acids that also make protein in meat so different from protein in beans.

Like carbohydrates and fats, proteins and their constituent amino acids are composed of carbon, hydrogen, and oxygen. However, proteins have one more element—nitrogen—which makes them unique from other energy nutrients.

Proteins: Their Makeup

Amino acids, the building blocks of proteins, are classified in groups based on the body's ability to produce them. Nine of these twenty amino acids are considered essential. Because the body can't make them, food choices must supply them. Their names may sound familiar: histidine, isoleucine, leucine, lysine, methionine, phenylalanine, threonine, tryptophan, and valine. While arginine isn't essential for adults, it is for young people.

Other amino acids are nonessential. The body can synthesize sufficient amounts. They're made by breaking other amino acids or nitrogen-containing compounds apart, then reusing the components. That's one of nature's great recycling projects! Alanine, aspartic acid (aspartate), asparagine, glutamic acid (glutamate), and serine are some nonessentials.

Six other nonessential amino acids have conditional status: arginine, cysteine, glutamine, glycine, proline, and tyrosine. The body makes them—if you consume enough essential amino acids and enough calories during the day from many different foods. For example, to make tyrosine you need to consume enough phenylalanine.

Amino acids are described as protein's building blocks. Like notes in a music scale or letters of the alphabet, they are arranged in countless ways; some combinations are used more often than others. The same music notes create symphonies, jazz, and pop hits, and the same twenty-six letters of the alphabet form thousands of words in many languages, each word with its own meaning. It's the same for amino acids. In a single body cell, ten thousand different proteins may exist. Short- or long-chain, intricately folded, each body protein has a unique arrangement of amino acids.

Just as words must be spelled correctly to express their intended meaning, the chains of amino acids that make up the unique proteins in different foods and in the body must be arranged in a precise number, combination, and order. In body cells, the genetic code (genes)—called DNA, or deoxyribonucleic acid—carries spelling instructions for making each protein. If an essential amino acid is limited, the body's ability to make certain proteins for muscles and all body tissues is limited, too. Your body can't store these essential amino acids, so you need a fresh supply daily.

They're in a constant state of turnover, always being made and broken down and made again. The pool of amino acids used for growth and repair comes from both proteins in food and from body proteins that are broken down and used for reconstruction.

To do this work your food choices must supply the essentials: essential amino acids, in sufficient amounts and in the right balance. Digestion releases amino acids from foods' proteins for absorption. When the right amino acids aren't available for protein synthesis, or for making new body proteins, the body may break down its own protein to get what it needs.

Protein to Regulate Body Functions

Protein does more than build muscle and body tissue. Of the possible one hundred thousand different proteins in your body, many help regulate body processes. Here are some examples:

● As enzymes and hormones, proteins help speed up or make many chemical reactions in the body happen. For example, a nonessential amino acid, L-arginine, may play a role in heart health by helping to keep blood vessels open. Insulin and glycogen are hormones

Proteins: What They Do

Nearly everything your body does requires protein! Not only do the amino acids in protein synthesize body proteins, as regulators, they're also part of body substances that make body processes happen. Protein is an energy nutrient, too.

Proteins for Growth and Repair

Proteins are part of every cell in your body. Except for bile and urine, they're also part of all body fluids. Amino acids are the raw materials needed to make and repair the many types of body proteins. Different tissues—skin, muscles, bone, blood, and organs, for example—are unique because the amino acid patterns of their proteins differ.

A constant protein supply is needed to make and repair body cells. You've experienced this process in action during times of growth—infancy, childhood, adolescence, and pregnancy—and when, for example, skin heals from a burn or blood gets replaced after bleeding. Not so obvious is the fact that the body also needs proteins to replace its cells as they wear out.

Proteins in Food: Complete and Incomplete

The quality of protein from food depends on the essential amino acids the food contains as well as on the digestibility. For that reason, proteins in foods are often defined as complete or incomplete.

Animal-based protein foods—meat, poultry, fish, eggs, milk, and milk products such as cheese and yogurt—supply all nine essential amino acids in proportions needed to make new body proteins. Proteins from soybeans and quinoa are the only plant-based foods that have them all, too. That's why all these foods are called sources of high-quality or complete proteins. *For more about soy protein, see "Soy Good?" in this chapter; quinoa is described in chapter 9.*

Almost all plant-based foods supply amino acids, too, but they lack one or more of the essentials. That's why their proteins are called incomplete. Still, beans and peas (legumes), seeds, and nuts do supply plenty of proteins. Grain products and most vegetables supply proteins, too, with smaller amounts of many essentials. Even fruit provides small but insignificant amounts.

that help maintain normal levels of blood glucose. Some of the body's proteins help regulate fluid balance in and out of body cells.

● Proteins are part of your body's defense mechanism. Skin, which is made of protein, is your first line of defense against bacteria and injury. Blood-clotting proteins limit blood loss from injury. And antibodies in your immune system help fight off disease-carrying bacteria and viruses.

● Actin and myosin, two muscle proteins, help muscles contract to help your body move. Your heart muscle also relies on proteins so it can contract and beat normally. Another amino acid, tyrosine, is part of epinephrine and norepinephrine, two neurotransmitters that relay messages in the nervous system. And tryptophan is a material needed for serotonin.

● Proteins are also in membranes, working as transport carriers. For example, hemoglobin is a protein that helps transport oxygen in blood to body cells. Lipoproteins carry lipids (fats) to body cells from the liver and intestines. Some vitamins need a protein carrier. Other body substances, including glucose, use proteins to help move across cell membranes.

Protein for Energy

Along with carbohydrate and fat, protein supplies energy: 4 calories per gram of protein. For comparison, carbohydrates also provide 4 calories per gram, and fats provide 9 calories per gram. When calorie (energy) intake from carbohydrates and fat is short, protein can be an energy source. Unlike fat, protein also can convert to glucose, the fuel for brain function.

Protein isn't the body's preferred fuel source, however. When carbohydrates and fats provide enough food energy, proteins are spared so they're available to do work that only protein can do: build and repair body cells and perform protein's many other body functions.

Protein: How Much for You?

How much protein do you need in a day? Actually, the optimal amount of protein—and even the types of protein—needed for health aren't fully understood. There's no one target amount.

The Dietary Reference Intakes (DRIs) advise a wide range of protein intake. That offers flexibility

Have You Ever Wondered ❓

... why protein foods seem to make meals more satisfying? Your satisfaction may come in part from what you define as a meal. Perhaps it's the protein food—such as meat, fish, poultry, eggs, or a soyburger that takes center plate—served with other foods (vegetables, fruit, whole-grain foods, and/or dairy foods). But the benefits of protein in meals extend beyond meal preferences.

Certainly your body needs enough high-quality protein that lean protein foods can provide. In addition, recent research indicates that protein may be more satiating than fat or carbohydrates. So a lean protein food may add satiety, or a feeling of fullness, to a meal. By helping to stave off hunger longer, protein foods may aid weight management if your calorie intake remains within your energy budget and your overall approach to eating is healthful. In other research, eating enough protein, along with adequate physical activity, also may help people lose fat, not muscle, as they manage weight. Look for more emerging research in these areas.

The bottom line: Include lean protein foods in sensible amounts in your meals. *MyPlate in chapters 10 and 11 offers a visual cue to the amount of protein foods on a meal plate.*

for your personal food preferences, needs, and eating patterns. For adults ages 19 and up, the Acceptable Macronutrient Distribution Range (AMDR) for protein is 10 to 35 percent of total calories; for children and teens ages 4 to 18 years, it's 10 to 30 percent of total calories; and for those ages 1 to 3 years, it's 5 to 20 percent of total calories. Most adults in the United States average about 15 percent of their calories from protein. As people lower their calorie intake for weight loss, their percent of calories from protein may rise— perhaps to 35 percent on a very-low-calorie diet—to meet protein recommendations. Consuming only the minimum amount from the AMDR range helps prevent protein deficiency, but that amount may not be enough for muscle growth.

Because they're growing so fast, kids need more protein for their body size than adults do. In fact, protein needs per pound of body weight for infants are the highest; consider that most babies double their birth weight by 6 months! As a child's growth rate slows, protein needs per pound of body weight decrease. That said, total protein need goes up as they grow taller, not only for their continued growth but also for the hormones, enzymes, and other ways the body uses protein. *See "How Much Protein?" below to learn more.*

Protein needs also increase during pregnancy, for the growing fetus and for the mother's increased blood volume, breast and uterine tissues, and placenta. During lactation, women need more protein to produce breast milk, which is high in protein.

How do the AMDR ranges translate to gram amounts of protein per day? The Recommended Dietary Allowance (RDA) for protein, set by the Institute of Medicine, is a minimum, based on body weight, age, and if you're female, whether you're pregnant or nursing.

- Ages 1 to 3: 13 grams
- Ages 4 to 8: 19 grams
- Ages 9 to 13: 34 grams
- Teen boys, ages 14 to 18: 52 grams
- Teen girls, ages 14 to 18: 46 grams
- Adult men, ages 19 or over: 56 grams
- Adult women ages 19 or over: 46 grams
- Pregnancy and breast-feeding: 71 grams

HOW MUCH PROTEIN?

The RDA for protein is based on ideal body weight. Here's how protein needs are figured based on body weight:

Tip: *Weight in kilograms = weight in pounds ÷ 2.2 pounds.*

AGE	PROTEIN (GRAMS/KILOGRAM BODY WEIGHT)	PROTEIN (GRAMS/POUND BODY WEIGHT)
0 to 6 months	1.52	0.69
6 to 12 months	1.2	0.55
1 to 3 years	1.05	0.48
4 to 13 years	0.95	0.43
14 to 18 years	0.85	0.39
≥ 19 years	0.8	0.37

Source: Dietary Reference Intakes, Institute of Medicine, 2005.

The RDA is the same for vegetarians and non-vegetarians.

To put this amount into food terms, one ounce of lean meat and plant-based protein foods each deliver about 7 grams of protein, and an 8-ounce glass of milk provides about 8 grams of protein.

The RDA is the amount needed to repair body proteins as they wear out and break down. In fact, these recommendations fall at the lower end of the AMDR—and may not be optimal levels to support muscle growth and other health benefits. The optimal level hasn't yet been determined.

Protein needs also may increase for healing after injury, burns, and surgery, or with some other health problems, including diabetes, significant muscle loss, and critical illness. Recommended amounts also may differ if you have diabetes or kidney disease. In these cases, talk to your doctor or registered dietitian.

Dietary Guidelines for Americans, 2010, has increased recommendations to 8 ounces or more of a variety of seafood per week, to provide about 20 percent of the total recommendation of protein foods. *For a food guide that helps you consume protein in recommended amounts, see chapter 10. To explore protein and protein supplements for competitive and weekend athletes, see chapter 20.*

Protein: Too Little?

When protein intake, especially that of high-quality protein, isn't sufficient, the body can't make or repair body cells. Instead, proteins in body tissues, including muscle, break down, releasing their pool of amino acids for recycling. With a lack of food energy (calories), the body uses its fat stores and perhaps its muscle protein for energy. With severe calorie restriction—common among those with anorexia—muscle loss is the outcome. *See chapter 2 to learn more about disordered eating.*

Most adults in the United States and other developed countries get enough protein. But where poverty or a limited food supply exists, protein deficiency is common. Growing children are at special risk. Kwashiorkor is a form of protein malnutrition; among its outcomes are loss of muscle, failure to grow, lower immunity, increased risk for disease, and weakened respiratory and cardiovascular systems. Marasmus, a type of severe protein-energy malnutrition, is a serious

Your Nutrition Checkup

How Do Protein Foods Fit in Your Eating Plans?

Look at protein-rich foods in your everyday food patterns. *Then refer to chapter 10 for a food guide to help you get the right amount to match your protein needs.*

	NEVER OR HARDLY EVER	ONCE OR TWICE A WEEK	EVERY OTHER DAY	MOST DAYS	A COUPLE OF TIMES A DAY
Meat, poultry, fish, eggs	_____	_____	_____	_____	_____
Milk, yogurt, cheese, cottage cheese	_____	_____	_____	_____	_____
Beans, lentils, nuts, nut butters	_____	_____	_____	_____	_____
Tempeh, tofu, soyburgers, other soy protein foods	_____	_____	_____	_____	_____

lack of food energy, causing a debilitating amount of muscle loss and often death.

Protein: Too Much?

No upper limit, or Tolerable Upper Intake Level (UL), for protein has been set in the Dietary Reference Intakes. The body doesn't store excess protein from food as a protein reserve. Instead it breaks down and converts to body fat or glycogen for energy storage. Its nitrogen-containing components, released in the process, are removed and excreted through the kidneys in urine. And if excess protein contributes to excess calories, it's one more factor that tips energy balance toward weight gain.

A high-protein diet and protein supplements can be risky for those with kidney disease. *See chapter 20 to learn about protein supplements.*

Completing the Equation

Consider this important combination: beans plus grains. That's a simple tactic for getting the most from the protein in foods from plant sources. Except for soybeans and quinoa, plant-based foods (beans, nuts, seeds, and grains) are limited in one or more amino acids. However, in combination they provide adequate amounts of all the essential amino acids, so they're often referred to as "complementary proteins."

To get the most out of the protein foods you eat,

remember to pair certain foods together, such as legumes plus grains. Four essential amino acids—cysteine, lysine, methionine, and tryptophan—are more often limited in the proteins of plant-based foods:

● Beans are high in lysine but limited in cysteine and methionine.

● Nuts, seeds, and grains are high in methionine and cysteine but limited in lysine.

● Rice is high in methionine but limited in lysine.

● Corn is a good methionine source but limited in lysine and tryptophan.

For your health, when eating protein foods . . .

● Eat a variety of protein foods, which include seafood, lean meat, poultry, eggs, beans and peas, soy products, and unsalted nuts and seeds.

● Increase the amount and variety of seafood consumed by choosing seafood in place of some meat and poultry.

● Replace protein foods that are higher in solid fats with choices that are lower in solid fats and calories and/or are sources of oils.

Source: Dietary Guidelines for Americans, 2010.

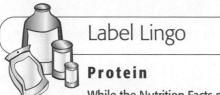

Label Lingo

Protein

While the Nutrition Facts panel on a food label gives the specific amount of protein in a label serving of food, "protein lingo" in nutrient content claims may offer a quick description. Look for these terms as you walk the supermarket aisles.

LABEL TERM . . .	MEANS . . .
High-protein	10 g or more per serving
Good source	5 to 9.9 g per serving
More, extra, plus, or added protein	At least 5 g more* per serving
Fortified or enriched with protein	At least 5 g more* per serving

*As compared with a standard serving size of the traditional food.

Combinations of these foods—for example, rice and beans, corn and beans, peanut butter on bread, and a bean burrito on a corn tortilla—form complete proteins.

If you choose a vegetarian eating style, here's good news: For complete proteins you don't need to combine specific plant-based foods with complementary proteins at each meal, as once thought. But you do need to eat a variety of plant-based foods—beans and peas, nuts, seeds, grains, vegetables, and fruits—and enough calories throughout the day. The amino acid or acids lacking in one food can come from other meals or snacks.

Proteins: Choose by the Company They Keep

It's not just the protein, but the nutrients packaged with protein that make a difference. Along with essential amino acids, beans and peas, lentils, nuts, and seeds provide fiber, certain vitamins and minerals, including nonheme iron, and more poly- and monounsaturated fats than animal sources of protein. Plant-based protein foods are cholesterol-free, too. Animal-based protein foods have more solid fats and contain cholesterol; seafood also contains beneficial omega-3 fatty acids (EPA and DHA). Milk, yogurt,

and cheese deliver calcium and vitamin D, among other important nutrients; their fat content varies. Heme iron and zinc are among the other nutrients in meat, poultry, and fish.

For kitchen nutrition, consider the whole nutrient package. Choose protein-rich foods with less fat and cholesterol. Trimming fat often trims calories, too.

- Choose lean meat; trim off any fat you see.
- For chicken and turkey, remove the skin to reduce the fat.
- Bake, broil, or grill meat, poultry, and fish, rather than fry them.
- Eat smaller portions of meat, and eat fish more often.

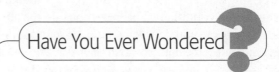

Have You Ever Wondered

. . . if you need a protein supplement, especially if you're physically active? Save your money. If you're healthy, you probably get all the protein you need from your everyday meals and snacks. Protein-rich foods, especially those from animal sources, have plenty of amino acids. Vegans likely don't need protein supplements either if they eat a variety of plant-based foods and enough calories in their day's meals and snacks. "Meatless" doesn't mean low-protein!

Protein supplements may be useful for some health conditions or for older adults who can't consume enough protein. However, talk to your healthcare provider before taking protein supplements. *For more about protein supplements see chapter 20.*

. . . what whey protein is? What casein is? They're the two high-quality proteins in dairy foods. While casein is about 80 percent of milk's protein, whey protein makes up the rest. Whey—composed of protein, lactose, other carbohydrates, minerals, fat, and other substances—is the liquid left after milk is separated and curdled to make cheese. At one time considered a waste by-product, today whey protein is recognized as an excellent source of high-quality protein. It's often used in protein bars, beverages, drink mixes, and yogurt. Whey protein contains all essential amino acids, including high concentrations of leucine, which may play an important role in glucose metabolism and insulin. Whey protein also may be efficient in helping to stimulate the synthesis of muscle protein.

- Choose low-fat or fat-free milk, yogurt, and cheese. Limit traditional cheese.
- Choose egg whites or pasteurized egg white products.
- Substitute pinto or black beans or soy products for meat in chili, tacos, and pasta sauces.

For more ways to buy and prepare protein-rich foods with less fat and fewer calories, see chapters 12 and 14.

Protein and Health

Considering protein's importance to health, there's surprisingly little research linking protein intake to many health conditions. The exceptions are the allergic reactions to some proteins in foods such as milk, eggs, peanuts, tree nuts, soy, fish, shellfish, and wheat. *See chapter 21 to learn about food allergies.* Increasingly, research questions are being raised to help address protein's links to many health issues, among them sarcopenia, overweight, obesity, osteoporosis, diabetes, heart health, and high blood pressure.

Do proteins from animal and plant sources make a difference? Most people consume both, so it's hard to know.

Protein and Sarcopenia

The term "sarcopenia" may be unfamiliar, but if you're an older adult or if you're caring for an aging person, you've likely observed this condition. It's the progressive decline in muscle mass and strength that happens naturally with aging. Among the reasons, the body doesn't convert amino acids to muscle tissue as efficiently.

For every decade of life after age thirty, sarcopenia results in a 3 to 8 percent reduction in lean muscle mass. In its advanced stages, it's seen as the frailty of age, associated with higher risks of falls and disability. As people age, preserving muscle is important for their physical endurance, for their ability to do the activities of everyday living such as lifting things and getting up from a chair, and for reducing their risk for falls.

Despite its prevalence, sarcopenia gets little attention. Yet for some people it may be slowed or partly

Animal-Based or Plant-Based: How Much Protein*?

FOOD	PROTEIN (G)
Sources of Animal-Based Proteins	
Chicken breast, meat only, roasted (½ breast)	27
Lean beef, sirloin, broiled (3 oz.)	26
Pork, lean, roasted (3 oz.)	23
Ground beef, 90% lean, broiled (3 oz.)	22
Salmon, sockeye, filet, baked (3 oz.)	22
Tuna, canned, drained (3 oz.)	20
Cottage cheese, low-fat (½ cup)	14
Yogurt, plain, low-fat, (8 oz.)	13
Cow's milk (1 cup)	8
Cheese, cheddar (1 oz.)	7
Egg, large (1)	6
*Sources of Plant-Based Proteins**	
Lentils, cooked (½ cup)	9
Peanut butter, smooth (2 tbsp.)	8
Kidney beans, cooked (½ cup)	8
Pumpkin seed kernels, roasted (1 oz.)	8
Soy beverage, unfortified (1 cup)	8
Hummus (⅓ cup)	6
Almonds (1 oz., 23 nuts)	6
Sunflower seeds, roasted (1 oz.)	5
Quinoa, cooked (½ cup)	4
Bulgur, kasha, oats, cooked (½ cup)	3
Pecans (1 oz., 19 halves)	3
Rice, white, cooked (½ cup)	2
Corn, yellow, cooked (½ cup)	2

* See page 96 for the protein content of soy foods.

Source: U.S. Department of Agriculture, National Nutrient Database for Standard Reference, Release 24, 2011.

reversed with sound nutrition and regular strength-building physical activity. Regular resistance exercise helps retain and build muscle strength and size. Emerging research suggests that consuming somewhat more protein than the RDA may help maintain muscle, and distributing it across meals may be beneficial. Most people in the United States consume more protein than the current RDA.

Protein intake often declines in later years, often because older people eat less food overall. As a result, they may not meet current recommendations (RDAs) for protein, and some older adults risk energy-protein malnutrition. Yet consuming enough protein, perhaps somewhat more than the current RDA, or a moderate increase in high-quality protein, may help older people retain muscle mass and strength. The research on this issue is evolving, however.

Protein and Weight Management

Is a higher-protein diet better for weight loss? Some research indicates a high-protein diet may help with initial weight loss if calories are reduced. However, over the long term, an eating pattern that's higher or lower in protein doesn't appear to make a difference in losing weight or maintaining weight loss. The protein source doesn't appear to make a difference either; if calories are controlled, vegetarian diets and meat-containing diets are comparable for weight loss. *The bottom line:* Weight loss and weight maintenance are all about calorie balance—calories in from any source and calories out through physical activity.

Protein may be linked to weight management in other ways. For one, protein is more thermogenic. In other words, it takes more energy to digest protein than carbohydrate and fat. Second, protein adds satiety, so you feel full longer after eating high-protein foods in a meal or a snack. It takes longer to move through the digestive tract. And that may help reduce the desire to overeat or to eat as often. And third, protein helps steady blood glucose levels and so helps control the brain signals for hunger.

Protein does contribute calories. Eating portions of protein-rich foods that exceed your needs do add up to more calories—and potentially to weight gain. Extra calories from protein-rich foods also may come from the company they keep. Extra calories from fat in a juicy steak, fried chicken, or full-fat cheese not only come from protein but also from their fat content. By choosing low-fat, fat-free, and lean protein foods for fewer calories, you also take care of your heart by eating fewer solid fats.

As an aside, preserving muscle mass has a weight management benefit. Ounce for ounce, muscle burns more calories than body fat.

See chapter 2 for the pros and cons of high-protein diets for weight management.

Protein and Bone Health

While calcium and vitamin D are well recognized for their roles in reducing the risks of osteoporosis, protein also plays a role in bone health. That's not surprising, since about 50 percent of bone volume is protein. Like other body tissues, bone tissue also undergoes ongoing repair.

How does protein impact bone density? Research isn't consistent or conclusive. Emerging studies suggest that there may be a positive link between higher protein intake and greater bone mass and fewer

---

Have You Ever Wondered

... if tryptophan in milk helps you sleep? Perhaps. Tryptophan is an amino acid used to make serotonin, a neurotransmitter (brain chemical) that helps control sleep patterns. However, it's more likely that drinking milk has a calming effect; the amount of tryptophan in milk is too small to make a difference. Similarly, tryptophan in turkey is often credited with drowsiness; however, the amount is comparable to that in most other meats. Feeling sleepy after a Thanksgiving dinner likely comes from many other factors, not feasting on turkey. As an aside, if you consider taking tryptophan as a dietary supplement, talk to your healthcare provider first, as it may have harmful side effects.

... why diet soda offers a warning about the amino acid phenylalanine? Diet sodas don't contain protein, but they're typically sweetened with aspartame, a nonnutritive sweetener that releases phenylalanine when digested. People with the rare genetic disease phenylketonuria (PKU) can't metabolize this amino acid properly; unmanaged PKU can cause tissue damage and brain damage in infants and young children. *See chapter 21 for more about PKU.*

... why beans have more protein than other vegetables? Kidney beans, black beans, red beans, soybeans, and other bean plants have a unique quality. Bacteria in their roots trap nitrogen. The plants not only fix nitrogen in the soil, but also contribute nitrogen, one element in protein, to the growing bean. Both the soil and the beans benefit!

Have You Ever Wondered ?

. . . how the protein in milk alternatives compares with cow's milk? The Nutrition Facts on food labels shows the protein content per 8-ounce serving. Like cow's milk, soy beverage, or soymilk, provides high-quality, complete protein. However, even though they're referred to as milk, rice milk and almond milk don't provide much protein, and their proteins lack some essential amino acids. While cow's milk and soymilk provide about 8 grams of protein per 8-ounce serving, almond milk and rice milk generally provide only about 1 gram or less of protein per 8 ounces. Since these milks are poor protein sources, labels on almond and rice milk state: "Not to be used as an infant formula." All these milk alternatives may be calcium- and vitamin D-fortified.

fractures—if calcium intake is also adequate. Other studies suggest that a high-protein diet over time may increase fracture risk. Along with calcium and vitamin D, more research is needed to determine protein's role in maintaining bone density and lowering fracture risk of older adults.

Protein and Other Chronic Conditions

Diabetes. While protein as an energy nutrient is included in diabetes management, no consistent evidence shows that protein intake from any source is linked to an increased risk. Any association between diabetes risk and protein-rich foods must factor in the calorie, fat, and fiber content.

Cancer. No consistent evidence links protein intake—from either plant-based or animal-based sources—to increased or lowered risk of most cancers. Some studies suggest a link between colon cancer and eating large amounts of red meat, especially processed meat such as ham, bacon, and hot dogs. However, the research is inconclusive. More studies are needed to show if there is any link to the type of meat, how it's prepared, how much, and whether other substances factor in. The best advice is moderation and to enjoy a variety of protein-rich foods.

Heart Disease and High Blood Pressure. Again, current research shows no consistent link to protein intake. Some research indicates that increased protein

may reduce heart disease risk when protein foods replace those high in carbohydrates. Protein may play a role in lowering blood lipids. Again, there's not yet enough research to offer advice.

Soy's Links to Health

Made into many food products, soybeans are very versatile and nutritious. Compared with many other legumes, soybeans are a rich, unique source of high-quality, plant-based protein—unique because soybeans contain complete protein, as does meat. Soybeans contain all nine essential amino acids needed to build and repair body cells. That's why many soy products make good protein alternatives in meatless meals! Soybean oil is not a protein source.

Beyond that, soybeans are a good source of B vitamins. A source of essential fatty acids (including ALAs, which convert to omega-3s), soybeans' fat is mostly poly- and monounsaturated. Tofu (made with calcium sulfate), calcium-fortified soymilk, and

Soy Protein: How Much?

FOODS WITH SOY PROTEIN (EXAMPLES)	AMOUNT OF SOY PROTEIN (GRAMS)
Tempeh (½ cup)	19.5
Soy bar (1)	14*
Soyburger patty (1)	13–14
Soy pasta, cooked (½ cup)	13
Soy nuts, roasted, unsalted (¼ cup)	11
Edamame (½ cup)	11
Soy breakfast patties (2)	11
Tofu (½ cup)	10
Soy nut butter (2 tbsp.)	7
Soy cereal (1¼ cups)	7
Fortified soymilk (1 cup)	6–7
Vanilla soy yogurt (1 cup)	6
Soy pudding (½ cup)	6
Miso (2 tbsp.)	4

*Varies by brand.
Source: United Soybean Board, 2010.

calcium-fortified soy yogurt deliver calcium, and they are often vitamin D-fortified, too.

Health benefits of soy may extend further, but research doesn't yet have a clear answer. Soy's isoflavones have been credited with helping to lower risks for some health issues, such as hot flashes and menopause symptoms, but evidence isn't consistent. Soy's two main isoflavones—genistein and daidzein—have weak estrogenlike effects.

Some evidence suggests that soy foods may be heart healthy, especially if they replace higher-fat options, since they're low in solid fat but provide fiber and polyunsaturated fat. Soy protein may have a small effect on lowering total and LDL cholesterol levels. Again, evidence isn't consistent; some experts advise reevaluation of the qualified health claim linking soy

Soy Good?

Fresh, canned, dried, or frozen, soybeans fit in soups, stews, casseroles, salads, pasta sauces, and Mexican dishes. The following are among the many products with soy protein:

- *Produce department:* tofu, tempeh, edamame (in the pod or shelled), soy sprouts
- *Grocery aisle:* canned black and yellow soybeans, dried soybeans, soy pasta (sold in many shapes), soy pudding, soy jerky, soynut butter (like peanut butter), soy cereal (soy flakes, granola, soy mixed with other cereals, soy grits), soy flour, soy baking mixes (for pancakes, muffins, brownies), textured soy protein (TSP) and soy beverage powders (to add to drinks and other foods), miso, seasoning mixes with soy for burgers, chili, and tacos
- *Dairy case:* soymilk, soy cheese, soy eggnog, soy yogurt, soy smoothies, dairy milk and dairy yogurt with added soy protein, soy beverage juice blends, and soy sour cream. (Although cholesterol-free, soy products differ in some culinary characteristics from milk products.)
- *Egg case:* egg replacers
- *Frozen foods:* edamame, soy entrées, soy sausage and patties, soy bacon, soy-based burgers, soy crumbles, soy ice cream
- *Meat case:* garden- or soyburgers, soy hot dogs
- *Snack aisle:* soynuts, soynut trail mix, soy protein bars

Have You Ever Wondered

... why soy products may carry a health claim on their food labels? A health claim, indicating a link between soy protein and the lowering of total and LDL cholesterol, was approved in the year 2000. The claim was based on the need for 25 grams of soy protein. For a label to carry the claim, a food must contain at least 6.25 grams of soy protein per serving. Since that time, research indicates that the effect may be smaller, from a greater soy protein intake, than once thought. Still, soy products are heart healthy.

... what textured soy protein, or TSP, is? Textured vegetable (soy) protein is a high-fiber, high-protein meat substitute that's made from soy flour. Often sold as granules, flakes, or chunks and either flavored or unflavored, it's used to boost the protein in some baked goods, casseroles, and other mixed dishes or to replace or extend meat or poultry. Vegetable burgers and sausages often are made with TSP.

protein and cardiovascular disease. Vegetable protein also may be linked to lower blood pressure, but other components of plant-based foods, such as fiber, might factor in; evidence doesn't consistently show that soy protein offers unique benefits for blood pressure control. With only limited evidence, vegetable protein doesn't appear to offer special protection from heart disease, type 2 diabetes, or some cancers.

Protein for Vegans

Vegetarians, especially vegans who consume no foods from animal sources, need to be mindful of protein. Carefully planned meals and snacks can provide enough protein and enough essential amino acids. That's easy for lacto- and lacto-ovo-vegetarians, who eat eggs and/or dairy foods. Vegans, including vegan athletes, need to consume a variety of plant-based foods because the amino acid content differs, and enough food energy each day. *See chapter 10 for food guidance for vegetarians.*

Amino acids from soybeans, for example, have the same health effects as amino acids from dairy foods or chicken. However, proteins from some plant-based foods, such as some cereals and legumes, may not be digested as well, so protein recommendations for vegans may be slightly higher than the RDA.

Because cereals are low in lysine, an essential amino acid, vegans may wisely consume more beans and soy products, which are good sources of lysine. Another option for vegans is to consume more protein from all sources of plant-based foods to make sure they consume enough lysine. To get enough protein, vegans need to consume a significant amount of beans; otherwise it's hard to get enough protein.

Generally, protein is only a concern for lacto-ovo-vegetarians, who eat dairy foods and eggs, when

FUNCTIONAL NUTRITION: A QUICK LOOK AT SOY PROTEIN

CLASS/ COMPONENTS	POTENTIAL BENEFIT	SOME FOOD SOURCES
Soy protein*	May reduce risk of cardiovascular disease	soybeans and soy-based foods such as milk, yogurt, cheese, and tofu

*The U.S. Food and Drug Administration has approved a health claim for this food component.

Source: Adapted from the International Food Information Council Foundation, 2011.

See chapter 6 to learn the functional benefits of phytoestrogens: isoflavones and lignan.

Have You Ever Wondered ?

. . . how much protein a vegan meal might have? Of course, that varies, but here's the protein in a sample meal: A 1-cup serving of rice and beans (half rice, half beans) supplies about 10 grams of protein. Add 1 cup of soymilk for about 8 grams of protein; a green vegetable side dish topped with nuts for 4 or 5 grams of protein; one whole-wheat roll, about 4 more grams of protein. That adds up to at least 26 grams of protein in just one meal (without dessert!).

. . . what tempeh is? Another soy food, tempeh is made from cooked, slightly fermented soybeans, perhaps grains, and spices or herbs, giving it a firm texture and a nutty flavor. Low in fat yet high in protein, it's a great meat substitute that's easy to slice or cube for stir-fries, chili, soup, and other mixed dishes.

calories are overly limited, when protein comes from a single source, or when calories come mostly from energy-dense, nutrient-poor foods and drinks. Vegans, who only consume plant-based foods, need to plan carefully to consume enough protein.

With careful planning, most vegetarians don't need a protein supplement. If you're vegan, check with your healthcare provider or a registered dietitian.

See chapter 10 for vegan and lacto-ovo-vegetarian food patterns.

CHAPTER 5

Fat Facts
Cholesterol, Too

For more than three decades, fats have been in the limelight, since the 1980 Dietary Guidelines linked dietary fat and cholesterol to heart disease. But current scientific evidence has revealed that the types of fat and their relationships to health are far more complex than once thought.

Dietary fat and cholesterol are key determinants of a major public health concern—cardiovascular disease—as noted in the 2010 Dietary Guidelines. Reducing solid fats (saturated fats and *trans* fats), and perhaps replacing them with unsaturated fats, appears to be more effective than just reducing total fat intake for decreasing the risk of cardiovascular disease. In fact, most fats in your meals and snacks should be unsaturated (liquid at room temperature). That includes omega-3s. What about dietary cholesterol? Unless you have diabetes, consuming moderate levels of cholesterol probably doesn't make much of an impact on your risk of heart disease.

Considering the growing obesity epidemic, cutting back on fat is certainly one way to reduce calories—but simply replacing fat with calories from carbohydrates and protein doesn't shift calorie balance toward weight loss. Without attention to calorie intake, cutting back on fat isn't a weight loss solution. From any source, all calories count. Evidence linking fat intake to increased cancer risk is still unclear.

So, as context for today's advice about dietary fats, let's first explore the fat facts.

Fats Matter

Suppose your doctor said, "You need to get your serum cholesterol level down. Your triglycerides are borderline high. And cut the fat, especially the solid fats, in your diet." Just what would this mean to you? And what would you do? To understand the role of fats in food, health, and chronic disease, let's start with the basics.

Fat: A Nutrient for Health

You may be surprised to learn that fats have fundamental health functions and positive benefits. Fat is a nutrient necessary for your health. In moderate amounts, fats perform a full workload of body functions. You actually can't live without them! That's why a fat-free diet isn't a healthful goal—and it's virtually impossible. There's more to healthful eating than simply cutting back on fats. In fact, the type of fat you eat may be just as important as the total amount of fat. Various types of fats in foods have different effects on health; some fats may offer health-protective benefits. So just how does fat help keep you healthy?

Fats: Essential Work

Fats and body chemicals that contain metabolites of fat are part of every cell in your body, including brain and nervous tissue. They're part of hormones that regulate many body functions, including muscle contraction, immune function, blood clotting, and blood pressure. A dietary fat may also carry essential vitamins; for example, soybean oil is a major source of vitamin E.

Fats work as partners in your body with other nutrients, too. Just as sugar dissolves in water, some vitamins dissolve in fat. That's how vitamins A, D, E, and K, as well as carotenoids, are carried in food and absorbed into and carried by your bloodstream. Without fats, these fat-soluble vitamins cannot fully nourish your body.

Certain fats are considered essential in your diet, specifically two fatty acids: linoleic acid (LA) and alpha-linolenic acid (ALA). Your body can't make them. (Fatty acids are the building blocks of fat.) For children to grow normally and for adults and children to maintain healthy skin, food choices must supply linoleic acid and alpha-linolenic acid.

Both linoleic acid and alpha-linolenic acid are widely available in food: for example, linoleic acid from vegetable oils and poultry fat, and alpha-linolenic acid from soybean oil, canola oil, nuts, and seeds. If your food choices are varied, getting enough of these fatty acids is easy.

You may know these types of fatty acids by other names: omega-3s and omega-6s. ALAs convert to EPA and DHA, which have their own unique and potential health benefits. Since ALAs don't convert readily, however, seafood is recommended as a good source of omega-3s. *See "Functional Nutrition: Eat Your Omega-3s and -6s" in this chapter.*

A "Power Source"

Like carbohydrates and proteins, fats supply energy, or calories, to power your physical activity and the many body processes that keep you alive. (*Remember:* A calorie is a unit of energy.) Also composed of carbon, hydrogen, and oxygen, fats are a concentrated energy source, supplying 9 calories per gram. To compare, carbohydrates and proteins provide 4 calories per gram. Although your body uses fat for energy, it's not the body's preferred fuel source.

Fats are part of the calorie balance equation, and so, along with other energy nutrients, play a role in body weight. If you consume more calories from any source (carbohydrate, fat, or protein) than your body needs, your body saves the extra in fatty tissues, mostly in

Have You Ever Wondered

. . . if a food that's "low-fat" is "low-calorie," too? Not necessarily. It's true that fat is a concentrated source of energy, or calories. However, cutting back on high-fat foods may not trim calories if too many carbohydrates or proteins take their place. The calorie content of the "regular" and "low-fat" version of a food may be similar because carbohydrate-containing ingredients often are added to help replace flavor that's lost when fat is removed. To find out, read the Nutrition Facts on the food label for packaged foods. Even if the calories are less, go easy on your amount of low-fat or fat-free foods. Eating a whole box of fat-free cookies isn't a "low-calorie" experience!

. . . if a reduced-fat food is always "low-fat"? Not necessarily. It just may have less fat (at least 25 percent less) than its full-fat counterpart. Check the Nutrition Facts on food labels to find out. *See "Label Lingo" later in this chapter to know what the terms mean.*

. . . if fish really is brain food? Today's science would say yes to that old wives' tale! DHA, the omega-3 fatty acid in oily fish, is found in the brain and throughout the body. Especially during pregnancy and nursing, omega-3s are important for brain and eye development. Because alpha-linolenic acid from plant sources converts to DHA ineffectively, consume seafood with omega-3s.

. . . if coconut oil has special health benefits? Despite the claims and testimonials, no clinical evidence shows that coconut oil is any healthier than other saturated fats. Neither the 2010 Dietary Guidelines nor the American Heart Association support these claims. In fact, coconut oil is 92 percent saturated fat—more than many sources of saturated fats. Saturated fats from any source should be limited to reduce heart disease risk.

fat cells. Body fat also is known as adipose tissue. When you need an extra energy supply, your body can draw on this stored fat. Other body cells and blood plasma have some fat, too.

Fat for Satiety

A little fat in food adds more than flavor. It also helps satisfy hunger by helping you feel full and by providing the mouthfeel that makes food so appealing.

See "Your 'Fat Tooth'" in this chapter. If low-fat food doesn't taste satisfying or if you don't feel full after eating, you may eat until you do feel full and satisfied. That may add more calories than those saved by choosing lower-fat foods.

Body Fat: Its Role

You need a certain amount of body fat: to cushion and position your body organs, to protect your bones from injury, and as a fat layer under your skin (subcutaneous fat), which offers insulation, helping you stay warm on a cold day. The soft fat pads on your buttocks and the palms of your hands protect your bones from bumps, bangs, and jolts. Fat that's stored around your organs isn't accessed for energy.

Why Foods Contain Fat

Fat offers sensory qualities that make food taste good. As an ingredient, fat carries flavor. It also gives a smooth, creamy texture to foods such as ice cream and peanut butter. When foods such as a brownie seem to melt in your mouth, that's just what's happening—the fat is melting! From meat to baked foods, fat makes many foods moist and tender, or brown and crispy.

Can you cut the fat in a recipe? To a certain extent, yes. The recipe may work if you use less. But eliminating fat altogether may not give the result you expect.

In baked foods. Fat tenderizes; adds moisture; holds in air so baked foods are light; and affects shape, for example, in cookies. With too little fat, baked goods might be tough or dry, or may not rise properly.

In sauces. Fat keeps sauces from curdling and forms part of an emulsion. An emulsion is a mixture of two substances, such as fat and water, that stay together instead of separating, as they normally would.

In other cooked foods. Fat helps conduct heat as food cooks—for example, when food is sautéed (cooked quickly in a small amount of fat) or fried.

In cooked meat, poultry, and fish. Fat seals in moisture as foods are basted, or brushed with liquid during cooking. Sometimes the surface gets dry if it isn't basted.

For foods cooked in a pan. Fat lubricates the pan so food won't stick.

In all kinds of food. Fat helps carry flavor and nutrients, provides texture (mouth feel), and adds satiety.

Sorting the Fats

The dictionary of fat terms seems endless and often confusing. In fact, there's no one kind of fat. Some terms describe fatlike substances in the body; others apply to different fats in food; and some to both. The

Your "Fat Tooth"

Have a craving for rich chocolates or desserts? Your "fat tooth," not your "sweet tooth," may account for that urge. In this world of high-fat foods, a preference for them may be culturally conditioned. Research suggests that happens early, when infants and young children learn through experience that fat is associated with satiety, a satisfying feeling of fullness.

A smooth, creamy milk shake; a flaky, tender pastry; and a juicy steak: The appeal of high-fat foods may come from qualities that fat imparts. Or perhaps the appeal stems from on-again, off-again dieting. Some studies say that dieting may amplify a fat craving, or more likely, the craving for sweetened fat like that found in many rich desserts.

No matter what the reason for a "fat tooth," you can overcome, or manage, your preference for fatty foods:

- Fool your tastebuds. Get a smooth, creamy consistency with low-fat and fat-free ingredients: low-fat yogurt in savory dips; thick, pureed fruit as a dessert sauce; and creamy buttermilk as a milk shake base.
- Indulge a "fat tooth." Share a rich dessert to cut your fat grams and calories in half.
- Gradually shift to lower-fat foods.

differences in the fatty acid makeup of food account for their differing effects on your health. Just what do all these terms really mean?

"Fat" Dictionary

Lipid. Scientific term that refers to all fats, cholesterol, and other fatlike substances; lipids do not dissolve in water.

Lipoproteins. Protein-coated packages that carry lipids, including cholesterol, in the bloodstream. Without the protein coating, lipids cannot travel through the bloodstream.

Cholesterol. Waxy, fatlike substance found in foods of animal origin and in every body cell. It's essential for cell building.

> *Blood (serum) cholesterol.* Cholesterol that travels in the bloodstream. The body manufactures most of its blood cholesterol; some is also absorbed from foods you eat.

> *Dietary cholesterol.* Cholesterol in food, found only in foods of animal origin, and never from plant sources, even if they contain fat.

> *HDL ("good") blood cholesterol.* Cholesterol carried by high-density lipoproteins (HDLs). HDLs carry cholesterol and other blood lipids away from body cells to the liver so they can be broken down and excreted. HDLs—with a higher ratio of protein to cholesterol—are made in the liver in response to physical activity and some foods. Food doesn't have them.

> *LDL ("bad") blood cholesterol.* Cholesterol carried by low-density lipoproteins (LDLs). LDLs circulate to body cells, carrying cholesterol and other lipids, where they may be used. LDL cholesterol may form deposits on artery and other blood vessel walls. LDLs—with a higher ratio of cholesterol to protein—are also manufactured in the liver. They are only in the body, not in food.

Fats. Group of compounds made of glycerol and fatty acids. Fats are one of three macronutrient groups that supply energy; the others are carbohydrates and proteins. Fats can be stored in the body.

> *Adipose tissue.* Scientific term for body fat.

> *Dietary fat.* Fats in food.

HOW MUCH OMEGA-3?

Oily fish, about 3 ounces, cooked	OMEGA-3S (GRAMS)	TOTAL FAT (GRAMS)
Atlantic herring	1.8	9.8
Anchovy, canned in oil, drained	1.8	8.3
Atlantic salmon, farmed	1.8	10.5
Chinook salmon	1.7	11.4
Atlantic mackerel	1.1	15.1
Rainbow trout, farmed	0.8	6.3
Less oily fish, about 3 ounces, cooked		
Tuna, white, canned in oil, drained	1.0	6.9
Tuna, white, canned in water, drained	0.7	2.5
Flounder	0.3	2.0
Halibut, Atlantic and Pacific	0.2	1.4
Tuna, light, canned in water, drained	0.2	0.7
Catfish, farmed	0.1	6.1
Cod, Atlantic	0.1	0.7

PLANT-BASED FOODS	ALA (CONVERTS TO EPA AND DHA) (GRAMS)*	TOTAL FAT (GRAMS)
Ground flaxseed, 2 tbsp.	3.2	6
Walnuts, 1 oz. (14 halves)	2.6	18.5
Canola oil, 1 tbsp.	1.3	14
Soy nuts, ¼ cup, dry roasted	0.6	9.3

Figures have been rounded.

*About 2 to 10 percent of ALA is converted to omega-3s.

Source: U.S. Department of Agriculture, National Nutrient Database for Standard Reference, Release 24, 2011.

Triglycerides. Scientific name for the common form of fat found both in the body and in foods. Most body fat is stored in the form of triglycerides; triglycerides also circulate in the blood. Triglycerides, made of three fatty acids and glycerol, act like saturated fat: they trigger the liver to make more cholesterol so levels of total and LDL cholesterol rise.

Functional Nutrition: Eat Your Omega-3s and -6s

No doubt about it: Seafood can be good for your health. Generally speaking, it has less total fat and less saturated fat than meat and poultry. For this reason, eating fish regularly may help lower your blood cholesterol levels. Moreover, seafood supplies several vitamins and minerals. The 2010 Dietary Guidelines recognizes the potential health benefits provided by the omega-3 fatty acids in fish!

Omega-3 fatty acids (EPA and DHA)—a type of polyunsaturated fatty acids—are found mostly in seafood, especially oily fish such as mackerel, albacore tuna, salmon, sardines, Atlantic herring, swordfish, and lake trout. Flaxseed oil, soybean oil, and canola oil, as well as walnuts, supply omega-3s, too, in the form of alpha-linolenic acid, some of which converts to EPA and DHA. Some eggs contribute significant amounts of omega-3s if the chicken feed supplied it.

Research suggests that omega-3s (EPA and DHA) may help thin blood and prevent blood platelets from clotting and sticking to artery walls. That, in turn, may help lower the risk for blocked blood vessels and heart attacks and strokes. These omega-3s may help prevent arteries from hardening, lower levels of triglycerides, and modestly reduce blood pressure levels. For those with cardiovascular disease, getting more ALAs from plant-based foods may offer benefits, but evidence is limited. In fact, more research is needed to know whether the amount of omega-3s produced from ALAs is sufficient to protect against heart disease.

Even if scientific evidence eventually completely explains the health benefits, omega-3 fatty acids by themselves aren't a magic remedy for heart disease—and you can't simply add them to your meals and snacks to get the potential benefits. Combined with eating less saturated fat in an overall healthful diet, they may have a protective effect.

Omega-3s, especially DHA, appear to have another benefit. Consuming two servings of fish (about eight ounces total) a week during pregnancy and nursing is linked to higher DHA levels in breast milk, as well as better cognitive development and vision in infants. The benefits outweigh potential risks of methyl mercury in some seafood. *Refer to chapter 13 for guidance on making educated seafood choices during pregnancy and nursing.*

Researchers are exploring other links between omega-3 fatty acids and health: eye health, rheumatoid arthritis, immunity and inflammation in the body that's linked to cardiovascular disease. Stay tuned!

To enjoy nutritional and omega-3s' benefits from some seafood, make fish a regular part of your eating style; eat oily fish twice weekly (8 ounces total per week). And try using foods with omega-3s in place of foods with more saturated fats.

How much omega-3s? The recommended amount isn't much; it adds up to 10 to 15 calories a day. The Institute of Medicine has set a daily Adequate Intake level: children ages four to eight years, 0.9 grams; boys ages nine to thirteen, 1.2 grams; girls ages nine to thirteen years, 1 gram; males ages fourteen years and older, 1.6 grams; females ages fourteen years and older, 1.1 grams; during pregnancy, 1.4 grams; and during breast-feeding, 1.3 grams. *Check the appendices for the Acceptable Macronutrient Distribution Range for omega-3s and omega-6s.*

Although fish oil supplements contain omega-3 fatty acids, they shouldn't be your first choice or be used in place of fish. Popping a fish oil capsule won't undo the effects of an otherwise unhealthful diet. Instead, enjoy fish for its nutritional benefits, flavor—and variety in your eating style. Remember food first. It's better to get omega-3s from food. For those with cardiovascular disease who don't consume enough omega-3s from food alone, the American Heart Association suggests talking to their doctor about fish oil supplements and safe dosages, especially for people with high triglycerides.

What about omega-6s (polyunsaturated fatty acids in vegetable oils)? They, too, may help reduce cardiovascular disease risk. Most people consume more than enough omega-6s. Some experts question if a substantial imbalance between omega-6s and omega-3s may interfere with the positive heart health benefits of omega-3s. However, more research is needed to determine this. Instead, focus on lowering saturated fats and replacing them with unsaturated fats for heart health benefits.

Another fatty acid—conjugated linoleic acid (CLA)—may offer functional benefits, too. CLAs, a type of *trans* fat, are naturally found in dairy foods and some meat products (beef, lamb). Research is exploring a potential link to decreased risk for certain cancers and a role in improved body composition. Little human research has yet been done.

Fatty acids. Basic units of fat molecules arranged as chains of carbon, hydrogen, and oxygen. Fats are mixtures of about sixteen different fatty acids, categorized by their structure. Each has its own unique physiological effect in your body. The terms "fats" and "fatty acids" are often used interchangeably.

Monounsaturated fatty acids (MUFAs). Chemically speaking, fatty acids missing one hydrogen pair on their chemical chain; they have one double bond. They trigger less total or LDL blood cholesterol, and more HDL blood cholesterol, production. Unsaturated fats are liquid at room temperature. Nuts, vegetable oils (such as canola oil, olive oil, high oleic safflower oil, and sunflower oil), and avocadoes are high in monounsaturated fatty acids.

Polyunsaturated fatty acids (PUFAs). Fatty acids missing two or more hydrogen pairs on their chemical chains; they have two or more double bonds. They also promote lower total blood cholesterol, as well as lower LDL and HDL cholesterol, production. Corn, safflower, soybean, sesame, and sunflower oils are high in polyunsaturated fatty acids. Fatty acids in seafood are mainly polyunsaturated, too.

Saturated fatty acids. Fatty acids that have all the hydrogen they can hold on their chemical chains; they have no double bonds. Except for stearic acid, saturated fats trigger the liver to make more total and LDL cholesterol than unsaturated fats do. In food, they come mainly from animal-based foods such as high-fat cuts of meat, butter, whole milk, whole milk products and cheese, and from coconut, palm, and palm kernel oils. Most saturated fats are solid at room temperature.

Oil. Fat in liquid form. They are mostly made of unsaturated fats.

Omega-3 fatty acids. Fatty acids (ALA, EPA or eicosapentaenoic acid, and DHA or docosahexaenoic acid) that are highly polyunsaturated. They may help reduce blood clotting in the arteries and protect from hardening of the arteries. Long-chain omega-3s (EPA and DHA) mostly come from seafood, especially oily fish such as albacore tuna, mackerel, and salmon; small amounts are converted from alpha-linolenic acid (a short-chain omega-3) in foods such as walnuts, and soybean, canola, and flaxseed oils.

Omega-6 fatty acids. Another group of polyunsaturated fatty acids. Linoleic acid is one type of omega-6 fatty acid. They, too, may help promote heart health by lowering total and LDL cholesterol. Vegetable oils—soybean, corn, safflower—are good sources.

Stearic acid. A type of saturated fatty acid that appears to have a neutral effect, neither raising nor lowering blood cholesterol levels. Dark chocolate and shea nut oil are high in stearic acid. It's also found in animal products, such as meat, milk, and milk products, and in some other plant-based foods.

Trans fatty acids. One type of fatty acid, formed during the process of partial hydrogenation. Although they're also found naturally in some

The "Good" and the "Bad"

Have you ever wondered what the terms "good" cholesterol and "bad" cholesterol really mean? They refer to cholesterol carried in your blood by two types of lipoproteins, and not to cholesterol in food.

Because cholesterol doesn't mix with water, it can't be carried alone in your bloodstream. Instead, it's combined in "packages" with fats and proteins. These packages, called lipoproteins, carry cholesterol both to and from your body cells.

The nicknames "good" and "bad" cholesterol relate to risk factors for heart disease. High levels of HDL, or "good," cholesterol are linked to *lower* heart disease risk; high levels of LDL, or "bad," cholesterol, to *higher* heart disease risk. Think "high" for health and "low" for less healthy. Total blood cholesterol consists of both HDL and LDL cholesterol.

Although HDL and LDL cholesterol aren't found in food, your food choices do influence LDL levels. If you lower the saturated fat and *trans* fat, and to a much smaller degree, cholesterol in your diet, you'll likely bring down LDL blood cholesterol levels. And if you're physically active, you'll likely lower your LDL cholesterol and keep your HDL blood cholesterol higher. What you eat and how active you are are just two of many factors that affect LDL, HDL, and total blood cholesterol levels. *Refer to "HDLs and LDLs: The Ups and the Downs" in chapter 22.*

foods, most *trans* fatty acids in the diet come from partially hydrogenated fats. In the body, man-made *trans* fats act like saturated fats and tend to raise blood cholesterol levels.

Hydrogenated fats. Unsaturated fats that are processed to make them more saturated, and stable and solid at room temperature—for example, in many packaged foods (such as crackers and cookies) and stick margarine. Hydrogen is added to their chemical makeup and makes them firmer and more saturated while extending their shelf life. The extent of hydrogenation determines whether there's a little or a lot of *trans* fats. An oil shown on a food label's ingredient list as "hydrogenated," rather than "partially hydrogenated," is fully saturated and has no *trans* fats. *See "About* Trans *Fats" in this chapter.*

Solid fats. This term is used in the 2010 Dietary Guidelines to refer to dietary fats that aren't liquid at room temperature. They contain more saturated fatty acids and/or *trans* fatty acids and less monounsaturated and polyunsaturated fatty acids than most oils do. Butter, stick margarine, suet (beef fat), and lard (pork fat) are solid fats. The top sources of solid fats in the U.S. diet include grain-based desserts; pizza; regular cheese; sausage, franks, bacon, and ribs; and fried potatoes.

AT A GLANCE: HOW DIETARY FAT AFFECTS BLOOD LIPIDS

TYPE OF FATTY ACIDS	EFFECTS ON BLOOD LIPIDS
Saturated	↑ total cholesterol, ↑ LDL cholesterol
Polyunsaturated	↓ total cholesterol, ↓ LDL cholesterol, ↓ HDL cholesterol*
Monounsaturated	↓ total cholesterol, ↓ LDL cholesterol, may ↑ HDL cholesterol*
Omega-3	↓ triglycerides, ↓ total cholesterol*
Trans	↑ total cholesterol, ↑ LDL cholesterol, may ↓ HDL cholesterol

*Unsaturated fatty acids may have a beneficial effect if they replace saturated fats, but not if they're simply added, making the diet higher in fat.

Have You Ever Wondered❓

. . . what trans-free spreads are? They're usually margarine-type products processed with little or no *trans* fatty acids. Their formulas differ and may contain fat replacers. Look for *trans* fat amounts on food labels.

. . . if melting a fat such as butter, stick margarine, or lard makes it less saturated? While unsaturated fats are liquid at room temperature, simply heating and melting doesn't change saturated fatty acids to unsaturated fatty acids. As soon as lard, margarine, or butter is cooled to room temperature, it's solid again.

. . . what high-oleic safflower and sunflower oils are? These oils, from high-oleic hybrid plants, are very high in monounsaturated fatty acids. They're used in baked goods, non-dairy creamers, crackers, cereals, and for frying as a substitute for saturated or *trans* fats. Without hydrogenation these oils are neutral in taste and very stable.

. . . why ground flaxseed often is recommended over whole flaxseed? Whole flaxseed passes through the GI tract without being digested. Unless it's ground, you miss out on the omega-3 benefits that flaxseed provides. Flaxseed oil is certainly a great option. However, it doesn't contain beneficial fiber and lignan supplied by ground flaxseeds. Buy ground flaxseed, or grind whole flaxseeds in a coffee grinder. Add them to smoothies, yogurt, sandwich spreads, baked goods, or your morning cereal.

. . . what shortening really is? It's simply another term that refers to fat. Solid at room temperature, shortening is vegetable oil (often partially hydrogenated soybean or cottonseed oil, palm oil, or coconut oil) sometimes combined with animal fat. As shortening is high in *"trans* fats" and perhaps "sat fats," go easy on foods made with shortening.

Fats: Not Created Equal

Whether solid or liquid, the fats that we consume are broken down into fatty acids and glycerol in the body. In turn, the body uses them to form other lipids, which are used for a variety of bodily functions. When fat is stored in your body, it's in the form of a triglyceride.

In scientific terms, fatty acids are chemical chains

of carbon, hydrogen, and oxygen. They may be saturated or unsaturated. The term "saturation" refers to how many hydrogen atoms link to each carbon in the chain.

● When carbon atoms have as many hydrogens attached as possible on the chain, a fatty acid is *saturated*.

● When hydrogen atoms are missing and a double bond forms between neighboring carbon atoms, the fatty acid is *unsaturated*. A polyunsaturated fatty acid has two or more missing hydrogen pairs; a monounsaturated fatty acid is missing one hydrogen pair on its chemical chain.

FATS AND OILS: HOW DO THEY COMPARE?

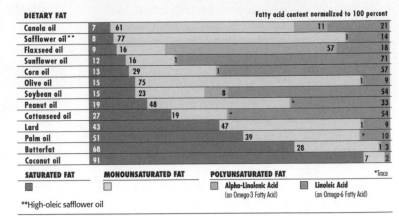

Fatty acid content normalized to 100 percent

DIETARY FAT	Saturated Fat	Monounsaturated Fat	Polyunsaturated Fat — Alpha-Linolenic Acid (an Omega-3 Fatty Acid)	Polyunsaturated Fat — Linoleic Acid (an Omega-6 Fatty Acid)
Canola oil	7	61	11	21
Safflower oil**	8	77	1	14
Flaxseed oil	9	16	57	18
Sunflower oil	12	16	1	71
Corn oil	13	29	1	57
Olive oil	15	75	1	9
Soybean oil	15	23	8	54
Peanut oil	19	48	*	33
Cottonseed oil	27	19	*	54
Lard	43	47	1	9
Palm oil	51	39	*	10
Butterfat	68	28	1	3
Coconut oil	91	7		2

*Trace
**High-oleic safflower oil

Source: Canolainfo/Canola Council of Canada, POS Pilot Plant Corporation.

Have You Ever Wondered

. . . if olive oil has fewer calories and less fat than butter? Because liquid oils are concentrated, and solid fats may contain a small amount of other ingredients besides fat, oils generally contain slightly more fat and calories than equal amounts of solid fat. Per tablespoon, olive oil contains about 14 grams of fat and 120 calories compared to butter, with about 12 grams of fat and 100 calories. The main difference is the types of fatty acids. Olive oil has a higher proportion of monounsaturated fatty acids; butter is more saturated.

. . . which has more solid fats: butter or margarine? One tablespoon of butter has about 7 grams of saturated plus about 0.5 grams *trans* fats; the same amount of some stick margarine usually has about 2 grams of saturated fat plus 2 to 3 grams of *trans* fats. Total fat is comparable.

Read the label to compare. Stick margarine has more *trans* fats; butter, more saturated fat. For less saturated and *trans* fats, tub margarine is an option.

. . . if foods made with fat replacers cause digestive discomfort? In the amounts generally consumed, likely not. However, consuming large amounts of fat-based replacers, such as olestra, and some carbohydrate-based fat replacers may cause short-term digestive discomfort, which comes from the added bulk from these ingredients.

Now what makes margarine different from vegetable oil? The fatty acid content. All foods with fats have a mixture of fatty acids: saturated, polyunsaturated, and monounsaturated. The proportion and differences in fatty acid content account for their varying characteristics—for example, liquid oil as compared with firm margarine. Their degree of saturation also has a significant role in how fatty acids from food affect health.

● Fats made mostly of saturated fatty acids usually are solid at room temperature. Animal-based foods and tropical vegetable oils (coconut, palm kernel, and palm) contain mainly saturated fatty acids. In general, harder and more stable fats are more saturated. They include butter, stick margarine, shortening, and the fat in cheese and meat.

● By contrast, fats that contain mostly polyunsaturated fatty acids usually are liquid at room temperature. Sunflower, corn, soybean, flaxseed, and cottonseed oils contain the highest amounts of polyunsaturated fats.

● Foods with mostly monounsaturated fatty acids are liquid at room temperature. They're found in more significant amounts in some vegetable oils, such as canola, olive, peanut, and high-oleic safflower oils.

Besides fats and oils, the proportion of fatty acids varies in other fat-containing foods. For example, seafood and meat both have saturated and unsaturated fatty acids. However, seafood has a higher proportion of polyunsaturated fatty acids; meat, more saturated fatty acids.

FAT, SATURATED FAT, AND CHOLESTEROL IN SOME FOODS*

	TOTAL FAT (G)	SATURATED FATTY ACIDS (G)	CHOLESTEROL (MG)	CALORIES
Grain Group				
Bread, 1 slice				
White (from refined wheat) (1 oz.)	1	Trace	0	75
Whole-wheat (1 oz.)	1	Trace	0	70
Egg bagel, ½ small (3-in. diameter)	1	Trace	8	95
Biscuit, homemade, 1 (2½-in. diameter)	10	3	2	210
Roll, dinner, 1 (1 oz.)	2	0.5	1	85
Croissant, 1 medium	12	7	38	230
Blueberry muffin, 1 (2¾-in. diameter)	13	2	26	260
Pancake, 1 (4-in. diameter)	1	0.2	5	75
Doughnut, yeast, glazed, 1 (3¾-in. diameter)	12	3.5	18	240
Danish pastry, cinnamon, 1 (4¼-in. diameter)	15	3.5	14	260
Oatmeal, cooked, ½ cup	2	0.4	0	85
Granola, homemade, ⅓ cup	10	1.5	0	195
Rice, white, cooked, ½ cup	Trace	Trace	0	105
Fried rice, restaurant, ½ cup	2	0.4	16	115
Dairy Group				
Milk, 1 cup				
Whole	8	4.5	24	150
2% reduced-fat	5	3	20	120
1% low-fat	2.5	1.5	12	100
Fat-free	Trace	Trace	5	85
Yogurt, 1 cup				
Low-fat plain	4	2.5	15	155
Cottage cheese, ½ cup				
Creamed	5	3	17	115
1% low-fat	1	1	5	80
Cheese, 1 oz.				
Natural Cheddar	9.5	6	30	115
Low-fat Cheddar	2	1	6	50
Mozzarella, part fat-free	6	3.5	15	85
Processed American	7	4.5	18	95
Vanilla ice cream, ½ cup	8	5	32	145
Frozen yogurt (not chocolate), ½ cup	3	2	11	110
Fruit Group				
Apple, 1 small (2¾-in. diameter)	Trace	Trace	0	75
Avocado, sliced, ½ cup	11	1.5	0	115
Olives, 5 large ripe	2.5	0.3	0	18

(continued)

Fat, Saturated Fat, and Cholesterol in Some Foods *(continued)*

	Total Fat (g)	Saturated Fatty Acids (g)	Cholesterol (mg)	Calories
Vegetable Group				
Potatoes				
Potato salad, homemade, ½ cup	10	2	85	180
French fries, 10 strips	5	1	0	205
Chips, 1 oz.	10	3	0	150
Coleslaw, homemade, ½ cup	2	0.5	5	50
Protein Foods Group				
Beef				
Lean cut (eye of round), roasted, 3 oz.				
Lean and fat, ⅛" trim	8	3	71	175
Lean only, ⅛" trim	4	1.5	65	145
Fattier cut (chuck blade), braised, 3 oz.				
Lean and fat, ⅛" trim	21	8.5	88	290
Lean only, 0" trim	11	4.5	90	215
Ground, cooked, 3 oz. patty				
70% lean	15	6	70	230
85% lean	13	5	76	210
95% extra lean	5	2	65	140
Pork center loin, roasted, 3 oz.				
Lean and fat	13	4	69	215
Lean	8.5	3	69	185
Beef liver, braised, 3 oz.	4.5	1.5	337	160
Chicken, breast, roasted, ½				
With skin	8	2	82	195
Without skin	3	1	73	140
Salmon, Atlantic, farmed, cooked, 3 oz.	10.5	2	54	175
Tuna, canned, 3 oz.				
In oil	7	1	26	160
In water	2.5	Trace	36	110
Shrimp, steamed or boiled, 8 large	0.5	Trace	93	52
Frankfurters, beef (48 g)	14	6	28	155
Dry beans, cooked, ½ cup	0.5	Trace	0	105
Peanut butter, 2 tbsp.	16	3	0	190
Sunflower seeds, 1 oz.	14	1.5	0	165
Egg, large, cooked, 1	4.5	1.5	185	72
yolk, 1	4.5	1.5	185	55
white, 1	Trace	0	0	17

	TOTAL FAT (G)	SATURATED FATTY ACIDS (G)	CHOLESTEROL (MG)	CALORIES
Solid Fats, Oils				
Butter, 1 tbsp.	11.5	7	31	100
Margarine, stick, 1 tbsp.	11.5	2	0	100
Vegetable oil (corn), 1 tbsp.	14	2	0	120
Salad dressing, 1 tbsp.				
Mayonnaise, regular	5	1	4	60
Mayonnaise, light	5	1	5	50
Italian	4	0.5	0	45
Italian, reduced-fat	1	Trace	1	10
Cream, 1 tbsp.				
Sour, regular	2.5	1.5	6	25
Light (table)	3	2	10	30
Cream cheese, 1 tbsp.	5	3	16	50
Sweetened Snacks, Desserts				
Cookie, chocolate chip, made with butter (2¼-in. diameter)	4.5	2.2	11	78
Cake, chocolate, frosted, 1 piece (¹⁄₁₂ of cake)	28	8	33	537
Pie, apple, ⅛ of 9-inch	19.5	5	0	410
Cheesecake, no-bake, ¹⁄₁₂ of 9-inch	12	7	29	270
Milk chocolate bar, 1.55 oz.	13	8	10	235

* Values are rounded.

Source: U.S. Department of Agriculture, Agricultural Research Service, 2005. U.S. Department of Agriculture, National Nutrient Database for Standard Reference, Release 24, 2011.

About Trans *Fats*

"Trans" refers to fatty acids with a certain chemical makeup. *Trans* fats are created when processing changes the structure of liquid oils with more unsaturated fatty acids to become semi-solid fats, which are more saturated and also more stable at room temperature. The process is called hydrogenation; hydrogen is added to fatty acid chains in their chemical makeup to make them more saturated. Usually hydrogenation is partial, making fat 5 to 60 percent saturated. The results are *trans* fatty acids.

Beef, pork, lamb, butter, and milk naturally have small amounts of *trans* fatty acids, too. The type, conjugated linoleic acid, has different physiological effects than most synthetic forms of *trans* fats.

Why hydrogenate the oil? Forty to fifty years ago, this process offered a way to provide food products that helped consumers follow advice of that time for heart health: simply to replace saturated with unsaturated fats. In those days, partially hydrogenated fats were considered healthier than animal fats; for example, stick margarine was recommended over butter. Back then, no scientific evidence showed that *trans* fats, created by hydrogenation, had their own health risks. With today's research evidence, *trans* fats are well known to increase heart disease risk.

Why hydrogenation? It gives desirable qualities to food. For example, because hydrogenated fats are more stable, they extend the shelf life of foods such as crackers and margarine so they don't develop a rancid flavor and odor as quickly. Hydrogenating the oil in peanut butter gives a creamy consistency; oil stays mixed in and doesn't rise to the top. Stick margarine and shortening remain firm at room temperature when partially hydrogenated.

Stick margarine is more hydrogenated than soft margarine sold in tubs or as "squeeze" margarine. Tub and squeeze margarines contain more water, and may have air whipped in so they may be lower in fat and calories.

Why the concern about *trans* fats? *Trans* fatty acids act like saturated fats, raising LDL ("bad") blood cholesterol levels and potentially decreasing HDL ("good") cholesterol. That, in turn, may increase the risk for fatty deposits on blood vessel walls and heart attacks. *Trans* fatty acids supply about 2 to 3 percent of total calories for American adults; saturated fat intake is more than 11 percent. Still, it's wise to be prudent, especially if you have high cholesterol levels already. You don't need *trans* fats for normal health.

As the 2010 Dietary Guidelines advises: *Keep* trans *fatty acid consumption as low as possible by limiting foods that contain synthetic sources of* trans *fats, such as partially hydrogenated oils, and by limiting other solid fats.* And at the same time, consume a healthful eating plan. Because they occur naturally in nutrient-rich foods such as beef and milk, you can't eliminate *trans* fats completely.

To cut back on *trans* fat, check food labels. As of 2006 *trans* fats were required on the Nutrition Facts panel, along with total and saturated fats. Why might a product with partially hydrogenated oil say "0 *trans* fats" on the label? Due to rounding, less than (<) 0.5 grams of *trans* fats is considered zero; food labels

must follow federal law. Go easy on foods with "partially hydrogenated vegetable oil" as one of the first ingredients: stick margarine, vegetable shortening, and many prepared foods, cakes, cookies, crackers, snack foods, and some commercially fried foods, including some fried fast foods.

Note: For nutrition labeling, FDA has excluded naturally occurring conjugated linoleic acid from its definition of *trans* fats.

Over the past few years many food manufacturers have reformulated their food products to reduce or remove *trans* fats without increasing saturated fats. In fact, many of today's chips, breakfast cereals, and granolas are *trans*-fat free. Read the label! In some parts of the United States, *trans* fat-containing cooking oils are banned; even fast food chains must use *trans* fat-free oils for frying.

Fat: More Than Meets the Eye!

Visible or not, almost all foods contain fat in varying amounts. Some are very high in fat; others have just trace amounts.

The fat content of some foods is obvious: for example, in butter, oil, and margarine. Even in certain cuts of meat and poultry with the skin on, fat is easy to see—and easy to trim off.

In most foods, however, clues to a food's fat content appear on food labels. The Nutrition Facts panel tells how much total, saturated, and *trans* fats per label serving. Salad dressings, many baked foods, chips, crackers, chocolate, nuts, avocados, sauces, meat, poultry, fish, cheese, dairy products, and egg yolks, for example, all contain varying amounts of fat. Obviously, fried foods contain more fat than those that are baked or steamed.

Which foods typically supply the most fat?

● On average, most fat in the American diet comes directly from fats and oils, as well as salad dressings, candy, gravies, and sauces.

● Animal-based foods provide varying amounts of total fat and saturated fat. With lean and fat-modified products on the market, check the Nutrition Facts on food labels to know how much and which types.

● Some major sources of solid fats (saturated and *trans* fats) in the U.S. diet are grain-based desserts, pizza, regular cheese, sausage, franks, bacon, ribs, and fried white potatoes.

● With only a few exceptions (avocados and olives), fruits and vegetables don't supply much fat naturally. That's true for most grain products, too—unless it's added during food preparation or processing; for example, in French fries, fried okra, croissants, and hush puppies.

About Fat Replacers . . .

Today's supermarkets sell options! Foods made with fat-reduction ingredients can help you consume less fat if they really replace full-fat products in your food choices. They can help you expand your food choices for healthy, flavorful eating as you control fat and/or calories, too. These foods have much of the taste, texture, and appearance of their higher-fat counterparts. Besides being lower in fat, they're usually, but not always, lower in saturated fat, cholesterol, and calories as well.

Fat gives unique characteristics to food, so when fat is removed from a "recipe," perhaps to make a low-fat cookie, many characteristics of the food change, too. Fat replacers can give these foods a familiar texture, appearance, and taste.

Ingredients used to replace fat are made from different building blocks, such as carbohydrates, fats, or proteins. Most contribute calories, although less than fat does. Because no fat replacer acts exactly like fat, most reduced-fat and fat-free products contain a mixture of fat replacers to get a desirable result. From a food safety standpoint, scientific research and review by the U.S. Food and Drug Administration (FDA) recognize fat replacers as safe. New products must go through thorough review.

Carbohydrate-Based Fat Replacers

These fat replacers combine with water to provide texture, appearance, and mouth feel similar to fat and to retain moisture. They include carrageenan, cellulose, gelatin, gellan gum, gels, guar gum, maltodextrins, polydextrose, starches, xanthum gum, and modified dietary fibers. Fat-free salad dressings, for example, contain carbohydrate-based substitutes. The calories in carbohydrate-

based replacers range from almost nothing to 4 calories per gram compared to 9 calories per gram of fat. The difference is that some, such as modified starches and dextrins, are digested; others, such as cellulose and other fibers, aren't digested, so they are essentially calorie free. Most of these fat replacers can withstand some heat; however, they can't be used for frying.

Pureed prunes (dried plums) and applesauce sometimes are used as fat replacers in baked foods. They're an easy fat substitute you can try yourself. Pureed prunes and applesauce add bulk, flavor, and nutrition.

Protein-Based Fat Replacers

Made with protein from egg whites or fat-free milk, these fat replacers provide a creamy sensation and

---

FAT REPLACERS: ONE WAY TO LOWER FAT AND CALORIES

Fat-modified foods can make a difference in the calories and fat of a meal. Foods with fat replacers may have more carbohydrates; that's why the percent of fat reduction may be higher than the percent of calorie reduction.

	CALORIES	FAT (GRAMS)
Regular Lunch		
2 slices bread	130	2
1 oz. American cheese	95	7
2 oz. bologna	175	14
1 tbsp. mayonnaise	100	11
Banana	105	0
2 chocolate chip cookies (30 g)	160	9
Total	765	43
Lunch with Fat-Modified Foods		
2 slices bread	130	2
l oz. reduced-fat cheese product	60	3
2 oz. fat-free bologna	45	0
1 tbsp. low-fat mayonnaise/dressing	50	5
Banana	105	0
2 reduced-fat chocolate chip cookies (30 g)	140	5
Total	530	15

Source: Adapted from International Food Information Council Foundation, ific.org, and U.S. Department of Agriculture, National Nutrient Database for Standard Reference, Release 24, 2011.

improve appearance and texture when fat is removed. Low-fat cheese made with a protein-based substitute gives an appearance and texture that come close to full-fat cheese. Most protein-based replacers aren't used in foods prepared at high temperatures. That's because the protein coagulates, and they no longer function in ways similar to fat. Whey protein concentrate, microparticulated egg white, and milk protein (Simplesse) fit in this category.

Protein-based replacers contribute 1 to 4 calories per gram, compared with 9 calories per fat gram. What accounts for the calorie range? These replacers may be blended with ingredients such as cellulose that can't be digested. Protein-based replacers provide small amounts of amino acids.

Fat-Based Replacers

These are made with fats that have been altered. They provide few or no calories as compared to fat because the body is unable to fully absorb the fatty acids. Because they're made from fats, their physical properties—taste, texture, and mouthfeel—are the same as fat. They may be used in baked foods, some fried foods, cake mixes, frosting, and dairy foods.

Olestra is a calorie-free fat replacer made from vegetable oils and sugar. It contributes no calories because it passes through the body without being digested and absorbed. Olestra provides the characteristics of fat in cooking, especially for frying and snack foods. Olean is the brand name for olestra that you'll see on food labels. Because olestra isn't digested, some vita-

Functional Nutrition: Plant Stanols and Sterols

Phytosterols (plant stanols and sterols) are found naturally in fruits, vegetables, vegetable oils, whole grains, nuts, and seeds. Although similar in structure to cholesterol, they function differently. Instead of raising blood cholesterol levels, they prevent cholesterol absorption in the intestines, which, in turn, helps to reduce blood levels of total and LDL ("bad") cholesterol—but they don't affect HDLs or triglycerides.

Getting enough phytosterols from food isn't easy. The average person consumes less than 500 milligrams (0.5 grams) of phytosterols a day, not enough to lower blood cholesterol levels. For that reason, food manufacturers are fortifying some food products with plant stanols and sterols: for example, some butterlike spreads, mayonnaise, yogurt beverages, milk, orange juice, cereals, chocolate, and snack bars. Check the ingredient list and label to know if they contain stanols and sterols, and how much. Studies show that stanols and sterols may lower LDL-cholesterol levels by about 6 percent on average, and for some people, perhaps as much as 14 percent in four weeks.

Two spreads—Promise active and Benecol—contain these unique dietary ingredients. Use them in food preparation, not only as a spread. Benecol regular spread (with plant stanol esters) can be used in cooking and baking without changing the flavor of food. Use it like any margarine, substituting it equally for the fat, oil, or shortening in a recipe. A spread with plant sterols (Promise active) isn't recommended for baking or frying; use it in foods that aren't cooked.

Foods fortified with plant stanols and sterols offer cholesterol-lowering benefits. Research shows that people with elevated cholesterol levels benefit most. The National Cholesterol Education Program of the National Institutes of Health recommends consuming two grams of plant stanol/sterols every day as part of an overall heart-healthy diet. For example, two to three tablespoons of margarine spread with plant stanols or sterols have that much, as do two cups of orange juice fortified with plant sterols.

As part of a low-fat eating plan, plant stanols and sterols appear to be equally effective in lowering LDL-cholesterol. They aren't meant to replace statin drug therapy, but they may help lower cholesterol further as part of a healthful eating plan.

The U.S. Food and Drug Administration (FDA)–approved health claim on phytosterols states: "Foods containing at least 0.65 gram per serving of vegetable oil plant sterol esters, eaten twice a day with meals for a daily total intake of at least 1.3 grams, as part of a diet low in saturated fat and cholesterol, may reduce the risk of heart disease." Read the package label for serving size.

Plant stanols and sterols in soft-gel form are available as supplements, but talk to your doctor before taking them.

Have You Ever Wondered

. . . if using olive oil and canola oil in your food prep is healthful? Sure—if you substitute them for solid fats. Both oils are high in monounsaturated fatty acids and low in saturated fatty acids. Fats higher in monounsaturated fatty acids may help lower blood cholesterol levels when they replace fats higher in unsaturated fatty acids. However, simply adding olive or canola oil to an already high-fat diet is not the point. These oils are still 100 percent fat, with about 120 calories per tablespoon.

. . . what is the source of canola oil? Extracted from the seeds of the canola plant, canola oil is healthy oil that is very low in saturated fat, yet a great source of mono- and polyunsaturated fats, including omega-3s. Its name derives from Canada oil, where it was originally developed. Canola oil differs from rapeseed oil in a significant way. To clarify a misperception, canola oil is extremely low in erucic acid. While erucic acid hasn't been shown to affect human health, it's been linked to cardiac abnormalities in experimental animals. The U.S. Food and Drug Administration deems canola oil safe in food. The Codex Alimentaris has defined the maximum amount of erucic acid and glucosinolates that may be found in a seed before it may be called canola.

. . . if cholesterol supplies calories? Often confused with fat, cholesterol isn't a source of energy, or calories. Unlike fats, carbohydrates, and proteins, cholesterol isn't broken down, so the body cannot derive any energy from it.

. . . what tropical oils are? And how they stack up for nutrition? Tropical oils (coconut, palm, palm kernel) come from the fruit or nuts of the tropical plants they're named for. Their fats are highly saturated. You may not think you consume coconut or palm oils, but they're often used in processed foods, imparting qualities similar to partially hydrogenated oils. Palm oil also has quite a bit of polyunsaturated fat; coconut oil contains a fatty acid, called lauric acid, with possible health benefits. Until more is known, read the ingredient list on food labels; limit foods made with tropical oils.

mins (A, D, E, and K) carried by fat in these foods aren't fully absorbed. For this reason, fat-soluble vitamins are added to make up for possible losses.

Salatrim, caprenin, and mono- and diglycerides are other fat-based replacers used in baked goods, dairy products, and confection-type products. Salatrim provides calories, but only 5 calories per gram (as compared to 9 calories per gram in fat) because it is only partially absorbed in the body.

What Foods Contain Fat Replacers?

Check the ingredient list on all kinds of reduced-fat, low-fat, or fat-free foods: for example, salad dressing, mayonnaise, cheese, sour cream, ice cream, yogurt, pudding, gravy, margarine, butter, processed meat, baked foods, and candy. A combination of fat replacers may be used for the best texture and taste in fat-reduced foods.

To some degree, fat replacers supply calories, so the energy contributed by fat-modified foods may or may not be less than the original food. For the calories and fat per serving, check the Nutrition Facts panel on the food label. And go easy. Less fat is no license to overeat!

The bottom line: Foods with fat replacers can be a safe and effective option for making meals and snacks appealing—and at the same time, for controlling the fat and energy in your food choices.

Cholesterol: Different from Fat

To clear up a common misperception, cholesterol is a fatlike substance, and not a fat. Cholesterol has a different structure from fat and performs different functions in the human body. Some functions promote health; some don't. Because fat and cholesterol often appear together in foods of animal origin, and because their roles in health are so intertwined, they're easily mixed up.

Based on its biochemical makeup, cholesterol is a sterol. However, it's quite different from phytosterols, or stanols and sterols that occur naturally in plant cells. *See "Functional Nutrition: Plant Stanols and Sterols" in this chapter.*

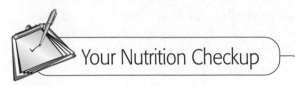

Your Nutrition Checkup

Fat Intake Audit

What's the fat and cholesterol quotient of your eating style? To be fat savvy, limit solid fats, as well as calories from total fat. *Remember:* Your overall fat intake over time is what counts—not each individual choice. Small steps to healthier eating add up.

☐ Choose lean meats, poultry, and seafood.

☐ Choose fat-free and low-fat milk and milk products.

☐ Eat fewer foods with solid fats, such as cakes, cookies, and other desserts made with butter, margarine, or shortening, as well as fewer sausages, hot dogs, bacon and ribs, regular cheese perhaps on pizza, and full-fat ice cream.

☐ When cooking, replace solid fats such as butter, beef fat, chicken fat, lard, stick margarine, and shortening with oils.

☐ Choose cooking methods that do not add fat.

☐ Choose baked, steamed, or broiled foods rather than fried foods most often.

☐ Read ingredient lists to limit foods with partially hydrogenated oils, a major source of *trans* fats, and choose foods that contain oils with more unsaturated fats.

☐ Check the Nutrition Facts on food labels to choose foods with little or no saturated fat and no *trans* fat.

☐ As a spread, choose soft margarines with zero *trans* fats.

☐ If you use butter, use just a small amount.

☐ Use vegetable oil, such as olive, canola, corn, safflower, or sunflower oil, rather than solid fats, such as stick margarine, butter, shortening, and lard, in cooking.

☐ Consider calories when adding oils to food or in cooking—only small amounts to control calories.

Like fat, cholesterol often gets a "bad rap," yet it's part of every body cell and of some hormones, including sex hormones such as estrogen. As part of a body chemical called bile, it helps the body digest and absorb fat, too. With the help of sunlight, a form of cholesterol in your skin can change to vitamin D, a nutrient essential for bone building. However, too much cholesterol in the bloodstream can lead to the buildup of fatty deposits in blood vessels. This in turn limits blood flow to arteries and can cause a heart attack.

Dietary vs. Blood Cholesterol

Confused about cholesterol? You're not alone! Actually, the term itself refers to two different types. Dietary cholesterol comes from food. Blood, or serum, cholesterol circulates in the bloodstream.

Cholesterol that circulates in your body comes from two sources:

● *Your body produces most of the cholesterol in your bloodstream*—enough for your needs. Your liver makes most of it, but every body cell can make cholesterol, too. In fact, when the body makes too much, the risk for heart disease goes up. Unlike adults, infants and young children don't produce enough cholesterol, so for children under age two, it's important that their food choices supply cholesterol.

● *Cholesterol also comes from foods and beverages of animal origin:* eggs, meat, poultry, fish, and dairy foods. Animals produce cholesterol, but plants don't. A diet high in cholesterol is one factor that elevates blood cholesterol levels for some people. That's why the Dietary Guidelines advises: *Consume less than 300 milligrams of cholesterol a day.* Dietary cholesterol doesn't automatically become blood cholesterol. Solid fats (saturated fat and *trans* fats) in your food choices affect blood cholesterol levels more than dietary cholesterol alone does.

Furthermore, because of genetic differences, individuals respond differently to the cholesterol in food. *See chapter 22 for more about cholesterol and risk factors for heart disease.*

Since the human body can make enough, no Dietary Reference Intakes for cholesterol have been established.

Cholesterol: In What Foods?

Only foods of animal origin contain cholesterol. Egg yolks and organ meats are especially high in cholesterol. And in varying amounts, meat, poultry, seafood, dairy products, and animal fats such as butter or lard all supply cholesterol, too. Cholesterol is not found in vegetable oils, margarine, or egg whites, or in plant-based foods such as grains, fruits, vegetables, beans, and peas.

As mentioned before, cholesterol and saturated fatty acids often occur together in animal-based foods. That's why they sometimes get confused. Sirloin steak, butter, and Cheddar cheese, for example, all contain both saturated fatty acids and cholesterol. On the other hand, shellfish and organ meats are high in cholesterol, yet they're low in saturated fatty acids.

In foods of animal origin, both lean and fatty tissues contain cholesterol. That's why some low-fat foods, such as squid and shrimp, can be relatively high in cholesterol. The sauce or butter they're dipped in can boost their cholesterol content, too.

Even though some plant-based foods (margarine, vegetable oil, nuts, and seeds) are high in fat or saturated fat, they have no cholesterol, even margarines made with *trans* fats.

So why do some vegetable dishes and grain-based baked goods contain cholesterol? It's the added ingredients: egg yolks, cheese, milk, meat, poultry, butter, or lard. Some common examples are refried beans made with lard, greens cooked with bacon, and muffins made with butter and egg yolks. The amount of cholesterol per serving varies with the recipe.

When shopping, if you spot a food that's labeled "no cholesterol" or "cholesterol-free," it cannot have any more than 2 grams of saturated fat. However, you'll want to read the rest of the food label to find out about the fat content; it could still be high in total fat or *trans* fat.

Too Much of a Good Thing?

An eating pattern that's high in fats, especially from solid fats, is linked to higher blood cholesterol levels and increases the risk of heart disease and type 2 diabetes.

Weight control is a good reason to go easy on fat since high-fat foods are often high in calories, too. And high-fat diets tend to be high in excess calories, as well as solid fats. Whether they're saturated or unsaturated, calories from fat are all alike. Every fat gram supplies 9 calories, or more than twice the amount provided by 1 gram of carbohydrate or protein. And excess calories, whether from fats, carbohydrates, or proteins, are stored in the body as fat. *Remember:* The total amount of calories eaten, not just the calories from fat, is the issue in weight management.

For more about the effects of fat, saturated fat, trans *fat, and cholesterol on heart disease and type 2 diabetes, see chapter 22.*

Fat and Cholesterol: Know Your Limits

How much fat is enough? That depends. The Dietary Reference Intakes recommend a range, not a single amount. The range is linked to a lower risk of chronic disease, yet allows for an eating plan with enough essential nutrients. Age is factored into the recommendations. And specific amounts depend on how many calories you consume overall. For adults, the 2010 Dietary Guidelines advises:

- *Consume less than 10 percent of calories from saturated fatty acids by replacing them with monounsaturated and polyunsaturated fatty acids.*

- *Consume less than 300 milligrams per day of dietary cholesterol.*

- *Keep* trans *fatty acid consumption as low as possible by limiting foods that contain synthetic sources of* trans *fats, such as partially hydrogenated oils, and by limiting other solid fats.*

- *Reduce the intake of solid fats and added sugars.*

What if you eat less than 20 percent of your calories from fat and oils? You might come up short on vitamin E, a fat-soluble vitamin with antioxidant powers that may be cardioprotective. Another possibility: missing out on essential fatty acids, which only food provides.

To clear up any confusion, advice for fat intake applies to your total diet, *not* to a single food or a single meal. Rather than focus on the percentage of fat within the 20 to 35 percent range, focus on the type of fat. Choose mostly mono- and polyunsaturated fats and fewer solid fats (saturated and *trans* fats). And the percent of calories you consume from fat—over several days—impacts your health. So don't worry or feel guilty if you occasionally eat more. Just make it up by eating less on other days.

In real numbers, how much is 20 to 35 percent calories from total fat—and less than 7 or 10 percent calories from "sat fat"? The specific amount depends on your energy needs. And that depends on your age, gender, body size, and activity level. *See "What's Your Limit on Fat and Saturated Fat?" in this chapter.* You can check the bottom of the Nutrition Facts panel on many food labels. For a 2,000- and a 2,500-calorie diet, it shows how many fat grams equal less than 30 percent of calories from fat. Guidelines for saturated fat from the American Heart Association are lower than the Dietary Guidelines. For heart health, the American Heart Association advises less than 7 percent of calories from saturated fatty acids. *See chapter 22.*

To guesstimate your calorie need, see "Your 'Weigh': Figuring Your Energy Needs" in chapter 2.

Fat in Your Food Choices

Do you consume too many calories from fat? Too many solid fats? From a health standpoint, spend your fat calories wisely; cut back if you need to and switch to oils!

To do that, the 2010 Dietary Guidelines not only advise more fruit and vegetables, which are naturally low in fat, they also advise:

● *Replace protein foods that are higher in solid fats with choices that are lower in solid fats and calories and/or are sources of oils.*

● *Limit the consumption of foods that contain refined grains, especially refined-grains foods that contain solid fats, added sugars, and sodium.*

● *Use oils to replace solid fats where possible and increase the intake of fat-free or low-fat milk and milk products.*

● *Increase the amount and variety of seafood consumed by choosing seafood in place of some meat and poultry.*

Cutting back on fat or switching solid fats to healthier unsaturated fats doesn't need to be a huge

---

Why Oils?

You know you need fat for health, energy, and for kids, growth. Most of it should be polyunsaturated or monounsaturated, the kinds you find in oils, such as canola, corn, olive, safflower, sunflower, and soybean oils.

All fats are made of saturated, polyunsaturated, and monounsaturated fatty acids, but the proportions differ; see *"Fats and Oils: How Do They Compare?"* earlier in this chapter. Their differences determine how they affect your health.

Polyunsaturated fats contain essential fatty acids, necessary for health. That's why the USDA Food Patterns have a category for oil; *refer to chapter 10 to learn more.* Besides their essential fatty acids, oils are the major source of vitamin E for most Americans. Another reason to consume oils in place of solid fats: neither monounsaturated nor polyunsaturated fats raise total or LDL ("bad") cholesterol levels in the blood. Oils are heart healthier.

That said, oils do provide calories: 120 calories per tablespoon, about the same as solid fats. You need to limit how much you consume to stay within your calorie budget; *see chapter 10.*

---

change. Even small changes add up. Often eating a smaller portion of a high-fat dessert, switching to lean meat and low-fat or fat-free dairy products, eating broiled rather than fried foods, and using soft tub instead of stick margarine can make a daily difference.

Remember that any type of fat is a concentrated source of calories. Rather than add fat to your eating plan, substitute unsaturated fats for solid fats (saturated and *trans* fats). You'll not only avoid added calories, but substituting rather than adding is a smart strategy for lowering risks for heart disease and type 2 diabetes.

Keep in mind that you can reduce fat, including solid fats, from your food choices in many ways. To start, try strategies listed here.

For Less Solid Fat . . .

Did you know that nearly 11 percent of the solid fat consumed in the United States comes from grain-based desserts? About 9 percent comes from pizza, regular cheese delivers more than 7 percent, and

What's Your Limit on Fat and Saturated Fat?

| | | LIMIT YOUR DAY'S SATURATED FAT INTAKE. | |
IF YOU CONSUME THIS AMOUNT OF CALORIES A DAY . . .	KEEP YOUR DAILY TOTAL FAT INTAKE WITHIN THIS RANGE (20 TO 35 PERCENT CALORIES)	SHORT-TERM GOAL: LESS THAN 10 PERCENT OF CALORIES	LONG-TERM GOAL: LESS THAN 7 PERCENT OF CALORIES
1,600	36 to 62 g	18 g or less	12 g or less
2,000	44 to 78 g	20 g or less	16 g or less
2,200	49 to 86 g	24 g or less	17 g or less
2,500	56 to 97 g	25 g or less	19 g or less
2,800	62 to 109 g	31 g or less	22 g or less

*Reflects 2010 Dietary Guidelines, adult recommendations.

sausage, franks, bacon, and ribs do, too. And fried white potatoes provide nearly 5 percent of solid fats. With that in mind, how might you trim solid fats in your food choices?

● Know where fat comes from. You can't cut back unless you know the sources of fat. *See "Fat, Saturated Fat, and Cholesterol in Some Foods" in this chapter.*

● Check the Nutrition Facts on food labels for how much fat, including saturated fat, *trans* fat, and cholesterol, a single label serving contains. *To learn how to best use the Nutrition Facts panel, see "Get All the Facts!" in chapter 12.*

● Look for nutrient content claims on the label, perhaps "low-fat" or "lean." As you shop, use these clues to help guide your food purchases. *To learn what these claims mean, see "Label Lingo: Fats and Cholesterol" in this chapter.*

● Choose lean meat (beef, veal, and/or pork) and skinless poultry. Loin and round cuts of meat have less fat. Trim visible fat from meat and poultry; remove skin from poultry. Lean meat isn't fat-free; it just has less fat.

Lean meat contains cholesterol in both the fat and in lean muscle tissue. Trimming the fat and buying lean cuts also reduce the cholesterol in meat but won't make it cholesterol-free.

● Make your meals "fishy." Enjoy seafood several times a week, prepared a low-fat way. Go for fish, preferably oily fish such as salmon, twice a week, 4 ounces cooked portion each, to get the potential omega-3 benefits.

● Eat plenty of fruits and vegetables. Besides being low in fat they fill you up and help curb your appetite.

● Go for grains—refined grain and whole-grain foods—with less fat. Choose lower-fat grain products—pasta, rice, breakfast cereal, bagels, tortillas, pita, and other lower-fat breads. Limit doughnuts, sweet rolls, higher-fat muffins, cakes, and cookies.

● Choose mostly low-fat or fat-free dairy products. The bone-building nutrients in fat-free, low-fat, and whole-milk products are about the same.

● Consider today's fat-modified foods on supermarket shelves: for example, fat-free salad dressing, low-fat snacks, *trans*-free spreads, and eggs with omega-3s. *Remember:* Many lower-fat processed foods have the same or more total calories than their traditional counterparts. Read the Nutrition Facts.

● Watch your "snack fats." Smart snacks fill in missing nutrient gaps, help control hunger, and can provide an energy boost between meals. But some popular snack foods are higher in fat, especially solid fats, than you may realize.

● Defat your cooking style without losing flavor. Broil, bake, boil, steam, stir-fry, or microwave foods, rather than fry.

● Add flavor with herbs and spices instead of high-fat sauces. Rub seasonings mixture of on tender cuts of meat before cooking. Use low-fat or fat-free marinades to tenderize and add flavor to lean cuts of meat.

● Watch your portion sizes. For higher-fat foods, the amount of fat and calories goes up when portions get bigger.

● Make beans the "main event" at meals occasionally. As the main protein source, most bean dishes are lower in total fat, saturated fat, and cholesterol—yet higher in starches (complex carbohydrates) and fiber—than dishes made with meat or cheese.

● Order "lean" when you order out. In a fast-food or table-service restaurant, look for menu clues that suggest less fat, such as "grilled" or "broiled." Ask questions about food prep. Go easy on foods that are fried, breaded, or prepared with rich sauces or gravy. *See chapter 15 for eating out tips.*

Have You Ever Wondered ?

. . . if nuts are heart healthy? There's some research evidence to suggest they are. If they're part of an overall eating pattern that's nutritionally adequate and without excess calories, they have a positive impact on risk factors for cardiovascular disease, especially blood lipid levels. Being a good source of protein, nuts are high in fat, but it's mostly unsaturated. An important reminder is to enjoy unsalted nuts in small portions, as they're high in calories and can contribute to weight gain. Like oils, different nuts have different amounts of various fats: total, saturated, mono-unsaturated, and polyunsaturated fats.

. . . how chocolate affects heart health? Chocolate is a gift from the heart, but the heart-healthy benefits and risks are minimal since chocolate is a small part of the diet. The main fat in chocolate is stearic acid, which doesn't raise blood cholesterol levels. And although product formulations vary, darker chocolate has less dairy fat and therefore somewhat less saturated fat. Heart healthy benefits may come from the flavonoids in chocolate; *see chapter 6 to learn more.* However, note that chocolate is often partnered with added sugars, and chocolate candy and desserts are typically high-calorie foods.

. . . if coconut milk is high in fat? One cup of canned coconut milk (made by combining grated coconut meat and coconut water) contains 445 calories and 48 fat grams (of which 43 fat grams are saturated). Coconut water, or liquid, drained from a fresh coconut—without any grated coconut meat—has just 46 calories and less than 1 fat gram per cup. Just ¼ cup of dried, sweetened coconut has 87 calories and 6 fat grams. Look for canned coconut milk with less fat.

. . . if air-popped popcorn is always low in fat? Not always. If you buy it ready-made, check the Nutrition Facts for total fat, saturated fat, and *trans* fat content. Although the package may say "air-popped," oil may be added after popping as a flavoring. For microwave popcorn, check the label to see if oil is added—and how much and what kind. The bucket of popcorn you buy in malls or movie theaters is usually loaded with fat. Satisfy your appetite with the small-size order.

. . . if ghee is a good substitute for butter? Common in the cuisine of India, ghee is clarified butter. It's been heated, then strained to remove milk solids so the fat is slightly concentrated—with more fat and calories per teaspoon. Why clarify butter? Without milk solids, it can be heated to a higher temperature without burning.

. . . how the fat in feta cheese compares with that in other cheeses? It's somewhat lower—but not much. An ounce of feta cheese has 6 grams of fat, which includes 4 grams of saturated fat. By comparison, 1 ounce of Cheddar cheese has 9 total fat grams, including 6 grams of saturated fat. With their intense flavors, small amounts of strong cheeses such as feta, Parmesan, and blue cheese go a long way in delivering flavor.

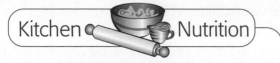

Kitchen Nutrition

Yogurt Cheese

Create your own "fat replacer": yogurt cheese as a thick spread, creamy dip, or baked potato topper. It's low in fat, yet high in calcium.

Line a strainer with a paper coffee filter, or use a strainer specially meant for making yogurt cheese. Place it over a deep bowl. Spoon gelatin-free yogurt (plain or flavored) in the strainer; cover. (Check the label to see if it contains gelatin.) Refrigerate. Drain the liquid whey for 2 to 24 hours, depending on the firmness you want. Drained for 24 hours, 32 ounces of yogurt yields about 1½ cups of yogurt cheese.

Add flavor with apricot preserves and chopped nuts; crumbled blue cheese and grated apple or pear; salmon and chopped green onion; or herb blend.

Source: St. Louis District Dairy Council.

To substitute unsaturated fats for solid fats (saturated and trans *fats) . . .*

● Switch from stick margarine or butter to soft margarine, perhaps with plant sterols.

● Cook with liquid oils instead of solid fats.

● Choose *trans*-fat free cookies and other snack foods.

● Compare the saturated fat on the food label, too. Look for foods with more mono- and polyunsaturated fats.

● Substitute foods and ingredients high in unsaturated fats for those high in solid fats. *See "Easy Substitutions for Less Total Fat, Solid Fats, and/or Cholesterol" in chapter 14.*

For example, choose soft tub or squeeze (liquid) margarine in place of stick margarine or butter. And try polyunsaturated or monounsaturated oil in recipes calling for melted shortening or butter. *Check "Lean Tips . . . for Baked Goods" in chapter 14 for substitutions with vegetable oil in baked goods.*

● Cut back on total fat. You'll likely reduce solid fats, too.

● Check the Nutrition Facts to compare fat, saturated fat, and *trans* fat in one label serving; choose foods

with less. Check the ingredient list, too. If any of these ingredients is among the first several listed, the food is likely higher in solid fats: butter, partially hydrogenated vegetable oil, coconut oil, palm oil, palm kernel oil, cocoa butter, meat fat, lard, egg yolks, whole milk solids, cream, or cheese.

CHECK OUT THE DIFFERENCE!

SNACKS	FAT (GRAMS)	CALORIES
Apple (1 medium)	0	70
Spiced applesauce (½ cup)	0	100
Apple pie (⅛ of 9-in.)	20	410
Banana (1)	0	105
Milk chocolate bar (1½ oz.)	13	235
Broccoli, raw (½ cup)	0	15
Chocolate chip cookie 2¼-in. (1)	4	80
Carrot (1 medium)	0	25
Carrot cake (1/12 of 9-in.)	11	240
Orange (1 medium)	0	60
Corn chips (1 oz.)	8	150
Strawberries (½ cup)	0	25
French fries (10)	5	200
Salsa (¼ cup)	0	20
Sour cream dip (¼ cup)	12	125
Saltines (10 crackers, or 1 oz.)	4	130
Potato chips (1 oz.)	11	155
Frozen yogurt (½ cup)	3	110
Ice cream, regular (½ cup)	8	145
Angel food cake (1/12 of cake)	0	130
Pound cake (1/16 of loaf cake)	13	230
Gingersnaps (4) (1 oz.)	3	120
Butter cookies 2-in. (6) (1 oz.)	6	135
Bagel, 3½-in., plain (1)	1	195
With 2 tbsp. jam	1	295
With 2 tbsp. part skim ricotta cheese	4	225
With 2 tbsp. cream cheese	11	285
Doughnut (1 glazed/sugared)	10	190

The fat smart strategies in this chapter can help give you a fat-savvy mind-set. For small action steps to manage fat in your meals and snacks, check here:

● Food shopping with fat savvy—see chapter 12.

● Preparing lean meals and snacks without giving up flavor—see chapter 14.

● Trimming fat in restaurant meals—see chapter 15.

● Managing dietary fat for heart disease, type 2 diabetes, and other health issues—see chapter 22.

For Less Cholesterol . . .

● Go easy on egg yolks, including eggs in prepared foods such as bread, cakes, and pancakes. The yolk has all the cholesterol—about 185 milligrams from a large egg. *Tip:* Substitute two whites for one whole egg in baked goods, or use an egg substitute.

● Go easy on organ meats such as liver. Even though they're nutritious, they're high in cholesterol.

● Look for lean meat, fish, poultry, and low-fat and fat-free dairy foods. You'll trim away some cholesterol along with fat.

● Check labels to find low-cholesterol or cholesterol-free foods. *See "Label Lingo: Fats and Cholesterol" in this chapter.*

FUNCTIONAL NUTRITION: A QUICK LOOK AT FATTY ACIDS, STANOLS, AND STEROLS

FATTY ACIDS: PLANTS STANOLS AND STEROLS	POTENTIAL BENEFIT	SOME FOOD SOURCES
Monounsaturated fatty acids (MUFAs)*	● May reduce risk of coronary heart disease (CHD)	● Tree nuts, canola oil, olive oil
Polyunsaturated fatty acids (PUFAs): omega-3 fatty acids—ALA	● Supports maintenance of heart and eye health ● Supports maintenance of mental function	● Walnuts, flaxseed, soy oil
PUFAs: omega-3 fatty acids—DHA/EPA*	● May reduce the risk of CHD ● Supports maintenance of eye health and mental function	● Salmon, tuna, marine, and other fish oils
Conjugated linoleic acid (CLA)	● Supports maintenance of desirable body composition and immune health	● Beef, lamb, some cheese
Free stanols/sterols*	● May reduce risk of CHD	● Corn, soy, wheat, fortified foods and beverages
Stanol/sterol esters*	● May reduce risk of CHD	● Stanol ester dietary supplements, fortified foods and beverages, including table spreads

* The U.S. Food and Drug Administration has approved a health claim for this food component.

Source: Adapted from the International Food Information Council Foundation, 2011.

For More Oils . . .

● Use vegetable oils—canola, corn, cottonseed, olive, safflower, soybean, sunflower—in place of stick margarine or butter. Mayonnaise, certain salad dressings, and soft (tub or squeeze) margarine with no *trans* fats are mainly oils, too.

● Fit nuts, olives, avocados, and oily fish into a healthful eating plan. *See "How Much Omega-3?" in this chapter.*

● Consider calories when adding oils to food or in cooking—add only small amounts to control calories.

Label Lingo

Fats and Cholesterol

Check food labels for clues about fat and cholesterol. You may find nutrient content claims.

LABEL TERM . . .	MEANS . . .
For Fat Content . . .	
Fat-free	Less than 0.5 gram fat per serving
Low-fat	3 grams or less of fat per serving
Reduced or less fat	At least 25% less fat* per serving
Light	⅓ fewer calories or 50% less fat* per serving
____ % fat-free	The food meets the definition of "low-fat" or "fat-free" if stated as 100% fat-free
Light meal	"Low-fat" (at least 50% less fat per serving*) or "low-calorie" meal (at least ⅓ fewer calories per serving*)
Low-fat meal	3 grams or less fat per 100 grams, and 30 percent or less calories from fat
For Saturated Fat Content . . .	
Saturated-fat-free	Less than 0.5 gram saturated fat and less than 0.5 gram *trans* fatty acids per serving
Low saturated fat	1 gram or less saturated fat per serving and no more than 15% of calories from saturated fat

LABEL TERM . .	MEANS . . .
Reduced or less saturated fat	At least 25% less saturated fat*
For Cholesterol Content . . .	
Cholesterol-free	Less than 2 milligrams cholesterol and 2 grams or less of saturated fat per serving
Low cholesterol	20 milligrams or less cholesterol and 2 grams or less of saturated fat per serving
Reduced or less cholesterol	At least 25% less cholesterol* and 2 grams or less of saturated fat per serving
For Fat, Saturated Fat, and Cholesterol Content . . .	
Lean†	Less than 10 grams total fat, 4.5 grams or less saturated fat, and 95 milligrams cholesterol per 3-ounce serving and per 100 grams
Extra lean†	Less than 5 grams total fat, 2 grams saturated fat, and 95 milligrams cholesterol per 3-ounce serving and per 100 grams

*Compared with a standard serving size of traditional food

†On packaged seafood or game meat, cooked meat, or cooked poultry

Note: Although not a nutrient content claim per se, look for packages that say "0 g *trans* fat" or "no *trans* fat."

CHAPTER 6

Vitamins, Minerals, and Phytonutrients
Variety on Your Plate!

Vitamins, minerals, and phytonutrients: your body needs them—*perhaps more of them*—for your good health. That's positive nutrition! Just how much do you need for optimal health? What foods are your best sources? And how do these food substances keep you fit?

Although headlines may seem confounding, there's plenty that's well known about the roles of vitamins, minerals, and phytonutrients (plant substances) in health. Over the last century, research unlocked puzzles related to widespread deficiencies. Today's nutrition breakthroughs focus less on cures and more on the roles of nutrients, phytonutrients, and other food components in health promotion and in protection from from weight gain, heart disease, cancer, and osteoporosis, among other health concerns.

● *Today,* more than forty nutrients, including vitamins and minerals, have been identified. Their functions, the amount you need at different stages of life, and their food sources are better understood. Today's vitamin and mineral research is extending well beyond their well-known, important roles in health, noted in this chapter.

● *Today,* we know more about the balance of vitamins and minerals—and the variety of foods—that allow the body to absorb and use them most efficiently. We're discovering what's enough, but not too much, for our unique, individual needs.

● *Today,* science is exploring a new frontier: food components, including phytonutrients, that offer health benefits beyond basic nourishment.

The bottom line? A variety of food—with plenty of vitamins, minerals, and phytonutrients—is part of your ticket to good health! In fact, it is . . . all about food!

Team Players!

Vitamins and minerals are key to every process that takes place in your body. They don't work alone, but instead in close partnership with other nutrients to make every body process happen normally: from helping carbohydrates, fats, and proteins produce energy, to assisting with protein synthesis (the creation of new proteins), to building your healthy bones, to helping you think about the words on this page.

● Vitamins are complex substances that regulate body processes. Often they act as coenzymes, or partners, with enzymes, the proteins that cause reactions to take place in your body.

● Minerals are part of many cells, including (but not only) the hard parts: bone, teeth, and nails. Minerals also are part of enzymes that trigger some of your body's reactions.

Compared with carbohydrates, proteins, and fats, your body needs vitamins and minerals in only small amounts, so they're called *micro*nutrients. Don't let these small amounts fool you, however. Vitamins and minerals don't supply energy directly. But they do regulate many processes that produce energy—and do a whole lot more!

The appendices give specific recommendations— Dietary Reference Intakes (DRIs)—for vitamins and minerals. Within this chapter, you'll learn about the vitamins and minerals that the Dietary Guidelines for Americans, 2010, regard as a public health concern since they often come up short : calcium, vitamin D, and potassium, and for some populations, iron, folate, and vitamin B_{12}. In addition, these are likely to be inadequate, too: for adults, vitamins A, C, E, and K, choline, and magnesium; for children (mostly notably adolescents), vitamins A, C, and E, phosphorus, and magnesium. Sodium is another public health concern; most people consume too much!

Alphabet Soup

Dietary Reference Intakes (DRIs). Daily nutrient recommendations—expressed as RDAs or AIs—based on age and gender; set at levels to decrease the risk of chronic disease.

Recommended Dietary Allowances (RDAs). Recommended daily levels of nutrients to meet the needs of almost all healthy individuals in a specific age, life stage, and gender group; used when there's scientific consensus for a firm nutrient recommendation.

Adequate Intakes (AIs). Similar to RDAs, and used for nutrients that lack sufficient scientific evidence to determine a firm RDA.

Tolerable Upper Intake Level (UL). Not a recommendation; maximum intake that most likely won't pose risks for health problems for almost all healthy people in that age and gender group based on current research findings.

Source: Institute of Medicine, National Academy of Sciences.

Daily Values (DVs) for nutrients aren't DRIs, although they are based on previous RDA values. DVs are used primarily for food labeling for a quick comparison to daily recommendations.

Vitamins: The Basics

Vitamins belong in two groups: fat-soluble and water-soluble. Their category describes how they are carried in food and transported in your body.

Fat-soluble vitamins (vitamins A, D, E, and K) dissolve in fat. That's how they're carried into your bloodstream and throughout your body—attached to substances within your body made with lipids, or fat. These vitamins are one reason why you need moderate amounts of fat in your overall food choices.

Your body can store fat-soluble vitamins in body fat, so consuming excessive amounts of any fat-soluble vitamins for too long can be harmful. Vitamins A and D, for example, can build up to harmful levels. High intakes of vitamins E and K usually aren't linked to unhealthy symptoms since higher levels are the least toxic of excess vitamins.

As their name implies, water-soluble vitamins (B-complex vitamins and vitamin C) dissolve in water. They're carried in your bloodstream. For the most part, water-soluble vitamins aren't stored in your body—at least not in significant amounts. Instead, your body uses what it needs, then excretes the extra through urine. Since they aren't stored, you need a ,

It's About the Food!

Think food—to get enough (and not too much) of the vitamins, minerals, and phytonutrients discussed in this chapter. You'll find practical food tips and how-tos throughout the book. Start here:

- Explore new-to-you fruits, vegetables, and grain products—see chapter 9.
- Plan a day's food choices that deliver enough vitamins and minerals and plenty of phytonutrients—see chapters 10 and 11.
- Scout for nutrient-rich, phytonutrient-rich foods when you shop—see chapter 12.
- Lock vitamins in, boost calcium, and cut sodium when you prepare food—see chapter 14.
- Enjoy the flavors and get the nutrient and phytonutrient benefits of fruits and vegetables—see chapters 14 and 15.
- Use nutrient supplements wisely—see chapter 23.

On the Label

Without looking, do you know which vitamins and minerals appear on food labels? The four required on the Nutrition Facts need your special attention: vitamins A and C, calcium, and iron. Consume enough of these nutrients to reduce your risk for some common health problems. Other nutrients may appear on the label: some voluntarily, others required if these nutrients are added.

Be aware: Daily Values (DVs) for nutrients, used with food labeling, may differ from today's DRIs. DVs for nutrients are based on previous RDAs. *See "% Daily Values: What Are They Based On?" in the appendices.*

Nutrition Facts	
Serving Size 1 cup (228g)	
Servings Per Container 2	

Amount Per Serving	
Calories 260	Calories from Fat 120

	% Daily Value*
Total Fat 13g	20%
Saturated Fat 5g	25%
Trans Fat 2g	
Cholesterol 30mg	10%
Sodium 660mg	28%
Total Carbohydrate 31g	10%
Dietary Fiber 0g	0%
Sugars 5g	
Protein 5g	

Vitamin A 4%	•	Vitamin C 2%
Calcium 15%	•	Iron 4%

* Percent Daily Values are based on a 2,000 calorie diet. Your Daily Values may be higher or lower depending on your calorie needs:

	Calories:	2,000	2,500
Total Fat	Less than	65g	80g
Sat Fat	Less than	20g	25g
Cholesterol	Less than	300mg	300mg
Sodium	Less than	2,400mg	2,400mg
Total Carbohydrate		300g	375g
Dietary Fiber		25g	30g

Calories per gram:			
Fat 9	•	Carbohydrate 4	•	Protein 4

regular supply of water-soluble vitamins from your food choices.

How much do you need? Enough, but not too much. Even though you excrete excess amounts of water-soluble vitamins, moderation is the best approach. For example, taking large doses of vitamin C from a dietary supplement may create extra work for your kidneys, which may result in kidney stones, as well as diarrhea. Likewise, too much niacin, vitamin B_6, folate, or pantothenic acid also may result in health risks.

Read on to find out how vitamins keep you healthy: their functions, effects of getting too little or too much, Dietary Reference Intakes (DRIs), and their food sources. *Note:* On the following pages, the amounts of vitamins in food have been rounded.

Fat-Soluble Vitamins

Vitamin A (and Carotenoids)

See also "Carotenoids: 'Color' Your Food Healthy" in this chapter.

What it does:

● Promotes normal vision, and helps your eyes see normally in the dark, helping adjust to the lower level of light.

● Promotes the growth and health of cells and tissues throughout your body; with pregnancy, important for reproduction and development of the embryo.

● Protects you from infections by keeping skin and tissues in your mouth, stomach, intestines, and respiratory, genital, and urinary tracts healthy.

● Helps regulate immune system.

● Works as an antioxidant in the form of carotenoids, and may reduce your risk for certain diseases of aging.

As antioxidants, some carotenoids (which form vitamin A) are thought to have other health benefits, *addressed later in this chapter.*

How much you need: From age fourteen on, the RDA is 900 micrograms Retinol Activity Equivalent (RAE) (3,000 IU) of vitamin A for males and 700 micrograms RAE (2,333 IU) for females. During pregnancy, the recommendation is 770 micrograms per day, and during breastfeeding, 1,200 micrograms RAE daily.

Note: The 2001 RDAs measure vitamin A in RAEs, reflecting retinol and carotenoid units. You might see vitamin A expressed in other ways: International Units

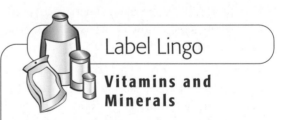

Label Lingo

Vitamins and Minerals

The lingo on the front of many food packages describes the amount of vitamins or minerals found in a single serving. For specific amounts of the nutrients described, check the Nutrition Facts on the label.

High, Rich in, Excellent source of means 20% or more of the Daily Value.

Good source, Contains, Provides means 10 to 19% of the Daily Value.

More, Enriched, Fortified, Added means 10% or more of the Daily Value.

(IU)—used for food labels and dietary supplements, or as Retinol Equivalents (RE)—used in the 1989 RDAs and many nutrient databases.

Convert Retinol Equivalents to Retinol Activity Equivalents. For vitamin A derived from:

- Animal-based foods   1 RE = 1 RAE
  or supplements
- Plant-based foods   1 RE divided by 2
                         = 1 RAE

If you don't consume enough: Night blindness; other eye problems; dry, scaly skin; problems with reproduction; diminished immunity, and poor growth are symptoms of a significant deficiency. The deficiency disease from too little vitamin A is called xerophthalmia.

If you consume excess amounts: Because it's stored in your body, large intakes of vitamin A, taken over time, can be quite harmful: headaches, dry and scaly skin, liver damage, bone and joint pain, vomiting or appetite loss, abnormal bone growth, nerve damage, and birth defects. These symptoms more likely result from high intakes of vitamin A from dietary supplements. High doses of beta-carotene supplements aren't advised for smokers. Beta carotene from fruits and vegetables is okay! Converting carotenoids to vitamin A decreases once the body stores enough vitamin A. High carotenoid intake may turn skin yellow, but that's not considered harmful. The Tolerable Upper Intake Level is 2,800 micrograms of RAE daily for ages fourteen to eighteen, and 3,000 micrograms

Vitamin A and Carotenoids: Good Picks

Besides supplying essential carotenoids, enjoy carotene-rich fruit or vegetables daily for the antioxidant power, too!

Vitamin A content is given below in two ways: in approximate Retinol Equivalents (currently used in many nutrient databases) and in approximate Retinol Activity Equivalents (used with 2001 RDAs for vitamin A).

Food	Retinol Equivalents (RE)* (Approximate)	Retinol Activity Equivalents (RAE)* (Approximate)
Beef liver, cooked (3 oz.)	8,025	8,025
Sweet potato, mashed (½ cup)	2,580	1,290
Carrot (1 medium)	1,030	515
Collards, frozen, boiled (½ cup)	980	490
Kale, boiled (½ cup)	890	445
Turnip greens, cooked (½ cup)	550	275
Cantaloupe (½ cup)	300	150
Spinach, raw (1 cup)	280	140
Romaine lettuce (1 cup)	270	135
Red bell pepper, raw (½ cup)	235	115
Apricot (3)	200	100

Food	Retinol Equivalents (RE)* (Approximate)	Retinol Activity Equivalents (RAE)* (Approximate)
Papaya, medium (½)	170	85
Milk, fat-free (1 cup)	150	150
Tomato, medium, raw (1)	105	50
Mango, medium (½)	80	40
Egg, large (1)	70	70
Milk, whole (1 cup)	70	70
Broccoli, raw (½ cup)	30	15
Green bell pepper, raw (½ cup)	30	15
Orange, medium (1)	30	15

Many fortified foods, including breakfast cereals, supply vitamin A, too. Read the Nutrition Facts on food labels to see how much.

*The % Daily Values—used on food labels and many dietary supplements—are based in International Units (IUs) for vitamin A (not REs or RAEs).

daily during adulthood. (Retinol, beta carotene, and other provitamin A carotenoids determine RAE.)

Where it's mostly found:

● In animal sources of foods, vitamin A, in the form of retinol, is completely made (or preformed). Vitamin A comes from liver, other organ meats, eggs, milk fortified with vitamin A, and other vitamin A-fortified foods such as breakfast cereal.

● Carotenoids, such as alpha carotene and beta carotene, come from foods of plant origin. Certain carotenoids form vitamin A (referred to as "provitamin A carotenoids") in your body. Carotenoids are found in red, yellow, orange, and many dark-green leafy vegetables. Plant sources of carotenoids are especially important to those who eat few animal-based foods.

Do you get most or all of your beta carotene (which turns to vitamin A) from fruits and vegetables? If so, you may need to eat more of them! According to the 2001 DRI report from the Institute of Medicine, the conversion of carotenoids to vitamin A was overestimated in the past. In fact, it takes twice the amount of carotene-rich foods to meet the body's vitamin A needs as once thought.

Click Here! Websites to Know . . .

How do your favorite foods stack up for vitamins and minerals? Other nutrients? Calories?

What more does science say about the vitamins and minerals discussed in this chapter? More in-depth information is just a click away.

● What's in the Food You Eat—Search Tool, U.S. Department of Agriculture, www.ars.usda/gov/foodsearch

● National Nutrient Database for Standard Reference, U.S. Department of Agriculture, www.ars.usda.gov/ba/bhnrc/ndl

● Dietary Supplement Fact Sheets (covering specific vitamins and minerals), Office of Dietary Supplements, National Institutes of Health, ods.od.nih.gov/supplements

Search these websites for apps, too!

Vitamin D

See "Vitamin D: Often Shortchanged!" in chapter 19.

What it does:

● Helps almost every part of the body.

● Promotes absorption of calcium and phosphorus; regulates how much calcium remains in blood.

● Helps deposit these minerals in bones and teeth and helps keep them strong and so reduces fracture risk.

● Helps regulate cell growth.

● Plays a role in immunity.

Compelling evidence shows that vitamin D is linked to bone health. Although studies are exploring the links to vitamin D's potential role in preventing cancer, diabetes, cardiovascular disease, and autoimmune conditions, among other health conditions, the evidence isn't sufficient to offer guidance.

How much you need: From age one to seventy years, the Recommended Dietary Allowance (RDA), updated in 2010, has been set at 600 IU, or 15 micrograms cholecalciferol, which is the form of vitamin D in an animal-based food (vitamin D from plant-based foods is in a different form), with no increased need during pregnancy or breast feeding. One microgram cholecalciferol = 40 IU vitamin D. Advice for vitamin D goes up to 800 IU or 20 micrograms cholecalciferol daily for adults over age seventy.

The RDA for vitamin D assumes little or no sunlight exposure. Vitamin D is unique because sunlight that touches skin lets the body make vitamin D *(continue reading to understand why vitamin D is known also as the "sunshine vitamin")*. The recommendation also allows for a margin of safety that recognizes differences in season, latitude, skin pigment, and genetic differences, among other factors, and considers risks for skin cancer with more sun exposure.

The 2010 Dietary Guidelines recognizes vitamin D as a nutrient that is low enough for many Americans to be a public health concern.

If you don't consume enough: This could occur if you don't consume or absorb enough vitamin D from food or if your sun exposure is limited. Another cause could be if your kidneys can't convert vitamin D to its active form. In your older years, you may have greater loss of bone mass (osteoporosis), and your risk of softening of the bones (osteomalacia) increases with insufficient vitamin D intake. Children with a significant vitamin D deficiency may develop rickets, or defective bone growth. Fortifying milk with vitamin D had virtually wiped out rickets in the United States. Rickets is reemerging as a concern, however, possibly related to regularly consuming juice or soft drinks in place of milk. That's happening even though some juices and other foods are vitamin D fortified.

In recent years there's been confusion about identifying a vitamin D deficiency because lab tests don't have standardized cutoffs to define a deficiency. According to data from the National Academy of Sciences, if your blood levels are at or above 20 nanograms per milliliter, you get enough vitamin D.

If you consume excess amounts: Because it's stored in your body, too much vitamin D can be toxic, possibly leading to confusion, problems with heart rhythm, and kidney stones or damage. Symptoms include poor appetite, weakness, constipation, nausea, and weight loss. An overdose usually comes from dietary supplements, not food. For that reason, an upper limit, or Tolerable Upper Intake Level (UL), of 4,000 International Units (IU), or 100 micrograms, per day for people ages nine and over was set. The UL for infants is 1,000 to 1,500 IU/day, and for children ages one to eight it is 2,500 to 3,000 IU/day. Because the body limits its own vitamin D production, excessive sun exposure won't result in vitamin D toxicity.

The "sunshine vitamin": Your body can make vitamin D after sunlight, or ultraviolet light, hits your skin, even on cloudy days. That's no excuse for overexposure to sun from sunbathing or a tanning booth. Skin makes less vitamin D on cloudy days, in shade, and with dark-colored skin, and little to none through indoor exposure from a window.

To lower your risk for skin cancer, wear protective clothing and apply sunscreen that is Broad Spectrum with an SPF (sun protection factor) 15 or more to exposed skin if you're out for more than a few minutes. Be aware that tanning beds not only cause the skin to make vitamin D, but also increase risks for skin cancer. Broad Spectrum protects against both ultraviolet A and ultraviolet B rays.

During cold months in the northern half of the

Vitamin-Rich Cures

Nutrition history is full of fascinating stories of nutrient-deficiency diseases that confounded doctors of the past.

- The scourge of *scurvy,* which plagued seafarers several hundred years ago, was finally cured by stocking ships with lemons, oranges, and limes; hence, British sailors were called "limeys." Scurvy is caused by a deficiency of vitamin C, a nutrient that citrus fruits provide in abundance.

- *Night blindness,* often caused by a deficiency of vitamin A, was known in ancient Egypt. The recommended cure of the day: eating ox or rooster livers. Today it's well known that liver contains more vitamin A than many other foods.

- Giving children cod liver oil to prevent *rickets* was practiced in the nineteenth century. But not until 1922, when vitamin D was discovered, did scientists know what substance in cod liver oil gave protection.

- *Beriberi,* a deficiency of thiamin, was noted in Asia as polished, or white, rice became more popular than unrefined, or brown, rice. The cure was discovered accidentally when chickens with symptoms of beriberi ate the part of rice that was discarded after polishing. It contained the vitamin-rich germ. Today the process of enrichment adds thiamin and other B vitamins back to polished rice; today rice is fortified with folic acid, too.

United States, the sun's energy isn't strong enough for your skin to make vitamin D.

If you avoid the sun, cover with sunscreen or clothing, or live in the northern half of the United States during the winter, consume good food sources of vitamin D and perhaps take a vitamin D supplement. The area above a line drawn between Boston and the northern border of California is the northern half of the United States for this purpose.

Where it's mostly found: Some oily fish naturally supply vitamin D—another reason to enjoy salmon and tuna. As a public health strategy, most milk is vitamin D fortified, with 100 IU of vitamin D in an 8-ounce serving. Today's supermarkets also carry many vitamin-D fortified foods: yogurt, cheese, juices, soy drinks, breakfast cereals, breads, and cereal bars, as well as eggs from hens raised on vitamin D-fortified feed. Mushrooms are another source. Some mushrooms that are newly on the market have been exposed to ultraviolet light to boost their vitamin D content.

Fortified foods and dietary supplements supply vitamin D in two different forms: D_2 (ergocalciferol) and D_3 (cholecalciferol). Both increase vitamin D in your bloodstream. Current research shows that vitamin D_3 and vitamin D_2 are equally good for bone health.

FOOD	VITAMIN D (INTERNATIONAL UNITS)
Salmon with bones, canned (3 oz.)	465
Milk, fat-free, 1%, 2% (1 cup)	115
Fortified ready-to-eat cereals (about 1 oz.)	35–100
Orange juice, vitamin D fortified (½ cup)	70
Shiitake mushrooms (½ cup)	25

Vitamin E

See also "Vitamin E: One Main Mission" in this chapter.

What it does:

● Neutralizes free radicals, which may damage cells.

● Works as an antioxidant, preventing the oxidation of LDL cholesterol, and perhaps lowering the risk for heart disease and stroke.

● May contribute to immune function.

● As an antioxidant, protects essential fatty acids and vitamin A. *See "Vitamins as Antioxidents" later in this chapter.*

How much you need: The RDA guideline for males and females age fourteen and over is 15 milligrams of alpha-tocopherol each day. Children need less, depending on their age. During pregnancy, women still need 15 milligrams daily; during breast-feeding the recommendation goes up to 19 milligrams daily.

If you don't consume enough: Many Americans consume enough vitamin E, yet it's still a nutrient that's often shortchanged, according to the Dietary Guidelines. Coming up short on vitamin E over time may cause nerve and muscle damage and make your body less able to fight off infection. Premature, very-low-

birth-weight infants and people with poor fat absorption, cystic fibrosis, or some other chronic health problems may be deficient in vitamin E. In these cases, the nervous system and immune response can be affected. Because vegetable oils are good sources of vitamin E, people who cut back on total fat may not get enough. Vitamin E-fortified cereal may be a good choice.

If you consume excess amounts: Eating plenty of vitamin E-rich foods doesn't appear problematic. However, taking large doses of vitamin E as a supplement hasn't been shown conclusively to have benefits—and isn't recommended. Too much may increase the risk of bleeding, may impair vitamin K action, and may increase the effect of anticoagulant medication.

That's why a Tolerable Upper Intake Level (UL) has been set: 800 milligrams daily for teens ages fourteen to eighteen; 1,000 milligrams of alpha-tocopherol daily for adults ages nineteen and over. If you take a supplement, 1,000 milligrams equal about 1,500 IU of natural vitamin E or 1,100 IU of dl-alpha-tocopherol synthetic vitamin E.

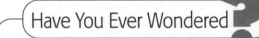

Have You Ever Wondered

. . . if hair analysis is a valid way to diagnose a vitamin or mineral deficiency? Except to detect poisonous elements such as lead or arsenic, hair analysis isn't a valid way to check your nutritional status. Why? Hair grows slowly; the condition of hair strands differs along their length. Chemicals used to clean and treat hair affect its composition. Differences in age and gender also affect the quality of hair. Too often, those who promote hair analysis for nutrition reasons are also trying to promote dietary supplements. Buyer, beware!

. . . if vitamin E or other nutrients in skin moisturizers gets rid of wrinkles? Vitamins, amino acids, cocoa butter, or other nutrients in skin creams and cosmetics can't remove or prevent aging skin. The possible exception is Retin-A, sold by prescription, which may slow the process. However, there's no research on its long-term effects. Protecting your skin from damage caused by ultraviolet light (sunshine) is the most important way you can slow the process of wrinkling. Moisturizing your skin daily with skin cream, preferably one containing a sun block of SPF 30 or more, will help, too. Healthful eating overall promotes healthy skin.

Where it's mostly found: The best sources of vitamin E are vegetable oil, for example, sunflower, cotton-seed, and safflower oils. That includes salad dressings, margarine, spreads, and other foods made with these oils. Nuts, especially almonds and hazelnuts, seeds (such as sunflower seeds), wheat germ—all high in oil—are good sources, too, as are peanut butter and some fortified breakfast cereals. Green leafy vegetables also supply small amounts.

Some oils and nuts are better sources of vitamin E than others. To boost vitamin E intake, make substitutions without increasing your calorie intake: for example, sunflower oil in place of soybean oil, and almonds or hazelnuts in place of cashews.

Note: Heating vegetable oils to high temperatures, as in frying, destroys vitamin E.

FOOD	VITAMIN E (MG ALPHA-TOCOPHEROL)
Fortified ready-to-eat cereals (about 1 oz.)	3–15
Sunflower seeds (1 oz.)	11
Almonds (1 oz. or 24 nuts)	7
Sunflower oil, high linoleic	6
Safflower oil, high oleic	5
Hazelnuts (1 oz.)	4
Peanut butter (2 tbsp.)	3
Corn oil (1 tbsp.)	2
Spinach, cooked (½ cup)	2–3
Turnip greens, cooked (½ cup)	2

Note: Vitamin E is a group of substances called tocopherols with different potencies. Alpha-tocopherol is its most potent form. On food and supplement labels, the amount is given in International Units (IU) of alpha-tocopherol, not in milligrams.

To make the conversion, 15 milligrams of alpha-tocopherol (the RDA for adults) equal:

- About 22 IU of d-alpha-tocopherol ("natural" vitamin E in some supplements)

- About 33 IU of dl-alpha-tocopherol (a synthetic form in fortified foods and some supplements)

The "natural" form of vitamin E is more fully used than the synthetic form. That's why there's a difference in the conversion factor.

Vitamin K

What it does:

- Makes proteins that cause your blood to coagulate, or clot, when you bleed. That way, bleeding stops.

- Regulates calcium metabolism.

- Plays a key role in cellular signaling and proliferation.

- Helps your body make some other body proteins for your blood, bones, and kidneys.

How much you need: The Adequate Intake (AI) advises 75 micrograms daily for teens ages fourteen to eighteen. During adulthood the intake goes up: 120 micrograms daily for men and 90 micrograms daily for women. Neither pregnancy nor breast-feeding increases the recommendation. To make sure infants have enough, newborns typically receive a shot of vitamin K.

If you don't get enough: Blood doesn't coagulate normally. Except for rare health problems, a deficiency of vitamin K is very unlikely. Prolonged use of antibiotics could be a problem since they destroy some bacteria in your intestines that produce vitamin K.

If you consume excess amounts: No symptoms have been observed, but moderation is still the best approach. People taking blood-thinning drugs, or anticoagulants, need to eat foods with vitamin K in moderation. Too much can make blood clot faster. No Tolerable Upper Intake Level (UL) is established.

Where it's mostly found: Like vitamin D, your body can produce vitamin K on its own—this time from certain bacteria in your intestines.

The best food sources are green, leafy vegetables such as spinach and broccoli. However, a variety of foods provide smaller amounts, including some fruits, vegetables, and nuts.

FOOD	VITAMIN K (MCG)
Spinach, raw (1 cup)	145
Broccoli, raw (½ cup)	45
Black-eyed peas, cooked (½ cup)	20
Canola oil (1 tbsp.)	17
Blueberries (½ cup)	15

FOOD	VITAMIN K (MCG)
Pine nuts (1 oz.)	15
Pistachios (1 oz.)	5
Raspberries (½ cup)	5

Water-Soluble Vitamins

Thiamin (vitamin B₁)

What it does:

- Is essential for producing energy from carbohydrates in all the cells of your body.

- May contribute to maintaining mental function.

- Helps regulate metabolism.

How much you need: The RDA for thiamin is tied to your energy needs: 1.2 milligrams daily for males age fourteen through adulthood. For females, the recommendation is 1.0 milligram daily from ages fourteen through eighteen and 1.1 milligrams daily from age nineteen on. During pregnancy and breast-feeding, the amount recommended goes up to 1.4 milligrams daily.

If you don't consume enough: Because most people consume many grain products, a thiamin deficiency is rare in the United States today, with one exception: Chronic alcoholics may not consume enough, or their body might not convert thiamin to a bioactive form. Symptoms include fatigue, weak muscles, and nerve damage. Before refined grains were enriched with thiamin, a deficiency was common, sometimes resulting in a disease called beriberi, which affects mainly the cardiovascular and nervous systems.

If you consume excess amounts: Your body excretes any excess amount you may consume. Contrary to popular claims, extra amounts have no energy-boosting effect.

Where it's mostly found: Whole-grain and enriched grain products such as bread, rice, pasta, tortillas, and fortified cereals provide much of the thiamin we eat. Enrichment adds back nutrients, including many B vitamins, lost when grains are refined. Pork, liver, and other organ meats provide significant amounts, too.

FOOD	THIAMIN (MG)
Pork, lean, broiled (3 oz.)	1.0
Beef liver, braised (3 oz.)	0.2
Enriched flour tortilla (1)	0.2
Enriched rice, cooked (½ cup)	0.2
Whole-grain bread (1 slice)	0.1

Riboflavin (vitamin B₂)

What it does:

- Helps produce energy in all cells of your body.

- Helps change the amino acid called tryptophan in your food to niacin.

- Helps support cell growth and antioxidant protection.

- Helps regulate metabolism.

How much you need: Like thiamin, the RDA for riboflavin is tied to your energy needs. Adult men need 1.3 milligrams daily and adult women need 1.1 milligrams daily. During pregnancy, the recommendation is 1.4 milligrams; during breast-feeding, the amount goes up to 1.6 milligrams daily.

If you don't consume enough: Except for people who are severely malnourished, a deficiency isn't likely. Deficiency symptoms include eye disorders (including cataracts); dry and flaky skin; and a sore, red tongue. Contrary to popular myth, riboflavin deficiency doesn't cause hair loss.

If you consume excess amounts: No reports suggest problems from consuming too much.

Have You Ever Wondered

. . . what B complex vitamins are? They're a "vitamin family" with related roles in health: thiamin (vitamin B₁), riboflavin (vitamin B₂), niacin, vitamin B₆, folate, vitamin B₁₂, biotin, and pantothenic acid. Besides their varied, unique body functions, most B vitamins help your body produce energy within its trillions of cells.

. . . how cooking affects the vitamin content of foods? Water-soluble vitamins are destroyed more easily during food preparation, processing, and storage than fat-soluble vitamins are. *For food handling tips to retain vitamins, see "Simple Ways to Keep Nutrients in Food" in chapter 14.*

Where it's mostly found: Milk and other dairy foods are major sources of riboflavin. Some organ meats—liver, kidney, and heart—are excellent sources. Enriched bread and other grain products; eggs; meat; green, leafy vegetables; and nuts supply smaller amounts. Because ultraviolet light, such as sunlight, destroys riboflavin, most milk is packed in opaque plastic or cardboard containers, not clear glass.

FOOD	RIBOFLAVIN (MG)
Beef liver, braised (3 oz.)	3.5
Yogurt, fat-free with dry milk solids (1 cup)	0.4
Milk, fat-free (1 cup)	0.4
Spinach, cooked (½ cup)	0.2
Egg, large (1)	0.2
Enriched corn tortilla (1)	0.1
Whole-grain bread (1 slice)	0.1

Niacin

What it does:

- Plays a key role in all aspects of metabolism, including cell growth and energy production.
- Helps enzymes function normally in your body.
- Helps your body use sugars and fatty acids.

How much you need: Niacin recommendations are given in NE, or niacin equivalents. That's because it comes from two sources: niacin itself and from the amino acid called tryptophan, part of which converts to niacin.

Like thiamin and riboflavin, the recommendation is tied to energy needs. The advice for adult males is 16 milligrams NE daily, and for adult females, 14 milligrams NE daily. During pregnancy, 18 milligrams NE is advised; during breast-feeding, 17 milligrams NE daily.

If you don't consume enough: For people who consume adequate amounts of protein-rich foods, a niacin deficiency isn't likely. Pellagra is caused by a significant niacin deficiency. Symptoms include diarrhea, mental disorientation, and skin problems.

If you consume excess amounts: Consuming excessive amounts, not likely from food, may cause flushed skin, rashes, or liver damage. The Tolerable Upper Intake Level (UL) is 35 milligrams daily for adults, and 30 milligrams daily for teens ages fourteen to eighteen. Self-prescribing large doses of niacin to lower blood cholesterol may lead to adverse effects—and may not give cholesterol-lowering benefits. If your doctor prescribes niacin, take it in the recommended dosage.

Where it's mostly found: Foods high in protein are typically good sources of niacin: poultry, fish, beef, peanut butter, and beans (legumes). Niacin is also added to many enriched and fortified grain products.

FOOD	NIACIN (MG NE)
Turkey breast, roasted, without skin (3 oz.)	6.0
Peanut butter (2 tbsp.)	4.0
Codfish, cooked (3 oz.)	2.0
Enriched flour tortilla (1)	1.5
Enriched spaghetti, cooked (½ cup)	1.0
Black-eyed peas, frozen, cooked (½ cup)	0.5
Lima beans, boiled (½ cup)	0.5
Yogurt, fat-free with dry milk solids (1 cup)	0.5

Have You Ever Wondered

. . . about the difference between the terms "enriched" and "fortified"? Both terms indicate that nutrients—usually vitamins or minerals—were added to make a food more nutritious. *Enriched* means adding back nutrients that were lost during food processing. For example, B vitamins, lost when wheat is processed, are added back to refined white flour. *Fortified* means adding nutrients that weren't present originally. For example, milk is fortified with vitamin D, a nutrient that helps your body absorb milk's calcium and phosphorus. Most enriched grain products are fortified with folic acid to reduce the incidence of certain birth defects.

. . . if microwave cooking destroys vitamins? Even if you cook foods properly, some water-soluble vitamins, such as B vitamins and vitamin C, can be destroyed. For several reasons, more vitamins are retained with microwave cooking than with most other methods: very short cooking time, covered cooking, and little or no cooking water.

Pyridoxine (vitamin B₆)

What it does:

● Helps your body make nonessential amino acids, or protein components, which are then used to make body cells.

● Helps turn the amino acid called tryptophan into two important body substances: niacin and serotonin (a messenger in your brain).

● Helps produce other body chemicals, including insulin, hemoglobin, and antibodies that fight infection.

● May contribute to maintaining healthy immune function.

● Helps regulate metabolism.

How much you need: The RDA is 1.3 milligrams daily for adult males and females through age fifty. After age fifty, the RDA increases to 1.7 milligrams daily for males and 1.5 milligrams for females. The amount increases to 1.9 milligrams daily during pregnancy and 2.0 milligrams daily during breast-feeding.

If you don't consume enough: A deficiency can cause confusion, mental convulsions, depression; a sore tongue, or greasy, flaky skin. For infants, breast milk and properly prepared infant formulas contain enough. A deficiency also may increase blood levels of homocysteine, an amino acid. Some evidence suggests that an elevated homocysteine level may increase the risk for heart disease and stroke.

If you consume excess amounts: Large doses, over time, can cause nerve damage. The Tolerable Upper Intake Level (UL) is 100 milligrams daily for adults; 80 milligrams daily for teens, fourteen to eighteen.

Where it's mostly found: Vitamin B₆ is found in a wide variety of foods including fortified cereals, beans, meat, poultry, fish, and some fruits and vegetables.

FOOD	PYRIDOXINE (MG)
Ready-to-eat cereal, 100% fortified, (¾ cup)	2.00
Potato, baked, flesh and skin (1 medium)	0.7
Banana, raw (1 medium)	0.7
Garbanzo beans, canned (½ cup)	0.6

FOOD	PYRIDOXINE (MG)
Chicken breast, meat only, cooked (3 oz.)	0.5
Pork loin, lean only, cooked (3 oz.)	0.4
Trout, rainbow, cooked (3 oz.)	0.3
Walnuts, English/Persian (1 oz.)	0.2
Peanut butter, smooth, (2 tbsp.)	0.2

Folate (folic acid or folacin)

What it does:

● Plays an essential role in making new body cells by helping to produce DNA and RNA, the cell's master plan for cell reproduction. It also helps prevent changes to DNA that may lead to cancer.

● Works with vitamin B₁₂ to form hemoglobin in red blood cells and prevent anemia.

● May help protect against heart disease.

● Helps lower the risk of delivering a baby with a brain or spinal-cord defect such as spina bifida.

● Helps control plasma homocysteine levels, linked to increased cardiovascular disease risk. *See chapter 22.*

How much you need: For folate, the RDA for males from age fourteen through adulthood is 400 micrograms daily. Folate can come from foods with naturally occurring folate, as well as from foods fortified with folic acid and from supplements.

The 2010 Dietary Guidelines advises *that women capable of becoming pregnant should consume 400 micrograms (mcg) per day of synthetic folic acid (from fortified foods and/or supplements) in addition to food forms of folate from a varied diet.* Pregnancy increases the recommended amount to 600 micrograms daily; during breast-feeding, 500 micrograms are advised.

If you don't consume enough: A deficiency affects normal cell division and protein synthesis, especially impairing growth. Anemia, caused by malformed blood cells that can't carry as much oxygen, may result from a folate deficiency. Other symptoms are subtle.

Pregnant women who don't get enough folate, especially during the first trimester, have a greater risk of delivering a baby with neural tube defects such as spina bifida.

If you consume excess amounts: Consuming too much can mask a vitamin B_{12} deficiency and may interfere with certain medications and offers no known benefits. For adults, the Tolerable Upper Intake Level (UL) is 1,000 micrograms daily of folic acid, the form of folate in fortified foods and supplements. For teens ages fourteen to eighteen, it's 800 micrograms daily. Adults over age fifty should talk to their doctor to check their vitamin B_{12} status before taking a supplement that contains folic acid (*see chapter 19 to learn more*). For this age group, the 2010 Dietary Guidelines Advisory Committee Report advises avoiding a supplement with more than 400 micrograms of folic acid.

Where it's mostly found: Orange juice, lentils, beans (legumes), spinach, broccoli, peanuts, and avocados are among the good sources of naturally occurring folate. Enriched grain products—such as most breads, flour, crackers, rice, macaroni, and noodles— must be fortified with folic acid, a form of folate. Some breakfast cereals are fully fortified at 400 micrograms per serving—100 percent of the daily recommendation for many people. Unenriched grain products, such as some imported pastas, may not be fortified with folic acid. Check the Nutrition Facts on the label of grain products to see if folic acid has been added and how much. Many whole-grain breads and other whole-grain products are not fortified with folic acid; check the label. If most of your grains are whole grain, then choose some that are folic-acid fortified.

FOOD	FOLATE (MCG)
Breakfast cereals, fortified with folic acid (¾–1 cup)	100–400
Spinach, boiled (½ cup)	130
Navy beans, boiled (½ cup)	125
Orange juice (1 cup)	110
Wheat germ (¼ cup)	100
Avocado (½)	80
Pasta, fortified with folic acid, cooked (½ cup)	50
Rice, fortified with folic acid, cooked (½ cup)	45
Peanuts, dry roasted (1 oz.)	40
Bread, fortified with folic acid (1 slice)	30
Romaine lettuce, shredded (½ cup)	30

Vitamin B_{12} (cobalamin)

What it does:

● Works with folate to make red blood cells.

● Serves as a vital part of many body chemicals and so occurs in every body cell.

● Helps your body use fatty acids and some amino acids.

● May contribute to maintaining mental function.

● Plays a critical role in cell division and growth.

How much you need: The RDA is 2.4 micrograms daily for adults. The recommendation increases to 2.6 micrograms daily during pregnancy and 2.8 micrograms daily during breast-feeding.

The 2010 Dietary Guidelines advises *those ages 50 years and older to consume foods fortified with vitamin B_{12}, such as fortified cereals or dietary supplements.* Although adults of this age on average do consume enough vitamin B_{12}, a significant number may have reduced ability to absorb naturally occurring vitamin B_{12}, but the crystalline form in fortified foods and supplements is well absorbed.

If you don't consume enough: A deficiency may result in anemia, fatigue, nerve damage, a smooth tongue, or very sensitive skin. A deficiency of vitamin B_{12} can be masked—and even progress—if extra folic acid is taken to treat or prevent anemia.

For either genetic or medical reasons, some people develop a deficiency—pernicious anemia—because they can't absorb vitamin B_{12}. They're missing a body chemical called intrinsic factor that comes from their stomach lining. This problem can be medically treated with injections of vitamin B_{12}.

Strict vegetarians, who eat no animal products, and the infants of vegan mothers are at risk for developing a vitamin B_{12} deficiency. This could cause severe anemia and irreversible nerve damage. The elderly also are at risk. Including foods fortified with vitamin B_{12} or dietary supplements can prevent vitamin B_{12} deficiency.

If you consume excess amounts: No symptoms are known, but taking extra vitamin B_{12} to boost energy has no basis in science.

Where it's mostly found: Vitamin B_{12} comes from animal products—meat, finfish, shellfish, poultry, eggs, milk, and other dairy foods. Some fortified foods may contain it.

FOOD	VITAMIN B$_{12}$ (MCG)
Salmon, cooked (3 oz.)	3.0
Beef tenderloin lean, broiled (3 oz.)	2.3
Yogurt, fat-free (1 cup)	1.5
Shrimp, cooked (3 oz.)	1.3
Milk (1 cup)	1.3
Egg, large (1)	0.7
Chicken, light meat, skinless, roasted (3 oz.)	0.3

Biotin

What it does:

- Helps your body produce energy in your cells.
- Helps metabolize (or use) proteins, fats, and carbohydrates from food.
- Helps regulate hormone synthesis.

How much you need: The Adequate Intake (AI) for biotin is 30 micrograms daily for adult males and females, including during pregnancy. The AI increases to 35 micrograms daily during breast-feeding.

If you don't consume enough: That's rarely a problem for healthy people who eat a healthful diet because the body also produces biotin from intestinal bacteria. In rare cases of deficiency, these symptoms may appear: heart abnormalities, appetite loss, fatigue, depression, or dry skin.

If you consume excess amounts: There are no reported effects of consuming excess amounts.

Where it's mostly found: Biotin is found in a wide variety of foods. Eggs, liver, yeast breads, and cereals are among the best sources.

FOOD	BIOTIN (MCG)
Egg, large (1)	11
Wheat germ (¼ cup)	5
Peanuts (½ cup)	5
Cottage cheese (½ cup)	5
Whole-grain bread (1 slice)	2

Pantothenic Acid

What it does:

- Helps your body cells produce energy.
- Helps metabolize (or use) proteins, fats, and carbohydrates from food.
- Helps regulate hormone synthesis.

How much you need: The Adequate Intake (AI) for pantothenic acid is 5 milligrams daily for teens ages fourteen to eighteen and for adults. During pregnancy and breast-feeding, the AI increases to 6 and 7 milligrams, respectively.

If you don't consume enough: That's rarely a problem for healthy people who eat a healthful diet.

If you consume excess amounts: The only apparent effects are occasional diarrhea and water retention.

Where it's mostly found: Pantothenic acid is widely available in food. Meat, poultry, fish, whole-grain cereals, and legumes are among the better sources. Milk, vegetables, and fruits also contain varying amounts.

FOOD	PANTOTHENIC ACID (MG)
Yogurt, fat-free (1 cup)	1.5
Salmon, cooked (3 oz.)	1.3
Sweet potato, mashed, cooked (½ cup)	1.0
Milk, fat-free (1 cup)	0.9
Chicken, light meat, skinless, roasted (3 oz.)	0.8
Corn, boiled (½ cup)	0.7
Egg, large (1)	0.7
Ham, lean (3 oz.)	0.5
Whole-wheat macaroni, cooked (½ cup)	0.3
Kidney beans, cooked (½ cup)	0.2

Choline

What it does: Choline, a vitaminlike substance, plays a role in many body processes.

- Promotes the transport of fats and helps make substances that form cell membranes.

● Helps make acetylcholine, which is a neuro-transmitter in your body needed for many functions, including muscle control and memory storage.

● Plays a role in liver function and reproductive health.

● Works with folic acid during pregnancy for the development of a baby's brain and nervous system.

How much you need: There is no RDA for choline. However, Adequate Intake (AI) levels were set in 1998: 550 milligrams daily for males ages fourteen and older; 400 milligrams daily for girls ages fourteen to eighteen; and 425 milligrams daily for women. During pregnancy and breast-feeding, the AI increases to 450 milligrams and 550 milligrams, respectively.

If you don't consume enough: Although there's little evidence of significant deficiencies in the United States, inadequate choline intake, common in the United States, may have health risks. A choline deficiency may be linked to an increased risk of heart disease because it results in increased homocysteine levels. *See chapter 22 to learn more.*

If you consume excess amounts: The Tolerable Upper Intake Level (UL) for adults is 3.5 grams of choline daily; for teens ages fourteen to eighteen, 3.0 grams daily.

Where it's mostly found: Choline, a natural food component, is widely distributed in food. Consuming modest amounts of eggs and eating beans (legumes) in place of some meat and poultry may provide enough. Eggs, soybeans, peanuts, and meat are especially good sources. Since nutrient content claims on food labels for choline are FDA-approved, you may find new choline-fortified products.

Food	Choline (mg)
Beef liver (3 oz.)	425
Egg yolk, large (1)	255
Beef, extra-lean (3 oz.)	85
Pistachios (1 oz.)	70

Vitamin C (ascorbic acid)

See "Vitamin C: More Jobs than You Think!" later in this chapter.

What it does:

● Helps produce collagen, a connective tissue that holds muscles, bones, and other tissues together.

● Helps keep capillary walls and blood vessels firm, and so protects you from bruising.

● Helps your body absorb iron and folate from plant sources of food.

● Helps keep your gums healthy so they don't bleed.

● Helps heal any cuts and wounds.

● Protects you from infection by stimulating the formation of antibodies and so boosting immunity.

● Works as an antioxidant to neutralize free radicals, which may inhibit damage to body cells.

Vitamin C works in partnership with iron, helping the body to absorb iron from plant sources of food. *See "Iron: The Power of Partnership" later in this chapter.* In fact, an adequate daily supply of vitamin C in your food choices can increase the absorption of nonheme iron (mostly from plant sources) by as much as two to four times. For those who get most of their iron from plant sources of food, including vegetarians, vitamin C is of special importance.

How much you need: The RDA for females and males ages fourteen to eighteen is 65 milligrams and 75 milligrams of vitamin C daily, respectively. Adult males need 90 milligrams daily; adult females, 75 milligrams of vitamin C daily (about the amount in ¾ cup of orange juice). Women need somewhat more during pregnancy (80 to 85 milligrams) and breast-feeding (115 to 120 milligrams).

For people who smoke, the RDA for vitamin C is increased by 35 milligrams daily to help counteract the oxidative damage from nicotine.

If you don't consume enough: Eventually, a severe deficiency of vitamin C leads to scurvy, a disease that causes loose teeth, excessive bleeding, and swollen gums. Wounds may not heal properly either. Because vitamin C-rich foods are widely available, scurvy is rare in the United States today.

If you consume an excess amount: Because vitamin C is water-soluble, your body excretes the excess; high levels of vitamin C in urine can mask the results of tests for diabetes. Very large doses may cause kidney stones and/or diarrhea, and for those with iron overload (hemochromatosis), excessive vitamin C (which enhances iron absorption) can make the problem worse. But the effects of taking large amounts for a long time isn't known. A Tolerable Upper Intake Level (UL) for vitamin C has been set: 2,000 milligrams daily for adults; 1,800 milligrams daily for teens ages fourteen to eighteen.

Where it's mostly found: Vitamin C mainly comes from plant sources of food. All citrus fruits, including oranges, grapefruits, and tangerines, are good sources. And many other fruits and vegetables listed below supply significant amounts, too.

FOOD	VITAMIN C (MG)
Red bell pepper (½ cup)	140
Papaya, medium (½)	95
Orange juice, 100 percent (¾ cup)	75
Green bell pepper (½ cup)	60
Broccoli, boiled (½ cup)	50
Strawberries (½ cup)	50
Grapefruit, white (½)	40
Tomato juice (¾ cup)	35
Cantaloupe (½ cup)	30
Mango, medium (½)	30
Cabbage, red, raw (½ cup)	25
Collard greens, frozen, boiled (½ cup)	25
Potato, medium, baked with skin (1)	20
Tomato, medium, raw (1)	15

Some fruit drinks, bottled waters, and other processed foods are fortified with vitamin C. Check the Nutrition Facts. If you rely only on fortified foods as your vitamin C source, you may miss out on other nutrients and compounds in foods with naturally occurring vitamin C.

Vitamins as Antioxidants

You've probably read the headlines "Antioxidants Promote Health!" or "Antioxidants Prevent Aging." Many food manufacturers are fortifying food with beta carotene (which forms vitamin A in the body), vitamin C, and vitamin E, as well as selenium (a mineral).

Antioxidants are a handful of vitamins, minerals, carotenoids, and polyphenols present in a variety of foods that significantly slow or prevent the oxidative (damage from oxygen) process and so prevent or repair damage to your body cells. They may also improve immune function and perhaps lower risk for infection and cancer.

What makes them unique? What foods supply them naturally? How might they work in your body? And how may antioxidants promote health and reduce chronic disease risk? Since antioxidants research is new, there's no conclusive evidence yet on their role in health.

Rounding Up Free Radicals

Just how do antioxidant vitamins work? First let's learn more about oxygen. To produce energy, every cell in your body needs a constant supply of oxygen. For this reason, oxygen is basic to life.

There's another side to the oxygen story. When body cells burn oxygen, they form free radicals, or oxygen by-products; a free radical is an unstable molecule with a missing electron. Free radicals can damage body cells and tissues, as well as the DNA, your body's master plan for reproducing cells. Environmental factors such as cigarette smoke and ultraviolet light also cause free radicals to form in your body.

Damage caused by oxidation is quite familiar: for example, the quick browning on a cut apple or pear, and rancidity in oils. However, if you dip your apple or pear in orange juice, which has vitamin C, it stays white. And if vitamin E is added as a preservative to vegetable oil, it doesn't turn rancid as fast.

In your body, the process is similar. Free radicals cause oxidation, or cell damage, as they "steal" an electron from body cells to become stable. Over time, that may lead to cell dysfunction and contribute to the

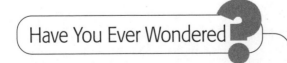
Have You Ever Wondered

. . . if bleeding gums mean you're not getting enough vitamin C? It's not likely unless you have a severe deficiency. Most cases of bleeding gums come from poor oral hygiene. Brushing and flossing regularly help keep your gums healthy. *For more about healthy gums, see chapter 22.*

onset of health problems such as cancer, artery and heart disease, cataracts, age-related macular degeneration, diabetes, Alzheimer's disease, and some deterioration that goes with aging. Antioxidants in your body counteract the action of free radicals.

Three antioxidant vitamins appear to neutralize free radicals: beta carotene and other carotenoids, vitamin C, and vitamin E. Some enzymes that have trace minerals—selenium, copper, zinc, and manganese—and some phytonutrients act as antioxidants, too. As scavengers, antioxidant vitamins mop up free radicals by donating an electron of their own. The result? Antioxidants may control free radicals or convert them to harmless waste products that get eliminated before they do damage. Antioxidants even may help undo some damage already done to body cells.

Each antioxidant has its own biological job description. Being water-soluble, vitamin C removes free radicals from fluids inside and outside of body cells. Beta carotene and vitamin E, because they're fat-soluble, are present in lipids and fat tissues in your body. Antioxidants seem to complement each other. Because they work together, an excess or a deficiency of one may inhibit the benefits of other antioxidants.

Scientific evidence can't promise that antioxidant nutrients provide a "safety shield" from chronic diseases. Their role and potential interactions in reducing the risks are among the many unknowns. And we don't know the potentially adverse affects of ongoing, high intakes of these nutrients from supplements, either. Still, a varied diet—that follows the food guide—with plenty of antioxidant-containing fruits, vegetables, and whole grains is smart eating! *See chapter 10.*

Carotenoids: "Color" Your Food Healthy

Imagine a beautiful autumn day. Leaves of red, orange, and yellow rustle in the branches overhead. The colors of the season belong to carotenoids, or plant pigments that generally are red, orange, and deep yellow.

The array of colors in fruits and vegetables also comes from carotenoids. The clues to their presence are obvious in the vibrant palette of produce in your supermarket. It's no surprise that apricots, cantaloupes, mangoes, carrots, red and yellow peppers, and sweet potatoes, for example, all contain carotene. Broccoli, kale, romaine lettuce, and spinach have carotene, too—even though they're dark green! The

Have You Ever Wondered

. . . if beta carotene supplements offer protection for smokers? No research supports any benefit. More importantly, a large study of smokers indicated that beta carotene supplements may be harmful to smokers. Smokers who used supplemental beta carotene had a higher incidence of lung cancer than those who didn't. For nonsmokers, it's still unknown whether higher intakes of beta carotene offer benefits.

orange-yellow color of their carotene gets hidden by the chlorophyll in the leaves. *For food sources of carotene see earlier in this chapter.*

Beta carotene is the carotenoid most familiar to us. Actually, the plant world has more than six hundred known carotenoids. Of those, only a few have been analyzed in fruits and vegetables: alpha carotene, beta carotene, beta cryptoxanthin, gamma carotene, lycopene, lutein, and zeaxanthin; even then, the data are limited.

Of the 563 identified carotenoids, only about 10 percent, including beta carotene, perform as precursors to vitamin A. Carotenoids also have other health-promoting functions. As antioxidants they offer protection from some diseases and degenerative changes that accompany aging.

For foods high in carotenoids, try to choose red, orange, deep-yellow, and some dark-green leafy vegetables every day. Color is a clue, not an assurance, that fruits and vegetables are good sources of beta carotene. For example, despite their color, neither corn nor snow peas have much beta carotene—but they do supply other nutrients and phytonutrients. *See vitamin A earlier in this chapter for sources.*

No Dietary Reference Intakes (no RDA, AI, or UL) specifically for carotenoids have been established yet except as precursors to vitamin A. Be cautious; consuming too much of them from dietary supplements may have an adverse effect. *See "Vitamin/Mineral Supplements: Benefits and Risks" in chapter 23.*

Vitamin C: More Jobs Than You Think!

Over the years, vitamin C, also known as ascorbic acid, developed celebrity status with claims that it can prevent or cure the common cold. Although those claims have been overblown, an adequate intake of vitamin C does play an important role in fighting infection; *see chapter 23*.

As an antioxidant, vitamin C may protect your body in much the same way that beta carotene and vitamin E do. However, vitamin C attacks free radicals in body fluids, not in fat tissue. Preliminary research is exploring a link to reduced risk of cataracts and cancer protection; no evidence exists to advise consuming more than the RDA for vitamin C.

Because vitamin C isn't stored in the body, you're wise to consume a vitamin C-rich food daily. If you habitually consume a vitamin C-rich fruit or juice with breakfast, you probably consume enough.

Fruits, Vegetables, Herbs, and Spices: Their Antioxidant Potential

A food's health-promoting benefits likely come from many antioxidants, not just a single antioxidant nutrient or food substance. With this in mind, a scientific scoring method—the ORAC (oxygen radical absorbency capacity) score—has been created to estimate the overall antioxidant potential of fruits, vegetables, spices, herbs, and other foods. The higher the ORAC score, the greater the antioxidant potential.

FRUIT (RAW)	TOTAL ORAC UNITS	VEGETABLES (RAW)	TOTAL ORAC UNITS	HERBS AND SPICES	TOTAL ORAC UNITS
Cranberries, chopped (½ cup)	5,000	Asparagus (½ cup)	1,508	Cinnamon, ground (1 tsp.)	3,417
Blackberries (½ cup)	4,252	Beets, sliced (½ cup)	1,208	Oregano, dried (1 tsp.)	3,155
Strawberries, sliced (½ cup)	3,571	Broccoli, chopped (½ cup)	680	Turmeric, ground (1 tsp.)	2,795
Blueberries (½ cup)	3,502	Sweet potatoes, cubes (½ cup)	595	Thyme, dried (1 tsp.)	2,203
Pomegranate juice (½ cup)	3,351	Corn (½ cup)	531	Rosemary, dried (1 tsp.)	1,983
Apple with skin, slices (½ cup)	1,677	Cauliflower, chopped (½ cup)	470	Curry powder (1 tsp.)	970
Peaches, sliced (½ cup)	1,479	Spinach (1 cup)	454	Ginger, ground (1 tsp.)	703
Red grapes (½ cup)	1,378	Carrots, sliced (½ cup)	446	Red pepper (paprika) (1 tsp.)	504
Dates, medjool (2)	1,145	Green bell pepper, sliced (½ cup)	430		
Orange juice (½ cup)	900	Red bell pepper, sliced (½ cup)	390		
Banana, small (1)	803	Tomatoes, chopped (½ cup)	348		
Green grapes (½ cup)	764	Onions, sliced (¼ cup)	262		
Cantaloupe, cubes (½ cup)	255				

*Total ORAC units are both water-soluble and fat-soluble antioxidant compounds. Scores for all foods have variability; the values here have been recalculated to provide foods in household measures and rounded.

Source: Oxygen Radical Absorbance Capacity (ORAC) of Selected Foods, Release 2 (2010) www.ars.usda.gov/Services/docs.htm?docid=15866

This database contains ORAC data for 326 food items and represents a collaboration between the Nutrient Data Laboratory, Beltsville Human Nutrition Research Center, and the Arkansas Children's Nutrition Center in Little Rock, Arkansas.

Remember: The ORAC score offers a scientific method for looking at food in a new way. No guidelines exist to suggest how many ORAC units you need. *Be aware:* A high ORAC value doesn't mean a food performs better as an antioxidant source; the ORAC score does not suggest bioavailability of these antioxidants, which cannot be measured at this time.

Vitamin E: One Main Mission

For years, vitamin E has been surrounded by pseudo-scientific myths. It's been misguidedly acclaimed as a cure for almost all that ails you: for example, improving sexual prowess, curing infertility, preventing aging, curing heart disease and cancer, and improving athletic performance, to name just a few. The benefits of vitamin E don't extend this far, but it does appear to play a broad role in promoting your health.

The main role of vitamin E—a fat-soluble vitamin—appears to be as an antioxidant. It may help prevent the oxidation of LDL ("bad") cholesterol, which contributes to plaque buildup in the arteries; although the jury's still out, that may help reduce the risk for heart disease and stroke. Vitamin E also may help protect from cell damage that can lead ultimately to health problems such as cancer. Vitamin E appears to work with other antioxidants such as vitamin C and selenium.

In vegetable oils, nuts, and seeds, vitamin E protects their unsaturated fats from oxidation. Typically, foods high in unsaturated fats also are good sources of vitamin E. *See "Vitamin E" earlier in this chapter for sources.*

A "Garden" of Antioxidants

Where should your antioxidant vitamins come from? An eating style with plenty of fruits and vegetables is undisputed as the wisest approach to good health. Eating plenty of whole-grain foods, as well as nuts, containing vitamin E provides them, too.

Many foods are fortified with antioxidant vitamins: C, E, and beta carotene. While they may not supply enough antioxidant vitamins for their possible protective benefits, they're often good sources. For carotenoids and vitamin C, fruits and vegetables still are the best sources, as they contain other phytonutrients that may help protect against some health problems such as some cancers and heart disease.

Antioxidant vitamins in fruits and vegetables may work together to reduce the risks of chronic disease. That's one more reason to eat a variety of them!

Antioxidants in Supplements

Even if a little is good, a lot may not be better. So far no research proves that taking beta carotene, vitamins C or E, or other antioxidant supplements reduces disease risk.

Have You Ever Wondered

. . . how tortillas made with corn could have calcium? Made in the traditional Mexican way, corn tortillas can supply significant amounts of calcium, especially to people who eat them as the main bread in their everyday diet. Corn itself doesn't have calcium. But to prepare corn for tortillas, it's first soaked in slaked lime to remove the hard coating on corn kernels. Not from citrus fruit, this lime is instead calcium hydroxide, which is safe to eat when used this way in food processing.

To date, scientists haven't pinpointed which antioxidants offer specific benefits, how much would be enough—or how long you'd need to take them. They don't know enough about side effects from taking supplemental antioxidants over long periods of time. Moreover, the mix of antioxidants in food, not just one or two from supplements, may offer positive and powerful antioxidant action.

Other antioxidant issues need research. For one, high doses from antioxidant supplements may be harmful, perhaps by working as pro-oxidants that promote, rather than neutralize, oxidation. Second, not all free radicals are harmful. Some protect by attacking harmful bacteria or cancer cells in the body. Very high intakes of antioxidants may destroy or hinder these protective free radicals.

Until more is known, enjoy a wide variety of fruits, vegetables, whole-grain products, and nuts and seeds, with their many naturally occurring antioxidants. And avoid high doses from supplements. *For more about dietary supplements, see chapter 23.*

Minerals—Not "Heavy Metal"

The term "minerals" may conjure up thoughts of rocks. But to your body, minerals are another group of essential nutrients, needed to both regulate body processes and give your body structure.

Like vitamins, minerals help trigger, or regulate, a myriad of processes that continually take place in your body, so they are essential to your life. For example, they regulate fluid balance, muscle contractions, and nerve impulses.

Even though they make up only about 4 percent of your weight, minerals help give your body structure. They not only give structure to bones and teeth, but muscles, blood, and other body tissues all contain minerals, too.

Unlike vitamins, minerals are inorganic. Minerals can't be destroyed by heat or other food-handling processes. In fact, if you've ever completely burned food, perhaps while cooking over a fire, the little bit of ash left over is its mineral content.

From a dietary perspective, minerals belong in two categories—major minerals and trace minerals—depending on how much you need. Regardless of amount, they're all essential.

● *Major minerals:* Major minerals are needed in greater amounts than trace minerals are—more than 250 milligrams are recommended daily for each one. Calcium, phosphorus, and magnesium fit in this category, along with three electrolytes—sodium, chloride, and potassium.

Electrolytes, grouped together because their work is interrelated, regulate body fluids in and out of every cell. Electrolytes also transmit nerve, or electrical, impulses. *To learn more, see "Sodium and Potassium: You Need Them!" in chapter 7.*

● *Trace minerals:* Your body needs just small amounts—fewer than 20 milligrams daily—for each of the trace minerals, or trace elements: chromium, copper, fluoride, iodine, iron, manganese, molybdenum, selenium, and zinc. Recommended Dietary Allowances have been set for only some: copper, iodine, iron, molybdenum, selenium, and zinc. Others are presented in the DRIs as Adequate Intake Levels (AIs).

Nutrition experts have reviewed research on other trace elements: arsenic, boron, nickel, silicon, and vanadium. They don't appear to have a role in human health. However, Tolerable Upper Intake Levels (UL) have been set for some: boron (20 milligrams a day), nickel (1.0 milligram a day), and vanadium (1.8 milligrams a day) for adult levels.

All minerals are absorbed in your intestines, then transported and stored in your body in different ways. Some pass directly into your bloodstream, where they're carried to cells; any excess passes out of the body through urine. Others attach to proteins and become part of your body structure; because they're stored, excess amounts can be harmful if the levels consumed are too high for too long.

Note: On the following pages, the amounts of minerals in foods have been rounded.

Major Minerals

Calcium

See "Hot Topic: Bone Health" later in this chapter.

What it does:

● Builds bones, in both length and strength, becoming part of bone tissue.

● Helps your bones remain strong by slowing the rate of bone loss as you age; reduces the risk of osteoporosis.

● Helps your muscles contract and your heart beat.

● Plays a key role in normal nerve function.

● Helps your blood clot if you're bleeding.

● May help control blood pressure. *See chapters 10 and 22 to learn about the DASH (Dietary Approaches to Stop Hypertension) Eating Plan and its calcium link.*

● Although research is limited, calcium or dairy foods may reduce the risk of breast cancer and may play a role in cardiovascular health.

How much you need: With recommendations updated in 2010, the Recommended Dietary Allowances (RDA) for children ages four to eight and for adults ages nineteen to fifty are set at 1,000 milligrams of calcium daily. For women ages fifty-one and above and for men over age seventy, the RDA goes up to 1,200 milligrams daily. From ages nine to eighteen the RDA is 1,300 milligrams. Calcium recommendations for women who are pregnant or breast-feeding are the same as for other women in their respective age group. Following RDA advice for vitamin D is essential, too, as these two nutrients work in partnership (*see "Vitamin D" earlier in this chapter*).

Like vitamin D, calcium is a nutrient cited by the 2010 Dietary Guidelines as a nutrient of public health concern.

As an extra safeguard, many doctors also recommend a calcium supplement, especially for menopausal and postmenopausal women to help slow bone

Hot Topic: Bone Health

The human body contains more calcium than any other mineral. For an average 130-pound adult, about 1,200 grams (almost 3 pounds) of the body is calcium. Your body composition, of course, depends on the size of your body frame, the density of your bones, and, if you're older, how much bone mass you've lost through aging.

About 99 percent of your body's calcium is in your bones. The remaining 1 percent is in other body fluids and cells. Calcium is as important to you as an adult as it was during your childhood. The reasons really aren't that different.

Your bones are in a constant state of change. Because bones are living tissue, calcium gets deposited and withdrawn daily from your skeleton, much like money in a bank, in a process called re-modeling. Older bone tissue is replaced with new bone tissue. To keep your bones strong and to reduce bone loss, you need to make regular calcium deposits to replace the losses—and even build up a little nest egg of calcium for when your food choices come up short.

Calcium doesn't work alone. It works in partnership with other nutrients, including phosphorus and vitamin D. Vitamin D helps absorb, carry, and deposit calcium in bones and teeth. Phosphorus is also an important part of the structure of bone.

If you don't consume enough calcium—or if your body doesn't adequately absorb it (perhaps because you're short on vitamin D)—your body may withdraw more calcium from your bones than you deposit. You need calcium, for example, for muscle contraction and for your heartbeat, too. This process gradually depletes bone, leaving a void in places where calcium otherwise would be deposited, eventually making bones more porous and fragile. (*Refer to "Which Bone Is Healthy?" in chapter 22 to compare healthy bone with osteoporotic bone*).

Regular, weight-bearing physical activities—such as walking, strength-training, dancing, kick-boxing, and tennis—are essential to bone health, too. They trigger nerve impulses that, in turn, activate other body chemicals to deposit calcium in bones. When you don't put weight on your bones because you're bedridden or very sedentary, it signals to your body that it doesn't need bone, which results in calcium excretion.

"Boning up " is a life-long process—starting at the moment of conception:

- During the childhood and teen years, bones grow long and wide. Forty percent or more of the body's bone mass is formed during adolescence. *See chapter 17 for more about calcium during the teen years.*

- By age twenty or so, that phase of bone building is complete. But building peak bone-mass continues until your early thirties. Bones become stronger and more dense as more calcium becomes part of the bone matrix.

- After age thirty or so, bones slowly lose minerals that give them strength. That's a natural part of aging. Whatever calcium a woman has stored away in her skeleton will be the amount in her bones when she enters menopause. Even then, consuming enough calcium and vitamin D can help women retain their bone density and lower the risk for osteoporosis later on.

- For women during their child-bearing years, the hormone estrogen appears to protect bones, keeping them strong. With the onset of menopause, bone loss speeds up as estrogen levels go down. If women achieve their peak bone mass as younger adults, their risk for osteoporosis, or brittle bone disease, is reduced later in life.

- For older adults ages fifty-one and over, calcium and vitamin D remain essential for building and maintaining healthy bones, as well as for protection from high blood pressure. Even if you start now, you can benefit from consuming more calcium and vitamin D. *See chapter 19 to learn more.*

Basic strategies for bone health:

- Consume adequate amounts of calcium and vitamin D—at every age and stage of life!

- Participate regularly in weight-bearing activities—at least three times weekly.

- Be careful about weight loss. Eating plans that severely restrict food often restrict calcium and vitamin D, too.

- Avoid smoking and excessive amounts of alcoholic beverages. Both interfere with bone health.

To review the many factors that relate to osteoporosis, refer to chapter 22.

loss that comes with hormonal changes. Many women simply don't consume enough calcium.

If you're advised to take calcium supplements, use them to fill the calcium gap—not to substitute for calcium-rich foods. *See "Calcium Supplements: A Bone Builder" in chapter 23.*

If you don't consume enough: For children, not getting enough calcium may interfere with growth; a severe deficiency may keep children from reaching their potential adult height. Even a mild deficiency over a lifetime can affect bone density and bone loss, increasing the risk for osteoporosis, or brittle bone disease.

If you consume excess amounts: Unless the doses are very large (more than 2,500 milligrams daily), adverse effects for adults are unlikely. Very large doses over a prolonged time may cause kidney stones and poor kidney function, and may affect the absorption of other minerals such as iron, magnesium, and zinc. Regular consumption of milk and milk products won't result in excessive amounts of calcium. The Tolerable Upper Intake Level (UL) from the Dietary Reference Intakes have been set at 2,500 milligrams for those

ages one to eight and ages nineteen to fifty. For those ages nine to eighteen, the UL is 3,000 milligrams of calcium; for those over age fifty, it's 2,000 milligrams. Chronic heartburn may result from consuming antacids with calcium in amounts beyond the recommended dosage.

Where it's mostly found: Milk and other dairy foods such as yogurt and most cheeses are the best sources of calcium. These foods and foods made from them provide about 72 percent of the calcium in the United States. In addition, some dark-green leafy vegetables (kale, broccoli, bok choy), fish with edible bones, calcium-fortified soy milk, and tofu made with calcium sulfate also supply significant amounts. Juice, bottled water, and bread may be calcium fortified.

Green, leafy vegetables and grain products supply some calcium. However, some vegetables such as spinach contain oxalates; grains may contain phytates. Both bind with some minerals, including calcium, magnesium, and iron, partially blocking their absorption. Caffeine slightly interferes with calcium absorption, as well.

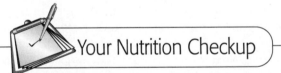

Your Nutrition Checkup

Do You Consume Enough Calcium?

Estimate your intake from food yesterday.

Step 1: Estimate calcium intake from calcium-rich foods.*

PRODUCT	SERVINGS/DAY		ESTIMATED CALCIUM/SERVING (MG)		CALCIUM (MG)
Milk (8 oz.)	_____	×	300	=	_____
Yogurt (6 oz.)	_____	×	300	=	_____
Cheese (1 oz. or 1 cubic in.)	_____	×	200	=	_____
Fortified foods or juices	_____	×	80 to 1,000**	=	_____

Step 2: Total calcium from Step 1 + 250 mg for nondairy sources = total dietary calcium = _____

About 75 to 80 percent of calcium consumed in the American diet is from dairy products. Although not included in this score, some other dairy foods such as ice cream, also provide some calcium.

**Calcium content of fortified foods varies.*

Source: Adapted and reprinted with permission from *Clinician's Guide to the Prevention and Treatment of Osteoporosis,* 2010, National Osteoporosis Foundation, Washington, D.C. 20037.

Food	Calcium (mg)
Yogurt, plain, low-fat (1 cup)	450
Tofu, regular (processed with calcium*) (½ cup)	435
Milk, fat-free (1 cup)	305
Chocolate milk, 1% (1 cup)	290
Swiss cheese, low-fat (1 oz.)	270
Calcium-fortified orange juice (¾ cup)	260
Calcium-fortified soy milk (8 oz.)	250–350
Cheese pizza† (⅛ of 15-in. pizza)	220
Cheddar cheese (1 oz.)	205
Salmon, canned with edible bones (3 oz.)	205
Pudding (½ cup)	160
Turnip greens, boiled (½ cup)	100
Frozen yogurt (½ cup)	90
Tempeh (½ cup)	90
Okra (½ cup)	90
Cottage cheese (½ cup)	75
Tofu, raw (processed without calcium*) (½ cup)	60
Mustard greens, boiled (½ cup)	50
Orange (1)	50
Tortillas (made from slaked lime-processed corn*)	45
Pinto beans, boiled (½ cup)	40

*Read the labels.
†The amount of calcium may vary, depending on the ingredients.

Have You Ever Wondered?

... if calcium supplements or calcium-fortified foods can substitute for dairy foods? For most people, fortified foods and supplements are meant to supplement, not replace, foods naturally rich in calcium.

Although they may fill the calcium gap, supplements and calcium-fortified foods (such as in some juice, cereal, pasta, and rice) don't supply all the other health-promoting nutrients and food substances found in dairy foods. Besides calcium, dairy group foods are key sources of protein, vitamins A, B_2 (riboflavin), B_{12}, and D (if fortified) and the minerals phosphorus, potassium, magnesium, and zinc. Beyond that, dairy foods offer substances with potential functional benefits: conjugated linoleic acid (CLA), sphingolipid, and butyric acid, which may help protect you from some cancers and other health conditions. *For more about CLA, see "Functional Nutrition: Eat Your Omega-3s and -6s" in chapter 5. See chapter 12 for more about calcium-fortified soy beverages.*

You can overdo calcium if you regularly consume calcium-fortified juice and/or calcium-fortified breakfast cereal—and take a calcium supplement as "insurance." What's the downside? Too much calcium, most likely from fortified foods and supplements, may limit the absorption of iron and zinc, two minerals that often come up short for many Americans.

... if eggs count as a calcium-rich dairy food? Although they're typically sold in the dairy case, eggs aren't a dairy food! Since you don't eat the shell (your body can't use that form of calcium), eggs supply very little calcium.

Phosphorus

What it does:

● Helps generate energy in every cell of your body.

● Acts as the main regulator of energy metabolism in your body's organs.

● Is a major component of bones and teeth, second only to calcium.

● Serves as part of DNA and RNA, which are your body's master plan for cell growth and repair.

How much you need: The RDA for phosphorus is 1,250 milligrams daily for ages nine through eighteen, then decreases to 700 milligrams daily for adults of all ages. Scientific evidence shows that people need less than previously thought.

If you don't consume enough: A deficiency is quite rare, except for small, premature babies who consume only breast milk, or for people who take an antacid with aluminum hydroxide for a long time. In those rare cases, the symptoms include bone loss, weakness, loss of appetite, and pain.

If you consume excess amounts: An excess amount may lower the level of calcium in the blood—a problem if calcium intake is low. As a result, bone loss may increase. Besides that, consuming too much phosphorus doesn't appear to be a problem in the United States. The Tolerable Upper Intake Level (UL) for phosphorus is 4,000 milligrams a day for people ages nine through seventy; after age seventy, it's 3,000 milligrams of phosphorus daily. For pregnancy, the level drops slightly, to 3,500 milligrams of phosphorus daily.

Where it's mostly found: Almost all foods contain phosphorus. Protein-rich foods—milk, meat, poultry, fish, and eggs—contain the most. Beans (legumes) and nuts are good sources as well. Even bread and other baked foods have some. You'll also find phosphorus in colas and other dark-colored soft drinks.

Food	Phosphorus (mg)
Milk, fat-free (1 cup)	245
Perch, cooked (3 oz.)	220
Lean ground beef, cooked (3 oz.)	195
Cheddar cheese (1 oz.)	145
Kidney beans, cooked (½ cup)	125
Tofu (½ cup)	120
Peanut butter (2 tbsp.)	115
Egg, large (1)	95
Cola (12 oz.)	40

Magnesium

What it does:

- Serves as an important part of more than three hundred body enzymes, body chemicals that regulate body functions, including producing energy, making body protein, and helping regulate blood glucose levels.
- Helps maintain body cells in nerves and muscles, signals muscles to relax and contract.
- Keeps heart rhythm steady, and promotes normal blood pressure.
- Serves as a component of bones.
- May help maintain immune response.

How much you need: The RDA for teenage boys is 410 milligrams of magnesium daily to age eighteen; for teenage girls, 360 milligrams daily. The RDA for adult males is 400 milligrams daily through age thirty, then

420 milligrams daily after that. For females, the recommendation is 310 milligrams daily through age thirty, then 320 milligrams daily after age thirty. Neither pregnancy nor breast-feeding increases the need for magnesium.

If you don't consume enough: A deficiency is rare except in diseases where the body doesn't absorb magnesium properly. Then symptoms might include irregular heartbeat, nausea, weakness, and/or mental derangement.

That said, many Americans don't consume enough and may not have enough magnesium stored in the body to protect against health problems such as heart disease and immune disorders.

If you consume an excess amount: Consuming too much magnesium from food probably won't do any harm—unless it can't be excreted properly due to kidney disease. The Tolerable Upper Intake Level is 350 milligrams a day; this amount is less than the RDA because it represents only the amount of magnesium in supplements or drugs, and not from food or drinks.

Where it's mostly found: Magnesium is found in varying amounts in all kinds of foods. The best sources are beans (legumes), nuts, and whole grains. Green vegetables are good sources, too, because chlorophyll contains magnesium.

Food	Magnesium (mg)
Spinach, boiled (½ cup)	80
Peanut butter (2 tbsp.)	50
Black-eyed peas, boiled (½ cup)	45
Pecans, dried (1 oz.)	40
Lima beans, boiled (½ cup)	40
Whole-wheat bread (1 slice)	25
Parsnips, boiled (½ cup)	25
Whole-wheat spaghetti, cooked (½ cup)	20

Major Minerals: Electrolytes

Chloride

What it does:

- Helps regulate fluids in and out of body cells.
- As a component of stomach acid, helps with

the digestion of your food and the absorption of nutrients.

● Helps transmit nerve impulses, or signals.

How much you need: The Adequate Intake for all aged nine to fifty (including during pregnancy and breast-feeding) is 2,300 milligrams a day. For ages fifty-one to seventy years, it goes down to 2,000 milligrams a day; after age seventy, it's 1,800 milligrams daily.

If you don't get enough: Because salt is such a common part of the diet, a deficiency of chloride isn't likely. If deficient, however, symptoms are similar to sodium deficiency.

If you consume excess amounts: For people who are sensitive, along with sodium, there may be a link to high blood pressure, but more study is needed. The Tolerable Upper Intake Level (UL) is 3,400 milligrams daily for kids ages nine to thirteen; after that, the UL is 3,600 milligrams daily for teens and adults.

Where it's mostly found: Salt is sodium plus chloride. Salt and salty foods are the main chloride sources: ¼ teaspoon of salt has 750 milligrams of chloride.

Potassium

See chapter 7, "Sodium and Potassium: A Salty Subject."

What it does:

● Helps regulate fluids and mineral balance in and out of body cells.

● Helps maintain your normal blood pressure by blunting sodium's effects on blood pressure.

● Helps transmit nerve impulses, or signals.

● Helps reduce the risk of kidney stones and decreased bone loss.

● Helps your muscles contract.

How much you need: The Adequate Intake (AI) level for potassium is 4,500 milligrams daily for those ages nine to thirteen. From ages fourteen on up, the AI is 4,700 milligrams daily, including pregnancy. For breast-feeding women, the AI is 5,100 milligrams. People with kidney disease and on some diuretics or heart disease medicines such as ACE inhibitors should check with their doctor for guidance on potassium intake. Current evidence suggests that African Amer-

icans and those with high blood pressure especially benefit from increasing their intake of potassium.

The 2010 Dietary Guidelines advises consuming more potassium from a variety of foods, notably vegetables, fruits, and dairy foods, to reach the recommended level for optimal health without over-consuming calories (energy).

If you don't consume enough: For healthy people, a potassium deficiency is rare. When vomiting, diarrhea, or laxative use goes on for too long, the body may lose excess amounts. Kidney problems also may cause severe loss. Deficiency symptoms include muscle cramps, weakness, appetite loss, nausea, and fatigue. You may need a potassium supplement if you're on medication for high blood pressure. Talk to your doctor.

If you consume excess amounts: Harmful effects from consuming too much from food are rare; excess amounts usually are excreted. If an excess can't be excreted, it can cause heart problems and possible sudden death. People with kidney problems may not be able to get rid of excess potassium and may be advised to limit potassium-containing foods and to avoid using potassium chloride as a salt substitute. There is no Tolerable Upper Intake Level for potassium.

Where it's mostly found: Potassium is found in a wide range of foods, especially fruits, many vegetables, beans (legumes), dairy foods, meat, poultry, fish and nuts. Less processed foods tend to have more potassium.

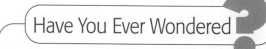

Have You Ever Wondered

. . . about sulfate—since it's considered an electrolyte? Inorganic sulfate is a nutrient with electrolyte properties. The Dietary Reference Intakes (DRIs) identify sulfate, but don't show an Adequate Intake (AI) level. Food, water, and the metabolic breakdown of amino acids in the body provide enough. Dried fruit and fruit juice, wine, beer, soy flour, bread, and meat supply sulfate. No Tolerable Upper Intake Level (UL) exists, either. The odor and off-flavor usually limit how much people consume. That said, when the water supply has a high level of sulfate, diarrhea may result.

FOOD	POTASSIUM (MG)
Banana, medium (1)	420
Milk, fat-free (1 cup)	380
Kidney beans, cooked (½ cup)	360
Haddock, cooked (3 oz.)	340
Dates, medjool (2)	335
Potato, baked, with skin (2 oz.)	330
Tomato, medium (1)	290
Orange, medium (1)	235
Turkey, light and dark meat, roasted, skinless (3 oz.)	225
Almonds (1 oz. or 24 almonds)	210
Spinach, raw (1 cup)	170
Okra, boiled (½ cup)	110

Sodium

Sodium is a nutrient of public health concern due to its link to high blood pressure. Many Americans consume significantly more sodium than the Tolerable Upper Intake Level (UL). *See chapter 7, "Sodium and Potassium: A Salty Subject."*

What it does:

- Helps regulate the movement of body fluids in and out of your body cells.
- Helps muscles, including your heart, relax.
- Helps transmit nerve impulses, or signals.
- Helps regulate your blood pressure.

How much you need: The Adequate Intake (AI) for males and females ages nine to fifty is 1,500 milligrams a day. The level stays the same during pregnancy and breast-feeding. For ages fifty to seventy, it goes down to 1,300 milligrams a day; after age seventy, it's 1,200 milligrams daily.

The 2010 Dietary Guidelines advises *reducing daily sodium intake to less than 2,300 milligrams (mg) and further reducing intake to 1,500 mg among people who are fifty-one and older and those of any age who are African American or have hypertension, diabetes, or chronic kidney disease.* The 1,500 mg recommendation applies to about half of the U.S. population, including children and the majority of adults.

If you don't consume enough: Unless you have prolonged diarrhea or vomiting, or have kidney problems, a sodium deficiency isn't likely. If it happens, symptoms might include nausea, dizziness, and muscle cramps.

If you consume an excess amount: For healthy people, excess sodium is excreted, but some kidney diseases interfere with sodium excretion, causing fluid retention and swelling. For people with sodium sensitivity, a high-sodium diet can increase blood pressure.

The UL is 2,200 milligrams daily for kids ages nine to thirteen; after that, the UL is 2,300 milligrams daily for teens and adults, including pregnant or breast-feeding women. This advice is set for people who don't have high blood pressure; the UL may be too high for those who already have it.

Where it's mostly found: Processed foods account for about 75 percent of the sodium in food. The rest comes from from salt added in cooking and at the table and the small amount that occurs naturally in food. As a point of reference, ¼ teaspoon of salt contains about 500 milligrams of sodium.

FOOD	SODIUM (MG)
Beef bologna (1 oz.)	310
Cheddar cheese (1 oz.)	175
Whole-wheat bread (1 slice)	150
Milk, fat-free (1 cup)	105

The Nutrition Facts on food labels tell how much sodium comes from a single label serving of food. *See "Get All the Facts!" in chapter 12 on food labeling.*

Trace Minerals

Chromium

What it does:

- Works with insulin to help your body use blood glucose, or blood sugar.
- May be involved in carbohydrate, fat, and protein metabolism.

How much you need: A level of Adequate Intake (AI) has been set for chromium: 35 micrograms per day for males ages fourteen to fifty, and 30 micrograms per day from age fifty-one on. For females, 24 micrograms daily from ages fourteen to eighteen; 25 micrograms daily from ages nineteen through fifty; and 20 micrograms daily from age fifty-one on. During pregnancy, the AI level is 5 micrograms daily higher; during breast-feeding, an additional 20 micrograms.

If you don't consume enough: Because chromium works closely with insulin, a deficiency can look like diabetes. *See "Diabetes: A Growing Concern" in chapter 22 for more about diabetes.*

If you consume excess amounts: Consuming harmful amounts from dietary sources is highly unlikely. No UL has been set for chromium; few serious adverse effects have been linked to high intakes of chromium.

Where it's mostly found: Meat, eggs, whole-grain products and some fruits and vegetables are all reasonable sources.

Food	Chromium (mcg)
Liver, braised (3 oz.)	42
Shredded wheat (1 oz.)	33
Peas (½ cup)	30
Egg, large (1)	26

Copper

What it does:

● Helps your body make hemoglobin, needed to carry oxygen in red blood cells.

● Serves as a part of many body enzymes.

● Helps your body develop connective tissue, myelin, and melanin.

● Helps your body produce energy in the cells.

How much you need: The RDA for copper is set at 890 micrograms per day for teens ages fourteen to eighteen, and 900 micrograms daily for adults. During pregnancy the level is 1,000 micrograms daily; during breast-feeding it's 1,300 micrograms daily.

If you don't consume enough: A deficiency rarely comes from a lack of copper, but instead from genetic problems. Another cause: excess zinc from supplement sources can hinder copper absorption.

If you consume excess amounts: Harmful effects of copper from dietary sources are extremely rare in the United States. The Tolerable Upper Intake Level (UL)

is 8,000 micrograms daily for teens ages fourteen to eighteen, and 10,000 micrograms daily for adults.

Where it's mostly found: Organ meats, especially liver; seafood; nuts; and seeds are the best sources. Cooking in copper pots increases the copper in food.

Food	Copper (mcg)
Beef liver, braised (3 oz.)	12,140
Clams, cooked (3 oz.)	590
Sunflower seeds, dry roasted (1 oz.)	520
Peanuts, dry roasted (1 oz.)	190
Mushrooms, canned (½ cup)	180

Fluoride

See "The Fluoride Connection" in chapter 8.

What it does:

● Helps harden tooth enamel and so helps protect your teeth from decay.

● May offer some protection from osteoporosis, or brittle bone disease, by helping to strengthen bones.

How much you need: An Adequate Intake (AI) for fluoride has been set. AI levels for children are as follows: ages four to eight, 1 milligram of fluoride daily, and ages nine to thirteen, 2 milligrams of fluoride daily. For teens the AI is set at 3 milligrams of fluoride daily. For adults, the guideline is 4 milligrams of fluoride daily for males and 3 milligrams daily for females. There are no increased needs during pregnancy or breast-feeding. A fluoride supplement may be prescribed by a dentist or doctor for some infants and children. *See "Vitamin and Mineral Supplements for Breast-Fed Babies" in chapter 16.*

If you don't consume enough: Tooth enamel may be weak with greater risk for cavities.

If you consume excess amounts: With excessive fluoride, teeth become mottled, or marked with brown stains, although teeth are healthy in every other way. This consition is called fluorosis. Be aware that these stains may have other causes as well. The Tolerable Upper Intake Level (UL) is 2.2 milligrams of fluoride daily for children ages four through eight; from age nine through adulthood, the UL is 10 milligrams of fluoride daily.

Where it's mostly found: Fluoride is not widely available in food. Two significant food sources are tea, especially if it's made with fluoridated water, and fish with edible bones, such as canned salmon. Many municipal water supplies are fluoridated; however, most bottled waters are not. The fluoride content in food varies and is affected by the environment in which the food originated. Based on current scientific reviews, the U.S. Department of Health and Human Services announced plans in 2011 to lower the recommended level of fluoride in drinking water. Fluorosis among youth is becoming more common, and studies also are exploring other health risks related to excess fluoride.

Iodine

What it does:

● Serves as part of thyroid hormones such as thyroxin, which regulate the rate at which your body uses energy.

● Plays an important role in fetal and infant development and proper health at all life stages.

How much you need: The RDA for iodine is 150 micrograms daily for adults. During pregnancy, the recommendation goes up to 220 micrograms; during breast-feeding, 290 micrograms daily.

If you don't consume enough: With an iodine deficiency, the body can't make enough thyroxin. As a result, the rate at which the body burns energy slows down, and weight gain may become a problem. Goiter, an enlarged thyroid gland, is the deficiency disease often caused by a lack of iodine. With the use of iodized salt, goiter and other serious health problems rarely are caused by an iodine deficiency.

If you consume excess amounts: Goiter also can be induced when people consume high levels of iodine—but not at levels consumed in the United States. Too much also can result in irregular heartbeat and confusion. The Tolerable Upper Intake Level (UL) is 900 micrograms daily for teens ages fourteen to eighteen, and 1,100 micrograms daily during adulthood.

Where it's mostly found: Iodine is found naturally in saltwater fish. Foods grown near coastal areas also contain iodine, but many people don't have access to these foods. For this reason, salt is iodized voluntarily, to help assure an adequate amount of iodine in the food supply, even if you consume only modest amounts of salt. One-half teaspoon of iodized salt provides almost enough iodine to reach the RDA for a day. Most salt intake in the United States comes from processed foods, which usually isn't iodized.

FOOD	IODINE (MCG)
Cod, cooked (3 oz.)	99
Table salt, iodized (¼ tsp.)	98
Potato, cooked (1 medium)	54
Turkey breast, baked (3 oz.)	34
Navy beans, cooked (½ cup)	31

Iron

What it does:

● Serves as an essential part of hemoglobin, which carries oxygen in your blood from your lungs to every body cell, and other enzymes.

● Helps change beta carotene to vitamin A, helps produce collagen (which holds body tissues together), and helps make body proteins (amino acids).

● Helps in brain development.

● Supports a healthy immune system.

Although iron has many biological functions, its main job is to carry oxygen in the hemoglobin of red blood cells. In fact, about two-thirds of your body's iron is in hemoglobin. Hemoglobin takes oxygen to your body cells, where it's used to produce energy. Iron in red blood cells also helps take away carbon dioxide, a by-product of energy production. Red blood cells have a "life span" of about four months. After that, some of their iron gets recycled; either it's stored or used immediately to make new red blood cells. This recycling action helps protect you from iron deficiency.

How much you need: Iron needs are highest during periods of rapid growth: childhood, adolescence, childbearing years for women, and pregnancy. Prior to menopause, women need enough iron to replace losses from menstrual flow. Iron needs also go up to support increases of blood volume during pregnancy. Not surprisingly, iron-deficiency anemia is most common among people at these ages and stages of life, too, when the dietary need for iron is highest. In fact, it's hard to get enough without taking an iron supplement.

With menopause, iron needs drop. That's the time to *stop* taking an iron supplement, especially for women at risk for hemochromatosis, a genetic disorder that results in high levels of stored iron in the body. Iron-rich foods can supply as much as most postmenopausal women need.

The RDA for teen males ages fourteen to eighteen is 11 milligrams of iron daily; for adult men it's 8 milligrams daily. For teen females to age eighteen, 15 milligrams of iron daily; for females ages nineteen to fifty, 18 milligrams are recommended daily. From age fifty-one on, women need about 8 milligrams of iron daily.

During pregnancy at every age the recommendation goes up to 27 milligrams daily; during breast-feeding, the RDA is 10 milligrams daily for females age eighteen and younger and 9 milligrams daily for females ages nineteen and over.

The 2010 Dietary Guidelines advises women *who are capable of becoming pregnant to choose foods that supply heme iron (which is more readily absorbed by the body), additional iron sources, and enhancers of iron absorption such as vitamin C-rich foods. Women who are pregnant are advised to take an iron supplement as recommended by an obstetrician or other healthcare provider.*

If you don't consume enough: When iron gets short-changed or when iron stores in your body get too low, red blood cells can't carry as much oxygen, likely making you feel tired and maybe weak, and less able to perform at peak efficiency. Although there may be other causes, an iron deficiency can lead to anemia. All interfere with a person's physical ability to perform at full potential. *See "Anemia: More Than One Cause" in chapter 22 to learn more.* Among women with regular menstrual loss, iron deficiency is more common. Many women capable of becoming pregnant, including adolescent girls, are deficient in iron.

If you consume excess amounts: Iron can build up to dangerous levels for people with a genetic problem called hemochromatosis, whereby the body absorbs and stores too much iron. That excess can cause an enlarged liver, bronze skin pigmentation, and diabetes, as well as pancreatic, liver, cardiac, and other organ

damage. Ten times more common in men, symptoms of hemochromatosis usually begin to appear in adulthood, often in the thirties.

Taking adult iron supplements can be dangerous for children. Children should get immediate medical attention if they take an overdose of iron supplements. The Tolerable Upper Intake Level (UL) is 45 milligrams of iron per day for ages fourteen and over.

Where it's mostly found: Iron is widely available from foods of both animal (heme iron) and plant (nonheme) sources.

Most iron from meat, poultry, and fish is heme iron. That name comes from the way it's carried in food—as part of the hemoglobin and myoglobin (similar to hemoglobin in humans) in animal tissue. Foods of plant origin contain only nonheme iron. And egg yolks have mostly nonheme iron.

The deep-red color of animal muscle comes from hemoglobin. The darker the color, the higher the heme

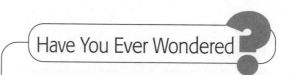

Have You Ever Wondered

. . . if spinach will make you strong, as the famous cartoon character Popeye believed? It's true that spinach contains iron. But another food component in spinach, called oxalic acid, binds with iron, impairing its absorption, so it's not the best source. Only physical activity, not iron or any other nutrient, builds muscle strength.

. . . if cooking in an iron skillet improves the iron content of food? It does. Before the days of aluminum and stainless steel cookware, great-great-grandma unknowingly supplemented her family's diet with iron from her iron pots and pans. If you have cast iron cookware, you can get the benefits, too. Foods with acids such as tomato juice, citrus juice, and vinegar help dissolve small amounts of iron from the pot into the cooking liquids—especially good for foods that simmer for a while.

. . . if you need more iron if you seem tired all the time? Maybe—or maybe you need more sleep, less stress, or perhaps more physical activity to increase your stamina! Fatigue is a symptom of anemia, however. Check with your physician for a blood test. *See "Anemia: 'Tired Blood'" in chapter 22 for more about anemia and blood testing.*

iron content. For example, beef liver, which is redder than roast beef, has more iron; dark turkey meat has more heme iron than the light meat.

FOOD	IRON (MG)
Sources of Mostly Heme Iron	
Beef liver, braised (3 oz.)	5.6
Lean sirloin, broiled (3 oz.)	2.9
Lean ground beef, broiled (3 oz.)	2.5
Skinless chicken, roasted dark meat (3 oz.)	1.1
Skinless chicken, roasted white meat (3 oz.)	0.9
Pork, lean, roasted (3 oz.)	0.9
Salmon, canned with bone (3 oz.)	0.7
Sources of Nonheme Iron	
Fortified breakfast cereal (1 cup)*	4.5–18
Pumpkin seed kernels (1 oz.)	4.2
Soybean nuts (½ cup)	3.4
Spinach, boiled (½ cup)	3.2
Wheat bran (½ cup)	3.0
Red kidney beans, cooked (½ cup)	2.6
Prune juice (¾ cup)	2.3
Lima beans, cooked (½ cup)	2.2
Enriched rice, cooked (½ cup)	1.4
Pretzels (1 oz.)	1.2
Dried plums (prunes) (5)	1.0
Whole-wheat bread (1 slice)	0.9
White bread made with enriched refined flour (1 slice)	0.9
Egg, large (1)	0.9
Raisins, seedless (¼ cup)	0.8
Peanut butter, (2 tbsp.)	0.6
Apricots, dried (3)	0.6
Egg white, large (1)	<0.1

Many foods on today's supermarket shelves are enriched or fortified with iron: iron-enriched flour (also used in baked goods and pasta) and iron-fortified breakfast cereals.

The amount varies. Read the Nutrition Facts on food labels.

Iron: The Power of Partnership

To help your body absorb more iron, pair foods like these at your meals and snacks. Meat, poultry, fish (all three with heme iron), and vitamin C-rich foods help release more nonheme iron from foods of plant origin and egg yolks.

ABSORPTION ENHANCERS	NONHEME IRON SOURCES
Sirloin strips	With spinach salad
Barbecued beef	With refried beans and tortillas
Ground beef	With a whole-grain roll
Pork	With bean soup
Chicken	With brown rice
Ham	With scrambled eggs
Grapefruit	With bran cereal
Strawberries	With oatmeal
Red bell pepper	With whole-grain pasta
Papaya	With whole-wheat toast
Orange	With a peanut butter sandwich on whole-wheat bread

Source: Adapted from National Cattlemen's Beef Association, *Iron in Human Nutrition* (Chicago, 1998).

Iron: Heme vs. Nonheme. What makes this difference nutritionally significant? First, consider that iron in food isn't absorbed efficiently. Much of the iron you consume never gets absorbed into your bloodstream. (Fortunately, the RDAs take this fact into account.) The amount of iron your body absorbs depends on several factors: among them, how much iron you consume and in what form (heme or nonheme); other nutrients in the meal or snack that can enhance or hinder its absorption; and how much iron your body has stored already. In fact, the bioavailability of iron in a mixed U.S. diet (animal- and plant-based foods) is about 18 percent; in a vegetarian diet, about 10 percent.

Heme iron is absorbed more readily than nonheme iron. Depending on how much you already have stored, 15 to 35 percent of heme iron gets absorbed. Only 2 to 20 percent of nonheme iron gets absorbed, even though foods with nonheme iron often contain more iron. Consuming vitamin C and foods such as meat with heme iron aids nonheme iron absorption.

Conversely, some phytonutrients—oxalic acid in spinach and chocolate; phytic acid in wheat bran and legumes; tannins in coffee and tea; and polyphenols in coffee—seem to inhibit nonheme iron absorption. Consuming vitamin C or iron from meat, fish, and poultry at the same time helps overcome these "inhibitors."

These quick nutrition tips can help your body better absorb iron (nonheme), especially important for vegetarians.

● Enjoy a vitamin C-rich food—such as an orange, cantaloupe, green pepper, or broccoli—along with it; for example, you get more iron from a peanut butter sandwich on whole-wheat bread if you eat it with orange juice. Add a little meat, poultry, or fish (with heme iron) to foods of plant origin and egg yolks; for example, include some ground beef in a pot of chili, or sliced lean ham in an omelette.

● Drink coffee or tea between meals—not with meals.

● Cook in an iron skillet.

For more combinations, see "Iron: The Power of Partnership" in this chapter.

Manganese

What it does:

● Serves as a partner of many enzymes, including RNA and DNA.

● Helps in bone formation.

● Helps in the metabolism of energy from carbohydrates, fats, and proteins.

How much you need: There is no RDA for manganese. However, the AI is set at 2.2 milligrams and 1.6 milligrams daily for males and females ages fourteen to eighteen, respectively. For adults the AI is 2.3 milligrams daily for males and 1.8 milligrams daily for females. During pregnancy (teens and adults), the AI is 2.0 milligrams daily; during breast-feeding, 2.6 milligrams daily.

If you don't consume enough: The chances of not getting enough are very low since manganese is so widely distributed in the food supply.

If you consume excess amounts: Consuming harmful levels from food is very rare, too. The Tolerable Upper Intake Level (UL) is set at 9 milligrams daily for teens

ages fourteen to eighteen, and at 11 milligrams daily during adulthood.

Where it's mostly found: Whole-grain products are the best sources of manganese, along with some fruits and vegetables. Tea also is a good source.

Food	Manganese (mg)
Pineapple, raw (½ cup)	1.2
Whole-wheat spaghetti, cooked (½ cup)	1
Tea, instant powder (1 tsp.)	0.9
Whole-wheat bread (1 slice)	0.7
Lentils, boiled (½ cup)	0.5
Kale, boiled (½ cup)	0.3
Strawberries (½ cup)	0.3

Molybdenum

What it does:

● Works with riboflavin to incorporate the iron stored in the body into hemoglobin for making red blood cells.

● Is part of many body enzymes.

How much you need: The RDA for molybdenum is 43 micrograms daily during the years fourteen to eighteen, and 45 micrograms daily during adulthood. During pregnancy and breast-feeding, the RDA level goes up to 50 micrograms daily for teen and adult women.

If you don't consume enough: With a normal diet, there's no need to worry about a deficiency. A deficiency of the enzymes made with molybdenum affects the nervous system, and in extreme cases may result in death.

If you consume excess amounts: Too much may have reproductive effects, but harmful levels are quite uncommon. The Tolerable Upper Intake Level (UL) is 1,700 micrograms daily during the years fourteen to eighteen, and 2,000 micrograms daily during adulthood.

Where it's mostly found: Molybdenum is found mostly in milk, beans (legumes), liver, breads, and grain products. The amount consumed in a typical eating pattern appears adequate. Little is known about the actual amounts in foods.

Selenium

What it does:

- Works as an antioxidant with vitamin E, to protect cells from damage that may lead to heart disease, and perhaps cancer and other health problems.
- Aids cell growth.
- Boosts immune function.

How much you need: The RDA is 55 micrograms daily for people ages fourteen and over. During pregnancy the recommendation remains the same, 55 micrograms daily; during breast-feeding it goes up to 70 micrograms daily.

If you don't consume enough: The general signs of a deficiency in humans aren't clear, but it may affect the heart muscle.

If you consume excess amounts: A normal diet with a variety of foods generally provides moderate levels of selenium. Very high levels from dietary supplements can be quite harmful. The Tolerable Upper Intake Level (UL) is set at 400 micrograms daily for people ages fourteen and over.

Where it's mostly found: The richest sources are seafood, liver, and kidney, as well as other meats. Grain products and seeds contain selenium, but the amount depends on the selenium content of the soil in which they're grown. Fruits and vegetables generally don't have much.

FOOD	SELENIUM (MCG)
Chicken, light meat, skinless (3 oz.)	24
Egg, large (1)	16
Brown rice, cooked (½ cup)	10
Whole-wheat bread (1 slice)	10
Peanuts (¼ cup)	3

Zinc

What it does:

- Promotes cell reproduction and tissue growth and repair. Adequate zinc intake is essential for growth.
- Associated with more than two hundred enzymes.
- Helps wounds heal; helps the immune system work properly.
- Promotes sensory responses (taste and smell).

- Helps your body use carbohydrates, proteins, and fats.

How much you need: The RDA for males is 11 milligrams daily for ages fourteen on. For females it's 9 milligrams daily for teens ages fourteen to eighteen, and 8 milligrams daily during adulthood. During pregnancy the recommendation increases to 13 milligrams daily for teens, and 11 milligrams daily for adults; during breast-feeding, 14 milligrams and 12 milligrams daily, respectively.

If you don't consume enough: A deficiency during childhood can impair growth, and during pregnancy can cause birth defects. Other symptoms include appetite loss, skin changes, and reduced resistance to infections.

If you consume excess amounts: Some symptoms can include nausea, diarrhea, and headaches. Over time, excess amounts can lead to low copper levels, lower immunity, and low levels of HDL ("good") cholesterol. The Tolerable Upper Intake Level (UL) for zinc is 34 milligrams daily for teens ages fourteen to eighteen, and 40 milligrams daily for adults.

Where it's mostly found: Good sources of zinc include foods of animal origin, including meat, poultry, seafood, and liver. Eggs and milk supply zinc in smaller amounts. Whole-grain products, beans (legumes), nuts, and fermented soybean paste (miso) also contain zinc, but it's in a form that's less available to the body.

FOOD	ZINC (MG)
Beef, ground lean (3 oz.)	5.5
Wheat germ (¼ cup)	4.7
Crab, canned (3 oz.)	3.5
Wheat bran (½ cup)	2
Sunflower seeds (1 oz.)	1.5
Black-eyed peas, frozen, boiled (½ cup)	1
Almonds (1 oz.)	1
Milk, fat-free (1 cup)	1
Tofu, raw (½ cup)	1
Peanut butter (2 tbsp.)	0.9
Tuna, canned, packed in water (3 oz.)	0.7
Egg, large (1)	0.6
Whole-wheat bread (1 slice)	0.5

Phytonutrients for Health

Besides nutrients, plant-based foods (beans and peas, vegetables, fruits, whole grains, nuts, seeds, and teas, as well as herbs and spices) have another "crop" of naturally occurring compounds with potential health benefits. Collectively they're called phytonutrients, or phytochemicals, meaning plant chemicals. "Phyto" means plant. Think *fight* for "phytos," since they appear to promote health by sparking body processes that fight, or reduce the risk for, the development of some diseases.

Why have phytonutrients captured our attention? Because of their potential for health promotion! Today consumers are interested in positive nutrition and self-care: adding (not avoiding) foods that may enhance health, boost immunity, slow aging, and prevent or slow the risks for chronic disease. In fact, consumer and media interest often is ahead of scientific evidence. Sound like you? Research on phytonutrients is the new frontier in nutrition, as exciting today as vitamin discoveries were a hundred years ago!

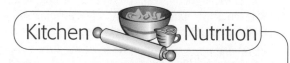

Boosting Phytonutrient Benefits

Research suggests that what you do in the kitchen can make a difference in food's phytonutrients benefits.

- Cooking or food processing may enhance the body's ability to use (bioavailability) some phytonutrients. Carotenoids (including lycopene) are one example. In addition, dietary fat may enhance the absorption of carotenoids; dietary fiber impedes it.

- Heat damages anthocyanins, which are flavonoids. On the flip side, the anthocyanin content may increase in fresh fruit if it's stored for a few days.

- Flaxseed needs to be crushed or ground to get the benefits.

- For the most benefit from tea's polyphenols, brew each cup fresh (preferably in water that's not hard) and drink it soon. Three to five minutes of brewing for one tea bag brings out 80 percent of the catechins, which are flavonoids.

- Chop garlic for about fifteen minutes before heating to allow allyl sulfides to fully develop.

Spice Up Your Health!

A pinch of this, a dash of that. Herbs and spices help define the flavors we enjoy. They contribute taste without salt, providing a strategy for reducing sodium. They offer a tasty way to cut back on fat and sugars in food prep. They add enticement to vegetables, fruits, whole grains, and other nutrient-rich foods, a positive strategy for weight management and following the dietary guidelines.

Moreover, their phytonutrients, including antioxidants, may have health-promoting potential, too. Among the range of benefits of herbs and spices being explored with animal studies are their possible abilities to promote immunity, reduce inflammation linked to heart disease, help to curb appetite, enhance satiety, boost metabolism, enhance insulin activity, and potentially protect against cancer.

Like fruits and vegetables, spices and herbs are sources of antioxidants, not surprising since they also come from plants. Many are phenolic phytonutrients. In fact, one-half teaspoon of cinnamon has slightly more antioxidant power than a half cup of raspberries, and a quarter-teaspoon of dried oregano has about twice as much as a half cup of chopped tomatoes. Since dry spices and herbs have water removed, the antioxidants are concentrated.

Among the common spices and herbs getting more research attention are cinnamon, ginger, oregano, red pepper (paprika), rosemary, thyme, and turmeric. *For more about antioxidants and the ORAC scores of some spices and herbs, see "Fruits, Vegetables, Herbs, and Spices: Their Antioxidant Potential" earlier in this chapter.*

For more about storing and preparing food with herbs and spices, refer to chapter 14.

Phytonutrients: What Role in Health?

Phytonutrients are among the many unique food components that offer functional benefits. The term "functional foods" refers to foods or their components that extend health benefits beyond basic nutrition (*see chapter 9 for more about functional foods*). In fact, their benefits are all about what you can eat, not what you can't!

Phytonutrients are bioactive compounds in food that promote your health by helping to slow the aging process or helping to reduce the risk for many diseases. Research is investigating how phytonutrients protect against some cancers, heart disease, stroke, high blood pressure, cataracts, osteoporosis, urinary tract infections, and other chronic health conditions.

Phytonutrients may serve as antioxidants, enhance immunity, enhance communication among body cells, cause cancer cells to die, detoxify carcinogens, and repair damage to DNA that's caused by smoking and other toxins. That said, the benefits and actions of phytonutrients are still uncertain. Do they work independently, together, with nutrients and fiber, or do their actions add up?

"Phytos": In a Class of Their Own

Neither vitamins nor minerals, phytonutrients are substances that plants produce naturally to protect them-

selves against viruses, bacteria, and fungi, as well as insects, drought, and even the sun. Beyond that, they provide the color, aroma, texture, and flavor that give food so much sensual appeal. Of the more than 25,000 phytonutrients, more than two thousand are plant pigments that put a rainbow of colors on your plate! *See "Paint Your Plate with Color!" in chapter 14.*

Like nutrients, phytonutrients are grouped according to their biochemical characteristics and probable protective functions. Only a few hundred have yet been studied. What we know today is merely the "appetizer."

Research has revealed a few things. Most fruits and vegetables contain phytonutrients. Different plant-based foods supply different kinds and amounts; some have a remarkable variety. An orange, for example, has

---

Functional Nutrition: Prebiotics and Probiotics—What Are They?

As other functional components of foods, prebiotics and probiotics may promote healthy bacteria, or microflora, in your intestines—and perhaps improve your health. *Prebiotics* stimulate or help activate bacteria growth; *probiotics* are the live cultures, or bacteria, themselves. Simply stated, prebiotics are food for probiotics. Consumed together, prebiotics and probiotics are synbiotics, working in a synergistic way.

- *Prebiotics* are nondigestible substances such as oligosaccharides, inulin, and polydextrose (indigestible carbohydrate) in food that promote the growth of normal, healthful bacteria that are already in your colon. Other substances in food, such as dietary fiber, starch, and sugar alcohols, may work as prebiotics, too. Prebiotics are found naturally in many fruits, vegetables, and whole-grain foods, such as oatmeal, flaxseed, beans (legumes), onions, dark-green leafy vegetables, and berries.

    Certain prebiotics also may enhance calcium and magnesium absorption, and may reduce risk factors for some intestinal problems. Further research is needed.

- *Probiotics* are active cultures, such as some strains of lactic acid bacteria, or foods that contain them, that help reintroduce or change bacteria in the intestine. *Lactobacilli* and *Bifidobacteria* in yogurt and other fermented dairy foods with live cultures and some nondairy foods have probiotic cultures.

Different bacterial strains, species, and genera (classifications) have different probiotic benefits, while some have no effect. *Lactobacilli and Bifidobacteria* in yogurt, kefir, and some other dairy foods with life active cultures may improve gastrointestinal health and promote immunity. *Streptococcus thermophilus* and *Saccharomyces* also are considered safe for the healthy population. Some non-dairy foods that may have probiotic cultures include tempeh, miso, kimchi, and sauerkraut.

Research suggests that probiotic cultures may help keep your immune system healthy and help maintain the "good" bacteria in your intestine. Some strains of probiotics also may help reduce the risk of some health problems—for example, shorten the duration of diarrhea, reduce the symptoms of lactose intolerance, decrease the risk of some cancers, help prevent some allergy symptoms, enhance immunity, and reduce symptoms of irritable bowel disease, among others.

There's more to learn, however, about the effectiveness, safety, strain, and amount of probiotics for specific health benefits. Although no health claims for prebiotics or probiotics are approved by the FDA, a structure-function claim may appear on the label, such as "promotes a healthy digestive system." It must be truthful and not misleading. Consult a registered dietitian to see if probiotics can help address your health needs, especially if you have a health condition with a compromised immune system.

FUNCTIONAL NUTRITION: A QUICK LOOK AT KEY PHYTONUTRIENTS

A HANDFUL OF PHYTONUTRIENTS	WHAT THEY APPEAR TO DO	WHERE THEY'RE FOUND (SOME FOOD SOURCES)
Carotenoids		
Beta carotene	● Neutralizes free radicals that may damage cells ● Bolsters cellular antioxidant defenses ● Can be made into vitamin A in the body	● *Yellow-orange fruits and vegetables* such as apricots, cantaloupes, papayas, carrots, pumpkins, sweet potatoes, winter squash ● *Green vegetables* such as broccoli, spinach, kale
Lutein, Zeaxanthin	● Supports maintenance of eye health	● *Green vegetables* such as asparagus, kale, spinach, collard greens, Swiss chard, Romaine lettuce, broccoli, Brussels sprouts ● Kiwifruit ● Egg yolks ● Corn, winter squash, citrus fruits (Eggs have a small amount of zeaxanthin, too.)
Lycopene	● Supports maintenance of prostate health	● *Most red fruits and vegetables* such as tomatoes, processed tomato products, pink grapefruit, guava, watermelon (*Note:* The red pigment in red peppers is from keto carotenoids, not lycopene.)
Flavonoids		
Anthocyanins: cyanidin, pelargonidin, delphinidin, malvidin	● Bolsters cellular antioxidant defenses ● Supports maintenance of healthy brain function	● Berries, cherries, red grapes
Flavanols: catechins, epicatechins, epigallocatechin	● Supports maintenance of heart health	● Apples, chocolate, cocoa, grapes, tea (black, oolong, or green)
Flavanones: hesperetin, naringenin	● Neutralizes free radicals which may damage cells ● Bolsters cellular antioxidant defenses	● Citrus fruit
Flavonols: quercetin: kaempferol isorhamnetin, myricetin	● Neutralizes free radicals which may damage cells ● Bolsters cellular antioxidant defenses	● Apples, broccoli, onions, tea
Procyanidins and Proanthocyanidins	● Supports maintenance of urinary tract health and heart health	● Apples, cinnamon, cocoa, cranberries, grapes, peanuts, strawberries, red wine, tea

(continued)

FUNCTIONAL NUTRITION: A QUICK LOOK AT KEY PHYTONUTRIENTS *(continued)*

A HANDFUL OF PHYTONUTRIENTS	WHAT THEY APPEAR TO DO	WHERE THEY'RE FOUND (SOME FOOD SOURCES)
Isothiocyanates Sulphoraphane	● May enhance detoxification of undesirable compounds ● Bolsters cellular antioxidant defenses	● Broccoli, broccoli sprouts, cabbage, cauliflower, kale, horseradish
Phenolic Acids Caffeic acid, ferulic acid	● Bolsters cellular antioxidant defenses ● Supports maintenance of eye and heart health	● Apples, citrus fruits, pears, some vegetables, coffee
Polyols Sugar alcohols*: lactitol, mannitol, sorbitol, xylitol	● May reduce risk of dental caries	● Some chewing gums ● Other food applications such as sugar-free candy
Phytoestrogens Isoflavones: daidzein, genestein	● For women, supports menopausal health ● Supports maintenance of bone and immune health, and healthy brain function	● Soybeans (edamame), soy-based foods such as tofu
Lignans	● Supports maintenance of heart health and immune health	● Broccoli, cauliflower, carrots, flaxseed (not flaxseed oil unless hull remains), lentils, rye, seeds and nuts, triticale
Prebiotics Inulin, fructo-oligosaccharides (FOS), polydextrose	● Supports maintenance of digestive health ● Supports calcium absorption	● Whole grains, onions, some fruits, garlic, honey, leeks, banana, fortified foods and beverages
Probiotics Yeast, *lactobacilli*, *bifidobacteria*, and other specific strains of beneficial bacteria	● Supports maintenance of digestive and immune health; benefits are strain specific	● Certain yogurts and other cultured dairy and non-dairy applications
Sulfides/Thiols Allyl methyl trisulfide, diallyl sulfide	● Supports maintenance of heart, immune, and digestive health ● May enhance detoxification of undesirable compound	● Garlic, onions, leeks, scallions
Dithiolthiones	● Supports maintenance of healthy immune function ● May enhance detoxification of undesirable compounds	● Cruciferous vegetables

(continued)

Source: Adapted from International Food Information Council Foundation, 2011.

*FDA-approved health claim established for component

**Probiotics are *not* phytonutrients, but they're listed here with prebiotics since some of their functions are interrelated.

Other phytonutrients are addressed elsewhere: fiber in chapter 3, stanols and sterols in chapter 5, and soy protein in chapter 4. Animal-based foods also contain some functional substances, e.g., some fatty acids; *see chapter 5.*

more than 170 different phytonutrients! In any fruit or vegetable, these substances appear to work together with nutrients and fiber for your good health.

For phytonutrients, food databases are limited, and include only a few key carotenoids (beta and alpha carotene, lycopene, lutein, and zeaxanthin), isoflavones, and proanthocyanidins. The USDA National Nutrient Database for Standard Reference has databases for these phytonutrients and can be accessed at www.ars.usda.gov/Services/docs.htm?docid=20958. However, no Dietary Reference Intakes exist for these phytonutrients yet. Healthy claims or qualified health claims have been approved by the FDA for some.

The bottom line: Already there's overwhelming evidence for the health benefits of plant-based foods: fruits, vegetables, legumes (including soy), nuts, seeds, and grains, especially whole grains. Research shows that you *lower the odds* for some cancers, heart disease, and other health problems by *eating more* fruits, vegetables, and whole grains.

To reap the potential benefits of the many phytonutrients, remember: food first! Supplements with just one or a few phytonutrients aren't likely as effective.

Functional Nutrition: More to Learn!

Phytonutrients aren't the only food substances with functional benefits. Check here to learn more:

- *"Prebiotics and Probiotics—What Are They?"* in this chapter.
- *"Soy's Links to Health"* in chapter 4.
- *"Functional Nutrition: Eat Your Omega-3s and -6s"* in chapter 5.
- *"Functional Nutrition: Plant Stanols and Sterols"* and *"Functional Nutrition: A Quick Look at Fatty Acids, Stanols, and Sterols"* in chapter 5.
- *"Sugar Replacers (aka Sugar Alcohols),"* about sugar alcohols, in chapter 3.
- *"Functional Nutrition: A Quick Look at Dietary Fiber,"* chapter 3.
- *"Teatime: Health Benefits?"* in chapter 8.
- *"Functional Foods: Benefits beyond Basics"* in chapter 9.
- *"A Toast to Heart Health"* in chapter 22.

CHAPTER 7

Sodium and Potassium
A Salty Subject

Your doctor, the media, and government experts have all spread the messages: "Check food labels for sodium." "Cook with less salt." "Put away the salt shaker." These are in today's headlines. Yet salt has made news for centuries!

Throughout recorded history, salt has played an important economic and political role—and has always been part of the world's food supply. Until the past two hundred years, salt was used heavily for preserving foods: meat, fish, vegetables, and even fruit. Cheese, too, was salted more than it is today. Especially in Mediterranean regions, cooks used herbs and spices to mask strong, salty flavors from preservation. Nations that controlled the salt trade also controlled distribution and preservation of food, especially in times of shortage.

Ancient Greeks valued salt so highly that they used it for currency. Salt was traded for slaves, hence the phrase "He's not worth his salt." Originally Roman soldiers were given a handful of salt every day. Later they received money to buy their own salt, which was referred to as *salarium argentum;* that means "salt money." The word "salary" is derived from this Latin term. Salad also derives from the Latin word "sal," meaning salt.

Because of its value, salt historically has been used symbolically. To the ancient Romans, salt given to a newborn symbolized the giving of wisdom. In Europe, a pinch of salt tossed three times over the left shoulder helped fend off evil. Even today, we reflect our doubts: "Take it with a grain of salt."

Until the late 1700s, salty flavors were common and came from food preservation. In the nineteenth century, tastes began to change, and people preferred less salty foods. Concurrently, other food preservation methods started: canning, freezing, and refrigeration. In the twentieth century salt and other sodium-containing ingredients performed different functions in food processing. Salt was deemed "generally recognized as safe" as an additive with no regulatory limits on its use

Did you know . . .

. . . 1 teaspoon of table salt contains 2,325 milligrams of sodium, or about a day's worth, according to the Dietary Guidelines? Two-thirds of a teaspoon of table salt provides about 1,500 milligrams of sodium for those ages 51 years and over?

. . . most sodium that Americans consume comes from processed or prepared food, not the salt shaker?

. . . a preference for salty foods is acquired?

. . . you can unlearn that preference by cutting back on salty foods gradually?

. . . for many people, the higher a person's sodium intake, the higher his or her blood pressure?

. . . by eating fewer calories you may also reduce sodium?

. . . by eating more fruits and veggies, you boost your potassium intake, which helps blunt the effect of sodium on blood pressure?

. . . you can cut back on salt in your food choices without giving up flavor?

(although this regulation has come under scrutiny and may be amended). Over the last century, sodium intake also rose significantly. While consumers cooked with fewer raw ingredients and more processed foods, they ate out more often and consumed more calories overall.

In ancient times, salt's ability to preserve food helped provide a varied supply of nutrients to the population. Any other health link, such as high blood pressure, was unknown. As science advanced, we learned that the blood pressure of some people may be sensitive to salt, or to the sodium it's made from. Now we recognize that the blood pressure link to nutrition may be more complex, with potassium, magnesium, and calcium also playing a role.

Sodium, Potassium, and Your Health

Salt . . . or sodium? Although we often refer to them in the same breath, salt and sodium aren't the same thing. Table salt is actually the common name for "sodium chloride." It's 40 percent sodium and 60 percent chloride. And potassium? Like sodium and chloride, it's an essential mineral, too.

Sodium and Potassium: You Need Them!

The link between sodium and high blood pressure is well publicized, yet few people know the flip side of the sodium story—why sodium is essential to health.

Sodium and potassium are minerals that occur naturally in food. Some of the most basic work your body does depends on these nutrients: maintaining proper fluid balance—controlling the movement of fluids in and out of your cells; regulating your blood pressure; transmitting nerve impulses; and helping your muscles, including your heart muscle, relax.

Sodium, along with other minerals such as chloride and potassium, are collectively called electrolytes, so named because they transmit electrical current in your body. Compare them to electrically charged particles, or ions, in flashlight batteries.

If you lick your upper lip after sweating a lot, you know that body fluids have salt. You can taste it! Sodium, chloride, and potassium dissolve in body fluids, where they become separate ions. With their electrical charge, they transmit nerve impulses throughout your body. And they send messages from your brain to your muscles, causing them to relax or to contract.

Have you ever sprinkled salt on a sliced eggplant or potato, then watched liquid come to its outer surface? That's because salt draws fluid out of the plant cells. That same reaction happens with electrolytes in your body. They control and regulate the balance of fluids in and out of cells. Sodium and chloride mostly work outside body cells, and potassium works mainly inside.

Fluid balance—moving fluid in and out of cells—has important health implications. Among them, electrolytes help move nutrients into cells and help take wastes away. Body fluids carry nutrients and wastes.

For more about these minerals, see "Major Minerals: Electrolytes" in chapter 6.

Keeping the Balance

Your kidneys regulate sodium and potassium levels in your body. If you're healthy, your body doesn't retain the excess sodium—even when you consume more than you need. And excess amounts don't get stored.

Instead your body rids itself of the extra. Excess sodium and potassium pass out through urine and, to a much lesser extent, sodium is released through perspiration. If, for example, you eat foods high in sodium, you may urinate more. Then you probably feel thirsty because you lost fluids, too.

Is extra sodium in the body always removed? No. When kidneys don't work properly, perhaps due to kidney disease, extra sodium isn't excreted. This causes swelling, often in the face, legs, and feet. In medical terms, this swelling is called edema.

For your health, when consuming sodium and potassium . . .

- Reduce sodium intake.
- Choose foods low in sodium and prepare foods with little salt.
- Increase potassium intake.

Source: Dietary Guidelines for Americans, 2010.

Can you have a sodium deficiency? Yes, but not likely, given that the average person in the United States consumes about 3,400 milligrams daily. That's another fifty percent more than the recommended 2,300 milligrams maximum level for adults whose blood pressure isn't sodium sensitive, and more than double the 1,500 milligrams daily advised for many people. Virtually all Americans consume more sodium than they need! However, if a person vomits or has diarrhea for a prolonged period, or if he or she has a kidney problem, sodium levels might get too low. Unless sweating is profuse and extended over a long time and the person drinks a lot of water, sodium levels will remain normal if healthy. Your body conserves sodium when your intake is low, but less effectively conserves potassium. Make up for it by eating more potassium-rich foods.

Links to Blood Pressure

High blood pressure, or hypertension, is a major risk factor for heart disease, stroke, kidney failure, and other conditions. In the United States about one-third of adults have it, and about one-third are prehypertensive. Increasingly more children are at risk, too. Yet, many don't know it. These are some factors linked to high blood pressure: family history of high blood pressure, overweight, excessive alcohol intake, advancing age, and smoking.

Why is attention given to sodium? There's a direct, progressive link between increased high blood pressure and sodium intake. On average, the higher the sodium intake, the higher a person's blood pressure. Conversely, especially for adults, as sodium intake decreases, so does blood pressure. High-sodium intake is one dietary factor linked to high blood pressure or perhaps its early prehypertension stage. On the flip side, reducing sodium intake may help to lower blood pressure if it's higher than normal. Normal blood pressure also lowers the risk of heart disease and kidney disease. Even a modest decrease in sodium can make a difference! *See chapter 22 for normal blood pressure ranges.*

Three other minerals may be important in regulating blood pressure: potassium from fruits, vegetables, milk, and yogurt; calcium from dairy foods and some vegetables; and magnesium from whole grains, legumes, nuts, green vegetables, and milk.

Although the scientific reasons aren't yet fully understood, foods high in potassium may help protect against high blood pressure. Potassium appears to blunt the effect of sodium on blood pressure.

In fact, the DASH (Dietary Approaches to Stop Hypertension) Eating Plan—that's low in fat, with low-fat and fat-free dairy foods and plenty of vegetables and fruits—may help lower blood pressure, even among people within the "normal" range. The reason is unclear; however, the DASH approach to eating is high in potassium, calcium, and magnesium. *See chapter 10 for the DASH Eating Plan.*

For some people, even 2,300 milligrams (the upper daily recommended level) for sodium may be too much. The DASH plan and lowering sodium intake to 1,500 milligrams daily have been shown to have even better blood-pressure-lowering results—especially for those with hypertension. *See "Blood Pressure: Under Control?" in chapter 22.*

Consider following the DASH plan whether or not you have high blood pressure. If you have it or some

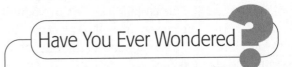

Have You Ever Wondered

... how you know if you're sodium-sensitive? There's no easy way yet to test blood pressure. Needing anti-hypertensive medications or diuretics isn't always an indicator. But about 20 percent of people are sodium sensitive; in other words, their blood pressure varies with sodium intake. Testing for salt sensitivity is highly controlled and takes several days; often it's done in a hospital setting. This test usually isn't done except for research. Because blood pressure rises with sodium intake, especially for those with salt sensitivity, and because many people don't know if they have hypertension or are salt sensitive, it's advised that everyone reduces sodium intake.

... if a high-salt diet is okay if you're not salt-sensitive? Moderation is always a better rule of thumb for anything you eat, so it's wise to reduce sodium and to consume foods with potassium. Choose and prepare foods with little salt, and hedge your bets with the DASH approach to eating: dairy foods, plenty of fruit and vegetables, whole-grain foods and low-fat foods. The body excretes more calcium in urine when salt intake is high. To help lower calcium loss, cut back on salt.

other health condition, your doctor might recommend less sodium than you consume now. Consult your doctor for the right sodium level for you, and a registered dietitian (RD) to help you follow this advice.

Research suggests high sodium intake may be linked to other health concerns, including gastric cancer, while inadequate potassium intake may increase the risks of kidney stones and perhaps osteoporosis. A possible benefit of cutting back on salt: less calcium loss from bone, and as a result, reduced risk of osteoporosis and bone fractures.

Sodium and Potassium: How Much Is Enough?

To keep your body running normally, you need sodium. But you likely consume more than enough. On average people in the United States consume about 3,400 milligrams of sodium (equivalent to 1½ teaspoons salt) daily. There's no known advantage to

consuming this much. Those at risk for or with high blood pressure are better off with less.

How much then? The Institute of Medicine's Daily Reference Intakes recommend a maximum for sodium intake: for the general public the Tolerable Upper Intake Level (UL) is 2,300 milligrams of sodium daily, and somewhat less for children ages thirteen and under. That's about the amount in 1 teaspoon of salt.

Less than 2,300 milligrams is better. In fact, for most healthy people ages nine to fifty, the Adequate Intake (AI) of 1,500 milligrams of sodium daily is enough and accounts for sweat losses. The AI is somewhat less for adults over age fifty and children eight years and under. Getting enough other nutrients, including potassium, may not be easy, however, in an eating plan at 1,500 milligrams of sodium daily.

When you sweat after strenuous physical activity, do you need extra salt—from the salt shaker, a salt tablet, or a sports drink? Probably not. Food eaten after exertion normally replenishes sodium lost in sweat. That said, sodium's AI level doesn't apply to highly active people, such as those doing endurance sports.

What's the potassium recommendation? For ages fourteen on up, the AI is 4,700 milligrams daily. However, on average, adult men take in only 3,200 milligrams of potassium per day; women, only 2,400 milligrams of potassium per day. Since excess potassium is excreted in urine, no UL is set for those with healthy kidney function. People with certain cardiac issues, such as arrhythmia, are advised to consume under 4,700 milligrams of potassium daily. Those with impaired kidneys also need to limit potassium. Some people with high blood pressure also have kidney (renal) failure.

Potassium: Another Reason for Fruits and Veggies!

Fruits and vegetables are among the best sources of potassium, a mineral that helps normalize blood pressure. Here are some good (at least 10% Daily Value) potassium sources :

Apricot	Parsnip
Avocado	Peach
Banana	Potato
Broccoli	Prunes (dried plums)
Cantaloupe	Raisins
Carrot	Spinach
Dates	Sweet potato
Kidney beans	Swiss chard
Lentils	Tomato
Mushrooms	Watermelon
Orange	Winter squash

Other good potassium sources: Dry beans, peas, almonds, and peanuts. Milk and yogurt supply calcium and potassium, perhaps protecting against high blood pressure.

Note: Potassium chloride, as a salt substitute, isn't recommended. Unless used under medical supervision, it can be harmful to health.

Advice . . . Even for Healthy People

As part of the healthful eating message, the Dietary Guidelines for Americans advises: *Reduce daily sodium intake to less than 2,300 milligrams sodium daily and further reduce intake to 1,500 milligrams among those who are age 51 years and older and those of any age who are African American or have hypertension, diabetes, or chronic kidney disease.* At the same time, the Guidelines advise choosing foods with potassium (such as fruits and vegetables), which is among the nutrients of concern in U.S. diets.

In 2010, the American Heart Association lowered its recommendation to no more than 1,500 milligrams of sodium daily for the general public.

Why is this advice given to healthy people? For one, you likely won't know if your blood pressure is sodium-sensitive. You may—or may not—develop high blood pressure from consuming too much sodium. Second, consuming less sodium or little salt certainly isn't harmful to healthy adults. Even if you don't have high blood pressure now, cutting back may offer protection, just in case. So stick to the recommendation.

Can your overall food choices be too low in sodium? With the sodium that occurs naturally in food and the current food supply, that won't happen.

Sodium in Your Food Choices

Salt and sodium—are they just in food for flavor? Or do they have other roles, too? It's easier to spot foods with salt or sodium if you know what they do.

Salt and Sodium: More Than Flavor

Why are salt and other sodium-containing ingredients added in food preparation and processing? Flavor probably comes to mind first. Just a few grains of salt can bring out food's natural flavors—even in sweet foods such as cakes and cookies or savory foods such as soup. A pinch of salt even helps disguise metallic or chemical aftertastes, such as in some soft drinks. However, sodium-containing ingredients play a broader role in the food supply.

● Before the days of refrigeration, people relied on salt to *preserve* many foods. Salt and sodium-containing ingredients preserve food by drawing water out of food and so inhibiting the growth of bacteria, yeast, and molds which need moisture to thrive—and so prevent food spoilage and foodborne illness.

Even today, many cured foods use salt or an ingredient made with sodium (such as sodium nitrate) as a preservative. For example, ham, sausage, prosciutto, corned beef, and Canadian bacon are cured meats. Another way to preserve vegetables is to soak them in

brine, or a solution of water and salt. Eat pickles? Cucumbers, peppers, and okra, and other veggies are pickled in brine, too.

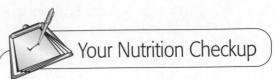

Your Nutrition Checkup

Sodium: A Healthful "Shake"

You know the guideline: *Choose and prepare foods with little salt.* How have you addressed this "salty issue"? Check the tips that apply to your approach to eating. *Do you . . .*

☐ Read Nutrition Facts on food labels to check the amount of sodium in food and buy foods with less?

☐ Shake a little salt on your food only *after* you taste it?

☐ Enjoy plenty of vegetables without added salt?

☐ Keep the salt shaker in the cabinet, not on the table or kitchen counter where it's easier to use?

☐ Eat smaller portions of high-sodium foods?

☐ Season food mostly with herbs, spices, and citrus?

☐ Consider the salt or sodium in restaurant food or fast food when you order restaurant food?

☐ Enjoy processed meats (corned beef, ham, bacon, bologna, salami, hot dogs, and pastrami) only occasionally?

☐ Buy prepared foods and snack foods that have reduced sodium or salt, or no added salt?

☐ Go easy on condiments such as mustard, ketchup, soy sauce, and tartar sauce, or use those with less sodium?

☐ Use half the seasoning packet in packaged rice, pasta, and soup mixes?

☐ Balance your food choices: If you enjoy some foods with more sodium, also eat others with less?

How many boxes did you check?

If you said yes to . . .

Nine to twelve items: You're likely conscious of consuming healthful amounts of sodium and salt. Read on for more ideas.

Six to eight items: You're controlling the sodium and salt in your food choices but may be able to "shake the sodium habit" even more. Read on.

Five or fewer items: It's time to read on and try the tips in this chapter to reduce the sodium and salt and boost the potassium in your food choices.

● In many foods, salt *affects the texture*. For example, yeast breads with salt have a finer texture; salt-free yeast breads tend to be coarser. Salt also reduces the dryness of crackers and pretzels.

● In some foods, such as cheese, bread dough, and sauerkraut, salt *controls the speed of fermentation*. Fermentation changes the chemistry of food, and as a result its appearance and flavor.

● In whipping egg whites or cream, a pinch of salt *increases and stabilizes the volume*.

● In processed meats, including sausage, salt and sodium-containing ingredients *help hold meat together*.

Some foods can't be produced without salt. Cheese is an example. Besides being critical for ripening cheese, it's needed for cheese texture, flavor, quality, shelf-life, and safety. That said, the "recipes" used to make the 300 or so types of cheese in the United States vary significantly. For example cheddar and mozzarella cheese have about half the sodium for the same portion that processed cheese has. Read the label!

Since salt and sodium-containing ingredients perform so many functions in food production besides adding flavor, lowering sodium in processed foods is

Have You Ever Wondered

. . . if draining and rinsing canned beans reduces the sodium content? If you drain and rinse canned beans under cool running water, you can reduce their sodium content by about 41 percent. If you drain only, sodium is reduced by about 36 percent. You also rinse away some nutrients, such as some B vitamins, that leach from vegetables into the canning liquid.

. . . if celery has a lot of sodium? Many people think so. But a celery stalk has just 35 milligrams of sodium.

. . . how can you spot chicken or turkey that isn't injected (marinated) with salt-water solution? Sometimes uncooked poultry is injected with a salt-water solution to keep it moist, tender, and flavorful. Usually fresh poultry has less sodium, but check. But read the label, or talk to your butcher to find out. Brining, sometimes done by chefs and home cooks, is done for similar reasons—and does increase the sodium content.

challenging. Yet many food companies are quietly adjusting the formulations in many food products to reduce salt and sodium, in fact, so gradually that your taste buds likely won't notice! The goal of the National Salt Reduction Initiative is to reduce salt in packaged and restaurant foods to achieve a 20 percent reduction of sodium intake between 2009 and 2014. As a consumer, periodically check the Nutrition Facts on food labels so you're up-to-date on the sodium content.

Where Does Sodium Come From?

Many people think their taste buds offer all the clues they need to the sodium content of food. That's because sodium is consumed mostly as salt. However, you can't always judge food's sodium content by its taste! Many foods with sodium don't have a salty flavor. Pizza, Mexican mixed dishes, pasta dishes, chicken and beef mixed dishes, and yeast breads are among the major sources of sodium.

A shake here and a shake there—the amount of salt sprinkled on food can add up, especially if you shake before you taste! The same is true for sodium-containing condiments such as soy sauce, mustard, and tartar sauce. However, only about 5 to 10 percent of the sodium in the food most people eat comes from the salt shaker or from salt added during cooking or at the table.

Processed foods are the main sources of sodium in the average American diet: about 75 to 80 percent. Because salt and sodium-containing ingredients serve several functions in the food supply, it's not surprising that processed foods contain varying levels of sodium. For example, two cookies or crackers vary, from 25 to 270 milligrams of sodium. A frozen dinner might vary from 550 to 1,300 milligrams of sodium. And two slices of bacon may deliver 500 to 800 milligrams of sodium. Even "reduced-sodium" foods may be higher in sodium than you think!

For clues to the sodium in processed foods, check the label for sodium-containing ingredients. If an ingredient has *Na, salt, soda,* or *sodium* in its name, that's a clue for sodium. ("Na" is the scientific symbol for sodium.) Foods described as "broth," "cured," "corned," "pickled," "smoked," "basted," "brined," and "marinated" usually contain sodium, too; cured ham often contains about 350 milligrams of sodium per ounce.

Because sodium occurs naturally, too, even unprocessed foods may contain sodium. But the amounts (about 10 percent of our overall sodium intake) aren't high enough for concern.

How do you know if a food has a lot of sodium, or a little? Check the amount of sodium in one label serving of a food, using the label's Nutrition Facts. If one serving contains 5 percent or less of the Daily Value (DV) for sodium, that's low. If it contains 20 percent or more DV, that's a lot. *Remember:* Two servings double the sodium. *For tips on using food labels, see "Today's Food Labels" in chapter 12.*

Which food groups have the most sodium? The sodium content of foods varies—even in very similar foods. The difference comes from the way foods are prepared and processed. Foods in every food group may contain sodium.

If you're ambitious enough to count sodium in your food choices, you can use food labels and websites that show nutrient content for various foods.

Salty Terms

When a recipe calls for salt, which one will you use? Most recipes call for table salt. How does table salt compare with other types of salt for nutrition and culinary uses?

- *Iodized salt:* table salt with iodine added. The body needs just small amounts of iodine. Using iodized salt, people get enough iodine—even when they go easy on salt. An important nutrient, iodine helps prevent goiter, a thyroid gland condition.

- *Kosher salt:* coarse grain salt that adds a crunchy texture to some dishes and drinks, such as margaritas. Kosher salt is used to prepare meat by religious Jews. "Kosher salt" may have anticaking additives.

   Tip: ¼ teaspoon of kosher salt has somewhat less sodium than ¼ teaspoon of table salt. That's because kosher salt has a coarser grain, so less fits in the spoon. For the same saltiness in a cooked dish, you need the same amount by *weight*— and that has the same amount of sodium, kosher or not.

- *Lite salt:* salt that is "50–50": half sodium chloride (regular salt) and half potassium chloride. It has less sodium than table salt, but it's not sodium-free.

- *Pickling salt:* fine-grained salt used to make brines for sauerkraut or pickles. Unlike table salt, it has no iodine or anticaking additives. Additives would make the brine cloudy or would settle to the bottom.

- *Popcorn salt:* very finely granulated salt that sticks well to popcorn, fries, and chips

- *Rock salt:* large, chunky crystals of salt used in a crank-style ice cream maker or as a "bed" for serving foods such as clams or oysters. Not commonly used in recipes, rock salt contains some harmless impurities.

- *Salt substitute:* made by substituting some or all of the sodium with potassium, magnesium, or another mineral. It may be recommended by a healthcare provider for people on a sodium-restricted diet.

- *Sea salt:* salt—either fine-grained or in larger crystals—produced by evaporation of seawater—for example, Black Sea, French (fleur de sel), Celtic, or Hawaiian sea salt. It has trace amounts of other minerals that may offer a somewhat different flavor. Still, it's sodium chloride. Even though sea salt is often promoted as a healthful alternative to ordinary table salt, the sodium content is comparable; the small amount of other minerals offers no known health advantages. As with other salts, use sea salt judiciously. If the grain is coarse, it may have less sodium per teaspoon, but not by weight.

   Tip: With canning, trace minerals in sea salt may discolor food.

- *Seasoned salt:* salt with herbs and other flavorings added, such as celery salt, garlic salt, onion salt, or other seasoned salts. Seasoned salt has less sodium than table salt but more than herbs alone.

   Tip: For less sodium in cooking, use just herbs— for example, celery seed, garlic powder, or onion flakes. Check the ingredient list for salt.

- *Table salt:* fine, granulated salt commonly used in cooking and in salt shakers. An anticaking additive— calcium silicate—helps table salt flow freely and not get lumpy.

Ingredients with Sodium	What They Do
Baking soda (sodium bicarbonate)	Leavening agent
Baking powder	Leavening agent
Brine (salt and water)	Preservative
Disodium phosphate	Emulsifier, stabilizer
Monosodium glutamate (MSG)	Flavor enhancer
NaCl (salt or sodium chloride)	Flavor enhancer, preservative
Sodium benzoate	Preservative
Sodium caseinate	Thickener, binder
Sodium citrate	Acid controller, stabilizer
Sodium erythorbate	Antioxidant
Sodium nitrate/nitrite	Preservative
Sodium propionate	Preservative, mold inhibitor
Sodium sulfite	Preservative for dried fruits
Soy sauce	Flavor enhancer
Teriyaki sauce	Flavor enhancer

Flavor . . . with Little Salt and Less Sodium

Do you like the taste of salty snacks? Does food seem to taste better after a few shakes of the salt shaker? Most people eat what they like. According to consumer research, taste ranks first in making food choices. Good news: You can enjoy plenty of flavorful foods prepared with *less* salt and sodium.

"Salty"–an Acquired Taste

A preference for strong, salty tastes is acquired, probably starting as early as infancy if a baby is exposed to salty tastes. It's the saltiness that people like, not the sodium. In fact, chloride in salt may have more to do with flavor than sodium does.

Except for the sensory experience, the body adjusts easily to eating less salt. Interestingly, when people gradually cut back and learn to go with less salt in their food choices, the desire for salty tastes declines, too. Over time, the less salt they consume, the less they want.

For taste perception, no other foods truly substitute for the taste of salt. Even salt substitutes, suggested for some people, don't give the same taste sensation. They may taste somewhat bitter or sharp.

About Salt Substitutes

Are salt substitutes good for moderating sodium intake? That depends. Salt substitutes aren't appropriate—and may not be healthful—for everyone.

Many salt substitutes contain potassium in place of all or some of the sodium. For some people, potassium consumed in excess can be harmful. For example, those with kidney problems may not be able to rid their bodies of excess levels of potassium. If you're under medical care—especially for a kidney problem—check with your doctor before using salt substitutes.

Rather than salt substitutes (potassium chloride), try herb-spice blends as a flavorful alternative to salt—or try lemon or lime juice to bring out the flavor. Today's supermarkets carry a variety of salt-free seasoning blends. Remember to read the ingredient list and the Nutrition Facts on the label. Some herb-spice blends are neither salt- nor sodium-free. As an alternative, make your own; *see "Kitchen Nutrition: Salt-Free Herb Blends" in this chapter. For more about the sensations of taste and flavor, see "What Is Flavor?" in chapter 14.*

Need more strategies to shake the salt habit? Check here for "how-tos":
- Shop for foods with less sodium—see chapter 12.
- Fit in more fruits and veggies (and more potassium)—see chapter 14.
- Cut salt in your cooking—see chapter 14.
- Give food a flavor burst with herbs and spices, not salt—see chapter 14.
- Order restaurant foods with less sodium—see chapter 15.
- Follow the DASH Eating Plan—see chapter 10.

MSG—Another Flavor Enhancer

You probably know about monosodium glutamate, or more simply, MSG. Common in some ethnic cooking, MSG enhances flavor. It blends well with salty or sour flavors . . . and brings out flavors of many prepared foods, such as "heat 'n' eat" meals, sauces, and canned soups.

MSG has nutrition-related benefits that may go unrecognized. Since a little goes a long way, MSG provides a bigger "bang" for the "shake." With only a third as much sodium as a comparable amount of table salt, it may be an option for controlling sodium intake. Using MSG instead of salt can lower the sodium in a recipe by 20 to 40 percent, while still enhancing flavor. In food preparation, one-half teaspoon of MSG is enough to season one pound of meat or four to six servings of vegetables.

Besides accenting the natural flavors, MSG adds a unique taste of its own. Called "umami," its taste is described as "meaty" or "brothlike." Studies show "umami" actually elicits a fifth taste sensation, distinctive in cheese, meat, and tomatoes. Sweet, sour, salty, and bitter are the other four taste sensations. *For more about taste, see "What Is Flavor?" in chapter 14.*

As its name implies, monosodium glutamate contains sodium and glutamate or glutamic acid. Glutamic acid is an amino acid found naturally in your body and in high-protein foods. Meat, fish, dairy foods, and some vegetables such as tomatoes and mushrooms, get their umami taste from glutamate.

Over the years, consumers have asked about the safety of MSG. The U.S. Food and Drug Administration considers MSG "generally recognized as safe" (GRAS) for consumption. Other GRAS substances include commonplace food "additives" such as sugar, salt, and baking soda. *See "Testing, Testing" in chapter 9 for more about the GRAS list. Also see "Have You Ever Wondered . . . if You Can Be Sensitive to MSG?" in chapter 21.*

Adding MSG to foods such as soups and stews may make eating more enjoyable for older adults. As we grow older, our sense of smell may weaken and our taste buds decrease in number. As a result, foods lose some of their "taste appeal." The decline in smell and taste often causes seniors to lose interest in eating, putting them at nutritional risk. Adding MSG to certain foods can perk up the flavor! *See "Aging with 'Taste'" in chapter 19 for more about taste and older adults.*

Taming Your Taste Buds

Enjoying what you eat is a top priority! Fortunately, a preference for salty foods isn't fixed; in other words you can learn to prefer foods with less salt! Moreover, healthful foods don't need to taste bland. And you don't need to give up your favorite high-sodium foods—just eat them in moderation. To slowly step down your sodium intake and your preference for saltiness:

● Cut back on high-sodium foods gradually if you prefer salty tastes. Because a preference for a salty taste is learned, it takes time to unlearn it, too—and to appreciate new flavor combinations.

● Taste before salting. Maybe food tastes great just as it is! Keep the salt shaker in the cabinet, not on the stove or the table. Use as needed—not as a habit.

● Enjoy more fruits and vegetables. Most contain only small amounts of sodium (unless added in processing), and they're rich in potassium. Eat them as low-sodium snacks!

● Choose food group foods that have less sodium: fresh meats, poultry, fish, dry beans (legumes), unsalted nuts, eggs, milk, and yogurt. Plain rice, pasta, and oatmeal don't have much sodium, either. Their sodium content goes up only if high-sodium ingredients are added during processing or food prep.

● Season with herbs, spices, herbed vinegars, herb rubs, and fruit juices instead of salt. *See "A Pinch of Flavor: Cooking with Herbs and Spices" in chapter 14. Or prepare the easy blends in this chapter to keep on hand.*

● Cook with less salt and high-sodium ingredients. For example, skip the salt in cooking water for pasta, rice, cereals, and vegetables. Salt toughens many vegetables, especially beans, as they're cooked. Salt draws water out of the plant cells. *See chapter 14, "Kitchen Nutrition: Cooking Matters."*

● Balance: If you eat high-sodium foods occasionally, choose other foods low in sodium to help lower your overall sodium intake. How much salt and sodium you consume over several days is what counts.

● Compare the sodium in processed and prepared foods such as soup, bread, and frozen meals. Read

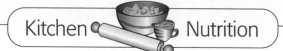

Kitchen Nutrition

Salt-Free Herb Blends

Enhance the flavor of food with salt-free herb and spice blends. Herbal seasonings don't taste like salt, but do add flavor to food! To make ½ cup, combine the ingredients in a jar. Cover tightly and shake. Keep in a cool, dark, dry place. Then rub or sprinkle them on food for flavor. *(Tip:* They make great gifts!)

Chinese five-spice . . . for chicken, fish, or pork.
> Blend ¼ cup of ground ginger, 2 tablespoons of ground cinnamon, 1 tablespoon each of ground allspice and anise seeds, and 2 teaspoons of ground cloves.

Mixed herb blend . . . for salads, pasta salads, steamed vegetables, vegetable soup, or fish.
> Blend ¼ cup of dried parsley flakes, 2 tablespoons of dried tarragon, and 1 tablespoon each of dried oregano, dill weed, and celery flakes.

Curry blend . . . for rice, lentil, and vegetable dishes, and chicken.
> Blend 2 tablespoons each of turmeric and ground coriander, 1 tablespoon of ground cumin, 2 teaspoons each of ground cardamom, ground ginger, and black pepper, and 1 teaspoon each of powdered cloves, cinnamon, and ground nutmeg.

Italian blend . . . for tomato-based soups and pasta dishes, chicken, pizza, focaccia, and herbed bread.
> Blend 2 tablespoons each of dried basil and dried marjoram, 1 tablespoon each of garlic powder and dried oregano, and 2 teaspoons each of thyme, crushed dried rosemary, and crushed red pepper.

Mexican chile blend . . . for chili with beans, enchiladas, tacos, fajitas, chicken, pork, and beef.
> Blend ¼ cup of chile powder, 1 tablespoon each of ground cumin and onion powder, 1 teaspoon each of dried oregano, garlic powder, and ground red pepper, and ½ teaspoon of cinnamon.

Greek blend . . . for seafood, poultry, and herbed bread.
> Blend 3 tablespoons each of garlic powder and dried lemon peel, 2 tablespoons of dried oregano, and 1 teaspoon of black pepper.

Easy dip blend . . . for mixing with cottage cheese, yogurt cheese *(see "Kitchen Nutrition: Yogurt Cheese" in chapter 5),* or low-fat sour cream; also nice on chicken and fish.
> Blend ¼ cup of dried dill weed and 1 tablespoon each of dried chives, garlic powder, dried lemon peel, and dried chervil.

food labels and look for sodium content in milligrams and % Daily Value (DV) for sodium per serving. Choose those with lower numbers. The DV is based on 2,400 milligrams sodium daily, which is higher than the 1,500 milligrams daily that's advised for many people.

● Read ingredient lists for hidden sodium and salt. For example, marinades, sauces, soy sauce, and meat marinades are high in sodium. *See page 165 in this chapter to learn more.*

● Scan the nutrient content claims on the front of food labels. From soup, canned fish, vegetables, and vegetable juice to crackers, popcorn, and snack foods, look for a "unsalted," "no salt added," "reduced sodium," "sodium-free," or "low in sodium" food

products. *To learn what these words mean, see "Label Lingo: Salt and Sodium" in this chapter.*

● Try lightly salted or unsalted nuts, popcorn, pretzels, crackers, and other dry snacks if an urge for a salty flavor strikes.

● Cut back on portions and calories to manage your weight. When calorie intake goes down, sodium intake may be reduced, too!

Eating Out

Unlike foods you buy at the supermarket, you usually don't know the sodium content of items on many restaurant menus. Yet, if you eat out a lot, the sodium from restaurant meals and snacks could be significant. To eat less salt from foods you order out:

● Move the salt shaker to another table, or taste before you shake. Ask for a lemon wedge, or bring your own herb blend to enhance the food's flavor.

● Recognize menu terms that may indicate a high sodium content: pickled, smoked, au jus, soy sauce, or in broth.

● Nibble on raw veggies rather than salty snacks.

● Go easy on condiments such as mustard, catsup, pickles, and tartar sauce for burgers, hot dogs, and sandwiches. Enjoy lettuce, onions, and tomatoes. Remember that bacon tends to be high in sodium.

● Ask the server to have your food prepared without added salt; ask for sauces and salad dressings on the side since they're often high in sodium. For a salad, use a twist of lemon, a splash of vinegar, or a light drizzle of dressing.

● Keep your order simple. Order broiled or grilled meat—without salty seasonings—rather than entrées cooked in sauces. Often special sauces and toppings add sodium.

● Look for sodium amounts in nutrition information for many larger restaurant chains. And know that many restaurants are cutting back quietly and gradually on salt in their menu items.

See chapter 15 for more on eating out.

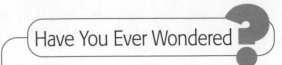

Have You Ever Wondered

. . . if drinking water has much sodium? The amount of sodium in drinking water varies from place to place. Unless you're on a sodium-restricted diet, you don't need to be too concerned. To know the sodium content, contact your local water department.

A water softener may add sodium to your water—but the contribution is typically small. Talk to the manufacturer of the water softener to find out how much sodium it adds to your water supply.

. . . if salting the cooking water speeds up the cooking? That's mostly urban legend. It's true that the boiling point of water may rise very slightly with added salt, but not enough for a noticeable difference. Salt added to cooking water will, however, make food a bit saltier.

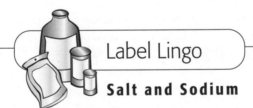

Label Lingo

Salt and Sodium

Does the term "sodium" or "salt" appear on the front of the food label? If so, here's what the descriptions mean.

For the specific sodium content in a standard serving, check the Nutrition Facts.

LABEL TERM	MEANS
Sodium-free	Less than 5 milligrams of sodium per serving
Very low sodium	35 milligrams or less of sodium per serving
Low sodium	140 milligrams or less of sodium per serving
Reduced or less sodium	At least 25% less sodium*
Light in sodium	50% less sodium*; restricted to foods with more than 40 calories per serving or more than 3 grams of fat per serving
Salt-free	Less than 5 milligrams of sodium per serving
Low-sodium meat	140 milligrams or less of sodium per 100 grams (3½ ounces)
Unsalted or butter, no added salt	No salt added during processing; does not necessarily mean sodium-free

*As compared with a standard serving size of the traditional food

CHAPTER 8

Fluids
Water and More!

Water? Unless your throat feels parched and sweat drips from your brow, you probably give little thought to water. Yet this clear, refreshing fluid is one of your body's most essential nutrients.

Water is vital. While you may survive for six weeks without food, you cannot live longer than a week or so without water. In fact, losing more than 10 percent of your body weight from dehydration, or water loss, causes extreme weakness and potential heat stroke. And a 20 percent loss is life-threatening. Water truly is the beverage of life!

A Fluid Asset

Water is the most abundant substance in the human body as well as the most common substance on earth. On average, body weight is 45 to 75 percent water—or for many, about 10 to 12 gallons of water. The percentage varies from person to person, relating to body composition, age, and gender, among other factors.

Compared with body fat, lean tissue holds much more water. The leaner you are, the higher proportion of water in your body. Males, with more muscle, carry a higher percentage of water in their bodies than females do. Younger people usually have more than older adults. Water accounts for about 75 percent of a newborn's weight, while the amount dwindles in the elderly to about 50 percent.

All body tissues contain water—some more than others. That blood contains water is certainly no surprise; your blood is about 83 percent water. Lean muscle tissue is about 73 percent water; body fat, about 25 percent. Even though bones seem hard, they, too, contain water, about 22 percent by weight.

Water: An Essential Nutrient

What does water do in your body? Far more than satisfy your thirst! Thirst is like a warning light that's flashing on your car's dashboard. This physical sensation signals that your body needs more fluid to perform its many functions. To satisfy thirst, you drink fluids.

Water itself is a simple substance, containing just one part oxygen and two parts hydrogen. It supplies no calories. Yet every body cell, tissue, and organ, and almost every life-sustaining body process, need water to function. In fact, water is the nutrient your body needs in the greatest amount.

Whether inside or surrounding your cells, nearly every body function takes place in a watery medium. Water regulates body temperature, keeping it constant at about 98.6° F. Many body processes produce heat, including any physical activity. Through perspiration, heat escapes as water evaporates on your skin.

Water dissolves nutrients and transports them, along with oxygen, to your body cells and carries waste products away. It moistens body tissues such as those in your mouth, eyes, and nose. Water is the main part of every body fluid, including blood, gastric (stomach) juice, saliva, amniotic fluid (for a developing fetus), and urine. By softening stools, water helps prevent constipation. It helps lubricate joints and cushion organs and tissues.

To keep your body functioning normally and to avoid dehydration, your body needs an ongoing water supply. During a strenuous workout, losing water weight is common, especially on hot, humid days. Losing just one or two pounds of your body's water weight can trigger thirst. With a little more fluid loss, the body loses strength and endurance; even mild dehydration can interfere with physical performance. With more water loss and prolonged exposure to high temperatures, a person may suffer from heat exhaustion or risk heat stroke. With a 20 percent drop in water weight, a person can barely survive.

Of all the nutrients in your diet, water is most abundant. Drinking water and other beverages are the main sources. But you "eat" quite a bit of water in solid foods, too—perhaps more than you think. Juicy fruits and vegetables such as celery, lettuce, tomatoes, and watermelon contain more than 90 percent water. Even dry foods, such as bread, supply some. *Check the chart "Food: A Water Source" in this chapter.*

Your body has still another water source. About 15 percent of your body's total water supply forms in your body cells when energy is produced from carbohydrates, proteins, and fats. Along with energy, water is an end product of metabolism.

Fluids: How Much Is Enough?

The average adult loses about 2½ quarts or more (about 10 or more cups) of water daily through perspiration (even when sitting), urination, bowel movements, and even breathing. During hot, humid weather or strenuous physical activity, fluid loss may be much higher. Unlike some other nutrients, the human body doesn't store extra water for times when you need more. To avoid dehydration and to keep your body working normally, replace lost fluids.

How much fluid do you need each day? The Dietary Reference Intakes from the Institute of Medicine (IOM) set the Adequate Intake (AI) level at 3.7 liters (125 ounces) of total water daily for males ages nineteen and over; for females nineteen and over, it's 2.7 liters (91 ounces) daily. (A liter is about 1 quart or

---

Dehydration: Body Signals!

The effects of dehydration, or loss of body water, can be significant and even lead to death. Watch for signals of water loss. All these steps won't happen in a single day.

PERCENT BODY WATER LOSS BY BODY WEIGHT	PROGRESSIVE EFFECTS OF DEHYDRATION (PARTIAL LIST)
0 to 1	Thirst
2 to 5	Dry mouth, flushed skin, fatigue, headache, impaired physical performance
6	Increased body temperature, breathing rate, pulse rate
8	Dizziness, increased weakness, labored breathing with exercise
10	Muscle spasms, swollen tongue, delirium, wakefulness
11	Poor blood circulation, failing kidney function

---

about 4 cups.) Teens and children need somewhat less; *refer to the appendices for recommended amounts.* The AI is for generally healthy people living in temperate climates. The IOM notes that people can be properly hydrated at higher or lower levels of water intake, too. In fact, the AI isn't a specific requirement or a recommended intake. It's based on the median total water intake, estimated from U.S. dietary surveys.

These amounts may seem like a lot, but "total water" comes from many sources—from drinking water, other beverages, and water in solid foods. If you're healthy and have access to drinking water and other beverages, you likely drink enough water. In fact, satisfying your thirst, along with a habit of drinking beverages with meals, is usually adequate. A little more than 8 cups of fluids a day, along with food, is generally enough to replace the fluids you lose.

Your own water needs vary from day to day. The amount depends on your level of physical activity, the climate, and your exposure to heat, along with other physical differences. Very hot weather increases the risk of dehydration for older adults. Other factors include:

● When you're exposed to extreme temperatures—very hot or very cold—your body uses more water to maintain its normal temperature.

● High altitudes (about 8,200 feet, or 2500 meters) may increase urine output and raise heart rate; both result in more water loss.

● With strenuous work or exercise, your body loses water through perspiration. Drink before physical activity. During exercise drink early and often. As a practical guide, check the color of your urine (*see below*). *For signs that you need to drink more, see "Dehydration Alert!" in chapter 20.*

● When you're exposed to heated or recirculated air for a long time, water evaporates from your skin. Dry, recirculated air on planes promotes dehydration.

● Pregnancy and breast-feeding increase the amount of fluid a woman's body needs. The AI level advised for pregnancy is 3 liters daily; for breast-feeding, 3.8 liters daily.

● Fever, diarrhea, and vomiting cause increased water loss. Follow the advice of your healthcare professional; drink plenty of water and other fluids to prevent dehydration. Depending on the illness, a doctor may advise an oral rehydration solution.

● On a high-fiber diet, your body needs extra water to process more roughage and prevent the chance of constipation.

In healthy people, water intake and water loss balance out. If you consume more than you need, your kidneys eliminate the excess, potentially 24 ounces of fluid an hour! You probably won't overdo on water. When you don't consume enough, your body may trigger thirst.

Thirst signals the need for fluids, but it isn't foolproof, especially for elderly people, children, and during illness, hot weather, or strenuous physical activity. Waiting until you feel thirsty to drink may be too long. By then, two or more cups of body fluids may be gone—even when you're healthy. *For more on fluids for older adults, see chapter 19.*

To see if you're drinking enough fluid, check your urine. A small volume of dark-colored urine indicates that you aren't consuming enough fluid.

Food: A Water Source

It's not easy to calculate how much water you consume each day. While drinks supply most of your water needs, solid food also provides a surprising amount.

Food	Percent Water by Weight
Lettuce, crisp head	96
Watermelon	91
Grapefruit, white	90
Broccoli, raw	89
Milk, lowfat	89
Orange juice	88
Carrot, raw	88
Apple, with skin	86
Yogurt, lowfat	85
Potato, baked with skin	75
Tuna, canned in water, drained	73
Rice, brown, cooked	73
Kidney beans, boiled	67
Chicken, roasted, no skin	65
Spaghetti, cooked	62
Whole-wheat bread	38
Cheddar cheese	37
Butter or margarine	16
Raisins	15
Pecans, dried	4
Vegetable oil	0

Source: U.S. Department of Agriculture, Agricultural Research Service, 2011. U.S. Department of Agriculture, National Nutrient Database for Standard Reference, Release 24, 2011.

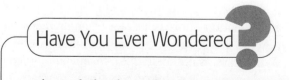 Have You Ever Wondered

... why you feel so thirsty after eating salty food? Salt is made of two minerals: sodium and chloride. When you eat a lot of salty foods, your body uses water to flush extra sodium away. With water loss, you feel thirsty, and you likely drink more. This explains why bars and cocktail lounges often serve salty snacks with drinks.

Water: In Balance

To maintain your body's fluid balance, replace the amount of water you lose each day. If you lose a little more, such as through perspiration, drink more to balance out.

Your body loses water daily through . . .

Urine	2 to 4 cups
Perspiration (lose through skin)	2 to 8 cups
Breath (expired air)	1 to 1½ cups
Feces	⅔ cup

You replace water in your body daily through . . .

Water and other fluids	9 to 12½ cups* (depending on gender)
Solid foods	2⅓ to 3 cups (depending on gender)
Water from metabolism	1 to 1½ cups

*Based on estimated minimum losses and production of water in healthy sedentary adults. If you consume a little more than your body needs, your body will excrete any extra.

Calculated from "Table: Estimation of Minimum Daily Water Losses and Production,: *Dietary References Intakes for Water, Potassium, Sodium, Chloride, and Sulfate*, 2004.

Besides feeling thirsty, this is your signal to drink more. Pale or almost colorless urine means you're drinking enough.

As another option, weigh yourself before and after strenuous physical activity. For every pound of weight you lose, replace it with two cups of fluid.

Caution: If you always seem thirsty or urinate too much, talk to your healthcare provider. This may signal diabetes or another serious health concern. Water retention, for reasons other than premenstrual syndrome, may suggest a kidney or a liver problem.

While rare, water toxicity can happen if someone drinks too much water, especially a problem for endurance athletes. Kidneys can't excrete enough urine; instead the mineral content of the blood gets diluted. The result can be hyponatremia, when sodium levels in the blood are too low. The effect can be life-threatening. Since it's so unlikely, a Tolerable Upper Intake Level for water wasn't set.

Drinking for Health

To keep your body well hydrated, consume enough water. Follow your thirst; drink beverages with meals. Because milk, juice, and some other beverages are mostly water, they count toward your daily water intake. So does water from solid foods, although you can't measure it. On average, moisture in food provides about 19 percent of total water intake.

Caffeinated beverages—coffee, tea, and some soft drinks—contribute to your day's total water intake, as noncaffeinated drinks do; consume them in moderation along with enough water. While a high intake of caffeine may have a diuretic effect, fluid from these beverages should offset any fluid loss. For that reason, they aren't dehydrating. Diuretic effect means water loss through increased urination. Any diuretic effect from alcoholic drinks appears to be short term, too; the effect may change during the day and may depend on how much water you drink before meals.

To increase your water intake . . .

● Drink mostly water and fluids with no or few calories.

● Take water breaks during the day instead of coffee breaks. If you're a mindless "sipper," keep a cup of water on your desk.

● When you buy a vending machine or convenience store drink, reach for bottled water.

● Complement meals and snacks with water, milk, or juice instead of soda. Occasionally, start your meals with soup.

● When you walk by a water fountain, drink!

● Snack on juice, milk, or sparkling water.

● Drink sparkling water at social gatherings.

● Before, during, and after any physical activity, drink water, especially in hot weather. Consume ½ to 2 cups of water every fifteen to twenty minutes while you exercise. Don't wait until you feel thirsty! *For more on fluids during exercise, see chapter 20.*

● Keep bottled water with you as you commute, while you work, as you run errands. Travel with bottled water, too, even for day outings. Airline travel promotes dehydration. Use clean, reusable water bottles when possible. *For tips on drinking fluids in flight, see chapter 15.*

Hydration for the Seasons

From the bone-chilling days of winter to the hot, sultry days of summer, your body needs water to maintain its normal temperature. Your body perspires as a cooling mechanism. Cooling down is harder in hot, humid weather than in hot, dry weather. That's because perspiration doesn't evaporate quickly from your skin. Instead your skin feels sticky and hot.

Dehydration may seem like just a summer issue. But keeping your body well hydrated during winter is just as important. When the weather turns chilly, most people head indoors. There heated air evaporates the moisture on your skin. Even in the cold outdoors, you may perspire . . . perhaps from the physical exertion of shoveling snow, skating or skiing, or from being bundled up with many layers of clothing.

What's to Drink?

Just plain water: It's the most available fluid around and often your best choice! Plain water has no calories or added sugars, and it's low in sodium. Watching your caffeine intake? Unlike many coffees, teas, and some soft drinks, water has no caffeine.

Juice and milk make good beverage options, too, since they supply other nutrients besides water. For

---

For your health, when consuming beverages . . .

● Cut back on drinks with added sugars or caloric sweeteners (sugar-sweetened beverages).

● Increase intake of fat-free and low-fat milk and fortified soy beverages.

● Replace higher fat milk with lower fat options.

● For adults of legal drinking age who choose to drink alcohol, consume it in moderation.

● Avoid alcohol in certain situations that can put you at risk.

Source: Dietary Guidelines for Americans, 2010.

---

example, juice offers vitamins A or C, or both, and milk is calcium- and vitamin D-rich. Other beverage choices—coffee, tea, soft drinks, and alcoholic drinks may quench your thirst but don't offer the nutrient benefits of milk, fortified soy beverage, or juice. And today there are more functional beverages than ever.

Do you know how many calories you drink each day? Beverage calories add up! Currently beverages provide an average of 400 calories daily for people ages two years and over. Some such as milk and 100 percent fruit juice are nutrient-rich. However, soda, energy drinks, sports drinks, and sugar-sweetened fruit drinks aren't; they're among the major sources of added sugars for Americans. To cut added sugars and, as a result, calories, replace them with beverages with few if any added sugars, such as water and unsweetened drinks.

Tap Water or Bottled Water?

Both are regulated stringently by the government—tap water by the Environmental Protection Agency (EPA) and commercial bottled water by the U.S. Food and Drug Administration (FDA). Especially from large municipal water systems, tap water is as safe for drinking as commercial bottled water.

Right from the Tap

Just turn on your faucet! Most drinking water in the United States comes right from the tap. Most of us take this for granted, but in many parts of the world,

---

"Wet" Your Appetite?

How much fluid do you drink during a typical day? How much from meals and snacks? Remember water you drank from a water fountain, tap, or refrigerator dispenser.

For good health, consume enough fluids: about 9 cups or more for women, and about 12½ cups or more for men. That adds up to about 80 percent of the AI for water. Drink more if you've been physically active or if it's a hot day. The rest of the water you consume (about 20 percent) comes from the food you eat.

Tip: With their mild diuretic effect, alcohol beverages don't provide a complete fluid-replacement benefit.

drinkable tap water is a luxury. If you live in an urban area, your tap water probably comes from a surface water source: river, lake, or reservoir, fed by a watershed, or land area. In a rural area, you likely drink groundwater that's pumped from an aquifer, an underground, natural reservoir. Either way, water must be treated with chemicals and filtered to ensure its quality and safety.

Treated: For Safety's Sake. No matter what the original source, water isn't naturally pure. Impurities dissolve or absorb in water as it flows through rivers and streams, filters through soil and rocks, and collects in lakes and reservoirs.

To make tap water safe to drink, the EPA has established standards for contaminants. Levels are set low enough to protect most people, including children. Treatment protects you from microbes such as bacteria and viruses, inorganic contaminants such as chemicals, and lead, arsenic, and other minerals.

To find out about a public water supply, ask for the annual report, or Consumer Confidence Report, from your community water supplier. It indicates the water source, the presence or level of contaminants, and what you can do to protect your drinking water.

Water may be disinfected chemically, or by a physical process such as ultraviolet light. Chlorination is a tried-and-true method for effectively treating water to protect against most immediate microbial reactions such as diarrhea and vomiting, and against outbreaks of cholera, hepatitis, dysentary, and other microbial diseases.

There's been some question about a by-product called trihalomethane (THM), created when chlorine breaks down organic matter in water. The very low amount of THM created in the process of making water safe to drink isn't enough to create a cancer risk. Protecting people from waterborne disease outbreaks far outweighs the insignificant effect of THM. If you or someone in your family is undergoing kidney dialysis, talk to your doctor about your water supply.

The Fluoride Connection

For children and adults, fluoride, a mineral, helps harden developing tooth enamel and so protects teeth from decay. It's also important for bone health. Many municipal water systems contain a natural supply of fluoride. But in areas where fluoride levels are low, the water system may be fluoridated.

The current recommended fluoride level, set in 1962, is 0.7 to 1.2 milligrams of fluoride per liter of water. However, in 2011 the U.S. Department of Health and Human Services proposed that the level be set at 0.7 milligrams of fluoride per liter of water. Why? Today the U.S. public has many fluoride sources besides water, including toothpaste, mouthwash, prescription fluoride supplements, and fluoride applied by dental professionals. A lower fluoride level in water would balance the decay-preventing benefits while limiting the possibility of fluorosis, or splotchy discoloration of teeth that can develop in the growing years.

If you're not sure about fluoride in your tap water, check with your local water department or public health department. If you have your own well, have it tested for fluoride.

In areas where water isn't fluoridated, dentists may prescribe fluoride supplements for children. "Topical" fluoride—applied directly to teeth with fluoride toothpaste, oral rinses, gels, foams, and treatments from a dental office—also helps strengthen tooth enamel. To reduce the chance for developing fluorosis, or brown spots, on permanent teeth, children shouldn't swallow fluoride toothpaste or rinses.

Consuming too much fluoride can cause fluorosis, even though teeth are healthy in other ways. That most likely happens with excessive supplement doses. The Tolerable Upper Intake Level for fluoride is 2.2 milligrams daily for children ages four through eight; from age nine through adulthood, it's 10 milligrams of fluoride daily.

People who drink mostly commercial bottled water may not consume enough decay-preventative fluoride. The fluoride content of commercial bottled water varies. It's hard to know how much fluoride it has since the U.S. FDA only requires fluoride labeling on bottled water if it's added in processing.

For more about fluoride and healthy teeth, see "Your Smile: Carbohydrates and Oral Health" in chapter 3 and "Caring for Baby Teeth" in chapter 16. Refer to chapter 6 for more on fluoride.

To know the THM level of your water, check your municipal water quality report; home testing is unreliable. The THM standard from the EPA is an average (per quarter of the year) of 80 parts per billion (ppb) as of January 2002. Home water filters can reduce these compounds in drinking water.

Water quality is assessed continually for safety. For example, in a few spots in the nation, low levels of arsenic in drinking water (from natural and commercial sources), consumed over time, were identified as a potential cancer risk. As of 2006, the arsenic level in water must be at a maximum level of 10 parts per billion (ppb). *For more information, check www.epa.gov/safewater/arsenic.html—EPA's website.*

Hard or Soft? Surprisingly, water itself may not be the only nutrient in drinking water. Unless distilled, or demineralized, drinking water may contain minerals in varying amounts, such as fluoride, calcium, sodium, iron, and magnesium. The water source and how it's processed determine the actual composition of drinking water. Water from underground wells, springs, and aquifers may contain high mineral concentrations. As water from rain and snow seeps through rocks, gravel, and sand, it picks up minerals along the way. That's how some underground water becomes naturally fluoridated.

Water may be "hard" or "soft" depending on its mineral content. Hard water contains more calcium and magnesium, which dissolves into rain water from

Have You Ever Wondered ?

. . . where to get your water tested? Whether you're checking for lead, trihalomethanes, or other contaminants, or having a private well tested, skip home testing kits. They're unreliable. Instead, contact the EPA or your local public health department.

. . . what you can do to help keep drinking water safe? Be environmentally conscious! Find out how to dispose of toxic trash such as household cleaners and batteries with lead or mercury. Your town may have a special collection site. Take used motor oil to a recycling center; don't discard it in your trash or storm sewer. Don't put any chemicals in places that seep into groundwater, such as septic systems, drainage wells, or dry wells.

Water: In Case of Emergencies

Disaster can hit anyone, anywhere! To ensure a safe water supply, disaster experts advise these precautions.

● Store a week's supply of bottled water for everyone in your family: about 1 gallon per person per day.

● Store containers of water in a cool, dry place away from direct sunlight.

● Label bottles of water with the date. Replace them every six months to ensure freshness.

the soil. Soft water has more sodium. With one exception there's essentially no difference in flavor between hard and soft water. Small amounts of iron give a metallic taste to hard water—but not enough to make it a significant source of dietary iron.

Where water is naturally hard, some consumers choose to use a water softener, which often replaces calcium and magnesium in water with sodium. The reason? Softening water can make soap work more efficiently, extend the life of a water heater, and avoid residue buildup in pipes. The amount of softening (salt added) depends on the hardness of the water. For well water that must be fully softened, the amount of sodium per cup of water is about 39 milligrams. Usually well water doesn't need to be fully softened; however, the average softened municipal water may contain less than 15 milligrams of sodium per cup. Again, your own water supply may not be softened. For most people, the amount of sodium in softened water isn't significant.

If you have a water softener, you might soften only hot water typically used for washing, not cooking or drinking. Then, if you're sodium-sensitive, you can drink unsoftened cold drinking water. Other options include buying demineralized water for cooking and drinking, or using a different type of water-purification system.

What about Bottled Water?

In recent years, consumption of bottled water has soared. Except for soft drinks, people living in the United States drink more bottled water than any other beverage! Since most tap water and bottled water are safe, why do some people choose bottled water? According to consumer research, some people prefer the taste. Bottled water usually doesn't contain chlorine, which can give water a slight flavor. It's convenient: portable for the office, a picnic, a drive, or a workout, and often easy to buy. You may buy bottled water instead of other bottled drinks for what it doesn't contain: calories, added sugars, caffeine, or alcohol.

About Bottled Water. Bottled water that's sold state to state is regulated by the FDA to assure its quality, safety, and accurate labeling. Terms on labels for bottled water, such as "spring water" or "mineral water," are defined legally. If bottled water comes from a municipal water supply, the label must state that fact, unless it's been processed to be purified water. By regulation, bottled water can't contain sweeteners or additives—besides flavors, extracts, or essences from food or spices (less than 1 percent by weight). And it must be calorie- and sugar-free.

Instead of chlorine, commercial bottled water usually is disinfected in other ways, including filtration; reverse osmosis; ultraviolet (UV) light; or ozone, a highly reactive form of oxygen. *See "Have You Ever Wondered?" in this chapter for more about water filtration systems.* Depending on the method, bottled water may or may not be 100 percent pathogen-free. If you have suppressed immune function, talk to your healthcare provider to find bottled water that's pathogen-free.

Ever see "NSF-certified" or "IBWA Bottler Member" on bottled water labels? IBWA stands for International Bottled Water Association. These label statements indicate that a voluntary inspection, using standards set by the National Sanitation Foundation, was conducted with the water source and the finished product and checked against FDA regulations. Safe water may not have a label since the inspection is voluntary. If you see "FDA-Approved" or "EPA-Certified," beware; neither agency conducts these inspections.

On bottled waters marketed for infants, look for the term "sterile." That means the water meets the FDA's standards for commercial sterilization, so it's safe from bacteria. If not, the label must state that the product isn't sterile and should be used to prepare infant formula only as directed by a doctor or according to infant formula preparation instructions. For

Label Lingo

Bottled Waters

Today's supermarket shelves offer bottled waters—some flavored, others plain. But what do the terms on the label mean? According to the FDA:

- *Artesian water* is a certain type of well water, collected without mechanical pumping. The well must tap a confined aquifer that has water standing much higher than the rock, gravel, or sand. An aquifer is an underground layer of rock or sand with water.

- *Well water* is collected from an underground aquifer, too, but with a mechanical pump.

- *Drinking water* is bottled water from an approved source. It must meet state and federal standards and go through minimal filtration and disinfection.

- *Mineral water* contains minerals at a standard level, no less than 250 parts per million (ppm) of total dissolved solids, or minerals. These minerals must be naturally present, not added. If the level is less than 500 ppm, it will be labeled "low mineral content"; if higher than 1,500 ppm, "high mineral content."

- *Purified water* has been processed to remove minerals and other solids. The process may be distillation, deionization, reverse osmosis, or another suitable process. *Tip:* "Purified" on the label doesn't mean that purified water is any more "pure" or better for you than tap water.

- *Distilled water,* which is one type of purified water, has been evaporated to steam, then recondensed to remove minerals.

- *Sparkling water* is water with a "fizz." Either carbon dioxide is added, or water is naturally carbonated. If carbon dioxide is added, it can't have any more than its naturally carbonated level. It can be labeled as natural sparkling water only if there's no added carbonation. Seltzer, tonic water, and club soda are considered soft drinks, not sparkling water, and may contain sugar and calories.

- *Spring water* comes from an underground source and naturally flows to the surface. It must be collected at the spring or through a bored hole that taps an underground source of the spring. If it's collected by an external (not natural force), it must have the same composition and physical qualities (perhaps carbonated) as the naturally flowing spring water.

safety, follow that guideline. Look for fluoridated bottled water if your child or infant consumes only bottled water.

Things to Consider about Bottled Water

● *Cost.* If you buy it, you may pay 240 to more than 10,000 times as much per gallon for bottled water that's no more healthful than most United States' tap water.

● *Nutrition and Safety.* From a nutritional standpoint, there's no significant difference, except that bottled water likely doesn't have as much fluoride, a concern for children and teens. In large municipal water systems, either bottled or tap water is safe and healthful. In fact, some bottled water *is* tap water, reprocessed to change its taste and composition.

Some commercial bottled waters may be a good beverage choice for those at high risk; *see "Drinking Water: For Special Health Needs" on this page.* In places where the lead or nitrate content of water is a concern, bottled water may be a good alternative, particularly for pregnant women or families with children. Bottled water doesn't contain lead.

In homes with lead pipes or lead solder, bottled water may be a good option in soups, stews, and other long-cooking dishes. During extended cooking, any lead in tap water may become more concentrated.

While potential risks are low, a few studies suggest that consuming food from plastic containers made with bisphenol A (BPA) may be a concern for infants and children. Many studies have found that BPA is at safe levels in food and beverage packaging. More research is needed. *For more about BPA refer to chapter 9.*

● *Taste.* Because the taste of tap water differs throughout the country, some people prefer commercial bottled water. Bottled and filtered waters usually don't contain chlorine, which may slightly alter the flavor of soups, stews, coffee, or tea. The appeal of flavored waters helps others drink more water, which is okay if it doesn't contain added sugars.

● *Environment.* Even if single-use plastic bottles are recycled, there's an environmental cost to making the bottle, transporting it with water inside, then handling waste. Thinner plastic bottles, as well as aluminum cans and paper containers—and tap water—are more eco-friendly.

For all these reasons, consider using a reuseable water bottle and look for water-refilling stations. Wash the bottle well with soapy water if you plan to reuse it; only refill bottles meant for reuse. Be aware that sipping from a bottle without cleaning it for several days increases risk of bacterial contamination.

Flavored and Nutrient-Added Water. Bottled water has been enhanced, sometimes just with flavorings, other times with added nutrients such as vitamins, electrolytes including sodium and potassium, and amino acids. For these waters, such as for spring water with berry flavor, the labels provide Nutrition Facts and an ingredient list, and the water itself must meet requirements for bottled water.

Safe Enough to Drink

For any nation, water safety is a top public health priority. In the United States, infectious disease spread by untreated water is almost nonexistent, except during

---

Drinking Water: For Special Health Needs

Some people are more vulnerable to microbial contaminants such as *Cryptosporidium* (or "crypto"), which isn't destroyed by chlorination. More often found in surface water than ground water, "crypto" may cause nausea, diarrhea, or stomach cramps when healthy people ingest it. For people who are more vulnerable, the symptoms may be more severe and perhaps life-threatening. That includes people with HIV/AIDS or other immune system disorders (such as lupus or Crohn's disease), organ transplants, the elderly, children, and those undergoing chemotherapy.

EPA standards put controls on disinfecting procedures for microbial contaminants, including "crypto," for surface water. However, at-risk people should still talk to their healthcare provider and take careful precautions.

Boiling tap water and pasteurizing bottled water destroy "crypto." Filters with an "absolute 1-micron" rating are relatively effective; see *"Have You Ever Wondered? . . . if you need a water filter"* in this chapter. Bottled waters—processed by distillation or reverse osmosis, or commercially filtered with an NSF International Standard 53 filter before bottling—are safe. Not all bottled waters are handled in this way.

natural disasters such as floods, earthquakes, or accidental contamination of wells or municipal water. These incidents can devastate a community's drinking water supply; you're wise to know what to do in a water emergency.

When the safety of your water supply is in doubt, don't drink it! Instead, take steps to make it safe.

● Report your concern to your water company or local public health department. They may test the water or refer you to a qualified private laboratory.

● If you rely on a private well or spring, have it tested annually by a certified water testing laboratory for coliform bacteria, nitrate, and perhaps other contaminants such as radon, pesticides, or industrial wastes. Do it more often if your sample exceeds the standard. People who draw their water from a private water source are responsible for its safety. For tips on how to protect a private water supply, www.epa.gov/safewater is the EPA's website.

● Purify contaminated drinking water by boiling tap water for at least one minute, then pouring the boiled water into a sterile container. At high altitudes, perhaps if you're camping, boil water longer. Why? At high altitudes water boils at a lower temperature, which may be less effective at killing bacteria.

● Use iodine or chlorine tablets to disinfect your water supply; strictly follow package directions. These products are available in camping stores. Campers, hikers, and others who rely on water supplied by wilderness lakes and streams might use water filtration and purification devices as well.

● Contact EPA's Safe Drinking Water Hotline or website; your state certification officer for referral to a certified water testing lab; or your local health department. *See "Resources You Can Use" in this book.*

In some countries, contaminated water is an ongoing problem, spreading diarrhea and even life-threatening diseases such as cholera and hepatitis. For globe-trotters, water is a common source of travelers' diarrhea. *See "What's Safe to Drink?" in chapter 15*

Have You Ever Wondered ?

. . . if you need a water filter? Probably not, unless you prefer the taste and smell of filtered water, or, although uncommon, if your water supply needs filtration or boiling for safety. If you buy one, read the manufacturer's information to see what it filters out. A water filter that meets National Sanitation Foundation (NSF) International Standard 53 for cyst removal or cyst reduction is the most effective. Using reverse osmosis (a type of filtration system), it has an "absolute 1 micron" rating given on the label, meaning that the pore size is 1 micron or less in diameter, with or without NSF testing. Filters rated as "nominal 1 micron" aren't reliable for removing bacteria, such as *Cryptosporidium.* Replace the filter cartridges regularly and properly, according to the manufacturer's instructions. A filter may not eliminate smaller bacteria.

. . . if seltzer and club soda are the same as bottled water? No. Still safe to drink, neither is required to meet the quality standards of bottled water. Some seltzer and club soda products contain sugar and sodium, whereas bottled water, by definition, cannot.

. . . what flavored waters really are? Flavored waters may have just a hint of flavor, derived from a natural fruit essence. Some may also contain sugar, or low-calorie sweeteners, and artificial flavors. Read labels to find out what's in beverages; remember, some flavored waters contain calories. Being clear doesn't mean that a beverage is simply water!

. . . if oxygen-enhanced drinks offer unique benefits such as a boost in athletic performance? No. It's just marketing hype. First, consider "oxygen-enhanced" water. Under pressure, only a tiny amount (about the amount in one breath) of oxygen can be forced into water. It quickly bubbles out as soon as you open the bottle.

Even if some "extra oxygen" in water made it to your mouth, your digestive tract would get it, not your lungs. Your lungs, not your intestines, process oxygen captured by the heme (iron) portion of blood. Fortunately, there's enough oxygen in the environment to sustain life.

for travelers. For added safety in less-developed areas, travel with a supply of iodine or chlorine tablets.

Get the Lead Out (and the Nitrates and Nitrites, Too)!

Since the spread of infectious disease from drinking water is under control in the United States, concerns have shifted.

Excessive lead in drinking and cooking water poses a serious health risk. Over time, too much lead consumed in food and beverages can build up in the body, potentially damaging the brain, nervous system, kidneys, reproductive system, and red blood cells. It can also lead to high blood pressure. Infants, children, and unborn babies are more vulnerable to lead poisoning.

Where does lead in the water supply come from? Often, from plumbing inside the home or from service lines. Many older houses and multifamily dwellings were constructed with water pipes, fittings, or fixtures made of lead. Additionally, lead service lines in older communities may connect a house with the municipal water system. According to 1996 amendments to the U.S. Safe Drinking Water Act, all pipe, fittings, and fixtures introduced into commerce must be lead-free.

If you are concerned, check your pipes and water supply; get your water tested. Even copper pipes might use lead solder in the joints; brass faucets and fittings may contain lead, too. Your local public health department or water utility company may have a free testing kit or may refer you to a government-certified laboratory that tests for water safety.

If the lead problem is severe, you might install a water filtering device or use bottled water for drinking and cooking. If less severe, follow these guidelines to help ensure water safety.

● Avoid drinking water that has been in lead plumbing for six hours or more.

● For drinking and cooking water, let the cold water run for sixty seconds or more to clear water in the pipes and faucet. This helps flush out water with the heaviest lead concentration.

● For cooking and baby formula preparation, use cold water from your tap or bottled water. Hot water dissolves lead from pipes more quickly than cold water does. Boiling water doesn't remove lead!

● To minimize lead in drinking and cooking water, install a water-softening system only on your hot-water faucet. Then for drinking and cooking use the hard water from your cold-water faucet. It won't pick up as much lead as soft water from your hot-water faucet. Use soft water for washing.

● Use bottled water for cooking and drinking.

As a precaution: The American Academy of Pediatrics and the Centers for Disease Control and Prevention (CDC) advise lead screening for infants and toddlers at ages one and two. If you have a young child between six months and three years old, talk to your doctor about possible sources of lead in your home or child care setting. *As a reminder about lead poisoning and kids, refer to chapter 17.* When lead in children's blood tests above 10 micrograms per deciliter, sources of lead in the child's environment should be identified and corrected, according to the CDC.

Another alert: If your water supplier alerts you to nitrate or nitrite levels that exceed EPA standards *and* if you have a child under six months of age, talk to your healthcare provider. Ingesting that water could cause "blue baby syndrome," which can be life-threatening without immediate medical attention. The symptoms are a bluish skin tone and shortness of breath.

Find a different and safe water source for preparing baby formula. Nitrates are inorganic and can't be destroyed as bacteria can be. As with lead, boiling water concentrates nitrates and so increases risk.

Water may become unsafe to drink for other reasons. Be aware of water alerts during natural disasters. Sanitize your refrigerator's icemaker and water disperser regularly, according to appliance guidelines. *For more about food and water safety, refer to chapter 13.*

Fruit Juice, Juice Drink, Fruit Drink?

When you're thirsty, a refreshing, fruity beverage often hits the spot. Which one will you reach for: fruit juice, juice drink, fruit drink, or fruit-flavored water? All provide fluid.

Depending on the fruits and perhaps the vegetables they're made from, juices and juice drinks supply varying amounts of vitamins A and C.

● *Fruit juice.* When it comes to terminology, only 100 percent juice can be called "juice."

● *Juice drink.* If juice is diluted (<100 percent juice), the product label must identify it with a different name: "juice drink," "juice beverage," or "juice cocktail"; these terms can be used interchangeably. Or it may be called "diluted _____ juice"—for example, diluted apple juice.

● *Fruit drink.* A "fruit drink" is simply flavored water (with no juice), perhaps fortified with vitamin C or other nutrients, phytonutrients, or herbs.

Does 100 percent juice have more vitamin C than a juice drink? Not necessarily. Some 100 percent fruit juices contain less than 100 percent of the Daily Value (DV) for vitamin C, while some juice drinks are fortified to supply at least 100 percent in a single label serving:

¾ CUP	% DAILY VALUE OF VITAMIN C
Orange juice	100
Fortified cranberry juice	100
Apple juice (unfortified)	3
Grape juice (unfortified)	0

Many of today's juices, juice blends, and juice drinks also are fortified with calcium, vitamin D, DHA, omega-3s, and more, as stated on the label.

To learn how to use Nutrition Facts, see "Today's Food Labels" in chapter 12; you'll also find advice on refrigerated juice safety.

All juice products contain water and sugar. Fruit juice contains naturally occurring fructose, or fruit sugar, whereas juice drinks have added sugars such as high-fructose corn syrup, as well as some fructose. *See chapter 3, "Carbs: Sugars, Starches, Fiber"* for more about natural and added sugars. Depending on the amount of added sugars, there may be a difference in the calorie amount per label serving between fruit drinks and fruit juices.

Some tart juices, such as cranberry, are blended with other juices, water, and sweeteners to make them more pleasing. A nutritional difference between fruit juices and fruit drinks is that fruit juices often contain more of other important nutrients and phytonutrients, such as folate in orange juice or antioxidants in blueberry juice.

Does fruit come to mind first when you think of juice? Give vegetable juice, such as tomato juice or a

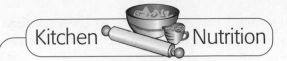

Kitchen Nutrition

Super Sippers

Hot-weather thirst quenchers:

● Combine grapefruit juice or cranberry-mango cocktail concentrate with chilled club soda. Serve with a sprig of fresh mint.

● Make a fruit smoothie. In a blender, puree berries, sliced kiwifruit, mango, or pineapple chunks with 100 percent juice and yogurt. Perhaps add fresh mint. For convenience, try canned and frozen fruit for smoothies!

● Create shakes. In a blender, puree melon chunks or peach slices with buttermilk, crushed ice, and a touch of ginger or cinnamon until smooth.

● Use silken tofu as a great nondairy alternative in a creamy shake. Add a little juice and frozen fruit; puree until smooth.

Cold-weather belly warmers:

● Simmer cranberry-apple juice with cinnamon, cloves, allspice, and orange peel for about twenty minutes. Strain. Stir in fat-free dry milk powder and vanilla extract. Heat through.

● Add anise seeds, ground cinnamon, and ground cloves to ground coffee. Prepare hot coffee using the spiced ground coffee. Lighten with warm milk.

● Scoop praline or chocolate frozen yogurt into a mug. Pour hot cocoa or coffee over the top. Stir with a cinnamon stick.

vegetable juice mixture, a try, too. For a hint of fruit flavor without adding calories, float citrus slices or berries in ice water.

One hundred percent juice counts toward your daily amount of fruit or vegetables. Consume most fruit as whole fruit; 100 percent juice lacks fiber and, when consumed in excess, can contribute extra calories.

For guidelines on fruit juice for infants and children, see chapters 16 and 17.

Juicing Fruits and Vegetables

Some juice-machine promoters may lead you to believe that juicing makes fruits and vegetables healthier. Of course, their juices are healthful, offering most of the vitamins, minerals, and phytonutrients found in the whole fruit or vegetables. However, juices typically have less fiber; it gets left behind in the pulp. In spite of "cure-all" claims, simply changing the form of food by juicing can't deliver added benefits. Enjoy juice as way to get the benefits of fruits and vegetables—but don't expect miracles!

If you decide to juice at home, consume the pulp for its fiber and because it helps you feel full.

Milk, Cocoa, and Flavored Milks: Calcium-Rich Choices

Like all beverages, milk supplies that essential nutrient water: about 89 percent by weight. As one of the best calcium sources, milk offers a lot more. Here's what just 1 cup (8 ounces) supplies. Just multiply by three for the amount from the recommended three cups (or the equivalent) daily.

NUTRIENTS IN 8 OUNCES	% DAILY VALUE
Calcium (305 mg)	30
Vitamin D (100 IU)	25
Vitamin A (500 IU)	10

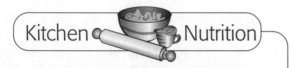

Kitchen Nutrition: Milk Plus

You say you're not a milk drinker? Just whisk one or two ingredients, such as those below, with one cup of milk—cold or hot, fat-free or whole—and give it a refreshing new flavor! (And enjoy the added benefits of 300 milligrams of calcium from a cup of milk.)

- ½ cup of fresh or frozen pureed berries: strawberries, raspberries, blackberries, or blueberries
- 2 tablespoons of fruit juice concentrate or 1 pureed peach and ½ teaspoon of flavor extract
- ¼ teaspoon of almond, anise, hazelnut, maple, or vanilla extract. Or try a flavored oil, perhaps cinnamon or peppermint: Use 2 drops of flavored oil in place of ¼ teaspoon of extract.
- ½ cup of cranberry juice cocktail and a small scoop of low-fat vanilla ice cream or frozen yogurt
- 1 tablespoon of creamy peanut butter and 2 tablespoons of chocolate syrup

Protein (8 g)	16
Potassium (380 mg)	11
Riboflavin (0.4 mg)	26
Vitamin B$_{12}$ (1.3 mcg)	22
Phosphorus (245 mg)	25
Niacin and niacin equivalents (2 NE)	10

Whole, 2 percent reduced-fat, 1 percent low-fat, and fat-free milks: the fat content varies, along with the calorie content. However, other nutrient contributions, including water, are about the same.

Flavored milk, including fat-free and low-fat options, can be a healthful choice. For flavored milk, the difference is about 30 more calories per 8-ounce serving from the added sweetener, and chocolate or cocoa. (Over the past five years, calories and added sugars in flavored milk have been lowered.) Whether it's flavored or unflavored, milk supplies the same amounts of calcium, phosphorus, protein, riboflavin, and vitamin D. *To compare the calories and nutrients in various milk, see "Milk: A Great Calcium and Vitamin D Source" in chapter 10.*

That many kids like flavored milk has prompted a question: Do the sugar and caffeine in chocolate milk cause hyperactivity? No scientific evidence suggests a link between sugar or caffeine and hyperactivity, mood swings, or academic performance. The amount of caffeine in the chocolate or cocoa is very small. Some soft drinks provide much more caffeine. *See "Caffeine: What Sources, How Much?" in this chapter.*

Among other dairy options: drinkable yogurt, smoothies, and hot cocoa made with milk. They, too, deliver calcium and often vitamin D; read the label's ingredient list and the Nutrition Facts to compare the calories and other nutrients. Drinkable yogurt and yogurt drinks may have active live cultures with probiotic benefits; check the label to find out.

Non-Dairy Alternates

Soy beverages that are calcium- and vitamin-D fortified can be nutrient-rich alternates for milk for those with milk allergies or for vegans. Beverages made from other plant-based foods—almonds, flaxseed, hemp, and rice milks—offer variety to beverage choices, but they don't provide all the nutrients in milk or fortified soy beverages. *For more about buying non-dairy alternates, see chapter 12.*

Drinks: With or without Caffeine?

Does coffee in the morning go with your "wakeup" routine? Caffeine, a mild stimulant, has been part of the human diet for centuries. As far back as five thousand years ago, records suggest that the Chinese were brewing tea. About twenty-five hundred years ago, highly valued coffee beans were used in Africa as currency. And in the Americas, the Aztecs enjoyed chocolate drinks. Today, caffeine-containing foods and beverages are a part of our food pattern.

A naturally occurring substance in plants, caffeine is found in leaves, seeds, and fruits of more than sixty plants, among them coffee and cocoa beans, tea leaves, and kola nuts. We consume these products as coffee, chocolate, tea, soft drinks, and energy drinks. Caffeine also is found in more than a thousand over-the-counter drugs as well as in prescription drugs, and as a subtle flavoring.

Have You Ever Wondered

... if sports drinks are good fluid replacers? The optimal drink for many sports is water! Sports drinks are meant to replace fluids, supply calories for energy, and replace sodium and potassium lost through perspiration. Most athletes don't need a sports drink unless they've exercised for an hour or more. Even then, the body mainly needs fluids. If you're more likely to drink a sports drink than water during physical activity, then do. Just be aware that these drinks contain added sugars, so they also supply calories. As a regular beverage choice, their calories can add up: often 50 to 100 calories per cup. *See chapter 20.*

... if coconut water is a good fluid replacement? Sure, if you like the flavor and find it thirst quenching. Coconut water (not coconut milk), which is the liquid inside young, green coconuts, is naturally rich in potassium. If unflavored, it's low in sugar and calories, so it might be a better choice than a soft drink. But it won't make you lose weight, detoxify, or be the perfect sports drink. Unlike commercial sports drinks, coconut water won't replace all the electrolytes lost through sweat—despite the claims.

Coffee remains the chief source of caffeine in the United States. That includes drinks made with coffee, such as latte, mocha, and cappuccino. The amount of caffeine varies depending on the type of coffee, the amount, and the brewing method.

Soft drink, teas, and many energy drinks are common sources of caffeine for children and teens. Among soft drinks, cola isn't the only beverage with caffeine; some citrus-flavored beverages contain caffeine as well.

As a mild stimulant to the central nervous system, caffeine helps people keep mentally alert, overcome fatigue, and sustain their attention. And it may help enhance mental and physical effort before someone gets tired. *For more about caffeine and physical performance, see chapter 20.*

Caffeine: A Health Connection?

Over the years many studies have explored the connection between caffeine and health. Growing research evidence suggests potential health benefits of moderate caffeine intake—beyond being more alert in the short-term. Among possible benefits linked to moderate caffeine intake are lower risks for type 2 diabetes, chronic liver disease, and some cancers, and perhaps helping to prevent cognitive decline associated with aging. Most research on caffeine has been done with coffee; many potential long-term benefits also may be linked to antioxidants, such as flavonoids or other components in coffee. More research is needed before recommendations can be made for treatment.

In addition, the scientific evidence does not link moderate caffeine intake to many increased health risks, including cancer (pancreatic, breast, or other types), fibrocystic breast disease (benign fibrous lumps), cardiovascular disease, blood cholesterol levels, ulcers, inflammatory bowel disease, infertility, birth defects, or osteoporosis.

Concerned about your blood pressure? Caffeine doesn't cause hypertension or a lasting increase in blood pressure. However, it may cause a temporary rise that lasts only a few hours and adds up to less than that from climbing stairs.

Caffeine may have a mild diuretic effect, increasing water loss through urination. However, fluid in the beverage usually cancels any loss. The diuretic effect depends on the amount of caffeine. Caffeinated drinks won't cause dehydration or electrolyte imbalance, either. If you have diarrhea, avoiding caffeine might be advised.

While caffeine can increase slightly the amount of calcium lost through urine and feces, this can be off-set by adding 1 tablespoon of milk to your daily cup of regular coffee. A 12-ounce caffe latte, made with fat-free milk and no added syrups or whipped cream, has about 400 milligrams of calcium and 110 calories. Moderate amounts of caffeine don't appear to raise the risk for osteoporosis. By the way, you don't need whole milk to get a foam on cappuccino. Low-fat or fat-free milk and soy beverage also will do the trick.

Chic coffee drinks? Adding shots of caramel, chocolate, fruit syrups, or cream to coffee bar bever-ages (lattes, mochas, cappuccinos, or other drinks) can up the added sugars, total fat, saturated fat, and calo-ries. The larger the size, the more calories they rack up! If you can customize your coffee drink, make it healthier. Ask for the smallest size. Request fat-free milk (no or less whipped cream) or soy beverage, and perhaps sugar-free syrup or a dusting of cocoa pow-der or cinnamon. Bottled coffee drinks may not have as much calcium as you think—and perhaps more added sugars and calories; read the Nutrition Facts.

Although many think coffee helps "sober up" someone who drinks too much alcohol, caffeine won't counteract its effects. Neither will a cold shower or a long walk. Only time can make someone sober.

In varying degrees, excessive caffeine intake may cause "coffee jitters," anxiety, or insomnia. Caffeine also may increase heart rate temporarily. These physical effects don't last long since caffeine doesn't accumulate in the body.

"Excessive" caffeine intake is subjective. One's caffeine sensitivity depends on the amount and fre-quency of caffeine intake, body weight, physical con-dition, and overall anxiety level, among other factors. Tolerance to caffeine develops over time. A regular coffee drinker may not notice the effects as quickly as someone who drinks an occasional cup. For most healthy people, moderate amounts of caffeine—300 milligrams a day, or about three 8 oz. cups of coffee—pose no problems. For kids, use common sense. No evidence shows that caffeine in levels normally found in food and beverages are harmful or that kids are any more sensitive to caffeine than adults. That said,

Did You Stop to Think

. . . that with so many bottled drinks sold today, you must read labels. Serving sizes aren't always the same. A single bottle may have two or more label servings, for at least twice the calories. And many flavored waters, teas, and coffee drinks are high in added sugars.

. . . that a large, regular soda (32 ounces) adds up to about 400 calories? Drinking one soda that size three times a week adds up to 1,200 calories per week, or about 60,000 calories over a fifty-week work year. A pound of body fat is about 3,500 calories. Do the math! That adds up to several pounds of extra body fat if you don't change in your food or lifestyle habits! Consider swapping out regular soda with low-calorie soda, low-fat or fat-free milk, or water. Small steps make a difference!

. . . that "slow sipping" a regular soft drink, sweetened ice tea, or juice drink bathes your teeth in cavity-promoting sugars? The effect continues for twenty or more minutes after your last sip!

. . . that 8 ounces of milk provide a quarter to almost a third of your day's calcium recommendation? Great for bones! A 12-ounce diet soda provides "zero" calcium.

current data show that kid's caffeine consumption is moderate and less than adults; soft drinks, which have less caffeine than coffee, are the main caffeine source for kids.

Can you become addicted to caffeine? No, but caf-feinated drinks may become a habit. If you drink them regularly, then suddenly stop, you may have short-term symptoms—drowsiness, headache, perhaps less concentration—that disappear in a day or two.

Is there a link between caffeine withdrawal and rebound headaches? Although some experts disagree, clinically significant symptoms from caffeine with-drawal aren't common.

According to the National Institutes of Health, caf-feine affects children and adults in the same way. No studies show that caffeine causes attention deficit dis-order or affects growth in children.

Sensitivity to caffeine varies among individuals. Some people feel its effects at very low levels, while others are unaffected and can consume more. After ingesting caffeine, it takes thirty to forty-five minutes to reach the bloodstream. The effect lasts about three to four hours, then it's excreted through urine. For smokers, it's slightly faster. Some people eliminate caffeine more slowly.

Sensitive groups of people such as pregnant women and those with a history of heart attack or high blood pressure should consult with their physician about their caffeine consumption.

● *If you're pregnant or nursing* . . . up to 300 milligrams of caffeine (about two to three 8 oz. cups of brewed coffee) doesn't appear to have adverse affects, and it doesn't affect fertility. Although most physicians agree on its safety, sensitivity to caffeine may increase during pregnancy. In breast milk, caffeine can pass to the baby, but the very small quantity in usual amounts isn't enough to affect the infant. During breast-feeding, limit caffeine drinks, advises the American Academy of Pediatrics; you don't need to avoid them.

● *If you have a medical problem* . . . ask your physician to guide you on caffeine intake, particularly if you suffer from gastritis, ulcers, or high blood pressure, or if you take beta-blockers. Caffeine doesn't cause gastric reflux disease (GERD). There's not enough evidence to advise all those with GERD to avoid caffeinated drinks.

● *At any age* . . . pay attention to how caffeine affects you, especially if coffee, tea, soft drinks, or energy drinks take the place of more nutritious foods or beverages.

For most people, two to three cups of coffee (or that amount of caffeine) are likely reasonable. To reduce your caffeine intake:

● Cut back gradually—if you've been ingesting a lot of caffeine—to get your body accustomed to consuming less. A gradual cutback helps avoid any temporary headaches or drowsiness.

● Mix half regular and half decaffeinated coffee.

● Drink decaffeinated coffee or tea, which has almost no caffeine at all, or caffeine-free herbal tea. Some bottled coffee drinks also are decaffeinated; check the label.

● Brew tea for a shorter time. A one-minute brew may contain just half the caffeine that a three-minute brew contains.

● Keep a cup of water handy to sip. If you drink coffee, tea, or soft drinks mindlessly, you may be drinking more caffeine than you realize.

● Read soft drink labels; many caffeinated soft drinks consumed in the United States are offered in decaffeinated form. Color doesn't indicate the presence of caffeine; both clear and caramel-colored soft drinks may have caffeine. Caffeine is listed in the ingredient list if it is present in the product.

● Go easy on energy drinks, and read the label. The caffeine content per label serving in energy drinks varies; a beverage container may contain more than

Caffeine: What Sources, How Much?

The amount of caffeine in foods or beverages depends on several factors: type of product, its preparation method, and portion size. Caffeine occurs naturally in some products, such as coffee and chocolate, and is added as a flavoring in some others, such as soft drinks.

BEVERAGE	CAFFEINE (MG)	
	TYPICAL	RANGE
Coffee* (8-oz. serving)		
Brewed, drip method	85	60–120
Instant	75	60–85
Decaffeinated	3	2–4
Espresso coffee (1-oz. serving)	40	30–50
Tea* (8-oz. serving)		
Brewed, major U.S. brands	40	20–90
Instant	28	24–31
Iced	25	9–50
Soft drinks cola (12 oz.)	40	30–60
Energy drinks (8.3 oz.)	80	50–160
Cocoa beverage (8 oz.)	6	3–32
Chocolate milk beverage (8 oz.)	5	2–7
Solid milk chocolate (1 oz.)	6	1–15
Solid dark chocolate, semisweet (1 oz.)	20	5-35
Baker's chocolate (1 oz.)	26	26
Chocolate-flavored syrup (1 oz.)	4	4

*For the coffee and tea products, the range varies due to brewing method, plant variety, brand formulation, etc.

Source: IFIC Foundation, 1998; *Food Chem. Toxicol*, 2004; Mayo Clinic, 2005.

one label serving. *See "Energy Drinks" later in this chapter to learn more.*

● Read medication labels carefully, or check with your pharmacist. One dose of an over-the-counter pain relief capsule can contain as much caffeine as one or two cups of coffee, which is amplified if you're consuming caffeinated foods or beverages.

● For those with insomnia, avoid coffee or other caffeine sources in the evening.

Take Time for Tea

Tea: Next to water, it's the most common beverage choice throughout the world. Whether it's black, green, or oolong tea, tea comes from the same plant, called *Camellia sinensis.* Differences in color and flavor depend on processing.

● For *black tea,* the most popular type in the United States, tea leaves are exposed to air. The natural biochemical process colors them a deep red-brown color and imparts a unique, rich flavor. Many flavored specialty teas start with black tea. *Note:* orange pekoe isn't made with orange flavor; instead "pekoe" or "orange pekoe" refers to the grade and size of tea leaves.

● For *green tea,* typically served in Chinese and Japanese restaurants, the tea leaves are not processed as much. Instead, they're just heated or steamed quickly to keep their green color and delicate flavor.

● *Oolong tea* is an "in-between" tea: between black and green tea.

Teatime: Health Benefits?

Whether black or green or oolong, tea appears to have potential health benefits, perhaps derived from its flavonoids. Flavonoids and other polyphenols, which are phytonutrients, work as antioxidants that may help protect body cells from damage done by free radicals. Using the oxygen radical absorbency capacity (ORAC) score, which ranks the antioxidant potential of plant-based foods, tea ranks as high as or higher than many fruits and vegetables. *To learn more about antioxidants and the ORAC score, see chapter 6.*

Can tea drinking help keep you healthy? Maybe, but the research evidence linking tea consumption and disease prevention isn't yet certain. And there's not

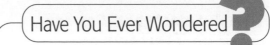

Have You Ever Wondered

. . . if a few cold beers on a hot day are as good as water to replace fluids? Not really. Alcohol is a mild diuretic, which increases urine output and so promotes dehydration—not the best fluid replacement when you're sweating! If you enjoy a beer, drink water, too.

. . . what's rooibos tea? Pronounced ROY-boss, rooibos is an herbal brew, not a tea. First popularized in South Africa, this red brew in nutty, flowery, and fruity flavors is purported to have antioxidant benefits. Research doesn't back up the advertised claims. Like other herbals, be cautious.

enough evidence for specific advice about tea drinking. Some promising areas of study suggest that tea or tea's flavonoids may reduce risk of gastric, esophageal, and skin cancers and may offer protection from heart disease and stroke—if you consume enough (four to six cups a day). Some studies are investigating whether tea plays a role in relaxation or mental performance or in lowering cholesterol, preventing diabetes, burning fat, and holding off dementia.

Tea may supply fluoride, which helps strengthen tooth enamel, if it's made with fluoridated water. Tea also may help fight cavities by reducing plaque formation and hindering cavity-forming bacteria. You still need to brush and floss!

For now, enjoy tea; steep it for at least three minutes to bring out the most flavonoids. Then stay tuned for science-based advice.

Creative Ways to Enjoy Tea

● Try bottled teas as a portable beverage choice. *Be aware:* Many bottled or canned ice tea drinks have as much added sugars and calories as regular sodas; read the label. Look for those flavored with low-calorie sweeteners.

● Watching calories? Enjoy unsweetened tea with no added sugars or honey. For a touch of flavor, add a slice of lemon or lime, fresh ginger, or fresh mint leaves.

● Add citrus juice for flavor and smart nutrition! Tea's flavonoids partly inhibit the absorption of nonheme iron (iron from legumes, grain products, and eggs).

Drink Smart—and Get Your Zzzzzzs!

Do you wake up with a sleep deficit? Do you regularly have trouble sleeping? Adequate rest, along with good nutrition and regular physical activity, are part of any fitness formula. For the "rest" of your life:

● If you're caffeine-sensitive, avoid caffeinated drinks six to eight hours before sleeptime. For meals and snacks later in the day, opt for milk, juice, water, or decaffeinated drinks.

● Don't expect a glass of wine or other alcoholic beverage to help you sleep well. A drink might help you feel drowsy at first, but even if you sip a drink two or three hours before bedtime, your sleep might be light instead of the deep, most restful sleep pattern.

An added note: Promote rest through regular physical activity. Being active actually helps your body relax and sleep soundly. Just refrain from exercise too close to bedtime. Exercise speeds up your metabolism for a while, perhaps keeping you "pumped up" and unable to sleep right away.

Will a glass of warm milk help you sleep? Perhaps. The reason is more likely the psychological impact of milk as a comfort food, not its relatively small tryptophan content.

A squeeze of vitamin C-rich lemon, orange, or lime juice in your tea can counteract some of the action.

● For more calcium and vitamin D, enjoy "milk tea": hot or cold tea added to milk. Some believe that adding milk to tea lowers tea's antioxidant power. However, no scientific evidence proves that milk binds to and inactivates polyphenols.

● Take milk tea up a notch; enjoy it as chai (rhymes with pie) or spiced milk tea! A favorite in India, chai blends black tea, milk, spices such as cardamom, cinnamon, ginger, cloves, and pepper, and a little sugar or honey to bring out the flavor of the spices. It's served iced or as a milkshake.

● Experiment with culinary uses of dried tea leaves: as a flavor rub for a roast, for tea-marinated meat, or in homemade sorbet.

● Use tea—perhaps flavored—in place of water in dough or batter for breads, cookies, cakes, and brownies.

● For the most potential benefit, drink your tea, rather than take a green tea extract as a dietary supplement. Tea itself may have health-promoting compounds that extracts don't have.

Pour an "Herbal" Tea?

Have a sip of apple-cinnamon tea, mint tea, or ginger tea. Interest in herbal teas has been rising for those seeking an alternative to caffeinated beverages—and for those hoping for other health benefits.

To clear up a misconception: Many branded herbal teas are really tea leaves with added herbs and perhaps fruit juice, honey, sweeteners, or flavor extracts; they have very small amounts of caffeine unless the label indicates "decaf." The ingredient list will include "tea." And some herbal teas on the market aren't tea at all. Instead, they're infusions made with herbs, flowers, roots, spices, or various other parts of many plants. The more correct term for them is "tisane," which means tealike substance.

For health benefits, herbal teas haven't been studied, so little is known. Some research suggests that their polyphenols, one type of phytonutrient, may bind iron before it can be absorbed. Most major branded herbal teas are considered safe to drink. Still, consume only common varieties sold by major manufacturers.

Some herbal teas interfere with over-the-counter or prescription medications. Talk to your doctor or pharmacist before drinking them if you're on medication.

Because of their potential harmful effects, be careful about using herbs to make "teas"—comfrey, lobelia, woodruff, tonka beans, melilot, sassafras root, and many others may be harmful in large amounts. For example, comfrey may cause liver damage. Woodruff, an anticoagulant, may cause bleeding. Lobelia may cause breathing problems. Even chamomile may cause an allergic reaction.

See "For Herbal and Other Botanical Supplements . . ." in chapter 23.

Functional Beverages

Improve your memory? Lift your mood? Build your immunity? Boost your energy? Aid weight loss? The popularity of functional beverages, promoted with benefits like these, is growing. However, they often displace nutrient-rich beverages, as well as water and soft drinks.

Functional beverages—energy drinks, herbal drinks, enhanced waters, juice, and more—are defined as being enhanced to provide health benefits beyond general nutrition. However, currently there's no regulatory definition. If they qualify, functional drinks may carry health, nutrient content, or structure-function claims. For example, juice, juice blends, and juice drinks that are fortified with calcium, vitamin D, or omega-3s might carry these claims. Depending on their ingredients (herbs, phytonutrients, nutrients, tea, and other), some are regulated as dietary supplements. S*ee chapter 23 to learn more.*

For many herbal drinks, such as acai berry drinks and noni juice (morinda), the scientific evidence for claims is limited and inconclusive. Many overpromise on what they can deliver. Some are high in added sugars. The amount of the herbal ingredient is neither standardized nor generally stated on the label. For safety, optimal amounts, interactions, and long-term consequences aren't known. Talk to your healthcare professional about using them.

Functional drinks do provide hydration. If you already eat smart, exercise regularly, manage stress, and get enough rest, they probably won't offer significant benefits. No functional beverage can counter the effects of dysfunctional eating or living.

Energy Drinks

For grab-and-go energy, energy drinks may give a short-term mental or physical boost. Yet they aren't meant to replace nourishing meal or snacks, even if they do contain some nutrients and food energy (calories).

Caffeine, often at very high levels, is the common ingredient in many energy drinks. *See "Drinks: With or without Caffeine?" in this chapter*. Unlike colas, caffeine levels in energy drinks aren't regulated. In addition, many energy drinks contain other ingredients—taurine (an amino acid), guarana (potent stimulant), ginseng, B vitamins, and carnitine—added for their purported roles in physical or mental performance. Scientific evidence, however, is inadequate to support these claims.

If you want the caffeine from an energy drink, look for the calorie and caffeine content per serving and the serving size on the label or product website. If the container has two to three servings, drinking the whole amount provides two to three times the calories and caffeine, too. Since energy drinks are often high in added sugars, their calories can add up. Choose energy drinks with less caffeine and added sugars, and drink them in moderation.

What about energy drinks for athletes? Their caffeine may give a physical boost at first. But performance may suffer with excessive caffeine intake; *refer to chapter 20 for more about drinks for sports.* Energy drinks with added sugars aren't the best fluid replacers, although some energy drinks specifically for athletic performance don't contain as much sugar. Concentrated sugar can slow the body's absorption of water. In addition, carbonated energy drinks may give a temporary sense of fullness, resulting in less fluid intake than needed.

Another caution is for energy drinks as mixers in alcoholic drinks. The stimulating effect of caffeine may mask the headache, weakness, and dry mouth that comes with consuming too much alcohol; less motor coordination and slower reaction time is still a potential danger! And what about caffeinated alcoholic drinks? The U.S. FDA hasn't approved caffeine in alcoholic beverages. Mixing caffeine and alcohol at home is not advised.

Caution: The American Academy of Pediatrics (AAP) advises against energy drinks for children and teens. The AAP poses concerns about potential health risks of stimulants for young people.

Sport drinks are different than energy drinks. *See chapter 20 for more information.*

Soft Drinks: Okay?

Flavored, carbonated drinks have been around for about two hundred years. The term "soft drink" originally was coined to distinguish these beverages from "hard" liquor. A hundred years ago, consumers asked for "pop," named for the sound made by popping open the bottle cap. Today, "soft drink"—or "soda" in some parts of the United States—refers to a beverage made with carbonated water and usually flavoring ingredients.

What's in soft drinks? Whether they're regular or diet varieties, soft drinks contain water: about 90 percent for regular soft drinks and about 99 percent for diet soft drinks. Carbon dioxide, added just before sealing the bottle or can, gives the fizz. Regular soft drinks are sweetened with sugar (perhaps high-fructose corn syrup); diet drinks, with saccharin, aspartame, and other low-calorie sweeteners; *see chapter 3*. Additional flavor comes from artificial and natural flavors. Acids such as citric acid and phosphoric acid give a tart taste and act as preservatives. Coloring may be added. Some caffeine may be added to enhance the flavor, while other ingredients may add consistency.

As soft drink consumption goes up, nutritional concerns do, too:

● Cut back on soft drinks as a way to reduce added sugars and calories. More than 35 percent of added sugars in the U.S. diet comes from soft drinks! If you are a soda drinker, drinking less regular soda may result in initial weight loss.

● Make soft drinks a sometimes beverage, not a replacement for nutrient-rich drinks such as low-fat and fat-free milk. Except for water and for carbohydrates in the form of sugars, soft drinks don't supply significant amounts of nutrients. A 12-ounce can of regular cola, for example, supplies water and about 150 calories (from almost 10 teaspoons of sugar), but little else. A 20-ounce bottle or cup has 250 calories! A diet soft drink is a source of water and has almost no calories.

● Soft drinks fortified with antioxidants? They don't provide the full array of nutrients and phytonutrients supplied by fruits and vegetables, so their potential benefits may be limited. *See "Vitamins as Antioxidants" in chapter 6.*

As your best guideline, enjoy soft drinks in moderation—if you also consume the nutrients you need from other sources and don't overdo on calories in your overall diet. *Remember:* Regular soft drinks deliver calories, but little else.

Alcoholic Beverages: In Moderation

No one's sure who first invented beer, wine, or spirits, but historians do know that societies have enjoyed these beverages throughout recorded history.

Today, moderate amounts still add pleasure to eating. For some, a single drink may be relaxing—perhaps in the company of another. The key to potential benefits is sensibility: moderation and understanding alcohol equivalency.

● *Moderation:* The 2010 Dietary Guidelines advises that *if alcohol is consumed, it should be consumed in moderation—up to one drink per day for women and two drinks per day for men—and only by adults of legal drinking age!*

The Dietary Guidelines defines heavy or high-risk drinking for women as more than three drinks on any day, or more than seven per week, and for men as more than four drinks on any day, or more than 14 per week. Binge drinking is four or more drinks within for hours for women; five drinks or more for men.

● *Equivalency of one drink:* 12 fluid ounces of regular (5%) beer (about 150 calories), *or* 5 ounces of fluid wine (12%) (about 100 calories), *or* 5 ounces of fluid wine (100 calories), *or* 1.5 fluid ounces of 80-proof distilled spirits (120 calories). Each con-

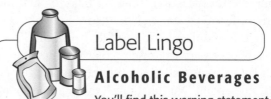

Label Lingo

Alcoholic Beverages

You'll find this warning statement on the label of beverages containing alcohol. On wine and beer labels, you may also find information on sulfite content. See *"For the Sulfite-Sensitive" in chapter 21.* (*Tip:* If you're sulfite-sensitive, distilled spirits and sake, a type of rice wine, don't contain sulfites.)

GOVERNMENT WARNING:

(1) ACCORDING TO THE SURGEON GENERAL, WOMEN SHOULD NOT DRINK ALCOHOLIC BEVERAGES DURING PREGNANCY BECAUSE OF THE RISK OF BIRTH DEFECTS. (2) CONSUMPTION OF ALCOHOLIC BEVERAGES IMPAIRS YOUR ABILITY TO DRIVE A CAR OR OPERATE MACHINERY, AND MAY CAUSE HEALTH PROBLEMS.

CONTAINS SULFITES found in most wines to protect flavor and color.

Currently the presence of major food allergens doesn't need to be disclosed on alcohol beverage labels. There is an interim rule, in effect since 2006, for optional allergen labeling statements.

tains the same amount of alcohol—approximately 14 grams (or 0.6 fluid ounces) of pure ethanol. Distilled spirits include bourbon, brandy, gin, rum, vodka, whisky, and liqueurs. *See the "Alcohol Calorie Calculator" later in this chapter.*

Note: A 750-milliliter bottle of wine contains about five 5-ounce glasses of wine.

Alcoholic Beverages: The Health Effects

For most adults, one alcohol-containing drink or two a day offers little risk for problems related to drinking. What are the risks? Are there benefits?

Unlike nutrients, most alcohol isn't broken down through digestion. Its "pathway" to body cells moves much faster, including directly through the stomach lining and wall of the small intestine. With no food in the stomach to slow it down, absorption into the bloodstream is even faster (within about twenty minutes). From the bloodstream, it goes to every cell of the body, to some degree depressing cell activity.

Although some people drink to be the "life of the party," alcohol actually is a depressant, not a stimulant. Any initial "lift" is short-lived. By dulling various brain centers, alcohol may reduce concentration, coordination, and response time; cause drowsiness and interfere with normal sleep patterns; and result in slurred speech and blurred vision. Because of the short-term diuretic effect, some people may feel thirsty after drinking a lot—perhaps the morning after.

Blood alcohol level depends on the amount of alcohol consumed over a period of time as well as body composition, body size, metabolism, and medications. A healthy liver detoxifies the alcohol at a rate of about $\frac{1}{2}$ ounce per hour. The higher the blood alcohol concentration level, the longer it takes. Two regular-size drinks consumed during a sixty-minute "happy hour" take about two to three hours to break down.

A single alcoholic drink affects women more than men, due in part to differences in body size and metabolism. Alcohol is carried in body fluids, not in

Have You Ever Wondered

. . . if a little "nip" of brandy will help fight a cold? On the contrary, if you have a cold or a chronic health problem that lowers your immunity, you're wise to abstain. Alcohol can impair the body's ability to fight infectious bacteria and may interfere with medication.

. . . if an alcoholic drink will warm you up in cold weather? No. Alcohol tends to increase the body's heat loss, making people more susceptible to cold. If you're ice fishing, cross-country skiing, or watching outside winter sports, an alcoholic drink won't keep you warm and may make you more vulnerable to the effects of cold.

. . . what the term "80 Proof" means on a bottle of liquor? The term "Proof" indicates the amount of alcohol. The proof is twice the alcohol content. If a label on a bottle of liquor states "80 Proof," this means that the liquor contains 40 percent alcohol. The proof will vary depending on the type of liquor.

. . . if a nightcap will help you sleep? It may put you to sleep, but not help you stay asleep—with the deep, rest-

ful sleep you need. A drink with dinner probably won't affect your sleep habits.

. . . how cooking wine compares to regular table wine? Cooking wine is usually high in sodium. From a flavor standpoint, regular wine may be better for cooking.

. . . how organic wine and beer are labeled? USDA organic labeling standards apply to alcoholic beverages, too. *See chapters 9 and 12.*

. . . what kombucha is? In general, it's a fermented beverage made of steeped tea, sugar, and yeast for fermentation. It may have fruit juice or other flavors added during production, too. Its alcoholic content varies, but if kombucha has at least 0.5 percent alcohol by volume, it's regulated as an alcoholic beverage.

. . . how to know the alcohol content of wine, beer, or distilled spirits? Check the label. Since not all beverages are required to list the alcohol content, check the bottler's website. For more help with label reading, check the U.S. Alcohol and Tobacco Tax and Trade Bureau, www.ttb.gov/consumer/labeling_advertising.shtml.

body fat. Women's bodies have a smaller volume of water than men's, so the same amount of alcohol is more concentrated in the bloodstream and potentially has a greater effect. The enzyme that helps metabolize alcohol is also less active in women. As a result, women are at greater risk for problems related to alcoholism.

The Risks. The Dietary Guidelines for Americans notes risks related to alcoholic beverage consumption. The hazards of heavy drinking are well known and include an increased risk for several health problems, including high blood pressure, liver cirrhosis, and several forms of cancer, as well as motor vehicle accidents, other injuries, violence, and death. During pregnancy, drinking increases the chances for birth defects. For women, moderate drinking may slightly increase the risk for breast cancer. Over time, excessive drinking is linked to increased body weight. For those with diabetes, alcohol intake must be managed; excessive amounts increase diabetes risks.

Heavy drinkers may have social and psychological problems: for example, altered judgment and a potential dependency. With both heavy drinking and episodes of binge drinking, mental function is impaired. Excessive drinking can lead to brain and heart damage, cirrhosis of the liver, and an inflamed pancreas. For children and teens, alcohol consumption increases the risks of drowning, car accidents, and traumatic injury and is the number-one cause of death in this age group. *Refer to "Drinking: For Some Not Advised" in this chapter.*

Potential Benefits? Moderate drinking may offer health benefits: lower risk for heart disease and all-cause mortality, mostly for middle-age and older adults. Healthful eating and active living are essential to the equation, too. The benefits appear to come from moderation of any alcoholic beverage: wine, beer, or distilled spirits.

An alcoholic drink before a meal may stimulate the appetite and make a meal more appealing. For older adults and people with some chronic illnesses, a drink before a meal may enhance appetite. Some evidence suggests that moderate drinking, along with a healthful eating pattern and regular physical activity, may help keep mental function intact with aging. Talk to your healthcare provider if you have a health problem

linked to appetite loss. That said, the potential benefits aren't reason enough to start drinking or to drink more frequently.

Watch the Calories, Mind Your Nutrients!

Alcohol is a fermentation product of carbohydrates: both sugars and starches. In beverages or food, alcohol supplies calories: 7 calories for every gram, compared with 4 calories per gram of carbohydrate and protein, and 9 calories per gram of fat. A 1½-ounce jigger or "shot" of vodka, for example, may be on average 40 percent alcohol, or up to 0.6 ounce of alcohol. That equals about 14 grams and contributes about 100 calories. Additional calories in beer, wine, or liqueurs come from carbohydrates; distilled spirits don't have carbohydrates.

Red Wine: Heart-Healthy?

Does red wine protect against heart disease? There's no conclusive answer. Research suggests that a moderate amount of alcoholic beverages—red wine as well as white wine, beer, and distilled spirits—may help lower the risk for heart disease. Possibly a small amount may help increase HDL ("good") blood cholesterol, and it may prevent LDL ("bad") cholesterol from forming. However, factors other than ethanol (alcohol) also may play a role.

Phytonutrients such as resveratrol and tannins in wine may offer heart-healthy benefits. Resveratrol, a flavonoid in the skins and seeds of grapes, has estrogenlike qualities that may help increase HDLs or increase the oxidation, or breakdown, of LDLs. (Grape skins are needed to make red wine.) Also speculated, resveratrol may boost the body's natural clot-dissolving enzyme; when blood platelets clot, they decrease blood flow, which can lead to a heart attack or a stroke. Tannins also may inhibit platelet clotting. However, research hasn't shown if these phytonutrients are bioavailable.

Scientists don't know enough to offer definitive advice, so if you don't drink, protecting your heart isn't a reason to start. If you do, a drink a day of any alcoholic beverage may offer a benefit. *Remember:* Other lifestyle habits—such as healthful eating, regular exercise, not smoking, and keeping a healthy weight—offer the most protection against heart disease! *See "A Toast to Heart Health" in chapter 22.*

The alcohol content of a single drink depends on the type of alcoholic beverage and the serving size. "Special" alcoholic drinks advertised on restaurant table tents usually contain more alcohol because they're bigger. The calorie content also is determined by the amount of alcohol and, for mixed drinks, the other ingredients in the drink. And as the alcohol content goes up, so do the calories. *See the "Alcohol Calorie Calculator" later in this chapter.*

Does drinking lead to weight gain? Not for moderate drinkers. In fact, a few scientific studies suggest that the body uses calories from alcohol differently than calories from other sources. But over time, heavier drinking—beyond two drinks a day—may lead to weight gain.

For some people who drink to excess, a "beer belly" is aptly named. Calories from alcoholic beverages can add up, contributing to excess overall body weight. For example, a six-pack of beer, consumed on a hot summer day, supplies 900 calories. To burn off those calories, a person would need to jog without a break for about two hours. A 5-ounce glass of dry wine before dinner supplies 100 calories, or 700 calories if consumed every day of the week. Within five weeks that can add a pound of body fat. (A pound of body fat equals 3,500 calories.) Mixers make calories add up even more, yet often add few nutrients; for example, the soft drink in a rum-and-cola drink, coconut cream in a pina colada, and sugar in a daiquiri or hot buttered rum.

Although it supplies calories, alcohol isn't a nutrient. On the contrary, because alcohol may interfere with nutrient absorption, heavy drinkers may not benefit from all the vitamins and minerals they consume. Unless juice or milk beverages are mixers, alcoholic beverages themselves supply few if any nutrients.

Moderate drinking isn't associated with poor nutrition. However, alcoholic beverages shouldn't take the place of nutritious foods and beverages—for example, when a glass of wine with dinner takes the place of calcium-rich milk. By moderating your intake of beer, wine, and spirits, there's room in your eating plan for more nutritious foods and drinks. For the casual or moderate drinker, this may not be much of a problem; malnutrition is a significant concern for very heavy drinkers.

Drinking: For Some Not Advised

Some people are wise to avoid alcohol entirely. Besides the risks mentioned earlier, avoid drinking . . .

. . . *if you're a teenager or a child.* Young people should not drink. That includes fortified fruit-flavored wines and hard (alcoholic) ciders. Since the risk of alcohol dependence goes up when drinking starts at an early age, kids who drink can set themselves up for the same health-related risks that adults have. Alcohol and inexperienced teenage driving is a very risky combination. Besides, buying alcoholic beverages is illegal in the United States for anyone under age twenty-one.

. . . *if you can't restrict your drinking to moderate levels.* As part of a lifelong commitment, recovering alcoholics and problem drinkers should abstain from any alcoholic drink. Because of the genetic link to alcoholism, people with alcoholism in their family are wise to moderate their intake of alcoholic beverages, too—or avoid them.

. . . *if your work requires attention, skill, or coordination.* Alcohol affects productivity, which can affect your work output and your personal safety. Even with moderate drinking—a glass of wine or beer—alcohol stays in your blood for about one hour, and two glasses, for two hours or more.

. . . *if you plan to drive or handle potentially dangerous equipment.* Even low levels of blood alcohol from a single drink can make you more accident-prone for an hour or so. If you plan to drink, designate another driver from the start who won't be drinking!

. . . *if you're pregnant, trying to get pregnant, or are unsure.* In the United States, drinking during pregnancy is the leading known cause of birth defects. Fetal alcohol syndrome is characterized by mental retardation, and by behavioral and psychosocial problems. While there's not enough proof that an occasional drink is harmful, even moderate drinking may have behavioral and mental consequences. No safe level has been established for a woman any time during pregnancy, including the first few weeks. Too often, women drink before they even know they're pregnant, potentially compromising their baby for life. *See "Pregnancy and Alcoholic Beverages Don't Mix!" in chapter 18 for more on fetal alcohol syndrome.* Heavy drinking may not be wise for dad, either. According to research, excessive alcohol may decrease sperm count and potency and so affect fertility.

. . . if you're breast-feeding. The level of alcohol in your breast milk will mirror that of your blood alcohol content if you consume alcoholic drinks. And even low to moderate drinking may adversely affect a baby's feeding and behavior—and may reduce the amount of breast milk. Although the data is limited, alcoholic drinks while nursing may be linked to a baby's sleep patterns, psychomotor patterns, or growth. Wait at least four hours after drinking alcohol before breast-feeding. Alcohol should not be consumed until consistent latching on and breast-feeding patterns are established.

. . . if you have certain medical conditions, such as liver disease, pancreatitis, or high triglyceride levels. Talk with your doctor.

. . . if you're on medication, even over-the-counter kinds. Alcohol may interact with certain medicines, making them either less effective or more potent. The medication itself may raise blood alcohol levels or increase its adverse affects on the brain. The result: A single drink may impair judgment, coordination, and skill faster. Check warnings on over-the-counter medications. Talk with your doctor, pharmacist, or healthcare provider about your prescribed and over-the-counter medications. *See "Food and Medicine" in chapter 22.*

. . . if you suffer from allergies. Sulfites in wine may trigger histamine production and allergy symptoms.

Taking Control: Drinking Responsibly!

If you choose to drink alcoholic beverages, always do so responsibly. Here's how you can moderate . . .

● Start with a nonalcoholic beverage. Satisfy your thirst first. Then drink an alcoholic beverage slowly.

● Don't drink on an empty stomach. Eating a little food helps slow the absorption of alcohol.

● Decide ahead to limit drinks, no more than one per day if you're a female or two per day if you're a male. If you choose to drink more, pace yourself. On average, the body can detoxify only one standard-size

drink (0.6 fluid ounces, or 14 grams of alcohol) per hour. The rest circulates until it's finally broken down.

● Slow your pace. Put your drink down. Socialize.

● If you have one alcoholic drink, make the next one nonalcoholic. When you do this, you consume less alcohol and give your body a chance to process the alcohol you've consumed already.

● Measure liquor for mixed drinks with a measured jigger so you know how much to pour from the bottle.

● Make an alcoholic drink last longer; you'll less likely order another. Learn to sip, not gulp; use a straw for mixed drinks. Dilute drinks with water, ice, club soda, or juice to increase the volume. Frozen drinks often take longer to sip.

● If you feel thirsty, drink bottled water or a soft drink instead. *Remember:* Alcohol actually has a diuretic effect.

● Prefer a wine cooler? Mix your own using less wine. For mixers, try sparkling water or fruit juice.

● Lighten up! Order low-alcohol beer, light wine, or a light distilled spirit instead. Each has somewhat less alcohol. Or try nonalcoholic beer or alcohol-free malt beverage.

● At the table, have a glass of water by your plate, too. You'll probably drink less alcohol.

● Skip the last round before the bar closes! As a host, don't feel a need to refresh your guests' drinks.

● Order a "virgin" cocktail: nonalcoholic mixers without the liquor. Mix in juice or carbonated water. Remember the garnish!

● Bring bottled water or soft drinks to a picnic or a sports event so you have a nonalcoholic option.

● Consider the calories in mixers as well as the alcohol.

● Know your triggers. If you tend to drink in certain situations, try to avoid them. For more tips, refer to *Rethinking Your Drinking* from the National Institute of Alcohol Abuse and Alcoholism and the National Institutes of Health.

Beer and Wine: What's in a Name?

Today these products appear on supermarket shelves. But just what do the descriptions mean, and how much alcohol do they contain?

Your Nutrition Checkup

Alcohol Calorie Calculator

Calories from alcohol add up, potentially contributing to unwanted weight gain. If you need to lose weight, your drinking habits may be a good place to start. Use the calculator below to figure how many calories you consume each week from alcoholic beverages. *For more about calories and weight control, refer to chapter 2.*

Although their calorie content differs, these standard-size drinks each supply about the same amount of alcohol—about 14 grams of pure ethanol. (*Note:* Alcoholic drinks are not 100 percent alcohol; that's why the volume differs.)

BEVERAGES	SERVING SIZE (FL. OZ.)	CALORIES (AVERAGE*) ×	AVERAGE NUMBER OF DRINKS PER WEEK =	CALORIES
Beer				
Regular	12	149	_____	_____
Light	12	110	_____	_____
*Distilled spirits***				
80-proof gin, rum, vodka, whiskey, tequila	1.5	98	_____	_____
Brandy, cognac	1.5	98	_____	_____
Liqueurs	1.5	188	_____	_____
Wine				
Red	5	96	_____	_____
Dry white	5	90	_____	_____
Sweet	5	126	_____	_____
Sherry	2	75	_____	_____
Port	2	90	_____	_____
Champagne	4	84	_____	_____
Vermouth, sweet	3	140	_____	_____
Vermouth, dry	3	105	_____	_____
Wine cooler	12	180	_____	_____
Cocktails				
Martini (traditional)	2.25	124	_____	_____
Martini (extra dry)	2.25	139	_____	_____
Cosmopolitan	2.75	146	_____	_____
Mojito	6	143	_____	_____
Margarita	4	168	_____	_____
Piña Colada	9	460	_____	_____
Manhattan	3.5	164	_____	_____
Daquiri	4	122	_____	_____
Whiskey sour	3	122	_____	_____
			Calories per week	_____

* Varies widely

** An added mixer, such as soft drink, adds more calories.

Remember that a pound of body fat adds up to about 3,500 calories!

Source: Adapted *from Rethinking Your Drinking,* National Institute on Alcohol Abuse and Alcoholism, U.S. National Institutes of Health, U.S. Department of Health and Human Services, 2009.

Near beer: Malt beverage that has an alcohol content below 0.5 percent by volume. It also can be labeled a "malt beverage," a "cereal beverage," or when the label says "contains less than 0.5 percent alcohol by volume" as "nonalcoholic."

Low-alcohol or reduced-alcohol beer: Malt beverage with less than 2.5 percent alcohol by volume.

Alcohol-free malt beverage: Malt beverage that contains no alcohol.

Flavored malt beverage: Malt beverage (beer, lager, ale, porter, stout) flavored after fermentation, perhaps with juice, fruit, or juice concentrate— for example berry-, lemon-, or orange-flavored beer.

Aperitif wine: Wine with an alcohol content of 15 to 24 percent by volume, made from grape wine and added brandy, or alcohol flavored with herbs or other natural aromatic flavorings.

Fortified wine: Wine that has brandy or distilled spirits added to it. Dessert wine has 14 to 24 percent alcohol by volume, more than table wine.

Table wine: Wine that has 7 to 14 percent alcohol by volume. Light wine, red wine, and sweet table wine are all types of table wine.

Low-alcohol wine: Wine, or fermented fruit beverage, that is less than 7 percent alcohol by volume. Low-alcohol wine isn't necessarily lower in calories; it may have more sugars than other wine.

Wine cooler: Diluted wine product (diluted with fruit juice, water, and/or added sugars) with an alcohol content of less than 7 percent by volume. Read the Nutrition Facts for calorie content. Wine coolers may have more alcohol and calories than you think since a serving is usually bigger: often 12 ounces, rather than a 5-fluid-ounce glass of table wine.

Sources: Bureau of Alcohol, Tobacco, and Firearms (2001); U.S. Food and Drug Administration (personal communication, 2001).

As an aside, an average, regular beer contains 5.0 to 5.5 percent alcohol by volume. In the United States and Europe, pale beer (usually a lager), rather than dark beer, may be called light beer. The alcohol content is about the same as in regular beer, but the calories are somewhat less. An alcoholic beverage with more than 24 percent alcohol by volume is defined (and taxed) as a distilled spirit.

Need more strategies to boost your fluid intake? Check here for "how-tos":

- Buy the type of milk, including soy beverage, that matches your needs—see chapter 12.
- Drink sensibly when you eat out—see chapter 15.
- Get enough fluids when you're physically active—see chapter 20.
- Know how to fit milk in if you're lactose intolerant—see chapter 21.

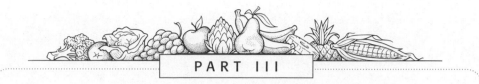

Food Choices
The Consumer Marketplace

What's on Today's Table?

With so many foods available for today's table, why do consumers choose one food over another? Consumer research says taste is the top reason, followed in varying order by nutrition, food safety, price, and convenience. How about you?

In the past decade or two there's been a change at the kitchen table. Perhaps you've noticed a shift to more health- or flavor-focused food products, more green and locally grown products, or changes in your own shopping and cooking patterns, lifestyles, and attitudes about food, health, and cooking. You may be eating smarter to promote health, or be more adventuresome with food and want more flavor. Or despite ever better kitchens and cooking equipment, convenience and speed may be top priorities.

The diversity of foods in today's marketplace reflects the diversity of today's consumers. Rather than selling just to the mass market, food producers know the value of providing different options for different people. As a result, a great variety of foods are produced and marketed to match the age, gender, health, lifestyle, ethnic or religious background, personal preferences and beliefs, and economic resources of different consumers.

Food: What's in Store for You?

Frozen skillet meals, bagged salad mixes, marinated ready-to-cook beef roast for convenience, almond milk, ostrich tenderloin, blue potatoes, doughnut-shaped peaches for something different, eggplant caponata, guava juice, pad Thai for ethnic variety, multigrain cereal with flaxseed, or juice with added antioxidants for health benefits—you'll find all these foods sold alongside traditional favorites in supermarkets today.

Every year U.S. consumers have more variety of foods to choose from and more ways to eat for health. A single supermarket stocks, on average, about fifty thousand different items, including nonfood items. In a typical year, about ten thousand new food products may launch. Yet only about 2 percent survive.

Away from home, you may notice that restaurants, even some fast-food menus, offer more variety these days, including more whole-grain, fruit, vegetable, seafood, and vegetarian items, and more grilled, broiled, steamed, and stir-fried choices. Many supermarkets sell fully prepared dishes and full meals to "heat and eat." Some sell "gourmet" takeout. Traditional restaurant menus and recipes for at-home cooking reflect interest in healthful eating, ethnic cuisine, flavor, local ingredients, and a blend (or fusion) of ingredients and cooking styles.

More choices mean more decisions—and more to learn about your food supply.

Healthy Foods

Packaging often promotes foods' health benefits with claims such as "lowers cholesterol," "promotes immunity," or "builds strong bones." Nutrition Facts on labels display the nutrition content per serving. Signs in many produce departments remind you to eat colorful fruits and vegetables. You can hardly walk through a supermarket without seeing a healthy eating message!

Better-for-You Foods: The Haves and the Have-Nots

Many traditional foods have been modified for health-conscious consumers. Breakfast cereals, bakery goods, pastas, prepared soups, cheese, salad dressings, milk, juice, and some other drinks, chips and snack foods are among them. Some provide more of the nutrients often short-changed. To alert you to those foods, you'll see nutrient content claims such as "more fiber," "more calcium," or "vitamin D added." Others deliver less of nutrients many people need to limit, such as less sodium, less added sugars, less saturated fat—or perhaps they're labeled as "trans-fat free."

To modify these foods, the ingredients or the processing methods are changed. For example, chips can keep their salty taste—with less sodium—when salt dusts the surface instead of being blended in.

That said, by lowering the nutrient content, a food's qualities may change. For example, to cut back on fat, the carbohydrate content from starch or added sugars may go up. Conversely, to lower carbs, fat may be bumped up. Modifications may change the flavor and the mouth feel of foods you're accustomed to. Formulating foods with less salt and sodium may make them less flavorful unless other flavor-intense ingredients, such as herbs or spices, are added.

Have You Ever Wondered

. . . what the term "superfood" means? No regulations define a superfood. And no individual food is a "magic bullet" for health—although high amounts of certain nutrients or phytonutrients in some foods may offer health benefits. Over time a "superdiet" will likely bring more health benefits. *Cautions:* Some foods marketed as superfoods are high in added sugars, solid fats, or sodium; nutrients or phytonutrients in others may have limited bioavailability, or available to the body.

Enjoy nutrient-modified foods in an overall way of eating that's varied, moderate, and balanced. But remember, "fat-free" doesn't mean calorie-free. And juice with "calcium and vitamin D added" doesn't make it a substitute for milk, although it may be a calcium-rich option for vegans or those with lactose intolerance. Check the Nutrition Facts on food labels. *See "Get All the Facts!" in chapter 12 to learn more.*

Functional Foods: Benefits beyond Basics

The term "functional foods" describes foods and beverages with health benefits beyond (and in addition to) basic nutrition. These foods or beverages may enhance your health, protect you from certain diseases, promote optimal health, or do all three.

Currently no legal definition for a functional food exists. Technically, all foods, in one way or another, are functional and provide health benefits. That includes traditional foods such as fruits, vegetables, yogurt, and whole grains, as well as foods fortified, enriched, or enhanced with nutrients, phytonutrients, or other health-promoting substances.

Why the interest? Attention to personal health is rising. Many people—perhaps you—want more control over their health. Especially as healthcare costs go up, an aging population seeks approaches for health promotion. Rapid advances in science provide a growing body of credible evidence for functional nutrition, and agricultural and food science technology can produce foods that offer more health benefits. In addition, changes in food regulation that began in the mid-1990s allow labels to provide health-related statements and claims; *see chapter 12.*

What foods may have functional benefits? Consider these examples:

- Many fruits, vegetables, and grain products naturally contain phytonutrients, or plant substances, such as carotenoids, flavonoids, isoflavones, or indoles, that may reduce the risk for certain diseases, including prostate cancer, heart disease, and macular degeneration. Phytonutrients that give health benefits also are the food components that deliver flavor and color.

- Strong scientific evidence supports the belief that oats help lower cholesterol levels.

Functional Nutrition: What's in a Name?

With the advent of functional foods, new terms have entered our vocabulary. Although not legally defined, here's what they generally mean and how they differ.

- *Functional foods:* foods that provide health benefits beyond basic nutrition
- *Phytonutrients:* substances in plant-based foods with physiologically active components that have functional food benefits; also called phytochemicals
- *Prebiotics:* nondigestible food substances that may stimulate the growth and activity of health-promoting, or "good," bacteria in the intestines
- *Probiotics:* live bacteria that may promote health by improving the balance of "good" bacteria in the intestines
- *Synbiotics:* products with both prebiotic and probiotic substances that work together to keep the balance of "good" bacteria in the intestines
- *Zoonutrients:* a term sometimes used for substances, such as omega-3 fatty acids, with physiologically active components, in animal-based foods; also called zoochemicals.

For more about phytonutrients, prebiotics, and probiotics, and substances in animal-based foods that promote health, see chapter 6.

- Prebiotics/probiotics such as fructo-oligosaccharides in shallots and *lactobacillus* in some dairy foods may improve the balance of good intestinal bacteria.
- Oily fish such as salmon have omega-3 fatty acids, which may help lower the risk for heart disease and improve mental performance.
- Dairy foods and some meat such as beef and lamb have another fatty acid, conjugated linoleic acid (CLA), which may help lower cancer risk.
- Calcium-rich dairy foods may help protect against high blood pressure and cardiovascular disease.
- Acai berries and pomegranates, which contain anthocyanins and flavonoids, may have some antioxidant benefits; *see chapter 6 to learn about antioxidants.*

Functional benefits probably come from several, perhaps many, food components. The heart-healthy benefits of oats not only come from its soluble fiber (beta glucan) but also from its antioxidants, amino acids, and natural plant sterols. Cancer protection from beans (legumes) may come from fiber as well as isoflavones, saponins, and protease inhibitors.

For more examples refer to chapters 3, 4, 5, and 6.

Different types. Tried and true, or innovative and new, functional foods belong in several categories:

- *Unmodified conventional whole foods* such as oats; carrots; tomatoes; grapes; blueberries; nuts; beans; salmon; and yogurt with live, active cultures, to name a few.

- *Modified foods,* including foods enriched or fortified with nutrients, such as calcium-fortified orange juice (for bone health) and folate-fortified breads (for proper fetal development), and foods enhanced with nutrients, phytonutrients, herbs, and other health focused-substances such as vegetable juice with added lutein, yogurt with DHA omega-3s, pasta with added fiber, and tea with ginkgo biloba. Through biotechnology, foods also are modified to provide more functional benefits, such as tomatoes with more lycopene and rice high in beta carotene. *Learn about food biotechnology in this chapter.*

- *Foods created for functional and other health benefits* such as shakes and snack bars with soy protein, omega-3s, and flaxseeds, spreads with plant

Click Here! Websites to Know . . .

- Know Your Farmer, Know Your Food, www.usda.gov/knowyourfarmer
- International Food Information Council Foundation, www.foodinsight.org/farmtofork.apsx www.foodinsight.org/understandingour food.aspx
- National Organic Program, www.ams.usda.giv/nop/indexIE.htm

See "Resources You Can Use" for more websites.

stanol or sterol esters that help lower blood cholesterol, and energy bars.

Functional foods are also: (1) medical foods for specific health problems such as a phenylalanine-free formula for an infant with PKU, as advised by a doctor and (2) foods for special dietary uses such infant foods, weight-loss foods, and gluten-free and lactose-free foods.

Fitting functional foods in. Credible research shows that along with overall healthful eating and regular physical activity, functional foods may help promote wellness, but they can't make up for poor eating habits or an unhealthy lifestyle. Although their bioactive components and their physiological action are full of unknowns, enjoy them for their potential benefits:

● Eat a variety of foods with potentially healthful benefits regularly, over time. Enjoy them as part of your health strategy, not in place of appropriate medical care or medications prescribed by your healthcare provider.

● Enjoy food first, rather than supplements. Food has many more functional components that likely work best together, as nature provided.

● Choose wisely. Foods fortified for functional benefits aren't always the best choice, especially if they aren't nutrient-rich, and instead have a lot of calories from added sugars or solid fats.

● Read food label claims to find foods that match your needs. *For what claims mean, see chapter 12.*

● Be savvy when you read about foods promoted with functional benefits. Junk science abounds! Nutrition research that's either misinterpreted or oversimplified often makes headlines. *To help you sort through the claims, see chapter 24.*

New Flavors

Global communications, travel, and food imports make the world of food highly connected. Just a few decades ago, bagels, pita bread, pastas of every shape, and tortillas were trendy; salsa and hummus were new flavor experiences, as were Cajun and California rolls (sushi). Today ethnic and regional foods such as these are supermarket mainstream.

Moroccan or Lebanese, Nuevo Latino or Thai, Indian or Ethiopian; many people want to go beyond ethnic basics such as Italian, Chinese, and Mexican. Regional ethnic foods—Tuscan, Liguria Roman, Calabrian, and Lazio (Italian); Sichuan, Peking, and Cantonese (Chinese); and Yucatán, Oaxacan, and Michoacan (Mexican)—have captured consumer interest, too, at least among foodies.

What sparks interest in and availability of ethnic and regional foods? Perhaps a sense of curiosity and adventure, and a desire to try nutritious, flavorful alternatives. Celebrity chefs entertain by preparing ethnic

Our Edible Heritage

"Ethnic food" isn't new. Throughout history, the foods of one culture have traveled to another, infusing cuisines with more variety and new flavors. Those foods also became new sources of nutrients and food energy.

The quest for flavor—exotic Eastern spices—launched the Age of Discovery and the exploration of the so-called New World. Among the discoveries: a vast array of foods! Among other foods, the Americas contributed tomatoes to Italy, potatoes to Ireland, peanuts (or groundnuts) to West Africa, and hot chiles to Thailand. And foods unknown to the Americas five hundred years ago came from all parts of the so-called Old World—for example, chickens, pigs, beef, wheat, oats, barley, okra, Asian rice, peaches, pears, watermelons, citrus fruits, bananas, and lettuce.

American cuisine has strong roots in its native foods: corn, legumes, pumpkins, peanuts, potatoes, tomatoes, peppers, pineapples, squash, wild rice, and turkey, among many others. Each immigrant wave has contributed its own ethnic cuisine. In time, many ethnic foods became "typically American"—for example, pizza, tacos, and chop suey. "Food immigration" continues as more recent waves of immigrants—mostly Latin Americans, Asians, East Europeans, and Middle Easterners—influence American cuisine today.

Regional specialties develop as people adapt their cooking style to available foods. And many foods once eaten as regional specialties have become nationally popular—for example, sweet potato pie, cooked collard greens, and black-eyed peas and rice from the South, created by African American cooks; crab cakes and clam chowder from the Atlantic coast; tamales, bean burritos, and cactus salad from the Southwest; and smoked salmon and berry cobblers from the Pacific Northwest.

foods and by taking us to global markets and kitchens. Travel, cooking classes, websites, blogs, print media, cookbooks, and restaurants expose us to unique ingredients, seasonings, and dishes. Supermarkets are stocked with ethnic and regionally inspired foods, partly to meet the demand from diverse populations and partly to match flavor trends. That offers you more food variety and more ways to fit whole grains, vegetables, beans and peas, fruit, seafood, and other nutrient-rich foods into your meals and snacks.

See "Vegetarian Dishes in the Global Kitchen" in chapter 15 and "Ethnic Table: For Variety, Health, and Eating Pleasure" in this chapter.

A Fusion of Flavor

The blending of cuisines, sometimes called fusion cuisine, is a culinary phenomenon. It combines the ingredients or cooking techniques of two or more cultures not geographically close together. The result is new cuisines such as Thai-French, Southwest-Asian, Cuban-French, and unique dishes such as Moroccan couscous topped with Chinese stir-fried vegetables. Even fast-food menus reflect fusion such as Mexican pizza, chili in a pita pocket, or a Thai wrap in a tortilla.

The fusion of ingredients and flavors isn't new. It has happened for centuries as people gradually adapted their cuisines to the available food supply, sometimes by choice and often by necessity. Consider how early American settlers substituted native ingredients such as cornmeal and squash in traditional English dishes. Interestingly, about 50 percent of foods eaten in the world today originated in the Americas.

Today, fusion cooking brings an explosion of new dishes to the table. In many cases, new fused dishes uniquely combine grain products, fruits, and vegetables.

Simply adding seasonings from an ethnic or a regional cuisine also creates fusion; perhaps a touch of curry powder from India in pumpkin soup, or basil and garlic, borrowed from Italian cooking, in beef stew. *See "Flavor Profile!" in chapter 14 for seasoning combinations.*

What's New Is What's Old, Too

What's new on the table is also what's old. Grandma's meat loaf, mashed potatoes, soup, and biscuits are dressed with today's seasonings such as sun-dried tomatoes, garlic, wasabi, lemongrass, and fresh herbs.

More often sold in farmers' markets, heirloom vegetables and fruits—with unique flavors, colors, shapes, and scents—provide variety. Heirlooms are open-pollinated (grown from seed) cultivars grown for at least fifty years. While generally not grown commercially, the unique genetics of heirloom varietals make them naturally resistant to certain pests and diseases—and a great gene bank for agriculture. You might find flavorful, pinkish-red Brandywine tomatoes (Amish); purple-striped Cherokee Trail of Tears pole beans (Native American); and sweet, lime-green Jenny Lind melons. If you're a gardener, try growing less-common and heirloom varietals!

Heritage grains, often fiber-rich with unique baking or cooking qualities, are finding their way back into breads and grain-based dishes, too. Consider emmer, millet, and amaranth. Heritage breeds of livestock and poultry are being conserved to help retain biodiversity in animal agriculture.

What Else Is New?

Supermarkets, superstores, wholesale grocery stores, farmers' markets, and restaurants feature foods that weren't easily available until recently:

● *More local and regional.* Committed to local food? Then call yourself a locavore! Local food is generally grown or produced close to where it's purchased, perhaps in the same state or closer; "local" isn't a defined and regulated term. Supporting local and regional agriculture, farm fresh food, and food producers offers a chance to learn about and enjoy foods produced in your region—and to connect with local farmers and food producers. *Refer to chapter 12 for more about farmers' markets and CSAs.*

● *More green.* Today's marketplace produces and distributes many environmentally friendly food products, plates and utensils, and kitchen equipment. Increasingly, social responsibility is part of the business bottom line. With the complexity of the issues, the term "green" is undefined and unregulated. Remember that because something is marketed with phrases about being better for the Earth doesn't necessarily mean that it is better for you.

Beware of "green washing" or "green sheen." These terms refer to misleading marketing practices that may suggest products are more environmentally friendly than they really are. To buy green, learn about the food, such as how and where it's grown and produced. *For starters, see "How Green Are You?" below.*

● *More organic foods. See "Organically Produced" later in this chapter.*

● *More convenience.* More prepackaged foods—fresh salad mixes, stew and stir-fry mixes, precooked meat and poultry, meal kits, speed-scratch meals, and takeout—may help you serve a nutritious home-served meal in record time.

● *More fruit and vegetable variety.* Produce departments—even the grocery and frozen-food aisles—stock a greater variety of fruits and vegetables year-round, including exotics and varietals. For exam-

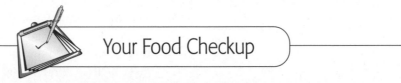

Your Food Checkup

How Green Are You?

Caring for the environment is everyone's responsibility! Check off ways you protect resources that bring food to your table. Then commit to taking more "green steps" yourself.

Yes No

- ☐ ☐ **1.** Buy, and eat, just what you need; reduce overconsumption.
- ☐ ☐ **2.** Minimize food waste.
- ☐ ☐ **3.** Compost vegetable and fruit scraps.
- ☐ ☐ **4.** Buy foods with recyclable packaging and less packaging overall.
- ☐ ☐ **5.** Recycle food packages. Most packaging today is recyclable.
- ☐ ☐ **6.** Carry water in a reusable water bottle, rather than always buy bottled water.
- ☐ ☐ **7.** Grow or raise fruit or vegetables in your backyard or container garden—perhaps share some with a friend or food bank.
- ☐ ☐ **8.** Take time to know your farmers at farmers' markets, farm stands, food co-ops, local farms, or pick-your-own farms. Learn about food they produce. Take children with you so they learn, too. Participate in a CSA (community supported agriculture) program; *see chapter 12 to learn more.*
- ☐ ☐ **9.** Volunteer at an urban or community garden, greenhouse, school garden, or food pantry.

Yes No

- ☐ ☐ **10.** Use Earth-friendly cleaning and gardening products. (Most household cleaning products are water-soluble, formulated for safe disposal, and don't contain ingredients in amounts harmful to the environment.)
- ☐ ☐ **11.** Walk or bike once a week, perhaps to a store or a farmers' market.
- ☐ ☐ **12.** Learn about land use issues, local drinking water, energy use, and local issues of air pollution.
- ☐ ☐ **13.** Conserve resources—water, energy, and more—at home, at work, and in your community.
- ☐ ☐ **14.** Support public policies that both conserve natural resources and protect the environment.
- ☐ ☐ **15.** Add your own green strategy to this list.

_____

For more ways to be a green consumer, see chapters 8, 12, and 14.

Be aware that some greener choices may come at a higher cost. The good news: Many conventional food products are being produced with less packaging and more environmentally friendly practices. You may be greener than you realize!

ple, a potato isn't just a potato anymore; it may be a Yukon Gold, a purple, or a fingerling. A peach may be a Babcock, a doughnut, or a Honey Baby. For specialty produce, look for different colors and miniatures, such as red carrots, okra, and corn; purple asparagus, artichokes, Brussels sprouts, kohlrabi, wax beans, and yams; white eggplant and sweet potato; yellow beets; golden kiwifruit; and miniature avocados, eggplant, squash, corn, bananas, bell peppers, and kiwifruit.

● *More grain variety, including whole grains.* Interest in breads has shifted to more coarse-textured, denser, whole-grain breads. Breakfast cereals are made with more whole grains—and not just corn, oats, or wheat. Salads, soups, and mixed dishes also feature whole grains of all kinds.

● *More "fresh."* Besides fresh fruits and vegetables, fresh options for seafood, pasta, salads, bakery, and more are available. Remember that "fresh" is mostly an unregulated marketing term. *See "Fresh vs. Processed: Both Ways to Good Nutrition" later in this chapter.*

● *More function and personal customization. "See Functional Foods: Benefits beyond Basics" earlier in this chapter.*

● *More plant-based (vegetarian) options.* You'll find more meatless, prepared entrées such as bean burritos and vegetarian lasagna, along with a greater variety of pasta, vegetables, and soy protein products for home-cooked vegetarian meals.

● *More specialty foods.* With growing food sophistication, more gourmet and unique foods are sold in mainstream stores. Being "gourmet" doesn't make food more nutritious. Read the label's Nutrition Facts.

● *More flavor.* The influence of—and interest in—ethnic cuisine, herbs, and other flavor ingredients have put more flavors in canned, pouched, frozen, and other prepared foods, recipes, and restaurant foods. Consider the many hot sauces!

● *More foods for special health needs.* For example, the gluten-free section is expanding in many grocery stores.

Garden of Eatin': Less Common Vegetables

Looking for new ways to enjoy a colorful variety of fruits and vegetables? Starting here, identify all the vegetables you've never tried. Then buy and try one or two of them the next time you shop or eat out.

● *Arugula (ah-ROO-gu-lah)* is a green, leafy vegetable with a distinctive flavor. Use it raw in mixed garden salads; cook and toss it with pasta or risotto.

● *Bok choy (BAHK choy) (or pak choi)* is a Chinese cabbage. It doesn't form a head but instead has several white, bunched stems with thick, green leaves. Eat it raw or cooked, and in stir-fry dishes.

● *Breadfruit* looks like a green, bumpy melon (brown when ripe) on the outside, and is creamy white on the inside. Like other starchy vegetables, it's peeled, then baked, boiled, fried, grilled, or cooked with stew and soup. Its flavor is somewhat sweet, yet mild. Some Caribbean dishes are made with breadfruit.

● *Broccoli raab* (also called rapini), with 6- to 9-inch stalks and small broccolilike buds, is strong and bitter. Use it raw in salads, cooked as a side dish, or in mixed dishes.

● *Cactus pads (nopales, or noh-PAH-lays)*, which are cactus leaves, are used in Mexican and Southwest dishes. Their thorns are removed before cooking them. Then they're usually sliced, then simmered or cooked in a microwave oven. Or buy canned nopales.

● *Cassava* (kah-SAH-vah) (manioc, or MA-nee-ahk; yuca, or YOO-kah, root), a starchy root vegetable, has a thick, brown peel; inside it's white or yellow like a potato. Cook it in dishes similar to the way you cook potatoes.

● *Celeriac (seh-LER-ee-ak)*, a member of the celery family, is enjoyed for its root, not its stalks. It has a fibrous, brown, bumpy peel and a sweet, celery flavor inside. Once peeled, enjoy it raw, perhaps in salads, or cooked—boiled, steamed, or fried. Use it in soups or stews, perhaps in place of celery.

● *Chard*, a white-rooted beet, is grown for its leaves and its creamy-white or red stalks. With its mild yet distinctive flavor, use it like spinach.

● *Chayote (cheye-OH-tay)* is a pale-green, pear-shaped vegetable with a mild flavor. Baked, boiled, braised, or stuffed, it complements the flavors of other ingredients in mixed dishes. Use it like squash.

Ethnic Table: For Variety, Health, and Eating Pleasure!

Enjoy the multicultural array of nutrient-rich foods on your table: perhaps Mediterranean tabouli (bulgur salad) or cucumber-yogurt dip; Brazilian black bean soup; Indian vegetable curries; Spanish paella (rice dish with meat, seafood, vegetables, and perhaps beans); Thai pad thai (a stir-fried dish with rice noodles, bean sprouts, eggs, peanuts, and shrimp, chicken, or tofu); or Ethiopian injera (bread) with meat and vegetable dishes. To be adventuresome:

- Try unfamiliar foods at an ethnic or regional restaurant, or local ethnic festival. *For restaurant tips see "Eating Out Ethnic Style" in chapter 15.*

- Be adventuresome with food when you travel, rather than head for familiar fast-food fare.

- For ethnic recipes, buy an ethnic cookbook or magazine, go online, or check food TV.

- Learn "hands on" from an ethnic cooking class, culinary trip or local tour, or friend who prepared his or her family's ethnic dishes.

- Shop the ethnic food section of your supermarket, or shop in an ethnic food store. Ask other customers or store staff for food preparation advice. Look for these foods:

	CUISINE*	SERVING/PREPARATION IDEAS
Grain Group		
Whole-wheat couscous (tiny, round pasta)	Moroccan	Serve hot with tomato sauce and Parmesan cheese, or serve cold as a salad with raisins, mandarin oranges, and spices.
Kasha (buckwheat kernels)	East European	Serve as a hot side dish with chicken or beef. Mix with pasta shapes.
Pozole (soup made with fermented corn kernels)	Mexican	Serve warm with diced onions, shredded cabbage, and a lime wedge.
Wonton wrappers (thin wheat dough used to wrap spring rolls)	Chinese, Vietnamese	Wrap thin strips of cooked lean barbecued pork or chicken, with shredded cabbage and carrots inside, then steam.
Vegetable Group		
Jicama	Mexican	Slice in thin strips, and dip into salsa or reduced-fat or fat-free ranch dressing. Use to replace water chestnuts in stir-fry dishes.
Collard greens	African American/ Southern	Boil greens with chopped, smoked turkey; vinegar; and seasonings.
Tomatillos	Mexican	Dice, and boil with jalapeño peppers for salsa. Dice, and combine with onions for an omelette
Shiitake mushrooms	Japanese	Add raw to salads and sandwiches, or toss in stir-fry dishes.
Fruit Group		
Lychee	Chinese	Serve on top of frozen yogurt.
Kumquat	Mexican, Central	Pack a few for snacking, or slice for fruit salad.

	CUISINE*	SERVING/PREPARATION IDEAS
Fruit Group (continued)		
Papaya	American	Blend with pineapple for tropical juices, dice and add to salsas, or simmer in a chutney recipe.
Plantain	Puerto Rican, Central American	Cube, and add to stews and soups.
Mango	Caribbean	Slice for fruit salads, or simmer in a chutney recipe.
Protein Foods Group		
Squid	Mediterranean, Asian	Slice in rings, and broil. Serve with marinara sauce. Or cook in stir-fry dishes.
Veal, lamb	Mediterranean	Marinate in Italian vinaigrette, then grill.
Hummus (mashed chickpeas)	Middle Eastern	Serve as a dip for raw vegetables or pita triangles.
Chorizo (sausage)	Mexican	Slice in bite-size pieces; add to omelettes or stews.
Tempeh	Japanese, Chinese	Slice for stir-fry dishes, or dice for salads or soups.
Black beans	Latin American	Use in place of red beans in chili or soup, mash for homemade refried beans, or mix with rice.
Dairy Group		
Plain yogurt	Middle Eastern	Top falafel sandwiches (chickpea- and vegetable-stuffed pita). Blend with mint as a dip or dressing for cucumbers.
Goat milk	Middle Eastern, African (some areas)	Drink goat milk plain. Make a thick drink by mixing with juice. Use it in place of cow's milk in baking.
Ricotta cheese	Italian	Use in lasagna, or stuffed jumbo pasta shells.
Queso blanco (white cheese)**	Mexican	Shred, and melt over enchiladas and quesadillas.

*These foods may be used in the dishes of many global cuisines.
**To reduce the risk of foodborne illness, look for queso blanco made from pasteurized milk.
Refer to chapter 15 for common food-group foods in Italian, Mexican, and Chinese cuisines.
Source: Adapted from the Academy of Nutrition and Dietetics.

● *Chicory (curly endive)* has a frizzy green leaf in a loose head of greens. Its bitter flavor adds a nice touch to salads in small amounts.

● *Daikon (DEYE-kuhn)* is a Japanese radish that looks like a smooth, white parsnip. It has a stronger, more bitter flavor than a red radish. Often it's used to make sushi (fish rolled with rice in seaweed) and in vegetable carvings.

● *Dasheen (dah-SHEEN)* is a large, round root vegetable with a coarse, brown peel, similar to taro. Usu-ally prepared boiled or baked, dasheen is starchy, somewhat like a potato.

● *Escarole (EHS-kah-role)* is a somewhat bitter salad green. Sometimes its green leaves have a reddish tinge. Unlike iceberg lettuce, it forms a loose head.

● *Fennel* looks like a squat bunch of celery with feathery leaves. Its flavor is like sweet, delicate anise. The bulb and stalks are often braised, steamed, sautéed, or used in soups. Use the feathery leaves in salads, as a herb, or as a garnish.

● *Jerusalem artichoke*—native to North America— has nothing in common with a globe artichoke. Like a potato, it's a tuber, which grows underground. But it's knobby and irregularly shaped, with a sweet flavor and a light-brown or purplish-red peel. It's often cooked in its peel; a little lemon juice in the cooking water keeps peeled Jerusalem artichokes from browning. Use it in dishes that call for potatoes, or eat it raw.

● *Jicama* (HEE-kah-mah), a root vegetable, is crisp and slightly sweet. Peel, slice, and eat it raw, perhaps in salads. Or cook it in stews and stir-fries.

● *Kale*, a leafy vegetable in the cabbage family, doesn't form a head. It has a curly, purple-tinged, green leaf. Use it in salads or prepare it like cooked spinach.

● *Kelp* is brown seaweed, often used in Japanese cooking and wrapped around sushi.

● *Kohlrabi* (KOLE-rah-bee), a member of the cabbage family, looks and tastes somewhat like a turnip. It's light green in color. Use it in recipes that call for turnips; slice and use it in stir-fry dishes; or peel and eat it raw or in salads.

● *Leeks* are onions. They look like a bigger, sturdier, flat-leaved version of green onions. Clean them well to remove soil that gets between the leaves. Slice the bulbs; steam them in soups or bake them in casseroles. Use the leaves in salads.

● *Lotus root*, the water lily root, has the texture of a potato and a flavor similar to fresh coconut. Peel, slice, then stir-fry, steam, or braise in mixed Chinese dishes.

● *Mushrooms* of all kinds include enoki, chanterelle, morel, oyster, porcini, portabello, shiitake, straw mushrooms, and wood ears. Each has a unique flavor and qualities. Some are sold dried.

● *Plantain* belongs to the banana family, but it's longer and thicker, starchier, and less sweet. Eat it at any stage—green, yellow, or black; it's sweetest when it's black. Eat it as a vegetable, cooked in or out of the peel. Bake, fry, or boil plantains, perhaps in a stew.

● *Radicchio (rah-DEE-chee-oh)* is a small, purplish head of leaves with white ribs. It's somewhat bitter. Use it in salad, pasta, and stir-fries.

● *Rutabaga (ROO-tuh-bay-guh)* is a root vegetable with a turniplike flavor and appearance. Use it in place of turnips in stews, soups, and casseroles.

● *Salsify* is a white root vegetable that tastes like delicate oysters. Eat it as a cooked side dish or perhaps in soups.

● *Seaphire* is a halophyte, or saltwater crop. With an asparagus-grass look, seaphire is crisp, crunchy, and salty. Since it's high in sodium, enjoy small amounts as a flavoring in salads, stir-fries, and vegetable dishes. Three ounces have 1,350 milligrams of sodium.

● *Seaweed*, used most often in Asian dishes and some Irish, Welsh, and Scottish dishes, has many varietals. Kelp may be the most common in the United States. Many Japanese dishes use nori (NOH-ree).

● *Taro (TAIR-oh)* is a rough, brown or purplish tuber that looks much like a yam, although some varieties look different. Peel taro and boil, bake, or fry it, much like potatoes. Hawaiian poi is made from taro. Its edible leaves, called callaloo in the Caribbean, are cooked as a soup.

● *Tomatillo (tohm-ah-TEE-oh)*, a member of the tomato family, has a paperlike husk. Under the husk it looks like a small green tomato. Often prepared like a green tomato, its flavor is citruslike. Use it in Southwest and Mexican dishes, including salsa and salads.

● *Winter squash*—acorn, bitter melon, buttermilk, crockneck, delicata, golden nugget, hubbard, kabocha, mini pumpkin, spaghetti (as a pasta alternative), sunburst, and turban—is used in cooked dishes.

Fresh Ideas: Uncommon Fruit

Rather than reach for fruit you know already, try something new! Many tropical and subtropical fruits aren't well known in the United States. Look for less common fruits in the produce department or as canned foods, or in Asian and Hispanic food stores.

Try different varietals of common fruits, too, such as red bananas, amnazano bananas, apple bananas, and plantains. Different varietals of apples, oranges, plums, and pears also offer unique flavors, textures, and perhaps cooking qualities.

● *African horned melon*, also known as kiwano, is spiked (yellow "horns"), oblong in shape, golden-orange in color, and with juicy green fruit inside that tastes like cucumber, banana, and lime. Mild in flavor, it's like a juicy, seed-filled cucumber. Scoop the pulp; enjoy it in salads, drinks, and sauces.

● *Asian pear* looks like a yellow apple and has a similar firm, crunchy texture. It's sweet, juicy, and eaten whole or cut for mixed salads.

● *Atemoya (a-teh-MOH-ee-yah)* is a cross between two fruits: cherimoya and sweetsop. With a green skin, it has a petal-like look. Inside, the cream-colored, custardlike pulp is studded with large black seeds and offers a mango-vanilla flavor.

● *Blood orange* is a tart yet sweet orange with flesh that's either bright red or white with red streaks.

● *Cherimoya (chair-ih-MOY-ah) (custard apple)* has a custardlike consistency and flavor. On the outside it looks like a little green pineapple without leaves. The inside has little black seeds. It tastes like a mix of strawberry, banana, pineapple, and mango. It's best eaten as whole fruit; cut it in half, remove the seeds, and scoop out the fruit.

● *Cape gooseberries* are juicy and bittersweet beneath their Chinese lantern skin. Serve them with meat, other savory dishes, and desserts.

● *Dates,* sold fresh and dried, are very sweet, with a shiny, thin skin. Enjoy them as a snack or in mixed-green dishes, sweet-savory sauces, and salad.

● *Dragon fruit*, in the cactus family, is yellow to shocking pink. Shaped like a hand grenade, it has spines on the outside; the fruit inside is juicy and grainy, with edible seeds that taste like kiwifruit or grapes. To enjoy, remove the peel or scoop out the flesh.

● *Feijoa (fay-YOH-ah, or fay-JOH-ah)* looks like a kiwifruit without fuzz. Inside, its cream-colored flesh is sweet, fragrant, and pearl-like. To eat it, remove the skin, which may be bitter, cut it in half, and scoop out the fruit. Use it as a recipe substitute for apples or bananas.

● *Guava (GWAH-vah) (guayaba, or gwey-AH-bah)* is a sweet, fragrant fruit that's about the size of a lemon. Its peel varies from yellow to purple; the fruit inside may be yellow, pink, or red. Eat guavas as whole fruit, or in sauces, salads, juices, frozen desserts, and jams.

● *Kumquat (KUHM-kwaht)*, a citrus fruit and looks like a small, olive-shaped orange. Kumquats are eaten with their thin peel on—either uncooked or cooked with meat, poultry, or fish. Slice them for a garnish or salads.

● *Longan (LONG-uhn)* is a small, round, cherry-sized fruit with a thick, nonedible brown shell. Inside, the white, juicy fruit surrounding the large black seed is sweet and fragrant.

● *Loquat (LOH-kwaht)*, a small, pear-shaped fruit, is light orange on the inside and the outside. Somewhat tart, it has a pit, which must be removed. Eat loquats whole, and perhaps in salads or in cooked poultry dishes.

● *Lychee (LEE-chee) (litchi)* is just 1 or 2 inches in diameter and has a pink to red shell. Inside, the fruit is white and sweet with a consistency like a grape. Its seed isn't edible. Eat lychees as a snack or a dessert just as they are.

● *Mango*, a sweet-tart and juicy fruit, ranges in size and shape. It can be about 6 ounces to 5 pounds, and round or long. Its inedible peel is orange when ripe, with orange fruit inside and a large seed. To easily eat a mango, either peel back the skin and eat it with a spoon, or remove both peel and seed and cut it into pieces. Use mangoes in fruit salads, smoothies, and desserts, and prepare them with cooked meat, poultry, rice, or grain dishes.

● *Mangosteen (MAN-goh-steen)*, small in size, has an inedible leathery brown skin. Inside, the soft, white, juicy fruit divides into segments. Buy it canned; it's rarely available fresh.

● *Papaya (pah-PEYE-ah) (pawpaw)* may weigh from 1 to 20 pounds in an elongated, oval shape. Its inedible peel is yellow or orange, with an orange fruit inside and many black seeds. Its tart, sweet flavor is delicious as is or mixed in salads.

● *Passion fruit (granadilla, or gra-nah-DEE-yah)* is a small, spherical fruit with a leathery peel, which may appear shriveled. It has a perfumelike, sweet-tart flavor. The color varies from light yellow to reddish-purple. Eat it as a whole fruit or add it to salads, sauces, desserts, or beverages.

● *Pepino (puh-PEE-noh)*, ranging in size from a plum to a papaya, is a fragrant melon with a smooth, golden skin that's streaked with purple. Inside, the yellow flesh is juicy sweet. Enjoy a peeled pepino whole, or cut it for salads or garnishes.

● *Persimmon (puhr-SIHM-uhn)* looks somewhat like an orange-red tomato with a pointy end. If it's ripe, it's sweet. If not, a persimmon is mouth-puckering, bitter, and sour. Eat it whole, or use it in desserts and baked foods.

● *Plumcot* is a cross between a plum and an apricot. It has an intensely sweet, fruity flavor.

● *Pomegranate (PAH-meh-gran-uht)* is unlike any other fruit. It has a red, leatherlike peel. Inside, membranes hold clusters of small, edible seeds with juicy red fruit around the seeds. The flavor is both tart and sweet. Use pomegranate seeds in salads and in many cooked dishes.

● *Pomelo (pom-EH-loh)*, a huge citrus fruit, can be as big as a watermelon! But it's more commonly the size of a cantaloupe. In many ways it looks and tastes like a grapefruit, but the sections are not as juicy.

● *Prickly pear (cactus pear)*, which is yellow-green to deep yellow, is the fruit of the cactus plant. It has a sweet, mild flavor. Peel and seed it before eating. It may have small hairs or needles in the peel that can be uncomfortable if they get into your skin. Eat the fruit whole or in salads, sauces, and other dishes.

● *Rambutan*, with its dark, bristlelike rind, is a small fruit. Peel away the rind; the translucent, grapelike flesh that surrounds the seed tastes like a lychee.

● *Sapodilla (sah-poh-DEE-yah)* is a small, egg-shaped fruit with a rough, brown peel. Only the creamy pulp inside is edible—when ripe. The flavor is mild, much like vanilla custard.

● *Starfruit (carambola, or kar-am-BOH-lah)*, with its unique shape, forms stars when the fruit is sliced. The flavor varies from sweet to tart. Eat it sliced, in salads, or as a garnish.

● *Tamarillo (tam-uh-RIH-yoh)*, with its tough but thin peel, is about the size and shape of a small egg. Being tart, it's often sweetened with sugar. Use it in baked or cooked foods.

● *Ugli (UH-glee)* fruit is a cross between a tangerine and a grapefruit. It's sectioned on the inside but looks like a small grapefruit on the outside.

● *Zapote (zah-POH-tay) (white sapote)* is a sweet, yellowish fruit about the size of an orange.

Today's Grains

Looking for creative ways to eat more grains? Most of today's new grains are really as old as the hills. Although less familiar in the United States, some are staples that nourish millions of people around the globe.

Grains, both whole and enriched refined grains, deliver health benefits; *see chapter 10 to learn more.* Seeds such as amaranth and wild rice are high in protein and often are used as grain substitutes.

● *Amaranth (AM-ah-ranth)*, a seed rather than a true grain, is a protein-rich food. Use the seeds as a cereal grain.

● *Arborio (ar-BOH-ree-oh)* rice, a plump medium- or long-grain rice, absorbs a lot of liquid. The result is a creamy-textured rice. Use it to make Italian risotto, a rice-based dish. It's usually cooked in broth.

● *Barley* is an ancient, hardy grain. Pearl barley with the bran removed is the polished and most common form; it's generally enriched with vitamins and minerals lost in processing. It makes a hearty addition to

Have You Ever Wondered

. . . if couscous is a grain? No, it's a form of pasta. Traditionally, couscous (made from ground millet) has been the pasta of northern Africa. In the United States it's made from ground semolina wheat and often used in salads, mixed with fruit, and in other grain dishes. Made from wheat, it's a good source of B vitamins. Look for whole-wheat couscous.

. . . what Quorn is? It's a mycoprotein, or a plant-based protein derived from the mushroom family. Sold in Europe for nearly two decades and now in the United States, this meat alternative is marketed as burgers, sausages, cold cuts, and other meat substitutes. Quorn supplies protein and fiber, with less fat and saturated fat than meat.

stews, soups, salads, and casseroles. Whole-grain barley, which is hulled, is sold, too. Barley typically is served in soups. Look for barley grits, flakes, and flour, which is hull-less, but still uses the whole-grain kernel.

● *Basmati (bahz-MAH-tee)* rice, a long-grained aromatic rice, has a distinctive nutlike, fruity flavor. Basmati rice may be polished or brown (whole-grain) rice. It's often used in Asian and Middle Eastern recipes and in salads because it's light and fluffy.

● *Brown rice* is whole-grain rice with only the inedible outer husk removed. Unlike refined white rice, brown rice contains the bran, germ, and endosperm of the grain. *For more about the nutrients in whole grains, see chapters 3 and 10.* Any variety of rice— long-, medium-, or short-grain—can be brown rice.

● *Buckwheat*, a whole grain, often is prepared like rice. The crushed, hulled kernels, called buckwheat groats, most commonly are used in dishes of Russian origin, such as kasha.

● *Bulgur*, whole-wheat kernels that have been parboiled, dried, and crushed, has a variety of textures— from coarse to fine. It provides a soft but chewy texture in many grain-based dishes such as pilaf and tabouli. Add it to bread dough, too. Bulgur isn't quite the same as cracked wheat.

● *Farro (emmer wheat)* dates back twenty thousand years! Used in bread, pasta, and risotto-type dishes, it's dense and chewy, rich, and nutty.

● *Glutinous rice*, either black or white, is very sticky because it's high in starch, making it easier to pick up with chopsticks. The grain is either short- or medium-grain. This type of rice is typically served in Japanese and Chinese restaurants.

● *Hominy (HAH-mih-nee)* is the dried corn kernel with the hull removed. It's usually soaked in liquid to soften, then cooked in stews, casseroles, or other mixed dishes. *Note:* Although corn is eaten as a vegetable, it's really a whole grain.

● *Jasmine (JAZ-mihn)* rice, another aromatic rice, is used in many Asian dishes. It's equally nice as a subtle "sweet" side dish, perhaps with pork or fruit-glazed poultry. A polished rice, it's often sold in specialty stores.

Need more strategies to enjoy the food varieties from today's marketplace? For how-tos:

● Use label claims to get clued in to foods' nutrient benefits—see chapter 12.

● Know how to fit all kinds of foods—including less common fruits, veggies, and grain products—into your eat-smart plan—see chapters 10 and 11.

● Add more food variety, perhaps functional ingredients, in your food prep—see chapter 14.

● Be more adventurous with food when you eat out—see chapter 15.

● *Kamut (kah-MOOT)*, a high-protein wheat, has a nutty flavor. Its contribution of other nutrients is higher than traditional wheat, too.

● *Millet*, a small, round, yellow grain, is a staple whole grain in Europe, Asia, and northern Africa. It's less common in the United States. Mild in flavor, millet cooks fast. Use it in mixed dishes such as pilaf or casseroles; as cooked cereal; and, when ground into flour, for bread such as roti from India.

● *Quinoa (KEEN-wah)*, a whole grain native to South America, cooks much like rice but faster. Nutritionally it stands out because it's higher in protein than other grains, and it's a good source of iron and magnesium. The grain is small, ivory in color, bead-shaped, and bland in flavor. Use quinoa in soups, salads, and casseroles, and in any dishes that call for rice.

● *Sorghum (or milo)*, a gluten-free whole grain, can be eaten as a cooked cereal or used as a flour for baked foods.

● *Spelt*, another ancient grain, is nutty and mellow in flavor. Among its benefits: it's easily digested and higher in protein than other grains. Substitute spelt flour for wheat flour in baking.

● *Texmati rice* (sometimes called popcorn rice), from Texas, is a cross between American long-grain rice and basmati rice. Less fragrant than basmati rice, it's an all-purpose aromatic rice.

• *Triticale (trih-tih-KAY-lee)* is a modern whole grain developed as a hybrid of both rye and wheat. The result: a nutty-flavored grain with more protein and less gluten than wheat alone. Cooked as a whole berry (not as flour), it's used in hearty grain-based salads, casseroles, and other grain dishes. Look for flaked and cracked varieties added to bread dough.

• *Waxy rice*, or sweet rice or sticky rice (opaque white or deep, dark purple in color) is moist and very sticky when cooked. The purple variety has a subtle fruity flavor.

• *Wehani rice*, a basmati rice, is sold with the bran intact. When cooked, it looks like wild rice.

• *Wheat berries* are whole grains that haven't been processed. They're often cooked and used in grain-based dishes. Cracked wheat isn't bulgur but instead is wheat berries that have been crushed. Also look for rye berries in specialty stores.

• *Wild rice* isn't a grain, but the seed of a water grass. With its nutlike flavor, it's often used in place of grains, or perhaps mixed with them. As a seed it's higher in protein and a good fiber source.

To learn how to prepare these grains, see "Cooking Grain by Grain" in chapter 14. For a list of whole grains, see chapter 3.

Ensuring the Food Supply

The United States' food supply is safe, affordable, and plentiful. Today's technology, methods of agriculture, and food processing, as well as transportation systems make safe, abundant food possible. In fact, the average U.S. farmer feeds you and about 154 others in the United States and around the world. Just 75 years ago, one U.S. farmer fed only about 20 people. Because this food system is efficient, Americans can engage in pursuits and careers other than farming if they choose.

Efficiency translates to economic benefits. In 2010 about 12.7 percent (7.5 percent for food at home and 5.2 percent for food away from home) of U.S. household spending was for food, according to the Bureau of Labor Statistics, compared with 25 percent in the 1930s. That's much less than in many other parts of the world—developed and less developed—

even in tough economic times. Looking forward, as the world's population increases, agricultural efficiency and increased production techniques will become increasingly important, as will urban farming and home gardening.

Processing: Making Food Available

Throughout much of recorded history, people have processed foods to make them edible and to preserve them for times of scarcity. In Europe and elsewhere 8,000 years ago, foods were smoked and dried. Cheesemaking developed 4,500 years ago in the Middle East to preserve milk. About 2,500 years ago, Egyptians and Europeans mastered skills for preserving foods with salt.

Modern processing methods began in the 1800s with canning, giving perishable food a longer shelf life. People could finally eat a variety of fruits and vegetables year-round. During the nineteenth century, pasteurization—a process of heating milk or other liquids to kill disease-causing bacteria—was developed. Today some foods are pasteurized, or perhaps ultrapasteurized at higher temperatures, to keep food safe and flavorful and to extend shelf life. Early-twentieth-century technology launched frozen foods. Later, lightweight, freeze-dried foods were developed for the space program; today backpackers and cyclists use them. Processing makes foods such as olive oil available that may not be grown, harvested, or produced where you live. In reality, most foods are processed in some way.

Processed foods include more than you think. It isn't a catchall term to mean foods with less nutrition, and it doesn't mean you need to avoid these foods. Instead, to quote the 2010 Dietary Guidelines Advisory Committee Report, processed foods, in part, are "any food other than a raw agricultural commodity." The amount of processing can be simply canning or freezing vegetables or fruit to preserve nutrients and extend freshness, or can be formulating a food product, perhaps for a health benefit or other quality.

Food processing, notes the 2010 report, includes washing, cleaning, milling, cutting, chopping, heating, pasteurizing, blanching, cooking, canning, freezing, drying, dehydrating, mixing, packaging, or other procedures that alter the food from its natural state.

Have You Ever Wondered

... why boxed fluid milk is sold on the grocery shelf, not the dairy case? Aseptic packaging, a relatively new food processing and packaging method in the United States, allows fluid milk to be stored at room temperature for up to a year without preservatives. Sterilization is the key to preventing spoilage. Food is first heated quickly (three to fifteen seconds) to ultrahigh temperatures to kill bacteria. Then it's packaged in a sterilized container, such as a box, within a sterile surrounding. Flash heating minimizes loss of nutrients, texture, color, and flavor—and extends shelf life. Besides milk, look for many other grocery items sold in aseptic packaging—for example, soup, tofu, liquid eggs, tomatoes, soy beverages, juice and juice drinks, syrup, nondairy creamers, and wine. In the future, you'll find even more!

... what sous vide is, and how it's used? Mostly for food processing and by restaurants, *sous vide* ("soo-veed") is a way to cook food at low temperatures in a vacuum pack and so extend the storage time. As a processing method, it may help food retain its sensory qualities longer—but it needs to be carefully controlled, since bacteria multiply at these lower temperatures.

Many of these processes are like what you do in your own kitchen. Processing also may include the addition of other ingredients, such as preservatives, flavors, nutrients, and other food additives or substances accepted for use in food products, such as salt, sugars, and fats. Processing, including the addition of ingredients, may reduce, increase, or leave unaffected the nutritional qualities of the unprocessed food.

Minimally processed foods keep most of their original physical, chemical, sensory, and nutritional qualities. They aren't fundamentally altered. Most are as nourishing as their unprocessed counterparts.

Some more highly processed foods are best enjoyed only occasionally since they're high in solid fats, added sugars, and sodium, and the processing method may minimize the nutritional value.

Many others have unique nutrition benefits, such as milk and juice fortified with calcium and vitamin D, and breakfast cereal with more fiber. Although you may give it little thought, food processing has made food safer, more convenient, better tasting, more consistent, of greater value—and often more nutrient-rich.

Many of today's newest contributions to food processing often have health-related goals—for example, adding substances for nutrient benefits or functional qualities; using new technologies to cut back on fat, added sugars, or sodium; and irradiating some foods for improved food safety.

Processing: A Continuum

Foods processing is really a continuum, from minimal to more complex:

- Minimally processed foods don't require much processing or production, perhaps just washing and simple "preprep" for convenience. These include washed and packed fruits and vegetables, bagged salads, and roasted and ground nuts.

- Foods are processed at their peak to keep and enhance the nutritional quality and freshness, such as with canned tuna, beans and tomatoes, frozen fruit and vegetables, and jarred baby foods.

- Ingredients are added to some foods for safety, flavor, and perhaps visual appeal. That includes sweeteners, spices, oils, flavors, colors, and preservatives in packaged foods such as instant potato mixes, jarred tomato sauces, spice mixes, salad dressings, sauces, and cake mixes.

- Ready-to-eat foods are processed so consumers have little or no food preparation. Some examples include breakfast cereal, crackers, yogurt, granola bars, rotisserie chicken, luncheon meats, ice cream, and carbonated drinks.

- And some processed foods are packaged for freshness and time saving, such as pizza, frozen meals, and prepared deli foods.

Fresh vs. Processed: Both Ways to Good Nutrition

The flavor of fresh produce in season is hard to beat: freshly picked, handled properly, and eaten right away. For convenience, their canned and frozen counterparts offer another option. Research shows that canned and frozen ingredients are comparable in nutrition to their cooked fresh counterparts.

The moment you pick fruit or vegetables, or catch

fish, or milk a cow, food starts to degrade in texture, taste, perhaps color, and nutrient content. That's why food producers usually process food as fast as possible, while nutrient content and overall quality are at their peak. Immediate processing, such as freezing, canning, and drying, helps lock these qualities into food. In canneries on board some fishing vessels, seafood is processed as it's brought in. Tomatoes may be canned just yards away from the fields. The same is true for commercially frozen foods.

If processed foods are handled properly—from the manufacturer, to store, to home—there's little nutrient loss.

A processing method called fortification (originally used to iodize salt to avoid goiter) increases the nutritional value of food by adding nutrients to food, such as vitamins or minerals, not present naturally. Milk and often yogurt and juice, for example, are fortified with vitamin D, which helps the body absorb calcium for bone-building. Many grain products are fortified with folic acid to reduce risk of birth defects. Some margarine and cooking oils are fortified with omega-3 fatty acids for heart health.

Food processing contributes to nutrition in other ways. By producing foods with fewer calories, or less sodium or less solid fat, no *trans* fats, or perhaps no allergens, lactose, or gluten, people on restricted diets have palatable and nourishing food options.

Whether food is fresh or processed, it's up to you to minimize nutrient loss from store to table. The nutritional quality of fresh fruit and vegetables depends on their care after harvest. Handled or cooked improperly or stored too long, they may not be quite as nutritious as their canned or frozen counterparts. *See "Food Prep: The Nutrition-Flavor Connection" in chapter 14.*

Protecting Food Safety and Quality

From farm to fork, food safety is top priority! Canning, freezing, and drying are traditional food processing methods that preserve food and destroy bacteria that cause foodborne illness and so keep food safe. Practices such as pasteurization and water treatment, along with certain additives, help ensure food safety. Today other food processing methods, such as food irradiation and antimicrobial washes and sprays, remove substances that may be harmful.

Although not risk-free, the U.S. food supply is among the safest in the world. Government regulations for food production and handling set out safeguards and minimize potential health risks. For example, a system called HACCP, or Hazard Analysis and Critical Control Points, used in food processing and food service, helps ensure food safety. It's used throughout food production, packaging, and distribution to better detect, reduce, eliminate, and track any foodborne pathogens. For some products, such as meat and juice, HACCP is mandatory; for others, its use is voluntary. Restaurants and other food service institutions use HACCP.

Canning. As a way to preserve food safely, canning has been around for 200 years. The processing method is simply cooking food in a can or a jar as it's sealed. The canning process (high temperatures and sterile containers) destroys organisms that would cause spoilage—with no need for preservatives. Any salt is there for flavor, not preserving. Lacking oxygen during storage, food quality and nutrient content remain relatively stable as long as the container and its seal or lid remain intact. Food inside the unopened can or jar has a long shelf life. Washing, peeling, and other steps before canning remove nearly all pesticide residues.

Foods sold in cans have another safety advantage: tamper-resistance. Any opening is clearly evident. Rust spots on the outer surface or dents don't affect the contents of the can as long as it doesn't bulge or leak.

While some nutrients are lost from the heating process, canned foods are as nutritious as their cooked fresh and frozen counterparts—and sometimes more so if fresh and frozen foods aren't handled properly. Heat from canning also makes lycopene in tomatoes and lutein in corn more bioavailable (available to the body). Similarly, the amount of beta carotene (vitamin A) in canned pumpkin is three times higher than in cooked fresh pumpkin. Heat in the canning process also increases the bioavailability of folate, thiamin, niacin, and vitamin B_6. Note that salt or added sugars may be used to enhance flavor in canned foods, not as a preservative. Look for those with no salt added or packed in natural juices.

Beyond that, canned products of all kinds are convenient, portable, and quick to prepare. They only need heating; they're already cooked in canning.

Freezing. Another food processing method, freezing keeps food safe by storing perishable food well below the temperature at which harmful microorganisms thrive. Freezing temperatures also help retain the quality and nutrition of foods over several weeks or months: longer than fresh, but not as long as canned and dried foods.

As consumed, frozen foods are comparable in nutrition to cooked fresh and canned foods—if properly stored, no longer than advised. *See chapter 13 for freezer storage times.* Frozen foods also offer convenience for busy consumers. Check the Nutrition Facts and the ingredient list to find those with less sodium, added sugars, and solid fats.

Drying. Drying is among the oldest methods of preserving food. By removing moisture from fruit, vegetables, beans, and nuts—even fish, meat, and poultry—bacteria no longer have one key condition to grow: water! In dry, covered conditions, even at room or cool temperatures, dried foods can remain safe. To keep dried protein-rich foods such as meat or fish safe, a preservative generally is used.

Irradiation. Irradiation, another newer method, extends the freshness of food, helping to retain quality and safety longer. Since it uses no heat, yet destroys disease-causing bacteria and other organisms, irradiation is sometimes called cold pasteurization. Poultry and beef can be irradiated to ensure that pathogens that are especially harmful to children, the elderly, and people with weak immune systems are destroyed. That includes *Escherichia coli* (*E. coli*) O157:H7, *Salmonella*, and *Campylobacter*. Irradiation also slows ripening and retards sprouting, for example, in potatoes.

Irradiation destroys bacteria, mold, fungi, and insects by passing food through a field of radiant energy, much like sunlight passes through a window or like microwaves pass through food. It leaves no residue. A small number of new compounds are formed when food is irradiated, just as new compounds are formed when food is exposed to heat. These changes are the same as those caused by roasting, steaming, pasteurization, and other cooking.

Irradiated foods generally retain their nutrient value. Like freezing, canning, drying, and pasteurization, irradiation results in minimal nutrient loss, often too insignificant to measure. Irradiation can't replace good food handling practices—nor improve the quality of food. As a consumer, you still need to store, prepare, and cook food in clean, safe ways to avoid foodborne illness.

Besides food safety, irradiation offers potential advantages. Agricultural losses caused by insects, parasites, or spoilage can be cut dramatically. Foods that stay fresh longer can mean less food waste in your kitchen. Like other processing methods, irradiation is regulated and approved by the U.S. Food and Drug Administration (FDA).

By law, whole foods that have been irradiated must be labeled on the package. Look for the international Radura symbol *(to the right)* and the phrase "Treated by Irradiation" or "Treated with Radiation." Irradiated ingredients in prepared, deli, or restaurant foods usually aren't labeled.

To control foodborne illness, irradiation—studied for safety by the FDA for forty years—was approved in 1997 by the FDA for fresh and frozen meats, including beef, pork, lamb, poultry, and seafood. The process protects these foods from contamination—for example, by *E. coli* O157:H7 and *Salmonella*—but doesn't compromise the nutritional quality of meat. For more about foodborne illness, *see chapter 13*. Irradiation also is used for some vegetables and fruit, wheat flour, beans, cereals, and spices. Research continues to evaluate irradiation as part of the overall system of ensuring food safety.

Additives: Safe at the Plate

Does it occur to you that most peanut butters don't separate? That prepared baking mixes rise in the oven? That ice cream is smooth and creamy? Or that milk is fortified with vitamin D for your bone health? Probably not. Most likely you take many desirable qualities of food for granted. And you may not attribute qualities you expect to food additives. Food additives are any substances added to food for purposes such as these.

What do they do? Additives help foods retain original qualities that might otherwise change through temperature changes, storage, oxidation, and contact with microbes. Benefits include nutritional value, freshness and safety, convenience, affordability, color, and flavor appeal.

Adding substances to food for preservation, flavor, or appearance is a centuries-old practice. Before refrigeration, salt preserved meat, fish, and poultry; vegetables were pickled in vinegar; and sugar was added to cut fruit to prevent spoilage. Ancient Egyptians used food colorings; Romans used sulfites to help preserve wine. The spice trade through Asia, the Middle East, and Europe flourished because people demanded flavors that spices added to food.

All additives are listed by name in the ingredient lists on food labels. Ingredient names may seem long and unfamiliar, but all foods—including fresh strawberries, sweet potatoes, and other fruits and vegetables—are made of chemical compounds, with chemical names, that provide their characteristic qualities.

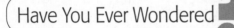

Have You Ever Wondered

. . . how natural and artificial additives differ? So-called natural ingredients come from natural sources such as soybeans or corn to make lecithin for product consistency, or beets to make food coloring. Others are man-made and can be produced with greater purity, consistent quality, and perhaps more economically. For example, vitamin C made in a lab or from fruit is the same. Whatever their source, additives must follow the same safety standards.

. . . if food additives are okay for everyone? Except for a very few people who may react, food additives are safe. In fact, a primary use of additives is protecting food quality and safety. For someone with an additive sensitivity, the reaction should be similar whether the additive is natural or synthetic, since the chemical makeup is similar. In those rare cases, people who react to an additive usually have asthma or a food allergy; they should see a board-certified allergist instead of self-diagnosing. *See "Sensitive to Additives? Maybe, Maybe Not" in chapter 21.*

. . . if people with gluten intolerance should avoid certain additives? Yes; they need to read food labels carefully to avoid additives with gluten. *For more about eating gluten-free, see chapter 21.*

Additives are subject to government review and safety regulations. Today more than three thousand substances are FDA-approved food additives, each with specific functions. Many are common household ingredients: sugar, salt, baking soda, vanilla, yeast, colors, and spices.

For Better Nutrition

Vitamins, minerals, or fiber are added to almost every category of processed foods to maintain or improve their nutrition and health-promoting qualities. Before the past eighty years or so, nutritional-deficiency diseases such as goiter, rickets, scurvy, and pellagra were relatively common. Adding nutrients to food has almost eliminated most nutrient deficiencies. Today nutrients are added to promote health, reduce risks of chronic disease, and contribute to a food's nutrient density—for optimal nutrition, too.

● *Enrichment* is replacing, or adding back, nutrients lost in processing. For example, refined grain products are enriched with B vitamins and iron.

● *Fortification* is adding nutrients that aren't present before processing: for example, vitamins A and D in milk and some soy beverages, folic acid in most refined grain products, calcium in some fruit juices, and fiber in breakfast cereal, some pasta, and other foods. Fortification adds nutrients often lacking in a typical eating pattern; for example, fortifying salt with iodine in the United States eliminated goiter. Today fortification also enhances food's functional qualities.

What nutrients and food substances are added? Check the food label. Any added nutrient shows up in two places: (1) the ingredient list and (2) the Nutrition Facts panel, telling the total amount or contribution (percent Daily Value) of that nutrient in a single serving. *See "Get All the Facts!" in chapter 12.*

For Freshness and Safety

Air, bacteria, fungi, mold, and yeast promote food spoilage. Some additives, called preservatives, slow spoilage and help maintain food's appeal and wholesome qualities. Some preservatives work as antioxidants, protecting food from chemical changes caused by contact with oxygen. Others are antimicrobials that inhibit the growth of mold, bacteria, and yeast. Some foods contain both. Antioxidants prevent rancidity or discoloration.

● *Tocopherols (vitamin E), BHA, and BHT* help delay or prevent vegetable oils and salad dressings from rancidity. Working as antioxidants, they help protect naturally present nutrients in foods: essential fatty acids (linoleic and alpha-linolenic acids) and fat-soluble vitamins (A, D, E, and K). Studies verify the safety of BHA and BHT; the FDA has deemed them GRAS ("generally recognized as safe") substances.

● *Citric acid*, a natural component of citrus fruits, works as an antioxidant, helping food keep its color. Coating sliced apples with lemon juice does the same thing, keeping them from turning brown. Ascorbic acid (vitamin C) does this, too.

● *Sulfites* help prevent color and flavor changes in dried fruits and vegetables. They're used to inhibit bacterial growth in wine and other fermented products. Some baked foods, snack foods, and condiments also may contain sulfites. Most people have no adverse reactions to sulfites. But packaged and processed foods containing sulfites are labeled for the small percentage who are sulfite-sensitive. *See "For the Sulfite-Sensitive . . ." in chapter 21.*

● *Calcium propionate*, produced naturally in Swiss cheese, is a preservative that keeps bread and other baked foods from getting moldy too quickly.

● *Sodium nitrite*, used as a preservative in processed meats such as ham, hot dogs, and lunch meat, keeps meat safe from the very harmful botulism bacteria. It also adds to the flavor and pink color. *For more on botulism and other food safety issues see "Bacteria: Hard Hitters" in chapter 13.*

For Food Preparation or Processing

From helping bread rise to keeping chocolate suspended in chocolate milk to keeping seasoning blends from clumping, food additives provide many of the food qualities or appeal that consumers want and expect.

● *Anticaking agents* prevent lumping and keep seasonings, baking powder, confectioners' sugar, table salt, and other powdered or granular products flowing freely. Because they keep food from absorbing moisture, it won't lump together. Calcium silicate and silicon dioxide are two anticaking agents.

● *Emulsifiers* distribute particles evenly. As mixers they keep ingredients and flavorings blended by holding fat on one end and water on the other end of their chemical structure. For example, they keep oil,

---

No Surprises

Additives in food are no secret to consumers. By reading ingredient lists on food labels, you can identify specific additives in any food. Note the "contains" statement for food allergen labeling.

Emulsifier
to keep ingredients blended

Flavoring
to add sweetness

INGREDIENTS: CRUST: WHEAT FLOUR WITH MALTED BARLEY FLOUR, WATER, PARTIALLY HYDROGENATED VEGETABLE OIL (SOYBEAN AND/OR COTTONSEED OIL) WITH SOY LECITHIN, ARTIFICIAL FLAVOR AND ARTIFICIAL COLOR (BETA CAROTENE), SOYBEAN OIL, YEAST, HIGH FRUCTOSE CORN SYRUP, SALT, CALCIUM PROPIONATE ADDED TO RETARD SPOILAGE OF CRUST, L-CYSTEINE MONOHYDROCHLORIDE; SAUCE: TOMATO PUREE (WATER, TOMATO PASTE), WATER GREEN PEPPERS, SALT, LACTOSE AND FLAVORING, SPICES, FOOD STARCH - MODIFIED, SUGAR, CORN OIL, XANTHAN GUM, GARLIC POWDER, TOPPING: LOW MOISTURE PART SKIM MOZZARELLA CHEESE (PASTEURIZED MILK, CHEESE CULTURES, SALT, ENZYMES). CONTAINS WHEAT, MILK, SOY.

Preservative
to retard spoilage

Thickener
to give a uniform texture

vinegar, and seasonings in salad dressings from separating. In peanut butter, emulsifiers keep peanuts and oil from separating. Even in baked foods, they help keep dough uniform. Some emulsifiers come from food itself: for example, lecithin (from soybeans, milk, and egg yolks), alginates (salts from algae), and mono- and diglycerides (from vegetables and beef tallow). Baked foods, bread, breakfast cereals, chocolate, chocolate milk, cocoa, frozen desserts, margarine, mayonnaise, and pie and pudding mixes also may contain emulsifiers.

● *Humectants* such as glycerine or sorbitol help foods stay moist and soft. Some examples: shredded coconut and marshmallows.

● *Leavening agents* help food rise. They create the light texture of waffles, bread, muffins, and other baked goods. Baking soda (sodium bicarbonate) and baking powder (sodium bicarbonate and acid salts) as well as yeast produce carbon dioxide that makes dough rise. Without them, the texture would be compact and heavy.

● *Maturing and bleaching agents* improve baking qualities of foods made with wheat flour and improve the appearance of certain cheeses. When the yellow pigment of wheat flour is bleached, dough becomes more elastic and results in better baking results. White curd in some cheeses, such as gorgonzola and blue cheese, comes from adding a bleaching agent to milk.

● *pH control agents* are used to adjust the acidity or alkalinity in food; this influences a food's texture, taste, and safety. Adding acids (acidulants) such as lactic acid or citric acid gives a tart taste to frozen desserts and beverages; they also inhibit bacterial growth in low-acid processed foods such as canned beets and help prevent discoloration and rancidity. Alkalizers neutralize acids in foods such as chocolate so the flavor is milder. Baked goods, chocolate, gelatin desserts, processed cheese, salad dressings, sauces, soft drinks, and vegetable oils may contain pH control agents.

● *Thickeners and stabilizers* give food a smooth, thick, uniform texture. In ice cream they keep the texture smooth without forming ice crystals. In chocolate milk they allow chocolate particles to stay in suspension. With stabilizers, oils that add flavor also stay in food. Proteins and carbohydrates—such as gelatin

from animal bones, carrageenan from seaweed, and pectin from fruit—commonly are used as thickeners and stabilizers. Baked goods, beverages, cream cheese, frozen desserts, jam, pie filling, pudding, salad dressings, sauces, and soups are among foods that often have these additives.

For Flavor and Appeal

Some additives add color, provide flavor or enhance it, or sweeten food.

● *Colorings* won't affect the nutrients, safety, or taste of food, but they make a nutritional contribution by making nourishing food look more appealing. Cheese and margarine often get their yellow coloring from annatto, which comes from the tropical annatto tree. Ice cream and many baked foods, yogurt, gelatin

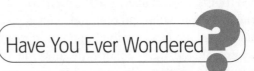

Have You Ever Wondered

. . . how nanotechnology might affect food in the future? Nanotechnology relates to extremely small particles of matter. In size, one nanometer equals about one millionth of a pinhead, or one blade of grass on a football field. As a science it's not new, but more potential applications are being identified regularly. Applied to agriculture, food processing, and food packaging, it's cutting edge. It also has potential applications in medicine and in helping the environment. Eventually nanotechnology may provide more benefits, including helping to make agricultural production more efficient, making functional foods more effective, making flavors more prominent, and even using food packaging to decrease any foodborne pathogens or contaminants. More research is needed before nanotechnology will be approved in food application to ensure its long-term safety. Stay tuned!

. . . how the food system may impact your carbon footprint? A carbon footprint is a measure of carbon emissions that seem to impact the environment. Some foods come with a greater carbon footprint than others, depending on how they're grown, produced, transported, and prepared. Food waste also contributes to the carbon imprint. To see how your food choices may impact your carbon footprint, check the Low Carbon Diet Calculator at www.eatlowcarbon.org.

mixes, specialty pasta, ice cream, jam, margarine, and pie and pudding fillings are among the many foods with added coloring.

Food colors may be added for many reasons: to offset any food color that's lost from exposure to light, air, temperature extremes, moisture, and storage; to correct natural color variations; to enhance natural colors; or to give color to fun or colorless foods for appeal.

Both natural and synthetic colors are used in food. Nine certified colors, such as FD&C Yellow #5 and Red #2, are approved in the United States. They offer intense, uniform color at a low cost, without undesirable flavor. More and more natural pigments from vegetables, minerals, and animal sources are being used as colorings, which can be more costly; they're exempt from certification, yet must meet safety and purity regulations. For example, look for foods with annatto extract, beet juice, paprika, carrot oil, beta carotene, grape skin extract, or saffron.

Only one food coloring is known to cause allergic reactions, in rare cases: FD&C Yellow #5, or tartrazine. *See "Coloring by Any Other Name!" in chapter 21.*

● *Flavorings*, which may be natural or synthetic, make up about seventeen hundred of the additives approved in the United States for use in food. They include spices, herbs, essential oils and their extracts, fruit juices, caffeine, and other seasonings. To make artificial flavorings, food scientists carefully study the makeup of natural flavors, then re-create the natural flavor. Natural flavors come from food itself after minimal processing. They're often taken from one food and added to another. The chemical structure of natural and artificial flavors is similar, although the taste may not be an exact match. Yogurt, milk, baked goods, gelatin pudding, salad dressing mix, sauces, and soft drinks are some foods with flavorings.

● *Flavor enhancers* don't add their own flavor. Instead, they heighten natural flavors already present in food. A well-known flavor enhancer is monosodium glutamate (MSG). MSG comes from a common amino acid, a protein called glutamic acid. MSG comes mostly from vegetable proteins. *See "MSG—Another Flavor Enhancer" in chapter 7.* Canned vegetables, processed meats, frozen meals, yogurt, sauce mixes, and soups are among the foods with flavor enhancers.

● *Sweeteners* are also flavorings, but they're grouped separately. Some, such as sucrose (table sugar), fructose, dextrose, and mannitol, are nutritive, meaning they add calories and produce energy in your body. Besides their sweet flavor, these sugars add mouth feel and work as browning agents in food. And they may be used as preservatives. Low-calorie, or intense, sweeteners such as saccharin, sucralose, stevia, and aspartame don't contribute calories. Sweeteners are used in baked foods, canned and frozen fruit, frozen desserts, fruit yogurt, fruit juice drinks, gelatin mixes, jam, pudding mixes, and soft drinks, among others. *For more about sugars and other sweeteners, see chapter 3.*

Testing, Testing

Did you know that new food additives must pass rigid safety tests before approval for use? During the past eighty or so years, the use of food additives has allowed a more varied and plentiful food supply. Beginning in 1938, government regulations have helped guide and ensure their safety in food.

Today food additives are regulated more tightly than ever—with safety as the primary goal. In 1958 the federal government passed the Food Additives Amendment, which gave the FDA responsibility for approving additive use in food. The FDA sets safety standards, determining whether a substance is safe for its intended use. If found to be safe, the FDA decides what types of foods the additive may be used in, in what amounts, and how it must be indicated on a food label.

Federal food laws distinguish among additives: those "generally recognized as safe" (GRAS), prior-approved additives, regulated additives, and color additives.

● *Generally recognized as safe* (GRAS). In 1959 the FDA established a list of about seven hundred additives that were exempt from regulation. This list—called the GRAS list—recognized that many additives had an extensive history or existing scientific evidence of safe use in food. Additives on the GRAS list include salt, sugar, spices, vitamins, caffeine, and monosodium glutamate.

From time to time, GRAS ingredients are reevaluated by the FDA, and perhaps removed from the list or reclassified. An example occurred in 1986, when research showed that some people are sensitive to sulfites. *See "For the Sulfite Sensitive . . ." in chapter 21.*

● *Prior-approved substances.* Before the 1958 Food Additives Amendment, some additives—such as nitrites used to preserve processed meats—had been approved by the FDA or the USDA. If used as originally approved, these substances didn't need to go through the approval process again; the government already had judged them safe.

As with the GRAS list, prior-approved substances are monitored continually. Current scientific evidence of their link to health is reviewed, recognizing that the statutes of prior-approved substances can be changed.

● *Regulated additives.* Any additive not considered as GRAS or prior-approved must be evaluated and approved by the FDA before it can be marketed and used in food. The evaluation addresses substance composition and qualities, amount typically consumed, immediate and long-term effects, and other safety factors. These are the regulatory steps:

● First, the manufacturer must prove that the additive is effective—that it does what it is supposed to do (for example, adds flavor or color) and that it can be detected and measured when put into a food.

● Second, the manufacturer must prove that large amounts of the food additive, when given to two kinds of test animals (usually rats and mice) over an extended time, won't cause cancer, birth defects, or neurological or other problems. Results of human studies may be submitted, also.

● The FDA reviews the results, then invites public response to the manufacturer's petition.

● If approval is given, the FDA establishes regulations for the types of foods in which the additive may be used, for what purposes, the maximum amount, and how the substance must be described on the label. The level approved is much lower than the amount that may have any expected adverse effect.

When a food industry proposes an additive for use in meat or poultry products, another approval also is required—this time from the USDA's Food Safety and Inspection Service (FSIS)—with standards that consider the unique characteristics of meat and poultry. For example, the FSIS doesn't allow sorbic acid, an approved additive, in meat salads because it could mask spoilage.

Color additives. The 1960 Color Additives Amendment requires that dyes used in foods, drugs, cosmetics, and medical devices be evaluated, with tests similar to those for regulated food additives.

Safety Check

Approval of food additives, including those on GRAS and prior-sanctioned lists, doesn't guarantee that they'll be used in food forever, nor does it infer absolute safety. No food can offer that. However, based on the best available science, FDA approval reflects reasonable certainty of no harm to consumers when the additive is used as intended. The FDA continues to review all categories of food additives, and judges them by the latest scientific standards and current consumption of that additive. Based on new evidence, approval is either continued or withdrawn.

As another safety check, the Food Additives Amendment also has a section called the Delaney Clause, which states that no additive known to cause cancer in animals or humans can be put in food in any amount. One artificial sweetener, called cyclamate, was removed from the GRAS list for that reason. Tests showed that large amounts were linked to cancer in test animals. The safety of cyclamate is being reevaluated; it is approved for use in some other countries.

To monitor and investigate complaints of adverse reactions to additives, the FDA also maintains the Adverse Reaction Monitoring System (ARMS), which records updated safety data. Incidences of allergic reactions to food and color additives and to dietary supplements, reported by individuals or their doctors, are recorded. These reports help determine whether further investigation is warranted—and if action is needed to maintain public health. *See "Sensitive to Additives? Maybe, Maybe Not" in chapter 21.*

Good Manufacturing Practices (GMP) regulations also limit additive use: only as much needed for the desired result.

Additives—Your Choice

With an array of foods available, consumers have choices about food additives. If you have a history of food-related allergies, you may need to limit or avoid foods with ingredients, including additives, that you're sensitive to. Read the ingredient lists on labels; see *"A Word about Ingredients . . ." in chapter 12.* If you have a food reaction and think it may be additive-related, talk to your doctor.

Pesticides: Carefully Controlled

The vast array of safe, nutritious foods available in your supermarket throughout the year doesn't happen by chance. Successful growers carefully manage their croplands and orchards to control about eighty thousand plant diseases, thirty thousand weed species, a thousand species of nematodes, and more than ten thousand insect species. In the United States alone, about $20 billion of crops (10 percent of our production) are lost yearly with these problems. If you've ever struggled with mildew, insects, weeds, and rodents in your own garden, just multiply the problem!

To produce high-quality produce with adequate yields, most farmers use some pesticides—either in the field or grove, or just after harvest—to prevent mold or insect damage during transport or storage.

Without prudent use of pesticides, many farmers couldn't control crop damage from disease, insects, molds and fungi, weeds, and other pests. And crop yields would be much lower. Yield is the amount of an agricultural crop, such as corn, produced in a season. Despite pesticide use, U.S. farmers annually lose a significant amount of crops from pest damage. That number would be far higher without careful pesticide use.

About Pesticides

Pesticides include a broad range of chemicals that protect crops. They're applied by dusting, fogging, spraying, or injecting them into the soil:

- *Herbicides* control weeds.
- *Fungicides* control mold, mildew, and fungi that cause plant disease, and inhibit molds that may be harmful to consumers.
- *Insecticides* control insects that damage crops or carry plant disease.
- *Rodenticides* control rodents in the field.
- *Disinfectants* act against bacteria and other disease-carrying microorganisms.

When people think of pesticides, synthetic chemicals often come to mind. However, naturally occurring chemicals in the environment, such as copper, nicotine, and sulfur, and some bacteria also are used to control pests. Many plants protect themselves by producing their own pesticides in low levels.

IPM—Best of Both Worlds

What does sex have to do with pest control? Interestingly, sex scents, called pheromones, can confuse pest mating patterns, allowing farmers to use less pesticides. It's part of a biological system of pest control.

IPM stands for integrated pest management—a farming approach that combines biological control, pesticides, farming practices, and biotechnology to reduce crop damage. As farmers work in partnership with nature, they apply pesticides on crops selectively, ultimately using less. This long-known technique, which may be set aside with monocrop (single crop) farming, has been reintroduced with successful results.

IPM incorporates several strategies to manage pests:

- Crop rotation—for example, switching from soybeans to corn—helps limit pest buildup because insects lose their natural food source. Mulch, spacing plants, tillage practices, and field sanitation are some other ways by which farmers can control pests. Today's technology, including computers and satellites, lets farmers apply only the pesticides, fertilizers, and irrigation water in the amount and locations needed.

- Farmers may use living organisms to help control pest diseases, or use pest predators (when "good" bugs eat "bad" bugs).

- Growers may choose plant varieties that are more pest-resistant. Traditional plant breeding and genetic engineering can help crops develop their own natural resistance. *See "Food Biotechnology: Enhanced Farming" in this chapter.*

- Computers can help growers forecast disease and weather conditions. The more they know, the more prudent farmers can be with pesticides.

Safety: Whose Job?

Pesticide safety starts with growers; most are prudent for many reasons. One is cost. Pesticides are expensive, so farmers must use them judiciously to remain profitable. Second, successful growers project toward the future. Using too much pesticide with one year's crop may cause crop damage in the future, since some pesticide residues remain in the soil. Third, today's farmers are more aware of the environmental impact—their livelihood depends on it. Most farmers are trained in the responsible, legal use of agricultural chemicals; some pesticides must be applied only by people certified or licensed to do so.

Pesticide manufacturers bear responsibility for the effects of pesticide use on consumers, farm workers, and the environment. If research indicates that pesticide use does not meet standards for toxicity, crop residues, or environmental impact, the Environmental

Have You Ever Wondered?

... what rBST is? First, BST, or bovine somatotropin, is a natural hormone in all milk, including breast milk, that helps increase milk production. As a supplement for dairy cows, rBST, or recombinant bovine somatotropin, is its synthetic form. Given as a supplement in small, controlled doses, it helps improve a cow's efficiency in producing milk. Even without a supplement, cows naturally produce small amounts of BST. There's no significant difference in the milk from cows that receive rBST and those that don't. The only difference: milk production goes up in cows that receive it.

BST and rBST have no effect on humans. No human studies link hormones in milk to early onset of puberty. Like other proteins, BST and rBST are broken down during digestion. In addition, there's no change in the flavor or nutrition of milk; either way, milk is an excellent source of calcium, protein, vitamins, and other nutrients.

In 1990, the National Institutes of Health reinforced that BST is safe for humans. In 1993 the FDA approved BST supplementation based on its safety for humans, cows, and the environment. Regulatory agencies around the world have authorized milk and meat from cows receiving BST as safe for people of all ages.

Since milk produced using rBST is identical to milk from untreated cows, there's no requirement for specially labeling. Most milk produced in the United States is *not* produced with rBST. That said, producers who don't use rBST may market their milk as "rBST-free."

... about the "dos and don'ts" surrounding BPA? First, a definition: Bisphenol A (BPA) is a compound used in some reusable plastic food and beverage containers, baby bottles, and can liners (as a barrier between the metal and the food inside). Having been researched and deemed safe for decades, it's being reviewed again for health issues, such as some cancers and certain hormone changes. Evidence shows no clear risk to human health, nor does it appear to build up in the human body. Any amount that migrates from plastic containers or cans to food is extremely low, many times lower than safe exposure levels set by the FDA and international regulatory agencies. Some cans and plastic containers are BPA-free. That said, as a concerned parent, you can buy BPA-free plastic or glass baby bottles. As a consumer, any risk is likely minimal, but you can hand-wash containers with BPA to avoid exposing them to high heat, or use stainless steel, glass, or porcelain bowls for hot foods or liquids instead.

... if wax on some fruits and vegetables is safe to eat? Yes—no need to peel waxed produce. Just wash it with water, no soap. You might use a brush to remove any dirt, bacteria, and pesticide residues. The thin, waxy coating on foods such as cucumbers and apples is applied after picking to replace natural wax that washes off after harvest and to help produce stay fresh and edible; a little fungicide often mixed with the wax helps control mold and rot. Wax helps retain moisture, protect food from bruising, and prevent spoilage. By long-standing federal law, waxed produce must be labeled.

... if you should avoid any specific fruit or vegetable to reduce exposure to pesticides? For any crop, pesticide use varies with the time of year, the soil conditions, the climate, and the presence of pests. There's no way you can tell the difference. *The best guideline:* Wash produce thoroughly, remove outer leaves on leafy greens—then enjoy the nutritional benefits that all fruits and vegetables provide. *See "What You Can Do" in this chapter.*

... if food grown in soil that's depleted of minerals or nitrogen is less nutritious? When soil lacks minerals or nitrogen, plants don't grow properly and may not produce their potential yield. If soil can grow crops or vegetables in your garden, the food produced is nutritious.

Protection Agency (EPA) can stop or change its use. Because pesticides can pose health risks, especially for children, regulations are essential. Several government agencies regulate and monitor pesticide safety in food:

● The *EPA* regulates pesticide manufacture, labeling, and use—and sets maximum levels, or tolerances, for pesticide residues. Before a pesticide can be used on crops, it must be thoroughly tested to assure its safety for the environment and human health. If approved, the EPA may limit its use—by amount used, frequency, or to specific crops—and require that these limitations be listed on the pesticide label. Growers who misuse pesticides, even mistakenly, risk having their crop seized or destroyed. The grower may be charged with a civil or a criminal lawsuit.

Regulations established in 1996 under the Food Quality Protection Act set even stricter safety standards. Among other measures, this law further protects children and infants from pesticide risk, requires testing and information about any estrogen-like effects of pesticide residues, and considers exposure of pesticides to drinking water.

● The *FDA* monitors pesticide residues in most foods (not meat, poultry, and eggs)—both raw and processed—and enforces tolerance levels set by the EPA. If residues exceed these levels, the food can be seized or destroyed, and a lawsuit may be filed. Residues remaining on produce skins or peels are minimal and must be within safe levels set by the EPA and the FDA. Washing produce at home before consuming it removes any pesticide residues that remain on raw foods.

● Like the FDA, the *USDA's Food Safety and Inspection Service* (FSIS) monitors pesticide residues and enforces tolerance levels for meat, poultry, and eggs.

● *Several states,* including California, that grow many fruits and vegetables have their own regulations, too.

Tolerances, or maximum levels, for pesticide residues are set in parts per million, parts per billion, and parts per trillion. For example, 1 part per million would mean 1 gram of residue is the maximum allowed in 1 million grams of food. That equates to 1 cherry in about 20,000 1-pound cans.

Tolerances for pesticide residues are legal limits. In most foods, levels are well below that. Tolerances are a hundred to a thousand times lower than the amount that might pose a health risk, so there's a very wide margin of safety. FDA testing has shown that foods rarely exceed limits; many samples are below the tolerance level or show no residues at all. To pass through U.S. customs, imported foods must meet the same stringent standards set for foods grown domestically.

Benefits vs. Risks

The presence of low levels of pesticide residues doesn't signal a risk. Tolerances are legal limits, not medical limits—set far below what is considered safe for the most sensitive part of the population, including infants and children. The Surgeon General and many health organizations, including the National Institutes of Health, the American Medical Association, the American Cancer Society, and the American Academy of Pediatrics, recognize that the health benefits of eating more fruits and vegetable far outweigh any possible pesticide-related risks.

In fact, pesticide use may reduce other food-related risks. For example, fungicides help control aflatoxin B_2, a naturally occurring toxin in grains and peanuts. Most important, prudent use of pesticides helps ensure a wide variety of fruits and vegetables, which supply important vitamins, minerals, fiber, and other phytonutrients for human health.

What You Can Do

Any pesticide residues in foods you buy are present at minimal levels. It's safe to say that they probably won't pose any health risk. You can add more to your safety net by the way you handle food in your kitchen and perhaps by the way you grow fruits and vegetables in your garden:

● Choose produce carefully. Avoid fruits and vegetables with cuts, insect holes, mold, or decay.

● Wash fresh fruits (including melons) and vegetables with water to remove residues on the surface and in the crevices. For foods such as carrots, squash, apples, and pears, use a vegetable brush to clean them even more if you eat the fiber-rich skin. Rinse well. Avoid soap, unless it's meant for produce; soap leaves its own residues. As an option, use a produce wash formulated to remove soil, wax, and pesticides. Rinse well after using a produce wash.

● Remove outer leaves of lettuce, cabbage, and other leafy vegetables.

● Although you could peel some fruits and vegetables, recognize what you'd be giving up—the nutrients and the fiber that the peel contains. Instead, wash them well.

● Eat a variety of foods. Not only do you get the nutritional benefits, but you also minimize pesticide risks.

Different crops require different pesticides, so variety limits exposure to any one type.

● If you're a home gardener, minimize your use of pesticides; follow directions for their safe use, storage, and disposal. Contact your county Cooperative Extension Service if you need guidance. *See "Resources You Can Use" to help locate your local Cooperative Extension Service.*

Have You Ever Wondered?

. . . what hydroponically grown foods are? They're foods from plants raised in water, not soil; "hydro" means water. The hydroponic solution—which varies by crop and environmental conditions—supplies roots with elements found in soil and fertilizer. With hydroponic farming, high-quality food can be produced almost anywhere: a desert, outer space, and areas with poor soil. Nutritionally, hydroponically grown foods are comparable to those grown in soil; undamaged by weather, they may look better.

A few more terms in modern agriculture: Aeroponics is a way to grow plants by spraying the roots with nutrient solution; aquaculture is raising fish in a controlled environment.

. . . about aquaculture and its role in food production? Growing globally, aquaculture is the breeding, rearing, and harvesting of both plants and animals in both fresh and salt water (ponds, rivers, lakes, and oceans). As with agriculture, it's done in both natural and man-made environments. About 50 percent of fish consumed around the world come from aquaculture. The Dietary Guidelines Advisory Committee Report in 2010 notes a need for more science-based evidence on aquaculture: its safety for the environment and its health implications. Stay tuned! Standards are being developed by the World Wildlife Fund for salmon aquaculture.

. . . if hormones used in beef production affect humans? The FDA and the FSIS work together to ensure the safe, proper use of hormones in cattle. In very small amounts, certain hormones have been approved by the FDA to improve feed efficiency or weight gain of beef cattle and sheep. Ready for market faster, animals have more lean muscle and less fat. The amount of growth-promoting hormones in treated meat must fit within the same range as for untreated animals. Producers must show that hormone levels in animals after treatment remain below a level that's too low to affect humans who consume the meat from those animals.

To put this in perspective, all meat, treated or not, contains hormones in very low levels; plant-based foods have them, too. A three-ounce serving of treated beef has 1.85 nanograms of estrogen, compared to 1.3 nanograms in the same amount of nontreated beef; one serving of many plant-based foods contains several hundred nanograms of estrogen, naturally. The human body produces thousands of nanograms of estrogen daily. One nanogram is very tiny: one billionth of a gram.

If you prefer meat from untreated animals, you have choices. Beef products may be labeled "no hormones administered"—if sufficient evidence is provided by the producer to the FSIS showing that hormones were not used to raise the animals. What about pork or chicken? Federal regulations prohibit using added hormones in raising hogs or poultry; the "no hormones added" claim can't be used on their labels.

. . . what a food desert is? It refers to geographic areas without access to affordable fruits, vegetables, whole grains, low-fat milk, and other foods that make up the full range of a healthful diet. The result? The ability to make nourishing food choices is limited, too. Since higher-calorie, lower-nutrient foods might be the options instead, food deserts may play a role in the obesity epidemic and some chronic health problems. Do you live in a food desert? There's no precise definition, but this government website offers insight: www.ers.usda.gov/data/fooddesert. Even if you do, you can take steps to eat healthy!

● Wash and sanitize refrigerator drawers frequently.

● Remember that just because a food is organic doesn't mean it's safe. Organic producers may use natural pesticides, which also can have health risks. Clean organic produce well.

Sustainable Food Production

There's a new buzzword these days in food production: sustainability. The 1990 Farm Bill defines sustainable agriculture as "an integrated system of plant and animal production practices having a site-specific application that will, over the long term:

● satisfy human food and fiber needs;

● enhance environmental quality and the natural resource base on which the agricultural economy depends;

● make the most efficient use of nonrenewable resources and on-farm resources and integrate, where appropriate, natural biological cycles and controls;

● sustain the economic viability of farm operations;

● enhance the quality of life for farmers and society as a whole."

To put it differently and more simply, sustainable agriculture is producing food in a way that doesn't jeopardize natural resources for the needs of the current generation, or compromise the needs of future generations. It's a system of producing and distributing enough food efficiently for a growing world population—with minimal use of natural resources (land, soil, energy, water, air, etc.) and minimal environmental impact. That includes managing waste, conserving and protecting resources and biodiversity, and using ecologically sound farming and food production practices. Among other outcomes: more food can be grown on less land. In that way valuable land such as rain forests won't be destroyed.

Sustainability is often viewed through a local lens—for example, recognizing local farmers and local farmers' markets. In fact, its strategies extend broadly to policies, regulations, and practices that involve food systems at every level: local, regional, national, and global. Since people live in concentrated areas, some less agriculturally productive, food must come from many sources, not just locally. A sustainable food system includes farms, food manufacturers, distributors, retailers, and restaurants—large and small, near and far—as well as consumers themselves. And it's a process, some say a journey, not a destination.

New science and agricultural technology help make food production more sustainable and help manage resources. For example, drip irrigation controls watering. Using satellites, farmers can plant and use pesticides and fertilizers more precisely. They also can match seeds and production practices to the soil type and climate, thus getting higher yield for lower cost and achieving more efficient fertilizer use. That can translate to lower food costs.

You can be part of creating a more sustainable food system. *See "How Green Are You?" in this chapter, and refer to "The 'Eco' Kitchen" in chapter 14 and "Shopping Green!" in chapter 12 to learn more. See supporting local growers through farmers' markets and community assisted agriculture in chapter 12.*

Organically Produced

Organic foods, once available mostly from health food stores, sell in most mainstream supermarkets. Organic farming is expanding fast—not only with fruits, vegetables, and grains, but also for eggs, dairy foods, meat, poultry, packaged foods, oils, baby foods, and even wine and beer! What are organic foods? And how do they compare with their conventionally produced counterparts?

All foods come from living organisms—plant and animal. Because all contain carbon, they're all organic. That said, foods referred to as "organic" are really organically grown or organically produced, with little or no synthetic fertilizers or pesticides and no antibiotics or hormones. The bottom line is that the term "organic" is legally defined and refers to a way of managing food production. It doesn't imply healthier or safer food. To clarify other misnomers, the marketing term "local" doesn't mean "organic," and "organic" doesn't mean "nutrient-rich."

Perspective: Organically Produced Foods

Using organic foods is an individual choice and another option for healthful food choices in the marketplace. Sold fresh, frozen, and canned, organic products have grown in quality, availability, and popularity.

Are organic foods pesticide-free? That depends. Organic farmers may use insects and crop rotation to control pests that damage crops. Certain insects, for example, are natural predators for other insects that cause crop damage. Or farmers may use chemicals found naturally in the environment, such as sulfur, nicotine, copper, or pyrethrins, as pesticides. When these methods don't work, organic farmers can use other substances (biological, botanical, or synthetic) from a list approved by the USDA's National Organic Program (NOP). With organic farming, manure, compost, and other organic wastes fertilize crops; there are some permitted synthetic fertilizers. Soil also is managed with crop rotation, tillage, and cover crops. Organic fertilizers are effective, yet plants can't distinguish them from synthetic fertilizers. Both types of fertilizer break down in the soil to nurture growing plants.

Criteria for organically raised livestock and poultry and for animals raised for milk and eggs are equally stringent. From the last third of gestation (or for poultry, the second day of life), animals are fed only 100 percent organic feed; they must have outdoor access and be humanely treated. (Organic or not, all livestock and poultry must be treated humanely.) Although vitamin and mineral supplements are allowed, hormones for growth and antibiotics to treat or prevent infection and disease are not. Any animal treated with medication can't become an organic food.

How do these foods compare for nutrition, taste, and appearance? So far, no conclusive scientific evidence shows that organically produced foods are healthier or safer. Based on current understanding, both approaches—organic and conventional farming—supply nutritionally comparable foods, although this is an issue of ongoing debate. For both farming methods, climate and soil conditions, genetic differences in plants, maturity at harvest, and the way food is handled affect the nutrient content of raw foods.

For taste and appearance, studies show no significant differences between organically and conventionally grown foods. Instead, these differences appear to come from food varietal, its growing conditions, its maturity at harvest, and how it is handled and perhaps packaged.

Organically produced foods often cost more. That's usually due to higher production costs (more labor, more management-intensive) and smaller scale (smaller farms or yields). However, organic produce purchased in season is often comparable in price to out-of-season produce grown conventionally. As a consumer, compare prices as you shop. You may elect conventional over organic if there is a big price gap, especially for produce you wouldn't consume with the skin or the peel on, which is the layer than would contain any pesticide residues. Either is a good option.

Today's organic farming alone can't produce enough food for the world's exploding population. Both conventional and organic farming are part of feeding today's world. Today both large food companies and small farmers offer organic food products.

Coming to Terms

The National Organic Program (NOP) ensures that the production, processing, and certification of organic foods meet expected standards. If you prefer organic foods, you can be confident of the food's organic status when you see the USDA's certified organic label.

Under the Organic Foods Production Act, federal regulations require consistent and uniform standards. Organic farming or processing operations that take in more than $5,000 gross per year must be certified. Even smaller, uncertified organic operations must abide by the standards and may label their products. Certification allows organic labeling with terms that have a consistent meaning: "100 percent organic," "organic," and "made with organic ingredients." The USDA organic seal may appear on any foods that contain at least 70 percent organic ingredients. In organic food production, food irradiation (to destroy foodborne bacteria), sewage sludge, and genetic engineering can't be used. A product with less than 70 percent organic ingredients can list only specific organically produced ingredients in the ingredient list. *For more about organic labeling, see chapter 12.*

Farmers may follow organic practices even if they don't choose to be certified. And those with traditional farming practices typically use many agricultural practices associated with organic farming. Organic or not, caring for natural resources helps ensure successful agriculture now and into the future.

Today's Meat

Through breeding, feeding, and farm management, hogs and beef cattle are leaner than ever. In addition, processing methods help create leaner meat. For example, pork cuts sold in the supermarket today have an average of 43 percent less fat than they did in 1983, and compared with the 1970s, beef has 27 percent less trimmable fat.

One reason for leaner hogs is genetics. Some of the eight major hog breeds in the United States carry genes that produce leaner, meatier hogs. With selective breeding, producers have changed the fat and muscle composition of hogs, gradually producing leaner animals over the past few decades.

As with humans, hogs' food and "lifestyle" affect their body composition. With a scientifically balanced diet matched to age, current weight, and nutrient needs, they're fed what they need without excess.

The next step in producing lean meat is with the meat packers or processors. They usually trim the fat surrounding meat cuts to ⅛ to ¹⁄₁₆ inch, rather than ½ to ¼ inch, as in the past. With beef, many cuts have no outside fat at all. Financial incentives may be offered by the packer to the farmer for producing lean animals. Even though many processed meats are produced with less fat and cholesterol than before, they're still tender, moist, and flavorful. Look for lean ground beef and low-fat pork sausages: just 5 fat grams and 6 fat grams, respectively, per 3-ounce serving. That's about 50 percent less than for regular meat.

Finally, it's up to you to keep lean meat lean and flavorful by using low-fat cooking methods, avoiding high-fat sauces, and cooking it to a safe internal temperature, without overcooking. *For more about leaner cuts and preparing meat, see chapter 14. For tips on buying lean meat, see chapter 12.*

Food Biotechnology: Enhanced Farming

In the twenty-first century your shopping cart will be filled with an array of new products, foods that include a greater variety of produce all year long, taste fresher and more flavorful, and have more health benefits. Today's food biotechnology has already put many of these foods on your table: canola, corn, soybean, and cottonseed oils along with new varietals of potatoes, squash, tomatoes, and papaya. This new science of farming offers other potential benefits as well, including improved food safety, reduced environmental impact, and a food system that's more sustainable. At the same time, its products need ongoing evaluation.

Modern biotechnology is simply applying plant science and genetics to enhance food production and food itself. Simply put, it's applied science.

Traditional biotechnology began perhaps ten thousand years ago, as farmers raised animals and grew plants to produce food with desirable traits: higher yields, new food varieties, better taste, faster ripening, and more drought resistance. Five thousand years ago in today's Peru, potatoes were grown selectively. In ancient Egypt—4,500 years ago—domesticated geese were fed to make them bigger and tastier. About 2,300 years ago, Greeks grafted trees, a technique that led to orchards and a more abundant fruit supply. In fact, products as commonplace as grapefruit and wine grapes came from traditional biotechnology, or traditional breeding and selection.

With traditional breeding, farmers changed the genetic makeup of plants and animals by selecting those with desirable traits. They then raised and selected again and again until a new, more desirable breed or food variety was established. Even in the old days, this breeding resulted in genetic change.

Over the years, farmers have replanted seeds or cross-pollinated from their best crops. They've bred new livestock from their best animals. For example, within the past few decades, hogs have been bred to be leaner, in turn producing lean cuts of pork for today's health-conscious consumers.

Traditional cross-breeding takes time. Often it's unpredictable. Each time one plant pollinates another, or one animal inseminates another, thousands of genes cross together. Along the way, less desirable traits—and the genes that cause them—may pass with desirable ones. Several generations of breeding, perhaps ten to twelve years, may go by before desirable traits get established and less desirable qualities are bred away.

Modern biotechnology offers new farming methods. It provides a faster, more precise way to provide foods with the qualities, or traits, that consumers expect, such as improved foods that are safe, nourishing, abundant, and flavorful, using environmentally friendly production methods.

Food Biotechnology Today: What's It All About?

In a nutshell, modern biotechnology refers to enhancing organisms—plants, animals, and bacteria—to develop new products, not just for food, but also for medical treatment, waste management, and alternative fuels, among other applications.

Today's food biotechnology started about four decades ago, as scientists learned more about DNA (deoxyribonucleic acid), genes, and the genetic code in living things, and applied this knowledge to plant and animal breeding. In fact, the latest advances in food biotechnology spawned a new vocabulary. For example, popular media may use "genetically improved" or "GM foods" to refer to these foods. Other terms, such as genetic engineering, gene slicing, cell culture, and recombinant DNA, refer to some methods of modern biotechnology. Recombinant DNA involves the process of inserting genes from one organism into the genetic code, or DNA, of another. That's how a trait is transferred.

To understand how this new science of farming works, think about writing a book on a computer. With a click of your mouse, you can copy a single quote from one document to another without merging the two, or you can highlight or delete a single phrase.

Likewise, agricultural scientists can pinpoint specific genes that carry traits they want, such as disease resistance, better nutrient quality, or flavor. Then they can transfer a single gene from one plant or from an unrelated species, such as a bacterium, to another. Or they can extract a certain gene, leaving undesirable traits behind. The latest advances in food biotechnol-ogy are more efficient, more predictable, and less time-consuming than traditional breeding.

Why Enhanced Farming?

Food biotechnology has developed new ways to improve crop yield, with a goal of reducing the impact certain crops have on the environment and of improving the nutritional quality. Foods are products of today's enhanced farming. As these new agricultural methods are used, new ways to assess the short- and long-range outcomes are needed, too.

Healthier crops, higher yields. Crops produced using biotechnology can thrive with less environmental impact. For farmers, that means lower production costs; for the environment, potentially more protection.

For example, some cotton and corn varieties have been enhanced through biotechnology to contain *Bacillus thuringiensis* (Bt), a common soil bacterium that lets corn protect itself from certain insects that eat and destroy plants. That lowers the use of insecticides. Bt itself isn't new, however. Organic and traditional farmers have used it on their crops for more than forty years. Its use has stirred controversy.

Contemporary farming is developing other crops to resist plant viruses and other diseases, or to require less insecticide or more environmentally friendly herbicides (glyphosate). Newly developed soybeans, as well as some corn, canola, cotton, and potatoes, flourish with the use of less insecticide.

Weather-resistant crops. Crops are being genetically improved to withstand severe weather, reducing crop loss and extending the growing season and region. That can make more fresh fruits, vegetables, and grains available year round.

Fresher foods, better flavor. By transferring desirable genetic traits, fruits and vegetables with different ripening qualities can be shipped longer and farther without spoilage or damage: bananas, pineapples, and strawberries, for example, that resist mold. This means better-tasting pro-

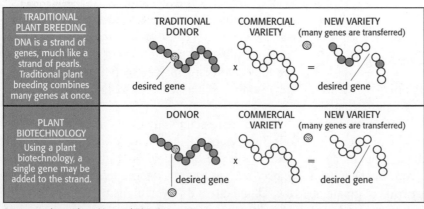

TRADITIONAL PLANT BREEDING			
DNA is a strand of genes, much like a strand of pearls. Traditional plant breeding combines many genes at once.	TRADITIONAL DONOR	COMMERCIAL VARIETY	NEW VARIETY (many genes are transferred)
	desired gene	x =	desired gene
PLANT BIOTECHNOLOGY	DONOR	COMMERCIAL VARIETY	NEW VARIETY (many genes are transferred)
Using a plant biotechnology, a single gene may be added to the strand.	desired gene	x =	desired gene

Source: Academy of Nutrition and Dietetics.

duce that stays fresh longer, such as sweeter peppers, or potatoes with fewer dark spots year round.

Healthier foods. Modern food biotechnology also may help to promote public health by providing fruits, vegetables, and grains with more nutrition benefits: More proteins, vitamins, and minerals, or less fat or saturated fat. In the future, fruits and vegetables such as sweet potatoes with higher levels of antioxidants (vitamins C and E, and beta carotene) may help reduce heart disease and cancer risk.

Already some vegetable oils have a better fatty acid profile—less solid fats (saturated fat and *trans* fat) and more monounsaturated fat—for heart health. Food biotechnology also has enhanced soybeans, canola, and other oil seeds so they have less saturated fat and more oleic acid, an unsaturated fatty acid that is beneficial

for heart health. Enhanced flaxseeds could bring more omega-3 benefits to vegetable-based cooking oils.

For those with food allergies, biotechnology may make it possible to reduce allergens in wheat, peanuts, and other crops.

In parts of the world, nutrient-enhanced crops may help to attack problems of malnutrition. For example, "golden rice" with beta carotene (vitamin A) and iron may address two health problems: blindness among children caused by a lack of vitamin A, and low iron intake, which is harmful to many children and women. Protein-rich potatoes and cassava (a staple in Africa) could help to eliminate malnutrition.

Safer foods. With food biotechnology, foodborne bacteria and viruses may be easier to detect, so potentially the risk of foodborne illnesses may decline.

Have You Ever Wondered?

. . . what nutrigenomics is, and what it may mean for you? Decoding the human genome, a remarkable feat completed within this new millennium, will offer a personalized way to approach health and nutrition decisions. Nutrigenomics is the study of genes and their link to nutrition. It's how nutrients and other food components interact with a person's genetic makeup, regulating particular genes to increase or decrease the risk for certain diseases.

Nutrigenomics, or personalized nutrition, offers a huge opportunity to customize what people eat for their unique genetic makeup and nutritional needs. The goal: the potential to slow and even prevent all kinds of diseases—some directly nutrition-related, such as celiac disease, diabetes, obesity, cancer, and heart disease, others not, such as sickle cell disease, cystic fibrosis, and Alzheimer's disease—for those at risk. Understanding functional foods and nutrigenomics goes hand in hand as science reveals unique ways in which foods' many substances work and interact within body cells.

That said, a great deal of research is needed before gene-based nutrition advice becomes a reality. But the first steps are being taken, already within our lifetime!

. . .if antibiotics used in agriculture affect human health? Antibiotics have been used in animal agriculture for many years to prevent or cure diseases in animals—

sometimes for just one animal, sometimes for the herd or flock if many animals are infected at the same time. The FDA and the FSIS work together to provide safe food by ensuring the proper use of animal antibiotics in agriculture. That includes type of antibiotic, the dose and its duration, and the time that the animal or animals must be withdrawn from the market before slaughter, or for dairy cows, from milking. USDA regulations require that antibiotic use must stop for at least sixty days before slaughter. The FDA regulates and monitors the use of animal antibiotics to ensure that any residues are minimal and at very safe levels. A dairy cow can't return to the milking herd until tests show that her milk is free of antibiotics. In addition, every tankload of milk is strictly tested for antibiotics; if it tests positive for an antibiotic, the milk is discarded without getting to the store.

Currently, questions have been posed about the possibility of "antibiotic resistance" in humans if animal antibiotics are used in cattle production. Definitive research is needed to determine any effect from the use of animal antibiotics on human health. (Penicillin, important to human health, is not used with cattle.) Meat and poultry may be labeled "no antibiotics added" or "raised without antibiotics" if there's enough substantiated proof to the FSIS that animals were raised without them.

Efficient food production, economic benefits. Foods can be grown in a better way to produce higher yields, reducing cost and effort for farmers. That needs to be balanced against the carbon footprint, too.

Food biotechnology also can use simple organisms to produce the same food components found in nature. One example is an additive called rennin. In fact, 70 percent of cheese produced in the United States is made with an enzyme available through biotechnology. Traditionally, rennet—an enzyme extracted from the lining of calves' stomachs—was used to form curds and whey from milk, a first step in making cheese. Through food biotechnology, scientists have transferred the calf gene into friendly bacteria to produce the same enzyme. This enzyme is more active and purer than rennet—and consistently available to food manufacturers.

New food varieties. Food biotechnology can extend to advances in traditional cross-breeding, allowing for new food varieties: for example, broccoflower (green cauliflower); single-serving, seedless melons; mini avocados; blood oranges; baby pineapples; doughnut peaches; and red sweet corn. By understanding the plant genome, traditional cross-breeding also can develop food varieties with better flavor, other agronomic qualities, and a better nutrient profile. And it can help scientists understand the thousands of edible plant species yet unexplored.

More food grown on less land. Food biotechnology can help grow more food on less land, allowing farmers to produce enough food to meet the world's rapidly growing population—expected to be about 9 billion by 2050. Within the next forty or so years, the world will need about 70 percent more food than needed today. To produce enough food, all food production methods and innovations are needed to provide enough nourishing and safe food!

Weather-resistant crops can turn regions with poor climate or soil conditions into productive agricultural land. Higher-yielding crops can feed more people, using less farmland, contributing to a more sustainable food supply.

Protection for the environment. With enhanced farming, greater crop yields may reduce the need to clear forests for farmland, thus protecting the environment. Better weed control with herbicide-tolerant crops

allows farmers to use no-till or other forms of conservation tillage. That leads to less erosion of valuable topsoil because soil isn't turned over as much; therefore there is less runoff and fewer greenhouse gas emissions. Crops with traits that repel pests require fewer pesticides. As a result, fewer residues pass into water supplies. With "environmentally friendly" animal feed, less unwanted phosphorus passes into manure, then into the water supply.

As another nonfood application, biotechnology may provide cost-effective options for renewable, nonpolluting fuel—for example, from corn. These fuel sources may reduce dependence on nonrenewable energy sources such as petroleum.

That said, the benefits and consequences of food biotechnology must be weighed against all outcomes for overall health and the environment.

Now about Food Safety

With any new technology, consumer safety is one of the first questions. The FDA subjects products of food biotechnology to the same stringent standards of labeling and safety as all foods sold in the United States.

Most foods enhanced through biotechnology don't differ in composition, nutritional quality, or safety from those that are conventionally produced—unless that's the trait specifically desired. Like other foods in the U.S. marketplace, any foods produced through biotechnology are rigorously tested and strictly regulated.

Who's responsible for safety? Several federal agencies and some state agencies regulate and ensure the safety of foods produced through biotechnology: the Food and Drug Administration (FDA), the Environmental Protection Agency (EPA), and the U.S. Department of Agriculture (USDA). The FDA's key role is assuring the safety of the product as a food for humans or as animal feed. The EPA regulates the safety of pest control properties of crops, including the impacts on the environment and the food supply. The USDA assesses the safety of crops growing in the field.

Seed manufacturers conduct thorough research and demonstrate proof of testing for every crop brought to market—for example, showing proper nutrient levels, status of allergens or natural toxins, how the improved crop functions as food or animal feed, scientific procedures for product development, environmental effects, and the history of safe use. For substances that differ significantly from existing foods and ingredients, special testing is required. Products are tested throughout their development before they reach consumers.

With new technology comes change, controversy, and more research questions to explore and answer. Current evaluation procedures used by manufacturers and regulators to ensure safety for consumers are endorsed internationally by the Food and Agriculture Organization (FAO) of the United Nations and the World Health Organization (WHO). In the United States, the National Academy of Sciences, the American Medical Association, the Society of Technology, and the Academy of Nutrition and Dietetics among others support the safety of foods produced by biotechnology. Stay tuned as more is learned.

Biotechnology Labeling: When You Need to Know

Most foods produced through biotechnology seem no different from foods you enjoy already. They taste good, look fresh, and are available throughout the year. In addition, most don't require special food labeling because they have been shown to be the same as other foods. Any labeling is voluntary.

Foods developed through biotechnology are subject to the same FDA labeling regulations and carry the same food labels, including allergen labeling, as any other foods. Additional labeling is required on biotech food and on foods with ingredients derived from biotechnology under some circumstances:

● If a known allergen is introduced into the food. Allergic reactions come from proteins in foods, and genes direct protein production. So if a gene is taken from a food known to cause allergic reactions (such as peanuts), then transferred to another food (such as potatoes or corn), the new food must be labeled as potentially containing that particular allergen. No foods introduced to the food supply to date are known to contain proteins from known allergenic foods. (*Note:* Through biotechnology, research is under way to remove known allergens from food—for example, to develop allergen-free or allergen-reduced peanuts.)

● If the nutritional content of the food changes. Foods that are enhanced to change their nutritional content

must be labeled. Perhaps rice with more protein or an orange with more vitamin C.

● If the food composition changes substantially. Perhaps it would be labeled with a new varietal name; or maybe, like broccoflower, a new identity.

According to federal regulations, manufacturers may label their foods voluntarily, as produced with or without the use of ingredients that are enhanced or produced through biotechnology. This labeling can be provided for the consumer's right to know. It must be truthful and not misleading. A recent American Medical Association report indicates no scientific reason for this labeling of most foods.

Growing Possibilities

Food biotechnology, to help feed a growing world, is developing globally, not just in the United States. Gradually you might find these foods in your supermarket:

● Tomatoes with more lycopene, an antioxidant that may protect against some cancers

Natural Toxins

Plants have built-in mechanisms for pest control: fungi, insects, and animal predators. Unlike animals, plants can't flee when they sense danger, so they produce natural compounds—actually, low levels of pesticides—to protect against these invading organisms.

Levels of natural toxins in food may be many times higher than any level of synthetic pesticide residue, according to the National Academy of Sciences. According to FDA estimates, Americans ingest ten thousand times (by weight) more natural pesticides than synthetic ones—with no apparent health risk.

Natural toxins are found in foods you eat every day—for example, oxalates in rhubarb, solanine in green potatoes, nitrates in broccoli, and cyanide in lima beans. At high levels, some might cause illness or may be carcinogenic (cancer-causing). However, in amounts normally eaten in a varied diet, none has been shown to pose a cancer risk.

Through advances in biotechnology, scientists can identify genes that produce natural toxins, then remove them or suppress their action, to provide a health benefit.

● Low-fat potato chips or French fries made from higher-starch potatoes that absorb less fat

● Vegetables and fruits with higher levels of antioxidants (vitamins C and E, and beta carotene) that may help reduce risks for some chronic diseases such as cancer and heart disease

● Rice with higher-quality protein (more amino acids) produced with genes from pea plants

● Vegetable oils—canola, corn, soybean, and others—with more stearate (a form of stearic acid, a saturated fat that doesn't appear to affect blood cholesterol levels) for use in margarine and spreads

● Garlic with more allicin, a phytonutrient that may help lower cholesterol levels

● Peanuts with less of the naturally occurring protein that causes allergic reactions

● Strawberries with more ellagic acid, a cancer-fighting phytonutrient

● Drought-resistant corn and rice for growing in regions with extreme heat and drought

● Fruits that can deliver vaccines in regions without adequate refrigeration to store vaccines

● Folate-rich grains

● As an ingredient, high linolenic acid soybean oil that is more stable, so fewer *trans* fats are formed during processing

CHAPTER 10

Planning to Eat Smart

Food, glorious food! We've explored how nutrients function in human health. But it's the wide array of food, not nutrients, that entices most people to eat. Aromas, flavors, textures, and the appearance of all kinds of foods stimulate your appetite, satisfy your taste buds, and give you the contented feeling that goes with a wonderful meal or a tasty snack.

These wise and flavorful decisions deliver much more, of course. The choices you make about food daily, along with physical activity, affect your health and how you feel today, tomorrow, and far into the future.

You're ready to harness the power of healthy eating. But how? The Dietary Guidelines for Americans, 2010—*summed up in chapter 1*—describes the principles of healthy eating:

● Balance calories with physical activity to manage weight.

● Consume more of certain foods such as fruits, vegetables, whole grains, fat-free and low-fat dairy products, and seafood, with nutrients that often come up short.

● Consume fewer foods with sodium (salt), saturated fats, *trans* fats, cholesterol, added sugars, and refined grains.

How do you put this advice into action?

Eating Patterns for a Healthy You!

Looking for a sensible guide for healthful eating—one that's meant for you? No matter what your food preferences or eating style, there's a pattern with enough flexibility to fit in foods that match your lifestyle, your food preferences, and your personal nutrition and health needs, and with options to match your cultural, ethnic, and traditional preferences, your food budget, and the foods available to you.

What is an eating pattern? Simply said, your own eating pattern is all the foods and beverages you consume over time. It's another way to say your total diet; diet doesn't necessarily mean weight loss. A healthy eating pattern is a flexible and intentional guide. It's meant to help individuals consume both favorite and available foods to meet their nutrient needs within their calorie limits for a day.

In this chapter you'll find several healthy eating patterns: USDA Food Patterns, their lacto-ovo-vegetarian and vegan adaptations, and the DASH Eating Plan. Each is a tool that translates advice from the Dietary Guidelines into a healthful way to eat. Pick one of these patterns. Then use it to make your own plan for healthy eating, or to assess your own food choices over a day or longer.

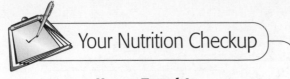

Your Nutrition Checkup

Keep Track!

How do your daily food and drink choices stack up? How can you make a healthy eating pattern work for you? Use the SuperTracker at www.ChooseMyPlate.gov to keep track in an interactive way!

With the SuperTracker you can identify food and physical activity recommendations right for you, track and compare your personal food choices with the 2010 Dietary Guidelines, check your total calorie intake as well as the empty calories you take in, track your physical activities and identify ways to improve, learn more about nutrients in food, keep a personal food and activity journal, and track your body weight history (great for weight management).

No matter which healthy eating pattern you choose, these are the basic recommendations to follow: plenty of vegetables and fruits, emphasis on whole grains, moderate amounts and variety of protein foods, low-fat and fat-free dairy foods, limited amounts of added sugars, and more oils than solid fats.

A Smart Food Plan: The Basics

The USDA Food Patterns, their vegetarian adaptations, and the DASH Eating Plan have many commonalities. First, each recognizes that one size doesn't fit all. Each offers a range of options, designed to be flexible. Individualize the one you choose to match your own food preferences and calorie needs. Beyond that, all share this guidance:

● Vary your choices. Why? Because no one food or food group supplies all the nutrients, fiber, and other components needed for energy, health, and, for kids, growth. Classifying foods and beverages into food groups, based on nutrient content, is the basis of a guide that can help you get the variety you need. Foods within each food group promote health in comparable ways. Yet, even within each food group, the nutrient content of foods isn't identical. That's why variety is so important!

So, consume a variety—among and within the food groups—to get the array of nutrients you need. Variety also adds flavor, interest, and pleasure to eating!

● Make your choices nutrient-rich. Nutrient-rich, or nutrient-dense, foods and beverages deliver

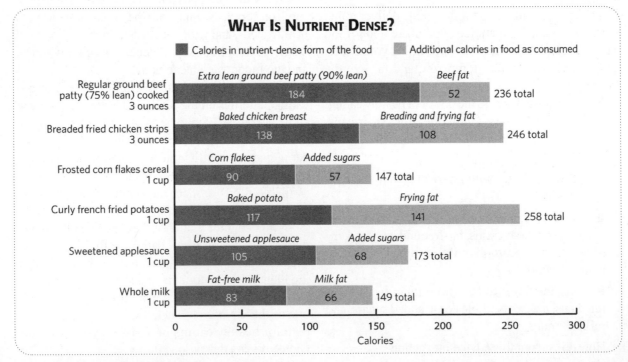

WHAT IS NUTRIENT DENSE?

■ Calories in nutrient-dense form of the food   ■ Additional calories in food as consumed

Food	Nutrient-dense portion	Additional calories	Total
Regular ground beef patty (75% lean) cooked 3 ounces	Extra lean ground beef patty (90% lean) — 184	Beef fat — 52	236 total
Breaded fried chicken strips 3 ounces	Baked chicken breast — 138	Breading and frying fat — 108	246 total
Frosted corn flakes cereal 1 cup	Corn flakes — 90	Added sugars — 57	147 total
Curly french fried potatoes 1 cup	Baked potato — 117	Frying fat — 141	258 total
Sweetened applesauce 1 cup	Unsweetened applesauce — 105	Added sugars — 68	173 total
Whole milk 1 cup	Fat-free milk — 83	Milk fat — 66	149 total

Calories: 0   50   100   150   200   250   300

Source: Dietary Guidelines for Americans, 2010.

MyPlate: Visual Cue for Healthful Eating

MyPlate is your reminder to eat foods from the five food groups. To learn how to choose a variety of foods and drinks for a day—in the right amounts for your calorie needs—click the website www.ChooseMyPlate.gov.

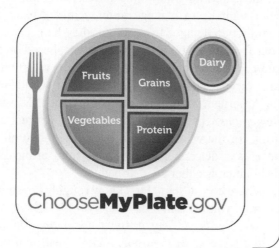

vitamins, minerals, and phytonutrients (including fiber) that may have health benefits, yet they have relatively few calories. They're mostly lean or low in solid fats, with minimized or no added sugars, starches, and sodium. What foods are defined this way? Vegetables, fruits, whole grains, seafood, eggs, beans and peas, unsalted nuts and seeds, fat-free and low-fat milk and milk products, and lean meats and poultry—if prepared without solid fats or added sugars. *See "What Is Nutrient-Dense?" in this chapter.*

● Think in proportions. You need more from some food groups than others to get the full variety of nutrients your body needs. For example, eat more vegetables than the amount of protein foods.

● Eat the right amounts. How much? The healthy eating patterns—USDA Food Patterns, the vegetarian adaptations, and the DASH Eating Plan—provide food group amounts for different calorie levels. For your calorie level, check overall daily amounts recommended for each food group. Look for advice for fats/oils and perhaps for added sugars, too. Food group amounts help you consider

how much you need and how much you eat over the course of a day.

● Right-size your portions. That helps you balance your calories to manage your weight and avoid overeating. Learn to estimate your food and drink portions (in cups and ounces). *See "A Visual Guide to Amounts" in this chapter and "Portion Distortion" in chapter 11.* That said, you don't need a tape measure or a kitchen scale to determine the size of each piece of fruit or vegetable!

No matter which eating pattern you choose, improve gradually. Take small steps to healthier eating. Small steps add up to big benefits. Remember to be physically active, too, a step at a time. It's the flip side of the calorie equation!

Save Calories, Spend Elsewhere

Before exploring healthy food patterns, consider this: Are some of your favorite foods higher in calories—perhaps from added sugars or solid fats? Rather than give them up, find ways to fit small amounts in occasionally. Your food choices and calories over the course of the day or several days are what count. For example, save in one meal to spend elsewhere. Make trade-offs! Try this:

● Skip the butter and sour cream on a baked potato to save for a small dish of ice cream.

● Make pizza with reduced-fat, rather than regular, mozzarella to save for a cookie later.

● Top French toast with sliced fresh peaches, rather than syrup, to save for sugar in your hot tea.

Click Here! Websites to Know . . .

● MyPlate, visual cue to healthful eating, www.ChooseMyPlate.gov

● Nutrient-Rich Foods Coalition, www.nutrientrichfoods.org/index.html

● DASH Eating Plan, www.nhlbi.nih.gov/health/public/heart/hbp/dash/new_dash.pdf

● Vegetarian Resource Group, www.vrg.org

To make meal budgeting easier, use information from the Nutrition Facts on food labels. Check the label's serving size and the calories per label-size serving. *See chapter 12 for label reading.*

Remember: Your goal isn't to eliminate foods, but to moderate and balance your day's meal and snack choices so the food pattern you choose works for you.

A VISUAL GUIDE TO AMOUNTS

What do 3 ounces of cooked meat, chicken, or seafood look like? How about ½ cup of vegetables, 1 cup of cooked pasta, 1½ ounces of cheese, or 1 teaspoon of spread on toast?

VISUAL CUES ARE ALWAYS "HAND-Y" EQUIVALENTS!	USE THEM TO GUESS-TIMATE FOOD AMOUNTS.
Average-size fist = 1 cup	cut-up vegetables sliced or whole fruit (equivalent to 1 medium apple, orange, or pear) cooked beans dry and cooked cereal cooked pasta, rice, other grains
Palm (no fingers) = 3 ounces	cooked meat cooked poultry cooked seafood
Small cupped handful = 1 ounce Large cupped handful = 2 ounces	nuts, seeds dry fruit, such as raisins pretzels, other dry snacks shredded cheese
Thumb (tip to base) = 1 ounce	cheese cube meat, fish, poultry
Thumb tip (to first joint) = 1 tablespoon	peanut butter
Fingertip (tip to first joint) = 1 teaspoon	butter, margarine, spreads mayonnaise, salad dressing vegetable oil sugar

---

A Food Guide for You

Local foods, ethnic foods, your favorite foods, restaurant foods, snack foods, foods you grow yourself, supermarket foods—all kinds of foods fit within the USDA Food Patterns. These patterns are meant to help you make smart choices from every food group, get the most nutrition from your calories, and control your calorie intake to manage your weight. Meant for healthy people ages two and up, they help you and your family put sound nutrition advice, based on the latest science, in action. Think of them as your practical, everyday guide for making the Dietary Guidelines for Americans and other nutrition standards work. *Remember:* It's your total diet—what you eat and drink for the whole day and over time—that either benefits or deters health. No single food, or meal for that matter, is either good or bad.

Where do you start? First know roughly how many calories you need in a day; r*efer to the "Estimated Calorie Needs per Day by Age, Gender, and Physical Activity Level" in the appendices.* Then plan your day's food and beverage choices to match.

For ease, the USDA Food Patterns provide twelve food-group plans, created for different calorie levels, from 1,000 to 3,200 calories. The amount advised from each food group and oils, to get enough essential nutrients, depends on your overall calorie needs. The more calories your body uses, the more calories you need. Calorie needs depend on age, gender, height and weight, and level of physical activity.

Recommended amounts are given in cups and ounces for a day, not in servings and serving sizes for a single meal or snack.

"USDA Food Patterns: In a Nutshell" in this chapter shows how you might spread out your food choices if you need 2,000 calories a day. "USDA Food Patterns" in the appendices gives amounts for each calorie level, or go to www.ChooseMyPlate.gov.

Now look inside the food groups for amounts and ideas to start you toward more healthful eating and to make your calories count for good nutrition. *Then check the rest of the book for pointers on food shopping (chapter 12), food prep (chapter 14), and eating out (chapter 15) at different ages and stages of life (chapters 17–19).*

To find the food groups and calories in a food, or to

USDA FOOD PATTERNS: IN A NUTSHELL

FOOD GROUP*	FOOD GROUP STRATEGIES **Steps for making smart food group choices appear throughout this book.**	HOW MUCH? **For a 2,000-calorie diet, you need this amount every day****
Fruits Focus on fruits.	● Increase fruit intake. ● Eat recommended amounts of fruits. ● Eat a variety of fruit. ● Choose whole or cut-up fruit more often than fruit juice.	2 cups
Vegetables Vary your veggies.	● Increase vegetable intake. ● Eat recommended amounts of vegetables. ● Include a variety of vegetables, especially vegetables, red and orange vegetables, and beans and peas.	2½ cups
Grains Make half your grains whole.	● Increase whole-grain intake. ● Consume at least half of all grains as whole grains. ● Whenever possible, replace refined grains with whole grains.	6-ounce equivalent
Protein Foods Go lean with protein.	● Choose a variety of foods from the protein foods group. ● Increase the amount and variety of seafood consumed by choosing seafood in place of some meat and poultry.	5½ ounces equivalent
Dairy Get your calcium-rich foods.	● Increase intake of fat-free and low-fat milk and milk products such as milk, yogurt, cheese, and milk alternatives such as fortified soy beverages. ● Replace higher-fat milk and milk products with lower-fat options.	3 cups

MORE ADVICE	MORE STRATEGIES	HOW MUCH? **For a 2,000-calorie diet, you need this amount every day****
*Oils and solid fats**	● Use oils instead of solid fats when possible. ● Cut back on solid fats. ● Choose foods with little solid fats and prepare foods to minimize the amount of solid fats. ● Limit saturated-fat intake and keep *trans* fat intake as low as possible.	27 grams (about 6 teaspoons) of oils
*Added sugars**	● Cut back on foods and drinks with added sugars or caloric sweeteners (sugar-sweetened beverages).	

* The maximum amount of solid fats and added sugars adds up to 258 calories on a 2,000- calorie-a-day eating plan.

** For the amounts that are right for your calorie level, check "USDA Food Patterns" in the appendices, or go to www.DietaryGuidelines.gov or www.ChooseMyPlate.gov.

Source: Dietary Guidelines for Americans, 2010.

compare two foods, check USDA's website: www.my foodapedia.gov.

Grain Group: Make at Least Half Your Grains Whole!

What's a grain product? It's any food made from wheat, rice, oats, cornmeal, barley, or another cereal grain. Bread, pasta, oatmeal, breakfast cereals, tortillas, and grits are among the many foods in the grain group. *You'll find more ideas in "Today's Grains" in chapter 9.*

Whatever grain products come to mind, they're all made with whole grains, refined grains, or perhaps both. In the food pattern, foods in the grain group fit into two subgroups:

● *Whole grains:* They're from the whole-grain kernel, with the bran, germ, and endosperm intact. *Refer to the list of whole-grain foods, including whole-wheat flour, bulgur, oatmeal, whole cornmeal, and brown rice, in chapter 3.*

● *Enriched and refined grains:* They're made from refined flour that's been milled for a finer texture or a longer shelf life. The bran and the germ are removed, taking dietary fiber, iron, and many B vitamins with them. White refined flour, degermed cornmeal, most white bread, and white rice are refined grain products.

Most refined grain products are enriched, meaning nutrients (thiamin, riboflavin, niacin, and iron) lost in processing are added back. Fiber isn't added back to enriched grains. Most refined grain products and some whole grains are also fortified with folic acid. The ingredient list on grain products is your way to find out if a grain product is enriched, fortified, or both; *see chapter 12 to learn more.*

Most Americans eat enough total grains. However, most are refined grains instead of whole grains. Many refined grain products are high in solid fats and added sugars.

Many grain products contain gluten, a type of protein. *Refer to chapter 21 for ways to manage gluten intolerance.*

Why Eat Grains, Especially Whole Grains?

Grain products, especially whole grains, offer a bundle of nutrients and phytonutrients vital for health and body maintenance benefits.

Key nutrients: Grain products deliver starches (complex carbohydrates), several B vitamins (thiamin, riboflavin, niacin, and folate), and iron, and additionally from whole-grain foods, magnesium, selenium, and in varying amounts, dietary fiber. *See chapters 3 and 6 to learn about these nutrients.*

Important health benefits: Grain's carbohydrates are your body's main energy source, and their B vitamins help your cells produce that energy. Their folic acid from fortified grains, consumed before and during pregnancy, helps protect against some birth defects. And switching to more whole grains, as part of healthful eating, may help reduce the risk of some chronic diseases, including heart disease, and may help you manage your weight, too. Whole grains that are higher in fiber have additional health benefits; limited evidence suggests a lower incidence of type 2 diabetes.

Grain Products: How Much?

Hit your carb goal with mostly whole-grain, nutrient-rich foods! Just how much do you need? Specific advice for you depends on your calorie need. If you need 2,000 calories a day, the recommended daily amount adds up to 3 ounces of whole grains and 3 ounces of enriched refined grain products. *Check "USDA Food Patterns" in the appendices for the amount that matches your calorie level.*

Make at least half of your daily grain choices whole grain. And replace many refined-grain foods with whole-grain foods that are nutrient-rich.

In general, 1 ounce of grain equals 1 slice of bread, or 1 cup of ready-to-eat cereal, or ½ cup of cooked rice, pasta, or cereal. *See "Grain Products: How Much Is One Ounce?" for more choices.*

Grain Group: Quick Tips

Eat more whole grains. Make at least half your choices whole grain for their fiber and other benefits. Do that by replacing refined grain products with whole grains when you can, not by adding more.

Choose grain products by the company they keep. Not only do whole grains provide unique nutrition benefits. By law most refined grains are fortified with folic acid, while folic acid fortification is voluntary in whole-grain products. That said, go easy on grain-based foods made with solid fats and added sugars,

GRAM PRODUCTS: HOW MUCH IS ONE OUNCE?

ONE OUNCE IS EQUIVALENT TO . . .	WHOLE GRAIN	REFINED GRAIN
1 regular (1 ounce) whole-grain or enriched bread slice, or 1 small slice French bread, or 4 snack-size slices rye	100% whole wheat	white, wheat, French, sourdough
1 mini bagel	100% whole wheat	plain, egg
½ English muffin	whole wheat	plain, raisin
1 small (2-inch-diameter) biscuit		baking powder, buttermilk
1 small (2½-inch-diameter) muffin	whole wheat	bran, corn, plain
1 small piece (2½ inches × 1¼ inches × 1¼ inches) cornbread		(is a refined grain)
5 whole-wheat crackers, or 2 rye crisp-breads, or 7 square or round crackers	100% whole wheat, rye	saltines, snack crackers
1 ounce ready-to-eat cereal (1 cup flakes or rounds, or 1¼ cup puffed)	toasted oat, whole wheat flakes	corn flakes, puffed rice
½ cup cooked, or 1 packet instant, or l ounce dry, regular, or quick oatmeal	(is a whole grain)	
½ cup cooked barley, bulgur, millet, quinoa, or other whole grains	(are whole grains)	
½ cup cooked (made from 1 ounce dry) rice or pasta	brown rice, wild rice, whole-wheat pasta	enriched rice, white rice, polished rice, enriched pasta, durum pasta
1 (6-inch) corn or flour tortilla	whole-wheat, whole-grain corn	flour, corn
3 cups popped popcorn	(is a whole grain)	
1 (4½-inch-diameter) pancake, or 2 small (3-inch-diameter) pancakes	whole wheat, buckwheat	buttermilk, plain

such as regular tortilla chips, croissants, pastries, doughnuts, hush puppies, and fried rice!

● Check the ingredient list on food labels for the words "whole" or "whole grain" before the grain's ingredient name. *Check chapter 3 for ways to identify whole-grain foods.* Use the Nutrition Facts to find whole grains that are good or excellent fiber sources. A good source has 10 to 19 percent Daily Value per serving; an excellent source has 20 percent or more.

● For more whole grains choose whole-grain versions of breakfast cereals, bread, crackers, rice, and pasta, perhaps whole-grain or oat bread for sandwiches and toast, oat breakfast cereal, brown rice with stir-fries, whole barley in soup, or bulgur in salads and casseroles.

● For refined grain products opt for bagels, bread sticks, English muffins, Italian bread, hamburger buns, pita bread, or corn and flour tortillas. Enriched and fortified pasta and white rice are other options. Ease up on croissants, doughnuts, and sweet rolls, which are high in solid fats and/or added sugars.

● Know that many grain products combine whole-grain and refined-grain ingredients. These don't count as a full whole-grain portion. Check the ingredient list;

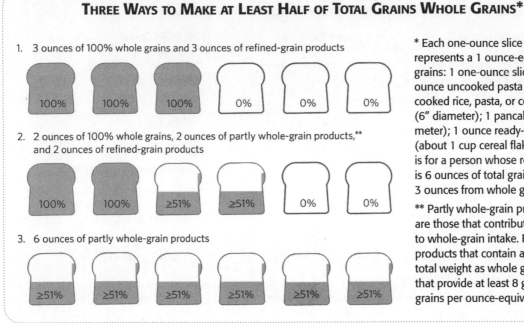

THREE WAYS TO MAKE AT LEAST HALF OF TOTAL GRAINS WHOLE GRAINS*

1. 3 ounces of 100% whole grains and 3 ounces of refined-grain products

    100% 100% 100% 0% 0% 0%

2. 2 ounces of 100% whole grains, 2 ounces of partly whole-grain products,**
    and 2 ounces of refined-grain products

    100% 100% ≥51% ≥51% 0% 0%

3. 6 ounces of partly whole-grain products

    ≥51% ≥51% ≥51% ≥51% ≥51% ≥51%

* Each one-ounce slice of bread represents a 1 ounce-equivalent to grains: 1 one-ounce slice bread; 1 ounce uncooked pasta or rice; ½ cup cooked rice, pasta, or cereal; 1 tortilla (6″ diameter); 1 pancake (5″ diameter); 1 ounce ready-to-eat cereal (about 1 cup cereal flakes). This chart is for a person whose recommendation is 6 ounces of total grains with at least 3 ounces from whole grains per day.

** Partly whole-grain products depicted are those that contribute substantially to whole-grain intake. For example, products that contain at least 51% of total weight as whole grains or those that provide at least 8 grams of whole grains per ounce-equivalent.

Source: Dietary Guidelines for Americans, 2010.

look for those with whole grain or whole wheat as the first ingredient. *See "Three Ways to Make at Least Half of Total Grains Whole Grains" above.*

● Try less common grains, perhaps quinoa, buckwheat, millet, or amaranth, or use couscous, in casseroles and grain-based salads, perhaps pasta salad, rice pilaf salad, or tabouli (made with bulgur). Or enjoy risotto (made with arborio rice) or polenta (made with cornmeal). *Refer to "Today's Grains" in chapter 9.*

● For snacks, choose whole grains such as air-popped popcorn, baked tortilla chips, and rye and whole-grain crackers. When eating refined grains, choose graham crackers, matzos, pretzels, rice cakes, saltines, baked pita chips, and bread sticks.

● For dessert consider angel food cake topped with fruit, graham crackers, and low-fat granola with a dollop of frozen yogurt more often than frosted cake, brownies, and pie, which are high in calories from solid fats and/or added sugars.

Vegetable Group: Vary Your Veggies!

Raw or cooked; fresh, frozen, canned, or dried/dehydrated; whole, cut-up, mashed, or juiced—no matter how you enjoy them, a colorful, bountiful array of vegetables fits within this food group. The more variety and color you eat, the better! *Check chapter 9, "Garden of Eatin': Less Common Vegetables," for more ideas.*

Fresh veggies aren't always available, but you have other healthful options. In fact, frozen or canned vegetables are picked and processed at their peak of quality. The nutrition in all these forms is comparable in their nutrient content to cooked fresh vegetables. *Refer to chapter 14 for tips on cooking veggies to retain nutrients.*

Why Eat Vegetables?

More than a colorful garnish on your plate or a crisp texture in a sandwich, vegetables are loaded with nutrients and phytonutrients, including fiber, vital for your body's health and maintenance. Eating a variety of vegetables as part of a healthy eating pattern overall may help reduce the risk for some chronic diseases.

Key nutrients. Vegetables are important sources of many nutrients, including carbohydrates, vitamins A, C, and E, folate, potassium, and dietary fiber.

Unless you add sauces and other seasonings, most vegetables are naturally low in fat and calories. None has cholesterol.

The nutrient content of vegetables' five subgroups differ somewhat; that's why you need variety. *Dark-green leafy vegetables* are great sources of beta carotene (forms vitamin A) as well as of vitamin C, folate, calcium, magnesium, and potassium. *Red and deep-orange vegetables* supply beta carotene. Some others have more vitamin C; many are rich in folate. Besides their complex carbohydrates, *starchy vegetables* supply niacin, vitamin B_6, zinc, and potassium. *Beans and peas (legumes)* provide protein as well as thiamin, folate, iron, magnesium, phosphorus, zinc, potassium, and fiber. *To learn about their vitamins, minerals, and phytonutrients, refer to "Different Vegetables and Fruits, Different Nutrients" in this chapter, "Phytonutrients for Health" in chapter 6, and "Paint Your Plate with Color!" in chapter 14.*

Important health benefits: Vegetables deliver many important health benefits. The vitamin C they contain not only helps to heal wounds and keep teeth and gums healthy, but also aids iron absorption. Their vitamin A keeps eyes and skin healthy and helps to protect against infections. Their vitamin E works as an antioxidant. Their folate helps form red blood cells and may help reduce the risk of some birth defects. Their potassium helps maintain healthy blood pressure. And their fiber may help maintain digestive health and possibly fill you up with fewer calories.

Vegetables in an overall healthy diet are linked to reduced risk of many chronic diseases, including reduced risk for stroke and heart disease. Some vegetables may be protective against certain cancers. Because vegetables are low in calories per cup compared to some higher-calorie food, they may be useful in lowering calorie intake.

Vegetables: How Much?

Make half your plate vegetables and fruit. The amount of vegetables advised for you depends on your calorie level. For 2,000 calories a day, the advice adds up to $2\frac{1}{2}$ cups of vegetables daily. Most people come up short. *Check "USDA Food Patterns" in the appendices for the amount that matches your calorie level.*

To get the nutrient variety that different vegetables

provide—and their varying health benefits—follow this weekly advice for the vegetable subgroups. If you need 2,000 calories a day, strive for:

- Dark-green vegetables $1\frac{1}{2}$ cups per week
- Red and orange vegetables $5\frac{1}{2}$ cups per week
- Beans and peas (legumes) $1\frac{1}{2}$ cups per week
- Starchy vegetables   5 cups per week
- Other vegetables   4 cups per week

One Cup of Vegetables Equals: For most vegetables, here's a rule of thumb: one cup is either: 1 cup of raw or cooked vegetables or vegetable juice, or 2 cups of raw, leafy greens. To extend the list, these are some vegetables that count as one cup:

Dark-green vegetables:

- 2 cups raw leafy greens (spinach, romaine, watercress, dark-green leafy lettuce, endive, escarole, other leafy greens)
- 1 cup cooked greens (collards, mustard greens, kale, spinach)
- 3 spears (5 inches long) or 1 cup chopped or florets broccoli

Red and orange vegetables:

- 1 cup cooked or raw (sliced or mashed) carrots, pumpkin, sweet potato, winter squash (acorn, butternut, hubbard), tomatoes, red peppers
- 1 large ($2\frac{1}{4}$-inch or more) baked sweet potato
- 1 large (3-inch) raw tomato
- 1 large (3-inch-diameter) red bell pepper
- 1 cup (12) baby carrots
- 1 cup tomato or mixed vegetable juice

Beans and peas:

- 1 cup whole or mashed, cooked dry beans or peas (black, garbanzo, kidney, pinto, or soybeans, or black-eyed peas or split peas)
- 1 cup tofu in $\frac{1}{2}$-inch cubes (about 8 ounces)

Starchy vegetables:

- 1 cup corn, green peas, or diced or mashed potatoes
- 1 large ear (8 to 9 inches) corn, yellow or white
- 1 medium ($2\frac{1}{2}$-to 3-inch-diameter) baked or boiled potato

● 20 medium to long (2½-to-4-inch) strips French fries (contains calories from solid fats)

Other vegetables:

● 1 cup chopped, mashed, or sliced other vegetables (cauliflower, celery, cucumbers, green or wax beans, green pepper, mushrooms, onion, summer squash, zucchini), cooked or raw

● 1 cup cooked bean sprouts

● 2 large stalks (11-to-12-inch) celery

● 2 cups raw iceberg or head lettuce, shredded or chopped

● 1 large (3-inch-diameter) green bell pepper

Vegetable Group: Quick Tips

Eat more veggies! Vary the types and colors—their nutrient and phytonutrient contents differ. Ease up on French fries and fried onion rings, or salads with heavy dressing; their preparation and/or toppings increase the calorie and fat content.

● Add more vegetables to meals. You might add some color and flavor to your pizza or pasta dishes with steamed, sliced vegetables such as zucchini, carrots, broccoli, and bell peppers. Add tomato or cucumber slices and spinach to sandwiches. Top baked potatoes with vegetable salsa or stir-fried veggies. Add spinach to hot soup.

● Try different greens and include dark, leafy greens such as arugula, beet greens, bibb lettuce, chicory, fennel greens, kale, leaf lettuce, romaine, spinach, and watercress in salads.

● Enjoy your vegetable favorites—just more of them! Broaden your vegetable repertoire. Besides green beans and broccoli, try okra, snow peas, or Brussels sprouts. Roast parsnips and beets with your carrots and potatoes. Shred fresh spinach for slaw. Need more ideas? Besides the vegetables noted in this chapter and in chapter 9, a walk through the produce department and grocery aisles may spark your creativity!

● Snack on veggies. Keep cleaned, raw veggies in the fridge, ready for a quick nibble. Tuck a can of 100 percent vegetable juice into your lunch or snack bag.

● As a sandwich side, enjoy broccoli florets, baby carrots, mini bell peppers, or bell pepper strips.

● Enjoy more beans and peas in soup (split peas or lentils), salads (kidney or garbanzo beans), and side dishes (baked beans or pinto beans). Or eat them as a main dish. They have a split personality—count them in either the vegetable group or the protein foods group, but the same bowl of beans can't count for both.

● Eating out? Order vegetables as a starter or side dish. Ask for slaw or a garden salad rather than fries with fast food.

● Shop and prep veggies for good nutrition. *Refer to chapters 12 and 14; you'll find more ways to fit veggies in, too.*

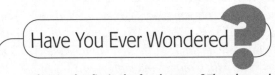

Have You Ever Wondered

. . . where salsa fits in the food groups? That depends on the ingredients. An all-vegetable salsa, perhaps made with beans, counts in the vegetable group. If the salsa has veggies, and perhaps mango or another fruit, your portion counts toward a little from both the fruit and the vegetable groups.

. . . what cruciferous vegetables are? Members of the cabbage family, they get their name from their four-petaled flowers, which look like a crucifer, or cross. They include a diverse variety: arugula, bok choy, broccoli, Brussels sprouts, cabbage, cauliflower, collards, kale, kohlrabi, mustard greens, radishes, rutabaga, Swiss chard, turnip, turnip greens, and watercress. Cruciferous vegetables contain nutrients, as well as phytonutrients with unique health-promoting benefits. This vegetable family has something else in common: a strong cooking aroma. Proper food handling enhances their flavor without intensifying the aroma: (1) eat them soon after you buy them—raw or cooked; (2) cook them quickly, just until tender-crisp; and (3) eat leftovers within a day.

. . . if MyPlate and the USDA Food Patterns apply to other cuisines or countries? These guidelines can apply to many cuisines you enjoy—perhaps Asian, Mediterranean, Latin American, Middle Eastern, and more. That said, many countries have their own food guides and healthy eating guidelines to match their foods, food-related health concerns, eating patterns, and culture. One example is Canada's Food Guide: www.health canada.gc.ca/foodguide.

Fruit Group: Focus on Fruits!

What's in the fruit bowl? All of America's favorites: apples, oranges, and bananas, as well as berries, melons, and some you may eat less often, such as cherries, mangoes, nectarines, pineapples, and kiwifruit. For more variety, fill your fruit bowl with less common fruits, too, such as lychees, loquats, and pomegranates! *Check "Fresh Ideas: Uncommon Fruit" in chapter 9.*

Any fruit or 100 percent fruit juice counts in the fruit group, whether it's fresh, canned, frozen, or dried. Fruit also may be whole, cut up, or pureed. Make most of your fruit choices whole fruit rather than juice. Fruit drinks, even if they provide 100 percent Daily Value for vitamin C, are considered sugar-sweetened beverages, not juice. *Refer to chapter 8 to know why 100 percent fruit juices are advised over fruit drinks.*

Fruit: How Much?

Sweeten your day with fruit! The specific amount depends on your age, gender, height, weight, and level of physical activity. For 2,000 calories a day, you need about 2 cups of fruit a day. Make most of your fruit choices whole fruit rather than juice. *Check "USDA Food Patterns" in the appendices for the amount that matches your calorie level.*

One Cup of Fruit Equals: As a rule of thumb, 1 cup of fruit is 1 cup of cut-up fruit, grapes, or berries or 100 percent fruit juice, or ½ cup of dried fruit. To limit added sugars, choose fruit canned in 100 percent juice instead of heavy syrup. Counting 1 cup with whole fruit takes more estimating:

- 1 cup cut-up fresh, frozen, or canned fruit (apples, bananas, melons, grapes, grapefruit or orange sections, peaches, pears, pineapples, plums, berries, other)
- 1 cup applesauce
- 1 small (2½-inch-diameter) apple
- ½ large (3¼-inch-diameter) apple
- 1 large (8-to-9-inch-long) banana
- 32 seedless grapes
- 1 medium (4-inch-diameter) grapefruit
- 1 large (3¹⁄₁₆-inch-diameter) orange
- 1 large (2¾-inch-diameter) peach

- 2 halves canned peaches
- 1 medium pear (2½ pears per pound)
- 3 medium or 2 large plums
- About 8 large strawberries
- 1 small wedge (1-inch-thick), equal to 1 cup diced (balls), watermelon
- ½ cup dried fruit (raisins, dried plums, dried apricots)
- 1 cup 100 percent fruit juice (orange, apple, grapefruit, other)

Why Eat Fruit?

Fit fruit into your meals and snacks because it tastes good and because fruit provides nutrients and phytonutrients for maintaining overall good health and reducing the risk of disease.

Key nutrients: Like vegetables, the nutrients in fruit vary—the reason for varying your choices! Overall fruit supplies carotenoids, including those that form vitamin A, as well as vitamin C, folate, potassium, fiber, and many other phytonutrients. *"Different Vegetables and Fruits, Different Nutrients" in this chapter shows some sources of each. To learn about the phytonutrients in fruit, refer to chapter 6, "Phytonutrients for Health," and to "Paint Your Plate with Color!" in chapter 14.*

Fruit's sweet flavor comes from its natural sugar, or fructose. Sometimes sugars are added to canned and frozen fruits and fruit juice to enhance flavor or to help maintain quality; choose mostly unsweetened fruit. Most fruits are low in fat, sodium, and calories, and all are cholesterol- free. Two fruits, avocados and olives, contain monounsaturated fat. Avocados also supply beta carotene (which forms vitamin A).

Most juices have little or no fiber, so choose whole or cut-up fruit more often.

Important health benefits: Fruits' vitamin C promotes growth and repair of all body tissues, helps heal cuts and wounds, and keeps teeth and gums healthy. Its fiber aids digestion. And its folate helps your body form red blood cells and, for many women, helps reduce the risk of birth defects.

As part of your overall healthy eating strategy, fruit is linked to some potential health benefits, such as

DIFFERENT VEGETABLES AND FRUITS, DIFFERENT NUTRIENTS

Sources of vitamin A

● Bright orange vegetables such as carrots, sweet potatoes, pumpkins

● Tomatoes, tomato products, and red sweet peppers

● Leafy greens such as spinach, collards, turnip greens, kale, beet and mustard greens, green-leaf lettuce, romaine

● Orange fruits such as mangoes, cantaloupe, apricots, and red or pink grapefruit

Sources of vitamin C

● Citrus fruits and juices, kiwifruit, strawberries, guava, papaya, cantaloupe

● Broccoli, peppers, tomatoes, cabbage (especially Chinese cabbage), Brussels sprouts, potatoes

● Leafy greens such as romaine, turnip greens, spinach

Sources of folate

● Cooked dry beans and peas

● Orange and orange juice

● Deep-green leaves such as spinach and mustard greens

Sources of potassium

● Baked white or sweet potatoes, cooked greens (such as spinach), winter (orange) squash

● Bananas, plantains, many dried fruits, oranges and orange juice, cantaloupe, and honeydew melons

● Cooked dry beans

● Soybeans (green and mature)

● Tomato products (sauce, pasta, puree)

● Beet greens

● Keep frozen, canned, and dried fruit on hand, especially when fresh fruits aren't in season. Choose canned fruit that's packed in juice for less added sugars and calories.

● Go beyond basics; enjoy variety and choose fruit such as prickly pear, papaya, mango, star fruit, figs, kiwifruit, or guava. Try new-to-you varieties of apples, pears, plums, or melons.

● Adapt food prep and recipes to include fresh fruits in season.

● Keep rinsed, fresh fruit and dried fruits handy for quick snacks. Cut up melon or pineapple so it's ready to eat, and store it in the refrigerator. Be aware that the cut surfaces of bananas, apples, and pears will turn brown, so slice them just before you're ready to eat them. (Hint: tossing these cut fruits with citrus juice delays browning.) Dried apricots, apple slices, cranberries, raisins, and prunes (dried plums) are great for pack-and-carry meals.

● Choose 100 percent fruit juice when choosing juice. Mix with sparkling water for a refreshing fizzy drink.

● Enjoy a fruit smoothie from a smoothie bar. Make one at home in your blender. Whirl cut-up fruit (canned, fresh, frozen), juice, and yogurt, frozen yogurt, or milk.

● Add fruit to leafy-green salads or slaw: mandarin orange segments, grape halves, berries, raisins, dried cranberries, chopped apples, or pomegranate seeds.

● Top breakfast cereal, pancakes, pudding, or frozen yogurt with cut-up or pureed fruit instead of sugar syrup or other sweet toppings.

● Blend dried fruits with stuffing and rice dishes. Mix them in muffin batter and bread dough.

● Enjoy fruit as an easy snack, salad, or sweet ending to your meals.

reduced risk for heart disease, and for some fruits, protection from some cancers. As a good potassium source, fruits may help maintain healthy blood pressure, and perhaps reduce the risk of developing kidney stones or possibly help reduce bone loss with age. Fruits' dietary fiber may help reduce heart disease risk, blood cholesterol levels, constipation, and diverticulosis in an overall healthful eating pattern.

Fruit is lower in calories per cup than many higher-calorie foods. For that reason, fruit may help lower calories in your meals and snacks. And fruit's fiber and water may help you feel full with fewer calories.

Fruit Group: Quick Tips

Eat more fruit! Enjoy a variety of fruits, and choose whole or cut-up fruits more often than 100 percent fruit juices.

Dairy Group: Get Your Calcium-Rich Foods!

Dairy foods, including milk, yogurt, and cheese, are calcium-rich! Fat-free and low-fat dairy foods are the most nutrient-rich. If you occasionally choose full-fat dairy foods, know that solid fats contribute to added calories. Added sugars in sweetened milk products, such as flavored milk, some yogurt and drinkable yogurt, and desserts, also contribute extra calories.

A few dairy foods—butter, cream, cream cheese, and sour cream—contribute fat but few other nutrients. They're made from the cream that naturally separates from unhomogenized milk and don't count as foods from the dairy group.

What about soy beverages? If they're fortified with calcium and vitamins A and D, they're considered part of the dairy group. From a nutrition standpoint and for their use in meals, they're similar to milk. However, they don't provide the same package of other nutrients found in milk and milk products. *See "The Vegetarian Way" later in this chapter for the vegan dairy group.*

Refer to chapter 21 for handling lactose maldigestion and intolerance.

Why Consume Dairy Foods?

For healthy bones, consume dairy foods! Over a lifetime, an adequate amount from the dairy group reduces the risk of low bone mass and osteoporosis. Any time is a good time to start consuming enough. Dairy is more than calcium. Milk's other nutrients also keep your body in good working order.

Key nutrients: Dairy foods are the body's best sources of calcium, vitamin D, and riboflavin. Without these foods, getting enough calcium and vitamin D for bone health isn't as easy. Many dairy foods are fortified with vitamin A, and most milk and yogurt are fortified with vitamin D. Dairy foods also are good sources of protein, magnesium, phosphorus, potassium, and vitamin B_{12}, a vitamin available only from animal sources of food. Milk is a better potassium source and lower in sodium than most cheese; in fact, without dairy foods, you may not get enough potassium. Low-fat and fat-free milk provide little or no solid fat. *To compare various types of milk, refer to "Milk: A Great Calcium and Vitamin D Source" in this chapter.*

The nutrient and calorie content of cheese varies. In general, cheese has more total fat, solid fat, cholesterol, and sodium than milk does. That said, fat-free and reduced-fat varieties are available; some have less sodium, too. Cheese with less fat usually has less

cholesterol. Regardless of the fat content, the amounts of other nutrients—calcium, protein, phosphorus, and vitamin D—are comparable.

Dairy foods may contain two types of sugars: naturally occurring lactose and added sugars. Any added sugars in dairy foods come from flavorings added to ice cream, flavored yogurt and milk, and other dairy foods.

Important health benefits: Eating patterns that include milk are generally higher in quality! The bone-health benefits—from childhood through adulthood—of milk and milk products are well known. Calcium in dairy foods is essential for building bones and teeth and for maintaining bone mass throughout life and reducing the risk of osteoporosis later in life. Milk's full nutrient package is vital for health and body maintenance. For example, vitamin D helps maintain proper levels of calcium and phosphorus, thereby helping to build and maintain bones. Its calcium and potassium, especially in yogurt and milk, too, helps maintain healthy blood pressure. These foods also provide cell-building protein.

More healthy eating tips: Most dairy group choices should be fat-free or low-fat, since they have little or no solid fat. To compare, cheese, whole milk, and products made from them are higher in solid fats and

Have You Ever Wondered?

... where fortified foods fit in the food groups? Fortified foods fit in the same food group as their unfortified counterparts. With their added nutrients, they simply provide a nutritional bonus. For example, a cup of calcium- and vitamin D-fortified orange juice can't replace a cup of milk; milk has other nutrients that juice doesn't have. Like any juice, calcium-fortified orange juice counts in the fruit group, with a calcium bonus. Fortified foods can provide a benefit: increasing the amount of certain nutrients or providing them in forms more available to the body.

... where dietary supplements fit in? All healthy people need to get their nutrients from food first. Food group advice doesn't change if you take a multivitamin/mineral supplement. Supplements are merely what their name implies; they're intended to supplement nutrients from the foods you eat, only if needed, not to replace nutrient-rich foods. *See chapter 23 for more about supplements.*

cholesterol. High intake of solid fats in particular raises LDL ("bad") cholesterol in blood, increasing heart disease risk. Using fat-free and low-fat dairy foods also helps you cut calories.

Besides its link to better bone health, consuming milk and milk products may have other health benefits, including reducing the risk of cardiovascular disease and type 2 diabetes and lowering blood pressure in adults.

Dairy Foods: How Much?

How do your dairy food choices stack up? The specific amount depends on your age, gender, height, weight, and level of physical activity. For moderately active kids ages seven and up, the recommended amount is equivalent to 3 cups of dairy foods daily. The advice for younger children is 2 to 2½ cups daily. Many people, teens and adult women especially, don't consume enough!

One Cup of Dairy Foods Equals. Figure 1 cup of milk or yogurt, or 1½ ounces of natural cheese, or 2 ounces of processed cheese as 1 cup from the dairy group. Choose fat-free or low-fat options most often.

- 1 cup or ½ pint container milk (flavored or unflavored) or buttermilk
- 1 cup (8 ounces) yogurt
- ½ cup evaporated milk
- 1½ ounces hard cheese (cheddar, mozzarella, Swiss, Parmesan)
- ⅓ cup shredded cheese
- 2 ounces processed cheese (American)
- ½ cup ricotta cheese
- 2 cups cottage cheese
- 1 cup pudding made with milk
- 1 cup frozen yogurt
- 1½ cups ice cream

Dairy Group: Quick Tips

Consume more fat-free or low-fat milk and milk products such as milk, yogurt, cheese, and/or milk

MILK: A GREAT CALCIUM AND VITAMIN D SOURCE

MILK		CALORIES	CALCIUM (MG)	VITAMIN D (IU)	FAT (G)	SATURATED FAT (G)	CHOLESTEROL (MG)
8 ounces . . .							
buttermilk	fat-free	90	300	0	<0.5	<0.5	5
	low-fat	100	285	0	2	1.5	10
unflavored milk	fat-free	85	300	115	<0.5	<0.5	5
	1% lowfat	100	290	115	2	1.5	10
	2% reduced-fat	120	285	120	5	3	20
	whole	150	275	130	8	4.5	25
flavored milk	fat-free	115*	300	115	<0.5	<0.5	5
	1% lowfat	130*	290	115	2	1.5	10
	2% reduced-fat	190	270	120	5	3	20
	whole	210	280	130	8	5	30
4 ounces . . .							
eggnog		170	165	60	10	5.5	75
evaporated milk	fat-free	100	370	100	<1	<0.5	5
	whole	170	330	100	10	5.5	35
sweetened condensed milk		490	435	10	13	8.5	50

(Figures are rounded.)
*With concerns about added sugars, many dairy producers have reduced added sugars in fat-free and low-fat milk by 38 percent, now with about 30 calories per 8 ounces more than in whole milk. U.S. Department of Agriculture, National Nutrient Database for Standard Reference, Release 24, 2011.

alternatives such as fortified soy beverages. And replace higher-fat milk and milk products with lower-fat versions. You'll cut calories but not calcium or other essential nutrients!

● Fit calcium-rich foods into meals and snacks: milk on cereal, yogurt dip with veggies, cottage cheese as a side dish, or pudding. Try flavored milk (chocolate, strawberry, other flavors) if you prefer.

● If you're lactose-intolerant, you don't need to give up dairy. Instead drink smaller amounts at a time; drink milk with a meal or a snack; and eat yogurt, which often is tolerated better. Or try lactose-free milk, or calcium- and vitamin D-fortified soy beverages. *See chapter 21 for more strategies.*

● Drink thick, creamy buttermilk, or use it in smoothies. Even with its buttery name, buttermilk is usually made from fat-free or low-fat milk. Or make your own fruity drinks by blending milk or yogurt with fruit and ice in a blender.

● Start your day with dairy: low-fat or fat-free yogurt or a yogurt-fruit smoothie with breakfast, or fat-free or low-fat milk on cereal or oatmeal.

● Buy milk to go with a deli or fast-food meal or snack.

● Make oatmeal, other instant cereal, and creamy soups with low-fat or fat-free milk rather than water.

● Lighten up your coffee or tea with low-fat or fat-free milk, not a powdered nondairy creamer. Drink cappuccino, latte, or chai made with fat-free or low-fat milk.

● Use evaporated fat-free milk instead of cream in coffee, on cereals, whipped as a topping, and in recipes calling for cream. Evaporated fat-free milk has a creamy texture and less fat than cream.

● Enjoy cheese on a sandwich, shredded cheese on soup or a salad, or cheese cubes for a snack. Try low-fat or fat-free cheese, or use a smaller amount of sharp cheese for less fat and calories.

● Use plain, low-fat, or fat-free yogurt or cottage cheese (pureed in a blender) as a sour cream substitute.

If you don't consume dairy foods, find other ways to get the calcium and vitamin D your body needs, perhaps from fortified soy beverages and yogurt, juice, cereal, and breads. Also, nondairy foods that contain calcium, but not as much as dairy foods, include canned salmon or sardines with edible bones, some leafy greens (collard and turnip greens, kale, bok choy), some beans (legumes), tempeh, lime-treated corn tortillas, almonds, and tofu processed with calcium salts.

Protein Foods Group: Go Lean with Protein!

Although we use a shortcut name, the protein foods group delivers many protein-rich foods: beef, veal, pork, chicken, turkey, finfish, shellfish, game, eggs, dry beans (legumes), lentils and peas, soybean products (tofu, tempeh, soyburgers, others), nuts, seeds, and nut butter. Beans actually lead a double life. They count toward the protein foods group or the vegetable group, but not both at the same time.

For good health, make most meat and poultry choices lean. Fish, nuts, and seeds contain oils, making them a great meat alternate. Eggs are an economical protein source. Enjoy meatless meals occasionally, too, with dry beans and peas as your lean protein choice.

Why Eat Protein Foods?

Meat, poultry, fish, dry beans and peas (legumes), eggs, nuts, and seeds: they're all protein-rich—and they deliver much more. Some are high in solid fats and cholesterol.

Key nutrients: Besides protein, foods in this group supply varying amounts of iron, zinc, magnesium, B vitamins (thiamin, niacin, vitamins B_6 and B_{12}), and vitamin E. Heme iron in meat, poultry, and fish is better absorbed than nonheme iron from eggs or plant sources of food. Vitamin B_{12} is available only from animal-based foods in the protein foods and dairy groups.

The fat and cholesterol contents within this food group vary. Lean meat and skinless (not fried) poultry are lower-fat choices, yet provide varying amounts of cholesterol. Many finfish have less fat, including less solid fat and cholesterol than meat and poultry do; shellfish tend to be low in solid fat but higher in cholesterol than finfish. Fish with more oil (such as salmon, mackerel, swordfish, and herring) have another benefit: more omega-3 fatty acids (EPA and DHA). *Refer to "Eat Your Omega-3s and -6s" in chapter 5.* By varying your choices and including fish, nuts, and seeds among your protein-rich choices, you boost mono- and polyunsaturated fats, too. Eggs are also a good choline source.

Soybeans contain high-quality proteins, with all essential amino acids. Other excellent protein sources— dry beans and seeds, and nuts—have nearly the high quality that meat, poultry, and fish have. Eating grain foods with these foods during the day completes the amino acid package. A great source of starches (complex carbohydrates), fiber, and other phytonutrients, beans and peas also are cholesterol-free and virtually fat-free. Nuts and nut butters are higher in fat (mostly oils) and calories than beans and peas.

Some nuts and seeds (flax, walnuts) are excellent sources of essential fatty acids, too. Some (sunflower seeds, almonds, hazelnuts) are good vitamin E sources.

Important health benefits: Protein provided by this food group not only builds body cells, enzymes, and hormones, it also supplies an energy source.

Protein foods have a vitamin and mineral package with more health benefits. For example, the B vitamins help with energy production, formation of blood cells and body tissues, and nervous system function. The iron helps carry oxygen in your blood. The magnesium aids in bone building and energy release in your muscles. The zinc not only helps your immune system function, it's part of other body processes, too.

The fat content of protein foods varies. Lean meat (including extra-lean, or at least 90 percent- lean ground beef), skinless poultry, and fish have less total and solid fats. Fatter cuts of beef, pork, and lamb; regular (75 to 85 percent lean) ground beef; regular sausages, hot dogs, and bacon; some luncheon meats such as regular bologna and salami; and some poultry such as duck have more fat. A diet high in solid fats raises LDL ("bad") cholesterol levels in the blood, which increases the risk for heart disease. While egg yolks contain cholesterol, egg whites are cholesterol-free. Organ meats such as liver and giblets also are high in cholesterol.

Fish, nuts, and seeds deliver mostly heart-healthier mono- and polyunsaturated fats. *See "Oils: Go for Healthful Fats" later in this chapter.*

Although nuts and seeds are higher in fat than many other protein foods, their fats are mostly oils. Nuts and seeds are cholesterol-free and provide good sources of

protein, phosphorus, zinc, and magnesium, as well as vitamin E and selenium (two antioxidant nutrients). Their phytonutrients may have other health benefits. As long as portions are small, they're a healthful choice. (*Note:* Peanuts are actually a legume, not a tree nut; their phytonutrient benefits differ.)

Protein Foods: How Much?

The recommended daily amount from the protein foods group is equivalent to about 5 to 7 ounces daily for most adults. This is often a surprise to those who sometimes eat more. That said, you may need to make your choices leaner and more varied!

How much you need depends on your age, gender, height, weight, and physical activity level. *Check "USDA Food Patterns" in the appendices for the amount of your calorie need.*

One Ounce of Protein Foods Is: An ounce is generally 1 ounce of meat, poultry, or fish, or ¼ cup of cooked dry beans, or 1 egg, or 1 tablespoon of peanut butter, or ½ ounce of nuts or seeds. For specifics:

- 1 ounce cooked lean beef, lean pork, or ham
- 1 ounce cooked chicken or turkey, without skin
- 1 sandwich slice (4½ × 2½ × ⅛ inches) turkey

Protein Foods: How Much Is a Portion?

A COMMON PORTION OF . . .	IS EQUIVALENT TO . .
1 steak, small eye or round, or filet	3 ½ to 4 ounces
1 small lean hamburger	2 to 3 ounces
1 small chicken breast half	3 ounces
½ Cornish game hen	4 ounces
1 small can tuna, drained	3 to 4 ounces
1 salmon steak	4 to 6 ounces
1 small trout	3 ounces
1 ounce nuts or seeds*	2 ounces
2 tablespoons peanut butter	2 ounces
1 cup split pea, lentil, or bean soup	2 ounces
1 soy- or beanburger patty	2 ounces

*1 ounce is 23 almonds, 14 walnut halves, or 21 whole hazelnuts.

- 1 ounce cooked fish or shellfish
- 1 egg
- ½ ounce nuts (12 almonds, 24 pistachios, 7 walnut halves)
- ½ ounce seeds (pumpkin, sunflower or squash seeds, hulled, roasted)
- 1 tablespoon peanut butter or almond butter
- ¼ cup cooked dry beans (such as black, kidney, pinto, or white beans)*
- ¼ cup cooked dry peas (such as chickpeas, cowpeas, lentils, split peas)
- ¼ cup baked beans or refried beans
- ¼ cup (about 2 ounces) tofu
- 1 ounce tempeh, cooked
- ¼ cup roasted soybeans
- 1 (4-ounce, 2 ¼-inch) falafel patty
- 2 tablespoons hummus

*Beans can count in either the vegetable group or the protein foods group, but not both. If beans count in the vegetable group, 1 cup of cooked beans is equivalent to 1 cup of vegetables.

See "Protein Foods: How Much Is a Portion?" in this chapter.

Protein Foods Group: Quick Tips

Fit in a variety of foods from the protein foods group—not just lean meat and skinless poultry, but fish, beans and peas, eggs, nuts, and seeds, too. In fact, eat more seafood by choosing a variety of seafood in place of some meat and poultry.

- Choose lean meat and poultry when you shop; *see chapter 12.*

- Prepare meat and poultry to keep them lean. Trim visible fat. Broil, grill, roast, or use other low-fat cooking methods; *see chapter 14.*

- Enjoy fish in place of meat or poultry twice a week. Include fish with more oils, such as salmon, herring, and trout. *Refer to chapter 13 for guidelines on eating fish during pregnancy and breast-feeding.*

- Be sensible with meat, poultry, and fish portions. A portion that fills about one quarter of your plate is enough. You probably need only about 5 to 7 ounces total from the protein foods group daily. Occasionally

it's okay to eat larger portions, but a 12- to 16-ounce steak is more than enough at one meal!

- Build menus around beans and peas, tofu, or tempeh several times a week. Try vegetarian chili or lasagna, vegetable tofu stir-fry, or bean soup. Or mix canned beans into a vegetable salad.

- Enjoy eggs in moderation. To control cholesterol, go easy on egg yolks and whole eggs to keep your total cholesterol intake under 300 milligrams daily. That includes eggs used in prepared and baked foods. Since egg whites and egg substitutes have no cholesterol and little or no fat, use them freely.

- Eat nuts, seeds, and nut butters. A small handful adds flavor and nutrition. Vary your choices—almonds, walnuts, sunflower seeds, and more—since their nutrients and phytonutrients differ.

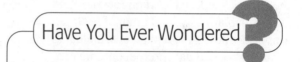

Have You Ever Wondered

. . . if frozen yogurt has the same nutrients as regular yogurt? No. Regular yogurt—plain or fruit-flavored—supplies a lot more calcium. The nutrient content of frozen yogurt varies, and it's similar to low-fat ice cream. No federal standards exist for frozen yogurt. Find the nutrient and calorie content on the food label.

Some regular and frozen yogurts contain active live cultures with possible health benefits; *see "Prebiotics and Probiotics: What Are They?" in chapter 6.* However, for frozen yogurt, very low temperatures slow the action of any live cultures. To find yogurt with live cultures, look for the seal from the National Yogurt Association.

. . . if venison, buffalo, and ostrich are good choices from the protein foods group? Sure. Their nutrient content is similar to that of other meat and poultry: good sources of protein and iron. Their fat content varies. Many types of game—venison, bison, elk, moose, squirrel—are quite lean.

Ostrich tastes like red meat, even though it's poultry. It's very lean—fewer than 3 grams of fat in 3 ounces, which is less than the same amount of beef round or chicken with skin.

● Vary your meals with other protein foods: perhaps tofu, tempeh, and veggie burgers. *For more about protein foods for vegetarian meals see "The Vegetarian Way" in this chapter.*

Oils: Go for Healthful Fats

Like the vegetable oils used in cooking, oils are simply fats that are liquid at room temperature. They come from two main sources: different plants and fish. Common oils include canola, corn, cottonseed, olive, safflower, soybean, and sunflower oils. Some others, such as walnut and sesame oils, make great flavorings. Several other foods are high in oils, too: avocados, nuts, olives, and oily fish such as salmon and tuna.

Mayonnaise, certain salad dressings, and soft (tub or squeeze) margarine are mainly oils without *trans* fats. Use Nutrition Facts labels to find soft margarines with 0 gram of *trans* fat.

Important note: A few plant oils, including coconut, palm, and palm kernel oils, are considered solid (saturated) fats. Other fats are solid at room temperature: butter, beef fat (tallow, suet), chicken fat, pork fat (lard), stick margarine made with hydrogenated fat, and shortening.

Why Consume Oils?

Fat: it's an essential nutrient. For their health benefits, most fats should be monounsaturated (MUFAs) and polyunsaturated (PUFAs), supplied mostly by foods' healthy oils. Some fatty acids in PUFAs are "essential"; *see chapter 5.*

Key nutrients: Not only high in heart-healthier monounsaturated or polyunsaturated fats, oils also are low in saturated fats. Coming from plant-based foods, including vegetable and nut oils, they're cholesterol-free. Oily fish supply another type of polyunsaturated fat: omega-3s. Many oils also supply vitamin E.

Important health benefits. What makes MUFAs and PUFAs healthful? They don't raise LDL ("bad") cholesterol levels in blood, as saturated fats do. Essential fatty acids (from some nuts and seeds) are important for a healthy nervous system and skin, and for kids, they help keep skin healthy. Oils, your body's main source of vitamin E, are important antioxidants. And the omega-3 fatty acids in oily fish may help promote heart health. Most of your fat should be MUFAs and PUFAs. Some PUFAs are essential for health since you're body can't make them from other fatty acids.

Oils: How Much?

The USDA Food Patterns offer specific advice for oils—get enough to provide essential fatty acids for health. Like most Americans, you likely consume

HOW ARE OILS COUNTED?

OILS/FOODS RICH IN OILS	PORTION	AMOUNT OF OIL	CALORIES FROM OIL	TOTAL CALORIES
Vegetable oil	1 tbsp.	3 tsp.	120	120
Margarine, soft (*trans* fat-free)	1 tbsp.	2½ tsp.	100	100
Mayonnaise	1 tbsp.	2½ tsp.	100	100
Mayonnaise-type salad dressing	1 tbsp.	1 tsp.	45	55
Italian dressing	2 tbsp.	2 tsp.	75	85
Thousand Island dressing	2 tbsp.	2½ tsp.	100	120
Olives, ripe, canned*	4 large	½ tsp.	15	20
Avocado*	½ medium	3 tsp.	130	160
Peanut butter*	2 tbsp.	4 tsp.	140	190
Peanuts, dry roasted*	1 oz.	3 tsp.	120	165
Mixed nuts, dry roasted*	1 oz.	3 tsp.	130	170
Cashews, dry roasted*	1 oz.	3 tsp.	115	165
Almonds, dry roasted*	1 oz	3 tsp.	130	170
Hazelnuts*	1 oz	4 tsp.	160	185
Sunflower seeds*	1 oz	3 tsp.	120	165

*Although they provide oils, avocados and olives fit in the fruit group, and nuts, including peanuts, and seeds fit in the protein foods group.
Source: www.ChooseMyPlate.gov.

enough in the foods you normally eat in nuts, fish, cooking oil, and salad dressing.

The recommended amount depends on you: your age, gender, height, weight, and physical activity level. If you need 2,000 calories a day, the recommended daily amount is 27 grams, or about 6 teaspoons, of oils. (One teaspoon of oil is about 4.5 grams.) *Check "USDA Food Patterns" in the appendices for the amount for your calorie need.* You need some healthy oils for health. Yet, like solid fats, they still contain calories, about 40 calories a teaspoon, or about 120 calories per tablespoon. Limit the amount to help balance your calorie intake with the calories your body uses.

One Teaspoon of Oils Equals: A teaspoon of vegetable oils (canola, corn, cottonseed, olive, peanut, safflower, soybean, and sunflower) is easy to measure. *See "How Are Oils Counted?" in this chapter to learn how other sources stack up.*

Oils: Quick Tips

Make the switch—use oils instead of solid fats when you can.

- Use mostly soft tub margarine with 0 *trans* fat in place of stick margarine or butter. If you use solid fats, use just a small amount.

- Consider calories! Use just small amounts of oil in cooking. Limit oil-based salad dressing to 1 or 2 tablespoons.

- Use vegetable oils in place of solid fats in food prep when you can. As a spread, try herbed olive oil or pesto.

- Top pizza with sliced olives, even nuts; use less shredded cheese.

- Use the Nutrition Facts on food labels to choose foods with less saturated and 0 *trans* fat.

Extras: Choose Wisely, within Your Calorie Budget!

Solid fats and added sugars? The USDA Food Patterns give advice for them, too: limit the amount and limit the calories!

Small amounts of solid fats and added sugars—sometimes called empty calories—in foods such as

---

Top Sources: Calories from Solid Fats and Added Sugars

Solid fats and added sugars can make a food or a beverage more appealing. However, they also can add a lot of calories. In some foods, like most candies and sodas, all the calories are empty calories. For Americans most empty calories come from:

- Cakes, cookies, pastries, and doughnuts (contain both solid fat and added sugars)
- Sodas, energy drinks, sports drinks, and fruit drinks (contain added sugars)
- Cheese (contains solid fat)
- Pizza (contains solid fat)
- Ice cream (contains both solid fat and added sugars)
- Sausages, hot dogs, bacon, and ribs (contain solid fat)

Source: www.ChooseMyPlate.gov.

---

breakfast cereal, an oatmeal cookie, or a small bacon slice on a BLT (bacon, lettuce, and tomato sandwich) add flavor. If you follow the food pattern for your calorie level, with nutrient-rich choices, you likely will have a little leeway to eat small amounts of foods with solid fats and/or added sugars—and still meet your calorie goal. (Remember that the term "nutrient-dense," or "nutrient-rich," refers to foods that are mostly fat-free, low-fat, lean, or have no added sugars.)

A small amount of empty calories is okay, but many Americans eat far more than is healthy. That's why the USDA Food Patterns have limits. For a 2,000-calorie-a-day eating plan, that's no more than about 260 calories from solid fats and added sugars—and/or from alcoholic drinks. Your limit is lower if your total calorie level is less than 2,000, and somewhat higher if your calorie level is more, perhaps because you're physically active. *See "USDA Food Patterns" in the appendices.*

How It Works

Empty calories, or those from solid fats and added sugars, are part of your total estimated calorie needs, not in addition to them. Assume that your calorie budget is 2,000 per day. Of these calories, you need to spend at least 1,740 calories on nutrient-rich foods for their nutrient essentials—doable with wise food-group choices. That leaves 260 more calories yet to spend. You can:

- Eat even more nutrient-rich foods from any food group.

- *Or* eat some higher-calorie versions of food-group foods, with more solid fats or added sugars. A few examples: whole milk, cheese, higher-fat meats, sausage, biscuits, sweetened cereal, sweetened baked foods, or sugar-sweetened yogurt.

- *Or* flavor your meals with some added fats or sweeteners, perhaps with sauces, salad dressings, sugar, syrup, or butter—or more healthy oils.

- *Or* enjoy a small portion of candy, soft drink, wine, beer, or other calorie-dense food or beverage.

- *Or* make trade-offs. *See "Save Calories, Spend Elsewhere" in this chapter.*

Whatever option, go easy. The calorie allowance from fats, added sugars, and alcoholic drinks isn't very big. Typically people have just 100 to 300 extra calories per day to spend, especially if they don't move much. The good news is that the more you get your

---

CALORIE DENSE VS. NUTRIENT DENSE

FOOD WITH SOME EMPTY CALORIES	FOOD WITH FEW OR NO EMPTY CALORIES
Sweetened applesauce (contains added sugars)	Unsweetened applesauce
Regular ground beef (75% lean) (contains solid fats)	Extra-lean ground beef (90% or more lean)
Fried chicken (contains solid fats from frying and skin)	Baked chicken breast without skin
Sugar-sweetened cereals (contain added sugars)	Unsweetened cereals
Whole milk (contains solid fats)	Fat-free milk

Source: www.ChooseMyPlate.gov.

---

body moving, the more extra calories you have to spend. Physical activity is the best way to increase your calorie budget overall, including calories from SoFAS (solid fats and added sugars)!

Eat More Food, Fewer Calories!

"More food, less calories" may sound great if you love to eat! In fact, fiber-rich, watery foods deliver more volume to your plate for fewer calories, so fit them into your food-group choices. Ounce per ounce, foods with more fat and with less fiber and water are more calorie-dense, with more calories per ounce. Calorie-dense foods add up to a lot less food for the same calories than those low in calorie density.

To compare, 1 cup of sliced raw carrots has 50 calories, and so does just 0.33 ounce of chips. (Even a small snack bag of chips is at least 1 ounce, or 150 calories.) And the carrots give you more nutrients and fiber, take longer to eat, and can leave you feeling satisfied with fewer calories. Other foods high in volume but low in calorie density include broth-based soups, fruits and vegetables, fat-free and low-fat milk and yogurt, and beans. *Refer to "Food: A Water Source" in chapter 8 for the percentage of water in common foods.*

Tip: a healthful eating pattern can include small amounts of calorie-dense foods such as olives and nuts.

Limiting Solid Fats and Added Sugars: Quick Tips

You can eat empty-calorie foods less often, or make the portions smaller.

Added sugars:

- Remember, beverages count! Drink few regular sodas, sports drinks, energy drinks, and fruit drinks, eat less cake, cookies, ice cream, other desserts, and candies—or just consume small portions. These foods and drinks are the major sources of added sugars for Americans.

- Choose fruit for dessert—and fewer high-calorie desserts.

- Drink water, fat-free milk, 100 percent juice, or unsweetened tea or coffee rather than sugar-sweetened drinks.

- Use the ingredient list on food labels to find foods with little or no added sugars. The total sugars in the Nutrition Facts on packaged foods is another clue, but total sugars also include sugars that are naturally present.

Solid fats:

- Ease up on the major sources of solid fats for Americans: cakes, cookies, and other desserts (often made with butter, margarine, or shortening); pizza, cheese; processed and fatty meats (sausage, hot dogs, bacon, ribs); and ice cream. Or switch to lower-fat versions such as low-fat cheese, lower-fat sausages and hot dogs, and lower-fat ice cream.

- Choose lean meat and poultry, and fat-free or low-fat dairy foods.

- Cook with oils, rather than butter, beef fat, chicken fat, lard, stick margarine, and shortening. Or cook without fat.

- Choose baked, broiled, steamed, or stir-fried foods more often than fried foods.

- Use Nutrition Facts on foods labels to choose foods with little or no saturated fat and no *trans* fat, and use ingredient lists to limit foods with partially hydrogenated oils, which contain *trans* fats.

Now . . . Make a Healthy Eating Plan Your Way!

Eating smart isn't just for today! For your good health and your healthy weight, you need to make wise food choices for a lifetime. For your health:

- *Choose an eating plan:* the USDA Food Patterns, or its vegetarian adaptations, or the DASH Eating Plan, *each described in this chapter.*

- *Make this eating plan yours.* Using your age, gender, and activity level, estimate your daily calorie needs; *see "Estimated Calories Needs per Day by Age,*

Pizza: What Food Group?

Pizza, fajitas, lasagna, and cioppino (fish stew) . . . many foods don't fit neatly into a single food group. Prepared with ingredients from several food groups, mixed foods can count toward your daily totals from two or more food groups. Use your best guesstimate to determine the amounts they represent. Be aware: some mixed dishes contain a lot of fat, oil, or sugar, which add calories.

The amounts of food group foods, fats and oils, and added sugars in any mixed dish depend on how it's prepared. Think about how you could change these dishes to add more vegetables and fruits, and perhaps lower the calories.

Food and Portion	Grain Group (oz. equivalents)	Vegetable Group (cups)	Fruit Group (cups)	Dairy Group (cups)	Protein Foods Group (oz. equivalents)	Calories (estimated)
Cheese pizza—thin crust (1 slice from medium pizza)	1	1/8	0	1/2	0	215
Lasagna (1 piece 3 1/2 inches by 4 inches)	2	1/2	0	1	1	445
Tuna noodle casserole (1 cup)	1 1/2	0	0	1/2	2	260
Bean and cheese burrito (1)	2 1/2	1/8	0	1	2	445
Beef stir-fry (1 cup)	0	1/2	0	0	1 1/2	185
Clam chowder—New England (1 cup)	1/2	1/8	0	1/2	2	165
Clam chowder—Manhattan (chunky—1 cup)	0	3/8	0	0	2	135
Apple pie (1 slice)	2	0	1/4	0	0	280
Pumpkin pie (1 slice)	1 1/2	1/8	0	1/4	1/4	240

Source: www.ChooseMyPlate.gov.

Gender, and Physical Activity Level" in the appendices. With the eating plan see how much you need from each food group for your calorie level. The beauty of these eating plans is their adaptability. As you get older or your activity level changes, adjust the plan for your new calorie target.

● *Get to know the food groups:* Foods in each food group, the recommended amounts, and easy ways to follow the advice.

● *Stay within your day's calorie budget.* Eat the right amounts of food to maintain your healthy weight. Balance calories consumed with calories used in physical activity; move more to spend more! Choose extra calories from solid fats and added sugars but keep within your calorie budget. And learn to fit foods you enjoy into your smart eating plan while sticking to your calorie budget.

● *Track your progress.* Go online, www.ChooseMy Plate.gov, to use the SuperTracker. Input what you eat and drink and your physical activity level to see how your food choices and physical activity stack up against your goals.

● *Take it one step at a time.* Modify your food choices, along with your physical activity level, gradually. That

Have You Ever Wondered ?

. . . where potato chips and corn chips fit in the food groups? Potato chips fit in the vegetable group; corn chips, within the grain group. Yet they supply more fat and more calories (less nutrient density) than most other foods in those groups. Eat them with discretion; try baked varieties, which have fewer calories and less fat. Count their calories as part of the extra calories you may have to spend if you've eaten enough nutrient-rich food group foods and you're still within your calorie budget.

. . . if potatoes can substitute for bread, since they're both high in starches? No. Potatoes are among the starchy vegetables in the vegetable group. Breadfruit, cassava, corn, green peas, hominy, rutabaga, taro, and yautia are some others. Although high in carbohydrates, starchy vegetables have different nutrients and phytonutrients than foods in the grain group. Potatoes, for example, supply vitamin C and potassium; grain group foods supply some B vitamins and iron.

Take Your Taste Buds to the Mediterranean

There's no single cuisine for regions that border the Mediterranean Sea. The dishes of Greece, southern Italy, Spain, southern France, Tunisia, Lebanon, Egypt, and Morocco, for example, are all distinctive, with no one eating pattern. Yet all of these eating patterns typically emphasize grain products (often whole grains), vegetables, beans and peas, nuts, and fruits; small amounts of meat, poultry, and full-fat dairy foods (including yogurt and cheese); more fish; and (except in Muslim areas) moderate amounts of wine. In general, the total fat intake of the Mediterranean diet isn't lower than that of the typical American diet. It's just shifted to more monounsaturated fat (mostly from olive oil).

Traditional Mediterranean eating may have several health benefits. Studies show reduced risk factors for cardiovascular disease, reduced incidence of cardiovascular disease, and a lower death rate. Incidence of these health problems has gone up among many Mediterranean populations who no longer eat in their traditional way. The reasons for this are not yet clear. Other dietary factors, not fully understood, may offer some protection.

Before you switch your eating style, be aware that the health benefits of Mediterranean-style eating may go well beyond food. Traditionally, the people studied in the region also were more physically active. Body weight and genetics are factors, too. And the overall lifestyle was more relaxed.

may be easier than overhauling your whole eating plan and lifestyle at one time. Perhaps start with a change in one meal or snack, just one food group, or one active living strategy today. Then move on gradually toward a healthier you.

DASH to Health

Another healthy eating plan may be right for you: the DASH Eating Plan. DASH stands for Dietary Approach to Stop Hypertension. Developed to help people prevent high blood pressure and other risk factors for heart disease, the DASH Eating Plan is consistent with the Dietary Guidelines. However, it's a guide to smart eating—even if you're not at risk for high blood pressure.

The DASH Eating Plan

Food Group	2,000 Calories	Serving Sizes	Significance for DASH Eating
Grains*	6 to 8	1 slice bread 1 oz. dry cereal ½ cup cooked rice, pasta, or cereal**	Major sources of energy and fiber
Vegetables	4 to 5	1 cup raw, leafy vegetable ½ cup cut-up raw or cooked vegetable ½ cup vegetable juice	Rich sources of potassium, magnesium, and fiber
Fruits	4 to 5	1 medium fruit ¼ cup dried fruit ½ cup fresh, frozen, or canned fruit ½ cup fruit juice	Important sources of potassium, magnesium, and fiber
Fat-free or low-fat milk and milk products	2 to 3	1 cup milk or yogurt 1 ½ oz. cheese	Major sources of calcium and protein
Lean meats, poultry, and fish	6 or less	1 oz. cooked meat, poultry, or fish 1 egg	Rich sources of protein and magnesium
Nuts, seeds, and legumes	4 to 5 per week	⅓ cup or 1 ½ oz. nuts 2 tbsp. or ½ oz. seeds 2 tbsp. peanut butter 2 tbsp. or ½ oz. seeds ½ cup cooked dry beans or peas (legumes)	Rich sources of energy, magnesium, potassium, protein, and fiber
Fat and oils ***	2 to 3	1 tsp. soft margarine 1 tsp. vegetable oil 1 tbsp. mayonnaise 1 tbsp. salad dressing	DASH has 27 percent of calories as fat (including fat in or added to foods)
Sweets and added sugars	5 or less per week	1 tbsp. sugar 1 tbsp. jelly or jam ½ cup sorbet, gelatin dessert 1 cup lemonade	Sweets should be low in fat
Maximum sodium limit****	2,300 mg per day		

* Whole grains are recommended for most grain servings.
** Serving sizes vary between ½ to 1 ¼ cups depending on cereal type. Check the Nutrition Facts on the label.
*** Fat content in different fats and oil varies: For example, 1 tbsp. of regular salad dressing equals 1 serving; 1 tbsp. of low-fat dressing equals ½ serving; 1 tbsp. of fat-free dressing equals 0 serving.
**** The DASH Eating Plan consists of patterns with a sodium limit of 2,300 mg and 1,500 mg per day.

Source: Dietary Guidelines for Americans, 2010.

Similar to the food patterns in the USDA Food Patterns, the DASH plan provides the nutrients needed for overall health. It limits saturated fats and cholesterol, and focuses on eating more foods that are rich in potassium, calcium, magnesium, protein, and fiber. Its approach: more fruit, vegetables, fat-free or low-fat milk and milk products, whole grains, fish, poultry, seeds, and nuts. The DASH plan advises less sodium, sweets, added sugars, sugary drinks, fats, and red meats than are found in the typical U.S. diet.

As a way to lower blood pressure, the DASH eating plan is a taste-appealing switch from just no-salt-added eating. It may be an alternative to medication. The DASH Eating Plan has several calorie levels. Daily food-group servings vary depending on calorie needs. *To see how a plan for 2,000 calories per day stacks up, see "The DASH Eating Plan" in this chapter. See the appendices for "The DASH Eating Plan at Various Calorie Levels."*

For more about blood pressure and the DASH plan, see chapter 22.

The Vegetarian Way

With today's focus on wellness, occasional meatless meals and vegetarian eating have become more mainstream. Among the reasons people cite are potential health benefits, concerns about the environment, animal welfare, and their belief in nonviolence. For some, religious, spiritual, or ethical reasons define their strict vegetarian lifestyle. Several religions advocate vegetarian eating—for example, Hinduism and the Seventh-Day Adventist Church. For some, vegetarian eating reflects their ethical approach to addressing world hunger. Others simply prefer the flavors and food mixtures of vegetarian dishes. And some may recognize that a plant-based diet may cost somewhat less. For all these reasons, eating for overall good health remains a common goal.

Vegetarian: What Type?

Being vegetarian may be a way of eating, or for some, a whole lifestyle. Nonvegetarians may just enjoy the flavors and want the health benefits of dishes made with beans, vegetables, and perhaps whole grains—regularly or as an occasional switch from everyday fare.

Broadly defined, a vegetarian diet means avoiding foods from animal sources. Instead, plant-based food sources—grains, beans and peas (legumes), vegetables, fruits, nuts, and seeds—form the basis of the diet. As a matter of choice, many vegetarians eat dairy products and perhaps eggs.

Vegetarians are described in these ways:

● *Lacto-ovo-vegetarian*, one who chooses an eating approach with dairy products and eggs but no beef, pork, poultry, or fish. The prefix "lacto" refers to milk; "ovo" refers to eggs. Most vegetarians in the United States fit within this category.

● *Lacto-vegetarian*, one who avoids beef, pork, poultry, fish, and eggs (and egg derivatives such as albumin or egg whites) but eats dairy products.

● *Strict vegetarian, or vegan*, one who eats no animal products: beef, pork poultry, fish, eggs, milk, cheese, or other dairy products. Vegans frequently also avoid foods with animal products as ingredients, too: for example, refried beans made with lard; fries cooked in beef tallow; baked goods made with butter, eggs, or albumin (from eggs); margarine made with whey or casein (from milk); foods flavored with meat extracts; and foods with gelatin (from animal bones and hooves). Some avoid honey, which is made by bees. *Fruitarian* diets are vegan diets based on fruits (including avocados and tomatoes, which are botanically fruits), nuts, and seeds.

● *Semivegetarian, also called flexitarian*, one who usually follows a vegetarian eating plan with limited amounts of poultry, fish and other seafood, pork, or beef, perhaps as a condiment or side dish. (*Note:* Many semivegetarians avoid beef.)

Health Benefits? Likely So!

Either approach, vegetarian or nonvegetarian, can be healthful—or not. Their health benefits depend on the foods chosen and the amounts eaten over time. If you plan well, vegetarian eating can match the healthy eating advice of the Dietary Guidelines, as well as the USDA Food Patterns.

Scientific research shows a positive link between vegetarian eating and health. It's associated with a lower body mass index, a reduced risk of cardiovascular disease and hypertension, and a lower overall cancer rate. Some studies link vegetarian eating to lower blood pressure, less risk for type 2 diabetes, and lower LDL ("bad") cholesterol levels, too.

What may account for the health benefits? Potential health-promoting benefits of vegetarian eating may come from the nutrients and phytonutrients (or plant components) in the overall food choices—and the bounty of plant-based foods! On average, vegetarians consume overall fewer calories; a smaller portion of calories from fat, especially saturated fat; and more fiber, potassium, and vitamin C. Their body mass index, an indicator of overweight and obesity, is generally lower. Lifestyle factors likely play a role, too; many vegetarians are physically active, avoid smoking, and drink alcoholic beverages in moderation.

A vegetarian eating approach isn't always healthier! Like any way of eating, it too can be high in calories as well as in total fat, solid fats, cholesterol, added sugars, and sodium. Poorly planned, with a heavy reliance on high-calorie foods, such as many quick-serve options, it also may come up short in fruits, vegetables, whole grains, and calcium-rich foods—without enough of the nutrients and fiber they provide.

Alert: Some women "go vegetarian" as a disguise for an undiagnosed eating disorder; *see chapter 2.*

Vegetarians: Nutrients to Focus On

Vegetarian eating plans can provide enough of all the nutrient essentials. Nutrient adequacy is just a matter of wise food choices and of following food group advice for your calorie level.

For vegetarians who consume dairy products and perhaps eggs, nutrition issues don't differ much from those of nonvegetarians. For vegans, however, getting enough calories to maintain a healthy weight may be a challenge, especially for growing children and teens. For vegetarians, nutrients that may need special attention include protein, iron, zinc, calcium, vitamin D, and vitamin B_{12}.

Protein. For vegetarians, questions about protein often arise. Why? Because vegetarians eat less—or perhaps no—foods of animal origin; lean meat, poultry, fish, eggs, and dairy foods are all sources of concentrated protein. Except for vegans, adequate protein generally isn't a concern. Almost every food of plant origin except fruit contains protein—at least a small amount. Beans, seeds, nuts, nut butters, and soy products (edamame, tofu, tempeh, textured vegetable protein, soyburgers) are good sources; for lacto-ovo vegetarians, eggs and dairy foods are, too.

An adequate supply of all essential amino acids comprise complete protein. Together they build and repair body cells and promote growth. Combining different protein sources at the same meal to make complete protein in the same meal isn't necessary. *See "Protein for Vegans" in chapter 4.*

Essential Fatty Acids. Somewhat like amino acids that comprise proteins, fats are made of fatty acids. Among them, alpha-linolenic acid (ALA), a type of omega-3, and linoleic acid, an omega-6, are essential to health, and for children, growth; the body can't make them. In the body, ALA converts to DHA and EPA, which are both omega-3 fatty acids. Besides maintaining a healthy nervous system and cell membranes, omega-3s may help protect against some chronic diseases, such as heart disease.

Vegetarian diets tend to be low in omega-3s, but often high in omega-6 fatty acids. The imbalance can interfere with the heart health benefits of omega-3s. Omega-6s come from corn, safflower, and sunflower oils.

Vegetarians are urged to consume alpha-linolenic acids from plant-based ingredients—for example, canola oil, soy oil, walnuts, ground flaxseed, and soybeans—since they convert to DHA and EPA omega-3s. Fatty fish and some eggs supply omega-3 fatty acids for some vegetarians.

Iron. Especially for vegetarian children, teens, and women of childbearing age, iron may be an issue. Iron carries oxygen in the blood. Foods of plant origin contain nonheme iron, a form that isn't as well absorbed as heme iron in meat and other foods (except eggs) of animal origin.

● Consume foods that contain nonheme iron: beans and peas, iron-fortified and whole-grain cereals and breads; some dark-green leafy vegetables (such as spinach or beet greens); seeds; prune juice; some dried fruits (dried apricots, prunes, raisins); and blackstrap molasses; and for lacto-ovo-vegetarians, eggs.

● To improve the absorption of nonheme iron sources

in meals, include vitamin C-rich food: for example, citrus fruits, 100 percent juice, broccoli, tomatoes, and bell peppers.

● If you're a semivegetarian, or flexitarian, eat a little poultry and fish. That too helps with nonheme iron absorption.

● If you cook foods in iron pots or skillets, some iron from the pots or skillets may pass into food—a good thing! That's especially true when ingredients being cooked are high in acid, such as tomatoes, and when you simmer foods (such as soups and stews) for a while.

Zinc. A mineral essential for many body processes, growth, and immunity, zinc may come up short in a vegetarian diet. For lacto-ovo-vegetarians, dairy foods and eggs provide zinc. In addition, many foods of plant origin contain zinc—but its bioavailability is less than from animal foods. For more zinc:

● Eat whole-grain foods, many types of beans (white beans, kidney beans, chickpeas), fortified breakfast cereals, seeds, and nuts. Grains lose zinc when processed to make refined flour. Fiber and phytates in plant-based foods can inhibit zinc absorption; however, phytates are broken down when yeast fermentation makes bread dough rise.

● Be cautious of zinc supplements. In large doses, they can have harmful side effects. If your doctor or registered dietitian recommends a supplement, stick with a vitamin-mineral combination with 100 percent or less Daily Value (DV) for zinc.

Calcium. Dairy foods are excellent calcium sources for lacto-vegetarians. Vegans can get enough calcium from calcium-fortified foods and some plant-based foods, but it may take more planning:

● Try tofu and tempeh processed with calcium, calcium-fortified soy or rice beverages, broccoli, almonds, soybeans, some greens (kale, collards, mustard greens), okra, rutabaga, bok choy, dried figs, or tortillas (made from slaked lime-processed corn).

● Look for calcium-fortified products: perhaps juice, bread, cereal bars, and cereal. Note that these grain products may not be vegan.

● Be aware: beet greens, rhubarb, spinach, Swiss chard, and a grain called amaranth supply calcium. However, these foods contain oxalates that bind cal-

cium, blocking its absorption. Some grain products also contain small amounts of calcium, but they may contain phytates that block calcium absorption, too.

● As a vegan, if you can't consume enough calcium from food, talk to your doctor or a registered dietitian about a calcium supplement with vitamin D.

Vitamin D. Lacto-vegetarians just need to consume enough vitamin D-fortified milk; some yogurt also is vitamin D-fortified. However, vegans need another vitamin D source. Your body needs enough vitamin D to absorb calcium effectively.

● If you're a vegan, check the Nutrition Facts on food labels—some breakfast cereals, some soy and rice beverages, some cereal bars, and some calcium-fortified juices are fortified with vitamin D.

● If you're in doubt, talk to your doctor or a registered dietitian about taking a vitamin D supplement at the level that's right for you. Choose one that contains 100 percent Daily Value (DV) per day.

Vitamin B_{12}. For vegetarians who consume dairy products or eggs, getting enough vitamin B_{12} isn't a concern; this vitamin is widely available in foods of animal origin. Plants supply vitamin B_{12} only when soil with vitamin B_{12}-producing microorganisms clings to fruits and vegetables. In the United States, fruits and vegetables are scrubbed clean before they're eaten.

Vegans need a reliable vitamin B_{12} source. Foods fortified with vitamin B_{12} or a vitamin B_{12} supplement are advised. Since vitamin B_{12} isn't absorbed as well with age, older vegetarians who consume dairy foods or eggs benefit by taking a supplement as well. A few tips:

● Look for vitamin B_{12}-fortified products: breakfast cereals, soy or rice beverages, or soy burger patties.

● Be aware that seaweed, algae, spirulina, and fermented plant foods such as tempeh and miso aren't good vitamin B_{12} sources, even if the package says so. Their vitamin B_{12} is inactive, or not in a form that the human body can use. Vitamin B_{12} in beer and other fermented foods isn't reliable, either.

● If your healthcare professional advises a supplement, find one with 100 percent DV for vitamin B_{12}. Check the Supplement Facts. Cyanocobalamin is the most bioavailable, or easily absorbed, form of vitamin

B$_{12}$. Vitamin B$_{12}$ in fortified foods and supplements is produced synthetically from bacteria, not from animal sources.

● Consider nutritional yeast if it's grown in a medium that's enriched with vitamin B$_{12}$, such as Red Star Vegetarian Support Formula Nutritional Yeast. Don't count on yeast to supply vitamin B$_{12}$; yeast typically used in baking doesn't supply any. Check the label.

See chapter 4 for more about protein, chapter 5 for more about essential fatty acids, and chapter 6 for more about calcium, iron, zinc, and vitamins B$_{12}$ and D and their food sources.

Food Patterns: Vegetarian-Style!

The USDA Food Patterns have two adaptations for vegetarians: for vegans with only plant-based foods, and for lacto-ovo-vegetarians with milk, milk products, and eggs. Planned carefully, both can provide enough nourishment needed for good health and for growing children and teens. Once you know how, being a smart vegetarian takes no more effort than any other approach to healthful eating. *See "USDA Food Patterns for Vegetarians" in this chapter.*

The general advice, *addressed in "A Food Guide for You" in this chapter,* applies to vegetarian eating, too. That includes ounce equivalents for amounts from the food groups. Read on for tips especially important for vegetarians.

Vegetarian Way: Grains

● Make grain dishes, especially whole grains, a centerpiece of your menu—perhaps tabouli, barley, rice pilaf, risotto, wild rice or buckwheat dishes, gnocchi, or polenta. Quinoa is a high-protein, grainlike seed that offers substantial benefits to vegetarian eating. Besides their other benefits, whole grains supply zinc, which may come up short for vegetarians.

● Add cooked grains to many foods. Stuff vegetables (eggplant, bell peppers, cabbage, zucchini) with cooked grain mixtures: rice, oats, and barley, among others. Blend cooked grains with shredded vegetables and perhaps tofu for vegetable patties or croquettes. Toss cooked grains, perhaps quinoa or whole-wheat pasta, with stir-fried vegetables. Add cooked bulgur, barley, and brown rice to soups, stews, and chili.

● Choose fortified breakfast cereals. Read the Nutri-

tion Facts panel on food labels for added nutrients, including iron, vitamin B$_{12}$, calcium, and zinc.

Vegetarian Way: Vegetables

● Vary your veggies! Especially if you're vegan, choose vegetables that have more calcium: dark-green leafy vegetables (such as kale, mustard, collard, or turnip greens), bok choy, and broccoli. Dark-green leafy vegetables also supply iron.

● Choose vegetables that are high in vitamin C—for example, broccoli, tomatoes, and green and red peppers. Vitamin C helps your body absorb iron in eggs and in plant-based sources of food. *See "Vitamin C: More Jobs Than You Think!" in chapter 6.*

● Plan meals with different vegetables, not just garden salads, baked potatoes, and fries. In that way you get the nutrient and phytonutrient benefits of variety.

Vegetarian Way: Fruits

● Enjoy a variety of fruits, including those rich in vitamin C, such as citrus fruits, melons, and berries. Among the other benefits, vitamin C-rich fruit is an important partner for the iron from eggs and plant-based foods. *For more about vitamin C, see chapter 6.*

● Look for calcium- and vitamin D-fortified juice, especially if you're a vegan.

Vegetarian Way: Dairy and Dairy Alternatives

● Choose low-fat and fat-free dairy foods if you're lacto-ovo-vegetarian, *as described for the dairy group earlier in this chapter.*

● Especially if you're vegan, choose soy beverages that are fortified with calcium and vitamins A and D. They can provide calcium in amounts similar to milk, and they're usually low in fat and cholesterol-free. *Important note:* Check for added sugars in soy beverages; many plain varieties use modest amounts of brown rice syrup, while flavored varieties such as vanilla and chocolate flavors use significantly more sweetener.

Read the Nutrition Facts on food labels to compare. Milk supplies about 300 milligrams of calcium per 8-ounce serving; choose soy beverages with at least this much. If soy-based products aren't calcium-fortified, they do not count as a dairy group option.

● Look for calcium-fortified soy yogurt and soy cheese, too.

● Avoid overloading on high-fat cheeses to replace meat in mixed dishes. Consider using lower-fat cheese, which is readily available in most grocery stores.

As an aside, calcium-fortified orange juice, rice milk, and other nondairy "milk" don't count in the dairy group.

Vegetarian Way: Protein Foods

● Eat beans and peas as one of your main protein foods. Besides protein, they're also good sources of iron and zinc, similar to meat, poultry, and fish. Beyond that, beans and peas are excellent sources of fiber, potassium, folate, and more. *For ways to cook them, see chapter 14.*

● Be creative with soy protein foods such as tofu, tempeh, textured vegetable protein, and gardenburgers. Try them in stir-fry dishes, casseroles, pasta dishes including lasagna, soups, and burger patties. Use these foods in place of beef. *See "Soy Good?" in chapter 4.*

● If you eat eggs, watch how many. For cardiovascular health, limit your cholesterol intake to fewer than 300 milligrams a day; one large egg yolk has about 185 milligrams of cholesterol. The American Heart Association notes that up to seven eggs a week is okay for heart health. Still, cut back on cholesterol from other sources, such as cheese, butter, and cream. Make egg-based dishes lower in cholesterol by substituting egg whites for some whole eggs. Examples of egg-based dishes include quiche, omelettes, frittata, scrambled eggs, French toast, egg salad, and egg foo yung.

For more about vegetarian eating, see

● "Going Meatless for Dinner"—chapter 11.

● "Stocking the Vegetarian Kitchen"— chapter 12.

● "Adapting Recipes for Vegetarians"— chapter 14.

● "Vegetarian Dishes in the Global Kitchen"— chapter 15.

● "For Vegetarian Babies . . ."—chapter 16.

● "Feeding Vegetarian Kids and Teens"—chapter 17.

● "The Vegetarian Mom"—chapter 18.

● "Vegetarian Fare for Older Adults"— chapter 19.

● "Vegetarian Athletes"—chapter 20, page 550.

Have You Ever Wondered

. . . how to adopt a vegetarian eating style? Start with small steps. For example, replace meat in meals with beans, tempeh, or tofu, perhaps in pizza, sandwiches, tacos, chili, soups, stews, and casseroles. Order a vegetarian meal when you eat out; get inspiration from many ethnic restaurants. Give meat alternatives, such as soy-burger patties and soy hot dogs, a try as you're learning to prepare more plant-based foods. If you're vegan, switch to soy: calcium- and vitamin D-fortified soy beverage and soy yogurt in place of cow's milk or yogurt. Take stock of your whole day's food choices—not just single foods or dishes—for overall nutrition.

. . . if "vegetarian" on a food label means "low-fat," too? No. Foods labeled as vegetarian on package labeling or restaurant menus may contain high-fat ingredients. Foods that can be higher in fat include textured soy patties, soy hot dogs, soy cheese, refried beans, and snack bars. Even tofu may have more fat than you'd think: 4 ounces (about ½ cup) have about 95 calories and 6 fat grams, mostly from polyunsaturated fats, compared with about 145 calories and 4 fat grams in 3 ounces of cooked lean beef round steak. Read the label's Nutrition Facts panel to compare calories and nutrients in a single serving.

. . . if a macrobiotic diet is nourishing? Like any approach, the answer lies in how the overall eating plan stacks up to today's healthful eating guidelines. A macrobiotic diet has been described as predominantly vegetarian, emphasizing fewer processed foods. Food choices are mostly grains (40 to 60 percent), vegetables (25 to 30 percent), and legumes (5 to 10 percent), with other foods, including miso soup, sea vegetables, seeds, nuts, and fruits, among other foods, eaten to a lesser extent. Some who follow a macrobiotic diet consume limited amounts of fish. For the record, the Zen macrobiotic diet, followed several decades ago typically for spiritual reasons, is different and highly restrictive.

● Include nuts, nut butters (almond butter, cashew butter, peanut butter), seeds, and seed spread (tahini, or sesame seed spread). They, too, supply protein and an array of phytonutrients. Since they're fairly high in fat, go easy even though most fat from nuts is unsaturated.

Vegetarian Way: Oils

● As for nonvegetarians, choose oils over solid fats; oil and tub margarine instead of stick margarine. Oils from nuts, seeds, avocados, and olives, as part of a vegetarian eating plan, are great sources.

● For vegans (who don't eat fish), consume plant-based foods—flaxseed, soybean, and canola oils, as well as walnuts, soy nuts, and ground flaxseed—with alpha-linolenic (ALA) fatty acids that convert to DHA and EPA fatty acids. *See chapter 5.*

Vegetarian Way: Solid Fats and Added Sugars

● A vegetarian eating plan doesn't automatically mean low in solid fats, added sugars, sodium, or calories. Follow the same advice for nonvegetarians *described earlier in this chapter.*

USDA FOOD PATTERNS FOR VEGETARIANS

Here's the daily advice for a 2,000-calorie-a-day eating plan. For a different calorie intake level, check the vegetarian adaptations of the USDA Food Patterns in the appendices.

	LACTO-OVO VEGETARIAN*	VEGAN*
Fruit	2 cups	2 cups
Vegetables	2½ cups, to eat as:	2½ cups, to eat as
Dark-green vegetables	1½ cups per week	1½ cups per week
Red and orange vegetables	5½ cups per week	5½ cups per week
Beans and peas (legumes)**	1½ cups per week	1½ cups per week
Starchy vegetables	5 cups per week	5 cups per week
Other vegetables	4 cups per week	4 cups per week
Grains	6 oz. equivalent, to eat as:	6 oz. equivalent, to eat as:
Whole grains	3 oz. equivalent	3 oz. equivalent
Refined grains	3 oz. equivalent	3 oz. equivalent
Protein foods	5½ oz. equivalent to eat as:	5½ oz. equivalent, to eat as:
Eggs	4 oz. per week	4 oz. per week
Beans and peas**	10 oz. per week	13 oz. per week
Soy products	12 oz. per week	10 oz. per week
Nuts and seeds	13 oz. per week	15 oz. per week
*Dairy***	3 cups	3 cups (vegan dairy)***
Oils	19 g. (about 4 teaspoons)	18 g. (about 4 teaspoons)
Maximum SoFAS (solid fats and added sugars)	258 calories	258 calories

*For ounce equivalents, see the food group discussion earlier in this chapter for the USDA Food Patterns.
**The total recommended amount for beans and peas is the sum from the vegetable and protein foods groups. For a 2,000-calories-a-day eating plan, that is 1½ cups + 10 ounces per week = about 4 cups cooked for lacto-ovo-vegetarians, and 1½ cups + 13 ounces per week = about 5 cups cooked for vegans. (An ounce-equivalent of beans and peas is ¼ cup.)
***The vegan dairy group is composed of calcium-fortified beverages and foods from plant sources such as calcium-fortified soy beverage, calcium-fortified ice milk, tofu made with calcium sulfate, and calcium-fortified soy yogurt.

Source: Dietary Guidelines for Americans, 2010.

CHAPTER 11

Meals and Snacks
Healthy Solutions!

Do you prefer a hearty breakfast or a light morning bite? A big meal at lunchtime or in the evening? Snacks or no snacks? Three meals a day or several minimeals?

No approach is healthier than another if you follow a healthful eating pattern matched to your calorie needs, *as described in chapter 10*. One meal, one snack, or one day of food choices won't make or break your health. And you don't need to eat foods from all food groups at every meal. What you eat consistently on most days over the long term is what counts!

As you make plans for breakfast, lunch, dinner, and snacks, consider how they fit into the big picture—a healthful eating pattern that's right for you. For these eating events, apply what you learned in chapter 10. *And refer to the "Sample Menus for a 2000-Calorie Food Pattern" for seven days in the appendices.*

Breakfast Matters

"No time," "nothing to eat," "woke up too late," and "on a diet": People give many reasons for breakfast skipping or skimping. Despite its benefits, breakfast may be the most neglected and skipped meal of the day. Some blame their body clock for not feeling hungry when they wake up. "Not hungry" may result from stress; stress hormones can affect hunger cues. With today's hectic lifestyles, others come up short on time and energy first thing in the morning—or they'd rather spend a few more minutes in bed. Some falsely believe

that skipping breakfast is effective for weight control.

Most people acknowledge that eating breakfast is the healthful way to start the day. Yet compared to even a decade ago, fewer people start their day with breakfast, notes research from the International Food Information Council Foundation.

So just what is breakfast? There's no one definition or breakfast food. You might say it's the first meal of the day, or food eaten before your daily routine kicks in, or what you eat within two hours of waking up, or anything eaten between 5:00 and 9:00 a.m., or perhaps before 10:00 a.m. Or maybe it's cereal, milk, and sliced banana, or eggs, toast, juice, and coffee. It can be all these, and more.

Why Breakfast?

Do you eat, skip, or skimp on breakfast? What you do likely affects the rest of your morning, and perhaps your day. According to research, breakfast eaters tend to have more strength and endurance, and better cocentration and problem-solving ability. Eating breakfast

---

Click Here! Websites to Know . . .

● Ten Tips Nutrition Education Series
  (with tips on menu planning),
  http://www.ChooseMyPlate.gov/
  tipsresources/tentips.html

See "Resources You Can Use" for more websites.

is linked to better attitudes toward work or school, and higher productivity in late morning, as well as better ability to handle tasks that require memory.

On the flip side, breakfast skippers are more likely tired, irritable, or restless in the morning. And breakfast skimpers? Eating even small food amounts helps restore blood glucose stores, but a heartier breakfast offers more benefits. Research supports many benefits for eating breakfast regularly.

An Energizing Start

Breakfast is your body's early morning refueling stop. After 8 to 12 hours without a meal or a snack, your body needs to replenish its glucose (blood sugar) with food. Because your brain has no stored reserves, it, too, needs a fresh supply of glucose, its main energy source. Sustained mental work—in school or at work—requires a large turnover of glucose in the brain. Your muscles also need a replenished blood glucose supply for physical activity—whether it's a morning workout or a walk from the bus stop to work or even from your desk to the printer—to get you through the day.

Your food choices for breakfast can make a difference in your morning's energy level. Eating a variety of food, with a mix of carbohydrates, proteins, and fats, provides a sustained release of energy. That delays hunger symptoms for several hours and helps maintain blood glucose levels. To compare, a breakfast of just fruit or fruit juice, or perhaps candy or a regular soft drink, provides quick blood glucose, causing an energy surge. After about an hour, blood glucose levels and energy decline, bringing on hunger symptoms.

The Nutrient Connection

Breakfast contributes more than calories or food energy. The good news is that total intake of vitamins, minerals, and fiber for the day is usually higher for those who eat a morning meal regularly.

Among its other benefits, breakfast provides a jump start for fitting enough fruit, vegetables, whole grains, and calcium-rich dairy foods into your day. For example, 100 percent orange juice provides more than vitamin C; it's also a good potassium source. Whole-grain and other fiber-rich cereals and breads boost your fiber intake; fortified ready-to-eat cereals and bread deliver folate, iron, and more. And cereal with milk or yogurt is a great way to fit calcium and vita-

min D into your day. To get the most out of your bowl of cereal, drink your cereal milk! A breakfast with whole-grain cereal, milk, and citrus juice can provide 100 percent of the vitamin C, 33 percent of the calcium, thiamin, and riboflavin, and a good supply of fiber, iron, folate, and other nutrients for a day.

On the other hand, breakfast skippers may not make up the nutrients they miss in the morning. If you have to skip a meal, try to make up what you missed in other meals or with snacks.

Breakfast and Learning

Breakfast may help prepare children and teens to learn. Although inconclusive, many studies indicate that kids who regularly eat a morning meal tend to perform better in school. The reasons? It may be linked to better memory, grades and test scores, school attendance, mood, and psychosocial behavior.

While adults may condition themselves to overcome symptoms caused by breakfast skipping, children probably can't. They experience the very real effects of short-term hunger.

Morning hunger may affect learning significantly by reducing concentration, problem-solving, and muscle coordination. That's especially hard on young children because basic skills—reading, writing, and arithmetic—are often taught first thing in the morning. Consider the long-term effect of transient hunger on learning. When children can't reach their learning potential day after day, they potentially can fall farther and farther behind.

Kids who eat breakfast are more likely to be present in class. Stomach aches or hunger pangs, caused by breakfast skipping or skimping, may result in morning visits to the school nurse. And breakfast skippers tend to be tardy or absent from school more often. Breakfast eaters often behave better in school, too.

Many schools provide breakfast. If your child doesn't eat breakfast at home, encourage school breakfast, if available. *See "For Kids Only—Today's School Meals" in chapter 17.*

Breakfast for Healthy Weight, Better Health

There are more reasons to eat breakfast beyond improved nutrient intake.

A morning meal is linked to weight loss and maintenance, although the reasons aren't clear. What's in the breakfast, or perhaps its timing, may make a difference. For example, a breakfast of cereal, including high-fiber cereal, and milk as a regular breakfast choice has been linked to healthy weight; one reason may be that it's satiating, or filling. Breakfasts that are very high in calories are associated with a higher body mass index (BMI). Compared to breakfast skippers, people who eat breakfast may not be overly hungry for a midmorning snack or lunch; the chance for impulsive snacking or eating more for lunch is less for those who eat breakfast. Breakfast skippers, including older children and teens, are at higher risk for overweight and obesity, have a higher BMI, and are more likely to gain weight.

Breakfast eating also may offer benefits for heart health, digestion, and bone health. Common breakfast foods—whole-grain breads and cereals, dairy products, fruit, and 100 percent fruit juice—and the nutrients, fiber, and pre- and probiotics they provide likely factor in. Emerging evidence suggests that breakfast eating also may have a positive effect on insulin levels and for reducing the risk of metabolic syndrome. Much more research is needed to explore these links.

Beating Breakfast Barriers

For you or for children, every excuse or apparent breakfast barrier has a solution! If you have kids, you're their best role model. Children who see their parents eat breakfast will more likely eat breakfast, too. To overcome these barriers to breakfast, try these tips, and *check the ideas in "One-Minute Breakfasts, Quick Lunch" on this page.*

Not Hungry When You Wake Up? Start with a light bite, perhaps 100 percent juice and whole-wheat toast. Later, perhaps midmorning, when you feel hungry, eat something more that adds variety to your food choices: perhaps a hard-cooked egg, low-fat or fat-free yogurt, or a fruit-yogurt smoothie.

No Time? Just Forgot? Get breakfast food, bowls, spoons, and juice cups ready the night before. And keep quick-to-fix foods on hand, such as ready-to-eat breakfast cereal, instant oatmeal, bagels, whole-grain toaster waffles, whole-grain bread for toast, yogurt, fresh fruit, canned fruit in juice, 100 percent juice, low-fat or fat-free milk, cheese, and cottage cheese. Also, set your alarm clock a few minutes earlier.

Too Much Effort? Plan on a breakfast that's easy to make and that goes with you: for example, a carton of yogurt; a whole-wheat bagel spread with peanut butter; or grapes, rye crackers, and cheese.

Want to Eat Less to Lose Weight? That probably won't work! In fact, skipped meals often lead to overeating later. A morning meal with a lean protein food and a whole-grain food actually may aid weight manage-

One-Minute Breakfasts, Quick Lunch

Each easy breakfast is packed with nutrients from three or more food groups. Good for a light lunch, too!

- ready-to-eat cereal topped with sliced banana, sunflower seeds, and low-fat yogurt
- bran muffin and low-fat yogurt topped with berries
- peanut butter or hummus on whole-wheat toast or soft tortilla, and fat-free milk or bottled yogurt drink
- cheese or lean-meat pizza slice and 100 percent orange juice
- instant oatmeal topped with dried cranberries and grated cheese
- breakfast smoothie (milk, fruit, and bran whirled in a blender)
- toasted whole-wheat waffle topped with fruit, nuts, and ricotta cheese
- granola topped with canned peaches (packed in juice) and low-fat yogurt
- whole-grain bagel topped with fruit chutney, baby carrots, and fat-free milk
- lean ham or deli meat on a toasted English whole-wheat muffin; vegetable juice
- low-fat yogurt with granola and cut-up fruit
- heated leftover rice mixed with beans, peppers, and cilantro, and vegetable juice or milk
- banana dipped in low-fat yogurt and rolled in granola or nuts
- heated leftover rice with chopped apples, nuts, and cinnamon, and 100 percent fruit juice
- breakfast wrap with cut-up fresh or canned fruit and yogurt cheese (*see chapter 5*) rolled in a whole-wheat tortilla, and chocolate low-fat milk
- whole-grain toast with nut butter and 100 percent juice

ment, so you won't be hungry by midmorning. *See "Breakfast for Healthy Weight, Better Health" earlier in this chapter.* Choose mostly whole-grain breakfast foods, fruits, 100 percent juice, lean meat, and low-fat or fat-free dairy foods. Limit bacon, breakfast sausage, hash browns, and biscuits with gravy; their higher fat content delivers calories!

Don't Like Breakfast Foods? That's okay. Breakfast can be any food you like, even soup, a chicken or lean-beef sandwich, or leftovers. If traditional breakfast foods seem boring, add interest with a new yogurt flavor, or an unusual fruit on your cereal. *For more ideas, refer to "Breakfast: Ready to Learn, Healthier Weight!" in chapter 17.*

For breakfast away from home, refer to "Break-FAST" and "Breakfast on the Road" in chapter 15.

Workplace Eating Dilemmas, Smart Solutions

Today's world of work demands high productivity. To reduce stress, and perhaps even increase your work output, eat for success! Remember, too, that your workday meals are regular meal events that need to deliver good nutrition to your overall eating pattern. *See chapter 10.*

● Start your workday with breakfast. You'll replenish the blood glucose stores you need for sustained mental work and physical activity. You'll also stave off midmorning hunger that may reduce your concentration. *See "Breakfast Matters" in this chapter.*

● Take short stress breaks: perhaps a brisk ten-minute walk. Stretch your muscles, and hold for 30 seconds. Relieve shoulder and neck tension by tilting your head from side to side and from front to back. Or switch tasks for a while. Avoid the urge to nibble for stress relief. Keep the candy bowl off of your desk!

● Take time for lunch—even when you're under time pressure. Eating lunch may help you avoid an afternoon dip in your energy level. That's especially true if your lunch provides a mix of foods, such as protein foods and whole grains, that have staying power.

Feel sleepy in the afternoon anyway? Your overall sleep habits, age, and body cycle may cause drowsi-

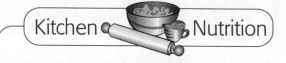

Jazz Up Cooked Cereal

For a great grain breakfast, add flavor and nutrition to cooked cereals (instant or not) such as oatmeal, cream of wheat, grits, brown rice, or whole-grain couscous:

● Use fruit juice—apple, orange, or other 100 percent juice—or low-fat or fat-free milk as the cooking liquid.

● To cooked cereal, blend in grated cheese (perhaps low-fat), chopped fruit (apple, peach, banana, kiwifruit), dried fruit (chopped apricots, papaya, dates, raisins), or nuts.

● Fortify cooked cereal with dry milk for more calcium.

● Liven it up with spices: ground cinnamon, nutmeg, allspice, or cloves.

● Top it with fresh fruit of any kind!

ness. New research also suggests that a midafternoon slump may be normal and induced by hormones. For some people, high-carbohydrate meals may increase serotonin, contributing to drowsiness. To stay alert all day, get enough regular sleep at night. If you feel sleepy in the afternoon, a 10-to-20-minute nap (if your workplace allows) might be enough to revive you.

● Carried lunch? *See chapter 13 for tips on a carried lunch packed with food safety in mind.*

● When you go out for lunch, think first before ordering an alcoholic drink, which may make you drowsy. Sparkling water with a lemon twist makes a great "cocktail" when you need to feel alert at work. When you handle potentially dangerous equipment or drive as part of your job, drinking and working is risky. Blood-alcohol levels from two drinks may stay with you the better part of the afternoon.

● Need a snack break? Bring snacks with you if your choices are limited at work. Choose single-serving (100-calorie) snack packs, or preportion your own at home to control amounts. Bring snacks to fill in food group snacks; *see "Snacks Count!" later in this chapter.* If your snacks are perishable, keep them in the workplace fridge or a cold-insulated container. And control any urge for mindless nibbling at the computer.

● Enjoy a cup of coffee or tea if that helps wake you up in the morning. Switch to decaf or water if caffeine bothers you.

● Reach for milk during your coffee break; perhaps bring it from home in a clean, insulated water bottle. Choosing milk as your snack (or coffee break) drink could help reduce your osteoporosis risk later in life.

● What about office parties? Enjoy just a small piece of cake or a single cookie. When it's your turn to bring doughnuts, bring bagels and fruit instead.

● Get your coworkers moving with you. Walk or take a fitness class over the lunch hour. Take time to use the workplace gym if it's an employee benefit. Team up for an after-work volleyball, softball, or bowling league.

Healthy Eating, Active Living from Your Home Office

Work from an office at home? Many do. If you're used to a company cafeteria or a nearby deli, you may need to redesign your eating approach.

● Keep a routine in your life. Instead of rolling out of bed and into your home office at the computer, start with breakfast, and perhaps a morning walk. Try to set a regular lunchtime.

● Stock your kitchen with food for nourishing, quick-to-prepare workday meals and snacks. A chef's salad, heated leftovers, or made-ahead chili with rye crackers and milk are easy to prepare.

● Occasionally change your lunch venue. Make a lunch date with others who work from home or who work in traditional settings. The social contact that goes with eating with others, and out of your home, is good for you.

● Take advantage of working at home for dinner food prep. As a break, start after-work meals. Perhaps simmer bean soup, or put a turkey breast, roast, or dinner casserole in the oven.

● Need a work break? Opt for a walk outside rather than a walk to the fridge.

● Make time to stay active. When you work at home, you miss the routine walk from the parking lot, bus, or train. However, you have unique opportunities for an action break, such as walking the dog, digging in the garden, or swimming in the neighborhood pool.

What's for Dinner?

No matter when you eat your big meal of the day or whether you have time to cook or eat out, or need to eat on the run, plan a meal to fit your overall eating plan. Tossing a quick salad, pouring a glass of low-fat milk, switching to whole-wheat bread, or topping ice cream with sliced fruit doesn't take effort, but each of these steps can make your dinner healthier and more flavorful.

To translate healthy eating advice into everyday dinners, or any meal, start with these planning tips. Then consider how you can make over your everyday meals.

● Avoid oversized portions. Eat the right amount of calories for you.

● Make half your plate fruits and vegetables. Eat red, orange, and dark-green vegetables, such as tomatoes, sweet potatoes, and broccoli, in main and side dishes. Plan fruit for dessert.

● Make half your grains whole grains. Try brown rice, and whole-grain pasta and bread. For the rest, choose enriched grains without much added sugars or solid fats.

● Switch to fat-free or low-fat milk. They have the same nutrient package as whole milk with less fat and calories.

● Vary your protein choices. Twice a week, make seafood the protein food on your plate. Eat beans, a great source of fiber, too.

● Base your meals on these foods: vegetables, fruits, whole and enriched grains, fat-free or low-fat milk and dairy products. Compare sodium in foods such as soup, bread, and frozen meals—and choose the foods with lower numbers.

● Drink water instead of sugar-sweetened drinks. A 12-ounce can of soda has about ten packets of sugar.

● Include these foods occasionally, not every day: cakes, cookies, ice cream, candies, sweetened drinks, pizza, and fatty meats.

● Enjoy your food, but eat less.

"What's on the Day's Menu for the Whole Family?"
in this chapter shows how each meal can fit into the

day's food choices. For the basics of meal planning, see "Start by Planning" in chapter 14.

Meals for Time-Pressed Lifestyles

Like many people, you may spend 45 minutes or less preparing a family meal (compared with 2½ hours 50 years ago). In fact, spending fewer than 15 minutes preparing a meal is all some people devote to dinner prep! And like others, you may not decide on the menu until the end of the workday. Sound familiar?

When time is short, don't give up on healthful eating. Just take shortcuts to save time and energy. A simple meal can be as healthful as one that takes more time. Make it easy!

● Buy foods for assembly, or speed-scratch, cooking: for example, precut stir-fry vegetables; shredded cabbage; prewashed salad greens or spinach; skinless chicken strips; and grated cheese. Even thin-sliced, lean deli meat is quick for stir-fried recipes.

● Plan ahead. Have a week's worth of meals in mind. Include plan-over meals, or meals made from leftovers of another meal, in your menu plan; for example, grilled chicken Caesar salad, made with sliced, leftover chicken breasts.

Four Quick-Assembly Meals Made with Foods on Hand

● *Chef's Salad.* Toss a chef salad with greens, any raw veggies on hand, lean deli meat, and vinaigrette. Serve with whole-grain bread, fresh or canned fruit in juice, and low-fat or fat-free milk.

● *Veggie Omelet.* Cook a vegetable omelet with leftover vegetables or no-salt-added canned vegetables and shredded cheese. Serve with whole-wheat toast and 100 percent fruit juice. (It's great for any meal of the day!)

● *Chicken Stir-Fry.* Stir-fry sliced chicken breast with frozen, canned, or fresh vegetables (perhaps mushrooms, peppers, carrots, beans, asparagus). Serve with brown rice or whole-wheat couscous, frozen yogurt with fruit for dessert, and unsweetened tea.

● *"Homemade Pizza."* Top a frozen pizza with any veggies on hand in any form—fresh, frozen, or canned. Serve with fruit and low-fat or fat-free milk. Or keep prepared pizza crust on hand to create your own.

● Have a backup meal waiting in the wings in case you get home too late to prepare a meal, or your original plan doesn't pan out as you hoped. It's okay to improvise with ingredients you have on hand. *See "Four Quick-Assembly Meals Made with Foods on Hand" on this page.*

● Prepare ingredients ahead of time. For example, wash and trim broccoli florets. Skewer kebobs with vegetable and meat pieces the night before. Cook lean ground meat ahead for soft tacos.

● Prepare meals that pack variety in just one dish. Try chicken fajitas in a soft taco. Stuff tuna, salmon, and vegetable salad into a pita. Prepare a ham and spinach quiche. Make a chef's salad with no cooking. Prepare risotto with seafood, Swiss chard, and shredded cheese, or stir-fry with noodles, tofu, and vegetables.

● Use quick cooking methods. Stir-frying, broiling, and microwaving are faster than baking or roasting. Slice meat and poultry thinly for faster cooking.

● Use cooking equipment to cut food preparation time. Rinse and dry vegetables in a salad spinner. Slice hard-cooked eggs and mash avocados with a pastry blender. Shred small amounts of cheese with a vegetable peeler. Thaw foods quickly in a microwave oven.

● Organize your pantry and refrigerator so healthful options are visible and in easy reach for you and your children.

● Keep your counters free of clutter and food so you have room to prepare meal with less stress.

● Serve assemble-your-own menus: perhaps deli sandwiches, minipizzas on English muffins, or burgers with veggies and cheese toppings that your family can assemble to personal preference.

● Prepare multiple batches. It's as easy to cook double or triple batches of ground beef; freeze the extra for tacos or spaghetti later. For example, simmer enough pasta for two days. Serve it hot one night with meat sauce, then chilled in a salad with tuna, parsley, and low-fat salad dressing the next.

● Cook on weekends and save food prep time on weekdays. Freeze leftovers in individual-meal containers for quick thawing midweek.

● Stock up with quick-to-fix foods: pasta, rice, frozen and canned vegetables and fruits, bread, lean deli meats, prewashed greens, presliced fruit or vegetables, salsa, canned beans, milk, yogurt, and cheese, among others. Check the Nutrition Facts to make healthier choices; *see chapter 12 for tips on label reading.* With a wide variety of great choices on hand, you won't need to worry about what's for dinner. *See chapter 14, "Stocking the Kitchen."*

● Although often more costly, buy prepared meals at your supermarkets. They simply need to be cooked, heated, or assembled on your plate. Just make a simple side dish, perhaps a tossed salad, and you're ready to eat. For example, buy a heat-and-eat pot roast sold in the meat case of the supermarket and serve with a microwaved potato and green beans. *For tips on take-out food, see chapter 15.*

● Involve everyone in the family from start to finish, from planning to serving. Preparing a meal can be everyone's responsibility. *For age-appropriate kitchen tasks for children, see chapter 17.*

● Time-strapped? Buy a rotisserie chicken. Serve it with salad, whole-grain bread, and low-fat or fat-free milk.

● Stay flexible. Switch your meal plans around if you need to accommodate unexpected family activities. You can always eat a breakfast menu for a light supper if time is short.

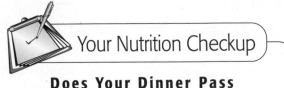

Your Nutrition Checkup

Does Your Dinner Pass These Tests?

☐ *Color-Crunch Test:* Try to choose fruits and vegetables with a variety of colors. Vary the textures, too!

☐ *Whole Test:* Serve a whole-grain version of the bread, rolls, rice, or pasta in your meal to help you make at least half of your grains whole.

☐ *½–¼–¼ Test:* Fill your plate half with vegetables and fruits, one quarter with grain foods (mostly whole grain), and one quarter with lean protein foods. (This general guideline isn't as easy to use with mixed dishes, but try.)

Use MyPlate as a visual cue to healthy eating. *See chapter 10 and www.ChooseMyPlate.gov.*

The Family Table

Can you get your family together at mealtime at least a few times a week? Research shows that family meals promote healthier eating—more fruits, vegetables, and fiber; less fried food; and often fewer calories. And they do far more than put healthful food on the table.

In our haste to get meals prepared, we may forget: Mealtime gives time to talk, listen, and build family relationships. And it's a chance for parents to be good role models for healthful eating. Try to make it routine.

● Set a regular family mealtime. Pick a time together.

● Enjoy more table time, less cooking time. Make quick, simple meals (even a sandwich, fruit, and milk) to give more table time together.

● Turn off the TV. Let phone messages go to voice mail. Focus mealtime on family talk.

● Keep table talk positive. Everyone gets to talk and to listen. Sitting around a table, not side by side at a counter, helps.

● Keep table time realistic—not so long that the pleasure goes away.

Source: R. L. Duyff, 365 Days of Healthy Eating from the American Dietetic Association, New York: John Wiley & Sons, Inc., 2004.

For more on the family table, see chapter 17.

Going Meatless for Dinner

Pasta salad with vegetables. Polenta topped with homemade tomato sauce and freshly grated Parmesan cheese. Bean burritos. Portobello mushroom sandwich layered with stir-fried onions and peppers. Split-pea soup with rye bread. Whether you choose a vegetarian eating style or not, these dishes add food variety, interest, and flavor to smart eating.

If you're planning a meatless meal:

● Build your meal around protein foods such as beans and peas, tofu or tempeh, or eggs if you eat them. Go easy on high-fat cheeses as a meat replacement.

● Experiment with vegetarian food products (soy protein or beans) created as meat alternatives. They're made to look and even taste like meat or poultry. For example, try veggie burgers in place of beef or turkey patties. For outdoor grilling, cook soy hot dogs, marinated tofu or tempeh, and veggie kabobs. These foods are usually lower in saturated fat and cholesterol-free.

● Adapt main dish recipes typically made with meat or poultry, such as lasagna and chili, into vegetarian dishes. It's a way to boost vegetables in your meal and

WHAT'S ON THE DAY'S MENU* FOR THE WHOLE FAMILY?

	1,600 Calories	2,000 Calories	2,400 Calories
Breakfast			
wheat-bran flakes topped with	1 cup	1 cup	1 cup
fat-free milk	½ cup	1 cup	1 cup
banana	½ small	½ small	1 medium
whole-wheat toast with	1 regular slice	1 regular slice	2 large slices
soft margarine	1 teaspoon	1 teaspoon	2 teaspoons
orange juice	¾ cup	¾ cup	1 cup
Lunch			
tuna fish sandwich with			
rye bread	2 regular slices	2 regular slices	2 regular slices
tuna, packed in water, drained	2 ounces	2 ounces	3 ounces
celery	1 (5-inch) stalk	1½ (5-inch) stalks	1½ (5-inch) stalks
romaine lettuce, shredded	¼ cup	¼ cup	¼ cup
tomato	1 medium slice	2 medium slices	2 medium slices
mayonnaise	½ packet	1 packet	½ packet
pear	½ medium	1 medium	1 medium
milk, fat-free	1 cup	1 cup	1 cup
Snack			
dried apricots	¼ cup	¼ cup	¼ cup
fruit yogurt, low-fat	½ cup	¾ cup	1 cup
whole-wheat crackers	4	4	6
peanut butter	½ tablespoon**	½ tablespoon**	1 tablespoon
baby carrots, raw	6	6	6
Dinner			
roasted chicken breast	1 small	1 small	3 ounces
(skinless, boneless)	(2½ ounces)	(2½ ounces)	
baked sweet potato, no peel	1 small	1 medium (5-inch)	1 large
peas and onions with	½ cup	¾ cup	¾ cup
soft margarine	1 teaspoon	1 teaspoon	1 teaspoon
leafy greens salad with	1 cup	1½ cups	1½ cups
sunflower oil and vinegar dressing	½ tablespoon**	1 tablespoon	1 tablespoon
whole-wheat roll with	1 medium	1 medium	1 medium
soft margarine	(2½-inch across)	(2½-inch across)	(2½-inch across)
	1 teaspoon	1 teaspoon	1 teaspoon
fat-free milk	1 cup	1 cup	1 cup

*Planned using the SuperTracker from www.ChooseMyPlate.gov.
**½ tablespoon = 1½ teaspoons

cut solid fats and cholesterol at the same time. *See chapter 14.*

For a full day's vegetarian menu that follows the USDA Food Pattern adapted for vegetarians, see "What's on the Vegetarian Menu?" on this page.

Snacks Count!

Snacking: Is it a type of food? An eating event? Or frequent eating? There's no single definition. With its many different definitions, the link between snacking and health is hard for research to discern.

Yet, at the office, in the car, by the TV or computer, at a sports event, in a movie theater—snacking is part of American life that can add to the nutrition bottom line, or contribute unneeded calories, solid fats, added sugars, and sodium. It's all about making smart snacking choices that work for you—and that takes planning!

Why Snack?

Carefully chosen, sensible snacks are part of a healthful eating pattern. They can supply foods and nutrients that often come up short during the day. Snacks offer

---

What's on the Vegetarian Menu?

To make food preparation fast and easy, choose dishes that everyone—vegetarians and non-vegetarians—around your table will enjoy. This vegetarian menu was planned for a 2,000-calorie-a-day eating plan, using the SuperTracker from www.ChooseMyPlate.gov.

Breakfast

1 cup oatmeal* made with ½ cup fat-free milk or calcium- and vitamin D-fortified soy beverage with ½ ounce (22 almonds) roasted almonds and 2 tablespoons raisins

1 regular slice whole-wheat toast with 1 tablespoon jelly

½ cup orange juice

8 ounces coffee or tea

Lunch

1½ cups hearty lentil soup

¼ cup carrot and ¼ cup green pepper sticks with ¼ cup salsa

1 small whole-wheat muffin

1 cup fat-free milk (or calcium- and vitamin D-fortified soy beverage)

Snack

½ small bagel with 1 tablespoon peanut butter

8 ounces unsweetened iced tea with fresh lemon slice

Dinner

Rice and beans made with ¾ cup kidney beans (no fat added), ½ cup rice (cooked without fat), and ¼ cup chopped, raw tomatoes

¾ cup steamed broccoli with 1 tablespoon lemon juice and 1 tablespoon sesame seeds

½ cup fresh fruit salad, no dressing

1 small slice Italian bread

1 cup fat-free milk (or calcium- and vitamin D-fortified soy beverage)

½ cup fruit sorbet

Snack

Fruit smoothie made with ½ cup plain, fat-free yogurt (or soy yogurt), and ½ cup sliced strawberries

Calories	1,962
Grains	7 ounces
Vegetables	2½ cups
Fruit	2½ cups
Dairy	3 cups
Protein Foods	5½ ounces
Oils	4 teaspoons

*or ready-to-eat breakfast cereal fortified with vitamins B₁₂ and D

Note: Rinse and drain canned kidney beans and choose reduced-sodium prepared foods to reduce sodium.

a great chance to eat more vegetables, fruits, whole-grain foods, and low-fat and fat-free dairy foods.

For active children and teens, snacks can supplement meals. Because their stomachs are smaller, children may need to eat more often to get the calories (food energy) they need—and to provide foods missing from their meals. Physically active, growing teens may need the added calories that snacks supply. No evidence shows that frequent eating is linked to overweight in very young children. *For more about snacking for kids and teens, refer to "Healthful, No-Cook Snacks for Kids" and "Great Snacking!" in chapter 17.*

For adults, a snack can provide an energy boost and satisfy midday hunger. If you haven't eaten for three or more hours, a snack may help bring up your blood glucose level; your body uses the stores in your liver in about 4 to 6 hours. A meal or a snack replaces them.

Older adults with small appetites or limited energy may find several small meals easier to handle. And many enjoy the social value of snacking with others. *See chapter 19 to learn more.*

For athletes of every age, snacks help fuel the increased energy demands of their sports. In fact, a light snack about two hours before exercise, rather than exercising on an empty stomach, may improve performance. A low-fat snack with carbohydrates and some protein is a good choice—perhaps low-fat yogurt with fruit; crackers and low-fat cheese; or a granola bar. Include fluid for hydration. Because timing is individual, adjust to what works best for you. *See chapter 20.*

That said, snacking often gets a bad rap, for good reason. Too often, people snack mainly on energy-dense, low-nutrient foods and drinks, then skimp on nutrient-rich foods and drinks at meals—or perhaps overdo on calories. Calcium-rich foods are a case in point. Compared with moderate snackers, research suggests that people who frequently consume a lot of added sugars in drinks or snacks tend to take in less calcium. It's likely that they're consuming these foods instead of calcium-rich dairy foods.

Myths about Snacking

Snacking: a smart habit—or not? Actually, there's no need to feel guilty about snacking. In fact, here's the truth behind common snacking myths.

Did You Know . . .

- munching on a handful of baby carrots can meet your day's vitamin A needs?
- preschoolers get nearly one third of their calories (food energy) from snacks?
- a planned snack can help prevent overeating?
- watching television tends to increase snacking—particularly high-calorie "goodies"?
- larger snack containers add up? People eat more when the package is bigger!

Source: Academy of Nutrition and Dietetics.

Myth: Snacks are fattening!

Fact: There's no direct link per se between snacking and body weight. The issue is total calories in and out that make a difference. Snacking may have weight-control advantages. Eaten during the stretch between meals, snacks help take the edge off hunger, helping you avoid overeating at meals. For smart snacking, choose foods carefully to fit within your day's calorie target; be sensible with megasize and empty-calorie snacks and drinks.

Myth: Snacking causes cavities.

Fact: Frequent snacking can promote cavities. The longer teeth come in contact with food, particularly any food with carbohydrates, the more time bacteria in plaque have to produce acids that damage tooth enamel. Foods with carbohydrates include grain products, fruit, vegetables, and milk, as well as regular sodas and candy.

To control a plaque attack, consume the whole snack at one time rather than constant nibbling. Choose snacks that aren't sticky. Brush and/or floss afterward to remove food that sticks to and between teeth, or rinse your mouth with water. Some cheeses have qualities that may protect against cavity formation. *For more about oral health, refer to "Your Smile: Carbohydrates and Oral Health" in chapter 3.*

Myth: Snack foods aren't good for you.

Fact: To the contrary, a snack can be any food! How healthful they are depends on what foods you choose. Choose snacks such as baby carrots or a tangerine and fill in the food-group gaps in your day's meal plan.

Ease up on those that are high in solid fats, added sugars, and calories, such as cupcakes, cookies, candy, and regular soft drinks.

Myth: Snacking isn't a good habit for kids to learn.

Fact: With their high-energy needs and small stomachs, most children need snacks. And so do teens. Three daily meals often aren't enough to provide all the nutrients and calories (food energy) they need. The advice for parents: help children learn good snacking habits. And keep nutrient-rich food-group snacks that kids enjoy easily available. Help them learn snack habits that satisfy hunger without overeating.

Myth: Snacks spoil your appetite.

Fact: It's all about timing! Eaten two to three hours before meals, a small snack, such as a banana or half a turkey sandwich, won't ruin your appetite. Snacks may quell hunger pangs so you are less likely to overeat at the next meal.

Myth: Healthful snacking means giving up fun foods.

Fact: Any food can be a snack—even sensible amounts of chips, candy, and soft drinks. *Again, use the USDA Food Patterns, described in chapter 10, as your guide.*

Two Food-Group Snacks

- whole-grain cereal and milk
- fruit smoothie (fruit or 100 percent juice with low-fat or fat-free milk or yogurt)
- yogurt and fresh fruit
- peanut butter on whole-wheat crackers
- pita bread and hummus (chickpea dip)
- apple or pear slices topped with cheese
- bagel chips (oven-baked) and salsa
- dried cranberry and peanut mix
- whole-wheat pita or tortilla stuffed with lettuce, tomato, cucumber, and low-fat dressing
- raw veggies with a cottage cheese or yogurt dip
- plain microwave popcorn and 100 percent fruit juice
- quesadilla (soft tortilla and cheese, folded and heated)
- flaked tuna or salmon and chopped celery with low-fat mayonnaise
- microwave-baked potato topped with salsa
- microwave-baked sweet potato topped with cheese shreds

If you eat a higher-calorie snack, balance it with less at mealtime. Remember, the more physically active you are, the bigger your calorie budget.

Snacking Smart: Plan!

Chosen wisely, snacks can work for you. Plan—to make between-meal eating a valuable part of your healthful eating style.

- Plan your snacks. Keep a variety of tasty, nutrient-rich, ready-to-eat snacks wherever you need a light bite to take the edge off hunger. Then you won't be limited to available snacks from vending machines, fast-food restaurants, convenience stores, or your own randomly stocked kitchen.

- Make snack calories count—without overspending. Choose foods to fill food-group gaps in your day's eating plan. Consider snacks as minimeals that can help you fit more fruit, vegetables, whole grains, and low-fat or fat-free dairy foods into your day. *Refer to "A Food Guide for You" in chapter 10, and "Two Food-Group Snacks" on this page.*

- Go easy on energy-dense snacks (candy, juice drinks, soft drinks, others) with more fat, especially solid fats and added sugars, and/or sodium. Make them occasional choices that fit your day's eating plan.

- Snack when you're hungry—not because you're bored, frustrated, or stressed. Feed an emotional urge to munch by walking the dog, checking your e-mail, or calling or texting someone instead.

- Snack on sensible portions. Choose a single-serve container; put a small helping in a bowl, rather than eating directly from the package; skip mega- or super-size drinks and snacks.

- Use food labels to make snack choices. If a snack package has two servings and you eat the whole amount, you double the calories, solid fats, and sodium in one label serving! *For more on label reading, refer to "Today's Food Labels" in chapter 12.*

- Make snacking a conscious activity. Overeating is all too easy if you mindlessly nibble as you watch TV or spend your time online.

- Eat small snacks well ahead of mealtime. A light bite two to three hours before a meal probably won't interfere with your appetite. Instead it may divert a temptation to snack heavily right before dinner. To stave off hunger longer, pick snacks with protein and fiber, such as peanut butter on celery, or cheese and whole-wheat crackers.

Snack Choices: Easy, Convenient, Nourishing

For any snacking situation, choose snacks by the calories and nutrients they supply.

● Make nutrient-rich snacks more easily available in your kitchen: whole fruit, washed and cut-up raw veggies, fat-free or low-fat yogurt and milk, cottage cheese, low-fat cheese, string cheese, lean deli meat, hummus or salsa, 100 percent fruit juice, frozen juice bars, frozen yogurt, whole-grain crackers, pita bread, dried fruit, nuts, or nut butter.

● Keep healthful snacks at work in case of late or busy workdays: mini-cans of water-packed tuna, instant oatmeal or couscous, dried fruit or single-serve fruit cups, whole-wheat crackers, snack-size cereal boxes, boxes of raisins, soy nuts, plain microwave popcorn, fat-free whole-grain granola or cereal bars. For bars, check the package label for calories per serving; choose those with whole grains, nuts, and dried fruit.

● Choose smart vending machine snacks: small bag of peanuts, pretzels, almonds, trail mix; dried fruit (raisins, cranberries, apricots); whole-grain granola or cereal bars; 100 percent fruit or vegetable juice; graham or animal crackers; whole-wheat crackers with peanut butter or cheese; microwaveable soup or oatmeal; and, if available, whole fruit, and low-fat or fat-free milk (flavored or unflavored).

● Pack nonperishable snacks to take: pretzels, soy nuts, sunflower seeds, air-popped popcorn, whole fruit, dried fruit, oatmeal-raisin cookies, fig bars, graham crackers, raisin-nut mixes, whole-wheat crackers and low-fat cheese, or canned or boxed 100 percent juice.

● Snack wisely from convenience stores or malls: soft pretzels, nuts, frozen yogurt, fruit smoothies (small size).

● Quench your thirst: water, low-fat or fat-free milk, 100 percent fruit juice or vegetable juice, juice spritzers (juice and mineral water), fruit smoothies (fruit or juice blended with milk or yogurt), hot chocolate. *Be aware:* Fruit-flavored waters may be high in added sugars; check the label.

FUNCTIONAL FOODS: FAST, EASY, DELICIOUS TIPS!

Foods from every food group have functional health benefits that go beyond basic nutrition. Try these quick, easy, and convenient ways to fit functional foods into everyday meals and snacks. *For more about functional foods, refer to "Phytonutrients for Health" in chapter 6 and "Functional Foods: Benefits beyond Basics" in chapter 9.*

BREAKFAST	HEALTHFUL LUNCH AND DINNER IDEAS	SNACK ON THE GO
● Top oatmeal with blueberries.	● Mix tuna salad with grated carrots, red peppers, onions, and garlic.	● Grab a piece of fresh fruit.
● Mix yogurt with whole-grain dry cereal.	● Serve whole-grain pasta with tomato sauce and fresh herbs.	● Mix soy nuts and dried fruit together and hit the trail.
● Spread soy nut butter on whole-grain toast.	● Cook leeks and onions with tomatoes as a side dish.	● Grab a glass or box of tomato, cranberry, or orange juice.
● Drink sparkling purple grape juice with breakfast.	● Grill salmon and serve with fresh greens and yogurt salad dressing.	● Try fresh broccoli, cauliflower, and carrots with a tofu dip.
● Blend soy beverage with fresh pineapple.	● Try low-fat cream of carrot, spinach, and broccoli soups.	● Mix bananas with fresh raspberries.
	● Enjoy green tea with a marinated tofu sandwich.	
	● Stir-fry fresh vegetables with garlic.	

Source: University of Illinois Functional Foods for Health Program.

Have You Ever Wondered

. . . if canned liquid supplements or meal replacements are good snacks? Despite advertising messages, you don't need pricey liquid nutrition to supplement your meals if you're healthy. Your kids don't, either. Food such as fruit, smoothies, whole-grain crackers, yogurt, and more provide nutrients and other beneficial substances that canned liquid meals lack. Sometimes, however, they may be a convenient, on-the-go option. If you think you need a supplement, talk to your healthcare provider about a multivitamin/mineral supplement tablet. For a fraction of the price you get the same nutrient benefits.

. . . what slow food is? It's a term used to refer to the slow food movement, or taking time to enjoy food and food traditions in your busy life. Consider how time at the table may add pleasure, great flavors, and social time to your lifestyle. Eating slower also may help you eat less as you pay attention to satiety cues. That's also called mindful eating! *See chapter 2 for more about mindful eating as a way to manage weight.*

Everyday Eating Challenges

Making healthful food choices often has its own challenges: lack of time, too much effort needed, and limited know-how. Sound familiar? And how about grazing and portion distortion? These are a few more issues to consider as you make plans to eat for health.

Grazing . . . Healthful or Not?

Many Americans have moved away from three square meals a day. Instead, their series of mini-meals, called grazing, matches their on-the-go lifestyle. That's okay—as long as healthy eating goals for smart eating and active living are met. The eating patterns, *described in chapter 10*, don't advocate a single meal and snack pattern. Instead, these patterns are meant for the entire day or for several days. Eating five or six minimeals can be as healthful as eating three meals a day.

Little meals—several small portions eaten throughout the day—are nothing new. Instead, they're part of the traditional eating style in many places outside the United States. A variety of small portions of traditional Spanish dishes are served as tapas. In Greece,

Turkey, and Egypt they're called mezze. A little meal, or spuntino, in Italy might be a minipizza, grilled bread with tomatoes and cheese, or small skewers of meat and vegetables. And dim sum, which means to do (or touch) the heart in Chinese, is a savory snack of spring rolls, pot stickers, and steamed dumplings, to name a few.

Eating several minimeals may have several benefits. Like traditional eating styles, minimeals can contribute nutrient-rich food-group foods. For some people, especially those with small appetites, little meals may match their personal needs and lifestyles. Eating fewer calories more frequently may burn a few extra calories; eating and digesting food have a thermogenic, or calorie-burning, effect for a short time. Some researchers also say that spreading the same number of calories over four to six meals throughout the day, rather than at three meals, may result in somewhat lower blood cholesterol levels, too. But these findings aren't conclusive.

For Healthful Grazing

Total it up. To avoid overeating, yet still satisfy your appetite, pay attention to your small helpings and to the overall amount you eat in all your minimeals.

● Choose appetizer-size portions in restaurants and at home. That's about right for mini-meals.

● Use the power of the USDA Food Patterns or the DASH Eating Plan to eat the right amount and food variety for you. Overgrazing can be a source of excess calories, solid fats, added sugars, and sodium.

For ways to avoid mindless eating or grazing, see chapter 2.

Portion Distortion

Large portions may seem to say "Eat until you feel stuffed, not just until you're satisfied." Because people listen less to hunger and fullness cues and eat what's on their plate, it's easy to see how they can lose their ability to regulate how much they eat. More food served on larger plates, bowls, bottles, and cups has changed perceptions of portion sizes. Many Americans underestimate how much they eat by 50 percent!

Large portions are linked to excess calorie intake. Besides potentially leading to overweight, diet-related health risks may go up as oversized portions "over-deliver" total fat, including solid fats, cholesterol, sodium, and added sugars. In contrast, research shows that smaller portions are linked to weight loss.

Be Portion-Savvy

How big is your bowl of pasta? Your favorite bakery-fresh blueberry muffin or bagel? Your fast-food drink? Perhaps bigger than you think! To find out, get out your measuring cups and a kitchen scale. For different foods or drinks, serve your normal portion on a plate or in a bowl or glass. Then measure or weigh them. Your amount may be bigger or smaller than you think! To right-size your portions:

- Know visual clues for portions. Use a hand comparison for a quick estimate: your fist is about 1 cup; your palm, about ½ cup, or 3 to 5 ounces; and your thumb, about 1 tablespoon. *See "A Visual Guide to Amounts" in chapter 10.*

- Use smaller serving utensils, dishes, bowls, mugs, and cups. A meal served on a lunch plate rather than a dinner plate looks like more!

- Let veggies, fruit, and grain products (mostly whole grain) fill most of your plate, with less plate space for meat, chicken, or fish.

- Eat from a plate, not a package, so you know how much you eat. Put the opened package out of sight to resist temptation.

- Repackage big packages of snack foods into several smaller containers—enough for one time. Or buy portion-controlled singles if that helps.

- Portion out foods before you eat. In that way you control the amount.

- For yourself or serving others, start with small helpings. Put the rest out of sight. Then eat slowly, paying attention to hunger and fullness cues. Go for seconds only if you're still truly hungry.

- Use the Nutrition Facts panel on a food label to gauge serving sizes. *"Get All the Facts!" in chapter 12 explains serving sizes on food labels.*

For more ways to overcome oversizing your portions, refer to tips in chapters 2 and 15.

PORTION DISTORTION: THE RECENT SHIFT

| | CALORIES IN PORTIONS | |
FOOD	MID-1980s	TODAY
Bagel	140 calories (3-inch-diameter)	350 calories (6-inch-diameter)
Fast-food cheeseburger	333 calories	590 calories
Spaghetti and meatballs	500 calories (1 cup spaghetti with sauce and 3 small meatballs)	1,025 calories (2 cups spaghetti and 3 large meatballs)
Bottle of soda	85 calories (6½ ounces)	250 calories (20 ounces)
Fast-food French fries	210 calories (2.4 ounces)	610 (6.9 ounces)
Turkey sandwich	320 calories	820 calories (10-inch sub)
Coffee	45 calories (8 ounces with whole milk and sugar)	350 calories (16 ounces mocha coffee with steamed whole milk and mocha syrup)
Blueberry muffin	201 calories (1½ ounces)	500 calories (5-ounce muffin)
Pepperoni slices	500 calories (2 slices)	850 calories (2 large slices)
Chicken Caesar salad	390 calories (1½ cups)	790 calories (3 cups)
Popcorn, movie theater	270 calories (5 cups)	630 calories (tub)
Cheesecake	260 calories (3 ounces)	640 calories (1 large)
Chocolate chip cookie	55 (1½-inch-diameter)	275 calories (1 large)
Chicken stir-fry, restaurant	435 (2 cups)	865 calories (enough for 2)

Source: Department of Health and Human Services, National Institutes of Health, hp2010.nhlbihin.net/portion. Accessed January 1, 2012. *Tip:* Check this website to see how long it would take to burn these extra calories with physical activity!

CHAPTER 12

Savvy Shopping

With about fifty thousand items available in today's supermarkets, it's no wonder you have so many decisions to make! From food labels, to brochures and food TV, to in-store consumer affairs professionals and computer kiosks, and food blogs, websites, and phone apps, you have more food facts at your fingertips than ever before. Food labels with Nutrition Facts are on almost all packaged foods, and many labels have claims about how that food can promote health.

Supermarkets comprise much of the retail food business, but that's not the only place where you can buy food. Today, specialty stores, warehouse and bulk food stores, wholesale clubs, health food stores, restaurants, convenience stores, gas stations, department stores, drugstores, mail order, and online shopping services sell food to eat at home. And farmers' markets and the ability to buy directly from farmers through farm stands and CSAs (Community Supported Agriculture) are growing by leaps and bounds.

Consider all the other tools stores provide these days to help you with nutrition, food safety, and creating a greener environment: cooking classes; product tastings; store or market tours and websites; healthy meal ideas and recipes; coupons for healthier products; ready-to-eat entrées, side dishes, and food bars; electronic newsletters and magazines; reward programs; shelf-label systems; and recycling programs. Some stores offer health screening services, in-store health seminars, discounts to local fitness clubs, personalized wellness plans, recipes for special health issues, and nutrition counseling. They can be a health destination in your neighborhood.

What matters to you as a savvy shopper? If you're like many other consumers, taste likely tops the list, notes 2011 consumer surveys from the International Food Information Council Foundation, followed by price, healthfulness, and convenience. And about half cited sustainability in the survey.

No matter where you shop for food or what matters most to you, look for qualities of excellence:

● The store or market should be clean—that means the display cases, the grocery shelves, and the floor. And it should have a pleasing smell.

● Produce, meat, poultry, fish, and dairy foods should show qualities of freshness. Read on for ways to spot the freshness signs.

● Refrigerated cases should be cold. Freezer compartments should keep food solidly frozen.

● Bulk bins, salad bars, and other self-serve areas should be clean and properly covered.

● Workers handling raw and unpackaged food should wear disposable gloves, and change them after handling nonfood items and again after handling raw food.

Now, let's shop!

Today's Food Labels

At the store, food labels are your best sources of consumer information. Food labels tell the basics. By law,

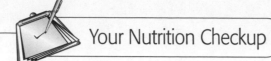
What's in Your Shopping Cart?

According to supermarket surveys done by the Food Marketing Institute and the International Food Information Council Foundation, consumers rank taste, nutrition, safety, storability, and convenience as important reasons for making decisions in the store. If that's true for you, just how do your "supermarket smarts" stack up? Check here before you read this chapter.

Do You . . .	ALWAYS (3 PTS.)	USUALLY (2 PTS.)	SOMETIMES (1 PT.)	NEVER (0 PT.)
For nutrition . . .				
Read the front-of-package nutrition information on a food label?	___	___	___	___
Use nutrient content claims and health claims to quickly spot foods you want?	___	___	___	___
Check the % Daily Values to get specific information after you read a nutrient content claim?	___	___	___	___
Use food labels to compare the nutrients and ingredients in similar foods?	___	___	___	___
Look for nutrition information displayed near fresh foods: produce, meat, poultry, and fish?	___	___	___	___
Know how to use the "5–20 guide" to quickly check Nutrition Facts?	___	___	___	___
Use Nutrition Facts including serving sizes on food labels to plan healthful meals and snacks?	___	___	___	___
Subtotal for nutrition	___	___	___	___
For safety . . .				
Look for dates printed on packages to buy foods at their peak?	___	___	___	___
Check packaging and cans to be sure they're clean and not damaged?	___	___	___	___
Take perishable foods home within thirty minutes of shopping, and immediately refrigerate or freeze them?	___	___	___	___
Check to be sure that frozen foods are solid and that refrigerated foods are cold?	___	___	___	___
Look for qualities of freshness in produce and raw meat, poultry, and fish?	___	___	___	___
Put fresh meat, poultry, and fish in separate bags when you can so they don't drip on other foods in your shopping cart?	___	___	___	___
Put foods that need to be refrigerated in separate bags to help maintain a cooler temperature when they're bagged?	___	___	___	___
Subtotal for safety	___	___	___	___
For cost savings . . .				
Use unit price codes on shelves to compare the cost of similar products?	___	___	___	___
Take advantage of cents-off coupons and in-store specials?	___	___	___	___
Buy only the amount you'll use to avoid waste?	___	___	___	___
Shop for seasonal produce?	___	___	___	___
Pay attention to the price as each item is scanned at checkout?	___	___	___	___
Consider carefully before buying a new food after you sample it or see an attractive display?	___	___	___	___
Subtotal for cost savings	___	___	___	___
For convenience . . .				
Keep a shopping list to use as you shop?	___	___	___	___
Shop during off-hours to save time and avoid crowds if possible?	___	___	___	___

275

Buy foods that are partly or fully prepared?	____	____	____	____
Buy single-portion or small-sized packages when you're feeding one or two?	____	____	____	____
Keep shopping trips to a minimum—no more than once or twice a week?	____	____	____	____
Subtotal for convenience	____	____	____	____

Count up your "supermarket smarts" category by category, then add up the total. *Total score* ____.

For nutrition and safety, a perfect score is 21 for each. For cost savings, it's 18; for convenience, 15. That adds up to 75 points.

If you come close to a perfect score in any category, count yourself as a smart food shopper in that area. And make it your goal to be a well-rounded shopper! *Read on to learn more about these and other ways to shop smart and boost your score.*

---

all packaged foods must identify the common name of the product, name and address of the food manufacturer, net contents (by weight, measure, or count), the ingredients, Nutrition Facts, and any common allergens in the product. Beyond that, the label may provide voluntary information, including safety guidelines, preparation and storage tips, and freshness dates. With this information you can make informed food choices for you and your family.

Shopping online for food products? When described on websites, food products are subject to the same regulations as for food labeling.

Nutrition on the Label

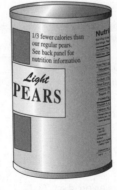

Wrapped around almost every packaged food in the supermarket you'll find nutrition and health information.

● *Nutrient content claims* such as "no salt added" or "high-fiber" help you easily find foods that meet your specific nutrition goals. *See "Label Lingo" in this and other chapters for specific nutrient content claims.*

● *Nutrition Facts* give specifics about the calories and nutrients in a single label serving of the food. This information must appear on virtually all food labels.

● *Ingredient list* gives an overview of the "recipe," with the ingredients listed from most to least by weight.

● *Health claims* describe the potential health benefits of a food, nutrient, or food substance, to reduce the risk of a chronic disease or condition.

● *Structure/function claims* describe the way a nutrient or a food substance maintains or supports a normal body function, such as "helps maintain bone health" or "supports a healthy immune system."

● *Allergen labeling* identifies common allergens in the product.

Nutrition Facts and the ingredient list appear on almost every packaged food. Today many fresh fruits and vegetables may be labeled voluntarily with nutrition information, too, either on the package or on a poster or a pamphlet displayed nearby. If you don't find this information, ask the store manager to start providing it.

Food labels can help you make nutrition-related decisions as you shop—and at home:

● Use Nutrition Facts to pick nutrient-rich foods and to compare calories and nutrients in similar foods.

● Use ingredient lists to identify allergens and other ingredients of interest—type of fat, added sugars, whole grains, and others.

The Language of Labels: Nutrient-Content Claims

Imagine rolling your shopping cart through the supermarket. Your eyes dart from one food product to another. Some canned peaches say "no added sugar." Certain breakfast cereals are "high in fiber"; others are "fortified." On packages of luncheon meat you see the term "lean." The words "high in calcium" on a milk carton or "excellent source of calcium and vitamin D" on a juice carton catch your eye. You can choose "lite" salad dressing. And a box of cookies says "fewer calories." What does all this label language mean?

Known as nutrient content claims, these terms describe the amount of nutrients, cholesterol, fiber, or calories in food. They often appear on the package front for quick comparisons. Some claims can say "contains [x amount] of [nutrient]."

A nutrient content claim can help you spot the right item; Nutrition Facts offer specifics. For example, suppose you're comparing the fat in hot dogs. Terms such as "lean" or "reduced fat" offer a general idea. For the amount of total fat—and saturated and *trans* fats—in one label serving, check the Nutrition Facts.

Nutrient content claims mean the same thing for all foods, no matter what food or manufacturer makes the

Label Lingo

What Nutrient Content Claims Mean

LABEL TERM ...	MEANS ...
Free	It's an amount so small that it probably won't have an effect on your body—for example, "calorie-free," "fat-free," "*trans*-fat free," or "sodium-free." *Other terms:* "no," "zero," "without," "trivial source of," "negligible source of," "dietarily insignificant source of," "non" (nonfat only).
Low	It's an amount specifically defined for each term, such as "low-calorie," "low-fat," or "low-cholesterol." *Other terms:* "few," "contains a small amount of," "low source of," "low in," "little," "a little."
Reduced	It's an amount describing a food with at least 25 percent less calories, fat, saturated fat, cholesterol, sugars, or sodium than a regular food. Look for information about the food it's being compared to. *Other terms:* "reduced in," "___% reduced," "fewer," "lower," "lower in," "less."
High	It's an amount that's 20 percent or more of the Daily Value* for a nutrient—for example, "high in vitamin C" or "high-calcium." *Other terms:* "excellent source of," "rich in."
Good source	It's an amount that's 10 to 19 percent of the Daily Value* for a nutrient—for example, "good source of fiber." *Other terms:* "contains," "provides."
More	It's an amount that's 10 percent or more of the Daily Value*—for example, "more fiber" or "more iron." You won't find it on meat or poultry products. *Other terms:* "enriched," "fortified," "added," "extra," "plus." *See chapter 9 for definitions of enrichment and fortification.*
Light	It's a food with a third fewer calories or 50 percent less fat than the traditional version. A "low-calorie" or "low-fat" food with 50 percent less sodium might also be called "light." *Other term:* "lite." When "light" describes a product characteristic, such as "light brown sugar," it isn't a nutrient content claim.
Healthy	It's a food that's low in fat and saturated fat, 60 milligrams or less cholesterol per serving, 480 milligrams or less sodium per serving, and at least 10 percent of the Daily Value per serving of vitamin A, vitamin C, calcium, iron, protein, or fiber. Fruits, vegetables and enriched cereal products can be labeled "healthy" without having 10 percent of the DV or more of these nutrients per serving. But they must meet low-fat, low-saturated-fat, cholesterol, and sodium criteria. A meal or main dish product must have 600 milligrams of sodium or less.

On seafood, meat, or poultry, look for:

Lean	It's a food with less than 10 grams total fat, 4.5 grams or less saturated fat, and less than 95 milligrams cholesterol per 3-ounce (and per 100 grams) cooked serving.
Extra lean	It's a food with less than 5 grams total fat, less than 2 grams saturated fat, and less than 95 milligrams cholesterol per 3-ounce (and per 100 grams) cooked serving.

*When compared with a label serving size of the traditional food.

product. That's because these claims are defined strictly by regulation. Like Nutrition Facts, nutrient content claims are defined for a single serving. That's a standard label serving size set by the government—not necessarily what *you* may consider to be one helping.

Nutrient content claims are optional. Many foods that meet the criteria don't carry these terms on the label. If you see a product with a nutrient content claim, use the % Daily Value in the Nutrition Facts to compare it to a similar food that doesn't carry a claim. *For definitions of nutrient content claims, see "Label Lingo" in this and other chapters.*

Click Here! Websites to Know . . .

● Labeling information, www.fda.gov/Food/LabelingNutrition/ConsumerInformation

● Farmers Market Search, apps.ams.usda.gov/FarmersMarkets

● What's in Season?, www.fruitsandveggiesmorematters.org

See "Resources You Can Use" for food buying advice from food industry groups; check websites for your local supermarket chain.

Front-of-Package Nutrition Labeling: What Does It Mean?

Many consumers want a quick way to identify and choose healthier foods. That's why nutrition information is appearing at point of purchase—and on the front of package (FOP) alongside U.S. FDA-regulated nutrient content or health claims.

The challenge: With many different symbols and systems, FOP labeling isn't consistent. Some FOP labeling simply brings information from the Nutrition Facts panel to the package front. Others use their own nutrient criteria (or scoring algorithms) to identify food products as better choices, or more nutrient-rich; their scoring systems differ, and they're often proprietary. Without consistency, some FOP systems may overrate products' healthful qualities, or may be more lenient with their own definitions.

In late 2011, many food packages began to carry Nutrition Keys, a voluntary FOP labeling initiative of the Grocery Manufacturers Association and the Food Marketing Institute. It's meant to help consumers decipher the nutrient and calorie content of food, especially calories, fat, sodium, and sugar content per serving, and see how a food fits into an overall eating plan. Some labels also show some nutrients that many consumers need more of.

Although currently there's no standardized, science-based criteria for FOP nutrition labeling, FDA regulations may come in the future. Until then, use FOP labeling as only one factor in your purchasing decision. Turn to the Nutrition Facts label, which is regulated by law, to make informed judgments about the calories and nutrients in food products.

Get All the Facts!

"Low-fat, "no added sugar," or "calcium-rich" as product claims do not mean the food is a healthy option! You've got to check the Nutrition Facts, along with the ingredient list, for specifics.

Nutrition Facts differ from nutrient content claims. Nutrition Facts specifically state the amount of key nutrients and calories in one label serving of a food, while claims such as "low in fat" or "more fiber" are quick-to-read descriptions. Read the Nutrition Facts:

● To compare similar foods for the calorie and nutrient content.

● To find foods with more fiber, vitamins A and C, calcium, iron, and, if listed, potassium.

● To find foods with less fat, saturated fat, *trans* fat, cholesterol, and sodium.

● To help you make food trade-offs. (If you want a high-fat snack, the label can help you trade off and find other foods with less fat.)

● To choose foods that match a special health need, such as to cut calories to manage weight, to limit sodium to manage blood pressure, or to count carbohydrates to manage diabetes.

This may surprise you: Fat-free products aren't always low in calories, and sugar-free products aren't always low in calories or low in fat! That's why you need to read and understand the Nutrition Facts! So where do you begin?

Step 1: Start with label servings . . . the serving size and number of servings per container. Standard

Metric conversion key:

- 28 grams (g) = 1 ounce
- 1,000 milligrams (mg) =1 gram

Use the "5–20 guide" as a quick guide to label reading. For any nutrient:

- *5% or less is low:* For nutrients you need to limit, look for foods with 5% or less Daily Value.
- *20% or more is high:* For nutrients you need more of, look for foods with 20% or higher Daily Value.

Note: The "5-20 guide"' doesn't define a food as good or bad. Instead it indicates how much.

serving sizes—set by government regulations—are expressed in familiar kitchen measures (e.g., teaspoon, tablespoon, cup) and in metric amounts. A label serving probably differs from portions you eat. In fact, studies show that most people underestimate portion sizes.

Nutrition Facts apply to the amount of food or beverage in one label serving, not necessarily to the whole container. Packaging—perhaps a 14-ounce can of ready-to-eat soup, or 1½ ounces of chips—may look like a single serving. However, Nutrition Facts may show it as more than one label serving.

By knowing the label serving and serving sizes in the Nutrition Facts, you won't be misled about the calories and the nutrient amounts in the whole container.

Step Two: Check the calories in a label serving. You'll also see how many of those calories come from fat. To help you manage your weight, know the calories per serving and in the portion you eat!

How to Read a Food Label

Macaroni & Cheese

Step Three: Note the nutrients. Unless their amounts are insignificant, some nutrients must appear in the label's Nutrition Facts: fat, saturated fat, *trans* fat, cholesterol, total carbohydrates, sugars, protein, vitamins A and C, calcium, and iron. Other nutrients may be listed, too: some voluntarily, others by law when a nutrient content claim is made. For example if the label says "fortified with vitamin D" or "high in folate," then vitamin D or folate must be listed in the Nutrition Facts.

Nutrients required are those that relate to major health issues. Most people need to limit total fats, saturated fats, *trans* fats, cholesterol, and sodium. Other nutrients often come up short: fiber, vitamins A and C, calcium, and iron. *Refer to earlier chapters to learn about these nutrients and their links to health.*

Step Four: Let the % Daily Value (DV) be your guide. The % DV is a guide for the amount of a nutrient in a single serving. Use it to decide how a food or a beverage may fit into your eating plan and to compare similar foods.

Generally speaking, % DVs show how one label serving of a food contributes to a typical 2,000-calorie-a-day diet for some nutrients. So if the label shows 15% DV for iron, that food has about 15 percent of the fiber needed for the day. That's the whole day, not a single meal or a snack. Daily Values are averages for healthy adults, not necessarily optimal nutrient amounts recommended for you. You may need more or less of the % DV for some nutrients.

Use Nutrition Facts to help you limit some nutrients and get enough of others. For example, to help get enough calcium for bone health, look for foods such as low-fat or fat-free milk or yogurt that have 20% DV or more for calcium. To limit salt, find foods with 5% DV or less for sodium. For heart health, choose foods with a lower combined "score of saturated and *trans* fats (solid fats)." For example, for the mac and cheese Nutrition Facts on the previous page, one cup has 6 grams of saturated and *trans* fats combined.

For Daily Values used in food labeling, see the appendices. To clarify, Daily Values aren't the same as the Dietary Reference Intakes (DRIs), *listed in the appendices. For more about DRIs refer to chapter 1.*

Have You Ever Wondered?

... why you don't see % Daily Values for protein? Getting enough protein isn't a health concern for many people age four and over, so it usually isn't listed with a % DV. Adjustments for protein's digestibility make calculating a % DV difficult. If the food is touted with a nutrient content claim—perhaps "high in protein"—then % DV for protein must be shown. Foods meant for infants and children under age four show % DV for protein on the Nutrition Facts.

... why a food with "no sugar added" shows grams of sugars on the Nutrition Facts? Fruits, vegetables, milk, grains, and beans (legumes) have naturally occurring sugars. "Sugars" in the Nutrition Facts include added and naturally occurring sugars. There's no DV for sugars because there's no daily recommendation. To find out about added sugars, check the ingredient list.

Corn syrup, invert sugar, and corn sweeteners are among the names for added sugars; *see chapter 3 for more about added sugars.*

... if a product labeled "zero grams trans *fats per serving" is really* trans-*fat-free?* A product with less than ½ gram *trans* fat per label serving can be labeled as "zero *trans fats.*"

... about nutrition labeling for meat and poultry? Starting in January 2012, Nutrition Facts were required for single-ingredient raw meat and poultry on packages or point-of-purchase signs. This labeling can help you compare different meat and poultry cuts and ground products. The Nutrition Facts are based on a label serving of 4 ounces (not the whole package) of raw meat or poultry as packaged—and not as cooked or eaten. These Nutrition Facts don't account for your food prep, such as removing poultry skin or draining away fat drippings.

To avoid confusion: The % DV for total fat is not the same as the dietary advice: "Eat 20 to 35 percent of total calories from fat." The latter applies to the DRIs for everything you eat and drink for the day, not to a single food, beverage, meal, or snack. The % DV for total fat shows if the food itself is high or low in fat. *See the explanation of % Daily Value.*

Note: No DVs are established for *trans* fats or sugars. Sugars in the Nutrition Facts reflect both natural and added sugars.

Step Five: Check the footnote. It shows Daily Values for some nutrients for two calorie levels—2,000 and 2,500 a day. They're maximum amounts for total fat, saturated fat, cholesterol, and sodium—and target amounts for total carbohydrate and fiber. The footnote is general advice and may not be right for you.

Step Six: Check the calories-per-gram conversion. That's just math to show the number of calories in 1 gram each of fat, carbohydrate, and protein. *Notice:* Fat supplies more than double the calories per gram (9 calories) than carbohydrate and protein do (4 calories per gram each).

Food labeling may change in the future as a tool to make healthful food choices in a marketplace. Stay tuned, stay informed!

A Word about Ingredients . . .

Imagine that you're reaching for a can of vegetable soup. The ingredient list, like a recipe, tells what's in the soup.

By regulation, any food with more than one ingredient must carry an ingredient list on the label. All ingredients are listed in descending order by weight, from most to least. For example, canned vegetable soup that lists tomatoes first contains more tomatoes by weight than anything else. Next time you reach for any mixed food, check what ingredients are listed first, second, and third on the label.

The ingredient list is also useful for people with special food needs; for example:

● A food allergy, perhaps to peanuts or eggs, or a food intolerance, perhaps to lactose (milk sugar) or sulfites. For those sensitive to artificial food color, the colors are named individually, not just listed as "coloring." If the ingredient list isn't clear to you, write or call the food manufacturer. *See chapter 21, "Sensitive to*

Food," for more about food sensitivities, and later in this chapter about food allergen labeling.

● Cultural or religious preferences, for example, those who avoid pork, shellfish, or other meat for religious or other reasons

● Vegetarians, including vegans, who choose to avoid foods made with ingredients from animal sources

A labeling definition for gluten-free is proposed. Until the label definition is regulated, the FDA allows its use on food products if it isn't misleading.

In some cases the ingredient list gives the ingredient source. For example, on the label for Mark's Cheese Pizza (*see below*), you'll see that "partially hydrogenated vegetable oil" is followed by "soybean and/or cottonseed oil" and that "tomato puree" is water and tomato paste. What is part-skim mozzarella cheese made from? The ingredient list says pasteurized milk, cheese cultures, salt, and enzymes.

See "Additives: Safe at the Plate" in chapter 9.

Health Claims on the Label

Another bit of nutrition information might appear on food labels: a health claim. Health claims link food—or food components—in your overall eating plan with a lowered risk for some chronic diseases. Since this information is optional, some foods that meet the

criteria don't carry any health claim on their label. Make shopping decisions using information from the whole label, not just the health claim. Read the Nutrition Facts to determine if the product is right for you.

Strictly regulated by the U.S. Food and Drug Administration (FDA), health claims are supported by scientific evidence. So far the following health claims have been approved:

● *Calcium* and osteoporosis

● *Calcium* and *vitamin D* and osteoporosis

● *Sodium* and hypertension

● *Dietary fat* and cancer

● *Dietary saturated fat and cholesterol* and the risk of coronary heart disease

● *Fiber-containing grain products, fruits, and vegetables* and cancer

● *Fruits, vegetables, and grain products that contain fiber, particularly soluble fiber,* and risk of coronary heart disease

● *Fruits and vegetables* and cancer

● *Folate* and neural tube defects

● *Dietary noncariogenic carbohydrate sweeteners* and dental caries (cavities)

● *Soluble fiber from certain foods* and the risk of coronary heart disease

● *Soy protein* and the risk of coronary heart disease

● *Plant sterol/stanol esters* and the risk of coronary heart disease

● *Whole-grain foods* and the risk of heart disease and certain cancers

● *Potassium* and the risk of high blood pressure and stroke

● *Fluoridated water* and reduced risk of dental caries

● *Saturated fat, cholesterol, and* trans *fat* and reduced risk of heart disease

(A few other health claims are approved for supplement labels; see chapter 23.) See the appendices for specifics.

With so much emerging science on nutrition and health, some approved qualified health claims also show the relationship between a food component and health or reduced disease risk. But a caveat, or qualifying language, must appear with it since supportive scientific evidence isn't conclusive. *Check the appendices for a website to find permitted qualified health claims.*

When you read health claims, remember: Your food choices are just one factor that can reduce your risk for certain health problems. Heredity, physical activity, and smoking are among other factors that affect your health and risks for disease.

Structure/Function Claims on the Label

Structure/function claims such as "helps promote urinary tract health" describe how a nutrient or a food substance may affect your health; these claims *cannot* suggest any link to lowered risk for disease. Unlike health claims, structure/function claims don't need prior FDA approval or review, but are still subject ot FDA enforcement. They must be truthful and not misleading.

Dietary Guidance Statements

Dietary Guidance statements describe the health benefits of broad categories of foods. For example, "Diets rich in fruits and vegetables may reduce the risk of some types of cancer and other chronic diseases."

Note: More specific Dietary Guidance statements are forthcoming from the FDA.

Food Labels: Food Safety and Handling Tips

For your good health, some food labels offer guidance on food safety and handling. To reduce the risk of foodborne illness, raw and partially cooked meat and poultry products must be labeled with guidelines for safe handling. *See the "Safe Handling Instructions" label.* Each of the simple graphics—a refrigerator, hand washing, fry pan, and meat thermometer— represents a safe handling tip.

Cartons of shell eggs also have safe-handling instructions (*see below*) to help control *Salmonella* contamination:

> SAFE HANDLING INSTRUCTIONS: To prevent illness from bacteria: keep eggs refrigerated, cook eggs until yolks are firm, and cook foods containing eggs thoroughly.

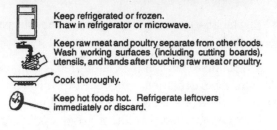

Safe Handling Instructions

This product was prepared from inspected and passed meat and/or poultry. Some food products may contain bacteria that could cause illness if the product is mishandled or cooked improperly. For your protection, follow these safe handling instructions.

Keep refrigerated or frozen.
Thaw in refrigerator or microwave.

Keep raw meat and poultry separate from other foods. Wash working surfaces (including cutting boards), utensils, and hands after touching raw meat or poultry.

Cook thoroughly.

Keep hot foods hot. Refrigerate leftovers immediately or discard.

Besides food safety, following these guidelines helps food retain its appealing flavor, texture, and appearance. *For in-depth information on food safety and handling, see chapter 13, "The Safe Kitchen."*

More Health-Focused Label "Info"

Food allergen labeling: Allergen labeling is required on foods containing a major food allergen or a protein from these allergens: milk, egg, fish, crustacean shellfish, tree nuts, wheat, peanuts, and soybeans. These allergens account for 90 percent of all food allergies. Allergen labeling may appear in the ingredient list or in a statement at the end of that list. Wherever, they must be identified by common names. For example, the label may say: "Contains milk, egg, peanuts." The label also might provide a disclaimer, such as "Made in a facility that also processes peanuts."

Health warnings for more conditions: Warnings for people with special needs include:

● Foods and beverages made with aspartame (a nonnutritive sweetener) offer a warning for people with phenylketonuria (PKU). Aspartame contains the amino acid phenylalanine, which people with PKU can't metabolize.

● You'll find "Contains Sulfites" on beer and wine labels and on dried fruit and some salad seasonings containing sulfites, too, for those who are sulfite-sensitive.

● Unpasteurized juice and juice products, including cider, must carry a safety warning if sold across state lines.

- Alcohol-containing beverages carry warnings for pregnant women.

See chapter 21 for more about allergen labeling and on PKU and other food sensitivities.

Food exchanges. Some foods provide food exchanges for help in managing diabetes or weight. The label probably will say that these exchanges are calculated based on exchange lists from the American Diabetes Association and the Academy of Nutrition and Dietetics (or the American Dietetic Association).

More Reading on the Food Label

Taking a few more moments with food labels teaches even more about the food inside the package.

Type of food. The product name tells what's in the container. Besides specifically naming the food, it tells the form, perhaps smooth or chunky, sliced or whole, or miniature—important to know when following a recipe.

Net contents. Food labels tell the total amount in the container, either in volume, count, or net weight. Net weight refers to the food amount inside the container, including any liquid.

For juice products, total percent juice content. Keep reading for the Nutrition Facts. Compare nutrients, along with sugars and calories, before making your selection.

A "100 percent juice" may—or may not—supply 100 percent of the Daily Value for vitamin C. That said, juices offer more nutrients and phytonutrients than just vitamin C. Many juices are fortified with additional nutrients, too.

Juice "drinks," "beverages," or "cocktails" (with some juice, but not 100 percent juice) may be fortified to provide 100 percent of the Daily Value for some nutrients. Typically these beverages have added sugars, but probably not the full array and amounts of nutrients and phytonutrients in 100 percent juice. *See "Fruit Juice, Juice Drink, Fruit Drink?" in chapter 8.*

Name and address of the manufacturer, packer, or distributor. Need to contact a food company with your consumer questions and concerns? Look for a consumer service phone number or website address. If the food is imported, the country of origin must be shown.

Food product dating. You can't see inside the package; how do you know if it's fresh? Many food packages, such as dairy products, have a date, often given as numbers, such as "12-15" or "1215" or "Dec. 15" to mean December 15. Food manufacturers and retailers use three types of dates:

- *"Sell by" or pull date:* That's the last day a food should be sold to remain fresh for home storage.

- *Pack date:* That's when the food was manufactured, processed, or packaged.

- *"Best if used by" date:* For optimal quality, use food by this date. For example, the label may say, "Best if used by 1-31-13." Depending on the food and if it has been stored properly, it likely will be safe beyond this date.

Remember these dates are for quality and optimum freshness—not for food safety. Safety depends on how these foods are handled until they reach your table!

Organic labeling. The Organic Foods Production Act and the National Organic Program ensure that the production, processing, and certification of organic foods are standardized. The term "organic" has legal label definitions. Foods also may bear the "USDA Organic" seal. On food labels "organic" means:

- *"100 percent organic"*: The product must contain only organically produced ingredients (except for water and salt).

- *"organic"*: The product must contain at least 95 percent organically produced ingredients (except for water and salt). The other 5 percent are ingredients that aren't available in organic form or that appear on an approved list.

- *"made with organic ingredients"*: Processed foods may bear this label if they contain at least 70 percent organic ingredients—for example, "soup made with organic peas, potatoes, and carrots." The regulation also identifies production methods that can't be used.

If it's labeled organic, the product's name and address of the certifying organization must appear—with an exception. Small farmers (less than $5,000 in organic sales), including those who may sell in small farmers' markets, don't need certification. Still, their label claims must be truthful and in compliance with organic labeling laws.

Organic labeling regulations don't change food labeling regulations, administered by the U.S. FDA and the U.S.D.A.'s Food Safety and Inspection Service.

Organic foods aren't necessarily more healthful or more nutritious than other foods. Using them is really a consumer preference. Terms such as "all-natural," "free-range," or "hormone-free" don't mean "organic." *For more about organically grown foods, see chapter 9.*

Grading and inspection symbols on some products. These symbols indicate that foods have met certain standards set by the government:

● *Inspection stamps* on meat, poultry, and packaged meats mean the food is wholesome and was slaughtered, packed, or processed under sanitary conditions.

● *Food grades*—for example, on some types of meat, poultry, eggs, dairy foods, and produce—suggest standards of appearance, texture, uniformity, and perhaps taste. With the exception of marbling fat in meat, food grading does not suggest nutrient value. *Grading for meat, poultry, and eggs appears later in this chapter.*

Preparation instructions. Some products suggest oven or microwave times and temperatures, or perhaps other preparation or serving tips. Some offer recipes.

Kosher symbols. The term "kosher" means "proper" or "fit" in Hebrew. Kosher symbols indicate that the food has met the standards of a Jewish food inspector, done in addition to government safety inspection. The kosher code, which may appear on foods throughout the store, doesn't imply any nutritional qualities.

Often the word "Pareve" is written next to these symbols, meaning the food has neither meat nor dairy ingredients. During March and April a large "P" next to the symbols means it's kosher for Passover.

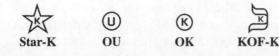

Halal and Zabiah Halal symbols. Products prepared by federally inspected meat packing plants and handled according to Islamic dietary law and under Islamic authority may bear Halal and Zabiah Halal references.

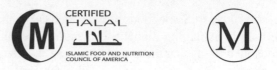

Universal Product Code (UPC). These black bars, which identify the manufacturer and the food, are used by the food industry for inventory control and price scanning.

Country of origin. As of 2009 most supermarkets were required to label many food commodities with country-of-origin labeling (COOL). Muscle-cut and ground meats (beef, veal, pork, lamb, goat, and chicken); wild and farm-raised fish and shellfish; fresh and frozen fruits and vegetables; peanuts, pecans, and macadamia nuts; and ginseng must be labeled. COOL *only* tells you where the food is from—not more, not less. It's not a food safety program. Specialty stores such as butcher shops and fish markets are exempt.

Labels—and You

What's the best way to shop for good nutrition? Start with a plan that helps you choose from a variety of foods—in the amounts you need. The food guides, *addressed in chapter 10*, provide flexible plans that

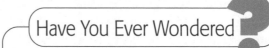

. . . what the code on the lid or the bottom of canned foods means? A series of letters or numbers identifies the plant location, exact date, and perhaps work shift or time of processing. Codes differ from one processor to another. If you can't read the code but wish to, contact the food company, using the toll-free number, website address, or address on the label.

. . . if tattoos on eggshells and on produce peels are safe? Imprinted with a laser light beam, the tattoos provide codes for inventory, pricing, freshness, and tracking. They're safe and don't affect the quality of the food.

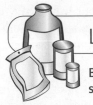

Label Lingo

Besides nutrition and health claims, some labels carry other label terms.

LABEL TERM . . .	REFERS TO . . .
Fresh	Food in its raw state. The term can't be used on food that has been frozen or heated, or on food that contains preservatives.
Frozen fresh or fresh frozen	Food that is quickly frozen while very fresh shortly after harvest
Quickly frozen	Frozen long enough with a system to freeze the center of the food fast, but with virtually no deterioration
Homogenized	Process of breaking up and separating milk fat. This makes the texture of milk smooth and uniform.
Natural	Product with no artificial ingredient or added color and that is minimally processed. The label must explain the use of the term "natural" (e.g., "no added colorings or artificial ingredients"; "minimally processed"). The term is only defined for meat and poulty.
Pasteurized	Process of heating foods such as raw milk, raw eggs, and fresh juice to a temperature high enough to destroy bacteria and inactivate most enzymes that cause spoilage
Ultrapasteurized	Process of heating food such as cream to a temperature higher than pasteurization. This extends the time it can be stored in the refrigerator or on the shelf.
UHT (Ultra-High Temperature)	Process similar to ultra-pasteurization. With high heat and sterilized containers, food can be stored unopened without refrigeration for up to three months. Once opened, it needs refrigeration.

can work for you. Then use food labels—nutrient content claims, health claims, ingredient lists, and Nutrition Facts—to choose nutrient-rich foods that fit your plan: your nutrient and health needs—and your calorie target!

With the Nutrition Facts, *always start with the serving size and the servings in the container,* considering your own portions, too. Then . . .

● Weight concerns? Compare the calories.

● Managing blood glucose (sugar)? Pay special attention to the carbohydrates, including added sugars, and the fiber content.

● At risk for heart disease or high blood pressure? Check the total fat, saturated fat, *trans* fat, cholesterol, and sodium content. Key in on fat (for heart health) and sodium (for blood pressure).

● Concerned about bone loss? Look at the % DV for calcium—and if provided, vitamin D.

For example, suppose you're buying spaghetti sauce. If you want to ease up on sodium, spot the product with a nutrient content claim "reduced sodium" or "low sodium." Then check the Nutrition Facts for the exact sodium content per label serving. Compare it to other spaghetti sauces before you buy. If you're curious, check the ingredient list to find the sodium-containing ingredients. And a granola bar? If you're watching calories, the calories in the Nutrition Facts apply to one serving, but see how many servings that package provides, then figure the calories in the amount you eat.

Nutrition Facts can also help you make trade-offs. For example, a switch from regular to lean hot dogs likely saves both total fat and saturated fat grams and calories without giving up protein. The label tells how much. Feeling indulgent? "Spend" some of those savings on ice cream for dessert. *See "Save Calories, Spend Elsewhere" in chapter 10.*

Maxing Your Food Dollar

Understanding food labels can help you shop for wellness and nutrition. Good news: You don't need to give up good nutrition for a reasonable grocery bill! But how do you save money, as well as time and hassle, when you shop for food?

Label Confusion?

Food packages may carry other attention-grabbing, marketing terms. But what do they really mean? There are no consistent definitions—and some may lead to shopper confusion. These are among the terms with no current government-regulated definitions for food labeling.

- doctor-recommended
- eco-friendly
- energy
- green
- natural (except for the term's regulated use on meat and poultry)
- naturally raised, naturally grown
- high-quality
- local
- no additives
- sustainable
- wholesome

Nutrition $ense

To get the most nutrition for your food dollars, be an educated consumer. Plan ahead. Know exactly what you need. And be aware of marketing ploys that may encourage you to buy beyond your shopping list.

Plan before you shop:

● Plan menus ahead. You'll more likely buy just what you need, avoid overbuying especially on perishable foods or foods you already have on hand, and prevent unneeded shopping trips. *See "Stocking the Kitchen" in chapter 14.*

● Know what you spend on food. Check and analyze your receipts. Create a food budget to help you get the most nutrition for your food dollar.

● Keep a shopping list. You might use a smartphone app or an online site to help maintain your routine purchases and any foods you need for a planned recipe. Stick to the list! A list jogs your memory, saves time and money at the store, and may keep you from buying what you don't need. A running list in your kitchen is another time saver. Organize your list by category to match the store layout—for example, produce department, dairy case, meat counter, deli, bakery, frozen, and grocery aisles.

● Check supermarket specials in store circulars, newspaper inserts, or online. Then plan menus around them. If the store runs out of an item on special, ask for a rain check. Be aware that "limit" signs ("limit three per customer") and messages such as "two for $5.00" (not "$2.50 each") are marketing ploys to get consumers to buy more. Research shows they work!

● Clip or download coupons, but only for items you really need. *Be alert:* Items with coupons aren't always the best buy. Another brand or a similar food might be cheaper and perhaps more nourishing, even without a coupon.

● Sign up for a frequent shopper program—if it offers benefits that match your needs and if your store has one. Besides the savings, you may get advance notice of in-store specials, cash-back offers, coupons, recipes, nutrition and health tips, and reminders of products you buy frequently.

● Take advantage of seasonal produce. In season, the price for fresh fruit and vegetables may be lower, and the produce more flavorful with more varietals. Depending on where you live, go directly to the farm or to a local farmers' market.

Time your shopping trip:

● Try to shop just once or twice a week. You'll spend less on impulse items—and save time and fuel cost, too.

● Eat first so you're not hungry! That helps you avoid impulse buys from store sampling and perhaps less nourishing snack and dessert items.

● Shop during off-hours if you can. In the early morning, late evening, or midweek rather than weekends, stores are often less crowded and shopping may be less stressful.

● Walk or bike to the store for a small purchase when you have time. If you need to carry food home, you'll be less likely to impulse-shop—and you'll fit in some exercise, too!

Shop smart:

● Use food labels to find foods that match your needs, and get the most nutrition for your food dollar. Use Nutrition Facts to compare.

● Decide what quality food you need. For example, if you're making a casserole, chunky tuna may be fine. But more expensive solid-pack tuna has more eye appeal in a tuna-vegetable salad.

● Buy the economy size or family packs only if it's cheaper and you can use that much. While warehouse stores may charge less, the need to buy large amounts may not be a savings, especially if food spoils and must be discarded. For foods that freeze, take time to repackage food into smaller amounts in freezer bags, then freeze for later use.

● Compare prices. Unit pricing on supermarket shelves makes comparisons easier, especially for similar foods in different-size containers. Prices are given as cost per unit rather than price per package or container. The unit might be an ounce, a quart, or some other measurement. If the foods and the units being compared are the same, the best value is the lowest price per unit.

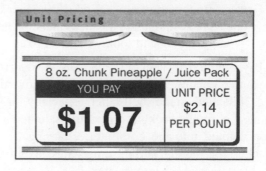

● Compare the prices of private-label brands, store brands, and generic brands. Store brands and generic products may cost less since they don't have the same promotional costs. And the quality is likely similar. Convenient, innovative packaging such as squirt bottles and ready-to-serve pouches often add to the cost; decide if the benefits are worth any extra cost.

● If available, and if you qualify, take advantage of senior citizen discount days.

● Stock up on canned and other nonperishable foods when they're on sale. At home, rotate your food supply so that the "first in" is the "first out."

● Buy perishable foods in amounts that will be consumed during their peak quality. An extra bunch of broccoli that spoils in the refrigerator is no savings.

● Buy from bulk bins. Without the expense of packaging or branding, bulk foods often cost less, and they're usually the same foods you find on supermarket shelves. The best advantage: You can buy just the amount you need. Foods such as dry fruits, rice, pasta, other grains, snack mixes, and spices are among those sold in bulk. And without packaging, it's eco-friendly!

● Consider the cost for convenience. Prepared, presliced, and precooked foods usually cost more. For example, ready-to-grill beef kebobs cost more than buying beef to make your own. However, depending on your schedule, labor-saving and step-saving ingredients may be worth the price.

● Remain flexible. If you see a better bargain or a new food (perhaps a vegetable or a fruit), adjust your menu.

● Plan menus that combine more costly ingredients with more affordable ingredients, such as whole grains, vegetables, fruits, and low-fat or fat-free dairy foods as the main feature. Use small amounts of lean meats.

COMPARE THE VALUE!

Limit or avoid expensive snack foods, desserts, and soft drinks that provide little or no nutrition value for your money.

WHAT YOU GET FOR ABOUT THE SAME COST*	NUTRITION VALUE FOR YOUR $$
1¼ pound carrots	Vitamins, minerals, fiber, antioxidants
4 oz. bag regular chips**	Calories from fat, salt
3 small (2¾ in) apples	Vitamins, minerals, fiber, antioxidants
2 typical cookies**	Calories from fat and added sugars
64 oz. 100% orange juice	Vitamins, minerals, antioxidants
2 liters regular soda	Calories from added sugars

*Prices are approximate and will vary depending on location, sales, coupons, etc.
**In varying amounts, these foods provide some other nutrients.
Adapted from: Produce for Better Health Foundation, 2011.

● Beware of marketing ploys. End-of-the-aisle displays and store sampling are meant as attention grabbers! When you stop and look, you more likely buy.

● Pay attention at checkout. Put down the magazine or your cell phone. See that prices scan as advertised or as indicated on the shelf label, especially for sale items. Common checkout errors are: sale items not programmed into the computer; charging for the weight of packaging; and in some states, taxing nontaxable items. Check your receipts.

● Be cautious with credit cards. Paying interest just adds to the cost of your groceries!

"Small-Household" Shopping

How do small households maximize their food dollars? Besides general cost-saving tips, you might save in other ways if you're a household of one or two:

● Buy frozen vegetables and fruit in bags, not boxes. As long as they aren't thawed, you can pour out as much as you need, then reseal and return the package to the freezer.

● Look for foods sold in single servings: juice, yogurt, frozen meals, soup, and pudding, among others. In that way you can have a greater variety of food on hand. "Singles" may help with portion control, too. Because small households are a big consumer market segment, more and more products now are available in single-size servings.

● To save with economy-size packages, share your food purchases with a friend.

● Decide if the bigger package with the lower unit price is really a saving. If you can't use it all, it's no savings. Get the smaller package.

● Shop from bulk bins for small amounts.

● At home repackage meat, poultry, and fish into single portions in freezer wrap or plastic freezer bags. Freeze these portions to use later.

● Ask the butcher or the produce manager for a smaller amount of prepackaged fresh meat, poultry, or produce. Usually they can repackage food.

● Buy produce that keeps longer in the refrigerator: broccoli, Brussels sprouts, cabbage, carrots, parsnips, potatoes, sweet potatoes, apples, grapefruit, melons, oranges, pears, and tangerines.

● Shop for convenience. Often mixed salad greens (perhaps from the salad bar) or raw vegetables, already cut and mixed for stir-fry dishes or salads, cost less than individual foods bought in quantity.

● Buy small loaves of bread, or wrap and freeze what you won't use right away.

Shopping for Health

Filling your shopping cart? Let's tour the supermarket, department by department, focusing on shopping tips for high-quality, nutritious, and safe foods—that match your needs. Certainly this "shopping trip" won't cover all the foods sold today. And new products, including more variety and more better-for-you products, constantly come on the market. However, some basics for each food category can help you make healthier shopping decisions. For more nutrition, try to choose mostly nutrient-rich food choices. *For more about food from farm to supermarket, refer to chapter 9.*

Produce Department

Today's supermarkets offer a great variety of fresh fruits and vegetables—about three hundred different types of produce in the average store. *See chapter 9 for new fruits and vegetables you might try.* Because fruit and vegetables are most nutritious and best-tasting at their peak quality, shop with savvy.

● Check the produce department. Besides being clean, organized, and appealing, fresh fruits and vegetables should be held at a proper temperature. Most are chilled; a fine mist helps keep greens crisp; being soggy promotes growth of mold or rot.

● For fresh fruits, consider ripeness before you bring them home. If you plan to eat them today, buy ripe! Some fruits—for example, bananas, apples, pears, and mangoes—ripen after picking; they sweeten as their starches convert to sugar. Avocados ripen only after picking. Apricots, blueberries, cantaloupe, honeydew, peaches, and nectarines don't get sweeter, but their juiciness, texture, and color ripen after picking. *Tip:* To hasten ripening, put them in a loosely closed paper bag at room temperature. Putting an apple or a banana

Shopping for Freshness!

For Fruit . . .

Apples: firm with smooth, clean skin and good color. Avoid fruit with bruises or decay spots.

Apricots: plump with as much golden-orange color as possible. Blemishes, unless they break the skin, will not affect flavor. Avoid fruit that is pale yellow, greenish-yellow, very firm, shriveled, or bruised.

Avocado: green to purplish-black, smooth to bumpy skin, and yellow-green, soft flesh. They're ripe when they yield to gentle pressure. Most are sold unripe.

Bananas: plump with uniform shape at desired ripeness level. Avoid produce with blemished or bruised skins.

Blueberries: plump, firm berries with a light-grayish bloom. The bloom is the thin coating on the surface.

Cantaloupes: slightly oval fruit, 5 inches or more in diameter, with yellow or golden (not green) background color. Signs of sweetness include pronounced netting on the rind and a few tiny cracks near the stem end. Smell the melon; it should be noticeably strong and sweet. At home, check for ripeness before you eat it; the stem area will be slightly soft when ripe.

Cherries: plump, bright-colored sweet or sour cherries. Sweet cherries with reddish-brown skin promise flavor. Avoid overly soft or shriveled cherries or those with dark stems.

Grapefruits: firm, thin-skinned fruit, full-colored, and heavy for their size. The best grapefruits are smooth, thin-skinned, and flat at both ends. Avoid fruit with a pointed end or thick, deeply pored skin.

Grapes: plump grapes firmly attached to pliable green stems. Color is the best indication of ripeness and flavor. Avoid soft or wrinkled fruits and those with bleached-looking areas at the stem end.

Honeydew melons: melons weighing at least 5 pounds, with waxy white rind barely tinged with green. Fully ripe fruit has a cream-colored rind; the blossom end should give to gentle pressure.

Kiwifruit: softness similar to a ripe peach. Choose evenly firm fruit.

Lemons: firm, heavy fruit. Generally, rough-textured lemons have thicker skins and less juice than fine-skinned varieties.

Mangoes: usually quite firm when sold and need to be ripened further at home before eating. Avoid those with shriveled or bruised skin. Once ripened, they will give to gentle pressure.

Nectarines: orange-yellow (not green) background color between areas of red. Ripe nectarines feel slightly soft with gentle handling, but not as soft as ripe peaches.

Oranges: thin-skinned, firm, bright-colored fruit. Avoid oranges with any hint of softness or whitish mold at the ends.

Papayas: fruit with the softness of peaches and more yellow than green in the skin. Most papayas need to be ripened further after purchase in a loosely closed paper bag at room temperature. Avoid bruised or shriveled fruit showing any signs of mold or deterioration.

Peaches: creamy or yellow background color. Ripe peaches feel slightly soft with gentle handling. Avoid green, extra-hard, or bruised fruit.

Pears: fruit with firm skin. Pears gradually ripen after picking.

Pineapples: large, plump, fresh-looking fruit with green leaves and a sweet smell. Avoid fruit with soft spots, areas of decay, or fermented odor.

Plums: full-colored fruit. Ripe plums are slightly soft at the tip end and feel somewhat soft when handled gently. Avoid fruit with broken or shriveled skin.

Raspberries or blackberries: firm, plump, well-shaped berries. If soft or discolored, they are overripe. Avoid baskets that look stained from overripe berries.

Strawberries: firm, plump berries that are full-colored.

Watermelons: fruit heavy for its size, well shaped, with rind and flesh colors characteristic of the variety. Ripe melons are fragrant and slightly soft at the blossom end. A melon that sloshes when shaken may be overripe. Stem should be dry and brown, not green. When thumped, you should hear a low-pitched sound, indicating a full, juicy interior.

For Vegetables . . .

Artichokes: tight, compact heads that feel heavy for their size. Surface brown spots don't affect quality.

Asparagus: firm, brittle spears that are bright green almost their entire length, with tightly closed tips.

Beans (green or waxed): slender, crisp beans that are bright and blemish-free. Avoid mature beans with large seeds and swollen pods.

Beets: firm, smooth-skinned, small to medium beets. Leaves should be deep green and fresh-looking.

Bok choy: heads with bright white stalks and glossy dark leaves. Avoid heads with slippery brown spots on the leaves.

Shopping for Freshness! *(continued)*

Broccoli: compact clusters of tightly closed, dark green florets. Avoid heads with yellow florets or thick, woody stems.

Brussels sprouts: firm, compact, fresh-looking bright green sprouts. They should be heavy for their size.

Cabbage: firm heads that feel heavy for their size. Outer leaves should have good color and be free of blemishes.

Carrots: firm, clean, well-shaped carrots with bright, orange-gold color. Carrots with their tops still attached are likely to be freshest.

Cauliflower: firm, compact, creamy-white heads (without brown spots), with florets pressed tightly together. A yellow tinge and spreading florets indicate overmaturity. Leaves should be crisp and bright green.

Celery: crisp, rigid, green stalks with fresh-looking leaves. Avoid celery with limp stalks.

Corn: fresh-looking ears with green husks, moist stems, and silk ends free of decay or worm injury. When pierced with a thumbnail, kernels should squirt some juice. Tough skins indicate overmaturity.

Cucumbers: firm, dark-green cucumbers that are slender but well shaped. Soft or yellow cukes are overmature.

Edamame (immature soybeans in the pod): bright green pods, no yellowing; tender

Eggplants: firm, heavy for their size, with taut, glassy, deeply colored skin. Stems should be bright green.

Fennel: fragrant, celery-like stalks with a bulbous base and feathery leaves

Greens: fresh, tender leaves that are free of blemishes. Avoid bunches with thick, coarse-veined leaves.

Jicama: firm, well-formed tubers free of blemishes. Size does not affect flavor, but larger roots do tend to have a coarse texture.

Kohlrabi: young, tender bulbs with fresh green leaves. Avoid those with scars and blemishes. The smaller the bulb, the more delicate the flavor and texture.

Leeks and green onions: clean, white bottoms and crisp, fresh-looking green tops.

Mushrooms: blemish-free mushrooms without slimy spots or signs of decay.

Okra: small to medium pods that are deep green and free of blemishes. Pods should snap or puncture easily with slight pressure.

Onions: green onions with crisp, bright green tops and clean white bottoms. Choose firm, dry onions with brittle outer skin, avoiding those with sprouting green shoots or dark spots.

Parsnips: small to medium, smooth, firm, and well shaped. Avoid large roots because they may have a woody core.

Peas: small, plump, bright-green pods that are firm, crisp, and well filled.

Peppers: bright, glossy, firm, and well shaped. Avoid those with soft spots or gashes.

Potatoes: firm, smooth, with no wrinkles, sprouts, cracks, bruises, decay, or bitter-green areas (caused by exposure to light).

Rutabagas: small to medium, smooth, firm, and heavy for their size.

Salad greens: crisp, deeply colored leaves free of brown spots, yellowed leaves, and decay.

Sprouts: crisp buds still attached.

Summer squash: yellow squash and zucchini of medium size with firm, smooth, glossy, tender skin. Squash should be heavy for their size.

Sweet potatoes and yams: firm, well shaped, with bright, uniformly colored skin.

Tomatoes: smooth, well formed, firm, not hard.

Turnips: firm, smooth, small to medium size, that are heavy for their size.

Winter squash: hard, thick-shelled.

Source: Adapted from M. J. Smith, *The Miracle Foods Cookbook* (Minneapolis: Chronimed Publishing, 1995). This material is used by permission of John Wiley & Sons, Inc.

in the bag, too, speeds the process; these fruits give off ethylene gas, a ripening agent.

Soft berries, cherries, citrus, grapes, pineapples, and watermelon won't ripen after picking.

● Buy only the amount you need since they're perishable. Produce at peak quality contains the most nutrients.

● Look for nutrition information. Packaged produce may carry Nutrition Facts. If not, check for a poster or a pamphlet nearby. Ask the store manager to provide this information if it's not available.

● Choose a colorful variety of fruits and vegetables. Rather than just the old standbys, buy a new fruit or vegetable each week or two; try some locally grown.

The store may have preparation and handling tips for unfamiliar produce.

Explore different varieties of a familiar food. For example, try different apples: perhaps Cortland, Granny Smith, Newtown Pippin, and Rome Beauty. Or choose one of each variety of plums: perhaps Laroda, Queen Ann, Santa Rosa, and Wickson.

● Look for signs of quality. Bruised or wilted produce suggests improper handling or produce that's past its peak. Some nutrients may be lost as a result. *Refer to the chart "Shopping for Freshness!" earlier in this chapter.*

● For flavor, buy small. Small fruit is often sweeter than larger pieces of the same fruit.

● Handle fresh fruits and vegetables gently. Damage and bruising hasten spoilage. Place produce in the shopping cart where it won't get bruised. At checkout, make sure it's packed on top or in separate bags.

● For convenience choose prewashed bags of salad greens, sliced stir-fry veggies, precut fruit, and packaged baby carrots and celery sticks for quick vegetables and fruit. Choose packaged, sliced fruit, such as melon and pineapple, without added sugars.

● For cost saving, buy unpackaged produce. Then you can pick out items at their peak of quality.

● Look for fresh herbs, herbs in jars, and sun-dried tomatoes in the produce department. Choose fresh herbs that look fresh, not wilted. They're sometimes found growing in a pot!

Have You Ever Wondered

… how Community Supported Agriculture (CSA) works? CSAs provide a way to buy local, seasonal food directly from farmers—often at a more affordable price. Farmers sell a set number of shares, or memberships, to consumers. The shares usually provide a container or containers of vegetables or other seasonal farm products on a weekly or biweekly schedule during the growing season, depending on growing conditions. CSAs provide a market for local farmers, and both fresh products and a farm connection for consumers. Find one near you: www.localharvest.org.

● Another option: Dried fruits are nonperishable, often sold in the produce department; they supply the same nutrients as fresh fruit. If you're sensitive to sulfites, check the label; sulfites prevent browning in many dried fruits.

Meat and Deli Case

Through advanced breeding and feeding practices, today's animals are leaner than ever. Leaner cuts also result from newer meat cuts and from closer trimming of beef, veal, pork, and lamb cuts. The average thickness of fat around the edge of steaks and roasts has trimmed down to less than ⅛ inch trim today. *See "Today's Meat" in chapter 9.* Choose mostly lean meat.

● Check Nutrition Facts on single-ingredient, raw meat to make lean choices. For example, in raw ground beef, a 4-ounce label serving of "80 percent lean" ground beef has about 290 calories and about 205 calories from fat, compared to just about 115 calories and about 50 calories from fat in 4 ounces of "95 percent lean" ground beef. The term "percent lean" in the description can be confusing; 80 percent lean ground beef has 20 percent fat, while 95 percent lean ground beef has 5 percent fat. *See page 280 for more on meat and poultry labeling.*

● *Shop for meat's lean cuts.* For lower-fat cuts of fresh meats, look for "round" or "loin" in the name when shopping for beef, and "loin" or "leg" when buying pork or lamb. Some lean cuts:

  ● *Beef:* eye of round, top round steak, top round roast, sirloin steak, top loin steak, tenderloin steak, flank steak, and chuck arm pot roast

  ● *Veal:* cutlet, blade or arm steak, rib roast, and rib or loin chop

  ● *Pork:* tenderloin, top loin roast, top loin chop, center loin chop, sirloin roast, loin rib chop, and shoulder blade steak

  ● *Lamb:* leg, loin chop, arm chop, and foreshanks.

Learn more about beef's lean cuts and pork's lean cuts in this chapter.

Unsure of the cut? Check the meat label. It identifies the kind and cut, along with the net weight, unit price, and cost per package.

● Choose leaner grades of meat. "Select" grades of beef have the least marbled fat (or thin streaks of fat between the muscle) followed by "choice," then "prime" beef grades. Veal and lamb use the same grading system; however, the term "good" is used instead of "select." Grading, determined by the U.S. Department of Agriculture, is based on fat content, appearance, texture, and the age of the animal. Pork is not graded.

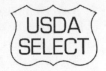

More costly "prime" grades of beef—more often found on restaurant menus than sold in supermarkets—have more marbled fat, which helps make meat juicy and flavorful. With proper methods of cooking and carving, leaner "select" and "choice" meats can be tender, juicy, and flavorful, too.

Shopping at a Farmers' Market?

With several thousand farmers' markets in operation in the United States and more every year, farmers' markets give you a chance to talk to growers and producers and perhaps find local products you can't find elsewhere: local varietals of vegetables and fruits; artisan cheeses; fresh or potted herbs; cut flowers; homemade sauces; oven-fresh baked goods; organically certified foods; locally produced poultry, eggs, or meat; or fresh fish. And it's a great shopping option for getting more fresh fruits and vegetables in your food plan!

Be aware that the produce sold may—or may not—be fresh from the field. Some markets feature only local growers. Others sell brokered products from the same commercial markets that supermarkets buy from. And some sell both. Ask the market manager.

For food safety and great shopping, bring a clean carry bag or two, perhaps insulated: separate ones for raw and cooked foods, or for meat, poultry, or fish. As you shop, pay attention to food safety practices of the vendor: cleanliness, gloves or clean utensils for food handling, covered garbage cans, clean bags. Go early for the best selection; check the market website ahead if there's one. Shop with flexibility; the market changes with the season and the local growers and vendors who come to market. Take time to talk to and learn from them. Many small farmers are eager to talk about their growing methods and how they care for their animals. They may even invite you for a farm visit! Pack your purchases so they don't crush; take perishables home right away. Check www.localharvest.org to find a local farmers' market.

Meat Buying Guide

How much raw meat should you buy? For about 3 ounces of cooked, lean meat per person, that's about 4 ounces of raw meat per person. For some meats you'll need to take the amount of bone and fat into account.

TYPE OF MEAT	SERVINGS PER POUND*
Boneless or ground meat	4
Meat with a minimum amount of bone (steaks, roasts, chops, etc.)	2 to 3
Meat with a large amount of bone (shoulder cuts, short ribs, neck, etc.)	1 to 2

*Three ounces of cooked trimmed meat equal one serving.

Nutritionally speaking, nutrients in meat—protein, thiamin, niacin, iron, and zinc, among others—are the same, regardless of grade.

● Buy well-trimmed meat: ⅛-inch fat trim or less. "Trim" refers to the fat layer surrounding a steak or other cut of meat. *Note:* Marbled fat cannot be trimmed away. Only cooking methods can remove some, but not all, marbled fat.

● Check the "numbers" for ground meat—look for packages that have the greatest percent lean to percent fat ratio. Ground beef labeled as 95 percent lean also may include the nutrition description "Lean" because it meets the definition of a lean product. *Note:* "Percent lean" refers to the weight of the lean meat in relation to the weight of the fat.

● Buy enough meat without overdoing portion sizes. For moderate-size portions (3 ounces cooked), figure 4 ounces of uncooked, boneless meat per person. *Refer to the chart "Meat Buying Guide" on this page to help you decide how much meat to buy.*

● Use nutrition labeling to find lean packaged meats. By regulation, packaged deli meats must carry Nutrition Facts. Use it to find hot dogs, luncheon meats, and sausage that are leaner and have less sodium.

Check for lean options from the deli case. For ready-to-slice luncheon meats from a deli, ask for nutrition information if you're unsure of its leanness. Some lean products will be identified with a nutrient content claim such as "low-fat," "____% fat-free," or "lean."

● Look for nutrition information for fresh meat, poultry, and seafood. Single-ingredient raw meat, poultry, and seafood soon may be labeled voluntarily with nutrition information.

● For bacon, try Canadian or turkey bacon. Canadian bacon is lean, much like ham. In contrast, traditional bacon is mainly fat, including saturated fat. Bacon counts as a solid fat, which should be limited, and not as a lean protein food. For bacon, check the label for sodium content, too.

● If you eat organ meats, also called variety meats, make them occasional choices. Brain, chitterlings (pig intestines), heart, kidney, liver, sweetbreads (thymus gland), tongue, and tripe (stomach lining of cattle) are all organ meats. Organ meats are good sources of many nutrients; liver, in particular, is high in iron. However, most are higher in cholesterol than lean meat. Some, such as chitterlings, sweetbreads, and tongue, have more fat.

● For convenience, look for meat that's already seasoned, prepared, and ready to cook, such as meat and vegetable kebobs or marinated pork loin. However, precooked, packaged heat-and-eat meats in the refrigerated case may be higher in sodium. Check the Nutrition Facts.

● Recognize the qualities of fresh meat. Color indicates freshness. Beef is typically bright red. Both young veal and pork are grayish-pink. Older veal is darker pink. Lamb can be light to darker pink, depending on the animal feed.

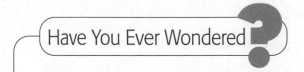

Have You Ever Wondered

... what is meant by grass-fed beef? It comes from beef cattle that graze in pastures their whole lives. It generally grades as "Select" meat. Conventional beef cattle graze most of their lives in the pasture, too, but they're finished on a balanced, grain-based diet in a feed lot. Grass-fed meat isn't necessarily organic.

... if free-range chickens have less fat? It's a common misperception that free-range chickens—those that "roam the barnyard and forage for food"—are always leaner than chickens raised in coops. Whether raised in a coop or a barnyard, their exercise level often is about the same. Genetic stock, age, and growth rate have more influence on fat levels. Older, larger chickens and those that grow faster tend to have more fat—no matter how they're raised.

According to the USDA's Food Safety and Inspection Service, which regulates poultry labeling, the terms "free-range" and "free-roaming" may be used on poultry labels if the producers can demonstrate that the poultry has been allowed access to the outside for a significant portion of their life. Free-range chickens usually cost more; blind taste tests don't show differences in flavor perception. That said, they are a nourishing option.

While free-range chickens are raised outdoors or have daily outdoor access, in reality, most stay indoors. Because free-range chickens may be exposed to outdoor pollutants, some food safety questions have been raised. Cage-free chickens aren't caged but may not have outdoor access. Mortality rates of these poultry are higher since they tend to peck at and injure each other.

... how the fat and cholesterol in surimi compare with crabmeat? Surimi is imitation crabmeat, made from pollock or another mild-flavored fish. The fish is processed by rolling "sheets" of fish and adding color so it looks like crab legs. The nutrient content reflects the fish it's made from. Surimi is comparable in fat content but lower in cholesterol than crabmeat.

Reading Meat Labels

1. The kind of meat—Listed on every label
2. The primal (wholesale) cut—Tells where the meat came from on the animal
3. The retail cut—Tells from what part of the primal cut the meat comes

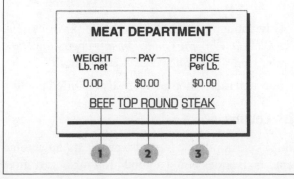

MEAT DEPARTMENT

WEIGHT Lb. net — PAY — PRICE Per Lb.

0.00 $0.00 $0.00

BEEF TOP ROUND STEAK

①   ②   ③

● Check the dating on meat. Only buy fresh and processed meats that still will be fresh when you're ready to eat them. Or plan to freeze immediately for later use.

● Notice the safe food handling label. *A sample label is shown in this chapter. For more about handling meat safely, see chapter 13.*

Poultry Counter

Besides being economical, chicken and turkey offer high-quality protein, and they're usually very lean. As you choose poultry:

● Choose mostly lean varieties of poultry—turkey and chicken. Check Nutrition Facts, *as noted earlier in this chapter.* Domesticated duck and goose are higher in fat. A 3½-ounce cooked portion of roasted, skinless chicken (light and dark meat) has about 7 fat grams compared with 11 fat grams in the same portion of roasted, skinless duck. Pheasant and quail, especially without the skin, are lean, too.

● To trim fat, shop for skinless poultry—chicken and turkey. Compared to skin-on, the grams of total fat and saturated fat are half. Or buy skin on poultry if it costs less. Remove the skin before or after cooking it. Either way, the fat content is comparable when eaten.

Poultry Buying Guide

How much poultry? Here's how many servings come from 1 pound of uncooked chicken, duck, goose, game hens, or turkey.

POULTRY	SERVINGS PER POUND*
Whole chicken (broiler-fryer or roaster)	2
Boneless chicken breast	4
Duck, whole	1
Goose, whole	1½ to 2
Rock Cornish game hen, whole	1
Whole turkey, bone in	2
Boneless turkey roast	3
Ground turkey	4

*Amounts are based on 3 ounces of cooked poultry without bone per serving.

For less fat, choose light meat such as the turkey or chicken breast. Compare: 3½ ounces of roasted, skinless, dark-meat chicken have about 10 fat grams and 3 grams of saturated fat; the same amount of roasted, skinless, light-meat chicken has about 3 fat grams and 1 gram of saturated fat. The cholesterol content is about the same.

● When you buy whole turkey, know that self-basting varieties are higher in fat and sodium. Self-basting turkeys are moist and flavorful because they're injected with fat—including saturated fatty acids and sodium. Instead, baste turkey with broth, juice, or juices from the poultry. *Hint:* Roasting any whole bird with the breast side up makes it more moist.

● Is ground meat on your shopping list? Try lean ground turkey breast. Ground turkey breast can be as lean as 99 percent fat-free. The fat content is higher if it's ground with dark meat and skin.

● Recognize the qualities of fresh poultry. Look for meaty birds with skin that's creamy-white to yellow and that are free of bruises, tiny feathers, and torn or dry skin. Check for product dating on food labels.

● Read the Nutrition Facts before you buy turkey dogs, turkey ham, or turkey bologna. They may—or may not—be low in fat. Compare the sodium content with that of traditional processed meats; processing typically adds sodium. For fresh cuts of meats and poultry, look for the Nutrition Facts, which may be posted on the package or in the retail case.

● Check the Nutrition Facts for sodium content. Uncooked poultry may be plumped, or injected with a saltwater solution, to keep in moisture, flavor, and tenderness. For less sodium, or salt, look for other poultry options.

● For cost savings, buy a whole bird and carve it yourself.

● Buy enough poultry for moderate portions. *The chart "Poultry Buying Guide" on this page shows how much to buy for 3-ounce cooked portions.*

● For food safety, don't buy fresh prestuffed poultry.

Fish Counter

Today's seafood sales are driven by its nutritional benefits. Besides being a good protein source, most seafood is low in fat, especially saturated fat. Fatty fish offers potential health benefits from omega-3 fatty acids. *See "Functional Nutrition: Eat Your Omega-3s and -6s" in chapter 5.*

Fifty to a hundred varieties of fish are commonly on the market today at any given time. Much of this fish is wild, coming from oceans and freshwater lakes, ponds, or rivers. As the demand for fish grows, aquaculture, or fish farming, has become a more important source, especially for catfish, trout, salmon, shrimp, and tilapia. *Refer to chapter 9 for more about aquaculture.*

A few definitions: Seafood includes both finfish and shellfish; catfish, cod, flounder, haddock, mahimahi, salmon, snapper, tilapia, tuna, and trout are among the many types. Shellfish are both crustaceans (crab, crayfish, lobster, and shrimp) and mollusks (clam, mussel, oyster, scallop, octopus, squid, abalone, conch, and snail). Learn to choose high-quality, safe seafood that also matches your personal needs and preferences.

● Check the fish counter. Always buy fresh or frozen seafood from a reputable source. Fresh seafood should be displayed for food safety properly iced, well refrigerated, and in clean display cases. To reduce the chance of spoilage, fish should be displayed "belly down" to drain away melting ice.

Check for general fish counter cleanliness: clean look and smell; free of insects; employees wearing disposable gloves (changed after handling nonfood and again after handling raw fish); and knowledgeable workers who can answer your questions about the freshness of the seafood. Ask when and how often fresh and flash-frozen fish come in. Be flexible; buy the freshest fish if you don't need a specific type.

● Recognize the fat content of various fish. In general, most fish has less fat than many other protein-rich foods, including meat and poultry with skin. And most fat in fish is polyunsaturated.

Fish that is firm and darker in color, such as king mackerel, salmon, and tuna, tends to have more fat and omega-3 fatty acids; omega-3s may offer heart-healthy benefits. Try to eat fatty fish at least twice a week.

● Choose fish that's best for the recipe. Lean fish is great for baking, microwaving, and poaching. Fish with more fat tends to be better for grilling and roasting because it doesn't dry out as quickly and because it holds its shape better. For example, salmon and tuna are better for kebobs. Mild-flavored fish, such as cod, flounder, haddock, sole, snapper, and tilapia, tends to be the lowest in fat, while fish with more fat usually has a fuller flavor.

● Know what form you need: finfish—fillets, steaks, whole fish, or dressed (head, tail, and fins removed), or shellfish—whole live or just "meat."

● Learn to recognize the qualities of *fresh* seafood.

● *Finfish.* At peak quality, whole finfish have a fresh ocean-breeze scent, not a fishy or ammonia-like smell. They're naturally firm to the touch, with stiff fins and scales that cling tightly to the skin. The skin is shiny and "metallic," not dull. The gills are pink or bright red and free from mucus or slime. If undamaged, their eyes are clear, bright, and protruding. Walleyes are among the few fish with naturally cloudy eyes. Fish fillets or steaks also have a mild scent, firm and moist flesh, a translucent appearance, and no browning around the edges. If wrapped, packaging should be tight and undamaged.

● *Shellfish.* Crustaceans and some mollusks are sold live. In fact, unless frozen, canned, or cooked, crabs, crayfish, and lobsters should be alive when sold. They'll move slightly if they're alive, and live lobsters curl their tails a bit when handled. For food safety, buy shellfish from a reputable source.

If their shells are still on, clams, mussels, and oysters must be sold alive, too, for food safety's sake; shells shouldn't be damaged. When these mollusks are alive, their shells are slightly open, but they close tightly when tapped. As another test, hold the shell between your thumb and forefinger; press so that one part of the shell slides across the other. If the shells move, it isn't fresh.

Freshly shucked mollusks (shells removed) have a mild, fresh scent. A somewhat clear liquid, not too milky or cloudy, should cover shucked "meat."

Scallops are removed from their shells at sea. They vary in size and color, from creamy white to light orange, tan, or somewhat pinkish. When fresh, they're not dry or darkened around the edges.

Fresh, raw shrimp will have a mild odor. For all fish—finfish and shellfish—use your nose. A strong "fishy" odor is a sign that fish is no longer fresh.

● Know the qualities of *frozen* fish. Frozen seafood should be solidly frozen, mild in odor, and free of ice crystals and freezer burn. Freezer burn is indicated by drying and discoloration. The package shouldn't be damaged or water-stained, and it should be stored below the frost line in the store's display freezer. These qualities apply to frozen fish and frozen prepared items such as crab cakes and breaded shrimp.

Note: "Previously frozen" (thawed for sale) fish—harvested and frozen in remote locations—may be superior in quality to fresh fish, transported for several days.

● Check the food product dating on the label of frozen fish. Choose packaged seafood that doesn't show signs of thawing, then refreezing. Check the "sell by" date, if it has one. *Read about product dating earlier in this chapter.*

● Choose *cooked* shrimp, lobsters, crabs, and crayfish that are moist with a mild odor and a characteristic color. The shells of cooked shrimp should be pink to reddish. For other crustaceans, the shells should be bright red. Some stores cook them for you.

● For safety, don't buy cooked seafood that's displayed alongside raw seafood. Bacteria from raw fish can contaminate cooked fish, creating a potential for foodborne illness. *For more about cross-contamination, see "Checklist for a Clean Kitchen" in chapter 13.*

● Choose *smoked* fish, such as smoked salmon or smoked trout, that is bright, glossy, and free of mold. Since it may not be cooked before serving, smoked fish should be wrapped and kept away from raw fish to avoid cross-contamination.

● Substitute one fish for another. When the store doesn't have the seafood you want or if it costs more than you anticipate, make a switch. Sometimes lesser-known species cost less. For example, when a recipe calls for flounder, almost any mild finfish (perhaps haddock, halibut, or perch) can take its place.

Be aware of differences in nutritional content when you make substitutions. Squid, shrimp, and lobsters, for example, have more cholesterol than clams, crabs, mussels, and scallops do. Three ounces of boiled shrimp supply about 165 milligrams of cho-

Seafood Buying Guide

TYPE OF SEAFOOD	APPROXIMATE AMOUNT OF RAW SEAFOOD NEEDED PER ADULT SERVING*
Whole fish	¾ pound
Dressed or pan-dressed fish	½ pound
Fish fillets	¼ to ⅓ pound
Fish steaks with bone	½ pound
Fish steaks without bone	⅓ pound
Live clams and oysters	6 to 8
Shucked clams and oysters	⅓ to ½ pint
Live lobsters and crabs	1 to 1½ pounds
Cooked lobster or crabmeat	¼ to ⅓ pound
Scallops	¼ to ⅓ pound
Shrimp, headless and unpeeled	⅓ to ½ pound
Shrimp, peeled and deveined	¼ to ⅓ pound

*The smaller amounts in the ranges shown provide a cooked portion that is approximately 3 ounces when prepared by most common cooking methods.
Source: New York Seafood Council, 2010.

lesterol; the same amount of scallops has about 55 milligrams.

● Whether it's sold from the seafood counter or the freezer, go easy on breaded items such as shrimp and fish sticks, often containing more calories and fat.

● For nutrition information check the Nutrition Facts on packaged seafood products. For fresh seafood you'll find this information displayed nearby.

● Buy only the amount of seafood you need. Because of waste, you need more when preparing whole or dressed fish. A dressed fish has the head, tail, and fins removed. Usually fish steaks, fillets, and shellfish, which have less waste, cost more per pound. Without the waste, the price may equal out. *The chart "Seafood Buying Guide" on this page helps you estimate how much for a cooked 3-ounce portion.*

Refrigerated Case

Although you'll find tortillas, refrigerator rolls, and biscuits among the many products in the refrigerated case, dairy foods, eggs, biscuits, and juice are prominent.

Dairy Foods

Milk:

Which milk for you? Because milk solids make up at least 8.25 percent for each type of milk, their protein, vitamin, and mineral content is about the same. (Milk solids are the part of milk that's neither milk fat nor water; percentages of milk fat refer to percent by weight, not by calories.)

● Consider milk's calorie and fat content. Choose mostly low-fat and fat-free. Check the Nutrition Facts; *refer to chapter 8 to see how different milk compares.*

  ● *Whole milk:* no less than 3.25 percent milk fat; usually vitamin D-fortified.

  ● *2% reduced-fat milk:* 2 percent milk fat; is vitamin A- and D-fortified.

  ● *1% low-fat milk (or light milk):* 1 percent milk fat; must be vitamin A- and D-fortified.

  ● *Fat-free (or nonfat or skim milk):* less than 0.5 percent milk fat; must be vitamins A- and D-fortified.

  ● *Flavored milk* (whole, 2 percent reduced fat, 1 percent low-fat, or fat-free); with added chocolate, cocoa, or fruit-flavoring, and sweetener. Look for those with added vitamin D. *For more about flavored milk, refer to chapter 8.*

● Lactose-sensitive? Try lactose-reduced or lactose-free milk (whole, low-fat, or fat-free). Lactase enzyme, added to milk, "predigests" lactose (sugar in milk), so you can enjoy milk without discomfort. Because lactose converts to simple sugars (glucose and galactose), it tastes slightly sweeter. To be "lactose-reduced," lactose must be reduced by 70 percent. Lactose-free milk is 100 percent lactose-reduced. *See chapter 21 for more on lactose intolerance and maldigestion.*

● Use Nutrition Facts to compare various nutrient-enhanced milks and those with added health benefits.

  ● *Protein-fortified milk* has added nonfat milk solids and perhaps thickeners. Enhancing fat-free or low-fat milk with milk solids adds a fuller flavor and creamier consistency, and more protein and calcium.

  ● *Skim deluxe or skim supreme milk* is fat-free but has the mouth feel (from some added fiber) of 2 percent reduced-fat milk.

● *Milk with functional benefits* may be enhanced with omega-3 fatty acids or with plant stanols or sterols to reduce heart disease risk. Other enhanced milks might have added DHA, a form of omega-3s, which may promote vision and the health of the nervous system.

● Enjoy acidophilus milk and kefir (a yogurt drink). They're made by adding "friendly" bacteria cultures, often to fat-free or low-fat milk. The bacteria culture produces their unique flavor, aroma, acidity, and thick texture. Salt may be added for flavor. Although research isn't conclusive, live active "friendly" bacteria

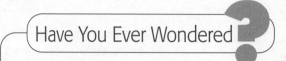

Have You Ever Wondered

. . . how cow's milk and soy beverage compare? The nutrient content of soy beverage isn't the same as in cow's milk. Unless fortified, soy beverage, made by pressing ground, cooked soybeans, is significantly lower in calcium. As a substitute for cow's milk, choose soy beverage that's calcium-fortified. Soy drinks range from 80 to 500 milligrams of calcium per cup; read the Nutrition Facts.

The calcium absorbed from fortified foods varies. For example, the calcium from 1 cup of milk and 1 cup of soy beverage fortified with calcium carbonate is about the same. However, to get the same amount from soy beverage with tricalcium phosphate, you'd need to drink 1⅓ cups; this form of calcium isn't absorbed as well in the body.

Compared with cow's milk, soy beverage is lower in protein and riboflavin, and has little vitamin A or D naturally; some soy beverages are fortified with vitamins A and D and riboflavin. As a phytonutrient, isoflavones in soy may offer unique benefits as phytoestrogens; *see "A Quick Look at Key Phytonutrients" in chapter 6.* Soy protein may have cardiovascular benefits. Soy beverage is cholesterol-free. The fat content of soy beverage is similar to 2 percent cow's milk. Also look for low-fat versions; they may have less protein too.

. . . why cottage cheese has less calcium than other cheese? During processing, the whey is drained away, along with 50 to 75 percent of the calcium. Check food labels for cottage cheese processed with extra calcium. Good news: It still provides plenty of protein and riboflavin, without much fat.

work as probiotics in fermented dairy foods and may help improve digestion and promote healthy bacteria in the gastrointestinal tract. The probiotic benefits are specific to the bacterial strain.

● Enjoy tangy, cultured buttermilk as another great source of calcium. It too is made with the action of "friendly" bacteria cultures but doesn't have probiotic benefits from live cultures. Despite its name, butter isn't added to cultured buttermilk! Sweet cream buttermilk is the by-product of churning cream into butter, but it's not available in stores.

● Looking for organic milk? It must comply with organic standards, *as explained earlier in this chapter and in chapter 9.*

● Try eggnog during the winter holidays. It's a blend of milk, pasteurized eggs, sugar, cream, and flavors. Because eggnog is higher in calories and fat, you might prefer eggnog-flavored milk, made with fat-free or reduced-fat milk. Vegans might enjoy soy eggnog.

Yogurt:

Fruit-flavored or plain, whole, low-fat, or nonfat, yogurt is another high-calcium, high-protein dairy food. It's made with "friendly" bacteria, which give a tangy taste and thick consistency.

Nutritionally speaking, 8 ounces of yogurt supply about 300 milligrams of calcium, as does 8 ounces of milk. If you're not a milk drinker, consider yogurt as a key calcium source. Yogurt's calorie and fat content reflect the milk it's made from. Yogurt also may be sweetened with fruit, fruit preserves, honey, or other sugars, or flavored with extracts such as vanilla or coffee. It may contain pectin, found naturally in fruit, or gelatin to make it thicker and creamier.

● For fewer calories and added sugars, reach for plain low-fat or fat-free yogurt, or perhaps yogurt flavored with a low-calorie sweetener such as aspartame, or both.

● Look for yogurt that's vitamin D-fortified, especially if you don't drink milk. *Remember:* Vitamin D is a nutrient often lacking in people's meals and snacks.

● Check the carton size—and Nutrition Facts. The smaller (4- or 6-ounce) carton of yogurt isn't a complete calcium swap for 8 ounces of milk.

● For potential immune-boosting benefits, look for the "Live and Active Cultures" seal from the National Yogurt Association on the label. The ingredient list shows the probiotic, or live, cultures used to make it: often *Lactobacillus acidophilus, L. casei, L. reuteri,* and *Bifidobacterium bifidum (Bifidus).* Yogurt with live cultures also may help the body digest milk's sugar. A label that says "made with active cultures" doesn't mean the cultures are live; heat from processing may destroy bacteria. Research on the health benefits of active, live cultures in yogurt isn't conclusive. *See chapter 6 for more on probiotics.*

● For the thick creaminess (without the high calories and fat) of sour cream, try Greek yogurt. It's made by straining whey from whole, low-fat, or fat-free yogurt.

● Enjoy flavored yogurt-juice beverages, drinkable yogurt, or kefir—other sources of calcium and perhaps vitamin D. Ingesting thick, frothy kefir is like drinking yogurt; some are high in added sugars.

Other yogurts: They may be enhanced nutritionally in other ways—for example, with DHA or with inulin, a prebiotic. Read the label's structure-function claim, the Nutrition Facts, and the ingredient list to learn more. While they may offer health benefits, these yogurts don't replace an overall healthy eating pattern. Organic yogurt? Like milk, it must comply with organic standards.

Cheese:

Cheese: It's milk in concentrated form—and more compact and portable, with a longer shelf life. That's why cheese is a great source of milk's naturally occurring nutrients. Many cheeses also have considerably more fat (including solid, or saturated, fat) per serving than a serving of milk does. Some are vitamin D-fortified.

Most cheese is made from cow's milk, but goat's and sheep's milk cheeses also are common. Many cheeses are made by coagulating the casein, a milk protein, then separating the solids and pressing them into their final form. Differences in style, texture, and flavor depend on the type of milk; its origin; its butterfat content; the bacteria or mold used; its processing; its aging time; and any herbs, spices, and perhaps wood smoke for flavoring.

● Buy cheese in well-sealed packaging. Check "use

by" or "sell by" dates on packaged cheese. On chunk cheese, make sure it has no cracks or surface mold. For fresh-cut cheese, ask about storage time.

● Try different types. Choose the right cheese for its use; handle properly. Check the Nutrition Facts since calorie and nutrient contents vary. For example, fat in double and triple cream soft cheeses is much higher.

● *Soft, semisoft, semihard, or hard cheeses.* Differences depend on moisture content and aging time. With less moisture, harder cheeses have a longer shelf life. Without preservatives, soft cheeses such as feta and ricotta spoil quickly. Semisoft cheeses such as Muenster and Monterey Jack are great for melting. Semihard cheeses such as Cheddar and Gouda are great for sandwiches. Very hard cheeses such as Parmesan are grating cheeses.

● *Processed cheeses.* They're blends of traditional cheeses that are shredded, mixed, and heated with emulsifying salts, and perhaps milk, preservatives, and food coloring. They melt well. Some, such as American cheese, are sold presliced.

● *Veined cheeses.* Either soft or hard, these cheeses, such as blue and Roquefort, get their strong, unique flavor from blue or green veins of "friendly" mold in the interior.

● *Soft-ripened cheeses.* They're firm to start with, but as they age, the center gets soft, the flavor gets more intense, and a white mold grows on the outside. Two examples: Brie and Camembert.

● For less fat, including saturated fat, and perhaps fewer calories, look for lower-fat cheeses such as low-fat ricotta, part-skim mozzarella, string cheese, or reduced-fat Cheddar. Made with reduced or fat-free milk, they usually have less fat and fewer calories.

● *Low-fat cheese* has 3 grams or less fat per serving; that's 1 ounce for most cheeses and 4 ounces for cottage cheese.

● *Reduced-fat cheese* has 25 percent less fat than the same full-fat cheese.

● *Fat-free cheese* has less than 0.5 gram of fat per serving.

Cheese with less fat usually has less cholesterol, too, but check the label to be sure.

● To savor the flavor but control the fat, use grated, shredded, and sharp-flavored cheeses. When grated, you may use less than if it's sliced or chunk cheese. Grate your own, or buy grated or shredded cheese, which likely costs more per ounce. With sharp cheeses such as sharp Cheddar, Provolone, or Parmesan, you get plenty of flavor with less cheese. Sharp flavor develops with aging.

● Look for reduced-sodium cheeses to lower sodium intake. Traditional cheese has sodium because it's a key ingredient in cheesemaking.

Note: Reduced-sodium cheese has a shorter shelf life.

Cream, Sour Cream, Spreads:

● Buy them—go easy on how much you use. Many are high in calories and fat and contain little calcium.

Read Nutrition Facts to compare calories and nutrients, including saturated and *trans* fats, in a label serving.

● Try lower-fat and fat-free products. Other options: half-and-half or fat-free half-and-half instead of coffee cream or heavy cream; and sour half-and-half or fat-free sour cream. An exception: To whip the cream in recipes, you'll need a carton of heavy or whipping cream.

● Know the differences. Both regular butter and stick margarine contain about 35 calories and 4 grams of total fat per teaspoon. Either way, they're mostly fat. Butter contains cholesterol and more saturated fats. Made from vegetable oil, stick (hard) margarine is cholesterol-free and has more poly- and monounsaturated fats; it's still high in *trans* fats. If the ingredient list says "partially hydrogenated vegetable oil," it has *trans* fats. Limit margarine with more than 2 grams of saturated fat per tablespoon.

● For spreads, buy soft tub, liquid, or spray margarines. They have less saturated fat and likely 0 grams of *trans* fat per serving. The first ingredient is probably liquid vegetable oil or water rather than partially hydrogenated vegetable oil.

● Consider whipped butter or margarine for spreads. They have less fat and calories per tablespoon because air adds volume. They can't be substituted for regular butter or margarine in recipes that require baking or

CREAM: FAT? CALORIES?

CREAM	% MILK FAT CONTENT	TOTAL FAT GRAMS	SATURATED FAT GRAMS	CALORIES
			PER TABLESPOON	
Half-and-half	10.5 to 18	2	1	20
Light or coffee cream	18 to 29	3	2	30
Light whipping cream	30 to 36	5	3	44
Heavy cream	36 or more	6	3	52
Cream in aerosol cans		1	.5	8

frying; they're fine for melting on veggies or bread. Because reduced-fat butter and margarine have more moisture, they're not suitable in some recipes.

● If you like buttery flavor, try blends of butter with olive or canola oil. They likely have less saturated fat and cholesterol. Read the label.

● Enjoy small amounts of cream cheese, but don't confuse its nutrient content with other cheese. Cream cheese is mainly milk fat, with very little milk solids. For a creamy texture with less fat, look for reduced-fat or fat-free cream cheese. Or buy regular cream cheese, then spread a little less on your morning bagel. Whipped cream cheese is often easier to spread, so you may be able to use less.

● As an alternative, look for cholesterol-lowering spreads with plant stanol and sterol esters. *See chapter 5.*

For fluid milk and other dairy foods, products that are properly refrigerated in the store won't spoil as quickly at home. Check the "sell by" date on the carton.

Nondairy Alternatives

Nondairy alternatives for vegans and for those with milk allergies are sold in the dairy case. Many are made with soy: soy beverages, soy yogurt, soy cheese, soy sour cream, soy eggnog, and soy smoothies. Although cholesterol-free, and likely lower in total and saturated fats, soy foods don't have the same characteristics as milk products. Their nutrient content varies, so read the label! *For more about the nutrition and health benefits of soybeans, refer to chapter 4. Other plant-based milk alternatives (from rice, almonds, other nuts, and grains), typically sold on store shelves, are addressed later in this chapter.*

Eggs

For an economical, convenient, and easy-to-prepare source of high-quality protein, try eggs. One egg supplies about 10 percent of the protein you need in a day, along with good amounts of vitamins A, D, and B_{12} choline, as well as phytonutrients (lutein and xeaxanthin). Although eggs are high in cholesterol, 185 milligrams per large egg, they have 5 grams of fat—no more than an ounce of cheese. Shell color—brown or white—doesn't affect the nutritional quality of eggs; the color varies with the breed of hen. Yolk color depends on the feed and doesn't affect the quality, flavor, nutritive value, or cooking characteristics.

From jumbo to small eggs: What size to buy? The bigger the egg, the more it has of everything: nutrients, cholesterol, calories. *As a shopping and food preparation tip:* Four jumbo eggs equal five large eggs or six small eggs. Most recipes are written for large eggs.

The size is different from the grade printed on the label. Eggs are graded AA, A, and B. Grading refers to the interior and exterior quality of eggs when they're packed. Most eggs sold in supermarkets are Grade A; they're almost the same as Grade AA eggs, which are considered slightly higher in quality.

● To check the freshness of shell eggs, find the date on the carton. If eggs come from a USDA-inspected plant, the carton will display a number (called a Julian date) for the packing date. A Julian date will be between 1 (January 1) and 365 (December 31). You can refrigerate fresh shell eggs for four to five weeks beyond the Julian date, in their carton, without losing quality. The carton also may carry an expiration date; after that it can't be sold. The yolks of fresher eggs hold their shape when they're cracked open. As eggs age, the white thins and the yolk flattens. However, the nutrition and functional qualities don't change.

● Open egg cartons before you buy, to be sure they're clean. Avoid cartons with cracked eggs. They may be contaminated with *Salmonella.*

● Buy eggs that are refrigerated, not kept at room temperature. Even though eggs are stored in their own natural package, unrefrigerated eggs spoil quickly.

● Need to limit yolks to cut cholesterol? Try cholesterol-free or reduced-cholesterol egg substitutes. The yolk, which contains the cholesterol, is left out. Other ingredients, such as nonfat milk, tofu, and vegetable oils, take its place; for coloring, it may contain beta carotene. Find egg substitutes, including soy-based egg replacers for vegans made with potato starch and lecithin, in the store's freezer or the refrigerated section.

Since cholesterol is in the yolk, not the white, you also can buy eggs and use just the whites to replace some or all of the whole eggs. *For more on cutting cholesterol in egg cookery, refer to chapter 14.*

● Want convenience? Consider frozen and refrigerated whole egg products. They're pasteurized, or heat-treated to kill potential *Salmonella* bacteria inside. The heat processing slightly lowers heat-sensitive nutrients, but not much. Use them immediately after opening the container.

● Also available in some stores: refrigerated, peeled, and ready-to-eat hard-cooked eggs.

Juice and Juice Drinks

Juice options are more than orange and grapefruit juices! You can find "lots of pulp" and "no pulp" juice; juice that's fortified with calcium, vitamin D, DHA, omega-3s, and more; juice blends; and juice drinks. *To compare these products, refer to chapter 8.*

● Read the label. Then choose the juice that's right for you. Remember that juice drinks have added sugars; 100 percent juice does not.

● Know that most packaged juices and juice drinks are pasteurized or processed to destroy harmful bacteria and naturally occurring enzymes that hasten spoilage.

If sold in interstate commerce, fresh juice and juice products that have *not been pasteurized* or appropriately treated must show this warning on the package label.

> WARNING: this product has not been pasteurized and, therefore, may contain harmful bacteria that can cause serious illness in children, the elderly, and persons with weakened immune systems.

Have You Ever Wondered

. . . if fertile eggs, organic eggs, free-range, or cage-free eggs have nutritional advantages? No, and they cost more. Fertile eggs, which can become chicks, won't keep as long. For organic eggs, produced by hens on organic rations, the nutrient content is the same regardless. Eggs from "free-range" or "cage-free" chickens have no extra nutritional benefits. Free-range chickens are raised outdoors or have daily outdoor access; in reality, most stay indoors.

. . . if modified-fat eggs or lower-cholesterol eggs are worth the extra cost? That depends on your food budget and overall food choices. Hens on feed with flaxseed, fish oil, or Maine algae can produce eggs with more omega-3 fatty acids; flaxseed is a great source of omega-3 fatty acids, which may offer health benefits. Eggs with more omega-3s also have more vitamin E. *See "Functional Nutrition: Eat Your Omega-3s and -6s" in chapter 5.* Shell eggs produced with less cholesterol are available as well; however, you may save money by buying whole eggs and tossing out some yolk. Look for other specialty eggs, including eggs high in lutein and vegetarian eggs, raised on feed with no animal by-products.

Juices made locally, such as apple cider from a nearby orchard, aren't required to provide this warning unless there is a state ruling. Juice bars and restaurants that sell freshly squeezed juice in glasses to drink right away don't need to provide this warning, either.

Tofu, Tempeh, and More

● As a plant-based protein alternative, try tofu, a cheeselike curd made from curdled soybean milk and pressed into soft cakes. Its calcium content is highest when calcium-fortified, often with calcium sulfate. Buy the form you need: *soft or silken tofu* for dressings, smoothies, soups, dips, and sauces; *medium-soft tofu* for puddings, cheesecakes, pie fillings, and salads; and *firm or extra-firm tofu* for grilling, marinating, slicing, and stir-frying and in casseroles, soups and sandwiches. Bought unpackaged or in water, refrigerate tofu in water, change the water daily, and use it within a week. Bought in aseptic packaging, tofu doesn't need refrigeration until it's opened. (For a chewier texture, freeze it for up to 3 months.) Try flavored tofu such as smoked, teriyaki, Mexican, and Italian tofu.

● Try another plant-based protein option with less calcium than tofu: tempeh. It's a rich, fermented soybean cake made from a mixture of soybeans, rice, millet, or other grain. Grilled or marinated, it adds a smoky or nutty flavor to soups, casseroles, chili, or spaghetti.

● Look for refrigerated spreads with more nutrients and less fat. One option: protein-rich hummus, made with chickpeas, soybeans, or other beans (legumes).

Freezer Case

Bagels and bread dough; waffles and cookies; fruit and fruit juice; pizza and burritos; vegetables and full dinners; fish, meat, and poultry; ice cream and frozen yogurt—the freezer case is stocked with nearly every kind of convenience food.

Frozen foods offer convenience, time saving, no food waste, consistent prices, year-round availability, and longer storage. Commercial quick freezing preserves freshness, flavor, color, and nutritional quality. Frozen at their peak, they're nutritionally comparable to cooked fresh products—if handled properly. Many are preportioned, or partly or fully cooked; prepare and serve them with little time or effort.

● Buy only clean, firm packages. Discoloring, frost, or ice may mean improper storage.

● For the best nutrition, choose those that are minimally processed. Read the Nutrition Facts and ingredient lists to compare.

Frozen Vegetables and Fruits

Stock up for quick, easy food prep!

● Choose frozen plain vegetables or those with low-fat sauces to control fat and perhaps calories. Some sauces mixed with frozen vegetables add total fat, solid (saturated) fats, and calories; check the Nutrition Facts.

● Consider frozen fruits, especially when fresh fruit isn't in season. Look for unsweetened varieties without added sugars. So it keeps its shape, serve it while still somewhat frozen.

● Buy frozen fruit and vegetables in loose-pack plastic bags. To serve, pour out only what you need; immediately return the rest to the freezer.

● Frozen juice? Buy 100 percent juice concentrate. It often costs a bit less than juice in cartons, and you can store it longer.

● Shop beyond fries and corn! Look for colorful frozen veggies, fruits, and legumes. Try frozen sweet potato fries, artichoke hearts, bell peppers, blueberries, peaches, mangoes, butter beans, and edamame.

● More convenience? Buy frozen sliced stir-fry veggies and mixed fruit or veggies.

● Buy frozen fruit bars as a nutrient-rich snack. Read the ingredient list to know if they're made with 100 percent juice, or instead with flavored water and sweeteners.

Frozen Meals, Entrées, Mixed Dishes

● Use nutrition labeling to compare frozen prepared meals, bowl meals, soups, stews, and entrées. Along with traditional foods, look for products with fewer calories; more fruit, vegetables, and whole grains; and with less fat, including solid fats (saturated fat and *trans* fats), cholesterol, and sodium—even pizza, lasagna, enchiladas, and burritos! When comparing one frozen dinner with another, check the label serving size. For example, some may be 7-ounce dinners; others, 11 ounces.

● Whether vegetables, fish, or poultry, go easy on breaded and fried frozen foods. They supply more calories and fat. Check the package directions for oven heating, rather than deep-fat frying, to control calories and fat.

● Be adventuresome. Try frozen entrées and sides that may be new to you, perhaps ethnic dishes. Although they'll cost more than homemade, they may introduce new foods and culinary experiences!

Frozen Desserts

Frozen yogurt, ice cream, sherbet, sorbet: Besides their many refreshing flavors, how do the calories and nutrients stack up? Check the Nutrition Facts. Remember, if your portion is bigger than the label serving, you consume more calories, fat, and added sugars, too.

● *Frozen yogurt (hard-frozen or soft):* Most frozen yogurt has less fat than ice cream does; however, the amount of fat and calories from fat depends on its main ingredient (whole, 1 percent low-fat, or fat-free milk). Although made with lactic acid cultures, frozen yogurt may or may not have active, live cultures; if present, freezing slows their action. Look for the "Live and Active Cultures" seal from the National Yogurt Association.

● *Ice cream:* The creamy texture and rich flavor of premium ice cream come with more fat and thus more calories than frozen yogurt. Enjoy, but cut calories and fat elsewhere, or eat a smaller helping. You also can find lower-fat ice cream. Slow- or double-churned ice cream, for example, has fewer calories; because the churning makes the fat particles and ice crystals smaller, it still has a creamy texture with less fat. In a half-cup serving:

● *Reduced-fat (2 percent) ice cream* has at least 25 percent less fat than regular ice cream.

● *Low-fat (1 percent) ice cream* has 3 grams or less of fat.

● *Light ice cream* has at least 50 percent less fat or 33 percent fewer calories.

● *Fat-free ice cream* has less than 0.5 fat grams per serving.

Special dietary needs? Although the flavor and mouth feel may differ, look for ice cream with sugar substitutes (labeled "no sugar added" or "sugar free"), with added calcium or other nutrients, or lactose-free, and for vegans, soy or nondairy ice cream. Prepackaged portions might be helpful for counting calories, carbohydrates, or fat grams. Remember that mix-ins such as cookies, brownies, candies, and cake add to the calories, added sugars, and fat content.

● *Frozen custard:* It's about the same as ice cream. The only difference is that more egg yolks are used in custard. It's also called semifreddo.

● *Sherbet:* It's made with sweetened fruit juice and water, 1 to 2 percent milk fat, and 2 to 5 percent milk solids, and stabilizers, such as egg white and gelatin. It has less fat but more sugar than ice cream.

● *Sorbet:* Whipped and frozen fruit juice, it can be counted in the fruit group. It's dairy-free and may be slightly sweetened.

● *Gelato:* Often served semifrozen, it has less milk fat than ice cream. It also contains egg yolks, sweeteners, and flavoring.

● *Whipped topping:* Frozen whipped toppings are convenient to keep in the freezer. Many have the same calories and contents as real whipped cream. If they're made with palm or coconut oils, frozen whipped toppings are high in solid (saturated) fats. If you enjoy the taste of whipped cream, buy it—then use just a dollop, not a heaping spoonful. Or look for light or low-calorie versions of frozen whipped toppings.

Grocery Aisles

Up and down the inside aisles of the supermarket, you'll find convenience foods, ethnic foods, baking ingredients, snack foods, seasonings, and beverages. Look for those that are nutrient-rich.

Canned, Jarred, and Dried Fruits and Vegetables

● For a nonperishable supply of fruit and vegetables, buy canned and jarred varieties. They're great to have on hand for boosting vegetables and fruits in mixed dishes and for convenience—especially when their fresh counterparts aren't in season. Besides common items, you'll find beets, collards, pumpkin, hominy, zucchini, blueberries, mangoes, and papaya, among others. Use them in mixed dishes such as in soups, stews, other cooked dishes, and smoothies. Look for flavorful, newer products, too, such as raspberry-flavored peaches, cinnamon-flavored pears, tomatoes with chilies or herbs, and corn with chopped peppers. Stock up on some special items—perhaps canned or jarred artichokes, olives, and roasted peppers.

● *Canned fruit:* Examine the label. You'll find descriptions such as "packed in its own juices," "packed in fruit juice," "unsweetened," "in light syrup," or "in heavy syrup." Fruits packed in juices have less added sugars and so fewer calories than fruits packed in syrup.

● *Juice, juice cocktail, or juice drinks:* Which should you buy? *See "More Reading on the Food Label" in this chapter and "Fruit Juice, Juice Drink, Fruit Drink?" in chapter 8.*

● *Canned vegetables:* If you're cutting back on sodium, read the Nutrition Facts for sodium content. Or look for descriptions such as "no salt added" and "reduced sodium." Sodium in canned vegetables is used as a flavoring, not a preservative. Heat from the canning process does the preserving. To help people follow the 2010 Dietary Guidelines for sodium, more canned foods with less sodium are appearing on store shelves.

● *Dried fruits:* Dried plums (prunes), berries, peaches, pears, apples, and more. Check the label for added sugars; for example, dried banana chips are often sugar- or honey-coated. To protect them from browning, some may contain sulfites. If you're sulfite-sensitive, look for sulfite-free or unsulfured options.

● *Fruit snacks that say "made with real fruit":* No regulation states how much fruit they need to contain. So read the ingredient list; added sugars and fruit flavoring may be key ingredients, with just a little real fruit.

Canned and Pouched Fish, Poultry, and Meat

● For convenience, keep canned or pouched fish on hand: tuna, salmon, sardines, clams, mackerel, and others. Some are packed in water; others in oil, typically canola, vegetable, or olive oil. Oil-packed fish, even when drained, have significantly more fat than water-packed varieties, but it's mostly unsaturated. In oil-packed fish, some heart-healthy omega-3 fatty acids transfer to the oil, which gets discarded when drained. *For more about omega-3s, refer to chapter 5.* Look for those that have reduced sodium content.

● For a milder flavor and a drier texture, choose fish packed in spring water. Also look for fish in shelf-stable pouches, often infused with lemon, herbs, or other flavorings.

● Compare the form and cost differences. "Chunk" tuna has many cut pieces and generally costs less; "solid" tuna is a portion that fits in the can. Buy the form to fit your use.

● For a calcium boost, buy canned fish (salmon and sardines) with edible bones. Three ounces of salmon eaten with the bones have about 200 milligrams of calcium, comparable to 6 ounces of milk. (Not all canned salmon has edible bones; check the ingredient list.) Canning softens bones, making them edible. Canned tuna and crabmeat don't have edible bones.

● Although tuna outsells other canned fish, enjoy a change in flavor with canned salmon or sardines. Salmon is higher in omega-3 fatty acids. Use it in salads, stir-fries, soups, and pizza toppings.

● More convenience? Buy canned chicken, turkey, or meat as a protein source to keep on hand and for emergencies. Check the Nutrition Facts. Some are water-packed, and some are reduced in sodium.

Soups, Stews, and Convenience Foods

Shelf-stable soups, stews, and other packaged foods are convenient but may be high in sodium, although many food manufacturers are gradually cutting back on sodium. Look for "less sodium" or "no salted added" products, especially if you eat them regularly. Use Nutrition Facts and the ingredient lists to compare them.

● On soups, stews, and chili (canned, jarred, or boxed), check the fat content, too! Clear soups and stews are usually lower in calories and fat than creamy varieties or stew with gravy. Many creamy soups, such as cream of celery and cream of mushroom soup, are sold in low-fat and fat-free versions.

● Ready-to-eat, condensed, or dehydrated? Buy the type that fits your needs; compare nutrition first. With ready-to-eat soups, stews, or entrées, such as pasta with meat or chow mein, just open the container, heat, then serve. For condensed and dehydrated soups add water, broth, or milk, then heat.

● To trim the fat, buy defatted broth with less fat, too. Another option: Put canned soup or stew in the refrigerator prior to use. The fat will congeal so you can skim it off.

● Know that many instant noodle (Asian-style) mixes, dehydrated soups, and entrée mixes (macaroni and cheese) are high in sodium. If you buy them, use half the seasoning packet to cut sodium; then for more flavor and nutrition, mix in chopped vegetables. For less fat, plan to use less butter or margarine than the directions call for, or use oil instead for less solid fat.

Pasta, Rice, and Other Grains

Pasta:

Buying pasta today is about more than just shape! Pasta itself is made with all kinds of grains: traditional durum wheat as well as whole wheat, rice, buckwheat, quinoa, kamut, spelt, flour-legume blend, and others. Noodles are part of ethnic cuisines around the world.

● Use food labels to compare. The fiber and nutrient

contents of pasta and noodles depend on the grains they're made from. Check both Nutrition Facts and the ingredient list; pay attention to portion size. When the first ingredient is semolina or durum flour, it's made mostly from refined white flour. Also notice the cooking instructions since they differ from one pasta to another.

● For meal appeal, buy a variety of pasta shapes. For thick sauces, use thicker pastas: fettuccine, lasagna, and tagliatelle. Chunky sauces are best with sturdy pasta shapes: fusilli (twists), farfalle (bow ties), macaroni, rigatoni, and ziti. With smooth, thin sauces, use thinner strands of pasta: cappellini (angel hair), vermicelli, and spaghetti. The refrigerated section of the store also sells fresh pasta; use it right away or freeze it.

● Look for whole-grain pasta: spaghetti, lasagna, macaroni, and fettuccine. Like traditional pasta, whole-wheat pasta is high in starches (complex carbohydrates). The fiber content is almost three times higher; half a cup of whole-wheat pasta has about 3 grams of fiber, compared with about 1 gram of fiber in traditional pasta. Another option: Some may blend whole-wheat flour with white flour for a more familiar texture.

● For more variety, savor the appeal of vegetable and herbed pasta. The addition of tomatoes, beets, carrots, spinach, and other vegetables adds a variety of colors and flavors to pasta itself. And herbs add a delicate flavor. What about the nutrients? Tomato pasta and spinach pasta don't count toward your vegetable intake. Nutrient amounts in the vegetable purees used to make commercially flavored pasta are quite small. It's the vegetables or tomato sauce tossed with pasta that carry extra nutrients.

● Experiment with Asian-style noodles. They're made with many ingredients besides wheat flour, including potato flour, soybean starch, rice flour, and buckwheat flour. Japanese soba noodles are made with buckwheat and wheat flour; Japanese wheat noodles are udon (thick noodles) and somen (thin noodles). Look for rice noodles, mung bean noodles, wonton wrappers (sheets of wheat dough), and rice paper (a thin dough used somewhat like a tortilla). Ramen noodles, which are Japanese instant-style deep-fried noodles, are often packaged with dehydrated vegetables and broth mix; the mix is typically high in sodium and solid (saturated) fats.

● Wonder about the fat in egg noodles? While pasta is made from flour and water, noodles also contain eggs, egg yolks, or egg whites. Non-egg pasta contains no cholesterol and very little fat. Egg noodles may have small amounts of cholesterol and a little more fat but still are low in fat and cholesterol.

● More options in the pasta aisle: soy pasta for soy protein health benefits; wheat-free or gluten-free pasta; and pasta with added fiber and perhaps protein for more health benefits. *For more about finding wheat-free and gluten-free products, refer to chapter 21.*

Rice:

● Try different forms of rice. Use the label to compare their nutrients. Brown rice contains the most nutrients, followed by polished white rice, then instant white rice. Because it's a whole grain, brown rice—with 1.5 grams of fiber per half cup—has about three times the fiber of white rice. When you read the label, check for uncooked and cooked rice; it may give the

How Much Pasta? How Much Rice?

Dry pasta and rice cook to a larger volume. Base the amount of dry pasta and rice you buy on their cooked volume. And remember, figure the nutritional contribution based on the amount you really eat!

PASTA OR RICE	UNCOOKED	EQUAL COOKED
Egg noodles	8 oz. (2 cups)	4 cups
Spaghetti, fettuccine, other long shapes	8 oz. (1½-in. diameter bunch)	4 cups
Macaroni, shells, bow ties, penne, other small to medium shapes	8 oz. (2 cups)	4 cups
Brown rice	½ lb. (1¼ cups)	4⅓ cups
Polished, long-grain white rice	½ lb. (1¼ cups)	3¾ cups
Converted white rice	7 oz. (1 cup)	3½ cups
Instant white or brown rice	8 oz. (2 cups)	4 cups

nutritional content for prepared rice with added butter or salt.

● Change the flavor and the texture with specialty rices. Jasmine and basmati rice have a fragrant flavor and aroma, especially nice with Thai and Indian food. Arborio rice, a short-grain rice, gives Italian risotto its creamy texture.

● What about rice mixes? If you need to watch sodium, consider using just half the dry seasoning mix.

Other grains:

● Despite its name, know that wild rice is actually a long-grain marsh grass. From a nutritional standpoint, wild rice has a little more protein, riboflavin, and zinc and a little less carbohydrate than brown rice. The fiber content is about 0.5 gram per half cup. For its nutty flavor, serve wild rice in salads, stir-fries, soups, stuffing, and side dishes. Or mix it 50–50 with regular or brown rice.

● Browse the grocery shelves for other grain products: barley, bulgur, couscous, kasha, and quinoa, to name a few. Try them! *See "Today's Grains" in chapter 9. In "Cooking Grain by Grain" in chapter 14 you'll find guidelines for cooking with other grains.*

Breakfast Cereals

Breakfast cereals vary from product to product and from brand to brand. They're made with different parts of the grain—bran, germ, and endosperm—in differing amounts, so their nutrient contents vary. Besides wheat, oats, corn, and rice, they're made with many other grains and seeds, too, such as flaxseed. Most are ready-to-eat; some are ready-to-cook. Many are fortified with vitamins, minerals, and fiber. Some contain dried fruit and nuts; others are gluten-free. Sweetened cereals are high in added sugars; some have more sodium or fat than you think! *The bottom line:* Read the label, and note that a portion size of cereal can go from ¾ cup to 2 cups.

Cereal labels often give the Nutrition Facts both for cereal only and for cereal with added milk. Why? Adding milk or yogurt makes cereal a great vehicle for delivering calcium and other nutrients in milk. *Tip:* During processing, fortified vitamins and minerals are often sprayed onto cereals. They may dissolve in milk. So drink your cereal milk—bottoms up!

● Unsweetened or sweetened cereals: Use the same criteria to compare calories; fats, including saturated and *trans* fats; fiber; vitamins; and minerals. For less added sugars, buy unsweetened cereals, then top with fruit (not table sugar) to sweeten. For oral health, sweetened cereals are no more cavity-promoting than unsweetened cereals; both contain starches and sugars that can linger on tooth surfaces.

● "Multigrain," "whole grain," "bran": Do they really have more fiber? Check the Nutrition Facts and ingredient list. *Refer to "Is It Really Whole Grain? Check the Label!" in this chapter.*

● Cereals that are good fiber sources supply at least 2.5 grams of fiber per serving; whole-grain cereals typically have more. The ingredient list reveals the whole grains and bran in the cereal's "recipe." Although high in fiber, bran lacks the vitamins and minerals supplied by the germ portion of grain.

● Check the nutrients in fortified cereals. Most supply about 25 percent of the Daily Value for vitamins and minerals. And some have much more—100 percent—making these cereals comparable to a dietary supplement. Remember, a variety of other foods supply these nutrients, too. Like any food, consider fortified cereal as part of your whole day's eating plan.

● Check the variety of cooked cereals, too: Cream of Rice, grits, rolled oats, and toasted wheat. Many are whole grain.

Think cooked cereals take too long to prepare? With today's packaging, you'll find microwave instructions for quick prep. Many to-be-cooked cereals—oatmeal, grits, Cream of Wheat—are "instant" varieties. The nutritional content is comparable to their traditional counterpart, although sodium may be higher in instant cereals. Read the label to compare.

● *Note:* "Natural" cereals or granola may have more fat, sugars, or sodium than you'd think; many are high in solid fats from palm and coconut oils. Instead try muesli, made with grains, nuts, and dried fruit, with less fat and added sugars.

Beans, Nuts, and Peanut Butter

● Add a variety of beans and lentils to your shopping list: adzuki, cannellini, garbanzos, navy and black beans, soybeans, and pinto beans, to name a few. With the demand for nutrient-rich, high-fiber recipes and the interest in ethnic cooking, today's stores stock a greater variety of beans and lentils—dry, canned, and frozen. You may find fresh dry beans in the produce department.

If the store doesn't carry the type you want, substitute another. For example, pinto, adzuki, and black beans can substitute for kidney beans, giving a dish a slightly different look. Cannellini, lima beans, and navy beans are the same color, just a different size. Nutritionally, most beans are about the same, even though their appearance, texture, and flavor differ somewhat. *To explore the varieties of legumes, see "Bean Bag" in chapter 14.*

● For freshness, look for these qualities in dry, uncooked (not canned) beans: no pinhole marks or discoloration, beans with a bright color, and bags that aren't torn.

● Stock up on canned beans (red, black, kidney, and more) for a quick way to fit fiber-rich beans in your meals. That's faster than soaking and cooking uncooked dry beans for hours. For less salt and sodium, buy reduced-sodium beans. Or buy regular canned beans, then drain and rinse them under cold running water to reduce sodium significantly.

● For less fat, buy vegetarian or fat-free baked beans and refried beans. Some are sodium-reduced, too. Some refried beans are made with lard, which contains saturated fat and cholesterol.

● Read labels on peanut butter, nut butter, and soynut butter. Peanut butter is simply roasted peanuts ground into a paste. The style—smooth, chunky, or crunchy—doesn't affect the nutritional content. All are good protein sources, but added ingredients may make a difference. Salt or small amounts of sugar may be added for flavor; unsalted and sugar-free varieties also are sold. Reduced-fat varieties may not be lower in calories; sugar and other ingredients may be added to enhance flavor and texture. The small amount of naturally occurring oils in peanut butter may be partially hydrogenated for spreadability, adding *trans* fats. *See "About* Trans *Fats" in chapter 5.*

To keep oil and solids from separating, stabilizers usually are added to peanut butter. However, in "natural" peanut butter, the oil separates out. At home, avoid the urge to make peanut butter lower in fat by pouring that fat away. Your peanut butter will become too stiff to spread. Instead mix it well, or turn the jar upside down to let the oil run through.

● Try a variety of tree nuts—almonds, cashews, hazlenuts, pecans, pine nuts, pistachios, walnuts, among others. Their nutrient and phytonutrient benefits differ, and their fats are mostly polyunsaturated. Be aware that nuts often are sold in salted and unsalted varieties. Some are sugar-coated. Unsalted nuts typically are found in the baking aisle; salted and sugared nuts, with snack foods.

Dry-roasted or oil-roasted nuts or peanuts: It's up to you. An ounce of dry- or oil-roasted tree nuts has about the same amount of fat and calories—almost 14 fat grams per ounce. Nuts and peanuts don't absorb much oil when they're roasted. The fat comes from the nuts and peanuts themselves. Either way they're a good protein source and provide fiber and varying amounts of different phytonutrients.

Beverages

● Enjoy flavored waters, but remember that waters in plastic bottles aren't the greenest beverage choice. Peach, lemon, mango, and other fruit-flavored waters are refreshing. For the "fizz," some are made of sparkling water and juice. Others are flavored with sweeteners but contain little juice. Unlike plain water, they may not be calorie-free. *See "What about Bottled Water?" in chapter 8.*

● For a no-calorie beverage, look for club soda, mineral water, and plain seltzer. Don't confuse these beverages with tonic or quinine water, which have 125 calories per 12 ounces.

● For carried meals, camping, and emergencies, stock up on boxed, or UHT, milk. Because boxed milk is ultrapasteurized, or heated to an ultrahigh temperature (UHT), then sealed in a sterile aseptic container, it can be stored unopened at room temperature for about three months without spoiling or nutrient loss. For added appeal, simply chill it before drinking. Once opened, UHT milk is as perishable as milk sold in the refrigerated dairy case.

● For more convenience, try nonfat dry milk or evaporated canned milk. They're both shelf-stable. When reconstituted, nonfat dry milk powder has the same amount of nutrients as fat-free fluid milk. *Tip:* For 1 cup of fluid milk, combine ¾ cup of water with ⅓ cup of dry milk powder. Use dry milk powder also to fortify casseroles and other mixed dishes with calcium and other nutrients from milk. It may cost less than fat-free fluid milk, too.

Evaporated milk has about 60 percent of the water removed, so its nutrients are more concentrated than in regular fluid milk. It's also fortified with vitamins A and D. If reconstituted, the nutrients are equivalent to the same-size serving. Evaporated milk may be whole or fat-free (skim). Sweetened condensed milk—whole or fat-free—is concentrated, too, but because sugars are added, it's higher in calories.

Tip: Once evaporated and condensed milks are opened and dry milk is reconstituted, all should be refrigerated.

● Alternatives to cow's milk? For vegans and those allergic to milk, look for plant-based products marketed as soy milk, rice milk, almond milk, flax milk, and others. They're often packaged in aseptic boxes and sold in the grocery aisle. Tastewise, their flavor differs from cow's milk; some are flavored. Look for alternatives fortified with calcium and vitamin D, yet remember, they don't provide all the nutrients in cow's milk, and except for fortified soy milk, they do not count in the dairy group. Some, like rice milk and almond milk, are typically low in protein. Check the Nutrition Facts. Rice milk is made with partly milled rice and water; almond milk, from finely ground almonds, water, and perhaps sugar. *To compare cow's milk to soy milk, refer to page 297 in this chapter.*

● *Note:* Nondairy creamers, either dry or liquid, may be high in solid fats (saturated fat or *trans* fat). Although nondairy creamers are made with vegetable oil, the fats—if coconut or palm oil—are highly saturated. To lighten your coffee or tea, nonfat dry milk or evaporated fat-free (skim) milk are both good substitutes from the grocery aisle—or use fluid milk or fat-free half-and-half instead.

● Sensitive to caffeine? Then look for decaffeinated coffee and tea, and caffeine-free soft drinks. Also, seltzer, sparkling water, and most fruit-flavored soft drinks have no caffeine. *See "Drinks: With or Without Caffeine?" in chapter 8.*

● *Note:* Flavored coffee mixes may contain added sugars and coconut oil, which are high in solid (saturated) fats.

● For soft drinks, know the calorie differences as you shop. A regular soda has 150 to 200 calories per 12-ounce can—with carbohydrates (from added sugars) and water as the only significant nutrients. Single soft drinks have gotten bigger; 20-ounce plastic bottles are common in vending machines. Do you need that much? Share! Buy sensibly sized cans or bottles, perhaps 8-ounce cans to control your portions. Diet sodas may quench thirst, too, and they're essentially calorie-free. *See "Soft Drinks: Okay?" in chapter 8.*

Soft drinks and other beverages with non-nutritive, or intense, sweeteners carry ingredient labeling. If you're sensitive to their non-nutritive sweetener, avoid these products. In moderation, non-nutritive sweeteners are fine. *See "Aspartame" in chapter 3.*

● Buy single-serving containers of juice and boxed milk, rather than rely on a vending machine. They're handy for packing along to lunch, meetings, or a spectator sport.

● If you enjoy the taste of alcohol-containing drinks but choose to cut back, look for low-alcohol versions of beer and wine. The taste compares favorably. For single serve, buy 12-ounce cans or small bottles of beer instead of a bigger size. For calories, check the label. *For more about alcoholic beverages, see "Alcoholic Beverages: In Moderation" in chapter 8.*

Crackers and Snack Foods

Store shelves display a growing array of crackers and dry snacks. Many promise "more fiber," "less fat," "0 gram trans fat," "less sodium," "gluten-free," "whole grains," and "fewer calories." To sort through the options, always check the serving size and servings per package, and compare the Nutrition Facts and the ingredient lists.

● To control calories, buy small, portion-controlled snacks (chips, crackers, dry snacks, and candy). They're often in 100-calorie packs. With them, it's not as easy to overindulge. Just limit yourself to one pack!

● Consider trail mix; buy the ingredients to make your own for less cost. The most nutrient-rich mixes combine dry fruit, nuts, and seeds, but no candy. Some have mini-pretzels.

● Many chips, crackers, and cookies are made with oil, but what kind? Those made with partially hydrogenated vegetables have more *trans* fats. Those with palm or coconut oil have more solid, or saturated, fats. For healthier fats, look for those made with nonhydrogenated soy, canola, corn, and peanut oils, or with high-oleic sunflower or canola oil, or low-linolenic soybean oil.

● Low-fat or even fat-free crackers? Try bread sticks, graham crackers, melba toast, rice crackers, matzos, rusk, saltines, and zwieback. Some may be made with whole grains; some may be lower in sodium.

● For a low-fat and crunchy snack, choose pretzels or plain popcorn. They're lower in fat than most snack chips, or buttered popcorn. Some are unsalted. Another option: oven-baked chips. One ounce of baked tortilla chips has about 1 fat gram compared with about 7 fat grams in the same amount of regular tortilla chips. Microwave popcorn often has high-fat flavorings.

● Less sodium? Look for chips and crackers with less salt, and unsalted peanuts and popcorn. Check the label to compare. One way chip manufacturers have cut the sodium is by sprinkling salt on the surface instead of baking the salt in, which changes the taste sensation.

● Buying cookies or candy? "Low-fat" and "sugar-free" don't mean "low-calorie"! Again, read the label. Animal crackers, fig bars, gingersnaps, and vanilla wafers are usually lower in calories, fat, and added sugars.

● Granola bars, breakfast bars, energy bars: sound healthy? They're often higher than you think in calories; fats, including solid fats; added sugars; and sodium! If you're looking for fiber or protein, that varies, too. *The bottom line:* Check the Nutrition Facts and ingredient list to find those with more fiber and less total and saturated fat. *Tip:* So-called energy bars are typically high in fat and added sugars.

Dressings, Sauces, Oils, and Condiments

● Mayonnaise or salad dressing? For less fat, choose "light," "reduced-fat," "low-calorie," or "fat-free" varieties. Fat-free dressings typically have 5 to 20 calories per tablespoon, compared with 75 calories and 6 to 8 fat grams in 1 tablespoon of regular salad dressing. Vinegar and water usually are the first two ingredients in fat-free dressing.

Have You Ever Wondered

. . . if snack foods labeled "0 grams trans fat per serving" are a better choice if made with palm oil? Probably not. In fact, palm oil and palm kernel oil are highly saturated. They're often used in place of partially hydrogenated oils to lower or to eliminate *trans* fats. But the switch doesn't make snacks healthier for your heart.

. . . if a beverage is made with corn syrup or high-fructose sweetener, does it have more calories? Used in the same amount, these sweeteners are equal in calories to table sugar, or sucrose. They are slightly sweeter than sucrose, however, so a little less might be used, perhaps resulting in somewhat fewer calories.

Another option: soy mayonnaise, typically made with tofu. For vegans, read the ingredient list to find out if it's made with eggs.

● Buy dry blends for mixing your own salad dressing. Then you can control the amount and type of oil and vinegar you add. Often you can use less oil and more vinegar, water, or other flavorful liquid than the package directions call for.

● Shopping for prepared pasta sauce? Alfredo, clam, meat, marinara, and primavera: you can tell the nutrient content by its name (although creamy sauces such as alfredo and clam usually have more fat). Read the Nutrition Facts. *See "Gourmet's Guide to Sauces" in chapter 15.*

● To cut back on sodium, look for reduced-sodium soy sauce, teriyaki sauce, chile sauce, and marinades. Their traditional counterparts may be quite high in sodium. Tamari is a wheat-free variety of soy sauce; shoyu is not.

● Buy oils to use in place of some stick margarine, butter, or other solid fats. Oils high in polyunsaturated fatty acids include corn, safflower, and sunflower oils. And those high in monounsaturates include olive, flaxseed, and canola oils. *See "Fats and Oils: How Do They Compare?" in chapter 3.*

● "Light" oil refers to the color or mild flavor, not the fat content.

● All vegetable oils contain the same amount of calories: about 120 calories per tablespoon. All are cholesterol-free.

● Look for oil (canola, olive, vegetable) sprays. With these sprays you can use less oil in a fry pan or casserole dish, or on a baking pan.

● Experiment with stronger-flavored oils: for example, sesame, walnut, herb-infused, or chile-flavored oils. These are finishing oils, not cooking oils. Just a splash adds a distinct flavor to salads, stir-fries, pasta, rice, and other dishes.

● Stock your kitchen with a variety of vinegars to pair with oils in salad-making: red wine vinegar, herb vinegars, apple cider vinegar, and fruit-flavored vinegars. The strong flavor of sweet balsamic vinegar complements salad greens. Vinegars are fat-free.

● Buy ketchup, mustard, and pickle relish as tasty spreads, with just 2 fat grams or less per tablespoon. Check the label for sodium content. Unless prepared with less salt or sodium, most of these condiments provide 150 to 200 milligrams of sodium per tablespoon. For more flavor with fewer calories, buy prepared horseradish. Look for chutney—a condiment with fruit or vegetables, vinegar, spices, and sugar—that's low in sodium and fat.

● Pickles, olives, sauerkraut, and other vegetables packed in brine: they too are high in sodium! If you buy them, plan to serve in just small amounts.

Have You Ever Wondered ?

. . . if virgin olive oil has fewer calories than pure olive oil? No matter what the type, olive oil is high in monounsaturated fatty acids, and the calories are the same. Terms that may confuse consumers, such as "virgin" and "extra virgin" olive oil, refer to the acid content—not the nutrient content. Extra virgin olive oil has less acid and a fruitier flavor than "pure" or "virgin" olive oil. Because it has more aroma and flavor, you can use less.

What about light olive oil? The term "light" refers to the color and fragrance, not to the calories, fat content, or if it has an olive-oil flavor.

● Remember salsas. They're low in calories and bursting with flavor but check the sodium. Experiment with the different levels of spiciness—usually labeled as mild, medium, or hot—to see which you like best Salsas have less fat then cheese dip or spreads.

● Fruit jams and jellies—nutritionally they're much the same. Check the label. Both have relatively small amounts of nutrients. *Hint:* Fruit jams and jellies supply extra calories from added sugars. Fruit spreads—sweetened with juice—can have the same number of calories as jam or jelly, or they may have less sugar. And they provide some nutrients. Check the label's Nutrition Facts.

Baking Aisle

Flour:

● Recognize different types and qualities of wheat flour before you buy. Whole-grain flour contains more fiber than refined wheat flour because the bran layer of the grain is still intact; that's where most of the fiber comes from. Whole-grain flour also contains the germ layer, which provides many vitamins and minerals. *See "What Is a Whole Grain?" in chapter 3.*

Refined flour, used in most baked goods, including most white bread, is made only from the endosperm of the grain. While the flour has a snowy-white appearance, almost all of the fiber and many of the vitamins and minerals are lost. Refined flour may be bleached or unbleached. Bleaching simply whitens the somewhat yellowish unbleached flour. From a nutritional standpoint, bleached and unbleached flours are almost the same.

When flour is enriched, four nutrients that were lost in processing—thiamin, riboflavin, niacin, and iron—are added back. Fiber is not. The amounts of these nutrients compare to those of whole-grain flour. Enriched flour also is fortified with folic acid and fiber; whole-wheat flour may or may not be folic acid fortified.

The label also may describe the flour as "all-purpose," "bread," "cake," or "self-rising."

● *All-purpose flour* is a mixture of high-gluten hard wheat and low-gluten soft wheat.

● *Bread flour* is mainly high-gluten hard wheat, suitable for yeast bread.

● *Cake, or pastry, flour* made from low-gluten soft wheat has a finer texture that makes pastry and cakes more tender.

● *Self-rising flour* is all-purpose flour with baking powder and salt added for making quick breads. *For ways to use whole-wheat flour in baking, refer to chapter 14.*

● Look for other types of whole-grain flour in the supermarket and specialty stores: barley, buckwheat, corn, oats, brown rice, rye, white, whole wheat, and triticale. Triticale flour, with less gluten than all-purpose flour, makes a denser bread; triticale is a blend of wheat and rye flour. To lighten the texture of baked goods, go "50–50" with triticale and bread flour. Corn flour, made from the whole kernel, is finely ground cornmeal; masa harina is a specialty corn flour used to make tortillas. Yellow corn flour—and other yellow cornmeal—have more vitamin A than white corn flour.

● Try other types of flour, such as corn, soy, almond, and rice flours, especially useful for people who have a wheat allergy or are sensitive to gluten. *See "Gluten Intolerance: Often a Lifelong Condition" in chapter 21. For tips on finding wheat- or gluten-free flour, see chapter 21.*

Sugar:

● Know the differences between various types of sugar. Most cooking and baking are done with granulated, refined sugar. Superfine sugars, more finely granulated, may be used in meringues or in recipes that call for granulated sugar. Powdered or confectioners' sugar is granulated sugar that's been crushed into a fine powder. *See chapter 3 for information on honey, brown sugar, and raw sugar as well as alternatives and to learn about non-nutritive sweeteners.*

Baking Mixes:

● Choose baking mixes—cakes, breads, waffles, muffins, etc.—that let you add ingredients. When you add the fat, eggs, and liquid, you can control the type you use. To watch cholesterol, add an egg substitute rather than an egg. Or to cut back on saturated fats, use soft margarine rather than butter. Perhaps add dry fruit and nuts. Check the label; some manufacturers provide tips for preparing mixes with less fat and less cholesterol. Whole-grain mixes have more fiber.

Have You Ever Wondered

… why some whole-wheat flour is white? White whole-wheat flour comes from a different type of wheat that's naturally lighter in color and milder in color than the red flour used to make traditional whole-wheat flour. For consumers who prefer products made with refined white flour, white whole-wheat products are appealing. Nutritionally speaking, they're comparable to traditional whole-wheat flour.

… why canned beans are often called dry beans? Beans such as pinto, cannellini, and kidney beans used for canning aren't picked until their fully mature in their dry pods. Canning is just cooking dry beans in the can; dry beans are also sold in dry form.

Breads and Bakery Items

● Make an effort to buy more "whole grain" and "whole wheat" bakery products. However, just because it's called "wheat bread" doesn't mean it's whole grain. Nearly all bread is made with wheat! "Stone ground," "multigrain," "cracked wheat," or "100 percent wheat" don't mean whole wheat either. And most store-bought rye and pumpernickel breads are made mostly from refined white flour. For more fiber, check the Nutrition Facts and the ingredient list for those made with mainly whole-wheat flour. Whole grains should be among the first ingredients. *See "Is It Really Whole Grain? Check the Label!" in this chapter.*

On the Nutrition Facts you'll see that a 1-ounce slice of whole-wheat bread has about 1.6 fiber grams compared to 0.5 to 1 gram of fiber in the same-size slice of enriched white bread. Bakery products that supply 2.5 or more grams of fiber per serving are a good fiber source. *Refer to chapter 3.*

● For white bread and rolls, look for "enriched." When the flour they've made from is enriched, B vitamins and iron are added back—but not fiber or other vitamins and minerals. Most products made with refined grains including bread, are fortified with folic acid.

● Choose mostly bread and other bakery products with less fat. Most Italian bread, French bread, bagels, pita bread, kaiser rolls, English muffins, rye bread, corn tortillas, and pumpernickel bread have 2 grams of fat or less per serving.

● Go easy on bakery products with more fat and perhaps added sugars: croissants, many muffins, doughnuts, sweet rolls, and many cookies and cakes. Half of a croissant has about 5 fat grams compared with 1 fat gram in half of an Italian roll. A doughnut has about 10 fat grams. Be portion-savvy; a small muffin is big enough.

● Use food labels—the ingredient list and the Nutrition Facts–to find bakery products with fewer calories and added sugars and less salt, too. Sensible, generally smaller-sized bagels and buns provide smaller amounts of calories, too.

Is It Really Whole Grain? Check the Label!

Finding whole-grain products can be tricky. Here's why. "Made with whole grains" on a label means it may have only a small amount of whole grains. "Wheat flour" or "100 percent wheat" doesn't mean *whole* wheat; it could be refined wheat. "Multigrain" can be flour from any combination of grains, refined or whole. Even products that are "good sources" of whole grains many not be high in fiber.

● Does the package claim link whole grains to a reduced risk for heart disease or some cancers? If so, the food must contain at least 51 percent whole grain by weight and meet specific levels for fat, cholesterol, and sodium. A FDA labeling guideline: a "whole-grain food" must contain the bran, endosperm, and germ in natural proportions.

● Is the first ingredient on the ingredient list whole grain? That's the ingredient in the greatest amount. That said, even if a refined grain is listed first, the sum of several whole grains listed next may add up to more by weight than refined grain. To help you, the package may have a voluntary Whole Grain Stamp sponsored by the Whole Grain Council, indicating whether one label serving of the food contains at least 8 grams of whole grain. To get the amount of fiber provided by the advice "Make at least half your grains whole," you'd need to eat at least 48 grams of whole grain daily. Some food companies have their own whole-grain symbol, too.

● Check the label's product date for freshness. Packaged bakery products, with preservatives added, may have a longer shelf life than those from the in-store bakery. *See "Additives: Safe at the Plate" in chapter 9.*

Seasonings: Dry or Fresh

Herbs and spices enhance the flavor of food without adding sodium. Dry or fresh, add them to your list.

● Buy herbs and spices in the amounts you need. Fresh herbs last in the refrigerator for only a short time. Dry herbs can be stored for up to a year to retain their peak flavors. *Tip:* Ethnic food stores often sell herbs and spices in bulk at lower prices.

● Know that seasoned salts are high in sodium. This includes garlic salt and onion salt. As an alternate, look for garlic powder and onion powder.

● Look for salt-free herb blends. Italian herb blend or herbs de Provence (typical in French cooking) take the guessing out of seasoning blends.

● Buy seasonings that may be new to you: perhaps sage for chicken soup, tarragon with peas, fresh ginger for sweet potatoes, or cumin in chili.

● Try liquid smoke. It adds the smoky flavor of cured meat without the salt that's added during curing.

See "Quick Reference: Herbs and Spices" in chapter 14; check "Salty Terms" in chapter 7 for more about types of salt.

Take-out Foods

Consumers increasingly shop at supermarkets for the most convenient home-served meals of all, foods that are ready to eat: salad bars, rotisserie chicken, steamed shrimp, sushi, and deli sandwiches, as well as a variety of heat-only main dishes, appetizers, and side dishes and cold salads.

If you're time-pressed, buy your main dish—or a whole meal—already prepared. Then just heat and serve as your own healthful eating solution on a hectic day! For food safety, eat them the same day you buy them. Guidelines for supermarket take-out foods are similar to buying and handling foods from a carry-out restaurant. *See "Safe Takeout" in chapter 15.*

Food Safety: Start at the Store

While the safety of the food supply has been monitored and regulated all along the food chain, it's your responsibility to select foods carefully at the store and to employ safe food handling practices at home.

● Only buy food from reputable food businesses that follow government regulations for food safety.

Note: Imported foods are subject to the same safety regulations as those produced domestically.

● Make a clean start. If provided, use the hand sanitizer at the store's entrance. Wipe the handle of the shopping cart with sanitizer, too.

Stocking the Vegetarian Kitchen

Today supermarkets sell all the foods needed for a healthful, vegetarian diet—even vegetarian convenience foods. Specialty stores may carry less common items, such as textured soy protein, quinoa, kosher gelatin, and wheat gluten.

Wherever you shop, follow the shopping-savvy advice in this chapter. The ingredient list helps identify animal-derived ingredients. As in any kitchen, stock up on fruits, vegetables, grain products, and seasonings, condiments, and other flavorings. For the vegetarian

kitchen, also stock up on meat and dairy alternatives. Plan to include foods that provide high-quality protein, iron, calcium, vitamin B_{12}, and other nutrients that may come up short; *see chapter 10.* The Vegan Awareness Foundation has a registered trademark Certified Vegan label for products that don't contain animal products and that have not been tested on animals.

Beans and Other Meat Alternatives
(Mostly with less fat and sodium)

● Canned, frozen, fresh, and dry beans such as pintos, black beans, split peas, soybeans, and garbanzos and lentils
● Vegetarian refried beans
● Dry bean mixes such as refried beans, falafel, and hummus (mashed chickpeas)
● Tofu and tempeh
● Miso
● Soy-protein patties, soy bacon, soy sausages
● Lentil or veggie burgers
● Falafel mix (for chickpea patties)
● Soy beverage, soy cheese, soy yogurt
● Soy nuts
● Soy flour, soy grits
● Textured soy protein
● Myco-protein (Quorn) meat alternatives sold as patties, sausages, and cold cuts
● Peanut butter
● Nut and seed spreads such as almond butter and tahini (sesame seed spread)
● Nuts such as pecans, almonds, walnuts, hazelnuts, and cashews

● Seeds such as sesame, pumpkin, and sunflower
● Eggs or egg substitute*

*For vegans, egg replacer powder made from tapioca starch and leavenings (not a meat alternative)

Grain Products

Read labels if you're vegan; some breads have ingredients derived from eggs, or they're brushed with eggs to make them shine.

Dairy and Dairy Alternatives
(Choose mostly with lowfat and fat-free.)

● Vitamin D-fortified milk, reduced-fat or fat-free
● Calcium- and vitamin D-fortified soy beverage
● Cheese (dairy or soy-based)
● Yogurt (dairy or soy-based)
● Dry milk powder
● Ice cream, frozen yogurt, or nondairy ice cream

Combination Foods
(Look for those with less sodium.)

● Canned and frozen vegetarian soups
● Frozen vegetarian entrées such as bean burritos or vegetable pot stickers
● Canned vegetarian dishes such as meatless chili
● Vegetable pizza

● Be careful of food sampling—unless you clean your hands first! If you plan to sample, bring moist towelettes or carry a bottle of hand sanitizer to use before you taste.

● Check food packages. They should have no holes, tears, or open corners. Frozen foods should be solid, and refrigerated foods should feel cold. Frozen foods shouldn't show signs of thawing.

● Check safety seals and buttons. Safety seals often appear on milk, yogurt, and cottage cheese. Jars of foods often are vacuum-sealed for safety. Check

their safety buttons or seals with your finger. If the indented safety button on the cap pulls down, it's still in place; if it's up, don't buy or use the food. Report a defective cap to the store manager.

● Reject cans that are swollen, damaged, rusted, or dented. These are warning signs for bacteria that cause botulism. Report these to the store manager, too. *See "Bacteria: Hard Hitters" in chapter 13.*

● If you suspect food tampering, report it to the store manager. Once you're home, contact your county public health department, the local police, or, for meat and poultry, the USDA's Meat and Poultry Hotline (800-535-4555), or, for other foods, the U.S. Food and Drug Administration (888-SAFEFOOD).

● When possible, put raw poultry, meat, and fish in separate plastic bags before placing them in your cart. Occasionally their packaging may leak and drip onto unprotected foods.

● Pay attention to "sell by" and "use by" dates on perishable foods. If the "sell by" date has passed, don't buy the product. The "use by" date applies to its use at home. Purchase only those that will be fresh when you're ready to eat them. *See "More Reading on the Food Label" earlier in this chapter for more about food product dating.*

● Select perishable foods such as frozen foods, meat, poultry, and seafood last before checkout, if possible.

● In the checkout line, pack cold foods together, preferably in paper bags, which keep foods cold longer than plastic bags do.

● Take groceries home immediately, and store them right away. If you must run a few quick errands, bring a cooler with chill packs for perishable foods if you'll be longer than thirty minutes. That's especially important in warm weather. The temperature of refrigerated food can go up 8 to 10 degrees Fahrenheit on a typical trip home from the store. That goes higher as the time gets longer. *For guidelines on keeping food safe at home, see chapter 13, "The Safe Kitchen."*

Shopping Green!

● Get reusable shopping bags. Keep them clean. Bring the bags when you shop!

● Recycle paper and plastic grocery bags, perhaps in the store's recycling program—or reuse them at home in your trash container. Either way it helps lessen the impact of 100 billion petroleum-based plastic bags, which often end up as litter and landfill, used annually in the United States.

● Buy products with less packaging. Or buy in bulk, and package them yourself. Be aware that single-serve products generally have more packaging per serving.

● Choose products in recyclable, recycled, or biodegradable packaging. Be aware that the "chasing arrows" symbol may mean (1) the package is made of recycled materials or (2) the package itself can be recycled. If just one claim is true, the manufacturer must say so. Even if a package carries the symbol, your community may not accept it for recycling. Check first. If it has a number, too, the lower the number, the more likely it can be recycled.

● Plan ahead; limit your shopping trips to save on gasoline. Walk to the store if you can.

● Buy only as much as you need without waste.

For more about food packaging refer to chapter 9.

The Safe Kitchen

America's food supply is among the world's safest. All those along the food chain—farmers, food manufacturers, supermarkets, and restaurants—are required by law to follow strict food safety regulations that minimize risks. However, once food leaves the store, the responsibility for food safety is up to you.

Like most people, you probably know the three basic food safety rules for serving, handling, and storage: Keep food clean, keep hot foods hot, and keep cold foods cold. But do you always practice food safety rules at home? Many people don't, even though they know better. To reduce the risks for foodborne illness, safe food handling must be observed farm-to-fork. Mishandling food—improper preparation, cooking, or storage—is the culprit for foodborne illness from most home kitchens.

Because of the health risks posed, the Dietary Guidelines for Americans provide advice for preparing and eating foods to reduce the risk of foodborne illness.

Foodborne illness is also an economic burden, linked to medical expenses, lost productivity, and even death. USDA's Economic Research Service (ERS) estimates that $6.9 billion annually are associated with five bacterial pathogens, *Campylobacter*, *Salmonella*, *Listeria monocytogenes*, *E. coli* O157:H7, and *E. coli* non-O157:H7 STEC.

Foodborne Illness: More Common Than You Think

An upset stomach, diarrhea, a fever—do you have the flu? Your illness actually may be foodborne illness.

Sometimes called food poisoning, foodborne illness is caused by eating contaminated food. Symptoms are often mistaken for other health problems. They vary from fatigue, dizziness, headaches, chills, a mild fever, an upset stomach, vomiting, and diarrhea, to dehydration, severe cramps, and vision problems, and even death can result. Although actual incidence is unknown, foodborne illness may be linked to a small percentage of some long-term health problems, including arthritis, acute kidney failure, and Guillain-Barré syndrome.

The ways in which people react to foodborne bacteria and contaminated food differ. Anyone can fall victim, but for some the risk is greater. One person

Click Here! Websites to Know . . .

- Home Food Safety,
  www.homefoodsafety.org
- Fight Bac, Partnership for Food Safety Education,
  www.fightbac.org
- Gateway to Federal Food Safety Information,
  www.foodsafety.gov

See "Resources You Can Use" for more websites.

may show no symptoms, while another may get very ill. The reaction depends on the type of bacteria or toxin, how extensively the food was contaminated, how much food was eaten, and the person's susceptibility. *See "Who Is at High Risk for Foodborne Illness?" in this chapter.*

How common is it? A 2011 Centers for Disease Control and Prevention (CDC) report estimates that 48 million Americans get sick, 128,000 are hospitalized, and 3,000 Americans die each year from foodborne illness. These data, says the CDC, are more accurate than—and cannot be compared to—previous estimates, from 1999.

Have You Ever Wondered ?

. . . if you need to worry about mayonnaise in picnic foods and brown-bag lunches? Mayonnaise is a perishable spread, so it must stay chilled. Homemade mayonnaise, made with uncooked eggs, is potentially more hazardous than its commercial counterpart and isn't considered appropriate for people at high risk. Commercial mayonnaise and salad dressings, made with pasteurized ingredients, contain salt and more acid, which slow bacteria growth. In unrefrigerated mayonnaise-based salads such as chicken, tuna, or egg salad, it's usually not the mayonnaise that poses the risk but the chicken, tuna, or eggs. That said, keep any mayonnaise in the fridge!

. . . if fish you catch are safe to eat? About 20 percent of fish eaten in the United States are caught for personal use. They're okay if caught in safe waters—and if properly cooked and not eaten raw. However, seafood toxins, which occur naturally in some waters, and fish contaminated by chemicals in the water pose health risks. Check with authorities from your local and state health department, state fishery agency, or Sea Grant office for a current safety status. Follow advisories.

. . . how food irradiation affects food safety? Food irradiation breaks down the DNA molecules in harmful organisms such as *Salmonella, E. coli*, and other foodborne bacteria. In that way it can dramatically reduce or eliminate disease-causing bacteria and other harmful bacteria and so reduce or prevent outbreaks of foodborne illness. Regardless, handle food properly to keep it safe. *See "Irradiation" on page 213.*

Actual incidence is unknown. While foodborne illness outbreaks from restaurant or grocery store food often get media attention, it's likely far more common from food prepared at home, where cases usually aren't reported. Foodborne illnesses that result in more severe symptoms or even death usually are diagnosed, but illnesses with less severe, nuisance symptoms often go unreported. Overall incidence is of concern, but the real issue is how you can prevent foodborne illness. Reducing foodborne illness by just 10 percent would keep 5 million people from getting sick!

Bacteria are the root of many cases of foodborne illness, usually due to improper food handling. Foods also can be contaminated by viruses, parasites, mold, and toxic chemicals, such as cleaning supplies stored near food and food preparation areas. With proper hand washing when preparing and handling food, nearly half of all cases of foodborne illness can be prevented. If you suspect that food is contaminated, don't even taste or smell it. Instead securely wrap the suspect food and discard it where neither humans nor animals can get at it. If you've just purchased the food, consider taking it back to the store for a replacement or a refund. Always make food safety your high priority.

Bacteria Basics

Life begins at 40! Between 40°F and 140°F, a single bacterium can multiply to become trillions in just twenty-four hours. Why the exponential leap? Under the right conditions, bacteria double in number every twenty or so minutes. The more harmful the bacteria are to start with, the greater the risk for getting sick.

Even with so many, you can't see bacteria without a microscope. Unlike microorganisms that cause food spoilage, you can't taste or smell most bacteria. Yet they live everywhere—in many foods, on your skin, under your fingernails, on other surfaces, and on pets and other live animals. Foods of animal origin—raw meat, poultry, fish, eggs, unpasteurized raw milk—are the most common food sources of bacteria. Although less common but equally important, harmful bacteria also can be transferred to fresh produce, perhaps through contaminated water or soil residue.

To survive and multiply, bacteria need time and the right conditions: food, moisture, and warm temperature. Many need oxygen, too. With their rich supply of nutrients and moist quality, many foods offer the perfect medium for bacteria to grow. Bacteria thrive on protein; that's why raw meat, poultry, fish, eggs, and milk are more likely linked to foodborne illness. The ideal temperatures for bacterial growth are between 40°F and 140°F. Above 160°F, heat destroys bacteria. Refrigerating foods below 40°F slows their growth. Freezing stops but doesn't kill bacteria. *Check "The Danger Zone" on this page.*

Most bacteria won't harm you. Some, such as those used to make yogurt, some cheeses, and vinegar, are helpful.

Harmful bacteria are among the main sources of foodborne illness in the United States. Because they're everywhere, you can't avoid harmful bacteria completely. Fortunately, from a food safety standpoint, most healthy adults don't need to worry about them—at least not in small numbers. Your body can handle small amounts with no health threat. However, risks for foodborne illness rise when bacteria multiply to very large numbers, which can happen with mishandled food. Note that even with small amounts of harmful bacteria, young children, pregnant women, older adults, and people whose immune systems don't function normally are at greater risk.

Bacteria: Hard Hitters

Although as many as a hundred bacteria cause foodborne illness, seven are among the worst troublemakers: *Salmonella* species, *Staphylococcus aureus*, *Campylobacter jejuni*, *Clostridium perfringens*, *Clostridium botulinum*, *Escherichia coli O157:H7*, and *Listeria monocytogenes*. You also may hear about *Bacillus cereus*, *Shigella*, *Vibrio vulnificus*, and *Yersinia enterocolitica*. Listed in alphabetical order:

● *Bacillus cereus* produces toxins that can cause diarrhea and perhaps vomiting. Contaminated meats, milk, vegetables, and fish, as well as some mixed foods such as sauces, puddings, casseroles, and salads, are sources.

● *Campylobacter jejuni* is estimated to be the major bacterial cause of diarrhea in the United States. Like *Salmonella*, *Campylobacter jejuni* grow in raw and undercooked poultry and meat, unpasteurized milk, and contaminated water.

The good news is that *Campylobacter jejuni* can

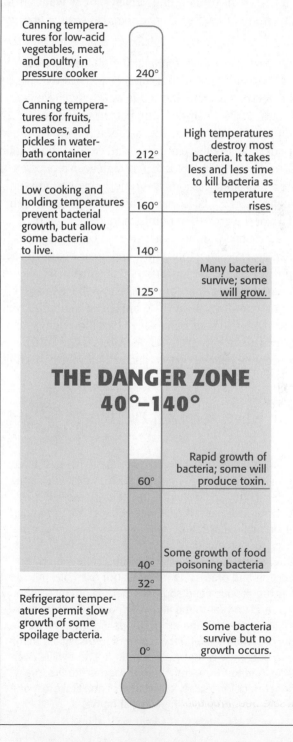

The Danger Zone

Effects of temperature (°F) on growth of bacteria in food. The most dangerous zone of temperature is between 40° and 140° F.

Canning temperatures for low-acid vegetables, meat, and poultry in pressure cooker — 240°

Canning temperatures for fruits, tomatoes, and pickles in water-bath container — 212°

Low cooking and holding temperatures prevent bacterial growth, but allow some bacteria to live. — 160°
— 140°

High temperatures destroy most bacteria. It takes less and less time to kill bacteria as temperature rises.

— 125°
Many bacteria survive; some will grow.

THE DANGER ZONE 40°–140°

— 60°
Rapid growth of bacteria; some will produce toxin.

— 40°
Some growth of food poisoning bacteria

— 32°

Refrigerator temperatures permit slow growth of some spoilage bacteria.

— 0°
Some bacteria survive but no growth occurs.

be destroyed easily through safe food handling and water treatment systems. To protect yourself, always cook food thoroughly and avoid cross-contamination by washing utensils, cutting boards, and hands after handling raw poultry or meat. Avoid unpasteurized milk. If you're camping, always treat water from streams or lakes. *See "Safe Enough to Drink" in chapter 8 for ways to treat unsafe water.*

● *Clostridium botulinum* contamination is rare. Yet, left untreated, botulism is often fatal. The toxin affects the nervous system and requires immediate medical attention. Botulism-causing bacteria can come from improperly home-canned or commercially canned foods. Usually these are low-acid canned foods such as meats and vegetables that haven't been processed or stored properly. Foods improperly canned at home, such as garlic, cheese sauce, and honey, pose a higher risk for the growth of botulism-causing bacteria.

Look for warning signs: swollen or leaking cans or lids, cracked jars, loose lids, and clear liquids turned milky. Beware of cans or jars that spurt when they're opened. Never eat—or even taste—these foods. For home canning, always use approved methods. Heat home-canned meats and vegetables thoroughly, about fifteen to twenty minutes, before serving. Serve or refrigerate baked potatoes and grilled vegetables right

Have You Ever Wondered❓

… why the spectrum of foodborne illness changes? Over the years food safety practices such as pasteurization, safe canning, and water treatment have resolved many foodborne diseases in the United States such as typhoid fever, tuberculosis, and cholera. Today new foodborne risks have emerged. Why? For one, the food supply has changed: a bigger global food supply; new food production and processing methods (for example, precut, bagged produce and sous vide packaging); and more demand for year-round and fresh produce and for minimally processed and ethnic foods. Second, the number of people at risk for foodborne illness is higher. Third, microorganisms themselves change and evolve over time. And fourth, according to consumer studies, many people lack food safety knowledge or don't take responsibility for proper food handling at home!

away. Food safety experts also advise that cooked root vegetables held at room temperature, instead of refrigerated, can be problems, too. That's especially true when they're wrapped in foil; *botulinum* spores thrive without air!

● *Clostridium perfringens* is present everywhere, growing where there's little or no oxygen. Sometimes called the buffet germ, it grows fastest in large portions—such as casseroles, stews, and gravies—held at low or room temperatures in the danger zone *shown in this chapter.* Chafing dishes that aren't hot enough and large portions that don't cool quickly in the refrigerator are breeding grounds. To slow bacterial growth, replace buffet food often, rather than put out large portions for an extended time. Refrigerate leftovers in shallow containers quickly.

● *Escherichia coli (E. coli)*, a common bacterium, is commonly found in the lower intestinal tract. For the most part, it's harmless. In fact, harmless strains in the normal flora of the intestine not only aid vitamin K production, they also help to keep harmful bacteria from being established there. Some strains of *E. coli*, however, are associated with foodborne illness. Travelers' diarrhea caused by contaminated drinking water, as well as with diarrhea among infants, are examples.

One strain—*E. coli O157:H7*—has received attention because its effects can be so severe. This strain, associated with eating raw or undercooked ground beef, or drinking unpasteurized milk or unpasteurized cider, has been known to cause life-threatening health problems such as hemorrhagic colitis with severe abdominal cramps, bloody diarrhea, nausea, and vomiting and perhaps hemolytic uremic syndrome (HUS), which may cause kidney failure, brain damage, strokes, seizures, and death, especially in young children and the elderly.

To combat harmful *E. coli* strains, cook and reheat meat thoroughly. Be especially careful of ground meat, for example, hamburgers; bacteria on the surface can get mixed into the center of the meat, which takes longer to cook. Keep cutting surfaces clean. Avoid cross-contamination; *see "Safe from Cross-Contamination" in this chapter.* Raw milk, cheese from raw milk, unpasteurized juice, and contaminated water also may be sources and should not be consumed.

● *Listeria monocytogenes* can cause a less common but *potentially fatal* foodborne illness called listeriosis. Pregnant women, infants, older adults, and those with weakened immune systems are more susceptible. In fact, pregnant women are twenty times more likely than other healthy adults to get this infection, which can lead to premature delivery or stillbirth.

Listeria are part of your surroundings, including

Who Is at High Risk for Foodborne Illness?

For those at high risk, follow general advice for food safety and avoid riskier foods. People at high risk include pregnant women and their unborn children; infants and young children; older adults; and people with weakened immune systems such as those living with cancer treatment, HIV/AIDS infection, organ transplants, and liver disease, among other chronic illnesses.

TYPE OF FOOD	HIGHER RISK	LOWER RISK
Meat and poultry	Raw or undercooked meat or poultry	Meat or poultry cooked to a safe minimum internal temperature
Seafood	Any raw or undercooked fish (such as sushi or seviche), refrigerated smoked fish (such as lox, jerky, kippered, and nova-style), precooked seafood (such as shrimp and crab)	
Milk	Unpasteurized milk	Pasteurized milk
Eggs	Foods that contain raw/undercooked eggs, such as Caesar salad dressings, homemade raw cookie dough, homemade eggnog (if premade from a grocery store, it's likely made with pasteurized eggs)	*At home:* Use pasteurized eggs/egg product when preparing recipes that call for raw or undercooked eggs *When eating out:* Ask if pasteurized eggs were used
Sprouts	Raw sprouts (alfalfa, bean, or any other sprouts)	Cooked sprouts
Vegetables	Unwashed fresh vegetables, including lettuce/salads	Washed fresh vegetables, including salads
Cheese	Soft cheeses made from unpasteurized milk, such as feta, Brie, Camembert, blue-veined, and Mexican-style soft cheeses such as *queso fresco* and Panela	Hard cheese, processed cheese, cream cheese, mozzarella, soft cheese that is clearly labeled "made from pasteurized milk"
Hot dogs and deli meats	Hot dogs, deli meats, and luncheon meats that have not been reheated	Hot dogs, deli meats, and luncheon meats reheated to steaming hot or 165°F to kill *Listeria*

Source: Food Safety and Inspection Service/USDA, 2010.

Information on food safety is constantly emerging. Recommendations and precautions for people at high risk are updated as scientists learn more about preventing foodborne illness. If you are among those at high risk, be aware of and follow the most current information on food safety. For the latest information and precautions, talk to your healthcare provider. Check the government's food safety website (http://www.foodsafety.gov), or call the government information numbers listed in the appendices. If you're at high risk, check here: www.fsis.usda.gov/factsheets/At_Risk_&_Underserved_Fact_Sheets/index.asp.

If you or someone you know is at high risk and needs help with meals, find out about services such as home-delivered meals in your community. Check their food safety ratings. *To find local services, see "To Find Food and Nutrition Services" in chapter 24.*

places where food is processed. It can grow even under proper refrigeration. Because it's common in unpasteurized milk and in cheese made from it, avoid eating any unpasteurized milk products. Raw and under-

Have You Ever Wondered?

. . . if you need to be concerned about red tide? No, unless you harvest your own shellfish. Red tide happens when marine algae are in a time of excessive growth. That's when they produce shellfish toxins that may cause illness. These areas are monitored carefully to protect the shellfish supply. Heed red tide warnings from local authorities if you harvest your own shellfish.

. . . if mercury in seafood is risky? Mercury is naturally present in all living things as well as in soil, air, and water. Pollution also releases into the air mercury that falls into water or on land, then washes into lakes, rivers, and oceans. Bacteria in water change mercury to methylmercury, which is toxic. Over time methylmercury can build up in long-lived larger, predatory fish.

The 2010 Dietary Guidelines advises that the health benefits to most healthy adults from consuming the amounts recommended—at least 8 ounces a week on a 2,000-calorie eating plan of a variety of cooked seafood—outweigh the risks linked to exposure from methylmercury. Consumers also should follow local seafood advisories and limit ingestion of large, predatory, long-lived fish. Because methylmercury is a potential risk to the developing nervous system of the fetus or the child, the U.S. Food and Drug Administration (FDA) and the Environmental Protection Agency advise that women who are pregnant or who might become pregnant, nursing mothers, and young children should avoid eating shark, swordfish, king mackerel, and tilefish.

To get the health benefits of seafood and limit methylmercury exposure, these women can eat up to 12 ounces (two average meals) a week of a variety of fish lower in mercury (for example, shrimp, canned light tuna, salmon, pollock, and catfish) and that can include up to 6 ounces of albacore (white) tuna.

Check local fishing advisories about fish you catch. No advice? You can eat up to 6 ounces of locally caught fish if that's all the fish you eat that week. This advice also applies to young children, but serve smaller portions. *Note:* Fish in fish sticks and fast-food sandwiches are usually made with fish that is low in mercury.

cooked meat, poultry, and seafood also may contain *Listeria*. As with any packaged food product, follow the label's "keep refrigerated" advice, the "use by" date on the package, and all reheating instructions. This is also why pregnant women are advised to avoid hot dogs, luncheon meats, or deli meats unless properly reheated to steaming hot (or 165°F).

To avoid *Listeria*, high-risk individuals are advised by the U.S. Food and Drug Administration (FDA) to avoid certain foods. *See "Who Is at High Risk for Foodborne Illness?" in this chapter.*

● *Salmonella*, the leading cause of estimated hospitalizations and deaths from foodborne illness, is found mostly in raw or undercooked poultry, meat, eggs, fish, and unpasteurized (raw) milk, cheese, and juice; and contaminated raw fruit and vegetables, such as melon and alfalfa sprouts. Control is simple enough: proper cooking kills *Salmonella*. Combat this bacterium by cooking raw foods thoroughly, especially eggs, poultry, and meat; by keeping foods clean; and by consuming only pasteurized milk.

● *Shigella*, one source of bacterial diarrhea, is transmitted through improper handling of food or water. It originates in the feces of infected humans and can pass easily through improper hand washing. Proper cooking eliminates it. Foods such as potato, tuna, or chicken salad are more likely sources because they're typically handled more during food preparation.

● *Staphylococcus aureus (staph)* spreads from someone handling food. It's carried on the skin, nose, and throat and in skin infections and on food preparation surfaces and equipment; then it spreads to food. Toxins, or poisons, produced by staph aren't killed by ordinary cooking. That's why personal hygiene and cleanliness in the kitchen are so important!

● *Vibrio* bacteria, which thrive in warmer waters, infect shellfish, especially raw or undercooked mollusks such as raw oysters. Pollution isn't a cause. These bacteria multiply even during refrigeration. Thoroughly cooking contaminated finfish and shellfish destroys them. For most healthy people *vibrio* are destroyed in the intestinal tract or in the immune system; however, *vibrio* infection can be very serious, even fatal within two days of developing it, for high-risk individuals. Symptoms include sudden chills, fever, nausea, vomiting, and stomach pain.

Have You Ever Wondered❓

... if your food is safe from foot-and-mouth disease and mad cow disease? These are different diseases. Although *foot-and-mouth disease* (FMD) is highly contagious among livestock and is economically disastrous, it poses no known risk to humans; FMD hasn't been found in U.S. livestock for about seventy-five years. Because travelers who visit agricultural areas can bring it back, the government prohibits import of agricultural products by people entering the United States who have been on a farm abroad or in contact with livestock abroad, and inspects their baggage.

Before returning to the United States from FMD-infected areas, the U.S. Department of Agriculture (USDA) advises: Avoid agricultural areas five days before returning; clean and disinfect footwear with detergent and bleach; wash or dry-clean clothing; avoid contact with livestock or wildlife for five days after returning.

As other safety measures, the USDA regularly monitors U.S. cattle herds and has banned animals and animal products from infected areas. *Note:* FMD is different from hand, foot, and mouth disease (HFMD), common among infants and children.

Mad cow disease, or bovine spongiform encephalopathy (BSE), affects the nervous system in cattle; it may be linked to a brain-wasting illness in humans known as Creutzfeldt-Jakob disease. To protect the U.S. food supply, government regulations have imposed import bans to make sure no live cattle or products from these animals are imported from areas where BSE is known to exist or is at risk, a ban on most mammalian protein in cattle feed, and a USDA surveillance program. A feed ban is in place to reduce the risk of BSE. Since 2004, the FDA and, similarly, USDA regulations have excluded potentially risky cattle products from human food, dietary supplements, and cosmetics. No research indicates that BSE is transmitted to cow's milk.

If you travel to Europe, where BSE is known to exist, your risk for getting this disease is very small according to the National Institutes of Health. If you're concerned, however, avoid beef or beef products, including brain, or eat only solid pieces of meat rather than ground-beef products such as burgers or sausage when you travel there.

● *Yersinia enterocolitica* is most often found in contaminated raw or undercooked pork products (including chitterlings, or pork intestines). The most common symptoms: for young children, fever, abdominal pain, and diarrhea, often bloody, and for older children and adults, fever and abdominal pain that feels like appendicitis. Unpasteurized milk or untreated water also may transmit this bacterium. In most cases the body can handle a yersiniosis infection without antibiotics. As prevention, avoid eating raw or undercooked pork and unpasteurized dairy foods, wash hands well, avoid cross-contamination, and dispose of animal feces in a sanitary way. If you're making chitterlings, have someone else care for your children. *For cooking pork, see "Safe Internal Temperatures" in this chapter.*

Parasites and Viruses, Too

Parasites and viruses—other tiny microorganisms—also can contaminate food. Parasites such as *Trichinella spiralis, Toxoplasma gondii, Cryptosporidium parvum, Taenia* (tapeworm), *Cyclospora, Entamoeba*

histolytica, and *Giardia lamblia* survive by drawing on nutrients in a living host. Viruses such as hepatitis A and Norovirus, or Norwalk virus, act like parasites. Through the food chain, parasites and viruses can infect humans.

● *Amebiasis (Entamoeba histolytica)* also comes from polluted water and vegetables grown in soil polluted with human feces. It's a problem mostly for travelers in less developed areas. Symptoms include intestinal cramps and diarrhea.

● *Cryptosporidium,* traditionally linked to travelers' diarrhea in developing nations, has become a more common parasitic illness in the United States. It enters the environment through the feces of warm-blooded animals, including humans. Contaminated water or ice is the usual source. Municipal water filtration controls this parasite; chlorine doesn't destroy it. Proper hand washing and food handling are extra control measures to take at home. People with compromised immune systems and children are among those at higher risk. *See "Drinking Water: For Special Health Needs" in chapter 8.*

● *Cyclospora cayetanensis* comes from consuming contaminated food or water. Prevent it at home with proper hand washing and by washing, peeling, and cooking raw fruits and beverages properly.

● *Giardiasis*, most often caused by drinking untreated water, also may be transmitted by uncooked food contaminated with *Giardia* or by passing the parasite from hand to hand on surfaces. In recent years, giardiasis has become one of the most common causes of waterborne disease among humans in the United States. Gastrointestinal symptoms more likely strike campers and hikers, travelers, diaper-age children who go to day-care centers, and others who drink untreated water from contaminated sources. Symptoms typically appear one to two weeks after infection and may last several weeks. Boiling destroys *Giardia* in water; chlorine may not if the chlorine concentration isn't high enough. Good hand-washing habits are essential to its control. If you travel or camp, drink only from a safe water supply; wash with safe water and peel produce before eating it.

What if there's a giardiasis outbreak in your child's day-care center? If it continues despite control efforts, children with or without symptoms might be screened and perhaps treated. If your child has symptoms (diarrhea, abdominal cramps, nausea), contact your healthcare provider. The American Academy of Pediatrics doesn't advise treatment for children diagnosed with giardiasis who don't have diarrhea unless poor appetite, weight loss, or fatigue are observed.

● *Hepatitis A* virus comes from food contaminated by feces. Conditions caused by hepatitis, such as jaundice and liver problems, can be severe. Sometimes hepatitis A comes through the food chain from shellfish harvested from contaminated waters—perhaps where raw sewage is dumped. More commonly, an infected person who handles food without proper hand washing can transmit the disease, most often in a food-service operation. Cooking may not kill the virus. As a precaution, always choose a restaurant known for cleanliness. Eat only well-cooked seafood. The CDC advises a hepatitis A vaccine for prevention; that is especially important for food service workers, who may be more susceptible.

● Norovirus, or Norwalk virus, is very common, resulting in about 60 percent of estimated foodborne

What Do You Do if You Suspect Foodborne Illness?

● Call or see a medical professional, especially if you have a fever. If it's a health emergency, call 911. Physicians and laboratories are responsible for contacting the appropriate health department to report diagnosis of foodborne illness. However, most cases of foodborne illness aren't diagnosed; the symptoms simply are treated to relieve discomfort. When diarrhea or vomiting are symptoms, drink plenty of fluids to avoid dehydration, and rest.

● If the suspected food came from a public place or a large gathering—a restaurant, sidewalk vendor, employee cafeteria, company picnic, or grocery store, among others—report the incident to your city, country, or state health department as soon as possible. You can contact the Centers for Disease Control and Prevention, 1-800-CDC-INFO (1-800-232-4636), or www.foodsafety.gov to report a foodborne illness, too.

● If you are reporting the incident, try to preserve the suspected food. Ask authorities for instructions for packaging and storing the food until it can be collected by them. If you can, keep the original packaging; it identifies where the product was produced. Mark it with a warning label so no one consumes it.

If you suspect food contamination from a household chemical:

● Check the label for an antidote or a remedy. Likely you'll find an 800 or other toll-free number for first-aid advice, too. Follow the advice.

● Call the national hotline to reach a poison control center: 1-800-222-1222. This number will automatically link you to the closest poison control center. Another option: Contact your local health department or use a local poison control center number. As a precaution, post their phone numbers by your telephone. You'll have them handy if needed.

illnesses but a much smaller proportion of severe illnesses. It causes acute gastrointestinal illness usually lasting two days. This virus is passed primarily from one infected person to another, often on the hands of kitchen workers who handle salads, sandwiches, and bakery products such as cream pies.

● *Taenia saginata* (beef tapeworm) and *Taenia solium* (pork tapeworm) are parasitic worms. Consuming undercooked beef or pork when traveling to places with poor sanitation increases the risk. The symptoms include abdominal pain, weight loss, digestive disturbances, and possible intestinal obstruction.

● *Toxoplasmosis* is caused by a parasite indirectly linked to raw and undercooked meat or poultry, unwashed fruits and vegetables, and contaminated water. It's also directly transferred to humans from cat feces. Pregnant women are at special risk because they can pass the parasite to their unborn baby. The disease can severely affect the central nervous system, causing mental impairment, visual disorders, and even death. To combat this parasite, cook meat, especially pork, lamb, and poultry, thoroughly. For pregnant women, avoid handling a cat's litter box; have some-

one else clean it daily. When possible, keep your cat indoors. If you do handle cats, wash your hands well with soap and water.

● *Trichinosis* is contracted by consuming undercooked pork or game that has been infested with trichina larvae. With careful food industry control and advancements in food processing, trichinosis is much less common today. However, still cook pork, game, and other meat to the recommended internal temperature to destroy any live trichina larvae. *See "Safe Internal Temperatures" in this chapter.*

Molds

Molds, or fungi that live on plant and animal matter, are another food safety issue. Why? Under the right conditions, some produce harmful mycotoxins.

Unlike bacteria, you can see some molds, such as the furry growth on food that's been forgotten in your fridge. But you can't always see the thin threads of mold branching and growing deep inside food, the mycotoxins that molds produce, or the bacteria that grow with mold. That's why simply cutting off surface mold may not remove the problem. Mold on certain cheeses may be handled differently; *for more about mold on cheese, see page 327.*

Like bacteria, most molds like warmer temperatures. But they also grow in the refrigerator. They tolerate salt and sugar, so jams and cured, salty meats can get moldy, too. Discard foods with obvious signs of mold. Cleanliness—in your refrigerator and with dishcloths, sponges, and cleaning utensils—is essential for controlling mold.

Checklist for a Clean Kitchen

Clean and sanitize! Cleaning is removing dirt; sanitizing is reducing microorganisms to safe levels. A clean, sanitized kitchen and eating space offer first-line defense against the spread of foodborne illness. Before handling food, eliminate breeding grounds for harmful bacteria, viruses, parasites, and mold. That includes your keyboard and desk if you eat while you work!

● *Hands.* Bacteria live and multiply on warm, moist hands. Hands pick up germs, spreading them from surface to surface, food to food, and person to person.

Should You Call Your Doctor?

Suppose you suspect foodborne illness. You or a family member has an upset stomach, diarrhea, vomiting, fatigue, abdominal discomfort, or a fever. Symptoms can appear from thirty minutes to three weeks after eating contaminated food. Most often, symptoms appear within four to forty-eight hours after eating, and usually pass within twenty-four to forty-eight hours. Rest and plenty of fluids are the best ways to treat most cases. Some foodborne illnesses can affect your health for weeks, months, or even years. Talk to your doctor or other healthcare provider if you think that food has made you sick. In some circumstances you need a doctor's care:

● Diarrhea is bloody. This may be a symptom of *E. coli O157:H7.*

● Diarrhea or vomiting is excessive. This may lead to dehydration if fluids aren't replaced.

● These three symptoms all appear: stiff neck, severe headache, and fever. The victim may have *Listeria*, which can be life-threatening.

● You suspect illness from *Clostridium botulinum* or *Vibrio*, which can be fatal.

● The victim is at high risk—perhaps a young child, an elderly person, or someone whose immune system is compromised due to illness.

● Signs of dehydration appear; *see "Dehydration: Body Signals" in chapter 8.*

● Symptoms persist for longer than three days.

Kitchen Safety

Are you food-safety savvy? Are you clean and careful enough to keep foodborne illness out of your kitchen? Take this kitchen safety checkup to find out:.

Do You . . .	Always	Usually	Sometimes	Never
Wash your hands for twenty seconds or more with warm, soapy water before and after handling food? Dry them with a clean cloth?				
Change your dishtowels and dishcloths every few days?	____	____	____	____
Clean up splatters in your microwave oven immediately with hot, soapy water?	____	____	____	____
Sanitize cutting boards after each use with a chlorine bleach-water solution?	____	____	____	____
Clean your refrigerator each week, discarding foods that are too old?	____	____	____	____
Wash fresh vegetables and fruit?	____	____	____	____
Thaw foods in the refrigerator, not on the counter?	____	____	____	____
Rotate foods in your freezer and cupboards, with the oldest foods in front?	____	____	____	____
Check foods in cans and jars for bulging or leaking before opening?	____	____	____	____
Marinate meat, poultry, and seafood in the refrigerator?	____	____	____	____
Grill food so it cooks evenly inside and outside?	____	____	____	____
Use a clean plate and fork to take cooked food from the grill to the table?	____	____	____	____
Clean your picnic cooler with hot, soapy water before you use it?	____	____	____	____
Use leftovers within three or four days? Heat leftovers until 165°F?	____	____	____	____
Remove stuffing from chicken and turkey before refrigerating leftovers?	____	____	____	____
Avoid the urge to use the stirring spoon for a quick taste?	____	____	____	____
Use a clean knife and cutting board for vegetables after cutting meat, poultry, or seafood?	____	____	____	____
Use a food thermometer to cook meat and poultry to a safe internal temperature? Cook eggs thoroughly?	____	____	____	____
Follow cooking instructions when microwaving packaged foods?	____	____	____	____
Put leftovers in the refrigerator within two hours of cooking?	____	____	____	____
Cook hamburger patties until they're 160°F and no longer pink inside?	____	____	____	____
Clean the outdoor grill after every use?	____	____	____	____
Remove perishable foods from a buffet after two hours?	____	____	____	____
Store poultry, meat, and fish on the bottom of your refrigerator in containers that won't leak?				
Use refrigerator and freezer thermometers to check their temperatures?	____	____	____	____
Subtotal	____	____	____	____

Now score yourself:

Always: 4 points
Usually: 3 points
Sometimes: 2 points
Never: 1 point
Your total score _____

When it comes to food safety, you need a perfect score: 100 points! Anything less and you're putting yourself—and anyone who eats with you—at risk for foodborne illness. It's safe to assume that the higher your score, the lower the risk.

If you scored 3 or less for any item, exert a conscious effort to change to always. Keep reading for more food safety advice!

Even while multitasking—desktop and drive-up dining—wash your hands before and after handling food. (Driving and eating don't mix anyway!)

Technique: Use soap and clean running water, warm if possible. Rub your hands to lather up for at least twenty seconds; wash front and back, between your fingers, under your fingernails. Rinse well under running water. Dry hands completely with a disposable paper towel or a clean cloth. Use the paper towel to turn off the faucet. Young kitchen helpers might sing "The Alphabet Song" or "Happy Birthday" while washing their hands; that takes about twenty seconds.

Hand sanitizers? Washing with soap and water is best; if unavailable, an alcohol-based, rinse-free hand sanitizer is okay. Apply it to the palm of one hand. Rub your hands and fingers together over all surfaces until they're dry.

What about wearing plastic gloves? They aren't enough for food safety. Although they are another barrier for foodborne contamination, even clean disposable gloves—used properly—can't substitute for regular, thorough hand washing and drying. The moist, warm conditions inside gloves are perfect breeding grounds for bacteria. If you use them, perhaps when handling food at a community event, wash and dry your hands properly before putting on clean, dry, disposable gloves. Change to new, clean gloves between food-preparation tasks and if they tear.

● *Work and eating surfaces.* Clean them often to remove food particles and spills, especially before food preparation. Use hot, soapy water and clean cloth towels or paper towels. Sanitize with a solution: 1 tablespoon of unscented liquid chlorine bleach to 1 gallon of water. Using any more bleach offers no

Need more strategies for food safety? Check here for "how-tos":

- Purify unsafe water—see chapter 8.
- Know about food safety in food production—see chapter 9.
- Shop with food safety in mind—see chapter 12.
- Learn to eat out safely—see chapter 15.
- Take food safety precautions when you travel—see chapter 15.

Wash Your Hands More Often!

Before you:
● handle or prepare food;
● eat meals;
● feed children.

After you:
● prepare food;
● touch raw food, especially meats and poultry;
● switch food preparation tasks;
● touch eggs and egg-rich foods;
● use the restroom;
● change a diaper;
● clean an appliance;
● handle garbage or dirty dishes;
● smoke a cigarette;
● pet animals and scoop animal feces;
● use the computer, phone, or other handheld device;
● touch face, hair, body, or other people;
● touch a cut or a sore, cough, or sneeze;
● clean or touch dirty laundry.

Adapted from: Home Food Safety . . . It's in Your Hands (Academy of Nutrition and Dietetics and ConAgra, Inc.).

advantage. In fact, sanitizing solutions that are too strong can be toxic and corrosive. Keep nonfood items—mail, newspapers, purses—off counters and away from food and utensils.

● *Utensils.* Wash dishes and cookware carefully in the dishwasher or in hot (at least 140°F), soapy water. Rinse well. Chipped dishes can collect bacteria.

● *Towels, dishcloths, sponges.* Change them often. Being damp, they're the perfect breeding grounds for bacteria; dry them between each use. Wash them in the hot cycle of your washing machine. Disinfect sponges in a bleach-water solution; replace worn sponges frequently.

● *Appliances.* Clean spills right away, including liquids from opened hot dog and deli meat packages. Clean splatters inside the microwave oven. Wash surfaces thoroughly with hot, soapy water or a bleach-chlorine solution; rinse. Remember to clean refrigerator and freezer shelves, sides, doors, knobs, handles, and food compartments—for example, meat and vegetables drawers. While cleaning and defrosting your refrigerator-freezer, pack perishables in coolers with ice. Scrub mold (usually black) on rubber casings of refrigerators with a bleach-water solution. Clean the outsides of appliances, too, with a soft cloth and a mild dishwashing detergent or an appliance cleaner.

Also remember to direct coughs and sneezes away from food. Cover your mouth and nose with tissue. Then wash your hands! No tissue? Cough or sneeze into your upper sleeve or elbow, not your hands.

Safe from Cross-Contamination

The term may be unfamiliar, but cross-contamination can happen in your kitchen. It's when bacteria from one food spread to another, often from a cutting board, knife, plate, spoon, or your hands. For example, drippings from raw meat, poultry, and seafood left on a cutting board can transfer bacteria to vegetables if

sliced next on the same cutting board that hasn't been properly washed.

● *Cutting boards.* Always use a clean cutting board—separate boards for fresh produce and for raw meat, poultry, and fish, especially if you prefer wooden cutting boards. Mark them—or get colored cutting boards—to avoid confusion.

Choose cutting boards that clean easily: smooth, hard maple, acrylic, plastic, or marble, free of cracks and crevices. Avoid boards made of soft, porous materials. Discard wooden boards with deep, hard-to-clean grooves and knife scars that can't be cleaned easily.

After each use, wash them in hot, soapy water, rinse, and dry well, perhaps in the dishwasher. That's especially important after using one to cut raw meat, poultry, or seafood. Rinsing or wiping isn't enough!

Sanitize cutting boards with a chlorine bleach-

Have You Ever Wondered?

... if you make any common food mistakes? Here they are: countertop thawing; leftovers left on the counter; unclean cutting board; store-to-refrigerator lag time; room-temperature marinating; grilling blunder (same platter for raw and grilled meats); "doggie bag" delay; stirring-and-tasting spoons; shared knife for trimming raw meat and chopping vegetables; and undercooking high-risk foods such as meat, poultry, fish, and eggs, including hide-and-eat Easter eggs.

... if lemon juice and salt can clean and sanitize a cutting board? No; you first need to wash it with hot water and soap and then sanitize with a diluted chlorine-bleach solution: 1 tablespoon bleach per gallon of water. You can sanitize a nonporous board but not a porous board, such as wood.

... if antibacterial cutting boards really minimize cross-contamination? Depending on the antibacterial rating, these cutting boards may reduce some common organisms, but research on their effectiveness is limited. These boards are treated with silver ions, which deliver some antimicrobial properties. If you use them, still follow food safety basics!

... if antimicrobial soap is a better choice? For long-term home use, wash with regular soap instead unless your

doctor advises otherwise. Over time microbes may resist antibacterial soaps.

... if you can catch bird flu from eating chicken? The U.S. Department of Agriculture (USDA) advises that proper food handling and cooking *(described in this chapter)* protect against avian influenza and other viruses and bacteria such as *Salmonella*. Cooking eggs properly and cooking poultry to safe internal temperatures of 165°F *(as noted in this chapter)* should destroy any possible foodborne virus. The chance of catching avian influenza from cooked poultry and eggs is extremely low. The USDA and other government agencies are working to protect poultry and eggs and prevent infected poultry and eggs from reaching consumers. If you travel to places affected by bird flu (avian influenza), check with the Centers for Disease Control and Prevention for current travelers' advice.

... if you can get H1N1 from eating pork? No. H1N1 is a respiratory disease spread by coughing and sneezing, not a foodborne illness. According to the Centers for Disease Control and Prevention, H1N1 isn't transmitted by food. For protection, wash your hands properly and avoid touching your eyes, nose, and mouth.

Keep Food Safe

1. **Clean:** Wash hands and surfaces often.
2. **Separate:** Don't cross-contaminate!
3. **Cook:** Cook foods to a proper temperature.
4. **Chill:** Refrigerate promptly.

Source: Fight BAC!, Partnership for Food Safety Education.

water solution after each use: Mix 1 tablespoon of liquid, unscented bleach in 1 gallon of water. Let the boards air-dry. Brush to reach grooves and other hard-to-reach places.

● *Utensils.* Unless it's cleaned well in between, avoid using the same knife to slice meat and chop vegetables.

Although hard to resist, remind everyone who ventures into the kitchen to never taste with the stirring spoon! If children reach for a finger-licking taste, be sure they wash their hands first. Another reason to resist tasting: If food (perhaps meat sauce) isn't cooked through yet, it still may harbor harmful bacteria!

● Other reminders: If you have an open cut or sore, wear latex gloves to handle food. Open food bags with a clean knife or scissors.

Safekeeping

Store food right: right container, right place, right temperature, right length of time. Foods keep their safety, quality, nutrients, and flavor longer when those are done. Besides, you stretch your food dollar when you don't need to discard spoiled food. *To determine the freshness of a packaged food, see chapter 12.*

In the Cupboard

How long do nonrefrigerated foods keep peak quality? That depends on how carefully they're stored. For safe, dry storage, use these guidelines:

● Keep your cupboards and pantry clean, dry, dark, and cool—preferably away from heat-producing appliances; 50°F to 70°F is the best temperature range. High storage temperatures (more than 100°F) lower the quality of canned foods.

● Organize your cupboards with older cans up front for first use. The good news is that canned foods have

Have You Ever Wondered?

. . . if molds on cheese are dangerous? That depends. Few molds on hard cheese produce toxins, or poisons. But to be safe, discard at least one inch of cheese on all sides where mold is visible. Keep the knife out of the mold. Recover the food with fresh, clean wrap. Soft cheeses such as cream cheese, Brie, and cottage cheese, and other foods with mold should be discarded. The exceptions are mold-ripened cheeses such as blue, Gorgonzola, Roquefort, and Stilton. Check the mold's color and pattern. If it's different from the usual blue or green veins and if you see furry spots or white, pink, blue, green, gray, or black flecks, cut off around and below the mold on cheese. For all types of crumbled, shredded, and sliced cheeses, discard if moldy.

. . . if raw milk is healthier than pasteurized milk? No; even if it's certified, raw milk can harbor *Salmonella*, *E. coli*, *Listeria*, and other harmful bacteria! Raw milk and unpasteurized cheese can be especially dangerous to those at risk, *as noted in this chapter*. In contrast, pasteurization, or heating milk quickly to high temperature, kills these harmful bacteria. To refute a few myths, pasteurization doesn't destroy nutrients. For those who are lactose-sensitive or have a milk allergy, the reaction to raw milk is the same as for pasteurized milk.

. . . is a raw-food diet safe? As consumers look for more minimally processed foods, this question may come up. Certainly raw fruits and vegetables are safe and nourishing if they're properly cleaned; if enjoyed at their peak, they can provide more heat-labile nutrients than their cooked counterparts.

Eating raw or uncooked meat, poultry, fish, and eggs is a different story. These foods provide perfect conditions for harboring and growing bacteria, *as discussed in this chapter.* A raw-food diet is especially risky for infants, young children, and those with impaired immune function.

. . . what to do about a food recall? The U.S. FDA and USDA monitor the safety of food products and issue recall announcements from the manufacturer or producer. That includes fresh fruits and vegetables. Get recall updates or report a food problem on www.recalls.gov/food, or download an app for your smartphone. *See chapter 12 for more about product codes on packages.*

a long shelf life. Stored properly, most unopened canned foods stay edible and keep their nutritional quality well beyond two years. Although the food is still safe to eat for longer, its color and texture may change after a while. Most dried fruit and vegetables can be stored for four to twelve months.

● Be alert for food spoilage. Never use food from cans that are cracked, bulging, or leaking or that spurt liquid when opened. Food may be contaminated with deadly botulism organisms. Toss—never taste!

● Store opened packages of dry food, such as rice and pasta, in dry, airtight containers. That keeps out insects and rodents and keeps food from absorbing odors.

● Store foods away from kitchen chemicals and household and kitchen trash. As important, keep chemicals and trash away from places where food is prepared and eaten.

In the Fridge

Do science experiments ever grow in your refrigerator? Is yesterday's meat loaf hiding behind tomorrow's juice carton? Has special cheese become as dry as old leather? With the pace of today's life, these things happen, even in the best kitchens! To keep perishable food safe and out of the danger zone, wrap and store it properly. Follow safe handling instructions on food packaging. For fresh meat and poultry labeling see *"Safe Handling Instructions" in chapter 12*.

● Keep your refrigerator cold—between 34°F and 40°F. Even at this temperature, bacteria that spoil food grow slowly. Keep a refrigerator thermometer inside on the middle shelf to check; buy the thermometer at the supermarket. Remind your family to make refrigerator raids quick so the door doesn't stay open too long. Twenty-three percent of consumer refrigerators aren't cold enough!

● Store all foods wrapped or in covered containers. Unless the package is torn, leave food in its store wrapping. If you rewrap, seal storage containers well to prevent moisture loss and absorption of off odors. Carefully date leftovers; use them within four days. Remove as much air as possible from storage bags to keep foods fresh longer. The less you handle food, the better. Store washed produce in a clean container.

● Store food quickly. Don't keep perishable foods and leftovers at room temperature for longer than two hours. Cool leftovers and food cooked for later use in the refrigerator or freezer, not on the counter.

● Keep leftovers where you see them, and use them right away. Discard after four days. If you can't remember when you stored them, toss! Once deli meat is opened, it's a leftover—even if its sell-by date is a week or more away.

● Avoid overloading your refrigerator. Cold air needs room to circulate.

● Eat perishable foods at peak quality. Once weekly, clean out the refrigerator. Discard foods, rather than risk foodborne illness, after they pass their prime.

Caution–Decorative Dishes

For years lead has been an ingredient in the glaze, or coating, on ceramic bowls, dishes, and pitchers. With proper firing, or heating in a kiln, glazes with lead are safe. However, when dishes are fired incorrectly or when copper is added to the glaze, hazardous amounts of lead can leach from dishes into food. Lead can collect in bones and some soft tissues. Among other problems, lead poisoning can cause learning disabilities, organ damage, and even death. Children and pregnant women are particularly sensitive to lead's toxic effects. *Check chapter 17.*

To be sure your dishes are safe enough for food, follow these guidelines:

● Inspect the surface of ceramic dishes. The surface that contacts food should be smooth and shiny, not rough or painted on top of the glaze.

● Check both sides of dishes, bowls, and pitchers. If it says "Not for Food Use" or "For Decorative Purposes Only," don't use it for food!

● Don't store food in ceramic dishes or leaded crystal. Lead can leach out when acidic foods and beverages such as coffee, juice, fruit, or wine come in contact with glaze or leaded crystal over time.

● Beware of ceramicware made by untrained potters and from foreign travel and older dishes, imported before government monitoring. Most of today's hobbyists know the problems of lead glazes.

If you're concerned about a possible lead hazard, have the item tested professionally. Check with the U.S. Consumer Product Safety Commission (CPSC) at www.cpsc.gov. Results from home lead test kits are unreliable.

● When in doubt about a food's safety, toss it out! Never trust its odor or appearance. Food may look, taste, and smell okay, even when no longer safe to eat. Sniffing moldy food may cause respiratory trouble.

● Discard moldy food in a bag or a wrapper so mold spores don't spread. Then clean the food's container, the refrigerator, or the pantry well to remove mold spores. Check items that moldy food might have touched; mold spreads fast in fruits and vegetables.

Meat, poultry, fish

● Keep packages of raw meat, poultry, and fish in separate plastic bags, in a bowl or a pan, on the lowest refrigerator shelf so juices won't drip onto other foods. The lowest shelf usually is coldest.

● Another option: Store them in the refrigerator's meat keeper. It's extra cold, so these foods stay fresher longer. Keep raw and cooked meat, poultry, and fish separate.

● Use fresh meat, poultry, and fish right away; *see "The Cold Truth: How Cold, How Long?" in this chapter.*

● Toss meat, poultry, and fish with an off odor, a sticky or slimy surface, and perhaps a color change.

● Live mollusks? For the very short time you keep them (within two days), refrigerate live mollusks in a container with a damp cloth on top. Be sure other foods don't drip on them. Don't store them in an airtight container or in water. They're saltwater fish that need air to stay alive. Scrub with a stiff brush just prior to shucking or cooking them.

Eggs

● Keep eggs in their carton, not in the egg tray or door shelf, to stay fresher longer.

● Use them within four to five weeks of the carton's Julian date. *See "Eggs" in chapter 12 to read the date on egg cartons.*

Fruit and vegetables

● Refrigerate perishable fresh fruits and vegetables such as berries, lettuce, and mushrooms, and herbs. Unless you dry them thoroughly with clean paper towels, wait to wash fresh produce until just before using it. Washing before storing can promote bacterial growth and speed spoilage if produce is still wet.

Have You Ever Wondered ?

. . . if freezer burn is harmful? The white, dried-out patches on improperly wrapped frozen food won't make you sick, but it will make food tough and tasteless. To prevent freezer burn, wrap food that hasn't been previously frozen in proper freezer wrap (aluminum foil, heavy freezer paper, or plastic freezer bags), push air out, then seal with freezer tape. Well-sealed freezer containers work, too; before putting on the lid, cover food with plastic wrap to avoid freezer burn from air in the container.

. . . if packaged ground beef that's red on the outside but grayish-brown on the inside is safe to eat? These color differences don't mean that the meat is spoiled or old. When oxygen from the air reacts with the meat pigments in freshly cut meat, they turn a bright red. You may see that on the surface of ground beef you buy at the store. The interior may be grayish-brown because no oxygen penetrates below the surface. Once exposed to air, meat will turn the familiar bright red.

. . . how to check refrigerator or freezer temperatures? For the fridge put a refrigerator thermometer on a middle shelf. Check in 5 to 8 hours. If it's not 38°F to 40°F, adjust the temperature control; check again in 5 to 8 hours. For the freezer put the freezer thermometer between frozen food packages. Check in 5 to 8 hours. If it's not 0°F to 2°F, adjust the temperature control; check again in 5 to 8 hours. Keep thermometers in your fridge and freezer all the time so you can check during a power outage.

For any produce you wash, store in clean bags or containers, not in the store's bag, which isn't clean.

● Keep produce in crisper bins in the refrigerator. That helps retain moisture. Keep fruit in a separate crisper from vegetables if you can; fruit gives off ethylene gas that can shorten their storage life.

● Refrigerate cut or peeled produce, or cooked fruit or vegetables, even if purchased precut or peeled.

For storing specific fresh fruits and vegetables, check the Produce for Better Health Foundation website: www.fruitsandveggiesmorematters.org.

Grain products

● Refrigerate or freeze whole-grain foods such as brown rice unless you plan to use them right away. They tend to get rancid faster than refined-grain products.

THE COLD TRUTH: HOW COLD, HOW LONG?

How long can refrigerated and frozen food keep safely and remain at top quality? Freezer and refrigerator times vary. As long as the food is properly packaged, these are basic guidelines:

FOOD	REFRIGERATOR (40° F)	FREEZER (0° F)
Eggs		
Fresh eggs, in shell	3 to 5 weeks	Don't freeze. Instead beat egg yolks and whites together, then freeze.
Hard-cooked eggs	1 week	Don't freeze
Liquid pasteurized eggs or egg substitutes,		
Opened	3 days	Don't freeze
Unopened	10 days	1 year
Dairy products		
Milk	1 week	3 months
Cottage cheese	1 week	Doesn't freeze well
Yogurt	1 to 2 weeks	1 to 2 months
Cheese, hard (such as Cheddar, Swiss)		
Opened	6 months	6 months
Unopened	6 months	6 months
Cheese, soft (such as Brie, Bel Paese)	1 week	6 months
Cream cheese	2 weeks	Doesn't freeze well
Butter	1 to 3 months	6 to 9 months
Commercial mayonnaise		
(refrigerate after opening)	2 months	Don't freeze
Hot Dogs*		
Opened package	1 week	1 to 2 months
Unopened package	2 weeks	1 to 2 months
Lunch Meats		
Opened package or deli-sliced	3 to 5 days	1 to 2 months
Unopened	2 weeks	1 to 2 months
Fresh Beef, Veal, Lamb, Pork		
Steaks	3 to 5 days	6 to 12 months
Chops	3 to 5 days	4 to 6 months
Roasts	3 to 5 days	4 to 12 months
Fresh Poultry		
Chicken or turkey, whole	1 to 2 days	1 year
Pieces	1 to 2 days	9 months
Giblets	1 to 2 days	3 to 4 months
Fresh Fish		
Lean fish (cod, flounder, etc.)	1 to 2 days	6 months
Fatty fish (salmon, etc.)	1 to 2 days	2 to 3 months
Smoked fish	14 days or date on vacuum package	2 months in vacuum package
Shellfish (shrimp, scallops, oysters, etc.)	1 to 2 days	3 to 6 months
Cooked shellfish	3 to 4 days	3 months

FOOD	REFRIGERATOR (40° F)	FREEZER (0° F)
Ham and Corned Beef		
Canned ham (label says keep refrigerated)	6 to 9 months	Don't freeze
Ham, fully cooked, half	3 to 5 days	1 to 2 months
Corned beef, in pouch with pickling juices	5 to 7 days	Drained, wrapped, 1 month
Hamburger, Ground, and Stew Meats		
Stew meats	1 to 2 days	3 to 4 months
Ground beef, turkey, veal, pork, lamb	1 to 2 days	3 to 4 months
Bacon and Sausage		
Bacon	1 week	1 month
Sausage, raw (pork, beef, turkey)	1 to 2 days	1 to 2 months
Precooked, smoked breakfast links, patties	1 week	1 to 2 months
Hard sausage (pepperoni, jerky sticks)	2 to 3 weeks	1 to 2 months
Variety Meats		
Tongue, brain, kidneys, liver, heart, chitterlings	1 to 2 days	1 month
Deli and Self-Serve Foods		
Salads: egg, ham, chicken, tuna, macaroni	3 to 5 days	Don't freeze
Entrées, cold or hot	3 to 4 days	2 to 3 months
Frozen Dinners and Casseroles		Keep frozen until ready to serve 3 to 4 months
Soups and Stews		
Vegetables or meat added	3 to 4 days	2 to 3 months
Leftovers		
Cooked meat or poultry	3 to 4 days	2 to 6 months
Chicken nuggets or patties	3 to 4 days	1 to 3 months
Pizza	3 to 4 days	1 month

Fresh Produce

● The quality of certain perishable fresh fruits and vegetables (such as strawberries, lettuce, and mushrooms) and herbs can be maintained best by refrigerator storage. If you're uncertain whether an item should be refrigerated to maintain quality, ask your grocer.

● All produce purchased precut or peeled should be refrigerated for safety as well as quality.

● Produce cut or peeled at home should be refrigerated within two hours.

● Any cut or peeled produce that is left at room temperature for more than two hours should be discarded.

For more about storing individual fruits and vegetables, refer to the Produce for Better Health Foundation website: www.fruitsandveggiesmorematters.org.

For specific foods, including condiments, as well as storage times for shelf-stable foods, check the Food Marketing Institute website: www.fmi.org/consumer/FoodKeeper/Food_Keeper_Brochure.pdf.

*Some may have package dates that are inconsistent with these guidelines.

Source: Adapted from www.foodsafety.gov, 2010.

Fresh dairy products

● Refrigerate promptly, preferably in the back of the fridge, where it's colder. Cover well so they don't pick up off odors. Pasteurization doesn't mean you can leave dairy foods at room temperature for a while.

● Once milk is poured, never return it to its original container. Pouring it back increases the chance of contaminating the milk with outside organisms that cause spoilage and foodborne illness.

Canned foods

Transfer opened canned food to a clean, covered container before refrigerating. You can refrigerate opened canned foods in the can if covered, but off flavors may develop.

Leftovers

● Refrigerate promptly—even if leftovers are still warm—to remove them from the danger zone. Today's refrigerators are powerful enough to cool food quickly. Store large amounts, such as soup or stew, in small, shallow containers to cool faster.

● Refrigerate them where you'll see them! Then use leftovers within three to four days. Toss if you can't remember when you stored them.

In the Freezer

In freezer storage, the colder, the better. Freezing extends the safety and quality of many foods. *For freezer storage times see "The Cold Truth: How Cold, How Long?" in this chapter.*

● Keep your freezer cold! For long-term storage, maintain a freezer temperature of 0°F or less. A freestanding freezer can stay that cold. However, the freezer compartment of most refrigerators usually can't; plan to use foods stored there more quickly. To check the temperature, install a freezer thermometer, available at kitchen stores or supermarkets.

● Store foods purchased frozen in their original packaging. Commercial packaging is usually airtight.

● Freezing home-prepared foods? Properly package them. Use freezer containers, moistureproof paper,

Have You Ever Wondered?

... how to handle sprouts for food safety? Sprouts tend to harbor *E. coli*, *Listeria*, and *Salmonella*; moist conditions that sprouts need to grow are perfect for breeding bacteria. The Centers for Disease Control and Prevention advise to thoroughly cook sprouts (alfalfa, clover, radish, mung, and other sprouts) before eating them to destroy bacteria, and for high-risk individuals, avoid sprouts! The FDA also recommends cooking sprouts. Even carefully washed sprouts can harbor bacteria. Especially if you're at high risk, ask for sandwiches and salads in restaurants made without raw sprouts.

To reduce your risk for foodborne illness if you choose to eat sprouts, handle raw sprouts with care: refrigerate to slow bacterial growth; wash under cold, running water; and buy them fresh with the buds on.

... about the safety of wild mushrooms? Stick with so-called exotic mushrooms from the store if you're a mushroom-lover. Telling the difference between edible and poisonous (some deadly) mushrooms takes expertise. Unless they're gathered by a trusted mushroom expert, avoid them.

... if blood spots on eggs are okay? Yes, they happen naturally while eggs are forming, sometimes when a blood vessel on the yolk ruptures. You can remove them.

... if using a vacuum sealer is a good way to store food longer? Yes, but only if done with food safety in mind. Freezing is as effective. A vacuum sealer shrink-wraps food, removing air (oxygen), and so preserves some qualities longer and potentially extends the storage time. Vacuum-sealing nonperishable dry foods such as dried nuts or crackers may be useful because their moisture content is so low that an airtight container works well.

Vacuum sealing doesn't ensure food safety and doesn't give the same long, shelf-stable benefits of home canning. Even vacuum-packaged perishable foods must be refrigerated or frozen, and handled (stored, thawed, etc.) like any other perishable foods to keep them safe. Removing oxygen may eliminate the growth of spoilage bacteria, but it doesn't eliminate bacteria that thrive in low-oxygen environments, such as *C. botulinum*, which give no visible indicators but can be deadly when consumed.

zippered plastic bags meant for freezing, or other freezer wraps. Traditional plastic wrap isn't suitable. Use freezer tape to help keep the package airtight and free of freezer burn. For storing fresh meat longer than a few days, rewrap or overwrap it.

● Before freezing, label each package with the food name, the date, and the amount. Freeze food in serving sizes appropriate for your meals or cooking needs.

● Organize your freezer. Rotate foods, keeping the oldest foods in front so they're used first. Stack similar foods together for an easier find.

● Remember that some foods don't freeze well: bananas, fresh tomatoes, lettuce, celery, gelatin salads, custard, mayonnaise, hard-cooked eggs, sour cream, cream (unless whipped), raw potatoes, unblanched vegetables, and foods made with these ingredients. Freezing affects quality, not safety.

● Blanch vegetables to lengthen freezer life: Immerse foods in boiling water for one to three minutes, then plunge them into cold water to stop the cooking. Freeze in airtight plastic bags after draining well. Blanching times vary; refer to the National Center for Home Food Preservation at www.uga.edu/nchfp for specific blanching times.

● Extra fresh eggs? Beat whole eggs until just blended, pour into freezer-safe containers, seal tightly, and freeze for up to a year. Label with the date and number of eggs in the container. Thaw in the fridge.

● Fresh milk? Freeze it while it's fresh, then thaw it in the refrigerator. Although still safe and nutritious, the flavor and the texture will change.

To Thaw for Safety

● Thaw foods in the refrigerator, not on the counter. Bacteria thrive at room temperature. Put food that's thawing into a plastic bag or on a plate to collect any juices. If you need a fast thaw, remove the store wrap first; put meat, poultry, or fish in a microwave-safe container; and defrost on low or defrost settings in your microwave oven. Or thaw frozen meat, poultry, or fish in cold water that's changed every thirty minutes. Cold water keeps the surface chilled. Then cook the food right away!

● Plan ahead to defrost frozen meat in the refrigerator. Here's how long it takes:

● Large roast—four to seven hours per pound

● Small roast—three to five hours per pound

● 1-inch-thick package of ground beef—twenty-four hours

● 1-inch-thick steak—twelve to fourteen hours

● To thaw, especially small amounts, in a microwave oven, use the defrost setting. The time for thawing depends on the amount of food you need to thaw.

Emergencies

Suppose a storm, an accident, or some other natural or man-made event shuts off power to your home—and your refrigerator and freezer. If you take precautions, maybe you won't need to toss food out.

Plan for Unexpected Emergencies

Wherever you live, keep a three-day emergency supply of food and water for you, your family, and your pets. *Refer to the "Disaster Planning: Emergency Supply Checklist" in this chapter.*

● Stock up on nonperishable foods: ready-to-eat canned meat, fruits, juices, milk, soups, and vegetables. Food in cans are better than in glass jars since cans won't break. Choose single-serving portions, too; you may have no way to keep leftovers cold. Keep high-energy foods on hand, such as peanut butter, nuts, and trail mix.

● Keep a manual can opener on your emergency shelf. No way to open canned food adds to any disaster! Keep an appliance thermometer in the refrigerator and freezer to check the temperature in case of a power outage.

● Plan for 1 gallon of water per person per day. Buy commercially bottled, well-sealed water, or store your own water in sanitized, food-grade containers (not milk cartons or jugs). *See "Safe Enough to Drink" in chapter 8 for making contaminated water safe to drink.*

● Rotate emergency food and water supplies every year or so. Then they're fresh when you need them.

When Your Power Goes Out

Keep refrigerator and freezer doors closed! Unopened, most refrigerators will keep food safely cold for about four hours if unopened, depending on the warmth of

Disaster Planning: Emergency Supply Checklist

Stocking up on emergency supplies—and rotating them regularly—can contribute safety and comfort during and after a disaster. Store enough supplies for at least seventy-two hours. If you're in a flood area, store foods and eating utensils where they'd likely be away from contaminated water in case of flooding.

FOOD AND WATER*

- Water: 1 gallon per person per day (for pets, too)
- Ready-to-eat canned meats (tuna, chicken, beef, chili), beans, soups, spaghetti
- Canned fruits, vegetables, juice; dried fruit, raisins; other dry foods
- Evaporated, powdered or ultrapasteurized milk
- Boxed soy beverage
- Crackers, ready-to-cereals, pretzels, instant oatmeal, pasta, rice
- Peanut butter, jelly, granola bars, trail mix, nuts
- Instant coffee, tea bags, hot chocolate, meals, pudding, cookies, candy
- Staples: sugar, salt, pepper, mustard, catsup, mayonnaise, creamer
- Ready-to-eat infant formula, infant foods, food for elderly people and those with special needs, if appropriate
- Pet food, if appropriate

Avoid salty foods since they'll make you thirsty, a problem when water is in short supply.

COOKING

- Barbecue grill, camp stove, pots/pans (*Warning:* Barbecue grills and camp stoves should not be used inside your home.)
- Fuel for cooking (charcoal, propane, etc.)
- Plastic knives, forks, spoons
- Paper plates and cups
- Paper towels
- Heavy-duty aluminum foil
- Matches in a waterproof container
- Can opener (manual)
- Appliance (refrigerator) thermometer

> The National Disaster Education Coalition provides more food and water related advice: www.disastereducation.org.

SANITATION SUPPLIES

- Large plastic trash bags for trash, waste, water protection
- Large trash cans
- Bar soap and liquid detergent
- Hand sanitizer, wet wipes
- Shampoo
- Toothpaste and toothbrushes
- Feminine and infant supplies
- Toilet paper
- Household bleach
- Newspaper (to wrap garbage and waste)

SAFETY AND COMFORT

- Sturdy shoes, socks
- Heavy gloves for clearing debris
- Candles and matches in a waterproof container
- Change of clothing, sweatshirts
- Knife or razor blades
- Garden hose for siphoning and firefighting

OTHER SUPPLIES

- Copies of personal identification, medication prescriptions, and credit cards
- Medication that doesn't need refrigeration
- Extra keys for car and house
- Map with places you could go and phone numbers
- First-aid kit—freshly stocked
- First-aid book
- Suntan lotion, hats
- Blankets or sleeping bags
- Portable battery-powered radio or television, flashlight, and spare fresh batteries
- Essential medication and spare glasses
- Fire extinguisher: A-B-C type
- Ax, shovel, broom
- Crescent wrench for turning off gas
- Screwdriver, pliers, hammer
- Coil of ½-inch rope
- Plastic tape
- Tent
- Money
- Essential medication for pets
- Toys for children

*In case distribution is disrupted after an emergency, store a two-week supply if you have special food or medical needs.

Sources: Adapted from American Red Cross WIC Program, San Diego, CA; "Emergency Supply Checklist;" Governor's Office on Emergency Services, Sacramento, CA; and the National Disaster Education Coalition.

your kitchen. If the power is out longer, dry ice or block ice can keep the refrigerator and freezer as cold as possible. Frozen foods can hold for about two days (forty-eight hours) in a full, freestanding freezer if it stays closed. Half full, a freezer remains cold for about one day (twenty-four hours) if the door stays closed. Freezers are well insulated; each frozen food package is an ice block, protecting foods around it.

Once the Power's Back On

Appearance or odor isn't a guide to food safety. Instead, follow these guidelines:

● If frozen foods still have ice crystals, or are at 40°F or less, refreeze them right away. Check with an appliance thermometer, then use them as soon as possible. Quality may be lost with refreezing; you might cook them first, then refreeze. If previously cooked foods are thawed in the refrigerator, you may refreeze the unused portion if it hasn't been left outside the refrigerator longer than 2 hours, 1 hour in temperatures above 90°F. Use these foods soon, within two to four months.

● If the power's been out for only a few hours, less perishable foods are likely fine. Fresh whole fruits and vegetables, hard and processed cheeses, condiments, butter, and stick margarine often keep for several days at room temperature. Although still safe, soft margarine (in tubs) loses its shape, texture, and flavor at room temperature and may get rancid. Toss food if it turns moldy or smells bad.

● Discard perishable foods if the power has been out for more than four hours: meat, poultry, fish, milk, soft cheese, eggs, leftovers, and deli items. In that time, bacteria can multiply enough to cause illness. Dispose of them safely, where animals can't eat them. For more about foods to keep and discard after an emergency, check the USDA website: www.fsis.usda.gov.

For more advice about handling and perhaps discarding food and kitchen equipment after disasters (fires, floods, hurricanes) and power outages, contact experts: U.S. FDA Food Safety Hotline (1-888-SAFE-FOOD), U.S. Department of Agriculture's Meat and Poultry Hotline (1-800-535-4555), your local American Red Cross, Cooperative Extension Service, Civil Defense, or emergency management office. Also check USDA fact sheets: www.fsis.usda.gov/Fact_Sheets/Preparing_for_Weather_Emergency/index.asp.

Safe Preparation and Service

Handle food properly from start to serving—for freshness and safety. Food is a delicate commodity. You can't fix it once those qualities are lost.

Prep It for Safety

Fresh fruits and vegetables

● Whether grown conventionally or organically—or gathered from your supermarket, farmers' market, or garden—wash produce, including bananas and oranges, thoroughly! Even if you peel it or discard peels or rinds, produce should be washed before cutting, cooking, or eating it. Cutting through unwashed produce can carry bacteria from its surface to the inside that you eat. Remove any outer leaves, too.

● Wash produce with clean, running water to remove any residue. Skip soap; porous surfaces on fresh produce can absorb soap's ingredients. On firm produce, such as melons and cucumbers, scrub with a clean brush. To debunk a myth: Misting produce at the grocery store doesn't wash it!

● Dry washed produce with a clean towel. If produce isn't eaten right away, moisture may attract bacteria and promote its growth.

● Remove bruised or damaged spots. They may harbor bacteria or mold. "Rust" spots on lettuce aren't harmful; they occur as cells in the leaf break down naturally after harvest.

● Check the package label on precut and packaged produce such as bagged lettuce. If it says "prewashed, ready to eat," it's safe without more washing if kept refrigerated and used by the "use by" date. In fact, you run the risk of cross-contamination by washing produce again. If you do choose to wash a product marked "pre-washed" and "ready-to-eat," use safe handling practices.

● A produce wash? Not necessary. If you use it, choose a produce wash meant for fresh fruits and vegetables, not hand or dishwashing soap.

Canned and jarred foods

● Check before opening. Safety buttons on jar lids should be depressed; canned goods shouldn't bulge or leak. Use the oldest cans and jars first.

● Wash lids before opening them so particles don't fall into food. Vacuum-packed canned foods may hiss softly when opened. That's probably the normal release of air pressure. But a loud hiss or spurting may indicate food spoilage.

● Wash can openers after each use.

Meat, poultry, and fish

● Skip an urge to wash raw meat, poultry, or fish. You can't rinse away all bacteria. Besides being unnecessary, it increases the chance of cross-contamination to other foods, utensils, and surfaces.

● Keep juices from raw meat, poultry, or fish from contact with other foods—cooked and raw. Use separate or thoroughly cleaned cutting boards, plates, trays, and utensils.

● Devein shrimp for cosmetic purposes. Cooking destroys any bacteria in the intestinal vein. In large shrimp the vein may contain a lot of grit.

● Marinate in covered glass or plastic containers—in the refrigerator! Marinades with acid-containing ingredients—wine, vinegar, and citrus juice—react with metals, which can migrate into food.

● To use marinade as a dip or sauce, double batch. Save half for serving time. Use the rest to marinate; discard it after marinating.

● Brush sauces onto cooked burger or ground meat patties when they're almost cooked. By mixing in dark-colored sauces (teriyaki, soy, barbecue, or Worcestershire sauces), it's hard to judge visual doneness of ground meat or poultry. That said, check with a food thermometer!

● Avoid eating raw seafood, meat, poultry, and eggs, or foods containing them. *See "Is Raw Seafood Safe to Eat?" in this chapter.*

Herbed oils

● If you infuse oil with herbs or garlic, use it right away; don't store it. Botulism has been linked to some home-prepared herb and garlic oils. Commercially prepared herb and garlic oils contain additives that prevent bacterial growth. For added precaution, always refrigerate commercial herb and garlic oil products.

Is Raw Seafood Safe to Eat?

With sushi bars and with seviche (a popular Mexican and Caribbean appetizer), many people enjoy raw and uncooked marinated seafood. However, lime juice in seviche doesn't guarantee safety! With careful control, these foods can be safe; read on to learn how.

Shellfish, especially mollusks (oysters, clams, mussels, scallops), may carry *Vibrio vulnificus* bacteria, which multiply even during refrigeration. Other viruses in uncooked or partly cooked mollusks also can cause severe diarrhea. *See the early part of this chapter for risks related to* Vibrio vulnificus.

Precautions to reduce the risks:

● High-risk individuals—those with HIV, impaired immune systems, liver and gastrointestinal disorders, kidney disease, inflammatory bowel disease, cancer, diabetes, hemochromatosis, stomach problems, or steroid dependency—should avoid eating any raw or partly cooked fish. Pregnant women and their unborn children, infants, young children, older adults, and those with alcohol problems also are considered at high risk.

● If you prepare raw fish at home, start with high-quality seafood—very, very fresh—and use it within two days. Buy from a licensed, reputable dealer. For mollusks (clams, mussels, oysters), ask to see the certified shipper's tag. If you harvest your own, make sure the waters of origin are certified for safety. Follow rules for safe food handling. Still, eating raw fish at home isn't advised. You're wiser to cook fish to an internal temperature of 145°F to destroy parasites, according to government food safety guidelines.

● If fish is sushi-grade or high-quality, sushi, sashimi, seviche, and oyster bars are generally safe for those not at risk. Reputable restaurants have highly trained chefs who know how to buy fish for safety and sanitation standards—and to handle fish safely.

See chapter 12 about buying fresh seafood.

Cook It for Safety

● Cook and hold cooked foods at temperatures higher than 140°F. High temperatures (160°F to 212°F) kill most bacteria. Temperatures between 140°F and 159°F prevent their growth, but bacteria may survive. You may need to set your over temperature higher than 140° F to keep food hot enough.

● Use a food thermometer to see when foods are cooked to a safe minimum internal temperature; an oven thermometer to check your oven heat; and a timer to cook accurately. Regularly check nondigital food thermometers; calibrate according to the manufacturer's directions.

● If you baste or brush sauces on food as it cooks, switch to a clean brush and fresh sauce for cooked foods. Then you won't transfer bacteria from raw to cooked foods. Discard marinade from raw meat, poultry, or fish, or boil it for a least one minute before using it on cooked food.

● Cook food thoroughly, all at one time; don't interrupt cooking. Food that's partly cooked and held, then cooked more, may not get hot enough inside for food safety. These conditions may encourage bacterial growth.

● Know how to use a slow cooker safely. Even though food is cooked at a lower temperature, usually between 170°F and 280°F, food prepared in a slow cooker is

---

Safe Internal Temperatures

Three numbers to remember for safe cooking: 145 for whole meats . . . 160 for ground meats . . . 165 for all poultry! These are safe internal temperatures; use a meat or "instant read" thermometer to check.

Food Item	Internal, Cooked Temperature (°F)	Food Item	Internal, Cooked Temperature (°F)
Beef, Veal, and Lamb		*Eggs and Egg Dishes*	
Ground meat and meat mixtures		Eggs	Cook until yolks and whites are firm.
Beef, pork, veal, lamb	160		
Turkey, chicken	165	Egg dishes	160
Fresh Beef, Lamb, Pork*, Veal		*Seafood*	
Roasts, steaks, chops		Fish	145 Cook fish until opaque milky white (opaque pink for salmon) and flakes with a fork.
Medium rare	145		
Medium**	160		
Well done**	170		
Fresh Pork		Shellfish	
All cuts, including ground products		Shrimp, lobster, scallops	Cook until flesh of shrimp and lobster are opaque color. Scallops should be opaque and firm.
Medium	160		
Well done	170		
Ham		Clams, mussels, oysters	Cook until shells open. Throw away any that were open already before cooking, as well as ones that did not open after cooking.
Fresh raw and precooked, ready-to-reheat	140		
Poultry			
Chicken and turkey, whole	165		
Poultry breasts, roasts, thighs, wings	165		
Duck and goose	165	*Casseroles and Reheated Leftovers*	165
Stuffing (cooked alone or in bird)	165		

*In May 2011, for food safety the USDA advised cooking pork steaks, chops, and roasts to an internal temperature of 145°F even if pink in the center, then allowing it to rest for at least three minutes before carving or consuming it. This is now the same safe internal temperature as for other whole cuts of meat.
**Not shown in 2010 Dietary Guidelines.
Source: Dietary Guidelines for Americans, 2010.

safe; lengthy moist heat is lethal to bacteria. Set the cooker on high until the food begins to bubble, then turn to simmer or low. Cover and check the internal temperature, which should be at least 160°F (165°F for chicken) when done. Always choose a recipe with a liquid. Use small, thawed pieces of meat or poultry. Fill the cooker from half to two-thirds full. Once cooked, food inside will be safe—if the cooker is on. If the power goes out on the cooker and you're not home, toss the food! *An added safety tip:* A slow cooker is not for reheating.

Meat and poultry

● Use a food thermometer to check the internal temperature of meat and poultry for doneness. *See "Safe Internal Temperatures" and "Using a Food Thermometer" in this chapter.* Even if you brine, check the internal temperature. After each use, wash the thermometer stem well in hot, soapy water. Don't immerse most thermometers. When properly cooked, juices from meat and poultry shouldn't be pink; poultry joints should move easily.

● Cook ground meat and poultry thoroughly—until the internal temperature reaches 160°F for meat and 165°F for poultry. Visual cues are inaccurate! You must use a food thermometer. Thorough cooking is especially important with ground meat and poultry; bacteria on the outside get mixed inside when they're ground and mixed. According to USDA research, one in four burgers browns on the outside before it reaches a safe internal temperature.

● Instead of rare, cook beef until medium rare (to an internal temperature of 145°F) for safety.

● Avoid very low oven temperatures (below 325°F) for roasting meat, or for long or overnight cooking for meat. Low oven temperatures for roasting encourage bacterial growth before the meat is cooked.

● When in doubt, cook ham. If the label says cooked ham, it's safe without cooking or heating. If not, don't take chances; cook it. Label terms such as "smoked," "aged," or "dried" are no guarantee of safety without cooking. The smoked flavor may come from added flavoring, not curing.

● If you stuff poultry, do so just before roasting; stuff loosely. Once roasted, the internal temperature of the bird and the center of the stuffing should reach 165°F before removing them from the oven. Another option is to cook the stuffing separately, especially if you don't have a food thermometer. Never cook stuffed

---

Where to Place the Food Thermometer?

Poultry (Whole Bird)
Insert the food thermometer or oven temperature probe into the inner thigh area, the wing, and the thickest part of the breast, but not touching bone; each area should reach 165°F. For personal preference, some consumers may choose to cook turkey to a higher internal temperature.
    If stuffed, the stuffing temperature must reach 165°F. Do this near and at the end of the stand time.

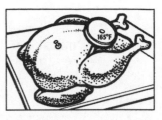

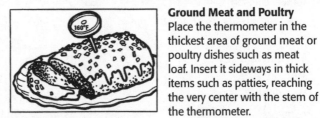

Ground Meat and Poultry
Place the thermometer in the thickest area of ground meat or poultry dishes such as meat loaf. Insert it sideways in thick items such as patties, reaching the very center with the stem of the thermometer.

Beef, Pork, Lamb, Veal, Ham (Roasts, Steaks, or Chops), and Poultry Pieces
Insert the thermometer or the oven temperature probe into the center of the thickest part, away from bone, fat, and gristle.

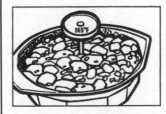

Casseroles and Egg Dishes
Insert the thermometer into the center or the thickest part.

Refer to "Safe Internal Temperatures" in this chapter to know what temperature your food should reach for safety.

poultry in a microwave oven. Refrigerate leftover poultry and stuffing separately.

Fish

● Follow the ten-minute rule for finfish—whole fish, steaks, and fillets. For every inch of thickness, cook for ten minutes at 425°F to 450°F. If it's cooking in a sauce or a foil wrap, cook for five minutes longer. The internal temperature should reach 145°F. If one end is thinner than another, fold it underneath so the thickness

For the Mile-High Cook

At an altitude of 1,000 feet or more, you may need to cook food longer to kill bacteria. At higher altitudes, water boils at a lower temperature, so it's less effective for killing bacteria. Most cooking and canning temperatures are based on food preparation at sea level. Check time and temperature adjustments for altitude in your canning book or recipe, or check the Food and Safety Inspection Service website: www.fsis.usda.gov/factsheet.

Using a Food Thermometer

The only way to know if meat, poultry, and egg dishes are done is to use a food thermometer! That takes the guesswork from cooking. Besides helping to reduce the risk for foodborne illness, a food thermometer helps to prevent overcooking. Use a food thermometer every time you cook poultry, roasts, ham, casseroles, meat loaves, and egg dishes. Check the temperature in several places for irregularly shaped meats or poultry, egg dishes, and ground meat and poultry. And give the thermometer reading enough time to respond.

Types of Food Thermometers

● *Dial oven-safe (bimetal):* Inserted 2 to 2½ inches deep in the thickest part of the food and can remain there throughout cooking. Reads in 1 to 2 minutes. Can be used in roasts, casseroles, and soups. Not appropriate for thin foods. Easy to read; placement is important. Some can be calibrated. Be aware that heat conduction of the metal stem can cause a false high reading.

● *Digital instant-read (thermistor):* Not designed to stay in food while cooking; reads in 10 seconds when the stem is inserted into the food about ½ inch deep. Can measure in thin and thick foods. Check at the end of cooking time. Some can be calibrated.

● *Dial instant-read (bimetal):* Not designed to stay in the food while cooking; reads in 15 to 20 seconds when the stem is inserted into the food about 2 to 2½ inches deep in the thickest part of the food. Can be used in roasts, casseroles, and soups. Not appropriate for thin foods unless inserted sideways. Check at the end of the cooking time. Some can be calibrated.

● *Pop-up:* Often found already inserted into poultry; pops up when the food reaches the final temperature for safety and doneness. Verify that the meat is done by checking the temperature with a conventional thermometer as well.

● *Thermometer-fork combination.* Not designed to stay in the food while cooking; reads in 2 to 10 seconds. Place at least ¼ inch deep in the thickest part of the food, with the sensor in the fork tine fully inserted. Can be used in most foods. Convenient for grilling. Check at the end of the cooking time. Cannot be calibrated.

● *Microwave-safe:* Designed for microwave ovens only.

● *Disposable temperature indicators:* Use once and toss. Reads in 5 to 10 seconds. Temperature-sensitive material changes color when the desired temperature is reached. Meant only for specific temperature ranges; for example, for burgers or chicken. Place about ½ inch deep, according to manufacturer's directions. Use only for the food intended. Useful for grilling at picnics and tailgate parties. They're inexpensive. Find them in the meat case of your supermarket. Use as directed by the manufacturer.

● Other types of food thermometers: An oven probe with cord, or a thermocouple. Use them according to the manufacturer's instructions.

Note: When buying a food thermometer, read the package label carefully to buy the type designed for use with meat, but not other food items such as candy. Look for a stainless steel thermometer with an easy-to-read dial and a shatterproof, clear lens.

Have You Ever Wondered

. . . if plenty of hot sauce kills harmful bacteria in fish such as raw oysters? No; neither does beer or vodka (for oyster shooters) "downed" with them. Only prolonged exposure to high enough cooking temperature kills bacteria. Love raw oysters? Don't rely on your senses as a safety gauge—even experienced oyster eaters can't tell. To refute a myth about raw oysters' seasonal safety: About 40 percent of cases of illnesses from *Vibrio vulnificus* bacteria happen from September to April, all months with the letter *r.*

is uniform. This rule applies to broiling, grilling, steaming, baking, and poaching. Cooking times for frying and microwaving are generally faster. If fish is cooked from a frozen state, double the cooking time. Most cooked finfish is opaque milky-white, or for salmon, opaque pink, and flakes easily with a fork.

● Cook shellfish properly. Scallops and shrimp take three to five minutes, depending on size. Scallops turn milky-white and firm; shrimp turn pink. Boiling lobsters takes five to six minutes per pound after the water comes back to a boil; when fully cooked, they turn bright red.

● Be sure that mollusks are still alive before cooking them. If the shells don't close tightly when tapped or if they're open, toss them! Cook them in a pot that's big enough to cook all them all thoroughly—even shells at the top or the middle. For live clams, mussels, and oysters: Boil water for three to five minutes after the shells open, or steam them for four to nine minutes. Cook until they open. Discard any that don't open during cooking.

If they're shucked:

   ● Bake them for about ten minutes at 450°F.

   ● Boil for at least three minutes or until the edges curl.

   ● Fry for at least ten minutes at 375°F.

   ● Broil them for at least three minutes.

"Egg-stra" Cooking Tips for Food Safety

If handled improperly, eggs and egg-rich foods are a perfect medium for *Salmonella* growth.

● Avoid washing eggs. You'll remove the coating that protects eggs from bacteria after they're washed during processing.

● Toss cracked or dirty eggs.

● Cook eggs until done—slowly over gentle heat until the yolks are firm. *See "How Do You Know When Cooked Eggs Are Done?" in this chapter.* For people with a compromised immune system, even lightly cooked egg dishes such as soft custards and French toast can be risky and should be avoided.

● Prepare soft meringues and mousse made with slightly cooked eggs to destroy any *Salmonella*. To prepare, put the egg whites in a double boiler or a heavy pan. Add 2 tablespoons of sugar for each egg white. Cook over low heat, beating on low speed as you cook, until the whites reach 160°F, then turn the speed to high and beat until soft peaks appear. Proceed with the recipe as directed.

● Avoid foods with raw eggs—such as homemade ice cream, mayonnaise, or eggnog; hollandaise sauce; and Caesar salad dressing—unless they're made with an unopened carton of pasteurized eggs. Once pasteurized eggs are open, treat them like other eggs; they can be contaminated by bacteria. How about eating homemade cookie dough? If it contains raw eggs, don't!

● As another option, use cooked yolks in recipes that call for raw eggs. Cook the yolks in a double boiler or a heavy skillet with liquid from the recipe: 2 tablespoons of liquid for each yolk. Beat while it cooks until the yolk coats a spoon, or bubbles form around the edges, and the temperature reaches 160°F.

● Pasteurized egg products? They're best used in cooked products, especially for people who are at risk for foodborne illness. Buy only pasteurized egg products with a USDA inspection mark.

● Keep eggs and egg-rich foods, including pumpkin and custard pies, at 40°F to 140°F for no longer than two hours, including serving time. Otherwise, refrigerate them. Use leftovers made with eggs within two or three days.

● Store Easter eggs in the refrigerator. Handle them carefully while decorating; cracked eggs invite bacte-

How Do You Know When Cooked Eggs Are Done?

Look for these doneness signs. When eggs are properly cooked, *Salmonella* are destroyed.

COOKING METHOD	SIGNS OF DONENESS
Scrambled, omelettes, frittata	No visible liquid egg remains
Poached, fried over easy, sunny side up	White completely set; yolk starting to thicken but not hard (*Hint:* For sunny-side up eggs, cover with lid to ensure adequate cooking.)
Soft-cooked	White completely set; yolk starting to thicken but not hard (Bring to a boil; turn off heat. Let eggs stand in water for four to five minutes.)
Hard-cooked	White and yolk are completely set (Bring to a boil; turn off heat. Let eggs stand in water for fifteen minutes.)
Stirred custard, including ice cream and eggnog	Mixture coats the spoon; temperature reaches 160° F
Baked custard, including quiche	Knife placed off center comes out clean (*Note:* Cheese in a properly cooked quiche will leave particles on the knife, too.)

ria. Hide them so they stay clean from pets, dirt, and other bacterial sources. Toss cracked or dirty eggs or those that aren't found until after two hours. Hard-cooked eggs don't keep as well as raw shell eggs; use hard-cooked eggs within a week. Like other high-protein foods, hard-cooked eggs shouldn't sit out at temperatures of 40°F or higher for longer than two hours. If they do, toss them!

Leftovers

● Heat leftovers to 165°F—and steaming hot. That includes precooked foods such as stuffed chicken breasts and preroasted chickens from takeout; eat them the same day you purchase them. Reheat sauces and gravies to a rolling boil for at least one minute.

Play It Microwave-Safe

Today microwave ovens are common, even at work, school, and in recreational vehicles and hotel rooms. Besides being convenient and speedy, microwaving has nutrition benefits. Faster cooking helps retain nutrients, and food can cook without adding fat.

General cooking guidelines apply to microwave cooking. In addition, take these food safety precautions:

● Use only microwave-safe containers. Check glass bowls, dishes, or cups for safety. Here's how: Place each container (empty) in the microwave oven with a separate cup of tap water. Microwave it on high for one minute. If the empty container stays cool, it's microwave-safe; slightly warm, use it for reheating only; and if it gets hot, it's not microwave-safe.

● Unless it says microwave-safe, avoid microwaving food in food packaging. That includes margarine or butter tubs, other plastic tubs, or polystyrene boxes or trays. Plastic bags, brown paper bags, paper towels, paper plates, and paper napkins aren't safe either. Chemicals from these products may migrate to food. Containers from store-bought microwave meals are meant for one-time use; toss them.

● Cut food for microwaving into same-size pieces. This helps ensure even cooking.

● Cover food well while cooking to keep it moist and promote even cooking. Use waxed paper, microwave-safe plastic wrap, or a lid that fits. For safety, allow a little space for some steam to escape.

● Rotate food for even cooking. Halfway through cooking, do one of the following: Turn the dish; stir or reposition the food on the plate or bowl; turn large foods over; or reposition the dish on the turntable. Check for cold spots.

● Be aware of differences in the power, or wattage, of microwave ovens. Cooking times may differ. In fact, check the wattage of your oven periodically; read the manual to know how.

● Allow standing time. Food keeps cooking after the microwave oven turns off, spreading heat more evenly. In fact, the internal temperature can go up several degrees as food stands. Without standing time, food may not be cooked to a safe temperature!

● Check for doneness—after the standing time. Then, as with food cooked in the oven, check the internal temperature. Check in several places but not near the bone.

● When preparing prepackaged, frozen microwaveable meals, read and follow all cooking instructions on the food packaging.

● Don't use your microwave oven for canning. Pressure that builds up in the jar may cause it to explode.

For more on microwave oven safety, see "Play It Safe: Warming Baby's Bottle and Food" in chapter 16 and "Microwave Oven Safety for Kids" in chapter 17.

REFRIGERATOR CALCULATOR: DO YOUR LEFTOVERS MAKE A SAFE MEAL?

PERISHABLE FOOD	KEEPS REFRIGERATED UP TO
Meat	
Cooked ground beef/turkey	3 to 4 days
Deli meat	3 to 5 days
Cooked beef, bison, lamb, pork, poultry	3 to 4 days
Seafood	
Raw (e.g., sushi, sashimi); must consume on day of purchase	
Cooked seafood	3 to 4 days
Soups and Chili	
Chili with or without meat	3 to 4 days
Soup, stews	3 to 4 days
Other Entrées	
Pizza	3 to 4 days
Pasta, rice	7 days
Casserole	3 to 4 days
Side Dishes	
Fresh salad	1 to 2 days
Pasta or potato salad	3 to 5 days
Deviled egg	3 to 4 days
Potato (any style)	3 to 5 days
Cooked vegetables	3 to 4 days
Hard-cooked egg	7 days
Dessert	
Cream pie, fruit pie	3 to 4 days
Pastries, cake, cheesecake	7 days

Source: "Home Food Safety . . . It's in Your Hands." Academy of Nutrition and Dietetics and ConAgra, Inc.,

Grill It for Safety

Before you put a burger on the grill, take these precautions:

● Clean the grill between each use with hot, soapy water. Removing charred food debris from the grill reduces exposure to bacteria.

● Adjust the grill so food cooks evenly—inside and out. When meat or poultry are too close to the heat source, the outside surfaces cook quickly and may appear done; the inside may not be cooked well enough.

● If you're grilling at a picnic site, do all the cooking there—from start to finish. Partly cooked meats transported to the picnic may still carry bacteria.

● Marinate to help keep meat, fish, and poultry from drying out.

● Grill on both sides. Turn meat, poultry, and fish over at least once for even cooking. If fish is less than ½ inch thick, you don't need to turn it.

● Grill meat, poultry, and fish until cooked through but not charred. High-heat cooking such as grilling can cause two potentially carcinogenic compounds to form: polycyclic aromatic hydrocarbons (PAHs), mostly from smoke, and heterocyclic amines (HCAs), mostly from charring, as in a well-done steak. These compounds form naturally during cooking and grilling. While research on the health effects isn't conclusive, the quality of the meat is better if you avoid the "black stuff." To reduce charring, especially if you grill a lot, be certain it reaches a safe internal temperature.

● Cook meat to medium, rather than well done; precook meat first, then quickly grill for flavor. Grill poultry and fish until the internal temperature reaches its target but the surface isn't blackened.

● Marinate. Emerging research indicates that marinating, especially with certain spices and herbs such as turmeric and rosemary, may reduce HCAs. *For more about safe marinating, refer to "Prep It for Safety" in this chapter.*

● Control hot coals to avoid flare-ups that cause smoke and charring. Trim away visible fat. Cook in the center of the grill—coals on the side—so fat and juices won't drip on them. Drain away high-fat marinades;

have a spray bottle with water ready for flare-ups. Never use water to control flames on a gas grill!

● Scrape off charred areas before eating the meat, poultry, or fish.

● Cooking in a smoker? It's a slow way to cook outdoors, good for less tender meat cuts—and it gives a smoky flavor. For safety's sake, make sure the smoker stays at 250°F to 300°F.

● Again, remember to transfer grilled or smoked food to a clean plate—not the unwashed plate used to bring raw food to the grill or the smoker. Use a clean utensil—not your fingers!

Plate It for Safety

● Use clean dishes and utensils for serving; use nothing that touched raw meat, fish, or poultry unless it was cleaned in hot, soapy water first.

● Avoid keeping perishable foods on a serving table or at room temperature for more than two hours (one hour at 90°F or above). That includes cooked meat, poultry, fish, eggs, and dishes made with them.

● For buffet-type service keep cold foods cold and hot foods hot. Serve cold foods on ice, at a temperature of 40°F or below. Use heated servers such as a chafing dish to keep hot foods hot. After two hours discard even these foods.

● When replenishing serving dishes, don't mix fresh food with food that's been sitting out. For more about *Clostridium perfringens* contamination on buffets, *see "Bacteria: Hard Hitters" earlier in this chapter.*

● Refrigerate leftovers as soon as you're done eating. That includes leftover pizza!

Carry It for Safety

Picnic Foods

Summer picnics, autumn tailgate parties—keep food fit to eat in your fresh-air kitchen. The basics: Keep food clean, keep hot food hot, and keep cold food cold. That includes proper hand washing!

● For perishables, use clean, insulated coolers chilled with ice or chemical cold packs. As a rule of thumb, pack your cooler with 75 percent food and 25 percent ice or frozen cold packs. Freeze cold packs at least

Have You Ever Wondered ?

. . . if liquid smoke is safe to eat? Bottled liquid smoke is sold alongside herbs and sauces in many supermarkets. It gives a smoky flavor without grilling. The flavoring is created by burning wood, then trapping the smoke; most potential carcinogens are removed. About 60 percent of processed meats sold in supermarkets are "smoked" with liquid smoke.

. . . if acrylamide is a health risk? In your own kitchen and in food processing, acrylamide forms naturally in foods such as fries, chips, coffee, browned breads, and toasted cereals. That happens when sugars react with certain amino acids as some foods are cooked at high temperatures—perhaps fried, baked, or toasted. The darker the browning, the more acrylamide forms. Likely around since cooking began, acrylamide has been detected only recently at very low levels in food. There's not enough research to conclude that acrylamide, in the small amounts consumed, is a human health risk. Yet the FDA is one of many institutions involved in long-term research. The best advice based on what's known now: There's no reason to change your food or cooking habits. Eat a variety of healthful foods, plenty of fruits and vegetables, and go easy on fatty and fried foods.

twenty-four hours ahead so they stay cold as long as possible. Chill the cooler ahead, too, with ice or cold packs. Secure the lid. Then keep it closed—no peeking!

● Store nonperishable foods in a clean basket, with heaviest foods on the bottom.

● Seal all foods tightly in bags, jars, or plastic containers. That keeps out moisture and bugs.

● Chill or freeze foods before packing them. Your cooler can't cool foods adequately if packed at room temperature. Pack perishables between ice or cold packs; they'll stay cold longer.

● Pack uncooked meat, poultry, or fish carefully—in well-sealed containers—for grilling at the picnic spot. Put them in the bottom of the cooler so any juices won't leak onto other foods. Bring a food thermometer in your picnic basket.

● Keep your cooler in a cool place (under a tree or a picnic table), not in the hot trunk or the sun.

● Keep ice for drinks in a sealed bag. Loose ice for chilling food and drinks isn't safe for drinks. If possible, keep drinks in a separate cooler since it may be opened frequently.

● Serve only the amount of food you'll eat right away. Return any perishable foods to the cooler immediately after serving.

● For picnics nearby when you'll eat right away, consider a hot dish—covered and wrapped well. Wrap the dish in several layers of newspaper, then in an insulated container. Baked beans are a great choice.

● Bring premoistened towelettes to wash up after handling meat, poultry, or chicken—or any food, for that matter. Or bring soap and a bottle filled with clean water to wash your hands and cooking surfaces. Another option: Bring a hand sanitizer, usually formulated with alcohol, which kills bacteria on your hands.

● Be prepared to clean the grill at the picnic site—unless you bring your own grill. Pack a brush, soap, and perhaps water. Make sure you have a safe water source for rinsing after washing the grill.

● After the picnic, toss perishable leftovers. Or repack them in a cold cooler if they have been out for less than two hours (one hour at 90°F or warmer) and are clean (no flies, dirt, or improper handling).

Carried Meals and Snacks

Whether you pack it at home or buy ready-to-eat takeout foods, any perishable foods left at room temperature for two hours or more are a risk for foodborne illness. That's especially true when food is stuffed in a school locker with a dirty gym bag or left on a warm windowsill at work! For safety's sake:

● Order take-out food just before lunch or dinner, then eat it right away, or keep it refrigerated.

● Use a clean insulated bag or a lunch box. Tuck in a small refreezable ice pack to keep food cold. Or freeze a juice box or small plastic container of water to keep the lunch box and the food cold. Pack a moist towelette or hand sanitizer, too, if there's no chance for hand washing with soap and water.

● For cold beverages, refrigerate an insulated vacuum bottle ahead. Then fill it with milk or juice. Or keep juice or milk in the fridge at work.

● Rinse raw produce, including peel-and-eat fruit, before packing it.

● For hot soups, stews, and chili, heat an insulated container ahead. Fill it with boiling water, then let it sit for several minutes before pouring it out. Then be sure the food is very hot when it's put into the container; keep the container closed until you eat the food.

● If you assemble your meal the night before, refrigerate perishables. Pack nonperishable foods, too: unopened canned soup or stew to heat up in the microwave oven at work, dried raisins or dried apple slices, crackers and peanut butter, boxed juice or milk, and beef jerky, to name a few. For canned foods with no pop top, tuck in a can opener!

● Keep carried, perishable food in an insulated container in a clean, cool place, away from sunlit windowsills, radiators, or warm vehicles. Or if a refrigerator is available, use it.

● Discard any perishable, carried food that isn't eaten. Remind your schoolkids, too!

● If your lunch is on your desk but work calls you away, put perishable food back in the refrigerator until you're ready to eat it.

● If you keep food in the office fridge, label and date it. Discard anything perishable, usually after three to four days. Check to make sure the refrigerator is regularly cleaned and is cold enough (40°F or less). You may need to initiate the cleaning!

● If you're in charge of cleaning the office kitchen, skip the corporate sponge. Use paper towels and hot, soapy water instead. Clean splatters in the microwave oven right away!

● If possible, keep a food thermometer handy at work to check the temperature when you reheat your lunch.

● Launder your lunch bag or wash your lunch box with soapy water after every use.

Ship It for Safety

Food safety is an issue if you buy food online or by mail order, get home-delivered groceries, or ship perishable-food gifts.

● To place an order, ask how and when perishable foods will be sent. Ask that food be packed with dry ice or cold packs; order for one-day delivery. Record the tracking number—just in case! Reputable mail-order companies take food safety seriously, but it's always wise to ask. Let the recipient know it's coming so it won't sit on the doorstep.

● If you're packing a perishable food gift, freeze it solid or refrigerate until cold before packing it. Pack food in an insulated cooler or a heavy corrugated box with cold packs or dry ice; talk to your shipper or the post office about proper forms, packing, and warning labels for shipping packages with dry ice. Mark the package as "Perishable—Keep Refrigerated." Use one-day delivery. Let the recipient know it's coming.

● If you receive a food gift, open it immediately. Some mail-order foods, such as dry-cured ham and hard salami, don't require refrigeration. Perishable meats (including most hams), poultry, fish, and other perishable foods should be packed in dry ice and arrive frozen. If cold enough, freeze or refrigerate the food. If not, toss it out; contact the mail-order company for a replacement or a refund.

Quick Tips for Injury Prevention

Kitchen safety is more than just preventing foodborne illness. Also keep safe from injury:

● Wipe up spills immediately so no one slips.

● Invest in a stable stool to reach a high cabinet.

● Keep cabinets, drawers, and doors closed so you don't bump into them. Put safety catches on drawers so they won't fall out when they're opened too far.

● Keep pot holders handy—and use them. Be careful if they get wet; water conducts heat.

● Turn handles on pots and pans inward and away from the stove's edge, where they may be knocked into or where children can grab them.

● Avoid overfilling pots and pans. Too much hot soup, stew, or pasta can burn you if it spills.

● Be careful with the hot water tap, especially if you have small children.

● Allow enough time for the pressure to release if you use a pressure cooker.

If You or Someone Else Is Choking

Perform the Heimlich Maneuver. If a victim can't talk, can't breathe, is turning blue in the face, or is clutching at his or her throat, get behind the person and wrap your arms around his or her waist. Making a fist, put the thumb side of the fist against the victim's upper abdomen, below the ribs and above the navel. Grasp your fist with your other hand and press into the victim's upper abdomen with a quick upward thrust. Repeat until the object is expelled. (Don't slap the victim's back—this can make matters worse.)

When you choke and no one is there to help, use the same technique as described above. You also can lean over a fixed horizontal object (a chair, a table edge, a railing), pressing your upper abdomen against the edge until the object is expelled.

Source: Courtesy of The Heimlich Institute, Cincinnati, Ohio.

Refer to chapter 16 for choking prevention for infants.

● Avoid dropping water into hot oil. Splatters may burn you. *Remember:* Water and oil don't mix!

● Douse grease fires at the base of the flames with baking soda—not water! Or put a lid on it to control flames.

● Keep electrical cords away from stove burners.

● Use a safety latch on cabinets with household chemicals, alcoholic beverages, matches, plastic bags, and sharp utensils (knives, toothpicks) so children can't reach them.

● Handle knives safely. Store them carefully, perhaps in a knife holder. Never leave them unseen in the kitchen drawer. Use sharp knives; dull knives are harder to use and promote injury. Always cut away from you—on a cutting board.

● Watch out for broken glass. If glass breaks in the sink, empty the water so you find all the pieces.

● Watch your fingers near your garbage disposal! Teach children to use it safely.

CHAPTER 14

Kitchen Nutrition
Cooking Matters

Kitchen nutrition—cooking for health—isn't new. About 150 years ago, *The Book of Household Management* described the kitchen as "the great laboratory of the household . . . much of the 'weal and woe' as far as regards bodily health, depends on the nature of the preparations concocted within its walls."

Throughout the decades, food preparation methods, recipes, and food itself have changed dramatically. Many of today's home cooks didn't grow up learning to cook from their parents. They have less time to prepare food, and use more convenience foods and time-saving appliances than previous generations. Despite the changes, the kitchen remains where foods can be transformed into the nourishing, flavorful dishes people enjoy. As a strategy for good nutrition: cooking skills matter—and so does flavor. And the family table? For health and more, it matters a lot! *See chapters 11 and 17 for benefits of the family table.*

Click Here! Websites to Know . . .

● Keep the Beat, Deliciously Healthy Eating, NHLBI/USHHS
http://hp2010.nhlbihin.net/healthyeating

See "Resources You Can Use" for more websites.

Cooking Essentials!

When you cook, you know about the nutrition and safety of food served at your table: the ingredients, their nutrient quality and calorie content, the ways you stored and cooked food, the flavors and visual appeal, and the portion sizes. You're in control.

What do you need to know to prepare food for your table?

Kitchen Basics!

Whether you cook from scratch or prefer speed-scratch cooking, having basic kitchen skills is key to successful, flavorful meals. Speed-scratch cooking is often just assembling partly prepared ingredients and perhaps cooking them. An example: triple-washed salad greens tossed with precooked chicken fingers and salad dressing for a quick main dish salad.

Start by Planning

Planning means having nutrient-rich ingredients on hand and deciding ahead how to use them. Along with better nutrition, planning can translate to time, effort, and money saved. Consider:

● *Your time and energy. Refer to "Meals for Time-Pressed Lifestyles" in chapter 11.*

● *Seasonality*. Seasonal produce is abundant and economical, with more varietals to pick from. It's also at peak flavor. Check local farmers' markets.

● *Your food budget. To maximize your food dollar and shop for seasonal food, see chapter 12.*

● *Food preferences and the health, age-related, and nutrient and calorie needs* of those eating. Plan sensible portions. *Refer to chapters 10 and 11 for planning a day's meals and snacks.*

● *Foods you have on hand* (pantry, refrigerator, and freezer). Check before you shop; make a shopping list. *Refer to "Stocking the Kitchen" in this chapter.*

● *Meal appeal. Refer to "Variety for Meal Appeal" in this chapter.*

● *Kitchen skills.* Simple speed-scratch cooking can be as nourishing and delicious as lengthy recipes. To learn more skills, take a local cooking class, get a step-by-step illustrated cookbook, or cook with a "foodie."

● *Kitchen equipment.* Mixing bowls and spoons, pots and pans, measuring cups and spoon, ladle, spatula, and cutting boards are basics. You don't need every kitchen gadget! *See "Well Equipped—for Healthful Cooking!" in this chapter.*

Prepare to Cook, Then Cook!

● Read the whole recipe *before* you start! Make sure you have all the ingredients.

● For recipes, look up terms you don't know. *See "Food Prep Skills to Know" and Cooking Methods to Know" in this chapter.*

● Get ingredients ready to cook: perhaps wash, chop, or slice. *Mise en place,* translated as "Everything in its place," as chefs say!

● Pick the right knife—for example, a paring knife for peeling and trimming vegetables and fruit, a serrated knife with a jagged edge for cutting bread, and a French knife for slicing and dicing all kinds of foods. Keep knives sharp. Use a clean cutting board. When cutting, be safe: Hold food so your fingertips are under your knuckles; cut away from yourself.

● Measure carefully. Although a pinch here or there may work in some recipes, exact measuring is critical in some recipes, such as in baked breads and cakes. Use liquid measuring cups for liquids; put the cup on a flat surface, and pour liquid to the line. Check at eye level; the correct measure is the bottom of the curve. Use graduated dry volume measuring cups for dry ingredients; fill to the top and level off with the back of a knife. For brown sugar and solid fats, you'll need to press or pack it firmly.

● Follow recipe instructions, cooking times, and temperatures! Substitute wisely.

Serve an Appealing Meal

● Serve sensible portions. For good nutrition fill half the plate with fruits and veggies, a quarter of the plate with whole-grain or enriched-grain foods, and another quarter of the plate with a lean protein food. Serve low-fat or fat-free milk or water.

● Serve food so it looks attractive. A simple fruit, vegetable, or herb garnish adds appeal yet few calories. *See "Beyond Parsley . . . Quick, Easy Garnishes" in this chapter.*

● Keep mealtime an event without distractions. To avoid mindless eating, turn off the television. Remove table clutter. Enjoy the food and table talk.

Variety for Meal Appeal

Like a well-decorated room or a beautifully landscaped garden, an appealing meal follows basic principles of design. Different foods add a variety of color, flavor, texture, shape, and temperature to meals or snacks. In fact, the more variety, the more satisfying the flavor experience! At the same time, food variety supplies different nutrients and phytonutrients.

Vary the color. Contrast visual differences: meat loaf, mashed potatoes with gravy, corn, and applesauce . . . compared with meat loaf, baked sweet potato with chopped chives, asparagus, and spinach salad with orange slices. Which one has more interest? The meal with an artist's palette of color! Phytonutrients that give fruits and vegetables their colorful appeal and health benefits also contribute different flavors.

Vary the flavors. Different ingredients and seasonings in a dish or meal add layers of flavor. Instead of sweet orange-glazed chicken, candied sweet potatoes, and fruit compote, complement chicken with wild rice pilaf and a crisp spinach salad with herbed balsamic dressing. Include sweet, sour, salty, bitter, and umami tastes. Other sensations, such as the "burn" of chiles and smoky aromas, add to flavor, too. *See "Flavor and Health" in this chapter.*

Vary the texture. Crunchy foods contrast soft foods—for example, chopped nuts in brown rice, or raw veggies with herbed yogurt dip. Variety of texture (soft, smooth, creamy, crunchy, crispy) adds appeal as much as variety of color!

Vary the shape and size. Round meatballs, round peas, round new potatoes, and round grapes may look some-what boring if plated together. Add variety to the plate with baby carrots or pea pods instead of peas, pasta spirals instead of potatoes, or sliced peaches instead of grapes.

Vary the temperature. Hot and cool in the same meal maximize the flavor perception of a meal. For example, a cold summer supper or a picnic from the cooler

---

Stocking the Kitchen

Keep a variety of nutrient-dense foods on hand—and make nutritious meals and snacks quick and easy to prepare. Buy fresh ingredients as you need them! Many of these foods are sold with reduced amounts of fat or sodium—or they're fat- or sodium-free. Decide which form to buy to fit your overall goals for your meal and snack choices.

To Store in Your Kitchen Cabinet . . .
  Whole-grain and fortified breakfast cereal
  Rice (brown and white)
  Brown and wild rice pilaf mix
  Pasta (spaghetti, macaroni, others, perhaps whole-grain or fiber-rich)
  Couscous (perhaps whole-wheat couscous)
  Bulgur or whole barley
  Gingersnaps or vanilla wafers
  Whole-wheat or mixed grain bread and rolls
  Beans (dry and canned)
  Peanut butter, nut butters (almond, cashew)
  Tuna or salmon (canned or vacuum-packed, packed in spring water)
  Refried beans (canned, fat-free, reduced-fat, vegetarian)
  Fruit (canned in own juice or light syrup, dried)
  Vegetables (canned, perhaps sodium-reduced)
  Vegetable soup (canned, perhaps sodium-reduced)
  Nonfat dry milk powder
  Evaporated fat-free (skim) milk
  Salsa or picante sauce
  Pasta sauce
  Chicken, beef, vegetable broth (canned, reduced sodium and fat)
  100 percent fruit spread
  Condiments (mustard, ketchup)
  Vinegar (balsamic, apple cider, rice)
  Vegetable or olive oil (peanut, canola, soybean, others)
  Salad dressing (perhaps reduced fat)
  Vegetable oil cooking spray
  Herbs and spices
  Flour (whole-wheat, bleached white, white whole-wheat)
  Sugar (granulated, brown, powdered)

  Cornstarch
  Baking ingredients (baking powder, baking soda, cocoa powder)

To Keep in a Cool, Dry Place . . .
  Potatoes, sweet potatoes
  Onions
  Garlic
  Shallots

To Store in Your Refrigerator . . . *
  Apples
  Oranges
  Carrots
  Tortillas
  Milk (fat-free, low-fat, perhaps whole milk)
  Yogurt (perhaps Greek yogurt)
  Parmesan cheese
  Cheese (regular, reduced-fat)
  Sliced turkey breast or chicken, deli meat
  Eggs (egg substitute in your freezer)

To Keep in Your Freezer . . . *
  Fruit juice concentrate (or fresh juice in your refrigerator, or juice boxes on the shelf)
  Frozen vegetables
  Frozen green pepper (chopped)
  Frozen onion (chopped)
  Frozen whole-wheat waffles or bagels
  Frozen fish fillets
  Lean ground beef
  Pork loin
  Skinless chicken breast or thighs
  Frozen yogurt or fruit sorbet

*Buy fresh produce, meat, poultry, and fish as you need them.

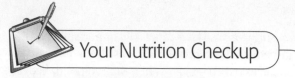

Your Nutrition Checkup

Cooking Literacy

How would you rate your cooking literacy? Enjoy learning more!

Do you know. . .

- ☐ Basic food preparation terms?
- ☐ Measuring and weighing skills?
- ☐ Knife skills and how to use knives safely?
- ☐ Basic food preparation techniques?
- ☐ Right techniques for specific ingredients (e.g., separating egg yolks and whites)?
- ☐ Dry- and moist-cooking methods?
- ☐ How to prepare basic savory and sweet sauces (with limited fat, sodium, and added sugars)?
- ☐ How to choose and use your home cooking equipment?

Techniques for . . .

- ☐ Retaining nutrients in food while cooking?
- ☐ Reducing saturated and *trans* fats, cholesterol, sodium, added sugars?
- ☐ Including oils, fruits, vegetables, and whole grains in food, meals, and menus?
- ☐ Cooking food to proper and safe temperatures for safety and food quality?
- ☐ Modifying recipes to change/improve nutritional value and control calories?
- ☐ Portion control as your serve a meal?
- ☐ Healthful use of convenience foods?
- ☐ Time management in the kitchen?
- ☐ Creating meals that are nourishing—and appealing?
- ☐ Keeping food safe as it's prepared?
- ☐ Kitchen ecology (less food, energy, and water waste; smart food packaging use)?

Source: Adapted from "Core Competencies," Food and Culinary Professionals Dietary Practice Group, Academy of Nutrition and Dietetics.

can be refreshing. However, a warm whole-wheat roll offers a nice contrast to a cool chef's salad. And frozen yogurt makes a nice ending to a hot dinner.

Recipes: Judge for Yourself!

Each year, hundreds of new cookbooks appear on bookstore shelves. Even more recipes appear in mag-azines and newspapers; on supermarket racks and package labels; and on websites, blogs, and phone apps. How can you pick the right recipes for your family meals?

● Look at the main ingredients and the portions. You'll get an idea of how just one recipe portion fits within your day's eating plan and how the nutrition stacks up. *Use the food guide described in chapter 10 for your healthy eating plan.*

● Check the nutrient analysis of the recipe—if it's provided. Unlike food labels, nutrition information and serving sizes for recipes aren't standardized. Recipes may list some, but not all, the nutrients you find on a label. When comparing nutrition information in similar recipes, be alert: Serving sizes vary from one recipe to another and may not be the same as one label-size serving of a frozen version.

● Choose recipes to complement the whole meal—and other meals and snacks for the whole day! Consider variety of color, flavor, texture, taste—and nutrition. If the recipe you choose has more calories, solid fat, added sugars, or sodium, plan your menu with other foods that have less.

● Most important, choose recipes that appeal to you and your family. No matter how nutritious a recipe sounds, it should be something you enjoy—or a food you're willing to experience, perhaps for the first time.

Recipe Makeovers

Chefs and test-kitchen experts change recipes all the time. There's nothing sacred about most recipes (except perhaps Mom's). Recipes get altered when new ingredients come on the market, when cooking equipment changes, when consumers want recipe shortcuts, when ingredients are in or out of season or become more or less costly, when consumers shift food preferences, and when nutrition and health issues arise.

In your own "test kitchen," you can modify recipes to improve the nutrient content or cut calories, often without much flavor change. You can change the ingredients, modify the cooking steps, cut portion sizes, or do all three. Experiment more dramatically by adding more fruits or vegetables, or switching to whole grains in recipes. Even one or two small recipe changes can net a significant nutrition difference. *This chapter has plenty of ideas!*

However you approach recipe makeovers, keep flavor, texture, and appeal as priorities. Remember that moderation in your overall food choices counts, not what's in one dish. For example, a single dish that's high in calories may not need a makeover—*if* you don't eat it often; *if* the rest of your day's choices have less calories, or *if* you eat just a small amount. To make over a recipe, you might:

1. *Change the ingredients or switch their proportions.* You might use less or more of one or more ingredients . . . or substitute one ingredient for another . . . or take an ingredient out entirely . . . or add something new.

● *Start by reviewing the recipe and the ingredient list.* Decide on ingredient changes to achieve your goals, perhaps switch the type of fat, boost fiber or calcium, add more vegetables, use leftovers, boost the flavor, take advantage of a supermarket sale, or match a family preference.

● *Consider the ingredients' functions before you switch.* For an appealing result use suitable substitutions and know how ingredients function in cooking. Learn more about ingredient functions: *see "Fats, Sugar, Salt: What They Do" in this chapter.*

Sometimes the switch is easy. For example, in meat, poultry, fish, and vegetable dishes, salt enhances taste; herbs make flavorful substitutes.

● *Reduce or eliminate some ingredients.* In some recipes you may cut back on sugar by a third and still enjoy good results. With sautéed foods, try less cooking oil. Optional ingredients are easy to take out; removing others may alter the appearance or the flavor. Season with extra herbs or spices if you cut back on salt.

● *Boost nutrients by adding ingredients.* Fortifying casseroles with wheat bran or dry milk powder may go unnoticed. Adding shredded carrots or mashed cauliflower to mashed potatoes, beans to salads, or dried cranberries to muesli gives extra flavor and color along with more nutrients and phytonutrients.

● *As easy substitutions, try modified ingredients.* For example, use cholesterol-free egg products, reduced-fat cheese, or sodium-reduced chicken broth in some recipes. Follow package directions if the product needs to be prepared differently.

● *Experiment a little at a time, perhaps with just*

one ingredient. That's especially important when the ingredient has functional purposes, such as eggs or sugar in baked foods. When the recipe makeover works, jot it down—in your cookbook or your file.

● *Make an ingredient switch,* perhaps to canola or olive oil for less solid fat. Regular ground beef is a key ingredient in hot chili, but lean ground beef or turkey works just as well. Low-fat yogurt can replace sour cream in dips, potato toppers, and some creamy sauce.

2. *Modify food prep.* Simple changes in cooking techniques may require little or no extra time investment—just know-how. For example, skim fat that

Food Prep Skills to Know

Cutting:

Slice: to cut through or across into slices

Chop: to cut food into smaller pieces of no particular size or shape

Cube: to cut foods into square pieces, usually ½ inch per side

Dice: to cut foods into small, square pieces, usually ¼ inch (or smaller) per side

Grate: to rub food against a serrated surface to create fine shreds

Julienne: to cut in matchlike strips

Mince: to cut food into very small pieces

Combining:

Beat: to mix briskly until the mixture is smooth with a spoon, whisk, or mixer

Cream: to soften fat with a spoon or mixer, perhaps with another ingredient, until smooth

Fold in: to blend ingredients gently, such as beaten egg whites or whipped cream, so volume remains and air bubbles don't break

Knead: to repeatedly fold, press, and turn dough by hand to mix ingredients and develop the gluten in dough

Mix: to combine ingredients so they're distributed evenly

Stir: to mix ingredients with a circular or figure-eight motion until evenly distributed or combined

Whip: to beat fast to incorporate air and increase volume

Other:

Marinate: to tenderize and add flavor by letting food, such as meat or chicken, remain in a flavor liquid, such as Italian dressing, for a period of time

Season: to add herbs, spices, salt, or pepper for flavor

Paint Your Plate with Color!

Toss blueberries in your yogurt. Garnish your salad with sliced beets. Tuck spinach leaves in your sandwich. Color offers much more than eye appeal to a wonderful meal! A rainbow of fruits and vegetables creates a palette of nutrients and phytonutrients on your plate, each with a different bundle of potential benefits in a healthful diet: from oxidizing free radicals that may damage healthy cells, to having anti-inflammatory qualities, to lowering LDL cholesterol. *See "Phytonutrients for Health" in chapter 6.*

● *Green: fruit*—avocado, green apples, green grapes, honeydew, kiwifruit, lime, green pears; *vegetables*—artichokes, asparagus, broccoli, Brussels sprouts, green beans, green cabbage, leafy greens, okra, green pepper, snow peas, zucchini. Their lutein and indoles have antioxidant potential and may help promote healthy vision and reduce cancer risks.

● *Orange and deep yellow: fruit*—apricot, cantaloupe, grapefruit, mango, papaya, peach, pineapple, yellow apple, yellow fig; *veggies*—carrot, yellow beets, yellow pepper, sweet corn, sweet potato, winter squash. Carotenoids, bioflavonoids, and the antioxidant vitamin C may promote a healthy heart, vision, immunity, and reduced risk for some cancers. The deeper the yellow/orange color, the more carotenoids these foods have!

● *Purple and blue: fruit*—blackberries, blueberries, plums, purple figs, raisins; *veggies*—eggplant, purple cabbage, purple-fleshed potato. Anthocyanins, which give a blue-purple color, and phenolics, may have antioxidant and anti-aging benefits, and may help with memory, urinary tract health, and reduced cancer risks.

● *Red: fruit*—cherries, cranberries, pomegranate, blood oranges, red/pink grapefruit; red grapes, strawberries, watermelon; *veggies*—beets, red onions, red peppers, red potatoes, rhubarb, tomatoes. This color group delivers lycopene, a powerful carotenoid, as well as anthocyanins. They may help maintain heart health, healthy vision, and immunity, and may reduce cancer risks. When cooked or canned, lycopene is more available to your body.

● *White, tan, brown: fruit*—banana, brown pear, dates, white peaches; *veggies*—cauliflower, jicama, kohlrabi, mushrooms, onions, parsnips, turnip, white-fleshed potato, white corn. Of particular interest: allicin in garlic and onion, and selenium in mushrooms may promote heart health and reduce cancer risks.

For more about vegetables and fruits, see chapter 10.

---

collects on stews, scrub rather than peel fiber-rich potato skins, or oven-bake frozen French fries rather than fry them. Shift proportions: for example, serve a bowl of fruit with a dollop of ice cream instead of a bowl of ice cream topped with a spoonful of fruit.

3. *Reduce portion sizes.* If a recipe is high in calories, fats, or sugars, serve less. For example, instead of ¼ cup of cheese sauce on a baked potato, use two tablespoons—and add some steamed, chopped vegetables and/or herbs for flavor. Trick the eye so less looks like more. Serve smaller portions on smaller plates.

Well Equipped—for Healthful Cooking!

To cook the healthful way, equip your kitchen.

Cheese grater. With a grater, a little cheese goes a longer way. When cheese is grated, a smaller portion still adds plenty of flavor. It's also a "grate" idea for shredding vegetables such as carrots and summer squash, or for grating citrus rinds for flavor.

Coffee grinder. It's great for grinding small amounts of nuts, seeds, and grains as well as dry herbs and spices.

Egg separator. An egg separator helps you easily separate the yolks from the whites. That's important when you're cutting back on dietary cholesterol. Using an egg separator has a food safety benefit, too. Compared to the technique of transferring the yolk back and forth between the two shell halves, using an egg separator reduces the chance of transferring bacteria from the outside of the shell to the uncooked egg.

Fat-separating pitcher. With the position of the spout, a fat-separating pitcher lets you pour out the liquid from the bottom, leaving the fat behind.

Food processor or blender. You can puree low-fat cottage cheese to the consistency of thick cream; chop, grate, or puree vegetables for use in soups, sauces, salads, and side dishes; or puree fruit, yogurt, and milk for a thick yet lower-calorie milk shake.

Hot-air popcorn popper. This popper requires no oil, so popcorn can be a quick, low-fat, low-calorie snack.

Immersion blender. This handheld blender makes it easy to prepare fruit smoothies and pureed fruit and vegetable soups.

Cooking Methods to Know

Bake: to cook food surrounded by hot air, usually in an oven

Boil: to cook food in liquid to a rapid boil

Braise: to brown or sear, then simmer over low heat in liquid—water, broth, or even fruit juice—in a covered pot for a lengthy time

Broil: to cook with direct heat, usually under a heating element in the oven

Deep-fry: to cook by submerging food in hot oil

Grill or barbecue: to cook with direct heat directly over hot coals or another heat source

Panbroil: to cook uncovered in a preheated, nonstick skillet without added fat or water

Pan-fry: to fry in fat

Poach: to cook gently in liquid, just below boiling

Reduce: to boil a stock, wine, or sauce until evaporation reduces the volume, the consistency thickens, and the flavor intensifies

Roast: to cook uncovered with dry heat in the oven

Sauté: to cook quickly in a small amount of fat, stirring so the food browns evenly

Sear: to cook, or caramelize, the surface (usually meat, poultry or fish) as part of grilling, baking, braising, roasting, etc., at a high temperature

Simmer: to cook slowly in liquid, just *below* boiling

Steam: to cook with steam heat over (not in) boiling water in a covered pot, or wrapped in foil or leaves (such as lettuce or banana leaves) packets, over boiling water or on a grill

Stew: to sear, then cook in liquid, such as water, juice, wine, broth, or stock, in a tightly covered pot over low heat

Stir-fry: to cook small pieces of meat, poultry, fish, seafood, and/or vegetables in a very small amount of oil, perhaps with added broth, over very high heat, stirring as you cook

Indoor grill. Indoor grills either fit over the burners on your stove, or they may be freestanding appliances. Either way, you can easily discard the excess fat, which drips through the grates into a drip pan.

Instant-read thermometer. An instant-read thermometer helps you cook food to a safe internal temperature. *See chapter 13 for tips on using a food thermometer.*

Kitchen scale. A scale that measures in ounces helps you figure portion sizes. If you have a hard time determining the size of your meat, poultry, fish, or cheese servings, a kitchen scale is helpful.

Kitchen scissors. Along with knives, kitchen scissors can trim visible fat from meat and poultry.

Knives. Good-quality for cutting fruit, vegetables, and more.

Microplane. This grater is useful for grating hard cheese, citrus peels, ginger, and more.

Microwave oven. A microwave oven cooks food fast, without the need for added fat. The fast cooking time also helps food retain vitamins and minerals. Why so speedy? Microwaves, which cause food molecules to vibrate and create friction, travel fast; the friction heats and cooks food.

Nonstick pots and pans. Some cookware is specially coated, allowing you to cook with little or no added fat. Although today's nonstick finishes last a long time, care for them properly. Use nonmetal utensils to prevent scratching; avoid abrasive cleaners that strip away coatings. Many are dishwasher-safe.

Pastry brush. A small pastry brush lets you just lightly coat meat, poultry, fish, and baked goods with oils.

Pressure cooker. To save time, you can cook dry beans in it quickly. (Cooked dry beans have less salt than canned beans.) It cooks food quickly without much water, helping with vitamin retention.

Pump spray bottle. A refillable oil pump can be filled with the type of oil you like, for use as a vegetable oil spray. By spraying olive oil on bread you may use less.

Ribbed frypan. The ribs on the bottom surface let meat or poultry cook above the fat drippings so less fat gets absorbed.

Rice cooker. With this countertop appliance, rice cooking is easy! Just add rice (white, brown, wild), the right amount of liquid of your choice (perhaps juice or broth), and perhaps herbs, and flip a switch. It turns off automatically when the rice is cooked.

Roasting pan with a grate. With a grate, roasted and broiled meat or poultry can't absorb fat drippings. They collect in the pan below.

Salad spinner. This plastic bowl with removable strainer and special top helps you easily remove excess water from fresh salad greens.

Slotted spoon. A slotted spoon allows you to lift food out of the pan, leaving any fat drippings behind.

For a Taste Lift

- Grill or roast your veggies in a very hot (450°F) oven or grill for a sweet, smoky flavor. Brush or spray them lightly with oil so they don't dry out. Sprinkle with herbs.
- Caramelize sliced onions to bring out their natural sugar flavor. Just cook them slowly over low heat in a small amount of oil. Use them to make a rich, dark sauce for meat or poultry.
- Enhance sauces, soups, and salads with a splash of flavored, balsamic, or rice vinegar. *See "Herbed Vinegars" in this chapter for ways to make your own herb and fruit vinegars.*
- Add a tangy taste with citrus juice or grated citrus peel: lemon, lime, or orange. Acidic ingredients help lift and balance flavor.
- Pep it up with peppers! Use red, green, and yellow peppers of all varieties—sweet, hot, and dried. Or add a dash of hot pepper sauce.
- Give a flavor burst with good-quality condiments such as horseradish, flavored mustard, chutney, wasabi, bean purees, tapenade, and salsas of all kinds!
- Simmer to make reduction sauces. Concentrate the flavors of meat, poultry, and fish stocks. Reduce the juices by heating them—don't boil! Then use them as a flavorful glaze or gravy.
- Intensify the flavors of meat, poultry, and fish with high-heat cooking techniques such as pan-searing, grilling, or broiling. These cooking techniques brown meat and add flavor.
- For their fuller flavors, incorporate more whole grains such as brown rice or quinoa, or experiment with amaranth and wild rice.
- Add small amounts of ingredients with bold flavors: pomegranate seeds, chipotle pepper, or cilantro.

More Taste Lifters

- For grains that absorb fluid (rice, buckwheat, and barley), cook them in defatted, perhaps reduced-sodium, chicken or beef broth. Risotto, an Italian rice specialty, typically is prepared by cooking arborio or white short-grain rice in broth, along with herbs and other ingredients.
- Blend herbs, spices, sun-dried tomatoes, and shredded cheese into bread dough before baking it.
- Experiment with herbs and spices: basil, chives, cilantro, rosemary, garlic, ginger, caraway, cumin. *See Quick Reference Herbs and Spices in this chapter.*
- Sharpen up the flavor with cheese. Add a little Parmesan, sharp Cheddar, Romano, feta, Asiago, or blue cheese—to vegetables, rice, or pasta.
- Intensify flavor with dried ingredients: sun-dried tomatoes, dried mushrooms, dried cranberries, dried apricots, dried plums (prunes), dried figs, and red pepper flakes. Plump sun-dried tomatoes and dried mushrooms in broth or cooking wine, and dried cranberries or dried plums in apple juice.
- Marinate with tangy, sweet, or savory sauces to infuse flavor from the outside in.
- Use a little nut oil: hazelnut, almond, or walnut oil. A little drizzle as a finishing oil will do!

Slow cooker. This countertop appliance cooks food with low, steady, moist heat. It can be used to make tougher cuts of meat more tender. Casserole-type dishes and soups work well in a slow cooker.

Steamer. Rather than fry foods, steam them. There are several kinds of steamers: an electric steamer for vegetables, rice, fish, or chicken; a stackable bamboo steamer set that fits in a wok or a stockpot; or a small aluminum vegetable steamer that fits in a saucepan.

Strainer. With a microwave-safe plastic strainer you can cook ground meat in a microwave oven, collecting fat drippings in a container underneath.

Wok. A wok's sloped sides allow food to cook fast without much oil. Unless it has a nonstick surface, "season" a new stainless-steel wok to keep food from sticking. Here's how: First coat the cooking surface with vegetable oil, then heat in a 350° F oven for about an hour. Oil will work its way into the porous surface.

Yogurt cheese strainer. A fine mesh strainer allows you to drain away the liquid in yogurt and use the thickened yogurt as a substitute for sour cream. *See chapter 5 for tips on making yogurt cheese.*

Beyond Parsley . . . Quick, Easy Garnishes

Garnishes do more than add eye appeal to food; they also offer flavor, color, and texture contrasts and some nutritional value. Garnish food with edibles that complement the ingredients in the food. For example, a sprig of basil goes with many Italian dishes; a slice of lemon or lime complements many seafood dishes; and a sliced vegetable garnish adds more veggies to a meal! Arrange the garnish artistically around, under, or on top of the food.

Parsley, which may be the most common garnish, dresses up a plate and serves as a natural breath freshener. While having less flavor than flat-leafed varieties, curly parsley adds texture to the plate, too, and both varieties have some beta carotene (which forms vitamin A) and vitamin C! To garnish, go beyond parsley and "paint your plate" with other foods, too:

On salads . . . rinsed capers; fennel slices; pomegranate seeds; red onion slices; red, green, and yellow pepper strips; toasted, chopped walnuts or pecans;

Give It a Little Salsa

Salsa is the Spanish word for "sauce." With today's cuisine, salsa has become a lot more sexy! By combining a variety of chopped vegetables, fruits, herbs, and even hot sauce, there's a salsa for every flavor mood.

Tomato salsa: Combine chopped plum tomatoes, onions, canned green chiles, cilantro, and lime juice. Add red pepper flakes or hot sauce for more zip. Chill. *Tip:* Plum tomatoes, especially when they're in season, often have more flavor than salad tomatoes.

Pineapple or mango salsa: Combine chopped, fresh, or canned pineapple or mango with chopped cilantro, fresh lime juice, and a touch of sugar and minced garlic. Chill.

Black bean salsa: Combine canned, drained and rinsed black beans with chopped tomato, chopped onion, chopped cilantro, and a little jalapeño and red wine vinegar. Chill.

For More Variety: Nuts, Seeds, Nut Butters

A small handful of nuts and seeds not only adds flavor; they're also sources of oils! Go easy since their calories can add up. Since their nutrients and phytonutrients differ, vary your choices:

- Cashews in stir-fries
- Pecans, almonds, or sunflower seeds in salads, waffles, or sweet potatoes
- Pine nuts or pistachios in pasta sauces and casseroles
- Sesame seeds on green veggies, soups, and stews
- Walnuts and macadamia nuts in quick breads
- Any nuts on cereal, yogurt, or in trail mix
- Nut butters and tahini (sesame paste) as a light spread

---

chopped apple (tossed with lemon juice to prevent browning); watercress; orange sections; blueberries or raspberries; grated cheese; snow peas; shredded jicama; or marigold petals. *For edible flowers as garnishes, see "Please Don't Eat the Daffodils" in this chapter.*

On soups . . . an avocado slice dipped in lemon; shredded carrot; minced chives; sprigs of herbs; minced fresh herbs; snow peas; a dollop of plain yogurt; orange peel strips; a lemon slice; croutons; pesto sauce; edible flowers; shredded green, yellow, and red peppers; grated cheese; or plain, air-popped popcorn.

On cooked vegetables . . . toasted, sliced almonds; toasted pine nuts; grated Parmesan cheese; stir-fried onion slices; stir-fried mushroom slices; chopped lean ham; chopped olives or pimiento; or fresh herbs.

In beverages . . . a mint sprig; scented geranium leaves; orange, lime, or lemon slices; fresh berries; sliced starfruit, apple, or kiwifruit; or a cinnamon stick.

With meat, poultry, or fish . . . tomato slices; a small bunch of grapes; lemon and lime wedges; crab apple slices; a grilled peach or pear half; baby corn; baby beets, squash, and carrots; or chutney or salsa in endive, a lettuce cup, or a lemon slice.

Please Don't Eat the Daffodils

Edible flowers add a distinctive flavor (*sweet* lilac, *spicy* nasturtium, *minty* bee balm) and a unique splash of color to foods. But you can't eat just any flower!

Some are poisonous; even edible flowers may be contaminated by chemicals if they weren't grown for eating. Don't eat flowers from a florist or a greenhouse—or that you pick along the road. Don't use them as a garnish, either. Flowers that aren't edible include buttercup, delphinium, lily of the valley, foxglove, goldenseal, periwinkle, oleander, sweet pea—and daffodils, to name a few!

For edible flowers, grow your own or buy them in the produce section of your store. They should be labeled as "edible flowers." Only eat flowers if you're *absolutely* sure of their safety! *Tip:* If you have hay fever, allergies, or asthma, be cautious about eating flowers.

Try growing edible flowers in your kitchen garden: bee balm, calendula (pot marigold), borage, chrysanthemum, day lilies, dianthus, marigolds, nasturtiums (enjoy leaves and blossoms), pansies, roses, scented geraniums, squash blossoms, sunflowers, tulips, and violets. Enjoy blossoms from any herb plant, try basil, chive, lavender, oregano, sage, savory, and thyme blossoms.

After harvesting, wash them well, and gently pat them dry. To keep edible flowers for a few days, refrigerate them. Just keep the stems in water, or put short-stemmed blossoms in a plastic bag or between damp paper towels. For most flowers, enjoy the petals.

Flavor and Health

Flavor is a bigger nutrition issue than many realize. According to consumer research, taste tops nutrition as the main reason why consumers buy one food over another. There's a lot wrapped up in why you prefer certain foods, including social, psychological (emotional), and health factors. In any case, the foods you enjoy are likely the ones you eat most. The more often you eat them, the more important their nutritional impact on your overall health.

For most Americans, enjoyment is an important reason for eating; it may even be *the* reason, so make food appeal a kitchen priority. When it comes to nutrition, think flavor . . . and when it comes to flavor, think nutrition!

What Is Flavor?

Imagine . . . the aroma of homemade, whole-wheat bread baking in your oven . . . the sweet, juicy taste of a ripe peach—just picked . . . the cool sensation of ice-cold milk . . . the crispy crunch of a raw carrot; the smooth, creamy texture of chocolate ice cream; or the fiery feeling of a hot chile pepper!

Foods that appeal to your senses are probably those you enjoy most! Sensory stimulation evokes food memories. The more senses a food or meal affects, the more vivid the flavor memory, positive or not. What is flavor? And how does it contribute to nutrition?

Flavor is several closely linked sensations: taste plus smell, as well as touch (temperature and mouth feel). Sound, perhaps the crunch of an apple, and sight contribute to flavor, too. With one sensation diminished, your flavor experience may be entirely different. As an experiment, hold your nose so you can't smell, then bite an onion. It may taste somewhat sweet, like an apple. Or think about how food tastes when your nose is stuffed up—not much flavor, not much pleasure either. About 80 percent of food's flavor is aroma.

As an average adult, you have about ten thousand taste buds, which respond to different tastes: sweet, sour, salty, bitter, and also umami (the brothy, meaty, and savory flavor of glutamate). You can sense *all* these tastes throughout your tongue and mouth. Some parts of the tongue may be especially sensitive to certain tastes. Even the lining of your mouth, the back of your throat, your tonsils (if you still have them), and your epiglottis (a flap of tissue that covers your larynx, preventing food and liquids from entering the airway) have some taste buds, especially in childhood.

Aromas that waft through the room get picked up by smell receptors in your nasal passages. Temperature, mouth feel, even the "irritation" from a jalapeño pepper or the "numbing" effect from a persimmon also affect your perceptions of food and its flavor—and what you may describe as its "taste."

Not surprisingly, we're born with an ability to perceive, and a preference for, sweet tastes. That's because amniotic fluid is sweet. To some degree, we can perceive all tastes at birth—sweet, sour, bitter, salty, and umami. Flavor preferences are learned—starting from the early years.

Are You a Supertaster?

Why do you like the foods you like? The reasons are partly genes, gender, and age. Even in the same family, people experience tastes differently. The intensity of taste depends partly on how many fungiform papillae (tiny, smooth red bumps with clusters of taste receptor cells, or tastebuds) a person has on his or her tongue.

Supertasters have a lot of papillae, experience the flavor of food more intensely, and tend to strongly like or dislike certain foods. They pick up bitter flavors, perhaps in pungent vegetables, tea, coffee, and grapefruit juice, and sweet flavors more intensely, too. Those with few papillae tend to be indifferent to one flavor over another, and those in the middle are likely to enjoy all kinds of food if prepared well.

Children have more papillae than adults, perhaps one of many reasons why a child may be a picky eater. Taste sensitivity seems to decline with age, which is explained by the decrease in the number of papillae.

Have you ever burned your tongue on steamy hot soup, or the roof of your mouth on cheese topping a hot pizza? Hot foods may damage papillae. Fortunately, your body repairs its papillae fairly quickly.

Are you a supertaster? Find out. First punch a hole (with a hole punch) in a small piece of wax paper. Put the hole on the tip of your tongue; wipe it with blue food coloring. With a mirror, magnifying glass, and flashlight, count the papillae. Nontasters have less than fifteen, but supertasters have dozens of them! (More women are supertasters than men are.)

Why does the same food taste too spicy for some but not for others? People sense the same foods differently. Among the factors that make a difference: saliva (affected by diet, heredity, and other factors), the number of taste buds, medications, some illnesses, and smoking. The senses of taste and smell diminish with age. That's partly why older people may say that foods just don't taste the way they remember. *For more about flavor and older adults, see chapter 19.*

Today, taste and smell are getting more attention in the scientific world. Since people eat for flavor, there's good reason to think of nutrition, taste, and aroma together. Research is being done, for example, to make food more flavorful for older adults; to find ways to magnify salty perception while lowering levels of sodium in food; and to develop more flavorful fruits and vegetables.

Food Prep: The Nutrition-Flavor Connection

Proper food handling and storage enhance the natural flavors of food and keep nutrient loss to a minimum. To maximize food's flavor and nutrition:

● Start with high-quality ingredients enjoyed at their peak quality. They don't need to be the most expensive foods—or served in big portions. *Refer to "Shopping for Freshness" in chapter 12.*

● Handle foods properly. Poor storage destroys flavor and quality. *Chapter 13, "The Safe Kitchen," offers tips to retaining freshness.*

● Cook to retain nutrients, flavor, color, texture, and overall appeal, *as described in this chapter.* Cooking can't improve poor-quality foods but it can enhance the flavors of high-quality foods. Overcooking destroys flavor and nutrients. *See "Simple Ways to Keep Nutrients in Food" in this chapter.*

● Use cooking techniques that enhance flavor. *For quick flavor enhancers see "For a Taste Lift" and "More Taste Lifters" in this chapter. For chef's flavor secrets see "Flavor on the Menu" in chapter 15.*

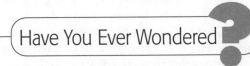

Have You Ever Wondered

. . . what makes chile peppers taste "hot"? Capsaicin in chile peppers stimulates pain receptors in your mouth. The irritation, or "heating" effect, depends on the amount of capsaicin, measured in Scoville heat units (SHU)—anywhere from 1 to 300,000 SHU (mild to very hot). A sweet bell (pimento) pepper is rated at 0 to 5; an anaheim pepper at 500 to 1,000; ancho or poblano pepper at 1,000 to 1,500; jalapeño or chipotle pepper at 2,500 to 5,000; a Serrano pepper at 5,000 to 15,000; and a habañero (Scotch bonnet) pepper from 80,000 to 300,000!

. . . how to reduce the "fire" caused by eating hot chile peppers? Try dairy foods! Caesin, the main protein in milk, washes away capsaicin that makes your mouth and throat "burn." Hot chile peppers do "fire up" the flavors of Thai dishes, Mexican salsas, and Cajun foods, among others. To tone down the heat, remove the seeds and inner membranes of hot chiles. To avoid a burning sensation on sensitive skin as you handle hot chiles, use rubber gloves. Never touch or rub your eyes—or any other sensitive areas—when you're handling them.

● Serve hot foods hot—and cold foods cold. Enticing flavors come partly from aromas released with heat. Coldness can give a refreshing mouth feel.

● When it's time to eat, take time to chew. Chewing stimulates saliva flow, enhancing flavor as food's components dissolve and blend. Textures change as you chew, too. And by taking time to savor the flavor, you may eat more slowly—and avoid overeating, too.

The bottom line: Flavor matters!

Healthful Cooking Techniques

Modifying recipes without compromising taste doesn't require extra time—just quick, easy kitchen know-how. Tips here offer many ways to make your food preparation flavorful, with more nutrient-rich fruit, vegetables, whole grains, low-fat and fat-free dairy foods, and lean protein foods. Here you'll also learn easy ways to prepare so-called whole foods that are less processed, how to cook to keep vitamins in, and how to trim calories, solid fats (saturated and *trans* fats), added sugars, and sodium. Now cook for the health (and flavor) of it!

Have You Ever Wondered

. . . if cooking ever makes vegetables or fruits more nutritious? Cooking won't add nutrients (unless ingredients are added) to a food, but can make food safer and perhaps more edible and appealing. For example, you probably prefer eating a potato that's cooked, not raw.

Sometimes cooking enhances nourishment. For example, lycopene, a phytonutrient in tomatoes, is absorbed in the body better from cooked or processed tomatoes; lycopene may offer some protection from some cancers. Carotenoids (form vitamin A) are more available for absorption when cooked, as is lutein, a phytonutrient in corn. Heat has also been shown to increase the bioavailability of thiamin, niacin, folate, and vitamin B_6.

. . . what's culinology? It's a term coined for bringing food science, food technology, and culinary arts together to create safe, more appealing food.

Fats, Sugar, Salt: What They Do

Fats, sugar, and salt are basic ingredients. While the Dietary Guidelines advises limits, each (in controlled amounts) also plays important culinary functions.

● *Cut the fat, not the flavor!* Fats carry, blend, and stabilize flavors. With less fat, flavors may be more volatile and may not hold up as long as you might like. In baked foods, fat tenderizes, adds moisture, holds air in so they're light, and affects the shape. In sauces, fats keep foods from curdling and form part of an emulsion so water and fats combine smoothly. Fat in recipes conducts heat—for example, when sautéeing and stir-frying. Fat lubricates so food doesn't stick to the pan and seals in moisture when foods are basted. Fat makes meat more moist and tender. Beyond that, fat also carries some nutrients from food into your body. In cooking, substitute healthy oils for solid fats. *See "Why Foods Contain Fat" in chapter 5.*

● *"Just a spoonful of sugar,"* notes Mary Poppins! Besides adding a sweet taste, sugar adds to the aroma, texture, color, and bulk of many foods. Sugar is the "food" for yeast that helps bread rise. In baked foods it contributes to the light brown color and to crisp textures. In canned jams and jellies sugar helps inhibit the growth of molds and yeasts. *See "Sugars: In Healthful Eating" in chapter 3.*

● *Salt: often just a pinch will do!* Salt brings out the flavor in food, but that's not its only culinary function. Among its roles, salt increases and stabilizes the volume of whipped cream and egg whites, controls the speed of fermentation in bread dough and cheese, and helps give yeast bread a finer texture. *See "Salt and Sodium: More than Flavor" in chapter 7.*

Fruits and Vegetables: Fit More In!

As a child, you probably enjoyed fruits and vegetables for their vibrant colors, crunch, and perhaps their different flavors. You probably also learned that fruits and vegetables were good for you. Today, science better understands why. Although their nutrient content varies, fruits and vegetables:

● Are nutrient-rich, providing relatively few calories for the nutrients they deliver. *See chapter 10 for the health benefits of fruits and vegetables, and for daily advice for fitting them into your meals and snacks.*

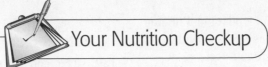

Healthful Cooking Techniques

Do you cook with good nutrition, as well as flavor, in mind? Test your kitchen nutrition IQ to see if what you know shows up in how you cook!

Do You . . .	Always	Usually	Sometimes	Never
Trim visible fat from meat and poultry?	____	____	____	____
Keep edible peels on fruits and vegetables—just wash, not peel them?	____	____	____	____
Remove the skin from poultry before eating it?	____	____	____	____
Use garnishes to make food look more appealing?	____	____	____	____
Cook vegetables only until they're just tender-crisp?	____	____	____	____
Plan meals with many different and colorful fruits and vegetables?	____	____	____	____
Cook mostly with healthy oils?	____	____	____	____
Cook with whole grains such as brown rice or whole-wheat pasta?	____	____	____	____
Try to include foods with different colors and tastes in a meal?	____	____	____	____
Add beans (legumes) to salads, soups, or other foods?	____	____	____	____
Sprinkle cheese on salads, soups, and vegetables for more calcium?	____	____	____	____
Cook vegetables with the lid on the pot—in just a small amount of liquid, or steam or microwave them?	____	____	____	____
Sweeten foods with fruit, fruit juice, or fruit purees?	____	____	____	____
Use ingredients with less fat, such as low-fat yogurt, lean ground meat, and defatted broth?	____	____	____	____
Boost calcium in creamy soups, cooked cereals, and casseroles with nonfat dry milk or calcium-fortified soy products?	____	____	____	____
Drain fat off meat after it's cooked?	____	____	____	____
Use herbs, spices, or lemon juice and ease up on salt to flavor food?	____	____	____	____
Use lower-fat cooking methods: broil, grill, roast, stir-fry, steam, microwave, or braise?	____	____	____	____
Taste before deciding to add salt to foods?	____	____	____	____
Use cooking water from vegetables for soups, stews, or sauces?	____	____	____	____
Subtotal	____	____	____	____

Now score yourself:

"Always": 3 points

"Usually": 2 points

"Sometimes": 1 points

"Never": 0 point

Your total score _____

With 50 to 60 points, you're "kitchen nutrition-savvy."

With 40 to 49 points, improving your food preparation skills would make a nutritious difference! Read on.

With 21 to 39 points, you're starting to get the hang of it. Now turn those "sometimes" answers to "usually" and "always." Read the rest of the chapter for "food prep" tips.

With 20 points or less, read the chapter. There's lots to learn!

● In varying amounts, deliver fiber, too, and they're loaded with phytonutrients.

Fruits and Veggies: Made Easy

● *Try "grate" ways.* Add grated, shredded, or chopped vegetables such as zucchini, spinach, and carrots to lasagna, meat loaf, mashed potatoes, and meat, poultry, pasta, rice, and other grain dishes. Try shredded carrot or zucchini in muffins and other quick breads. Add grated apples to pancakes.

● *Stuff an omelette with veggies.* For a hearty meal, fill it with crisp, tasty vegetables like broccoli, squash, carrots, peppers, tomatoes, spinach, or onions.

● *Toss a vegetable salad.* Add colorful vegetables, beans (legumes), and fruits (such as berries, kiwifruit,

---

Simple Ways to Keep Nutrients in Food

Proper cooking techniques keep nutrient loss to a minimum and food quality at its peak. Some minerals and water-soluble vitamins dissolve in cooking water; they're lost when cooking water is discarded. High temperatures and long cooking times can destroy heat-sensitive nutrients such as B vitamins including folate and vitamin C.

● Clean thick-skinned vegetables and fruits well with a soft brush and water. Avoid soaking them as you wash. Some vitamins dissolve in water.

● Leave edible skins on vegetables and fruits—for example, on carrots, potatoes, or pears. And trim away as little as possible. Most vitamins and minerals are found in the outer leaves, skin, and area just below the skin—not in the center. Peels also are natural barriers that help protect against nutrient loss.

● Cook vegetables or fruits in a small amount of water—or better yet, steam them in a vegetable steamer or a microwave oven. Steaming retains most of the nutrients because vegetables usually don't come in contact with cooking liquids.

● Cut vegetables that need to be cooked longer into larger pieces. With fewer surfaces exposed, less vitamins are lost.

● Eat vegetables and fruits raw; clean properly first! Or cook many vegetables, such as asparagus, green beans, broccoli, and snow peas, quickly—just until tender-crisp. Some nutrients, such as B vitamins and vitamin C, are destroyed easily by heat. The shorter the cooking time, the more nutrients are retained.

Short cooking times help vegetables keep their bright color and flavor, too. The flavors of strong-flavored vegetables, such as Brussels sprouts and turnips, can get even stronger when overcooked.

● Cook vegetables and fruits in a covered pot. Steam doesn't escape, and cooking time is faster.

● Just reheat canned vegetables on the stovetop or in the microwave oven. Canning is cooking, so canned vegetables don't need to be cooked again. They would lose flavor and nutrients!

● Save liquid from cooking vegetables for soups, stews, and sauces; perhaps freeze it for later use. That's one way to "recycle" water-soluble vitamins and minerals that otherwise would be tossed with the cooking water.

● For beets and red cabbage, add a little lemon juice or vinegar to the cooking water. This helps retain their bright-red color. Don't add baking soda! Although the alkali in baking soda keeps vegetables looking greener, it also destroys vitamin C and make them mushy due to cellulose breakdown. *Tip:* Adding acid (lemon juice) to green vegetables while cooking turns them olive green; add juice or sauce after cooking.

● Keep edible peels on fruits and vegetables. A medium baked potato with the skin on has about twice the fiber of a "naked" potato: 5 fiber grams compared to 2.5 fiber grams!

● Microwave! Why? First, because microwaving is so fast, heat-sensitive nutrients aren't subjected to heat for long. Second, microwaving doesn't require added fat. There's a flavor advantage, too: Unless overcooked, vegetables retain the color and tender-crisp qualities that make them appealing.

● Keep milk in opaque containers in the fridge. Leaving it in a clear, glass pitcher on the table allows some riboflavin to be destroyed by sunlight.

● Skip the urge to rinse grains, such as rice, before cooking. That may wash nutrients down the drain.

or mandarin oranges). Even if you prefer iceberg lettuce, which delivers less nutrients than other greens, pair it with other veggies—sliced beets, shredded red cabbage, spinach leaves, baby carrots. Adding half a medium-size carrot as a salad topper adds 1 gram of fiber, too.

● *Get creative with pizza.* Order or make it "deluxe" with vegetable toppings: asparagus, broccoli florets, mushrooms, carrot shreds, thinly sliced zucchini, chopped spinach, red and green bell pepper strips, chopped tomatoes, roasted peppers, or other firm veggies! For extra flavor, roast them first.

● *Bake with fruits and vegetables.* Use pureed fruit such as applesauce, dried plums (prunes), bananas, or peaches in place of about half the fat in recipes for homemade breads, muffins, pancakes, and other baked goods. Experiment first, because this substitution may alter the texture or volume of the end result. For flavor, texture, and nutrients, blend in shredded zucchini, carrots, or dried fruits.

● *"Sandwich" in fruit and vegetables.* Layer sliced pineapple, apple, raisins, peppers, cucumbers, sprouts, or tomatoes into sandwiches.

● *Add veggies or fruit.* Make a quick stir-fry or combine pasta or rice with just about any vegetables, or add them to soups, casseroles, and pasta and rice dishes—great ways to use fresh vegetables before they spoil. For example, adding ½ cup of broccoli to a pasta dish adds 2 grams of fiber. A quarter cup of cooked spinach, mixed in soup or risotto, adds 2 grams of fiber. Add apricots, pineapple, dates, other fruit, or fruit chutney to meat or poultry dishes. *Hint:* Add canned, frozen, or cooked beans (legumes).

● *Experiment.* Substitute a new-to-you fruit or vegetable in a favorite recipe. Try broccoli rabe (broccoli variety with smaller heads, also called rapini) in stir-fries, fennel in salad, or parsnips (a starchy vegetable) in stew. Or try a new fruit or vegetable recipe.

● *Take a fruit to lunch!* Make a habit of tucking an apple, a tangerine, plums or kiwifruit, grapes, cherries, dried fruits, or other fruit into your briefcase, tote, or lunch bag. Fruit is a great traveling snack.

● *Be saucy with fruit and vegetables.* Puree berries, apples, peaches, or pears for a thick, sweet sauce on grilled or broiled seafood or poultry, pancakes, French toast, or waffles. Add pureed broccoli to pasta sauce.

● *Flip the dessert.* For example, serve sliced fruit and berries with a shortbread garnish on top, rather than shortbread with a spoonful of fruit.

● *Make dips and spreads with vegetables and fruit.* Spicy salsas can be made with tomato, bell peppers, onions, and cilantro. For a tangy twist, also look for salsas with pineapples, mangoes, papayas, or peaches. Try hummus, made with mashed chickpeas; or caponata, made with eggplant and tomato; or baba ghanouj, made with eggplant.

● *Toss in dried fruits:* dried cranberries, apples, dried plums (prunes), bananas, papayas, mangoes, apricots, pears, pineapples, dates, or raisins. They're great in stuffing, rice dishes, salads, main dish salads, homemade breads, and casseroles; even cookie dough and desserts! One-quarter cup of raisins adds 2 grams of fiber; three dried plums have almost as much.

● *Focus on veggies and fruit.* Enjoy 3-ounce cooked portions of meat, poultry, and fish; fill the rest of the plate with vegetables, fruits, and grain products. Let meat, poultry, or fish add flavor rather than take center stage. A vegetable-meat kebob is one way to do it. It's great for grilling!

● *Stock up.* Fill your fridge with raw vegetables and fruits—"nature's fast food"—cleaned, cut up, and ready to eat. Try baby carrots! Keep canned and frozen vegetables and fruit on hand for convenience.

Refer to "Simple Ways to Keep Nutrients In Food" in this chapter. For more ideas, see "Garden of Eatin': Uncommon Vegetables" and "Fresh Ideas: Uncommon Fruit" in chapter 9.

Beans and Other Legumes: Enjoy More

Legumes—dried beans, peas, and lentils—are packed with fiber! A half-cup serving of cooked legumes supplies 4 to 10 grams of fiber. (As a healthy adult, you need 21 to 38 grams of total fiber a day, depending on your age and gender.) Legumes also are packed with protein, other nutrients, and phytonutrients, yet little fat and no cholesterol. So adding them to meals and snacks several times each week is well worth it. Canned beans take little effort.

When boiled and served plain, beans don't have much flavor. But when combined with other foods, they're versatile, taking on flavor.

BEAN BAG

Beans of all kinds are sold as dried, canned, frozen, and fresh. Each type has a distinctive appearance and flavor, varying cooking times, and somewhat different uses. Combine a variety of beans for a more interesting dish!

On average, 1 pound of dry beans equals about 2¼ cups of dry beans, or 5 to 6 cups of cooked beans. The yield for lentils is less; for 2¼ cups of dry lentils, figure about 3½ to 4 cups cooked. One can (15½ ounces) of drained, canned beans or lentils equals about 1⅔ cups cooked. Draining and rinsing canned beans reduces the sodium content by about 40 percent.

Note: Soak beans, not lentils or split peas, before simmering; *see "Cooking a Pot o' Beans" in this chapter.*

BEANS AND PEAS	SIZE AND COLOR	FLAVOR	SIMMERING TIME (HOURS)*	COMMON USES†
Adzuki or azuki bean	Small, red, shiny	Slightly sweet	½ to 1	Salads, poultry stuffing, casseroles, soups
Black bean	Small, black, shiny, kidney-shaped	Slightly sweet	1½ to 2	Stew, soup, Brazilian *feijoada,* Cuban rice and beans
Black-eyed pea or cowpea	Small, cream-colored, ovals with black spots	Vegetablelike, full-flavored	1 to 1½	Southern dishes with ham or rice, bean cakes, curries, *Hoppin' John*
Cannellini or white kidney bean	Elongated, slender, creamy white	Mild	2	Soups, stews, salads, casseroles, Italian side dishes, *pasta e fagioli*
Chickpea, or garbanzo bean	Golden, hard, pea-shaped	Nutty	2¼ to 4	Casseroles, cooked with couscous, soups, stews, *hummus, caldo gallego*
Fava or broad bean	Broad, large, oval, light brown	Nutty	1½ to 2	Stews, side dishes
Flageolet or green haricot bean	Small to medium, pale green	Nutty	1½ to 2	Mixed bean salads, vegetable side dish
Great northern	Large, white	Mild	1 to 1½	Soups, casseroles, mixed bean dishes
Lentils‡	Yellow, green, or orange	Earthy	¾	Soup, English pease pudding, Indian *dhal,* curry dishes
Lima bean	Large or small, creamy white or pale green, kidney-shaped	Like chestnuts	1½	Casseroles, soups, salads, Southern *succotash*
Mung bean	Small, olive green	Earthy	1	Soups, casseroles, purees, Asian and Indian dishes, "sprouted" for salads
Navy bean	Small, oval, white	Mild	1 to 1½	*Boston baked beans*
Pigeon pea	Small, round, slightly flat, beige, brown flecks	Mild	¾ to 1	Caribbean peas and rice
Pinto bean	Orange-pink, with rust-colored flecks, oval	Earthy, full-flavored	1 to 1½	*Mexican rice and beans, refried beans,* stew
Red kidney bean	Dark, red-brown, kidney-shaped	Full-flavored, "meaty"	1½ to 2	Stew, mixed bean salad, Cajun bean dishes, *chili con carne*
Soybean	Small, yellow or black	Full-flavored	3½ to 4	Side dish, soups, used to make tofu (bean curd), "sprouted" for salads

*Simmering time for uncooked dry beans.
†Traditional and ethnic dishes, italicized throughout the chart, commonly use the type of bean indicated.
‡Lentils don't require soaking, only shorter cooking times.

● Make minestrone soup with drained, canned kidney or garbanzo beans and vegetables. Add beef or chicken broth or canned tomatoes for flavor.

● Fill tacos or burritos with drained, cooked or canned pinto beans. Accent the flavor with a little grated cheese and lots of salsa, tomatoes, onions, and/or chopped lettuce or cabbage.

● Top green salads with drained, canned or cooked beans. Or mix up a three-, four-, or five-bean salad!

● For an easy lunch, serve split pea, navy bean, or lentil soup. Top with shredded carrot or apple!

● Add cooked, canned, or frozen beans, peas, or lentils to salads, casseroles, and pasta dishes. Puree cooked beans to use as a low-fat, high-fiber base or thickener in spreads, sauces, and soups.

● As an easy side dish, baked potato topping, or pasta sauce, simply heat frozen or canned beans with a tasty sauce of tomatoes, molasses, or jalapeño peppers.

● Use beans as a meat substitute in many mixed dishes: kidney beans in chili, lentils in meat loaf, pinto beans in enchiladas, black beans in chunky soups, mashed kidney or pinto beans in meatballs, soybeans in casseroles, and white beans in stews. *See "Adapting Recipes for Vegetarians" in this chapter.*

● Create a high-fiber pasta sauce that's low in fat. Puree cooked or drained, canned beans with beef or chicken stock. White cannellini beans make a creamy white sauce, but any variety of beans will do. Add fresh herbs: basil, chives, garlic, marjoram, and oregano, among others. Fresh tomatoes or tomato sauce add flavor and color.

Cooking a Pot o' Beans

If you're short on time, go for canned, frozen, or fresh beans. If not, try the traditional way, by soaking dry beans first. *Tip:* Uncooked dry legumes need soaking; lentils or split peas don't.

To soak beans, do this:

- ● Leisurely method. Reduce cooking time by up to half by soaking beans for at least four hours or overnight in a pot filled with room-temperature water. Choose a pot that's big enough; beans expand!

- ● Quick method. Time short? Then bring water to a boil, and let beans soak in hot water for one to four hours, depending on the variety of beans.

To reduce the intestinal gas you might experience, rinse beans, discard the soaking water and any debris, and cook in fresh water. Not to worry—beans, not the soaking water, retain most of the essential nutrients.

To cook, cover beans with fresh water: about 6 cups of fresh water for each pound of dry beans. Add seasonings to the cooking water. Salt toughens beans by taking out the moisture; and acid foods, such as tomatoes or vinegar, slow their softening. Wait until the end of the cooking time to add these ingredients.

Cover the pot partially. To keep legumes from foaming as they cook, add a little cooking oil (1/4 teaspoon) to the water. Simmer beans until they're cooked. *See the chart "Bean Bag" in this chapter for simmering times.* Add cooked beans or peas to your favorite dish.

Whole Grains: Boost Fiber

Does your plate lack much fiber? You're not alone. With so many refined grain ingredients in breads, pasta, and other grain products and too few fruits and vegetables, many people come up short. Your cooking style can boost your fiber factor—and add interest and flavor, too!

Why boost fiber? Besides fiber's many health benefits, it's often bundled with other important nutrients and phytonutrients. And many fiber-rich foods have fewer calories and less fat. *To learn more, see "Fiber: Your Body's Broom" in chapter 3.*

Make at least half your grains whole! Although fiber content varies, many whole grains are great sources of fiber (and they deliver many more nutrient and phytonutrient benefits, too). You may use whole grains in place of some reduced grains in your food prep. *See chapter 3, "Carbs: Sugars, Starches, Fiber."*

● Substitute whole-grain and other high-fiber pasta—lasagna noodles, macaroni, spaghetti, and other whole-grain pastas—in all kinds of dishes. Use brown or wild rice (2 grams and 1.5 grams of fiber, respectively, per 1/2 cup cooked) in place of white rice (<0.5 fiber grams per 1/2 cup cooked), too—or use a combination.

● For refined grains, look for enriched and perhaps fiber-fortified pasta, cereal, and other grain products.

COOKING GRAIN BY GRAIN

Wonder how to cook whole grains? You can use the same simple steps for all these whole grains. Bring the cooking water to a boil; stir in the grain. Cover, reduce heat, and simmer. Let stand, covered, if indicated below. Then use these wonderful cooked grains in salads; as side dishes flavored with sauces or seasonings; or in soups.

1 Cup Uncooked Grain	Cooking Water (Cups)	Cooking Time (Minutes)	Standing Time (Minutes)	Yield (Cups)	Common Uses
Amaranth	3	25	—	3½	Cereal, side dish
Buckwheat (kasha)	2	20	10	3	Side dish (buckwheat groats flour also used in baked foods)
Bulgur	1½	*	30	2½	Side dish, stew, salad (tabbouleh)
Hominy (corn) (soak 8 hours)	4	30	5	3½	Side dish, stew, soup, cereal
Millet	2¾	30	15	3	Side dish, bread
Pearl barley	3	40	5	3½	Side dish, cereal, soup
Quinoa (rinsed)	2	15	—	3	Side dish, stuffing, soup, salad, stew
Rice, brown	2½	45	5	3	Wherever rice is used
Rice, wild[†]	3	55	—	3½	Side dish, stuffing, soup, salad
Rye berries	2	60	—	2¾	Side dish, bread
Triticale (wheat and rye) (soak overnight)	2½	40	—	4	Side dish, soup, cereal, bread
Wheat berries (soak overnight)	2	45	—	2½	Side dish, bread

*Bulgur isn't cooked. Put bulgur in a bowl, pour boiling water over it, and let it stand until the water is absorbed.

[†]Wild rice is actually a seed, not rice.

Sources: Compiled from *L. C. Peterson, "The ABC's of Whole Grains," Food Management* (March 1993):108; J. E. Brody, *Jane Brody's Good Food Book* (New York: Bantam Books, 1987).

● Try brown rice, bulgur, kasha, quinoa, or whole-grain couscous instead of white rice in some recipes.

Refer to "Today's Grains" in chapter 9. The chart "Cooking Grain by Grain" on this page shows how to prepare them.

● In dough and batter, substitute whole-wheat flour for half of the refined white flour. Don't go 100 percent, though; the texture will be too dense. Try white whole-grain flour.

● Try oat flour in baking, too. Whirl dry oatmeal in a blender to make oat flour. Use it to replace up to ⅓ of white flour in a recipe.

● When substituting a whole-grain (graham, stone ground, whole-wheat) or specialty flour (bread flour, semolina flour, durum flour) for traditional white flour, find out if you need to adjust the recipe to get an acceptable result. The compositions of flour differ.

● Stack your sandwiches with whole-grain goodness. Use whole-grain breads, whole-grain English muffins, and whole-grain pita pockets.

● Add wheat or oat bran to casseroles, meat loaf, and dry or cooked cereal. Or blend some with yogurt for a little crunch. Each tablespoon of bran adds a little more than 1 gram of fiber.

● Add oatmeal, nuts, and seeds (sesame, poppy) to mixed dishes: pudding and fruit toppings, meat loaf, stuffing, salmon patties, crab cakes,and burgers.

● For bread crumbs: Use toasted wheat germ or bran or whole-wheat bread crumbs.

Have You Ever Wondered?

. . . how to cook with flaxseed? To get all the benefits of flaxseed, you need to grind it in a blender, food processor, or coffee grinder. Then add it to dough and batter, or use it as a topping on puddings, cereal, and other food. Flaxseed is high in fiber and supplies omega-3 fatty acids, yet has little saturated fat.

. . . if you should soak ham, bacon, or salt pork to get rid of some salt? No. Very little salt is removed. More important, for food safety, washing meat is not advised.

Meat, Poultry, Fish, Eggs: Cooking Lean!

Good cooking and good health rely on moderate amounts of total fat and limited solid fats and cholesterol. To keep meat, poultry, and fish dishes lean and flavorful, follow these cooking healthy tips:

● Cook with lean meats (*shown on this page*), skinless poultry, and fish. *See chapter 12 for buying tips. For how to cook them, see "Meat, Poultry, and Fish: Lean Cuts and Low-Fat Cooking Methods" in this chapter.*

● Use smaller amounts of processed meats that tend to have more fat: bacon, hot dogs, and luncheon meats. Or use leaner versions, at least "90 percent lean."

● When recipes call for bacon, use lean ham, Canadian bacon, or smoked turkey for the smoky flavor.

● Trim off visible, solid fat on meat and poultry before cooking. Even on lean meat, you'll find some fat. Trimming fat from the edges removes some, but not all the cholesterol; cholesterol is in both the lean tissue and the fat in meat, poultry, and fish.

● Go "skinless" on poultry. Under the skin there's a layer of fat. Remove the skin before or after cooking to cut the fat content about in half; there's not much difference, as long as you remove the skin before you eat it! On whole birds most fat

HOW MUCH "SAT-FAT" AND FAT IN LEAN** BEEF, PORK, AND POULTRY CUTS?

	CALORIES	SATURATED FAT (GRAMS)	TOTAL FAT (GRAMS)
Beef Cuts			
Eye round roast and steak	169	1.6	4.7
Sirloin tip side steak	168	1.9	4.8
Top round roast and steak*	199	1.7	5.0
Bottom round roast and steak*	216	2.7	7.7
Top sirloin steak	178	2.2	5.8
Brisket, flat half	213	3.2	8.0
93% lean ground beef	209	4.0	9.5
Round tip roast and steak*	174	2.2	6.2
Shank cross cuts	201	2.3	6.4
Sirloin tip center roast and steak*	177	2.5	6.8
Chuck shoulder steak	175	2.5	5.8
Bottom round (Western Griller) steak	182	2.5	7.1
Top loin (strip) steak	189	2.7	7.1
Shoulder petite tender and medallions	177	2.8	7.2
Flank steak	186	3.1	7.4
Shoulder center (ranch) steak	182	2.8	7.7
Tri-tip roast and steak	182	3.1	8.3
Tenderloin roast and steak	193	3.0	7.9
T-bone steak	189	3.1	8.7
Pork Cuts			
Tenderloin	187	2.2	6.3
Boneless top loin chop	170	1.7	4.3
Boneless top loin roast	173	1.9	6.3
Bone-in center loin chop	200	2.7	7.9
Bone-in rib chop	208	2.6	9.3
Bone-in sirloin roast	204	2.9	9.4
Chicken Cuts			
Skinless chicken thigh	177	2.3	8.3
Skinless chicken leg	174	2.1	7.8
Skinless chicken breast	165	1.0	3.6
Turkey Cuts			
Skinless turkey, light meat	149	0.6	2.1
Skinless turkey, dark meat	159	1.3	3.8

*Cuts combined for illustration purposes

**Less than 10 grams of total fat, 4.5 grams or less of saturated fat, and less than 95 milligrams of cholesterol per 3-ounce cooked serving (per 100 grams)

Calories and fat are based on 3-ounce cooked servings, visible fat removed.

Source: U.S. Department of Agriculture, Agricultural Research Service, 2011. U.S. Department of Agriculture, National Nutrient Database for Standard Reference, Release 24, 2011. Nutrient Data Laboratory homepage www.nal.usda.gov/fnic/foodcomp.

appears near the cavity opening. *Tip:* Cooking poultry with the skin on helps keep it tender and moist. The same is true for beef and pork; trim remaining fat after cooking.

● Drain off fat from ground-meat crumbles as they're cooked. To reduce fat further, transfer cooked ground-meat crumbles to a large plate lined with 3 layers of white, recycled paper towels. Blot the top of meat, and let it sit one minute. Place meat in a strainer or a colander. Pour about 1 quart of hot tap water over the meat. Drain five minutes. You can rinse away 2 to 5 grams of fat per 3-ounce cooked serving.

● Blot cooked ground-meat burgers, meatballs, and meat loaf with several layers of clean paper towels.

● Brown meat, poultry, and seafood in a nonstick skillet with little or no added fat, except for vegetable oil spray, or use a little oil. Compare: 2 tablespoons of oil to brown meat carry an extra 240 calories from 28 fat grams, compared with less than 10 calories (1 fat gram) from oil spray. Browning adds flavor.

Meat, Poultry, and Fish: Lean Cuts and Low-Fat Cooking Methods

| | Dry Heat | | | | | Moist Heat | | | |
	Roast	Broil	Grill	Panbroil	Stir-fry	Braise	Stew	Steam	Poach
Beef									
Eye round*		X				X	X		
Top round*	X	X	X	X	X				
Round tip*	X	X	X	X	X	X	X		
Bottom round*	X					X	X		
Sirloin	X	X	X	X	X				
Top loin	X	X	X	X	X				
Tenderloin	X	X	X	X	X				
Flank*		X	X		X				
95% lean ground beef	X	X	X	X	X				
Pork									
Tenderloin	X	X	X	X	X				
Boneless top loin roast	X	X	X						
Loin chop		X	X	X					
Loin strips					X				
Boneless sirloin chop		X	X	X					
Boneless rib roast	X		X			X	X		
Rib chop		X	X	X					
Boneless ham	X	X	X	X	X				
Poultry†									
Whole chicken	X		X			X	X		
Whole turkey	X		X			X			
Cornish game hen	X		X			X	X		
Breast	X	X	X	X	X				X
Drumstick	X	X	X						
Fish									
Cod	X	X	X	X	X		X	X	X
Flounder	X	X	X	X				X	X
Halibut	X	X	X	X	X		X	X	X
Orange roughy		X	X	X	X			X	X
Shrimp		X	X	X	X		X	X	X

*May be cooked by dry heat methods if they are tenderized first by marinating or pounding.
†White meat has less fat than dark meat. Skin should be removed before eating.
Source: ©Cattlemen's Beef Board and National Cattlemen's Beef Association Culinary Center.

● Grill, broil, or roast meat and poultry on a rack so fat drips through and drippings aren't reabsorbed. Drain away any fat that appears during cooking.

● Marinate meat, poultry, and fish in marinades with little or no fat: orange, lime, or lemon juice; defatted broth; wine; tomato juice; salsas; fat-free or reduced-fat salad dressings; plain, low-fat yogurt; or buttermilk. Add fresh herbs to the marinade.

● To keep fish or chicken moist, steam fillets in heavy aluminum foil with fruit, herbs, onions, vegetables, and other flavorings. Secure the "package" and then bake it in the oven or on the grill. For the oven, you can also wrap and cook meat, fish, or poultry in parchment paper (chefs call this *en papillote,* or paper package) or leaf packets (such as banana leaves).

● Oven-fry fish or chicken. Dip it first in egg whites, then coat with seasoned bread crumbs. Bake on a non-stick baking pan coated with vegetable oil spray.

Cookery: Dry-Heat Methods in Three Easy Steps

Roasting

1. Heat oven to recommended temperature (varies based on cut of meat).
2. Place roast (straight from refrigerator) fat side up, on rack in shallow roasting pan. Season before cooking as desired. Insert an ovenproof food thermometer so tip is centered in thickest part of roast, not resting in fat or touching bone. Do not add water; do not cover.
3. For beef, pork, veal, and lamb, roast to 5 to 10° F below desired doneness.* Transfer to carving board; tent loosely with aluminum foil. Let stand fifteen to twenty minutes. (Temperature will continue to rise 5 to 10° F to reach desired doneness.) For whole poultry, cook until desired temperature is reached.*

Broiling

1. Preheat broiler for ten minutes.
2. Place meat, poultry, or fish on rack in broiler pan. Season with herbs or spices as desired. Position thinner pieces (¾ to 1 inch) so that surface of meat is 2 to 3 inches from the heat; thicker pieces, 3 to 6 inches from the heat.
3. Broil to desired doneness, turning once.* After cooking, season with salt if desired.

Grilling

1. For gas grilling, set heat to medium. For charcoal grilling, coals should be ash-covered and medium temperature; allow about thirty minutes. (To test cooking temperature for charcoal grill: Spread coals out in single layer. Carefully hold palm of hand above the coals at cooking height. Count the number of seconds you can hold your hand in that position before the heat forces you to pull it away—approximately four seconds for medium heat.)
2. Season meat, poultry, or fish with herbs or spices as desired. For smaller pieces of meat, poultry, or fish (chops, steaks, burgers, breasts, fillets, or kebobs), place on cooking grid directly over coals. For roasts, thick steaks or chops, whole chicken or turkey, the meat is placed on the grill, with coals or heat source on each side.
3. Grill to desired doneness, turning occasionally.* After cooking, season with salt if desired.

Panbroiling

1. Heat heavy nonstick skillet over medium heat (meats ¾ inch or thicker) or medium high heat (meats ½ inch or thinner) until hot, about five minutes.
2. Season meat, poultry, or fish with herbs or spices as desired. Place in preheated skillet. Do not crowd. Do not add oil or water. Do not cover.
3. Cook to desired doneness, turning once.* For thicker pieces, turn occasionally. Remove excess drippings as they accumulate. After cooking, season with salt if desired.

Stir-Frying

1. Partially freeze meat, poultry, or fish (about 30 minutes) for easier slicing. Cut into thin, uniform strips or pieces. Marinate to add flavor or tenderize while preparing other ingredients if desired.
2. Heat small amount of oil in wok or large heavy nonstick skillet over medium high heat until hot.
3. Stir-fry in ½-pound batches (do not overcrowd), continuously turning with a scooping motion, until cooked to desired doneness. Add additional oil for each batch if necessary. (Cook meat and vegetables separately, then combine and heat through.)

See "Safe Internal Temperatures" in chapter 13.
These cooking methods apply to fruits and vegetables, too.

Source: ©Cattlemen's Beef Board and National Cattlemen's Beef Association Culinary Center.

● Bake fish with a splash of white wine, tomatoes, and fresh herbs, or poach fish in a flavorful broth rather than cooking it in oil.

A great meat alternative, eggs supply protein, iron, choline, and lutein to the diet. While nutritious, health experts advise healthy Americans to eat whole eggs and yolks in moderation to control dietary cholesterol (to keep cholesterol intake less than 300 milligrams daily).

Egg yolks, not whites, contain fat and cholesterol. (A yolk from one large egg has about 185 milligrams of cholesterol.) That's why you can use egg whites liberally in place of egg yolks in many foods. Here's how to enjoy eggs in moderation:

Have You Ever Wondered ?

... how the fat content of deep-fried turkey compares to roasted turkey? If the cooking oil stays high enough—350ºF for the entire frying process—it makes little difference. A 3½-ounce portion of deep-fried turkey with the skin on has about 12 grams of fat, compared with 10 grams in a 3½-ounce portion of roasted turkey (white and dark meat) with the skin on. However, if the cooking oil remains at 340ºF or less, more oil seeps into the turkey meat, adding to the fat content. For the record, without the skin, the same amount of roasted turkey (white and dark meat) has 5 fat grams.

Cookery: Moist-Heat Methods in Three Easy Steps

Braising

1. Slowly brown meat or poultry on all sides in small amount of oil in heavy pan. Pour off drippings. Season as desired.
2. Add small amount (½ cup to 2 cups) of liquid such as broth, water, juice, beer, or wine.
3. Cover tightly and simmer gently over low heat on top of the range or in a preheated 325° F oven until meat or poultry is fork-tender. (The cooking liquid may be reduced or thickened for a sauce after removing fat as desired.)

Stewing

1. Lightly coat meat, poultry, or fish with seasoned flour if desired. Slowly brown on all sides, in small amount of oil, if necessary, in heavy pan. Pour off drippings. Season as desired.
2. Add liquid such as defatted broth, water, juice, beer, and/or wine to pan. (Use ½ cup to 2 cups liquid for chili type/shredded beef dishes; enough liquid to cover for stews and soups.) Bring to a boil; reduce heat.
3. Cover tightly and simmer gently over low heat on top of the range, or in a preheated 325° F oven until meat, poultry, or fish is fork-tender. (Cooking soups in the oven is not practical.) Thicken or reduce defatted liquid as desired.

Poaching

1. Season meat, poultry, or fish as desired. For roasts, tie with heavy string at 2-inch intervals if needed. Brown on all sides in nonstick pan. Pour off excess drippings.
2. Cover meat, poultry, or fish with liquid such as defatted broth, juice, water, beer, or wine. Season with additional ingredients if desired.
3. Bring to a boil. Reduce heat, cover, and simmer until fork-tender.

Steaming

1. Place fish on a steamer pan or a perforated tray. Vegetables, such as onions, leeks, celery, and bok choy, can be added.
2. Set steamer into pan above simmering liquid.
3. Cover pan and continue simmering over low heat until fish flakes.

Microwaving

1. Place fish in a microwave-safe dish in spoke fashion for even cooking.
2. Add a small amount of liquid or seasoned vegetables if desired. (Some vegetables may take longer to cook; choose vegetables with similar cooking times, or cook vegetables separately.)
3. Cover with microwave-safe plastic wrap, venting or lifting one corner.
4. Following manufacturer's directions, microwave on high until fish flakes and any added vegetables are tender.

Source: ©Cattlemen's Beef Board and National Cattlemen's Beef Association Culinary Center.

Degreasing Pan Juices, Soups, and Gravies

Remember your science lessons? Fat rises to the top because it's lighter than water. The same thing happens in cooking. Fat in pan juices, soups, gravies, and canned broth collects on top, making it easy to skim off. Every tablespoon of fat you discard removes about 120 calories and 13 fat grams from the dish you're preparing.

- Remove fat from meat and poultry juices with a wide-mouthed spoon or a fat-separating pitcher.
- Refrigerate soups and stews before they're served. Do the same with homemade and canned broth, soups, and chili. Fat, which hardens when chilled, is easy to remove with a spoon.
- When time is short, add a few ice cubes to the broth. Fat will rise and congeal around the ice, but the ice may dilute the broth slightly and cool it down.

● Use two egg whites in place of one whole egg in breads, pancakes, casseroles, French toast, cookies, cheesecake, pudding, and other recipes that call for whole eggs. Although one egg white can substitute for one yolk, recipes that require egg yolks, such as puff pastry, are best made with whole eggs.

● In recipes that call for two or more eggs, substitute just some of the whole eggs with egg whites. For example, for two whole eggs, instead use two egg whites and one whole egg. That way you'll get the color and the flavor of the yolk, but less cholesterol and less fat. This idea works well for scrambled eggs, quiche, and omelettes.

Have You Ever Wondered

. . . if pizza can be healthier? Pizza is among the top contributors of solid fats in the American diet, notes the Dietary Guidelines for Americans, 2010. To easily make over your homemade pizza, top it with chicken, Canadian bacon, or seafood instead of pepperoni, salami, sausage, or regular ground beef. Use less meat and more vegetables, and even some fruit such as pineapple, as well as reduced-fat cheese, or less cheese instead of extra regular cheese.

● Use a cholesterol-free liquid egg product in place of whole eggs. Usually ¼ cup egg product equals one whole egg; check the package label.

Soups, Salads, Sides, Desserts, and More: Reduce Fat or Switch

To trim saturated and *trans* fats and calories, too, cook with more oils and fewer solid fats, low-fat or fat-free dairy foods. With these changes, you can cut or switch the fat without losing flavor.

● Use cooking methods that require little or no added fat; try to boil, broil, grill, roast, braise, stew, steam, poach, stir-fry, or microwave foods, rather than fry them, most of the time. *For more about these cooking techniques, see "Cooking Methods to Know," "Cookery: Moist-Heat Methods in Three Easy Steps," and "Cookery: Dry-Heat Methods in Three Easy Steps" in this chapter.*

● Stretch higher-fat ingredients. For example, grate cheese so less looks like more. Spread 1, not 2, tablespoons of peanut butter on toast.

● Use tempeh, tofu, or beans (legumes) as a low-fat but high-protein ingredient in stews, soups, pasta dishes, and other mixed foods. *For more about tempeh and tofu, see "Soy Good?" in chapter 4.*

● Substitute reduced-fat and fat-free products. *See chapter 12, "Savvy Shopping," for suggestions throughout the supermarket.*

● Coat pans with a thin layer of oil, then wipe with a paper towel. Two tablespoons of oil add 240 calories and 28 fat grams; a thin coating of vegetable oil spray has just 10 calories and 1 fat gram. Using nonstick pans makes it easier to use less fat.

● Substitute yogurt cheese or Greek yogurt for higher-calorie, higher-fat sour cream or cream cheese. *To learn to make yogurt cheese, see chapter 5.*

● Skip or limit breading, which adds fat and calories. It makes food soak up more fat during frying.

● Drain pan-fried foods on a paper towel to absorb extra grease. Go easy on the oil.

● When adding ingredients to packaged mixes (such as macaroni and cheese, scalloped potatoes, or brownies), try soft margarine or oil instead of stick margarine or butter. Or use half the fat, 95% lean ground beef in casserole mixes, or fat-free milk in brownies or instant pudding.

● In place of butter only, use half butter and half oil for less saturated fat.

● Match the right cooking oil to your recipe needs. Canola, corn, peanut, safflower, and soybean oils have high smoking points. They can be used for stir-frying and frying, but don't let them smoke! Olive and sesame oils are not appropriate for high-heat cooking; they have lower smoking points. The unique flavor of extra virgin olive oil may not be appropriate for some foods; a mild-flavored oil such as canola oil is versatile. Hazelnut, walnut, and other specialty oils are nice "finishing oils" to add a splash of flavor at the end of cooking.

Lean Tips . . . for Vegetables

● For vegetables, sauté with just a little oil. Or cook them in a little defatted broth, juice, wine, or water in a covered, nonstick pan. It's great for sautéing onions and mushrooms.

● Steam, stir-fry (in a nonstick wok or skillet), simmer, or microwave vegetables. If you really enjoy the crispiness of French fries and fried onion rings, oven-bake instead of fry them. Skip added fat, such as bacon, on beans (legumes) and other vegetables.

● Puree or mash potatoes, sweet potatoes, and other vegetables with milk, reduced-sodium broth, or liquid from cooking potatoes. Go easy on butter or margarine. Boost the flavor and the nutrients by blending in shredded carrots or zucchini or a little olive oil!

● For flavor on vegetables, add a small amount of butter—but just before serving. (Add herbs and garlic, too.) Cooking dilutes the flavor. You need less butter if you add it last.

● Sprinkle some Parmesan or Romano cheese on vegetables for flavor but not too much fat or calories.

● Roast or grill vegetables and fruit (sliced eggplant, pineapple slices, bell pepper chunks, sliced zucchini) as a low-fat way to bring out the flavor. They're great as kebobs! Coat them lightly with vegetable oil spray or olive oil. Then roast in the oven at 400° F or grill for about 15 minutes until tender-crisp.

Lean Tips . . . for Salads

● Adjust the proportions in homemade vinaigrette. Make it with three parts vinegar to one part oil (e.g., ¾ cup vinegar to ¼ cup oil) instead of the other way around, if you'd like. If it's too acidic, dilute the vinegar with broth or juice. That said, vinaigrette is a way to enjoy healthy oils. Experiment with different types of flavored oils and vinegars or make your own herbed vinegars. *See "Herbed Vinegars" later in this chapter.*

● On taco salads, use lots of salsa with tomatoes, chiles, onions, herbs, and lime juice. Use a lighter touch with sour cream by going "50–50": 50 percent sour cream, 50 percent plain, low-fat yogurt (or perhaps Greek yogurt). Or use reduced-fat or fat-free sour cream.

● Instead of creamy coleslaw made with regular mayonnaise, moisten cabbage and other shredded vegetables with low-fat or fat-free yogurt or mayonnaise with seasonings. Or use vinaigrette dressing.

Lean Tips . . . for Grain Dishes and Breads

● Skip the oil or use just a little when cooking pasta, but use plenty of water. Don't rinse, just drain cooked pasta; toss with sauce immediately so pasta won't stick together; use a lower-fat sauce such as tomato-based or other vegetable sauces. For more flavor, add herbs or spices such as basil or garlic.

● Cook couscous, rice, and other grains with herbs, defatted broth, or juice instead of fat. (*Tip*: Don't rinse rice; you'll wash away some vitamins, especially B vitamins, added to enriched and fortified grain products.)

● Serve breads, rolls, muffins, bagels, and biscuits with low-fat spreads—fruit butter, chutney, jam, mustard, reduced-fat margarine spread, nonfat mayonnaise, reduced-fat or nonfat cream cheese, or pureed beans such as hummus.

Lean Tips . . . for Soups, Stews, and Sauces

● Skip gravy and rich sauces; enhance flavors with fat-free ingredients: garlic, ginger, lemon juice, onions, tomatoes, herbs, and spices, among others. Before cooking, use a herb rub on meat, poultry, or fish; for a spicy taste, rub a mixture of cumin, chile powder, coriander, red and black peppers, and cinnamon on a

EASY SUBSTITUTIONS FOR LESS TOTAL FAT, SOLID FATS, AND/OR CHOLESTEROL

WHEN COOKING CALLS FOR . . .	USE . . .
Sour cream	Plain low-fat yogurt, or ½ cup cottage cheese blended with 1½ tsp. lemon juice, or light or fat-free sour cream, or Greek yogurt
Whipped cream	Chilled, whipped evaporated fat-free (skim) milk, or nondairy whipped topping
Cream	Evaporated fat-free (skim) milk, fat-free half-and-half
Whole milk	Fat-free (skim), 1 percent, or 2 percent milk as a beverage or in recipes
Full-fat cheese	Low-fat, part skim-milk cheese, cheese with less than 5 grams of fat per ounce, or fat-free cheese (be aware that cooking qualities differ), or use less full-fat cheese
Ricotta cheese	Low-fat or fat-free cottage cheese or nonfat or low-fat ricotta cheese
Ice cream	Low-fat or fat-free ice cream, or frozen low-fat or fat-free yogurt, frozen fruit juice products such as sorbet
Ground beef	95% lean ground beef, or lean ground turkey or chicken, or crumbled tempeh, or beans (legumes)
Bacon	Canadian bacon, lean ham, or smoked deli turkey
Sausage	Lean ground turkey, or 95% fat-free sausage
Whole egg	Two egg whites, or ¼ cup liquid egg substitute, or 1 egg white plus 2 tsp. oil
One egg yolk	One egg white
One egg (as thickener)	1 tbsp. flour
Ramen noodles	Rice or pasta (spaghetti, etc.)
Mayonnaise	Low-fat, reduced-fat, or fat-free mayonnaise or whipped salad dressing, or plain low-fat yogurt combined with pureed low-fat cottage cheese
Salad dressings	Low-fat or fat-free dressings, or homemade dressing made with less saturated oil (peanut, soy, olive, canola, others), water, and vinegar or lemon juice
Cream soups	Defatted broths, or broth-based or fat-free milk-based soups, evaporated fat-free milk
1 ounce unsweetened baking chocolate	3 tbsp. cocoa powder and 1 tbsp. oil
Butter, lard, stick margarine	Soft, tub margarine, squeeze margarine, or oil (canola, olive, vegetable, other)

pork roast. Or coat meat, poultry, or fish with salsas or chutneys. *See "Rub Combos" in this chapter.*

● Cut back on oil in homemade marinades. Or marinate with reduced-fat or fat-free salad dressing (may be high in sodium, however).

● Use pureed vegetables or reduction sauces rather than cream-based sauces. For a creamy texture, add milk, yogurt, or Greek yogurt as you puree vegetables. Reheat gently.

● For a "creamy" sauce, blend fresh dill or other herbs into fat-free, plain yogurt as a sauce for seafood or chicken. Blend horseradish with plain yogurt to serve with lean beef.

● Skim fat from pan juices, soups, and stews. *For quick techniques, see "Degreasing Pan Juices, Soups, and Gravies" in this chapter.*

● Thicken soups and stews with pureed beans, low-fat refried beans, potatoes, or other vegetables and nonfat dry milk. Or puree part of the soup and add it back as a thickener. Added vegetables can boost the vitamin and phytonutrient content; adding dry milk powder "ups" the calcium. Neither adds fat. For another "creamy" ingredient, try buttermilk or evaporated fat-free (skim) milk.

● If the recipe calls for a rich sauce, go easy. You want to add flavor, not overwhelm the food, with sauce.

Lean Tips . . . for Baked Goods

● Experiment a little. Take out some fat—but not all. In baked breads, cakes, muffins, and brownies, try substituting an equal amount of applesauce, mashed bananas or dried plums (prunes), other pureed fruit, mashed garbanzos, or cottage cheese for at least half the oil, margarine, or butter in recipes. Make sure they are well pureed or mashed. For bar and drop cookies, this substitution often works well.

Try buttermilk or nonfat or low-fat yogurt in place of sour cream, butter, and margarine in biscuits, muffins, and other breads. Some recipes work well with less fat; others don't. For example, with less fat, baked goods may not brown as well. Shortbread, butter cakes, butter cookies, and many pound cakes need fat for the flavor and texture you expect.

● Enjoy a nutty flavor? So less nuts taste like more, toast or chop them; toasting brings out the flavor. For even more flavor yet no more fat, mix in chopped dried fruits, too: dried apricots, dried apples, raisins, dried cranberries, or dried plums (prunes).

● Coat baking pans very lightly with nonstick vegetable oil spray rather than margarine, butter, or oil.

● Instead of whipped cream toppings, whip chilled evaporated fat-free milk—with a touch of sugar—for a creamy topping. Serve it right away since it's less stable and may get runny! Evaporated fat-free milk can be substituted for heavy cream in some recipes.

● Skip the frosting, or frost cake lightly, or dust it with powdered sugar, or top with fresh fruit or fruit puree.

● Instead of flaky pastry shells with their high-fat content, make desserts with graham cracker crumb crusts. Prepare crumb crusts with half the margarine or butter called for in the recipe. If the crumbs seem dry, add just a little liquid such as water or juice to moisten.

● Prepare single-crust pies. Either make an open-face pie, or arrange the fruit in the pie pan first, then put the crust on top. *Another tip:* Top with uncooked oatmeal mixed with a few finely chopped nuts.

● As easy substitutions, use low-fat and fat-free dairy products to trim calories, too, *as listed in this chapter.*

● To cut down on solid fats, experiment with cooking oil instead of margarine, butter, or lard. However, the texture of baked goods will differ, being coarser,

mealier, and perhaps more oily. This substitution isn't suggested for quick breads, pastry, or sweet baked goods that are higher in fat to start.

Oil has more shortening power than solid fat. When you substitute, the recipe probably needs less oil than the amount of solid fat called for.

FOR SOLID FAT . . .	TRY LIQUID OIL . . .
1 tbsp.	¾ tbsp.
⅓ cup	4 tbsp. (¼ cup)
½ cup	6 tbsp.
¾ cup	9 tbsp.
1 cup	12 tbsp. (¾ cup)

● Replace some (not all) whole eggs with whites. Baked goods can be rubbery with only whites.

Dairy and More: Boost Calcium

If you're like many Americans, the calcium and vitamin D in your diet need a boost! People of all ages need these nutrients for healthy bones and teeth, and for other body functions. Yet too many of us just don't consume enough calcium- and vitamin D-rich foods, especially milk and other dairy foods. *See chapter 6 for daily recommendations for calcium.*

Calcium and Vitamin D . . . From Dairy Foods

Use these food preparation tips to add a little more calcium and vitamin D. Fat-free and lower-fat products are good choices.

● Fortify mashed potatoes, casseroles, vegetable purees, and thick soups with nonfat dry milk, evaporated fat-free milk, or plain yogurt. Dry milk in meat loaf won't be noticed! One-quarter cup of dry milk powder adds 375 milligrams of calcium to a recipe.

● Sprinkle shredded cheese on salads, soups, stews, baked potatoes, and vegetables. One ounce (¼ cup) of Cheddar cheese has 200 milligrams of calcium.

● Make oatmeal, hot cereal, and hot cocoa with milk instead of water. One-half cup of milk adds 150 milligrams of calcium to your meal. You might fortify them with extra nonfat dry milk powder, too. Calcium-fortified soy beverage also adds calcium.

● Puree cottage cheese in a food processor or a blender. Add herbs; use it as a dip or a spread.

. . . where buttermilk got its name? The term "buttermilk" sounds like a misnomer. Its name refers to the way buttermilk was first made—from the whey, or liquid, left after butter was churned from cream. Today most buttermilk is made from fat-free or low-fat milk.

● Instead of black coffee (regular or decaffeinated) in the morning, try caffe latte (made with steamed milk, perhaps fat-free). One-half cup (4 ounces) of milk added to coffee adds 150 milligrams of calcium. Or drink chai (tea with milk).

● Use plain yogurt for some or all of the mayonnaise in salad dressings, sandwich spreads, and dips.

● If you boost calcium with reduced-fat or fat-free cheese, recognize that it doesn't blend or melt as well as whole-milk cheese. For best results shred lower-fat cheeses finely or use them in a mixture with whole-milk cheese. Blend them with other ingredients rather than just sprinkling them on top.

● Boost calcium, not fat, with yogurt cheese or Greek yogurt. Made by draining the whey from the solids, yogurt cheese may substitute for cream cheese or sour cream. *See "Kitchen Nutrition: Yogurt Cheese" in chapter 5.*

If you're lactose-intolerant, refer to "Lactose: Tips for Tolerance" in chapter 21.

● For something different, try goat cheese. It has a strong and unique flavor. A half-ounce portion of semisoft goat cheese has about 42 milligrams of calcium. Serve it on crackers, on salads, or as a vegetable garnish. A half ounce of hard goat cheese has 127 milligrams of calcium. *Hint:* You might find herb-flavored goat cheese in your supermarket.

How Much Cheese?

1 cup shredded cheese = 4 ounces*
1 cup grated cheese (Parmesan, Romano) = 3 ounces

*Eight ounces of milk is equivalent to ½ cup (2 ounces) of shredded processed cheese, or about ⅓ cup (1½ ounces) of natural cheese such as Cheddar or mozzarella.

Calcium . . . From Other Foods

● Add vegetables that have more calcium to many dishes: soups, salads, and stews, for example. One serving of broccoli, collard greens, kale, mustard greens, okra, and turnip greens all provide calcium, although not as much as milk.

● For main dish salads, casseroles, pasta dishes, salmon cakes, other mixed dishes, and sandwich spreads use salmon with bones as an occasional change from tuna. Fish with edible bones—salmon, sardines, perch—all supply calcium to the diet.

● Make salads, casseroles, chili, stir-fries, dips, smoothies, and other dishes with tofu (soybean curd), preferably made with calcium sulfate. One-quarter cup of tofu with calcium sulfate has about 130 milligrams of calcium. The same amount of tofu without calcium sulfate has 65 milligrams of calcium.

● Blend a delicious fruit smoothie with calcium-fortified beverages: soy beverage and/or orange juice. *See chapter 8 for more on calcium-fortified soy beverages.*

Salt "Shakers"

Cooking with salt may seem so natural that it goes unnoticed. As an average American, about 5 to 10 percent of your sodium comes from food prep or salt you add at the table. A salt preference and the habit of cooking with salt are learned. You can relearn a healthier approach, too.

You don't need to eliminate sodium from your cooking. In fact, you probably can't—and you shouldn't! Sodium occurs naturally in many foods. Just a pinch of salt may enhance the flavor. *See chapter 7, "Sodium and Potassium: A Salty Subject."*

Learn to choose and prepare food with little salt. Do so gradually . . . especially if you're a salt lover. After a while, your taste for salt probably will change. You might be surprised when some foods seem too salty! Except for recipes with yeast, you can cut back on salt, in most traditional recipes, by as much as 50 percent—or even eliminate it. Baked goods made with yeast need salt to control the rising of the dough.

● Taste before you reach for the salt shaker. Food may taste great just as it is!

Try This: Give It a Shake!

How much salt do you typically add to food? Take the "shaker test" to find out. Cover a plate or a bowl with foil or plastic wrap. Now pretend your dinner is on the plate—or that the bowl is filled with popcorn. Salt your "food" just as you would if the bowl or plate was full of food. Now measure how much salt you added. If you shook as much as ¼ teaspoon of salt, you added almost 600 milligrams of sodium to your meal or popcorn.

Be aware: Brining increases the sodium content of chicken or turkey significantly! The amount depends on the type of meat or poultry, the length of brining time, the salt concentration of the brine, and how much surface is covered.

● Remove the salt shaker from the kitchen counter and the table. A ⅛-teaspoon "salt shake" adds about 300 milligrams of sodium to your dish.

● Instead of added salt, spark up the flavor with herbs and spices, garlic, onions, balsamic vinegar, or citrus juice. *See "A Pinch of Flavor: Cooking with Herbs and Spices" in this chapter.*

● Make a little salt go further. Salt your food lightly just before serving. When it's on the surface of food, the salty taste seems more intense. Get a bigger flavor burst (and use *less* salt) with a large-granule, coarse salt, such as kosher or sea salt.

● Instead of salt, add a touch of flavor with foods that contain some salt and a little fat, such as olives, Parmesan or Romano cheese, and salted nuts. The fat helps keep the salty taste in your mouth longer.

● Drain liquid and rinse some canned vegetables such as canned beans to reduce salt. Cook in tap water or defatted sodium-free or reduced-sodium broth. Add herbs for more flavor.

● Reduce or skip salt in cooking water . . . even if a package label says to add it. Salt won't make water boil any faster. Instead, season pasta, rice, vegetables, and cereals with spices or herbs *after* they're cooked.

● Use prepared ingredients with less sodium—perhaps low-sodium broth, no-salt-added canned vegetables, light soy sauce, and salt-free seasoning mixes. Read the label. If foods have ingredients with salt or sodium already, you likely don't need more in a recipe.

Sugar Savers

Before you change the sugar amount in a food you're preparing, think about its function and whether reducing or eliminating sugars will give the baking or cooking result you want. *Refer to "Fats, Sugar, Salt: What They Do" in this chapter.* Then if you need to cut calories, use sugars in moderation in your cooking:

● In cakes, cookies, breads, and other baked goods, try using less sugar. Often you can reduce sugar by a fourth to a third, yet hardly notice the difference. *Be aware:* Many recipes already have done this. *Check "Baking with Sugar" on this page as your guide.*

● Instead of frosting, top cake with pureed fruit, sliced fresh fruit, or a dusting of powdered sugar. A half cup of strawberries and a half peach (skin on) each add 2 grams of fiber!

● "Sweeten" recipes with extracts such as vanilla or peppermint, or so-called sweet spices such as cinnamon or allspice. This enhances the sweetness of food. Warm spicy foods; they'll taste sweeter! Other spices that give the sweet perception include cardamom, coriander, ginger, mace, and nutmeg. *For more tips, see "Kitchen Nutrition: Sweet Seasons" in chapter 3.*

● Briefly broil or microwave peach, pear, or grapefruit halves. Sprinkle with a small amount of sweetener or "sweet" spice . . . or just enjoy the natural flavor. The warm temperature enhances their sweet flavors!

● Sweeten with fruit pureed in a blender or a food processor. Too thick? Add a little fruit juice. Fruit purees are great on pancakes, waffles, French toast, fruit salads, angel food cake, and frozen desserts.

BAKING WITH SUGAR

To ensure good results when reducing sugar in baked foods, use this guideline.

BAKED FOODS	FOR EACH CUP OF FLOUR USE
Cakes and cakelike cookies (cookies made with juice, milk, water)	½ cup sugar
Muffins and quick breads	1 tbsp. sugar
Yeast breads	1 tsp. sugar

SUBSTITUTIONS FOR ALCOHOLIC INGREDIENTS

Baby back ribs, chicken, or seafood tenderized in a beer marinade, a touch of distilled spirits to enhance the flavor of cooking juices, light biscuits or bread made with beer, chicken braised in wine. Wine, beer, and distilled spirits can add to the flavor, tenderness, and texture of your culinary creations.

If you choose to avoid wine, beer, or distilled spirits, it's easy to make a quick, flavorful substitution. To equal the amount of liquid from the alcoholic ingredient, you may need to add water, broth, or apple or white grape juice. (*Note:* Extracts may have small amounts of alcohol.) Adjust the recipe, as the flavor may be affected by ingredient substitutions.

IN A RECIPE THAT CALLS FOR . . .	USE THIS INSTEAD . . .
¼ cup or more white wine	Equal amount of: *In any dish:* white grape juice, apple juice, nonalcoholic wine* *In salad dressings:* lemon juice *In marinades:* vinegar *For savory dishes:* chicken, vegetable, or clam broth (Use ⅞ cup broth plus 2 tbsp. lemon juice or vinegar.) (*Add 1 tbsp. vinegar to balance sweetness.)
¼ cup or more red wine	Equal amount of: *In any dish:* red grape juice, cranberry juice, nonalcoholic wine* *In salad dressings:* lemon juice *In marinades:* vinegar *For savory dishes:* tomato juice, fruit-flavored vinegar, or beef, chicken, or vegetable broth (*Add 1 tbsp. vinegar to balance sweetness.)
¼ cup or more port wine, rum, brandy, sweet sherry	Equal amount of apple or apple juice plus 1 tsp. vanilla extract
¼ cup or more beer	*For soups, stews, and other cooked dishes:* Equal amount of nonalcoholic beer, apple cider, or broth
2 tbsp. almond-flavored liqueur, such as Amaretto	¼ to ½ tsp. almond extract
2 tbsp. bourbon	1 to 2 tsp. vanilla extract
2 tbsp. coffee liqueur, such as Kahlua	2 tbsp. double-strength espresso *or* 2 tbsp. instant coffee, made with 4 to 6 times the usual amount in a cup of coffee
2 tbsp. orange-flavored liqueur, such as Grand Marnier	2 tbsp. orange juice concentrate *or* 2 tbsp. orange juice plus a little orange rind
2 tbsp. chocolate/coffee-flavored liqueur	½ to 1 tsp. chocolate extract plus ½ to 1 tsp. instant coffee in 2 tbsp. water
1 tbsp. dry vermouth	1 tbsp. apple cider
2 tbsp. dry sherry or bourbon	2 tbsp. orange or pineapple juice *or* 1 to 2 tsp. vanilla extract
2 tbsp. rum or brandy	½ to 1 tsp. vanilla, rum, or brandy extract *or* 2 tbsp. orange or pineapple juice

They're also a tasty glaze for meat, fish, and poultry! Use applesauce or pureed baby-food fruits, too.

● Instead of fruit-flavored yogurt, add your own fruit flavoring to plain yogurt with fresh, canned, or frozen fruit. Blend in chopped fruit, berries, or fruit puree.

● Instead of pie, enjoy a baked apple or a pear for dessert, poached in fruit juice and any "sweet" spice.

● In some foods you can use intense sweeteners such as aspartame or saccharin. They're almost calorie-free! However, because they don't function in food like sugars do, their use is limited. *See "Cooking with Low-Calorie Sweeteners" in chapter 3 for more about cooking with these sweeteners.*

● Making a gelatin salad or a dessert? Rather than using flavored gelatin, dissolve unflavored gelatin in fruit juice. Then sweeten with an intense sweetener.

Adapting Recipes for Vegetarians

Looking for vegetarian recipes? Check the bookstore and magazine racks for many flavor-filled dishes from vegetarian cookbooks and publications. Go online! Or with just a few changes, adapt recipes from almost any cookbook or magazine for vegetarian-style eating—even if you choose to avoid eggs and dairy products. Try these recipe hints for adjusting recipes.

Instead of Meat, Poultry, or Fish . . .

● In casseroles, stews, soups, lasagna, and chili, substitute cooked or canned beans (legumes) for meat: perhaps kidney beans in chili or stew, or red lentils in spaghetti sauce or stuffed cabbage rolls, or refried beans in burritos, tacos, and enchiladas. Or add textured soy protein, often sold in granular form.

● In stir-fry dishes, use firm tofu, tempeh, soyburgers, or sausage, cooked beans, nuts, or sesame seeds in place of meat, poultry, or seafood. *Hint:* For more flavor, marinate tofu before adding it to dishes.

● For grilling, cube and skewer firm tofu and tempeh with vegetables.

● On pizza, hot sandwiches, sloppy joes, and other dishes that typically call for meat, use soy-protein alternatives: patties (gardenburgers or beanburgers), bacon, hot dogs, or sausage links.

● Prepare pasta sauces, pizza, soups, stews, and other mixed dishes as always—but skip meat. Add more chopped vegetables and beans. If you eat dairy products, top with cheese for more protein and calcium.

Instead of Eggs . . .

Eggs offer functional qualities to recipes—for example, thickening, binding ingredients together, clarifying stock, coating breaded foods, and leavening. A leavener lightens the texture and increases the volume of baked goods. Without eggs, the qualities of food often change. So experiment!

● Try these ingredients in place of eggs—but know that the results may differ from the original recipe. In place of one egg:

½ mashed banana (in breads, muffins, or pancakes)

2 tablespoons of cornstarch or arrowroot

¼ cup of tofu (Blend it with liquid ingredients until smooth; then add it to dry ingredients.)

¼ cup of pureed fruit, applesauce, or canned pureed pumpkin

Egg replacer powder, or vegetarian egg replacement (often sold in specialty stores)

¼ cup of cooked oatmeal, mashed potatoes, mashed beans, or tofu (in vegetarian burgers or loaves)

● Try scrambled tofu with herbs for breakfast!

Instead of Dairy Foods . . .

● For vegans, use soy margarine in place of butter or other margarines. Most margarine contains some ingredients derived from milk, such as whey or casein. Cookies, pastries, and other baked goods made with margarine may have a different texture than those made with butter. Remember that lard is another fat of animal origin and that stick margarine contains *trans* fatty acids; use mostly soft or liquid margarine.

● Enjoy thick, creamy fruit shakes? If you're a lacto-vegetarian, make them with milk, ice cream, or frozen yogurt. If you're a vegan, blend fruit instead with soft tofu, soy beverage, soy yogurt, or nondairy ice cream—or make all-fruit smoothies!

● Use tofu, soy beverage, soy cheese, and soy yogurt in place of dairy products. Crumbled tofu, for example, can replace ricotta cheese in lasagna. Soft tofu is great in dip or sauce; blend it with other ingredients. In baked foods, 1 cup of soy beverage plus 1 tablespoon of vinegar may replace 1 cup of buttermilk.

● Enjoy fruit sorbet in place of sherbet and ice cream.

Instead of Gelatin . . .

● Use kosher gelatin, made from a sea vegetable. Find it in a specialty food shop.

Spices–and Herbs, Too!

With today's cuisine, we've discovered a new world of taste. Innovative uses of herbs and spices offer a flavor advantage as we trim fat and sodium from cooking. And the result is a new fusion of flavors!

Herbs and spices have a long culinary tradition. If you're a history buff, you know that spices have been traded throughout the Mediterranean and the Middle East for more than two thousand years. In the first century, Apicus, who was a Roman epicure, described herb combinations to enhance flavor. Spices were a motive for Christopher Columbus's forays across the ocean. Now, with our nutrition interest and a flavor

Have You Ever Wondered?

. . . what a flavor extract really is? Extracts are concentrated flavorings from foods and plants dissolved in alcohol. Some are made by distilling fruits, seeds, or leaves; anise, vanilla, peppermint, and almond extracts are made this way. Because they are so concentrated, use just a few drops. Meat, poultry, and vegetable extracts (such as Kitchen Bouquet) are made by concentrating the stock, or cooking juices; use them in marinades and sauces. Flavoring oils are even more concentrated!

. . . how much alcohol burns off or evaporates in cooking? That depends on the cooking time, the temperature, and the amount of distilled spirits, wine, or beer used. Added to uncooked foods, the alcohol content doesn't change. However, added to boiling liquid at the end of cooking, about 85 percent of the alcohol may be retained, compared to only about 5 percent if the dish was braised for 2½ hours. A flamed (flambé) dish may retain about 75 percent of its alcohol content.

Flavor Profile!

Would you combine tomato with basil, or with cinnamon, or with chile powder? The subtle blend of the two ingredients often defines the distinctive flavor of an ethnic cuisine . . . in this case, Italian, or Middle Eastern, or Mexican. These are common in ethnic dishes.

China	Soy sauce, rice wine, and ginger
France	Thyme, rosemary, sage, marjoram, and tomato
Greece	Olive oil, lemon, and oregano
Hungary	Onion and paprika
India	Curry, cumin, ginger, and garlic
Italy	Tomato, olive oil, garlic, and basil
Mexico	Tomato and chile
Middle East	Lemon and parsley
Morocco	Cinnamon, cumin, coriander, ginger, and fruit
West Africa	Tomato, peanut, and chile

world that's smaller than ever, we use more herbs and spices—in new combinations—than ever before.

Many people confuse the terms "spice" and "herb." Spices, which grow in tropical areas, come from the bark, buds, fruit, roots, seeds, or stems of plants and trees. Usually they're dried; garlic and gingerroot are two common exceptions. Herbs, which grow in temperate climates, are the fragrant leaves of plants. The same plant may supply both. For example, the seeds of coriander are used in curry powder, while the leaves of the same plant are called cilantro, a favorite seasoning in Mexican dishes. *To learn about the potential health and phytonutrient benefits of herbs and spices, refer to chapter 6.*

Locking in Flavor: Storing Herbs and Spices

Your herbs and spices won't keep indefinitely—even dried! To lock in the aromatic flavors, store carefully.

● Store dry herbs and spices in tightly covered containers—in a cool, dry, dark place (not the refrigerator). Avoid placing your spice rack near a window or above the stove. Heat, bright light, and air destroy flavor. Moisture can promote mold.

● Date dry herbs and spices when you buy them. Then use them preferably within a year or less. After a while, even properly stored seasonings lose their full "bouquet."

● To check the freshness, rub seasonings between your fingers, and smell the aroma. If there's not much, get a new supply. Buy just enough dry herbs for a few months for the most freshness and flavor.

● To keep fresh herbs longer, treat them like a bouquet of flowers! Snip the stem ends, then stand them in water. Cover them with a plastic bag, and store in the fridge. Change the water every couple of days.

● Growing your own herbs? Preserve them for those long, cold weather months. Either freeze, dry, or add fresh herbs to vinegars. Be aware that some herbs are better dried—for example, bay leaves, marjoram, oregano, and summer savory.

● *To freeze herbs* . . . Wash and dry them well; then seal them in plastic freezer bags. Or snip herbs, then freeze them in water in ice cube trays. Adding a "herb ice cube" to soups and stews is easy! Basil, chives, dill, fennel, parsley, rosemary, and tarragon are among the herbs that freeze well.

● *To dry herbs in the oven* . . . Wash the herbs first, blot them dry or spin in a salad spinner, and remove the leaves from the stems. Place the herbs on baking trays in a single layer. Heat them in the oven at 100° F for several hours with the door slightly open. Remove the leaves before they get browned. Cool, crumble, then store in tightly covered containers.

● *To dry herbs in the microwave oven* . . . Wash the leaves first, then place them between paper towels. Then dry the herbs on the lowest setting for two or three minutes.

A Pinch of Flavor: Cooking with Herbs and Spices

Add a pinch of this and a pinch of that. Used carefully, herbs and spices make many foods distinctive and "simply flavorful"!

Dry or fresh—which herbs should you use? Nothing beats the delicate flavor of fresh herbs. But they're not always available. And unless you have your own herb garden, fresh herbs can be expensive. Whether you use fresh or dry seasonings, use them carefully for their best flavor advantage:

● Before using fresh herbs, wash them! Then pat them dry with paper towels.

● If fresh herbs have woody stems, strip off the leaves before using them. Discard damaged leaves. If the stems are soft and pliable, use them, too. Stems often carry a lot of flavor and aroma.

● To harvest herbs, pick them at their peak of flavor. That's just before they bloom. *Remember:* The flowers on many herb plants are very flavorful, too.

● To release more flavor and aroma, crumble dry, leaf herbs—basil, oregano, savory, and tarragon, among others—between your fingers. Or use a mortar and pestle or coffee grinder. Finely chop fresh herbs.

Herbed Vinegars

Although today's supermarket shelves are stocked with herbed vinegars, why not make your own? They're less costly—and very satisfying to make. They also make great gifts from your kitchen!

● To sterilize, simmer the bottle for ten minutes, and let it cool. Wash the cap or obtain a clean cork.

● Insert a combination of fresh herbs (stems and leaves) and spices into the bottle. Three or four herb sprigs per pint are usually enough.

● Fill the bottle with vinegar. You can use any vinegar as a base: white, red wine, or cider vinegar. Herbs and spices may go better with some vinegars than others. For example, try tarragon and garlic cloves in red or white wine vinegar, and delicate herbs in distilled white vinegar.

  Is wine or rice wine vinegar okay to use? Be aware that a protein they contain may promote bacteria growth if the herbed vinegar isn't stored properly.

● Put on the cap, or insert the cork. Store the bottle in a cool, dark place. Allow the flavor to develop for two to three weeks.

● Try these flavorful combinations: fresh tarragon in cider vinegar; garlic cloves, fresh rosemary or sage, and lemon peel in white wine vinegar; and fresh mint and orange peel in cider vinegar. For fun, make herbed vinegar with edible flowers—for example, nasturtiums with peppercorns, garlic cloves, whole cloves, and cider vinegar.

● In dishes that require a long cooking time, such as soups, stews, and braised dishes, add herbs toward the end of cooking. In that way their flavor won't cook out.

● For chilled foods such as salads and dips, add seasonings several hours ahead so flavors blend.

● When substituting fresh for dry herbs, figure: 1 tablespoon of fresh herb equals 1 teaspoon of dried herb. Dry herbs are stronger than fresh; powdered herbs are stronger than crumbled herbs.

● Add dry herbs and spices to liquid ingredients. They need moisture to bring out their flavors.

● Chop fresh herbs very fine. Kitchen shears are great for mincing and snipping. With more cut surfaces, more flavor and aroma are released.

● Use seasonings with care—especially if you're not familiar with their flavor. They should enhance, not disguise, the aroma and taste of food. Start with ¼ teaspoon of dry herbs for 1 pound of meat or 1 pint of sauce. You can always add more herbs and spices, but you can't take them away!

● Avoid overwhelming a dish with seasonings. A few simple herbs and spices bring out the flavor of food without confusing your taste buds.

● If you're doubling a recipe, you may not need to double the herbs or spices. Use just 50 percent more. If you triple the recipe, start by doubling the seasonings.

● Toast dry spices in a dry nonstick skillet to enhance their flavor.

● Use seasoning blends, including curry, fine herbes, and bouquet garni. Each one is really a blend of herbs—and maybe spices, too. *Curry powder* is a pulverized mixture of as many as twenty different spices, herbs, and seeds. The spice turmeric is the ingredient

Rub Combos

Experiment with your own favorite blend of herbs and spices for all sorts of great rubs. You don't need a recipe; just combine flavors that taste good to you. Use rubs on tender cuts of meat, poultry, and fish. To apply the rub, gently press the mixture onto the surface of the meat prior to cooking. Flavors usually become more pronounced the longer the seasoning is on the meat.

Citrus rub. Combine grated lemon, orange, and/or lime peel with minced garlic and cracked pepper.

Pepper-garlic rub. Combine garlic powder, cracked black pepper, and cayenne pepper.

Italian rub. Combine fresh or dried oregano, basil, and rosemary with minced Italian parsley and garlic.

Herb rub. Combine fresh or dried marjoram, thyme, and basil.

that makes curried dishes yellow. *For a recipe to make your own curry blend, see "Kitchen Nutrition: Salt-Free Herb Blends" in chapter 7. Fine herbes* usually refers to a mixture of chopped herbs, such as chervil, chives, parsley, and tarragon. *Bouquet garni* is a bundle of fresh and/or dried herbs, often parsley, bay leaf, and thyme, that's added to soups, stews, and braised meat or poultry. Usually they're tied up in cheesecloth or placed in a metal teaball to easily remove later.

● If you grow herbs, experiment with less common varieties: pineapple sage, orange mint, burnet, lemon basil, culinary lavender, and coriander, among others.

● Grow scented geraniums: lemon-, peppermint-, and rose-scented geraniums, to name a few. Their aromatic leaves and flowers offer a nice garnish and flavor to sauces, salads, vinegars, and baked foods.

See "Flavor Profile!" in this chapter for seasonings that define various ethnic cuisines.

Foods for All "Seasons"!

Use herbs and spices in food preparation.

● For baked chicken, fill the cavity with herbs and citrus peel—perhaps rosemary and sliced lemon—then roast it in the oven. Lemongrass or lemon-scented geranium leaves are nice, too.

● Cook strong-flavored vegetables, such as cabbage,

Have You Ever Wondered

. . . if homemade herbed oils and garlic oils can pose a food safety risk? Yes, for *Clostridium botulinum* bacteria! *(See chapter 13.)* If you make them at home, use immediately! The U.S. Food and Drug Administration advises that home-prepared mixtures of garlic in oil be made fresh for any meal or snack and not be left at room temperatures. Refrigerate and use leftovers within ten days; after that, discard.

Quick Reference: Herbs and Spices

Not sure what herbs and spices to use? Use this quick reference to enhance the flavor of foods in every part of your meal. This is just a partial list—add your flavor creativity to this list, too.

IN THESE FOODS . . .	TRY THESE HERBS AND SPICES!
Bread	
Sweet breads, rolls	Allspice, cinnamon, cloves, ginger, lavender, nutmeg
Other breads, rolls	Any herb, spice, or seed
Eggs	Basil, black pepper, chervil, chives, cilantro, garlic marjoram, oregano, paprika, tarragon, thyme
Fish and Seafood	
Finfish	Basil, bay leaf, chile powder, dill, fennel, ginger, oregano, paprika, sage, tarragon, thyme
Shellfish	Basil, black pepper, curry powder, dill, garlic, ginger, tarragon
Fruit	Cinnamon, cloves, ginger, lavender, mint, nutmeg, rosemary
Meat	
Beef	Bay leaf, basil, black pepper, celery seeds, curry powder, fennel (in sausage dishes), marjoram, oregano, onion, savory, thyme
Ham	Cloves, ginger, mustard seeds, tarragon
Lamb	Garlic, marjoram, mint, oregano, rosemary
Liver	Onion, garlic, thyme
Pork	Cayenne pepper, chile powder, cinnamon, cloves, fennel (in sausage dishes), sage, thyme
Veal	Basil, curry powder, lemongrass, oregano, rosemary, sage, thyme
Poultry	
Chicken, turkey	Curry powder, ginger, marjoram, paprika, sage, tarragon
Stuffing	Basil, marjoram, onion, parsley, sage, savory
Pasta, Rice	
Pasta (including couscous)	Basil, chives, marjoram, oregano, saffron
Rice (white)	Cinnamon, cumin, fennel, onion, parsley, saffron, turmeric
Rice (brown and wild)	Ginger, onion, parsley
Salads	
Chicken or turkey	Chives, celery seeds, oregano, tarragon
Egg	Marjoram, onion, parsley, paprika, tarragon
Fish or seafood	Chives, curry, powder, ginger, marjoram, oregano, tarragon
Fruit	Cinnamon, ginger, lavender, mint
Greens	Basil, black pepper, chervil, chives, cilantro, garlic, marjoram, mint, onion, parsley, tarragon, thyme
Vegetables or legumes	Basil, oregano, onion, parsley, tarragon
Sauces	
Cheese	Chervil, chile powder, chives, paprika, parsley, smoked paprika
Cream (milk-based)	Basil, curry powder, marjoram, tarragon, thyme
Tomato	Basil, bay leaf, cayenne pepper, cilantro, fennel seed, oregano, paprika, parsley, sage, thyme
Soups	
Chicken or poultry	Bay leaf, lemongrass, mace, marjoram, paprika, parsley, sage, savory, thyme
Clear broth	Basil, lemongrass, paprika, parsley
Cream (or milk based)	Chervil, chives, rosemary, sage, tarragon, white pepper

(continued)

Quick Reference: Herbs and Spices *(continued)*

IN THESE FOODS . . .	TRY THESE HERBS AND SPICES!
Soups (continued)	
Fish or seafood	Bay leaf, celery seeds, chives, curry powder, ginger, saffron, tarragon, thyme
Bean (legume)	Bay leaf, celery seeds, saffron, tarragon, thyme
Meat	Basil, clove, coriander (cilantro), oregano, rosemary, savory, thyme, smoked paprika
Mushroom	Basil, bay leaf, garlic, marjoram, onion, oregano, parsley, tarragon, thyme
Potato	Chives, curry powder, dill
Vegetable	Allspice, basil, bay leaf, black pepper, cloves, garlic, marjoram, sage
Vegetables	
Asparagus	Chervil, savory
Baked beans	Allspice, chile powder, cinnamon, cloves, mace, parsley, red pepper
Broccoli	Oregano
Brussels sprouts and cabbage	Caraway, celery seeds, dill, marjoram, mint, sage, savory, tarragon
Carrots	Basil, bay leaf, ginger, marjoram, mint, oregano, parsley, thyme
Cauliflower	Marjoram, nutmeg, parsley
Corn	Chile powder, chives, smoked paprika
Green beans	Basil, cloves, marjoram, parsley, sage, savory
Lima beans	Marjoram, sage, savory
Mushrooms	Marjoram, oregano, parsley, tarragon, thyme
Onions	Basil, oregano, sage, thyme
Peas	Basil, chervil, marjoram, mint, oregano, parsley, sage, tarragon, thyme
Potatoes	Basil, caraway, chives, dill, garlic, parsley
Spinach	Marjoram, ginger, nutmeg, parsley, savory
Tomatoes	Basil, bay leaf, cilantro, cloves, marjoram, nutmeg, oregano, sage
Winter squash and sweet potatoes	Allspice, cinnamon, cloves, ginger, nutmeg, savory, thyme
Sweet desserts	Allspice, cinnamon, cloves, ginger, lavender, mace, mint, nutmeg

with savory to cut down on the strong aroma yet enhance the flavor.

● Add flavor with herb and spice rubs. *See "Rub Combos" in this chapter.* For a simple rub, just combine garlic and lemon pepper or try smoked paprika.

Looking for more food preparation tips for healthy eating? Check here for "how-tos:"

● Find more creative food "prep" ideas—*see "Kitchen Nutrition" in many chapters.*

● Add nutrition to speed scratch meals—*see chapter 11.*

● Cook healthy and "small" for one or two—*see chapter 19.*

● Cook with kids—*see chapter 17.*

Use herbed yogurt as a flavorful dip or vegetable topping. To get started, blend dill, parsley, chives, and garlic into low-fat yogurt.

● Make no-fat marinades with an acid ingredient—vinegar or fruit juice—and herbs or spices. For example, combine orange juice and nutmeg. Splash herbed vinegar on salads and soups.

● Flavor mineral water, iced tea, lemonade, and spritzers with the leaves of scented geraniums, sprigs of fresh herbs, or edible flowers. Allow enough time for the flavor infusion. *For more about edible flowers, see "Please Don't Eat the Daffodils" in this chapter.*

● "Reverse" the flavors. Use a "sweet spice" with meat or poultry, and a savory herb in dessert. Try cinnamon in tomato sauce and rosemary in pound cake.

The "Eco Kitchen"

Go green in your kitchen—conserving fuel and water and minimizing waste. *See "How 'Green' Are You?" in chapter 9.*

Water in the "Eco Kitchen"

● Choose the proper-size pots and pans for what you're cooking. Equipment that's too big uses more cooking water.

● Cook in a microwave oven or a pressure cooker to conserve water—and time.

● Time foods that need to boil or simmer so you don't waste water through evaporation.

● Keep cold water in the fridge rather than run the faucet until the water is cold.

● Washing dishes? Turn the faucet on and off as you rinse, rather than allowing the water to run continually.

● Run your dishwasher only when full. Scrape soiled dishes; don't rinse them.

● Repair your faucet if it leaks. A drop a second can add up to 700 gallons of water a year!

Energy Savers

● Preheat your oven, but only right before you use it. Turn if off when cooking is done.

● Use equipment that cooks faster, such as a microwave or a convection oven, a pressure cooker, or ovens that also use radiant or halogen heat. Use small appliances when you can: a toaster oven rather than the standard oven.

● Trim the flame. Use a burner that matches the cooking pot.

● Cook the whole meal in the oven at the same time: for example, meat loaf, baked potatoes, and roasted vegetables.

● Arrange baking pans in the oven so air circulates. You'll get more even baking, and your food will cook faster and more efficiently.

● Use the old-fashioned approach: Mix by hand when you can. (You burn calories, too!)

● Turn off lights when you leave the kitchen.

● Avoid the habit of leaving the heat under the coffeepot all day. Turn it off when you're done. Better yet, unplug your coffee maker and other appliances that suck energy from the grid for clocks and light displays.

● Buy Energy Star–certified appliances if you need new major appliances; they also draw less energy for clocks and lights in their "off" mode. Dishwashers that use less hot water save energy, too; use the energy-saving cycle if available.

● Keep the oven and the refrigerator doors shut. Each time you peek inside, your appliance uses more power to regain its set temperature. For the refrigerator, decide what you want before you open the door; keep foods you need often in easy reach. When using the oven, use a timer. *Tip:* An open oven isn't efficient or safe for heating your kitchen!

● For energy efficiency, defrost your freezer regularly if it isn't self-defrosting.

● Keep appliances clean and in good condition: Tighten gaskets around the oven and refrigerator doors; clean refrigerator coils regularly. For efficiency, a gas stove should burn with a blue, not a yellowish, flame in the pilot light.

● Use the self-cleaning feature on your oven judiciously—only when it needs cleaning. For a head start, start it while the oven is still hot from baking.

More Resource Conservation

● Resist the urge to buy food you don't need. Buy only the amount you or your family will eat.

● Buy basic kitchen tools you need, but decide if you really need specialty kitchen gadgets.

● Limit disposables. Look for products in less packaging or recyclable packaging, such as aluminum cans, steel cans, glass containers, recyclable plastic, and paperboard cartons. On plastic containers, look for the recycling symbol with a number in the center. Lower numbers are recycled more easily.

● Keep a recycling bin. Dispose of recyclables according to municipal regulations and services.

● Reuse glass and some plastic food packages. Clean them well with hot, soapy water if used for food storage.

● Compost kitchen waste outside or in an indoor compost pail—for example, corn husks and melon rinds.

● Check your refrigerator regularly. Use perishable foods and leftovers before they spoil and need to be discarded.

CHAPTER 15

Your Food Away from Home

A fast-food meal, lunch in the company cafeteria, a delivered pizza, a casual dinner at a family restaurant, or an elegant evening of fine dining in a relaxing atmosphere: eating out is part of life! Food service includes any food that's not prepared in the home kitchen.

So what's cooking—and who's cooking for us?

The explosion of eating-out experiences offers traditional family menus and gourmet dining; regional, ethnic, and fusion cuisine; vegetarian choices; sushi, tapas, and other small plates; quick foods of all kinds; breakfast bagels and doughnuts to go; and specialty coffees, teas, and smoothies, to name a few.

Whether you're hungry or not, food bombards your senses nearly everywhere you go. Besides sit-down, buffet-style, and quick-service, or fast-food, restaurants, supermarket cafés let us "take out" to "eat in"— at home or at the store. Convenience stores, bookstores, drugstores, recreational centers, institutions (schools, hospitals, businesses, and others), sports and cultural events, and vending machines provide easily available food to eat away from home.

According to the National Restaurant Association, in 2010 a total of 44 percent of adults said that restaurants are part of their lifestyles. In fact, restaurants provided more than 70 billion meal and snack occasions in 2010! Overall, the restaurant industry share of the U.S. food dollar was 49 percent, compared to 25 percent in 1955. For 2011, total restaurant sales (food and drinks) are projected at more than $600 billion! Compare that to about $43 billion in current dollars in 1970.

In growing numbers, consumers want fast, convenient, easy, and flavorful food to fit their busy lifestyles. Take-out, delivered food, and fast-food restaurants allow time to do other things besides cook. In the late 1970s, fast-food sales were about $9 billion annually in the United States. In 2011 sales at quick-service restaurants are projected at nearly $168 billion.

What about full-service restaurants? Those sales may reach nearly $195 billion in 2011. They give people chances to socialize with family, friends, and coworkers; to enjoy leisure time; to celebrate; and to experience flavors that typically aren't prepared at home.

All these data show that eating out is a way of life today. So there's good reason to know how to make smart food and beverage choices away from home. Eating out together can also be a way to enjoy and get the benefits of family mealtime.

Where do you typically eat out, how often, and what do you order? The more you eat away from home, the greater the impact that food-service meals and snacks make on your overall food choices—and your overall health and well-being.

Dining Out for Health and Pleasure

Eating out? You've got choices—plenty of them! With forethought, culinary knowledge, and menu savvy, you can retain control of the food and beverages you consume away from home. Make your choices great-tasting, enjoyable, even adventuresome. And think about choosing healthy options when you eat out!

Dining Out Tip List

What are your eating-out challenges: Too-large portions? The urge to splurge? A food allergy or intolerance to certain ingredients? A need to cut back on calories or sodium? Limited options? Do you want ethnic cuisine, local foods, smaller portions, unique dishes, or lighter cuisine?

No matter where you eat out or what you'd like to order, apply smart eating strategies to restaurant dining: Plan ahead, consider the menu, ask questions, and order wisely.

Plan Ahead

Going prepared, with a smart-eating mind-set, can help you stick to a healthy eating goal. To fit your restaurant choices into your whole day's eating plan—without overdoing on calories or underdoing on vegetables, fruit, whole grains, or low-fat milk, and to enjoy the variety of foods offered in today's restaurant scene—check beforehand if you have time:

● Check your restaurant and menu options. Decide on healthful menu items to order. Perhaps start online by checking restaurant websites, blogs, or Facebook pages, or by using a restaurant app on a smartphone. Try a search engine such as www.HealthyDining finder.com to find healthier restaurant menu options in your zip code.

● Use calorie information for menus. Many restaurants post nutrition information for their menus, perhaps online. *See "Nutrition on the Menu: Your Right to Know" in this chapter.*

● Plan a light dinner out if you ate a big lunch. Or decide ahead to split a dessert, even before you see the menu. If you know ahead that your restaurant meal will have more calories, just trade off: cut back during other meals that day or the next.

● Save up for a special restaurant dinner. Eat small meals earlier, but don't skip breakfast or lunch. A meal-skipping strategy often backfires. Overindulging at a restaurant may result from being overly hungry.

Did You Know

. . . chef-dietitians are blending flavor and healthful eating into restaurant menus?

. . . many adult restaurantgoers like display or open cooking, where they can see their food prepared?

. . . personal chefs have been a growing trend for busy professional families for ten years? It's one way to match food preferences and plan for healthful eating while offering a convenient and time-saving alternative to eating out.

. . . the restaurant trend toward simple foods and local flavors is putting basic, "comfort" foods back on the table—more stews, mashed potatoes, steamed or grilled vegetables, macaroni and cheese, and meat loaf?

. . . chefs and farmers are collaborating to put more local and regional foods on restaurant menus? That includes a trend toward restaurant gardens.

. . . a cooking class can be a great way to dine out, sharpen your culinary skills—and help you learn more ways to prepare the flavors of good health?

. . . many restaurants are "going green" as they make kitchens and guest areas more environmentally friendly? Many also support local charities, for example through customer events, volunteer "chef-ing" in local schools, and culinary education projects.

. . . vegetables are "restaurant-trendy"? Meatless and vegetarian items are common. Microgreens and mini-vegetables, root vegetables (parsnips, rutabaga), fresh fava beans, purple potatoes, beet tops and kale, and sunchokes are among those appearing on menus.

. . . "pop up" and mobile truck restaurants are moving restaurant service to customers?

. . . restaurants contribute significant amounts of nourishing food to food banks and soup kitchens as part of their social responsibility commitment?

● To save time, order ahead: online, by phone, or perhaps by fax. Then the kitchen will have your food ready. Or make reservations ahead, perhaps online, in the restaurant's website or other websites, such as www.opentable.com.

● Call ahead to see if you can make special requests. If food can be prepared to order, you have more control.

Restaurants increasingly provide menu items that are gluten-free and food-allergy-friendly. Many of today's chefs, cooks, and servers are trained to be food-allergy- and gluten-free-aware. Some restaurants participate in the Gluten-Free Restaurant Awareness Program; look for this sign.

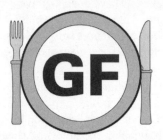

Source: Gluten Intolerance Group, 2011. Used with permission

Some states are considering legislation for posting allergen posters in restaurants, and for requiring servers to ask patrons if they have a known food allergy. *See chapter 21 for more advice on managing allergies and other food sensitivities when you eat out.*

Learn Menu Language

Primavera, béarnaise, al dente: What do they mean? Knowing menu terms and cooking basics makes ordering easier, especially for controlling calories, sodium, solid fats, and other nutrients, or for handling a food sensitivity such as a food allergy or intolerance.

Click Here! Websites to Know . . .

- Healthy Dining Finder, as partner with the National Restaurant Association, www.healthydiningfinder.com/

- Portion Distortion, U.S. Department of Health and Human Services, hp2010.nhlbihin.net/portion/

- Interactive Fast Food Menu, University of Missouri/Lincoln University, www.extension.org/pages/Interactive_Fast_Food_Menu

- DietFacts.com (nutrition information for many chain restaurant menus), http://www.dietfacts.com/fastfood.asp

See "Resources You Can Use" for more websites.

On the Leaner Side

Not sure what to order? For lower-calorie cuisine, try this:

Appetizers	Fresh fruit plate, broth-based soup, fruit or vegetable juice, marinated vegetables, crudités, or raw vegetables, with hummus or salsa dip, seafood cocktail
Breads	Hard rolls or whole-wheat buns, French or Italian bread, bread sticks, melba toast, or saltine crackers
Salads	Dressing on the side
Vegetables	Steamed vegetables, plain or with a lemon wedge, grilled, roasted, or dry-sautéed vegetables
Entrées	Lean meat, fish, and poultry that are broiled, grilled, or roasted, with any sauces served on the side (remove visible fat and poultry skin); vegetarian dishes that go easy on cheese or cheese sauces. *See chapter 14 for lean meat cuts.*
Desserts	Fruit or Italian ice or sorbet, fresh fruit, angel food cake with fruit, low-fat frozen yogurt

Menu literacy also makes eating out more fun! *For terms, check "Menu Language" in this chapter.*

For fewer calories look for foods with simple preparation, such as steamed vegetables or broiled chicken. The term "al dente" describes how pasta and vegetables are cooked: only until firm when bitten, not soft or overdone. Literally translated, it means "to the tooth." Vegetables cooked al dente retain more nutrients.

Have It Your Way!

As a restaurant patron, you have the right to request a substitute or a customized order. Be assertive, ask menu questions, make special requests, and be realistic about what you request. Service-oriented restaurants usually are eager to please if they can. They want you back!

- Ask about ingredients, if you can make substitutions, or how the food is prepared or served. That's especially useful if the description isn't clear or the food is unfamiliar. Since today's restaurant patrons often are food-savvy, servers expect questions and are generally willing to find out if they don't know the answers. You might ask:

● How are the vegetables seasoned? Can you prepare it without adding salt? Can you prepare it without butter, or just a little butter?

● Is the fish grilled or broiled? Breaded and fried, or cooked in butter, margarine, or some other fat, it has more calories.

● How is the sauce prepared? What is the difference between béarnaise and bolognese sauce? Which has fewer calories? What's a reduction sauce? *For a quick description, see "Gourmet's Guide to Sauces" in this chapter.*

● Can I have the sauce (or salad dressing or whipped topping) on the side? You control the amount.

● Is the soup clear (broth) or cream-based? Clear soups have fewer calories.

● Can I substitute a baked potato, rice, vegetables, or a salad for the fries or chips? Any extra cost may be worth the nutrition benefit.

● Can I substitute vegetables or salsa for cheese or cheese sauce?

● What is mole (in a Mexican dish)? Galangal (in a Thai dish)? Cassava (in a Caribbean dish)?

● Does the dessert have nuts (if you're allergic to them)?

● Can I share? Have a small plate portion? A to-go box?

Have You Ever Wondered

. . . if eating out makes you fat? That depends on your food and beverage choices. While some research shows a link between frequency of eating out and overweight, the real issue is how much and what you eat away from home (at home, too)—and how physically active you are. Use the tips in this chapter to order foods with fewer calories, and eat sensible restaurant portions. Keep a right-sized mind-set at home, too, rather than allow restaurant portions to redefine the amount of food on your "home plate."

Nutrition on the Menu: Your Right to Know

When restaurants prepare your food, providing the calorie and nutrient content of a menu item isn't required. Now with a federal menu label law, targeted for 2012 enforcement, many restaurant chains, including vending machines, need to provide calorie information for menu items.

By law, if a restaurant or retail eating establishment is part of a chain of twenty or more locations with the same name, menus must provide calorie information, at least for all standard menu items sold for at least sixty days of the year. The requirement: calorie information for standard menu items on the menu board or drive-through board. Other nutrition information besides calories that is available on request may include calories from fat, total fat, saturated fat, cholesterol, sodium, carbohydrates, sugars, fiber, and protein. Restaurants with fewer than twenty locations also can provide this same information on a voluntary basis.

Nutrient content claims such as "lean," low-fat," and "light" may appear voluntarily on menus. If so, their use must meet the code of federal regulations (CFR). They should have roughly the same meaning as these same terms on food labels. *For definitions of these terms see "Label Lingo" in chapter 12.*

● Be specific about a special menu request. For example, ask if the chef can "broil fish without butter," "bring dry toast," or "serve dressing on the side."

● Ask about portion sizes. Large portions may not mean better value. A 12-ounce or a 6-ounce filet mignon? A 5-to-6-ounce meat portion probably is enough, especially if you eat other protein foods during the day. *See "Restaurant Portions: You're in Control!" in this chapter.*

● At a steakhouse request leaner cuts of meat (for example, filet mignon, tenderloin, sirloin tip, flat iron, round or flank steak) for less total and solid fat rather than a rib eye or ribs, which have more calories and fat. On fatty cuts ask if visible fat can be trimmed before cooking.

● Nothing on the menu that's right for you? Ask if you can order "off the menu." For fewer calories and less solid fat, you might request broiled fish or chicken breast seasoned with herbs and lemon juice, or fresh fruit for dessert, or low-fat or fat-free milk. *See "On the Leaner Side" in this chapter for common menu items with fewer calories and less fat.*

● If you don't plan to eat a side dish or sauce, ask to have it left off your plate. Perhaps skip tartar sauce served with fish, or chips served with a sandwich.

● If you choose a higher-calorie entrée, balance it with a lower-calorie side dish and dessert. Perhaps balance fettuccine alfredo, which is high in calories and solid fat, with fresh fruit to end the meal.

● If the food isn't prepared as you ordered, politely ask to have it prepared correctly. Ask for something else if necessary.

Help Yourself

Practice the art of enjoying food variety, balance, and moderation when you eat out.

● Choose dishes with vegetables, fruit, beans, and whole grains. Ask if whole-wheat pasta or brown rice is available.

● Can't resist the urge to overindulge on tortilla chips or bread served when you're seated? Do you nibble mindlessly on pretzels, nuts, and chips brought with a beverage order? Take a few on a plate or napkin; choose one slice of bread. Then ask to have the rest removed from the table.

● Go easy on dipping oils, even though they're usually olive oils (healthy oils). A slice of bread may soak up 3 or 4 teaspoons of oil, or 14 to 19 fat grams.

● To curb a big appetite, start with a salad, broth-based soup, or appetizer crudités (raw vegetables). Go easy on dressings and dips.

● Eat slowly. Stop eating before you feel too full. That gives you time to get in touch with your satiety cues.

MAY I TAKE YOUR ORDER?

The choices on the left have less fat and calories than their counterparts on the right.

ENJOY MORE OFTEN . . .	ENJOY LESS OFTEN . . .
Consommé, gazpacho, clear soups	Cream soups, soups topped with cheese, bisques
Vegetable plate with salsa; steamed, grilled or roasted vegetables	Pâté, quiche, stuffed appetizers
Garden, tossed, or spinach salad with dressing on the side, crisp and crunchy vegetables	Salads with large amounts of dressing, bacon, cheese, and croutons, and mayonnaise-laden salads such as potato, macaroni, and tuna
Grilled, broiled, or flame-cooked meats	Breaded or batter-dipped meat, chicken, or fish, or extra gravy
Broiled, steamed, poached, roasted, baked, Cajun, or blackened	Breaded, fried, sautéed, au gratin, escalloped, en croûte, creamed, en casserole, or Kiev entrées
4-to-8-ounce steak, filet mignon, or flat iron steak	More than 8-ounce steak, rib eye steak, or ribs
Au jus, marinara, Provençal, or fruit sauces	Gravy, alfredo, béarnaise, béchamel, beurre blanc, carbonara, hollandaise, pesto, and velouté sauces
Baked potatoes (plain or with a small amount of butter, margarine, or sour cream), redskin potatoes	Home-fried and deep-fried potatoes, twice-baked potatoes, croquettes, butter noodles, mashed potatoes with gravy, fries, fried onion rings
Sandwiches on whole-wheat, pita, or rye with mustard or low-fat mayonnaise	Sandwiches on croissants or biscuits
Plain whole-wheat or multigrain rolls or bread sticks	Garlic bread, cheese spreads, flavored butters
Fruit, fruit sorbet	Cheesecake, French pastries, pie, ice cream, crème brûlée

Ask the server to remove your plate when you're done, even if a little food is left.

● If you drink wine, beer, or other alcoholic beverages, do so in moderation. *See chapter 8 for guidelines on alcoholic beverages.* A drink or two not only provide calories but also may increase your appetite and lessen your personal discipline at the table.

MENU LANGUAGE

Looking for foods with fewer calories, or less fat or sodium? Check the menu. Although they offer no guarantees, descriptive terms often give clues.

Menu Clues: Fewer Calories and Less Fat

Baked	Grilled
Braised	Lightly sautéed
Broiled	Poached
Cooked in its own juices	Roasted
Dry broiled (in wine or	Steamed
lemon juice)	Stir-fried

Menu Clues: More Calories and Fat

Au gratin or in cheese sauce	French-fried
Batter fried	Hollandaise
Béarnaise	Lightly fried
Breaded	Marinated (in oil)
Beurre blanc	Pan-fried
Buttered	Pastry
Creamed	Prime
Crispy	Rich
Deep-fried	Sautéed
Double crust	Scalloped (escalloped)
En croûte	With gravy
Escalloped	With mayonnaise
Flash-fried	With cream sauce

Sometimes "extreme" or "explosion" should be an alert!

Menu Clues: More Sodium

Barbecued	Smoked
Cured	Teriyaki
In broth	With Creole sauce
Marinated	With cocktail sauce
Pickled	With soy sauce

● As a drink option, order mineral water or club soda with a twist of lemon or lime. Also nonalcoholic: agua fresca ("fresh water" in Spanish). Made with a water-sugar base, it's flavored with fruit such as fresh melon, mango, guava, papaya, and strawberries. Since it's made with sugar water, enjoy, but in small amounts.

● What about wine or beer pairings with a meal, or flights (several smaller portions of wine, beer, sake, or other distilled spirits)? Go easy. Drink slowly with your meal; share if you can. Have a designated driver.

● Enjoy the flavors of desserts in trendy bite-size and miniportions for fewer calories.

● If you can't resist rich desserts, don't even peek at the dessert tray. If you're tempted, share one with someone else. Order seasonal fruit, cappuccino, or sorbet instead.

Enjoy, Enjoy, Enjoy!

Eating can nourish the soul as well as the body. In fact, eating out can be one of life's pleasures.

● Take your palate on a taste adventure. Order something you've never tried—or that you usually don't eat at home. Cautious about a new food or dish? Try an appetizer portion.

● Savor each bite. Enjoy food—and the layers of flavor—at a leisurely pace, rather than the abundance of food on a plate.

● If you eat with others, enjoy the social time. It can be a relaxing time with family and friends. *Check "Eating Out with Kids" in chapter 17.*

● Seize the chance for culinary insights. Eating out is a great time to learn about ingredients, flavors, and preparation of dishes on the menu. *See "Flavor on the Menu" below for healthful culinary techniques in restaurants.*

Flavor on the Menu

Dining out offers easy access to unique, delicious flavors. More than ever, chefs use culinary techniques to enhance foods' natural flavors while retaining their nourishing qualities. This phenomenon isn't reserved for table-service or upscale restaurants. Gradually it's happening in many fast-food, deli, casual-dining, and family restaurants, too.

Restaurant Portions: You're in Control!

If restaurant portions seem too big, remember that you have choices. You control portions—and calories—by what you order and how you handle what comes on your plate.

● First think, just how hungry are you?

● Order before your meal companions do, if possible. Then you won't be influenced by their orders.

● Choose the portion size you want. Many restaurants offer appetizer portions, half portions, and full portions. Or try tapas, "little plates," mezzes, or dim sum. Order one or two dishes to share at a time.

● Split a dish with someone. Ask for two plates.

● Order two appetizers, or an appetizer and a salad, instead of the full entrée and other courses.

● Order à la carte. À la carte means that each item is separately ordered and priced. Then you may not be tempted by more food than you need.

● Turn today's dinner into tomorrow's lunch. Most restaurants have to-go containers—a time-saver for your next meal. *Tip:* Store perishable foods in the refrigerator within 2 hours, or within 1 hour if the temperature is more than 90°F.

● For double benefits, look for early-bird specials. They may offer smaller portions at a lower price. Or eat out at midday for a lunch-size portion.

● Leave some food on the plate. Why pay twice, with your pocketbook and your waistline?

● Plan ahead for a multicourse tasting menu. Enjoying many small portions can add up to a lot of food!

● Pass on all-you-can-eat specials, buffets, and unlimited salad and food bars if you tend to eat too much.

● If buffet-style eating is your choice, fill up on salad (easy on dressing) and vegetables first to appease your appetite. Take only two trips to the buffet: one for veggies, fruit, and salads; one for anything else. Use a small plate, which holds less.

● Sit facing away from the buffet, and as far away as you can.

● Before your food is served, ask your server to put half in a take-away container.

Look for these techniques on menus that add flavor while promoting good nutrition. These culinary secrets can work in your kitchen, too.

● Poaching fish, poultry, or meat in flavorful broth, rather than cooking them in oil, or poaching fruit in juice rather than cooking in sugary syrup

● Intensifying flavors with high-heat cooking, such as pan-searing, grilling, or broiling, to brown the meat and seal in the juices

● Grilling or roasting vegetables, then featuring them center stage as an entrée

● Adding fuller flavors with more whole grains, including brown rice, amaranth, and quinoa, as well as wild rice

● Flavoring and adding volume and color to plates with creative fruit and vegetable sides and garnishes, often with less common fruits and vegetables

● Serving bean purees or tapenade (anchovy-olive spread) instead of butter or margarine as table condiments

● Using salsa, chutney, vinaigrette, reduction sauces, or fruit and vegetable purees in place of rich sauces

● Adding hazelnuts, pecans, or almonds

● Flavoring creatively with herbs and spices: perhaps a sweet spice, such as cinnamon, with meat, or a savory herb, such as rosemary, with fruit or desserts

● Using big, bold flavor ingredients, but perhaps small amounts, such as feta or blue cheese, pomegranate seeds, chipotle pepper (with a smoky taste), cilantro, or bitter broccoli rabe

● Layering flavors, with a variety of ingredients of contrasting flavors—as easy as a mixture of many greens, citrus fruit, and nuts in a salad

● Varying and balancing flavors in a dish or meal—for example, a fruit sauce for fish with mango (sweet), tarragon (bitter), vinegar (sour), broth (umami), and a touch of salt

● Infusing oils with herbs or garlic for more flavor

● Experimenting with unique ingredients, including flavorful local or ethnic foods and seasonings such as smoked paprika or sichuan pepper

For more about food and flavor, refer to "Flavor and Health" in chapter 14.

Gourmet's Guide to Sauces

What's in the sauce? Tomato- and other vegetable-based sauces are typically lower in calories and fat than cream-based sauces. And they count as another vegetable in your day's food choices!

Alfredo. Creamy Italian sauce, typically prepared with butter, heavy cream, and Parmesan cheese.

Béarnaise. Thick French sauce made with white wine, tarragon, vinegar, shallots, egg yolks, and butter.

Béchamel. Basic white sauce made with flour, milk, and butter, and flavored with onion.

Bolognese. Italian meat sauce made with ground beef and sometimes pork and ham and sautéed in a small amount of butter and/or olive oil with tomatoes, other vegetables, herbs, and sometimes wine. Also referred to as ragú bolognese sauce.

*Bourguignonne.** French sauce made with red wine, carrots, onions, flour, and a little bacon.

Buerre blanc. Thick, smooth sauce whisked with wine, vinegar, shallot reduction, and cold butter.

Carbonara. Italian sauce made of cream, eggs, Parmesan cheese, and bits of bacon.

*Coulis.** Thick puree or sauce, such as tomato or squash coulis.

*Demi-glace.** Reduction sauce that gets its intense flavor by slowly cooking beef stock and Madeira or sherry to a thick glaze.

Hollandaise. Thick sauce with white wine, vinegar, or water, egg yolks, melted butter, and lemon juice.

*Marinara.** Italian tomato sauce made with tomato and basil and perhaps other seasonings such as onions, garlic, and oregano.

Pesto. Uncooked sauce made of fresh basil, garlic, pine nuts, Parmesan or Pecorino cheese, and olive oil. It's a favorite with Italian pasta.

*Reduction sauce.** Sauce of usually broth or pan juices boiled down to concentrate the flavor and thicken the consistency. Unlike in many other sauces, flour or other starches aren't used as thickeners.

*Sweet-and-sour.** Sugar and vinegar added to a variety of sauces; typically added to Chinese and German dishes.

Velouté. Light, stock-based white sauce. Stock is the broth left from cooking meat, poultry, fish, or vegetables. It's thickened with flour and butter; sometimes egg yolks and cream are added.

*Vinaigrette.** Oil-and-vinegar combination.

*These sauces tend to be lower in calories and fat. But the ingredients vary, and so do the calorie and fat contents.

Sizing Up Salad and Other Food Bars

A salad bar can serve up a healthful meal all by itself—or as a great side dish. The rainbow of vegetables and fruits is not only a calorie bargain, it's also often loaded with vitamins A and C, folate, fiber, and an array of phytonutrients, with antioxidant potential.

That said, an average salad bar plate can top out at more than 1,000 calories, depending on your choices and portions—more than some fast-food meals. Where do excessive calories come from? Not from lettuce, tomatoes, cucumbers, and other fresh vegetables. Depending on the amount, regular salad dressings, along with many higher-fat toppings such as cheese, croutons, bacon bits, and fried onions, can heap calories on a bed of raw vegetables. Dressed side dishes (potato salad, pasta salad, ambrosia, and macaroni salad), creamy soups, cheese and crackers, even desserts—all with more calories—line up on the salad bar, too.

To control salad bar calories and solid fats:

● Pace yourself. Check out the salad bar from end to end before you fill your plate.

● Use a small salad plate, not a dinner plate, if you're tempted to overdo.

● Start with greens. Dark-green leafy vegetables such as spinach and romaine supply more nutrients and phytonutrients than iceberg lettuce does.

● Spoon on plenty of brightly colored vegetables (broccoli, peppers, beets, or carrots, to name a few), beans (such as kidney and garbanzo beans), and fruits.

● Make it a hearty salad with protein-rich ingredients: beans (legumes), lean meat, turkey, crabmeat or surimi, tuna, eggs, and cheese (perhaps low-fat). Cottage cheese, other cheese, and yogurt on the salad bar also add calcium.

BUILD A HEALTHFUL SALAD

Imagine a salad bar with bowls and bowls of fruits, vegetables, and lean protein foods. How would you build your salad?

Choose ingredients wisely from the following list. Choose sensible amounts. Be mindful of the calories from dressings and higher-fat ingredients such as regular cheese, mixed salads with mayonnaise, and bacon bits.

FOOD	AMOUNT	CALORIES*	FAT (G)	FOOD	AMOUNT	CALORIES*	FAT (G)
Greens				*Meat, Poultry, Fish, and Eggs*			
Bean sprouts	¼ cup	8	trace†	Eggs, chopped	2 tbsp.	25	2
Lettuce	1 cup	8	trace	Lean ham, chopped	1 oz.	40	2
Spinach	1 cup	7	trace	Popcorn shrimp	1 oz.	30	<1
Other Veggies				Surimi	1 oz.	30	<1
Artichoke hearts	¼ cup	20	trace	Tuna in spring water	1 oz.	35	<1
Beets	¼ cup	20	0	Turkey in strips	1 oz.	40	<1
Bell peppers	2 tbsp.	5	trace	*Cheese*			
Broccoli	¼ cup	8	trace	Cheddar cheese, grated	2 tbsp.	55	5
Carrots, shredded	¼ cup	10	trace	Cottage cheese, creamed	¼ cup	60	2
Cauliflowers	¼ cup	6	trace	Cottage cheese, 1% low-fat	¼ cup	40	<1
Cucumbers	¼ cup	4	trace	Feta cheese	2 tbsp.	50	4
Green peas	2 tbsp.	15	trace	Mozzarella cheese, grated (part skim)	2 tbsp.	45	3
Mushrooms	¼ cup	4	trace	Parmesan cheese	2 tbsp.	45	3
Onions	1 tbsp.	4	0	*Others*			
Radishes	2 tbsp.	2	trace	Bacon bits	1 tbsp.	25	2
Tomatoes	¼ cup	8	trace	Chow mein noodles	1 tbsp.	15	<1
Fruits				Croutons, seasoned	2 tbsp.	25	1
Avocados	¼ cup	60	6	*Mixed Salads*			
Canned peaches, in juices	¼ cup	25	trace	Potato (with mayonnaise)	¼ cup	90	5
Fresh melons	¼ cup	15	trace	Three-bean (in vinaigrette)	¼ cup	60	0
Fresh strawberries	¼ cup	10	trace	Tuna salad (with mayonnaise)	¼ cup	95	5
Mandarin oranges, segments in juice	¼ cup	20	trace	*Dressings*			
Olives, ripe	2 tbsp.	20	2	Blue cheese, regular	2 tbsp.	150	16
Raisins	2 tbsp.	60	trace	French, regular	2 tbsp.	145	14
Beans, Nuts, and Seeds				Italian, fat-free	2 tbsp.	15	<1
Almonds, sliced	1 tbsp.	55	5	Italian, regular	2 tbsp.	85	8
Chickpeas	¼ cup	65	1	Lemon juice	2 tbsp.	6	0
Kidney beans	¼ cup	55	trace	Oil and vinegar	2 tbsp.	145	16
Sunflower seeds	1 tbsp.	45	4	Thousand Island, regular	2 tbsp.	120	11
Tofu (raw, firm)	¼ cup (about 3 oz.)	90	6	Vinegar	2 tbsp.	6	0

*Nutrient values have been rounded.

†"Trace" on all the vegetables and fruits is about .05 to 0.2 gram of fat.

Source: U.S. Department of Agriculture, Agricultural Research Service, 2011. U.S. Department of Agriculture, National Nutrient Database for Standard Reference, Release 24, 2011.

● Include fiber-rich mixed dishes not only made with beans. Look for those made with brown rice and other whole grains.

● Take small amounts of higher-fat toppings and mayonnaise-based side salads.

● Dress your salad lightly! A 2-tablespoon ladle of French, Italian, blue cheese, or Thousand Island dressing adds about 150 calories to an otherwise low-calorie salad. Doubling or tripling that amount loads on calories and overpowers the delicate flavor of salad ingredients. Choose a low-fat or fat-free dressing, or sprinkle on just a splash of flavored vinegar or lemon juice.

Make healthful choices in other food bars, too, such as baked potato bars and pasta bars.

Eating Out Safely

Almost nothing can ruin a trip or a pleasant meal out more than foodborne illness. Although restaurants in the United States, Canada, and many other developed nations must operate under strict public health regulations, any restaurant can have an occasional sanitation lapse. In some parts of the world these regulations may not exist. Hotel staff or the concierge often can recommend restaurants with high standards.

These tips can help ensure that the meal you eat away from home won't come back to bite you:

● Check for cleanliness. Although you probably can't see into the kitchen, just looking at the public areas tells a lot about a restaurant. Look for:

● tables that are wiped clean, using clean cloths;

● well-groomed servers;

● clean silverware, tablecloths, glasses, and dishes;

● adequate screening over windows and doors to keep out insects;

● no flies or roaches, which can spread disease;

● clean restrooms with soap, hot water, and paper towels or air dryers;

● clean exterior with no uncovered garbage.

● Be cautious about raw meat and fish; they may carry bacteria and parasites. These menu items are served raw: steak tartare (raw ground beef and raw eggs), carpaccio (thin-sliced raw beef), and sashimi

(raw fish). Sushi, often made with raw fish, is popular among many restaurant goers. *See "Is Raw Seafood Safe to Eat?" in chapter 13 for guidance on sashimi.*

● Check your burger. It should be cooked until the center is no longer pink and the juices run clear. If it's not cooked thoroughly, send it back!

Safe Food Bar

● Use the hand sanitizer if available.

● Select food from food bars, buffets, and displays only if the food is properly covered with a sneeze guard or a hood. This includes dessert and appetizer displays.

● Check the temperature. A hot buffet should be piping hot. A cold salad bar should be well chilled or placed on ice.

● Use a clean plate when returning to the food bar.

● Get assistance if you can't handle serving utensils properly.

● *If you have a food allergy or intolerance, see chapter 21.*

Safe Takeout

From restaurants, delis, and supermarkets, many buy-and-go foods are perishable. Handle them carefully to avoid foodborne illness. Keep hot takeout foods hot, and cold takeout foods cold.

If takeout food is hot already . . .

● Eat it right away: within two hours, or within one hour if the air temperature is 90°F or more. Longer than that, toss!

● If it won't be eaten for more than two hours, refrigerate it in shallow, covered containers. Then reheat it to a temperature of 165°F, or until it's hot and steaming. Check the temperature with a food thermometer. *See "Using a Food Thermometer" in chapter 13.* Or reheat it, covered and rotated for even heating, in a microwave oven. Then let the food stand for two minutes for more thorough heating.

● Keep hot takeout food in your oven or slow cooker at 140°F or above—but for not much longer than two hours. Food loses its appeal if it's held longer. Cover it with foil to keep it moist. Check the temperature with a food thermometer.

For cold takeout food . . .

● If you don't eat it right away, refrigerate or store it in a chilled, insulated cooler until meal- or snacktime.

● For deli platters that stay on the buffet, keep the platters on bowls of ice.

● For takeout food that requires heating or cooking, follow food safety precautions. *See chapter 13, "The Safe Kitchen."*

Eating Out: Vegetarian Style

Today's restaurant menus offer creative, flavorful vegetarian options. Many traditional restaurants and cafeterias cater to vegetarians. Fast-food restaurants serve meatless main dish salads, as well as vegetarian deli sandwiches, pita pockets, pizzas, and tacos. And many ethnic restaurants (for example, Indo-Pakistani, other Asian, and Middle Eastern) feature vegetarian dishes among their specialties.

Whether you're vegetarian or simply enjoy an occasional vegetarian meal, consider these tips:

● Before ordering, ask your server about the ingredients in menu items. Most restaurants can modify a dish.

● If you're vegan, even ask about ingredients in vegetarian dishes prepared with no eggs and dairy products. For chain restaurants, contact the company to ask about ingredients if you frequently dine there.

● Ask for meatless sauces. Omit meat from stir-fries; add vegetables, beans, or pasta in its place. It's easier to substitute at restaurants that make food to order.

● If the menu doesn't offer a vegetarian entrée, order a salad with vegetable soup and perhaps bread, or several vegetable appetizers. A fruit plate—with or without cheese or yogurt—makes a great entrée.

● For a salad bar, toss with kidney beans, chickpeas, and a few sunflower seeds, as well as vegetables with more vitamin C. (Vitamin C helps your body absorb iron from plant sources of food.) If you're lacto-ovo-vegetarian, spoon on cottage cheese, shredded cheese, and chopped hard-cooked eggs. If you're vegan, find out if the dressing has ingredients derived from eggs; if so, vinegar and oil are great!

● Choose an ethnic restaurant that's likely to have vegetarian options. Perhaps try cuisines of the Middle East, Greece, India, China, Mexico, or parts of Africa. (*A tip for vegans:* Ghee, used in many dishes from India, is melted, clarified butter.) *See "Vegetarian Dishes in the Global Kitchen" below.*

● Ask for a vegetarian meal when you book long international airline flights. If needed, find out ahead if the meal is egg- and dairy-free. For airlines without vegetarian meals, request a fruit plate or bring your own snacks. *See "Dining at 35,000 Feet" later in this chapter.*

● For organized meal functions, request a vegetarian meal ahead of time.

Vegetarian Dishes in the Global Kitchen

Delicious and nutritious—vegetarian dishes are typical fare in many parts of the world. As you flip the pages of ethnic cookbooks or glance through the menu of an ethnic restaurant, build your meal around dishes such as these. They're typically made without meat, poultry, or fish—but check. Internationally, rice and beans—a high-protein food combination—is typical nearly everywhere, but uniquely prepared and seasoned in different cuisines.

Caribbean
  Callaloo: one-pot meal (stew) made with dark-green leafy vegetables, a variety of other vegetables, peppers, and seasonings
  Black-eyed pea patties: black-eyed peas mashed with eggs and seasonings, then quickly pan-fried in a small amount of oil
  Pois et ris: kidney beans and rice flavored with smoked meat and seasonings
  Gunga: pigeon peas and rice

China
  Vegetable-tofu stir-fry: variety of thinly sliced vegetables and cubed bean curd, stir-fried with soy sauce and perhaps vegetable broth

Vegetarian Dishes in the Global Kitchen *(continued)*

Egg foo yung: frittata-like dish made by combining slightly whipped eggs with sliced vegetables, then frying in a skillet until browned; also may be prepared with meat or poultry

Hot and sour soup: hot soup with tofu

Vegetable pot stickers: steamed vegetable dumplings

Soybean cakes: stir-fried tofu with steamed rice

East Africa

Kunde (bean and groundnut stew): stew made of black-eyed peas, peanuts (groundnuts), tomatoes, and onions; a similar stew is made in West Africa, often without peanuts

Injera and lentil stew: flat bread served with cooked lentils; this is an Ethiopian dish

France

Vegetable quiche: pie with a custard of egg and cheese mixed with chopped vegetables such as leeks, spinach, asparagus, and mushrooms

Ratatouille: soup or stew made of eggplant, tomatoes, onions, green peppers, and other vegetables; enjoy with crusty French bread

Greece

Tzatziki (cucumber-yogurt salad): plain yogurt mixed with shredded cucumber, garlic, and perhaps black olives; served with crusty bread

Vegetable-stuffed eggplant: eggplant hollowed and filled with chopped vegetables, cooked grains, and sometimes nuts

Spanakopita (spinach pie): pita made with a phyllo-dough crust and filled with a mixture of spinach, feta cheese, and eggs

India

Dohkla: steamed cakes made of rice and beans

Vegetable curry dishes: combination of chopped vegetables and lentils flavored with a curry mix and perhaps served with basmati rice

Idli or dhoka: steamed bean and rice cakes

Indonesia

Gado-gado: cooked vegetable salad with a peanut sauce; often seasoned with chiles

Italy

Pasta primavera: cooked pasta tossed with lightly cooked vegetables, with or without Parmesan cheese

Vegetable risotto: arborio rice, cooked in vegetable broth and combined with cooked vegetables and perhaps cooked beans or nuts, with or without grated cheese

Eggplant parmesan: sliced eggplant prepared by dipping it into a mixture of eggs and milk, coating it with bread crumbs and Parmesan cheese, and sautéeing it; serve with tomato sauce

Pasta e fagioli: pasta and white bean "stew" seasoned with herbs; usually prepared without meat

Mexico

Bean burrito: vegetarian refried beans wrapped in a soft tortilla, with or without cheese topping

Chiles relleños: poblano peppers stuffed with cheese, dipped in an egg batter, and baked or fried; if they're fried, they're high in fat

Huevos rancheros (Mexican eggs): scrambled eggs prepared with onions and served with tomato salsa, vegetarian refried beans, and tortillas

Vegetable fajitas: stir-fried vegetables and perhaps tofu rolled in a soft tortilla; often served with guacamole

Middle East

Falafel sandwich: ground chickpea patties (fried) tucked in pita bread with lettuce shreds and chopped tomato, topped with tahini (sesame seed spread)

Tabouli: salad made with bulgur, tomatoes, parsley, mint or chives, lemon juice, and perhaps cooked white beans

Ful: brown bean casserole made with tomatoes, lemons, parsley, and eggs

Mujadarah: lentils and rice seasoned with cumin, onions, and lemon

Native American Southwest

Maricopa bean stew: stew made of corn, beans, and cholla buds

South America

Ochos rios: kidney beans and rice flavored with shredded coconut

Spain

Tortilla à la española (Spanish omelet): egg omelet made with potatoes, onions, and other vegetables

Vegetable paella: saffron-flavored rice dish with tomatoes and other vegetables

Switzerland

Cheese fondue: cheese melted with wine and served with chunks of crusty bread

Raclette: cheese "scraped" from a melted piece of hard cheese, then spread on a boiled potato or dark bread

Fast Food, Healthful Food

Dependence on quick meals goes back thousands of years. In the Roman Forum more than two thousand years ago, urban consumers ate sausages and honey cakes. The Chinese ate stuffed buns in the twelfth century. Five hundred years ago, Spaniards encountered tacos in the markets of today's Mexico.

Quick service, or fast food, has been part of American food culture for many more years than most people realize. If your great-grandparents traveled by train in the early 1900s, they likely devoured quick meals, or fast food, from the dining car. When the automobile took over, the dining-car concept was reinvented as fast-food restaurants dotted the roadside. Eating in the car isn't new; the popular drive-in restaurant of the 1950s evolved into the drive-through window.

As known today, the so-called fast-food chain, or quick-service restaurant, is a phenomenon that's only about sixty years old, launched for a post–World War II, fast-oriented, mobile society. At that time, eating out also became more than an occasional treat. At the start, fast food was limited to mainly fried chicken, hamburgers, French fries, ice cream, shakes, and soft drinks.

Today's fast-food menus offer many "fast" options. From grilled chicken sandwiches, paninis, wraps, and broiled fish, to main dish salads, to low-fat and fat-free milk and fruit smoothies, you have plenty to choose from, including lower-calorie, lower-fat, and fresh menu items. Pizza, seafood, pasta, Tex-Mex food, stuffed baked potatoes, noodles, and deli items along with quick ethnic cuisine are commonly found. Breakfast also is big fast-food business. Even convenience stores where you gas up your car sell fast food—truly the "dining car" of the highway! And mobile truck restaurants with "street food" bring more food variety—often ethnic—to changing locations!

Because fast-food menus and portion sizes are varied, no overall comment can describe their nutritional value. Traditional meals—a large burger, large fries, a fried fruit turnover, and a regular soft drink, or fried chicken, a biscuit, creamy slaw, and mashed potatoes with gravy—remain high in calories and fat, including solid fats, and sodium, but low in vitamins A and C, calcium, and fiber, and short on fruits, vegetables, whole grains, and often dairy foods. In addition, many

Have You Ever Wondered **?**

. . . how to feel comfortable when you dine alone? Any discomfort from eating alone shouldn't make you skip a meal. In reality, you're likely the only one who notices that you're a solo diner. If you feel conspicuous, ask for a table off to the side. Take an avid interest in your surroundings. Talk with the server; study the menu and the decor. While you wait, be productive: Read, make notes on your to-do list, do a little office work, or simply reflect on your day. Once your meal is served, put down your book, turn off your handheld device, or put work away; eat slowly and savor the flavors. When you're traveling and truly need to wind down and be alone, choose a hotel with room service!

. . . what spa cuisine is? Although the term isn't regulated, spa cuisine often refers to health-positioned food preparation, perhaps in resorts or health club cafés. On a menu that offers spa cuisine you may find foods with fewer calories, more fruits, vegetables, and fiber-rich grains, or perhaps smaller portions. Like any cuisine, ask about the menu; order with consumer savvy.

of today's fast-food restaurants also offer more vegetables and fruits; grilled or broiled chicken or fish; whole-grain breads; low-fat and fat-free milk; smaller portions; and much more.

Fast-Food Pointers

If you're a fast-food regular, keep these pointers in mind. Check the calorie and nutrient information of fast-food items to identify the healthiest choices. You'll find this information on the restaurant's website and often posted on the menu board, near the counter, on a tray liner, in a pamphlet, or even on the receipt.

Watch Your Portions

● Choose the right-size portion for you. Fast-food portions may be larger than you need; "deluxe," "super," and "mega" are typically different sizes of "big." Whether it's a sandwich, fries, a shake, or another option, bigger portions mean more calories and likely more fat, cholesterol, added sugars, and sodium. For most people, the small or regular size is enough.

● Choose smaller portions of side items and snacks. A large order of fries and a large soft drink can add up to a hefty 650 or more calories!

● Split your order. Halve the calories, and double the pleasure. Share your fries or sandwich with a friend!

● Think before you buy. Order takers often promote with marketing questions such as "Would you like fries with that?" or "Do you want the value size?" Just say "No, thank you" if you don't want any particular item or items.

● Before you order, decide if the "value meal" is a good deal. If you don't need the extra food, there's no extra value; smaller may cost less. Sharing may be a better deal.

Order More Food Variety

● Consider the other foods you eat during the day. Try to fill in your own food group gaps. This is a great time for low-fat or fat-free milk!

● Order fruits, vegetables, calcium-rich foods, and even whole grains when you can.

● Select a side of salad or raw vegetables for added vitamins A and C and for fiber. Boost your calcium intake with reduced-fat, low-fat, or fat-free milk.

● Try different types of fast foods, not the same foods every time.

Eating and Driving: A Safety Issue?

When time is short, many people assume that the fastest food comes from the drive-up window. Not so. Many times the wait in a drive-through line is longer than that for counter service. Beyond that, eating or sipping while driving not only can be messy, it's also dangerous when one hand is on the wheel and the other hand is holding a burger or a steaming hot beverage. If the cell phone rings or a text message comes in at the same time, you really may be in trouble!

If you do eat in the car, pull over in a parking lot or a city park, or by the curb. Then enjoy those few minutes of eating without thinking about driving, too. Better yet, relax with your food in a mall or on a park bench. Then take a brisk walk.

● Enjoy fast-food outlets that serve ethnic foods: perhaps Chinese stir-fry dishes, a Mexican burrito, Japanese domburi, or a vegetable-stuffed pita with cucumber-yogurt dressing. Often food courts in shopping malls allow you to travel the world of flavor without leaving home. In the search for variety, portion sizes and calories still count!

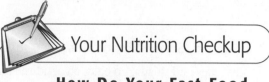 **Your Nutrition Checkup**

How Do Your Fast-Food Meals Stack Up?

Reflect on your last fast-food meal or snack. What did you order? Take a moment to rate your choices. Did you . . .

Yes No

☐ ☐ Order the regular size: burgers, fries, shakes, and drinks?

☐ ☐ Ask for whole grain: whole-wheat and other whole-grain buns or bread?

☐ ☐ Make it a single: single meat patty, no bacon?

☐ ☐ Layer on veggies: lettuce, tomato, bell peppers, shredded carrots, and more on burgers and sandwiches?

☐ ☐ Lighten the spread: less, or no, mayonnaise or sauce?

☐ ☐ Go for grilled: grilled (not fried or breaded) chicken sandwich (same for a fish sandwich)?

☐ ☐ Swap: a side salad, fruit, or baked potato instead of fries or onion rings?

☐ ☐ Substitute: water, 100 percent juice, or fat-free or low-fat milk rather than regular soda or sugar-sweetened tea?

☐ ☐ Order a sweet and healthy ending: fruit or low-fat frozen yogurt rather than a fruit pie or a sundae?

The best fast-food meals or snacks for you depend on you—your needs, your health, and your overall food choices for the day. Tips in this chapter can help you make better choices for your overall health—especially if you're a fast-food regular!

TOTAL: Nine "yes" answers add up to nine ways to make fast-food eating healthier!

Fast Food: Beyond Burgers

If you're in a fast-food rut, look around for some quick and different approaches to fast-food eating:

- Sushi bar
- Wrap restaurant
- Noodle shop
- Submarine sandwich spot
- Bakery-shop deli

Trim the Calories, Solid Fats, and Added Sugars

- In sandwiches and salads, go easy on condiments, special sauces, and dressings. One packet of mayonnaise (about 1 tablespoon) adds about 60 calories and 5 fat grams. The same size packet of tartar sauce has about 70 calories and 8 fat grams. And a 1½-ounce packet of French dressing contains about 185 calories and 17 fat grams. Ask for mustard, catsup, salsa, or low-fat or fat-free condiments, spreads, and dressings (mayonnaise, sour cream, or cream cheese).

- For fried foods, pay attention to the oil used for frying. Most fast-food chains use 100 percent vegetable oil, which may be identified on the menu. Vegetable oil is cholesterol-free and high in polyunsaturated fatty acids.

- Better yet, choose fried foods only as "sometimes" foods. Rely mostly on grilled, broiled, steamed, or microwaved fast foods instead.

- Go for the fruit cup; skip the fruit pie.

Lighten Up on Salt

Fast foods can be high in sodium. For less salt and sodium, ask for unsalted fries. Limit special sauces, pickles, olives, relish, bacon, sausage, ham, and deli meat. Taste before salting fries.

Break-FAST

With the more hectic pace today, more people buy breakfast on the run: a quick breakfast sandwich from the drive-up window; a sit-down meal of eggs and hash browns, or pancakes from the fast-food counter; or coffee latte and a deli muffin or a bagel to eat at the desk. When these quick breakfasts become a regular eating pattern, it's time to take stock of their nutritional impact!

Because fast-food restaurants usually offer fewer options for breakfast than for lunch and dinner, it's challenging to find healthier options. Many breakfast choices are high in calories, fat including solid fats, cholesterol, added sugars, and sodium.

For a Healthful, Quick Breakfast

- Order the fastest breakfast of all: ready-to-eat cereal with fat-free or low-fat milk. Cereal delivers starches (complex carbohydrates), B vitamins, iron, and almost no fat. A whole-grain or bran cereal provides fiber, too. And an 8-ounce carton of milk supplies about 300 milligrams of calcium, or about 25 to 30 percent of the calcium you need daily. Pour some on your cereal, perhaps some in your coffee or tea, and drink the rest!

- Order oatmeal. Top it with raisins, dried fruit, and a handful of nuts. Oatmeal is a whole grain!

- Look for other options: perhaps fruit, yogurt, and a small bagel. At a deli? Ask for yogurt to go with your bagel and juice. An 8-ounce carton of low-fat fruit yogurt supplies about 315 milligrams of calcium, 225 calories, and just 2 to 3 fat grams. Or order a fruit cup.

- Order 100 percent fruit juice as your breakfast beverage. With an 8-ounce carton of orange juice, you'll get more than 100 percent of the vitamin C you need in a day.

For Bakery Items

- Order an English muffin, bagel, toast, or plain, soft-baked pretzel. Doughnuts, sweet rolls, and croissants can deliver a lot of solid fats and added sugars.

- For bakery items, order small (small bagels and muffins) or share. Large muffins can be higher in calories or fat than you'd think. A typical 2-ounce muffin has about 5 fat grams—10 to 15 fat grams or more if it's jumbo-size! A large bakery bagel can count as 6 ounces (and 500 calories) from the grain group, enough for the day; eat half, save the rest for later.

- Biscuits and gravy? Skip the gravy; use a light, soft spread instead.

- Ask for spreads—cream cheese, margarine, jam, or jelly—on the side; then spread it lightly. Or ask for a low-fat cream cheese or margarine spread.

For Breakfast Sandwiches and Eggs

A typical bacon, egg, and cheese biscuit sandwich has about 440 calories, 24 fat grams, and 1,250 milligrams of sodium. A breakfast (bean and cheese) burrito has about 375 calories and 12 fat grams, yet 1,170 milligrams of sodium.

● Skip bacon or sausage on your breakfast sandwich. Or substitute ham or Canadian bacon for less fat.

● Order your sandwich on a whole-grain English muffin, bagel, or even a hamburger bun, whole grain if available. A typical fast-food breakfast biscuit can have about 18 fat grams and a croissant about 10 fat grams, compared to 1 fat gram in an English muffin.

● Try a breakfast burrito to fit beans in. Go easy on cheese.

● If you're a fast-food regular, ease up on egg entrées. A two-egg breakfast has about 370 milligrams of cholesterol (about 185 milligrams of cholesterol per 1 large egg). The 2010 Dietary Guidelines advises consuming fewer than 300 milligrams of cholesterol per day from all sources. Since cholesterol is only in the yolk, ask for an omelet or scrambled eggs made with egg whites only, or with 1 whole egg and 1 white, or ask for an egg substitute.

See "Breakfast on the Road" in this chapter for more tips.

Burgers, Chicken, or Fish?

Hamburgers may be America's all-time favorite fast food. But chicken and fish have gained a significant market share, in part because consumers perceive them as lower in calories and fat. Chicken and fish sometimes have a lean advantage. However, in fast-food preparation, breading, battering, and frying bump up the calorie and fat content significantly. A fried fish or fried chicken sandwich may supply more calories and fat than a burger!

For Hot Sandwiches

● Top all kinds of hot sandwiches—burgers, chicken, or fish—with tomato slices and other vegetables. If you're short on calcium, add cheese.

● For a fiber boost, ask for a whole-wheat bun if available.

● Cut calories by ordering sandwiches with no higher-fat condiments and special sauces, such as mayonnaise-based spreads and tartar sauce. Instead use mustard, relish, or ketchup. As a rule of thumb, calories go up with the number of extras.

● Skip the super-size or double-meat sandwich; go for the regular, junior, or single-size instead. The bigger size can about double everything, including the calories, fat, and sodium. A large hamburger, for example, can supply about 510 calories and 28 fat grams compared with 275 calories and 12 fat grams in a regular hamburger. Double patties are bigger still.

● Skip the bacon on a sandwich. While it adds flavor, bacon also boosts calories, solid fat, and sodium.

● Choose a grilled chicken sandwich most often. It has fewer calories and solid fats than breaded chicken.

For Fried Chicken

● Order "regular" rather than "extra-crispy," which soaks up more oil when cooked. The batter or the breading may have a high-sodium seasoning, too; lower the calories and sodium by removing the crust. Chicken nuggets are usually fried and may contain skin and meat (white and dark).

● Get a single-piece, rather than a two- or three-piece, order.

● Remove the crispy crust from fried chicken and the skin from rotisserie chicken. Poultry skin is high in fat.

For Fish

● Choose broiled, grilled, or baked fish and seafood if you have a choice. Be aware that the fillets on most fish sandwiches are battered and fried.

● Go easy on tartar sauce. Ask for tomato-based cocktail sauce instead. Better yet, just use a squeeze of lemon, which has no added sodium.

Deli Sandwiches and Wraps

Sandwiches, subs, and wraps, as well as yogurt, fruit, salads, soups, bagels and muffins, milk, flavored waters, coffee, and tea—the deli sells an array. But sandwiches take center stage. The great thing is that you often can order a deli sandwich just as you want it!

● *Bread:* Choose a whole-grain bread, roll, or pita pocket for more fiber. Get a sandwich "wrap" in a soft tortilla. Or try a thin-sliced bagel, flatbread, or herbed foccacia.

● *Spread:* Choose a spread that adds flavor, such as mustard, light mayonnaise, or fat-free dressing. To control fat and calories, ask the server to go easy on higher-fat spreads.

● *Filling:* With 2 to 3 ounces of lean meat or poultry, contribute protein, iron, and other nutrients.

  ● For less fat, order lean roast beef, ham, chicken breast, or turkey. Some delis use meats that are 90 percent or more fat-free. Ask.

  ● Request tuna, ham, or egg salad made with less mayonnaise or with reduced-fat or fat-free dressing if possible.

  ● Add a slice of cheese, perhaps low-fat, to boost the calcium content.

  ● Layer on vegetables—red or green peppers, jalapeños, tomatoes, sprouts, cucumbers, carrot shreds, onions, or grilled veggies. They're low in fat and supply vitamins A and C, fiber, and other nutrients.

  ● Enjoy wrap fillings that typically are low in fat. They may be brown or white rice blended with seafood, shredded chicken, or vegetables, or grilled vegetables and chicken breast.

● *Sides:* To cut down on fat, ask for carrot or green pepper sticks rather than chips or creamy slaw. For less sodium, enjoy a cucumber spear instead of a pickle.

For large sandwiches, subs, and wraps, buy one to share. Or keep half in the fridge for the next day.

Pizza—as You Like It!

Pizza is nutritious fast food. Pizza provides nutrition benefits from three or more food groups. The crust supplies starches and B vitamins, the cheese is a good source of calcium and protein, and the tomato sauce and vegetable toppings add vitamins A and C, potassium, and phytonutrients. Meat or seafood toppers add protein, iron, and some vitamins, too. Yet it's easy to consume too many slices in one meal.

Be Your Own Pizza Architect

Control the toppings and the type of crust, along with the nutrient and calorie content and the flavor, of the pizza you order:

● Consider the crust. For more fiber, build your pizza on a whole-wheat crust. To trim the calories, order a thin-crust pizza rather than a thick-crust or deep-dish pizza. A stuffed-crust pizza can have considerably more calories and fat than a thinner-crust pizza. For example, 1 slice of a large stuffed-crust pizza may have 20 fat grams or more, and 450 calories or more.

● Top with vegetables and even fruit. Again it may offer a nutrient and fiber boost, perhaps with fewer calories than from some other toppings. Some pizza parlors offer vegetables, such as artichoke hearts, broccoli florets, eggplant, red bell peppers, asparagus spears, shredded carrots, and pineapple chunks as well as mushrooms, sun-dried tomatoes, onions, and green peppers. *Check out "Pizza Toppings" below for lower-calorie choices.*

● Limit higher-fat toppings—bacon, pepperoni, prosciutto, sausage, and extra cheese. If you like higher-

---

PIZZA TOPPINGS

ENJOY MORE OFTEN			ENJOY LESS OFTEN
Artichoke hearts	Crabmeat	Pineapple chunks	Anchovies
Beans (legumes)	Eggplant slices	Shrimp	Bacon
Bell peppers	Green onions, chopped	Spinach	Extra cheese
Broccoli florets	Jalapeño peppers	Tomato slices	Olives
Canadian bacon or lean ham	Lean ground meat	Tuna or salmon	Pepperoni
Chicken	Mushroom slices	Zucchini slices	Prosciutto
	Onion slices		Sausage

fat toppings, stick with one. These foods add sodium, too. Many combination or deluxe pizzas have several high-fat toppings.

● Choose a lean protein topping: chicken, lean ham, Canadian bacon, tuna, salmon, shrimp, or beans (legumes).

● Want more flavor? Sprinkle on hot pepper flakes or herbs for no calories but lots of flavor. Enjoy wood-oven-baked pizza, or pizza with a regional twist: perhaps a Southwest pizza; a Cajun-style pizza; or a Hawaiian pizza with pineapple and lean ham.

● Go halfsies. Order half the pizza your way if someone else prefers toppings with more fat. In that way you both get what you want.

Pizza: Size Wise

● Order a reasonably sized pizza. Limit yourself to two or three slices—or just one slice if you're really watching calories. Calories from any pizza, even a veggie pizza, add up! A typical slice—an eighth of a 12-inch thin-crust meat and cheese pizza—supplies about 185 calories.

● If a bigger size is the better deal, wrap the extra before you start eating. Store it in the fridge. You'll enjoy your pizza again—and save time making or buying lunch—the next day. Leftover pizza is great for breakfast, too!

● Order a salad to complement your pizza. Salad not only adds nutrients and fiber, it also helps you fill up. You may be less likely to eat another pizza slice.

On the Side

Food variety adds nutrients, so round out your fast-food meal with veggies, fruit, and calcium-rich foods—perhaps a salad, baked potato, carrot sticks, fruit, 100 percent fruit juice, low-fat or fat-free milk, or frozen yogurt. Get the most nutrition mileage from the options you have.

Spuds

● Order a baked potato, mashed potatoes, or baked sweet potato rather than fries as a side dish, or even as an entrée—if you have the option. Served plain, a baked potato is fat-free and cholesterol-free, with almost no sodium. It also supplies complex carbohy-drates including fiber, vitamin C, and other vitamins and minerals.

● Go easy on higher-fat toppings—bacon, sour cream, and butter. For more nutrients and usually fewer calories and fat, top with broccoli, salsa, or cottage cheese. Chili as a topping? The calories and fat content depend on the ingredients; check nutrition information on the menu. Along with a salad and milk, a broccoli-cheese spud or a chili spud make a nutritious meal!

● For mashed potatoes, ask for gravy on the side to control how much you add. Gravy is high in calories! Find out how mashed potatoes with gravy are prepared, such as with butter; check the nutrition information if it's posted.

● Ask for a small, not a large, order of fries to limit calories and fat, especially in an already higher-fat meal. Then share. French fries provide some vitamin C. Sweet potato fries supply beta carotene (vitamin A).

● As an alternative to fries, fried onion rings, fried okra, and hush puppies, order corn on the cob, green beans, or baked beans. For corn, ease up on butter and salt.

Salads

● Order a garden salad with dressing on the side. Use reduced-fat or fat-free dressing if you have a choice. *For salad bar tips see "Sizing Up Salad and Other Food Bars" in this chapter.*

● Go easy on prepared salads with a lot of mayonnaise or salad dressing, such as creamy coleslaw, potato salad, or macaroni salad. They have more fat than salads with a vinaigrette dressing, such as coleslaw or three-bean salad.

● Order raw veggies or fruit chunks, or whole fruit if you can.

● Enjoy flavorful entrée salads (easy on the dressing) from most fast-food chains.

Beverages

● Make beverages count! For flavor and nutrients, round out your meal with low-fat or fat-free milk or 100 percent juice. For a flavor switch, try chocolate or other flavored milk; ask if it can be low-fat or fat-free.

● An 8-ounce carton of milk supplies about 300 milligrams of calcium as well as protein, riboflavin, vitamin D, and other nutrients.

● An 8-ounce carton of 100 percent orange juice supplies 75 milligrams of vitamin C, which more than meets your daily need.

● Go easy on regular soft drinks. Reasonable amounts are okay sometimes for their fluids, food energy (calories), and enjoyment. Unlike milk or 100 percent juice, they don't, however, contribute other nutrients supplied. Large-size drinks can add up to a lot of calories: 150 for every 12 ounces of regular soft drinks, and 400 calories for a 32-ounce cup! Diet drinks supply essentially no calories—and no nutrients (except water); to reduce added sugars, they are good alternatives to regular soda.

● If you can fit their calories in your eating plan, order a small milk shake. In any flavor it's a good calcium source—if it's made from milk. *Be aware:* A 10-ounce strawberry shake contains about 320 calories; let it serve double duty, as both beverage and dessert. Super-size shakes, with their 18 ounces, may supply a hefty 575 calories. *Another option:* Ask to have your shake made with low-fat or fat-free milk, or fat-free ice cream, if possible.

● Go to a smoothie bar for a thick blend of juice, fruit, and perhaps yogurt. Consider size. A smoothie that's 20 ounces or more may supply more than you need, including calories! Some smoothies are made with fruit syrup that adds sugar, but not all the nutrients that fruit contains. Ask about the ingredients before ordering.

● For coffee and tea drinks, order a latte, cappuccino, or coffee or hot tea (chai) with low-fat or fat-free milk—and get the calcium and vitamin D benefits. Milk, rather than cream, is a calcium booster. Creamers are typically high in solid fats, too. *Remember:* Sweetened ice tea and many flavored coffee and tea drinks can be high in calories and have added sugars.

Opt for sugar-free syrup and unsweetened tea. If you don't want to substitute lower-calorie ingredients, order a small, not a large, drink.

● For an ideal thirst quencher, choose water. For added flavor, add a lemon wedge. Unless bottled, water is usually offered free as a customer service. Ask!

Desserts

● Go easy on fried fruit fritters or turnovers. Eat them only if they fit within your daily calorie and fat budget. They usually have more added sugars and solid fats than fruit.

● Check to see if fresh whole or cut-up fruit is available.

● For a cold dessert, enjoy frozen yogurt or a scoop of ice cream or sherbet. You may find low-fat versions on the menu. Either way, the small or kid's portion offers a taste without indulging.

● For fewer calories, go easy on fudge sauce, candy pieces or mix-ins, or syrup toppings. A little of these toppings goes a long way. Ask for cut-up or dried fruit, nuts, or granola instead.

Eating Out Ethnic Style

As a nation of mostly immigrants, the United States always has been home to ethnic cuisine. The real interest in foreign-themed restaurants grew in the 1960s with pizza parlors and Japanese tabletop cooking. From there, exposure to a variety of ethnic foods became more sophisticated. We added Mexican and more Asian flavors to our restaurant repertoire. Today, ethnic restaurants offer far more culinary diversity.

What ethnic cuisines are most popular? Italian, Mexican, and Chinese (Cantonese) are so mainstream that they're no longer considered ethnic. French and fine Italian cuisines have been upscale restaurant cuisines for years. Appreciation for ethnic flavors continues to grow, with Japanese (sushi), Thai, Vietnamese, Caribbean, Indo-Pakistani, Nuevo Latino, and Middle Eastern restaurants among the many to enjoy. From every corner of the globe, urban areas offer even more ethnic flavors!

For fun, find the restaurant websites in your locale. Now count. How many different ethnic cuisines could

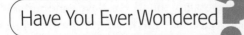

Have You Ever Wondered

. . . about herbal mix-ins in smoothies? Bee pollen, ginseng, and other herbal mix-ins may cost extra in smoothies, yet not offer the benefits you think. *See "Herbals and Botanicals: Help or Harm?" in chapter 23.*

you enjoy? To expand the variety in your eating style, try a new cuisine the next time you eat out!

Remember, the calorie and nutrient content, even for the same menu item from different restaurants, differs! That includes the fat, sodium, and added sugar content.

Italian . . . Not Just Pizza and Pasta!

With foods from every region, Italian foods are simple, flavorful, and nourishing. And they're not just pizza and pasta! The cuisine relies on small meat and seafood portions. Cheese is used to flavor many dishes. The pasta, risotto (rice dish), polenta (cornmeal dish), and crusty bread deliver complex carbohydrates (starches). Salads are among the typical ways in which veggies fit in.

Particularly with the foods of southern Italy, olive oil is the primary cooking fat, in contrast to butter, used in many northern Italian dishes. High in heart-healthier monounsaturated fatty acids, olive oil has nutritional benefits. Regardless, go easy; any oil is still fat, with the same number of calories per ounce as margarine and butter. *See "Take Your Taste Buds to the Mediterranean" in chapter 10.*

When you eat out in an Italian restaurant:

● Enjoy crusty Italian bread—a slice or two, but not the whole basket! For less fat, go easy on butter or on olive oil for dipping, or enjoy the flavor of fresh bread as it is, without a spread. *Hint:* Garlic bread usually is lathered in high-fat spreads, Parmesan cheese, and garlic before it arrives at your table. Plain bread is a lower-calorie, lower-fat choice.

● Go easy on antipasto. "Antipasto" means "before the pasta." It usually refers to a variety of hot or cold appetizers. In the Italian tradition, they include cheese, olives, smoked meats, and marinated vegetables and fish. While they're nutritious, some may be high in calories and sodium. Nibbling appetizers, followed by a heavy meal, may add up to more calories than you expect.

● Order a fresh garden salad, or insalata, to round out your meal, with salad dressing, perhaps herbed vinegar and olive oil, served on the side. Salads in Italian restaurants often are tossed with a variety of raw vegetables and mixed greens, including arugula,

Have You Ever Wondered ⍰

. . . what "primavera" and "fresco" on menus mean? Translated from Italian, "primavera" means "spring style." In cooking terms it refers to dishes prepared with raw or lightly cooked fresh vegetables. "Fresco" means fresh.

radicchio, bell peppers, tomatoes, and onions. As an entrée, salad with bread makes a nice, light meal.

● Look for traditional bean and vegetable dishes. Minestrone is a hearty, tomato-based soup with beans, vegetables, and pasta. White beans, called fagioli, are featured in soups, pasta fagioli, and risotto (rice dishes). Florentine dishes are prepared with spinach.

● Know menu lingo. For example, dishes described as fritto (fried) or crema (creamed) are higher in fat. Primavera refers to dishes prepared with fresh vegetables and herbs. Sometimes primavera dishes are served with a creamy sauce; ask your server.

● For enjoyment, order different types of pasta dishes—in shapes and sizes you may not find on supermarket shelves. Made of flour and water, pasta is a carbohydrate-rich food. Fat, and perhaps higher calories, come from the sauces and other ingredients tossed with pasta.

Did you know that a tomato-based sauce usually has fewer calories than a creamy white pasta sauce or a pesto sauce? Look for marinara and other tomato-based sauces that usually have more vegetables and fewer calories and less fat, too, than creamy white sauces such as alfredo and carbonara. *See "Gourmet's Guide to Sauces" in this chapter.*

● For polenta, gnocchi, or risotto, ask how they're made before ordering.

● *Polenta*, similar to a cornmeal mush, typically is served with sauce, vegetables, and meat; some ingredients may have more fat.

● *Gnocchi*, usually made from potatoes or flour, means dumplings. Sometimes eggs, cheese, or chopped vegetables are mixed into the dough. After they're cooked in boiling water they may be baked or fried, then served with a flavorful sauce.

● *Risotto*, typically made from arborio rice, usually is cooked in broth and perhaps butter, often with meat, seafood, cheese, and vegetables. Be aware that the broth may be salty.

● For another option, order ravioli, or square "pillows" of pasta filled with meat, seafood, cheese, or vegetables. Usually they're served with a sauce. Ask about preparation before you order; as appetizers, they may be fried.

● To watch calories and fat, go easy on veal scaloppini, and chicken or veal parmigiana, which are sautéed or pan-fried. Parmigiana entrées—made with Parmesan cheese—also are breaded, so they absorb more fat. As an alternative and a lower-fat option, order chicken or veal cacciatore, marsala, or piccata. Cacciatore is a tomato-based sauce; marsala is broth-based and cooked with wine; and piccata is pan drippings, lemon juice, and chopped parsley.

From the Italian Menu

Enjoy more often:

● Minestrone soup

● Pasta fagioli
● Roasted peppers
● Garden salad
● Bread sticks
● Vinegar and oil dressing
● Pasta with red sauce, such as marinara
● Cacciatore, piccata, and marsala dishes
● Cappuccino (Ask your server to have it made with fat-free or low-fat milk.)
● Italian fruit ice or fruit

Enjoy less often:

● Antipasto plates
● Fried croutons
● Buttered garlic bread
● Creamy Italian dressing
● Pasta with butter or white sauce such as alfredo or carbonara
● Italian sausage and prosciutto
● Parmigiana and scallopine dishes
● Tiramisu

POPULAR ITALIAN FARE: FITTING WITHIN THE FOOD GROUPS

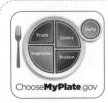
ChooseMyPlate.gov

Grains
Bread sticks
Gnocchi (dumpling)
Italian bread
Polenta (cornmeal mush)
Risotto (rice specialty)
Spaghetti, linguini, other pasta

Vegetables
Artichokes
Beans (white kidney, fava, garbanzo)*
Bell peppers
Eggplants
Grape leaves

Greens
Mushrooms
Tomatoes, tomato sauces
Spinach

Fruits
Dates
Figs
Grapefruit
Grapes
Olives
Oranges
Pomegranates
Dried fruits

Dairy
Cheese: mozzarella, pecorino, ricotta, others
Gelato

Milk
Yogurt

Protein Foods
Beef
Chicken
Fish (anchovies, tuna, others)
Beans (white kidney, fava, garbanzo)*
Nuts (pine nuts, almonds)
Sausage, proscuitto, ham
Shellfish (clams, shrimp, calamari)
Veal

Oils
Olive oil
Oils in nuts, olives, anchovies, tuna, other oily fish

*Beans (legumes) fit in either food group, vegetables or protein foods.

● Cannoli (Cannoli, cannelloni, and cannellini often get mixed up. Cannoli are deep-fried pastry shells filled with ricotta cheese or whipped cream and perhaps chocolate bits, nuts, and candied fruit. Cannelloni are pasta tubes filled with meat and cheese and topped with sauce. Cannellini are white kidney beans.)

It's Greek Food to Me!

Another popular Mediterranean cuisine is Greek food. For many people, experience with Greek restaurants comes from fast-food courts in shopping malls. The popular gyros (sandwich), souvlaki, Greek salad, rice pilaf, moussaka, and baklava are best known. Like other cuisines, full-service restaurants offer far more variety. To order smarter, consider these menu tips:

● For a creamy dressing on salads, or a sauce on pita sandwiches, enjoy tzatziki. It's made with yogurt, garlic, and cucumbers. Sometimes tzatziki is listed on the menu as a salad. Try tzatziki as an appetizer dip with pita bread, too. Watch the amount!

● Enjoy small amounts of baba ghanouj, a higher-fat dip with eggplant and olive oil, and of hummus with mashed chickpeas and sesame seed paste.

● Flavorful olive oil for dipping often is served with a basket of pita bread. Again, go easy. Although high in monounsaturated fat, low in saturated fat, and cholesterol-free, olive oil contains just as much fat as butter or margarine. Bread can soak up a lot of oil!

● Ordering saganaki as an appetizer? Saganaki is thick kasseri cheese that's fried and sometimes flamed in brandy. For fewer calories and less fat, share with someone.

● For nutritious fast food, order pita bread stuffed with Greek salad, lean meat, tabouli, or other ingredients. Tabouli is bulgur wheat mixed with chopped tomatoes, parsley, mint, olive oil, and lemon juice. For more fiber ask for whole-wheat pita. Another popular use of pita is the gyro, which is minced lamb molded and roasted vertically. When cooked, lamb is sliced and tucked into pita bread with grilled onions, bell peppers, and tzatziki sauce.

● As a main dish, look for broiled and grilled meat, poultry, and seafood: perhaps shish kebob, which is skewered and broiled meat and vegetables; souvlaki, which is lamb marinated in lemon juice, olive oil, and herbs, then skewered and grilled; or plaki, or fish broiled with tomato sauce and garlic.

● Try dolmades, or stuffed vegetables. Grape leaves are commonly stuffed with ground meat; other vegetables, such as bell peppers, cabbage leaves, eggplant, and squash, are stuffed with mixtures of ground meat, rice, dried fruit, and pine nuts. Because they're steamed or baked, fat usually isn't added with cooking.

● To boost fiber, order dishes made with beans (legumes). In a full-service restaurant you'll likely find mixed dishes and soups made with fava beans and other beans.

● Order a Greek salad with dressing on the side. Go easy on higher-fat, higher-sodium ingredients: anchovies, kalamata olives, and feta cheese.

● Go easy also on rich Greek desserts such as baklava. Made with phyllo and plenty of butter, honey or sugar, and nuts, this sweet, compact pastry is very high in calories, fat, and sugar. It tastes wonderful, but a small serving is enough to satisfy a sweet tooth!

From the Greek Menu

Enjoy more often:
- Broiled, grilled, simmered, or stewed dishes
- Greek salad
- Tabouli
- Dolmades
- Tzatziki
- Fresh fruit
- Pita bread
- Pita sandwiches

Enjoy less often:
- Pan-fried dishes
- Vegetable pies such as spanakopita and tyropita
- Baba ghanouj (Middle Eastern dish on some Greek menus)
- Baklava and phyllo pastry dishes
- Deep-fried falafel and calamari
- Gyro
- Moussaka and other creamy casseroles

Mexican Food: Tacos, Tamales, and More

From fast-food establishments to casual dining to full-service restaurants, Mexican food and its Tex-Mex offspring are among America's favorite ethnic foods. Mexican flavors now appear in pizzas, entrée salads, wraps, and stir-fries, too. The staples—tortillas, beans, and rice—are great sources of complex carbohydrates, and pinto or black beans supply protein and fiber as well. Moderate portions of meat and poultry contribute adequate amounts of protein. Beans and rice, or beans and tortillas, when eaten together, also supply high-quality protein.

Depending on the choices, Mexican or Tex-Mex cuisine can be high in fat—and sodium. In most restaurants, vegetable oil (no longer lard) is the fat used in cooking (except perhaps in refried beans). Cooked with vegetable oil, the solid fat may be lower than in the past, but not the calories or the total fat. As with foods of every culture, enjoy variety, but go easy on foods with more total fat, especially solid fats, cholesterol, and sodium.

● Order guacamole and sour cream on the side to control the amount. Or ask for low-fat or fat-free sour cream. For more vitamins A and C and potassium, use a heavy hand with tomato-based salsa. Made with tomatoes, onions, chiles, and herbs, it's virtually fat-free, yet bursting with flavor. So are the cilantro, hot sauce, and peppers!

● Ask for soft tacos. Crispy tacos and tostadas are deep-fried. Corn tortillas have a little less calories and fat than flour tortillas.

● Ordering a taco salad? Enjoy, but go easy on the big, crisp tortilla shell it's served in—or the taco chips on top—to trim calories and fat. Instead enjoy warmed, soft tortillas on the side. Dress the salad with salsa!

● Go easy on nachos and cheese, or chile con queso, especially if it's just your appetizer. To cut in half the calories and the solid fats from cheese, ask for half a ladle of cheese sauce, or half as much cheese shreds. For the starter of chips and salsa, enjoy one basket or less, then have it taken away if you can't resist, or skip the tortilla chip basket altogether.

● Order a low-fat appetizer in a cup (not a bowl): gazpacho (chilled tomato soup), jicama and salsa, tortilla soup, or black bean soup.

Mexican Menu Language

Learn to speak Mexican menu talk. Look for descriptions that offer clues to the fat content.

Menu clues—less fat and perhaps calories:

● Asada (grilled)
● Mole sauce (chile-chocolate sauce)
● Served with salsa verde (green chile sauce)
● Simmered
● Tomato sauce, picante
● Topped with lettuce and tomato
● Veracruz-style (tomato sauce)
● With chiles
● Wrapped in a soft tortilla

Menu clues—more fat and perhaps calories:

● Crispy
● Fried
● Layered with refried beans
● Mixed with chorizo (Mexican sausage)
● Served in a crisp tortilla basket
● Smothered in cheese sauce
● Topped with guacamole and sour cream
● Chile con queso

● Since portions in Mexican meals tend to be large, choose the regular plate, not the "deluxe combo" plate. For most people, the regular plate is plenty! To fill your plate, ask for more shredded lettuce and tomato instead.

● Choose mostly baked or stir-fried entrées such as enchiladas or fajitas with vegetables on a soft tortilla. Go easy on fried dishes such as chiles relleños, chimichangas, or flautas.

● Although tacos, tamales, enchiladas, and burritos are among the most popular items, especially in Tex-Mex restaurants, Mexican and Southwestern restaurants offer a far broader menu, especially in authentic restaurants. Check the menu for salads with nopales, or cactus pads; chayote and jicama, which are starchy vegetables; and tomatillos, or green tomatoes. For prepared foods look for Veracruz-style seafood dishes, which are cooked in a herbed tomato sauce; or chile verde, which is pork simmered with vegetables and green chiles.

● Want a margarita? "On the rocks" has fewer calories than "frozen." Skip the salt or sugar around the rim of the glass to reduce sodium or calories, respectively.

From the Mexican Menu

Enjoy more often:

- Jicama with fresh lime juice
- Salsa, pico de gallo
- Soft tacos
- Burritos, enchiladas, tamales, fajitas
- Red beans and rice*
- Spanish rice*
- Refried beans (no lard) or frijoles à la charra
- Steamed vegetables
- Black bean soup, menudo (spicy soup made with tripe and hominy), gazpacho
- Arroz con pollo (chicken with rice)
- Fajitas
- Taco salad (without sour cream; perhaps a few tortilla chips or strips instead of the taco shell)

- Fruit for dessert such as guava, papaya, or mango
- Flan, or pudding
- Grilled meat, poultry, fish

*The fat and calorie content varies depending on the ingredients and the preparation method.

Enjoy less often:

- Guacamole dip with taco chips
- Nachos with cheese sauce
- Sour cream and extra cheese
- Crispy, fried tortillas
- Crispy tacos
- Tostadas, chiles relleños, quesadillas, chimichangas, chalupas, flautas
- Refried beans (cooked in lard)
- Honey-sweetened pastry and sopapillas
- Chicharonnes (fried pork rinds)
- Fried ice cream
- Chorizo (sausage)
- Carnitas (fried pork or beef)

POPULAR MEXICAN FARE: FITTING WITHIN THE FOOD GROUPS

ChooseMyPlate.gov

Grains
Posole (soup made with corn kernels)
Rice
Sopa (thick rice soup)
Taco shells
Tortillas, flour and corn

Fruits
Avocados
Mangoes
Papayas
Platanos (cooking bananas)
Zapotes (sweet yellow fruit)

Vegetables
Beans and peas (pigeon peas, garbanzos, black, kidney, red beans)*
Chayote
Corn
Jicama
Nopales
Peppers
Refried beans*
Salsa
Tomatoes
Tomatillos

Dairy
Coffee con leche (with milk)
Flan (custard)
Jack cheese

Leche (milk)
Queso blanco (cheese)

Protein Foods
Beans and peas (pigeon peas, garbanzos, black, kidney, red beans)*
Beef
Chicken
Chorizo sausages
Eggs
Fish
Shrimp
Refried beans*

Oils
Corn oil
Vegetable oil

*Beans (legumes) fit in either food group, vegetables or protein foods.

Chinese Fare

Chinese cuisine, complex and highly developed, contributes significantly to the world's food experiences. With its focus on vegetables, rice, and noodles, Asian-style cooking has earned its place as a nutritious option for healthful eating.

The cuisine represents many cooking styles, ingredients, and flavorings from China's many regions. Restaurants may specialize in foods from Canton, Hunan, Peking (Beijing), Shanghai, or Szechuan. Cantonese-style cooking is the most popular in the United States, largely due to Cantonese immigrants in the mid-1800s who brought their cooking styles with them. Cantonese cuisine of southeastern China features roasted and grilled meat, steamed dishes, stir-fried dishes, and mild flavors. Szechuan and Hunan foods tend to be hot and spicy, and perhaps higher in fat. Peking cuisine, from northeastern China, is noted for skillful, subtle uses of seasonings. Shanghai-style has more seafood. The term "Mandarin" on menus usually refers to aristocratic cuisine, featuring the finest aspects of all regional cuisines.

Chinese meals emphasize rice or noodles, and vegetables, with their contribution of complex carbohydrates. Vegetables are good sources of fiber, beta carotene (which forms vitamin A) and vitamin C, and phytonutrients, too. Meat, poultry, and seafood are served in small portions, often sliced and cooked with vegetables. Tofu, or soybean curd, is a common, high-protein, low-fat, cholesterol-free ingredient. Many Chinese dishes are roasted, simmered, steamed, or stir-fried.

From a nutritional standpoint, Chinese cuisine can be high in fat and sodium. Deep-fat frying is a common cooking technique. Sometimes foods are stir-fried in large amounts of oil. For those who are sodium-sensitive, be aware of two ingredients with sodium—monosodium glutamate (MSG) and soy sauce, often used as a flavoring. MSG, however, has a third the sodium of table salt. *See "MSG—Another Flavor Enhancer" in chapter 7.*

Calcium-rich foods are limited on Chinese menus since milk, cheese, and yogurt aren't part of traditional cuisines. Most calcium comes from fish with edible bones and from vegetables such as broccoli and greens, although the amount of calcium per half cup portion is much lower than in eight ounces of milk.

Whether you eat in or carry out, keep these ordering tips in mind at a Chinese restaurant:

● Enjoy flavorful soup as a starter or a main dish. Many are made with clear broth with small amounts of meat and vegetables. Made by cooking eggs in the broth, egg drop soup and hot-and-sour soup are higher in cholesterol; the amount, however, is small, since there's not much egg in a single serving.

● Go easy on fried appetizers. Fried wontons, crab rangoon, and many egg rolls are deep-fat-fried. As an option, order steamed spring rolls, egg rolls, wontons, or dumplings.

● Enjoy the vegetable variety in Chinese dishes! Besides familiar bell peppers, broccoli, cabbage, carrots, chile peppers, green onions, mushrooms, and bean sprouts, Chinese dishes feature bamboo shoots, bok choy, lily pods, napa, snow peas, and other vegetables. Flip to the vegetarian section of the menu for dishes featuring tofu and beans (legumes).

● For less fat look for braised, roasted, simmered, steamed, and stir-fried dishes. Ask that stir-fried dishes be cooked in just a small amount of oil.

● Order plain rice and noodles rather than fried versions. Plain rice and noodles usually are lower in sodium than fried versions, which are flavored with soy sauce. Crispy skin on poultry dishes such as Peking duck is high in fat.

● Check the menu for steamed fare. Some Chinese restaurants offer dishes with your choice of protein food (chicken, shrimp, tofu), mixed with vegetables and sauce on the side.

● Be aware that the meat, poultry, or fish in sweet-and-sour dishes is typically breaded and deep-fat-fried. Instead, ask for roasted or grilled meat with sweet-and-sour sauce to cut down on fat.

● For less sodium, go easy on foods prepared with MSG, soy sauce, or high-sodium sauces such as black bean, Hoisin, and oyster sauce. Ask to have your dish prepared without high-sodium seasonings or sauces. You might ask for light or reduced-sodium soy sauce to add yourself. Or instead, choose dishes prepared with hot-mustard, sweet-and-sour, plum, or duck sauce, which have less sodium.

● For a small bite, enjoy dim sum. Translated as "little heart," these small portions include steamed dumplings and steamed spring rolls. Go easy on fried dim sum dishes. To order dim sum, you choose your dishes from a server, who passes your table with one dish after another. As a result, you can easily overeat!

● Enjoy your fortune cookie—and the fortune inside! A single cookie has just 15 calories and 0 grams of fat. Typically, Chinese meals don't give much attention to sweet desserts. Usually you can have ice cream, fresh fruit, or almond cookies.

● Control the urge to overeat. In Chinese restaurants portions are often quite ample. For a sit-down meal order the amount you need, not necessarily the meal "special" with several courses. Ask for half a portion if you can. Plan to share a dish; perhaps order two or three dishes to serve four people. Or take leftovers home. Skip popular Chinese buffets, or go easy.

From the Chinese Menu

Enjoy more often:

● Wonton soup, hot-and-sour soup
● Steamed spring rolls
● Chicken, scallops, or shrimp with vegetables
● Whole steamed fish
● Steamed rice (perhaps brown rice)
● Steamed dumplings and other dim sum
● Soft noodles
● Stir-fried dishes*
● Steamed and simmered dishes
● Tofu
● Fortune cookies

*If cooked in just small amounts of oil, they can be quite low in fat. Stir-fry dishes, however, can be quite oily (for example, lo mein).

Enjoy less often:

● Fried wontons

POPULAR CHINESE FARE: FITTING WITHIN THE FOOD GROUPS

Grains:
Fortune cookies
Dumplings (pot stickers, others)
Noodles
Rice
Rice noodles, rice sticks
Rice congee (rice soup)
Wonton or eggroll wrappers

Fruits
Guavas
Kumquats
Lychees
Oranges, mandarin oranges
Persimmons
Pineapples
Pummelos (large citrus fruit)

Vegetables
Asparagus
Baby corn
Bamboo shoots
Bean sprouts
Bell peppers
Bok choy
Broccoli
Carrots
Chives
Long beans
Mushrooms (straw, wood ear, others)
Napa cabbage
Pea pods
Tofu*
Water chestnuts

Dairy
Milk

Soy cheese (calcium-fortified)
Soy beverage (calcium-fortified)

Protein Foods
Beef
Cashews
Chicken
Eggs
Fish
Mung beans
Pork
Tofu*
Shellfish (shrimp, crab, lobster, scallops, octopus)

Oils
Peanut oil
Sesame oil
Vegetable (soybean) oil
Healthy oils from cashews, oily fish

*Beans (legumes) fit in either food group, vegetables or protein foods.

- Fried egg rolls or spring rolls
- Peking duck
- Fried fish with lobster sauce
- Fried rice
- Fried dim sum
- Fried noodles
- Fried "crispy" dishes, sweet-and sour dishes with breaded, deep-fried ingredients

Thai and Vietnamese Cuisine

For restaurant patrons who enjoy an Asian kitchen, "spicy hot" defines many Thai dishes. Although similar to Thai dishes, Vietnamese dishes are not known for spiciness. Both cuisines are noted for plenty of fruits, vegetables, rice, and noodles. Their unique flavors come from contrasting seasonings, unique herbs and spices, and fresh ingredients.

Rice is a staple that's simply cooked or enjoyed as an ingredient in rice noodles, rice flour, and rice "paper." Enjoy plain rice: long-grained jasmine rice with its perfumelike flavor; or sticky, plump rice. Try chopped, cooked vegetables, meat, seafood, or poultry, and fresh herbs, wrapped in moistened rice paper. Or order translucent rice noodles, tossed in salads and stir-fries. You'll find wheat flour noodles on the menu, too.

Vegetables and fruits add flavor, nutrients, and interest to Thai salads, soups, and mixed dishes. Look for dishes made with less familiar fruits and vegetables such as bamboo shoots, banana blossoms, bananas, bitter melons, green mangoes, pomelos, or straw mushrooms, as well as the familiar: cucumbers, bean sprouts, eggplant, green peppers, or snow peas. For Asian cuisine Thai restaurants are unique because you can order a salad, which is often a cooked salad.

In these dishes of mixed ingredients, meat, poultry, and seafood portions are reasonable. Look for all kinds of seafood, including shrimp, mussels, and scallops, as well as beef, pork, chicken, and duck.

Meatless dishes may feature tofu or egg, or combinations of noodles or rice, and vegetables. Popular pad Thai (with noodles, sprouts, tofu, eggs, scallions, and peanuts) may be a good choice. *Ask:* Pad Thai can be high in fat, depending on preparation and portion size.

What's the special flavor in Thai cooking? Menu descriptions may identify a unique variety of herbs native to Thailand that add flavor but no sodium: coriander, ginger, galangal, kaffir lime leaves (citrus leaf), lemongrass, and Thai basil. Look for spices in curry dishes. Peanuts and cashews, common to Thai cooking, may add texture and flavor as well as protein. The distinctive flavors of Thai curries come from a blend of nam bla (Thai fish sauce) combined with chiles, garlic, and seasonings such as coriander, cumin, and turmeric in Indian-type curries, or gingerroot, lemongrass, and shrimp paste.

Small, green or red bird's eye chiles (*prik kii noo suan*) are viciously hot and distinctively Thai. But they aren't the only chiles used in Thai cooking. Check the menu for clues to the "heat." If you can't take the heat, ask for "toned-down Thai." Many dishes can be prepared to suit your taste.

Consider the nutritional bounty in Thai cuisine—especially because it can have fewer calories, less fat and sodium, and great flavor! Keep these points in mind:

- If you enjoy Thai food often, go easy on soups, curries, desserts, and other dishes made with a Thai staple: coconut milk or cream. The fat in regular coconut milk is highly saturated and high in calories. The popular satay (grilled chicken or meat skewers) usually is marinated in curried coconut milk and served with a sauce of peanuts and coconut milk. To control the amount, ask for the peanut sauce on the side.

- Look for stir-fried, sautéed, braised, grilled, and steamed dishes. In Thai cooking you'll also find deep-fried foods and heavy sauces. Go easy.

- Ask about the oil the kitchen uses. If it's lard or coconut oil, ask for stir-fried and sautéed dishes cooked in vegetable oil instead.

- Ask for a light touch with nam bla, a high-sodium sauce, and with soy sauce. Or see if they can use light (low-sodium) soy sauce instead.

- Go easy on dishes made with salty condiments such as salty eggs, dried shrimp, and fish paste. Ask to have MSG left out to further cut sodium.

If you pick a Vietnamese restaurant, the cuisine is similar, also based on rice, noodles, similar vegetables, seafood, and meat; order with the same mind-set. Vietnamese cuisine also is flavored with fish sauce but contains more fresh coriander root and leaf (cilantro) and less garlic and chile pepper.

From the Thai and Vietnamese Menu

Enjoy more often:

- Broth-based soups such as tom yum koong
- Spring rolls in moistened rice paper
- Stir-fried noodle dishes such as pad Thai (The fat and calorie content varies depending on the preparation method.)
- Stir-fried or sautéed vegetables with meat, poultry, fish, or tofu
- Broiled or steamed dishes
- Steamed rice, sweet sticky rice
- Tropical fruits and juices
- Grilled or charbroiled meat, chicken, or seafood
- Fruit ice
- Lychees

Enjoy less often:

- Soups made with coconut milk such as tom ka gai
- Fried spring rolls
- Peanut-coconut milk sauce
- Fried shrimp toast
- Dishes (including curries) made with coconut milk
- Deep-fried tofu or eggplant
- Dishes with deep-fried fish, duck, or meat
- Fried rice and fried noodles
- Fried bananas
- Desserts made with coconut milk such as coconut flan

Japanese Cuisine

Interest in Japanese-style restaurants started with the Japanese steakhouse. There, Americans experienced the flair of tabletop, stir-fry cooking, seated around the grill. In either full-service or fast-food restaurants, today's Japanese menu offers more variety—and plenty of sushi!

With its use of rice, noodles, tofu, vegetables, seafood, and small meat portions as staples, and lim-ited use of oils, Japanese cooking is noted for being low in fat. Glazes and sauces typically are made with ingredients that are low in fat: broth, soy sauce, rice vinegar, and sake (rice wine). While some foods are fried, more common cooking methods are low in fat and include braising, broiling, grilling, simmering, and steaming. Rice, noodles, and vegetables contribute complex carbohydrates, and vegetables supply fiber, beta carotene, and vitamin C. Meat, poultry, seafood, and tofu are high-protein ingredients usually served in moderate-size portions. Calcium-rich foods are limited. For those trying to reduce sodium, high-sodium flavorings are a nutrition concern.

To the Japanese cook, artistry ranks as important as nourishment. Edible garnishes of ginger or vegetables, or seaweed carefully wrapped around raw fish and rice, or an artful food arrangement on a plate, are among the aesthetic touches that make Japanese food beautiful. Enjoyment of food has always been an important dietary guideline in the Japanese diet!

The language of a Japanese menu might be new to you. To sharpen your menu savvy:

- Know that tempura is a popular battered, fried dish. Agemono and katsu dishes also are breaded and fried. To control calories and fat, go easy on fried dishes, but don't avoid them altogether or you'll miss some outstanding taste treats! Just eat small portions, and balance these foods with other, lower-calorie and lower-fat choices.

- Look for menu terms that suggest less fat, such as *nimono* (simmered), *yaki* (broiled), and *yaki-mono* (grilled). Two examples for meat, poultry, or fish: yakitori, which is skewered, then grilled or broiled; and teriyaki, which is marinated in soy sauce and mirin (rice wine), then grilled.

- Looking for another low-fat choice? Try sashimi (raw fish) or sushi (vinegared, sweetened rice prepared with seaweed, raw fish, and/or vegetables). For less sodium, go easy on the soy sauce for dipping. *See "Is Raw Seafood Safe to Eat?" in chapter 13 for choosing a sushi restaurant and for advice to those who need to avoid raw fish.*

- As another bowl meal, try domburi, or rice covered with vegetables, meat, or poultry, and perhaps egg.

PASSPORT TO FLAVOR: SIX MORE ETHNIC CUISINES

When you eat out, try these cuisines for variety and adventure, too! Enjoy menu items with fewer calories more often. If you prefer a higher-calorie food, share or have a smaller portion.

ENJOY MORE OFTEN

Caribbean
- Beans and rice dishes
- Chicken and rice
- Grilled meat and chicken (jerk chicken or goat)
- Vegetable stews (callaloo)

Middle Eastern
- Bean and bulgur salad
- Cold yogurt soup
- Couscous
- Fatoosh (bread salad)
- Lamb and vegetable stew
- Rice and lentil/bean dishes

German
- Cooked cabbage
- Dumplings
- Potato salad with a sweet-sour dressing
- Roast pork (lean) with gravy on the side

French
- Broth-based fish soup (bouillabaisse)
- Demiglace, Bordelaise, and other wine sauces
- Poached fruit
- Provençal dishes (with tomatoes)
- Roasted or braised meat, poultry, or fish
- Salad greens with vinaigrette
- Steamed or sautéed vegetables
- Vegetable casserole (ratatouille)

Russian
- Boiled or baked dumplings (pelmeni)
- Broiled meat skewers (shaslyk)
- Kasha
- Meat-stuffed cabbage
- Whole-grain breads

Indo-Pakistani
- Baked roti (bread, such as naan), chapati
- Chicken or beef tikka (roasted with mild spices)
- Dishes prepared with yogurt
- Fragrant steamed rice
- Lassi (mango-yogurt smoothie)

ENJOY LESS OFTEN

- Fried fish
- Fritters (conch fritters)
- Fried plantain

- Baba ghanouj
- Fried chickpea cakes (falafel)
- Fried meat-bulgur patties (kibbeh)
- Rich pastries, often with honey (baklava)

- Breaded and fried meat and poultry (schnitzel)
- Creamy soup
- Noodle and cheese dishes
- Sausages
- Thick, creamy gravy

- Cheese
- Cream soups
- Creamy sauces (see *"Gourmet's Guide to Sauces"* in this chapter)
- Croissants
- Liver paté
- French fries (pommes frites), au gratin potatoes
- Rich desserts (mousse, Napoleon)
- Soups with gratinée (cheese)

- Blini
- Dishes made with sour cream gravy (stroganoff)
- Fried dumplings
- Salads with mayonnaise or sour cream
- Soups made with cream or sour cream (borscht)

- Dishes, such as curry dishes, made with coconut milk, coconut oil, or cream
- Fried bread (poori, paratha, pakora)
- Fried dishes (samosa, shami)
- Ghee (clarified butter)

410

ENJOY MORE OFTEN

Indo-Pakistani (continued)
- Lentil dishes, curries with vegetable or lentil sauce
- Papadum (lentil wafers)
- Rice pilaf with peas
- Roasted chicken or fish dishes with vegetable sauces; grilled kebobs
- Tandoori cooked chicken or fish

ENJOY LESS OFTEN

- Korma (meat dish with rich cream sauce)
- Sauced rice dishes

If you get even more adventuresome with new ingredients, new flavors, new cuisines, and new ways to fit nutrient-rich foods in, look for ethnic restaurants that are getting more attention these days: Nuevo Latino, Cuban, Peruvian, Malaysian, Korean, Spanish, North African (Moroccan), and Ethiopian. Or try regional American food, perhaps Cajun, Southwest, or California-style cuisine!

- To cut back on sodium, go easy on sauces such as soy sauce, miso sauce, or teriyaki sauce, as well as broth and pickled vegetables. Many dishes, such as soup, noodle dishes, and stir-fried dishes, also are flavored with soy sauce. Or instead, ask for dishes prepared without soy sauce—for example, shabu shabu, steamed seafood, or foods that aren't marinated; you can dip them in a low-sodium soy sauce if you choose. A little shredded or mashed green wasabi adds flavor, but no sodium. *Beware:* The very strong, hot-horseradish flavor of a little wasabi goes a long way!

- For more vegetables, order salad as a side dish. Try edamame (fresh, steamed soybeans, often in the pod). For less sodium, ask for a lemon slice to squeeze on top, rather than miso dressing. Miso, a common flavoring in Japanese cooking, is derived from fermented soybean paste and is high in sodium.

- Enjoy Japanese noodles—udon (wheat noodles) or soba (buckwheat noodles). Noodles often are served with cooked dishes such as sukiyaki or in soups.

- Order fresh fruit for dessert. Japanese menus typically don't offer rich pastries.

- Take time to enjoy the aesthetics of a Japanese meal. Learn to use chopsticks. They may slow your eating, and that can be a good part of the dining experience!

From the Japanese Menu

Enjoy more often:
- Stir-fried dishes such as sukiyaki
- Simmered dishes such as shabu shabu
- Grilled dishes such as yakitori
- Stir-fried tofu
- Clear soups such as miso and suimono
- Steamed rice
- Noodles and broth
- Steamed vegetables
- Sashimi and sushi

Enjoy less often:
- Deep-fried dishes such as tempura
- Breaded and fried dishes such as tonkatsu
- Fried tofu

Have You Ever Wondered

... how to make healthier choices from the kids' menu? Many restaurants now feature more vegetables and fruits, and other healthful options, on children's menus—with kid's meals of 600 calories or less, and limits on total fat, saturated fat, *trans* fat, and sodium. To go with the common grilled cheese sandwiches, chicken nuggets, hot dogs, and burgers, encourage an order of steamed broccoli, a fruit cup, carrot sticks, other fruit and vegetable side dishes, and low-fat or fat-free milk. Or offer something from the adult menu, perhaps to share. *See "Eating Out with Kids" in chapter 17.*

Eating for Travelers

Does eating on the road challenge your waistline and good nutrition sense? Overdoing is all too easy when eating out, especially when portions are big; the desserts are rich; and the menus, tantalizing. Dehydration and food safety also demand thought and action for many travelers.

Dining at 35,000 Feet

Airline food service? That depends on the carrier, where you sit on the plane, and the length and time of your flight. As airlines cut back to control costs, food service on most domestic flights have become just a beverage and a pack of crackers, cookies, pretzels, or peanuts—or no food at all. On some airlines, you can opt to buy a sandwich or a snack in-flight. So except for long (usually international) flights, don't count on an airline meal.

Whether you're a frequent flier or an occasional passenger, plan ahead for food to eat on board or at the airport.

● Check your flight confirmation or ask the airline or your travel agent about the type of food service. Find out if you can buy food on board. Many airlines realize that people want healthier options. They may offer hummus, pita chips, dried fruit, fresh fruit, nuts, or yogurt, among other options.

● If you or someone you're traveling with has a peanut allergy, advise the airline ahead. In that case, a different dry snack can be served to all passengers in-flight.

● Want a special meal on a long international flight, or perhaps in first or business class on some long domestic flights? That may be possible on major carriers—if you or your travel agent make a request at least twenty-four hours before your flight, or better yet, with your flight reservation. If the flight has meal service, vegetarian, kosher, low-calorie, low-fat, low-sodium, diabetic, and fruit plate, and perhaps meals for infants and children, may be available for no extra cost. Some carriers offer Hindu, Muslim, or Asian meals.

● If you take food on board, make portable, safe choices. Especially if you travel with small children, bringing a simple snack is a good idea. Dried fruit such as apricots, an apple or a banana, raw vegetables, pack-aged crackers and sliced cheese, muffins, bagels, pretzels, and protein bars travel well. For safety's sake, don't keep a sandwich with meat or another perishable food for too long at cabin temperature—no more than two hours. That includes transit time from your kitchen if food comes from home.

● If you bring food from home or outside the secured area of the airport, remember: Drinks, water, and some foods such as yogurt aren't allowed through security.

● If you buy airport food to take on board or eat as you wait, try to order sensibly—as noted earlier in this chapter—even if choices are limited.

● Rather than sit as you wait for a flight, exercise: Walk the concourses, skip people movers!

● Especially on a long trip, drink plenty of liquids before, during, and after flying—8 ounces every hour of your flight—even if you aren't thirsty. With the low humidity and recirculating air in the pressurized cabin,

---

Your Anti–Jet Lag Plan

Best advice: Organize ahead so you're well rested and relaxed before traveling. Avoid skipping meals as you rush to pack. On your trip, stick to healthful eating.

Being dehydrated actually promotes jet lag. To minimize the effects, drink a glass of water or 100 percent juice before your airline flight, then each hour in-flight. Alcoholic beverages also can promote dehydration and may increase jet lag. Go easy if you drink them. During long flights, get up, stretch, and walk around the cabin.

On the ground, keep drinking fluids. After a long flight, drink extra fluids for several days. Immediately adjust your meals and sleep to the new time if you've traveled over several time zones. If your body clock skips from late afternoon to early morning and you lose the night (as you often do with overseas flights), take a short nap when you arrive, then continue with a normal day—lunch, dinner, and an early evening. If you leave in the morning and arrive at night, have dinner and go to bed—even if your body clock says it's midday.

No evidence shows that anti–jet lag formulas or diets are effective. You may have heard anti–jet lag claims about a dietary supplement called melatonin. While this claim may be partially true, the amount of melatonin that may promote sleep is far less than the amount in over-the-counter products. *For more information on melatonin and other supplements, see chapter 23.*

airline travel can be dehydrating; you lose body fluids through evaporation on your skin. Dehydration causes fatigue. Good beverage choices: water, club soda, and 100 percent fruit juice. Pack an empty water bottle in your carry-on bag to fill—or buy bottled water after passing through security.

● When the beverage cart rolls by, consider calories as well as overall nutrition. Instead of regular soda, ask for 100 percent fruit juice, tomato juice, or low-fat milk. That said, it's okay to say no to the beverage cart. You don't need to take a snack or a soda just because it's offered.

● Want to relax or sleep on the flight? If you're sensitive to caffeine, avoid caffeinated beverages: coffee, tea, and colas. For some people, too much caffeine can promote sleeplessness, anxiety, and overstimulation, especially for those anxious about flying.

● If you drink alcoholic beverages, go easy—even if you have free drink coupons or you're in first class, where drinks are free. Stop after one or two drinks. On a long flight, wine or cocktails may not help you sleep or relax. Instead, larger amounts may have the opposite effect, making you more restless.

● Especially on a long flight, get out of your seat, and move a little as allowed by flight attendants. Even a brief walk in the aisle will help you feel better than just sinking into your seat with your headset and computer on or with a good book.

Travel Fare—on the Ground

For business travelers, eating on the road can present challenges. For leisure travelers, calories add up, too, especially when food is a main event. Eating just 500 extra calories a day as you travel can deliver 3,500 extra calories a week. Unless you compensate with more physical activity, those 3,500 extra calories can turn into about 1 pound of body fat as your souvenir!

● Continue to be a wise restaurant patron. *See "Dining Out Tip List" and "Fast Food, Healthful Food" in this chapter.*

● On an expense account? Avoid the urge to overeat just because you don't pay the bill. Promising to cut down when you get home may not be enough to keep trim, especially if you travel frequently.

Have You Ever Wondered

... how to enjoy the floating feast on a cruise ship without overdoing or feeling guilty? Use the ship's outer deck as a running or walking track, or take advantage of the ship's fitness center, pool, or workout classes so you can indulge a little more. Take advantage of the built-in variety on cruise ship menus. Many of today's cruise ships offer lighter or spa fare. If you stay up to enjoy late-night food, balance it by going easy at other meals. If you can't resist the urge to order another course, ask for a small portion. Just because your meals are prepaid doesn't mean you must order everything on the menu. Don't feel forced to order a beverage when you sit down to an evening show or sit around the pool.

Problem with seasickness? Skipping food entirely isn't the answer. Instead, ask the passenger desk for motion sickness medication; eat something light, perhaps crackers, to keep something in your stomach.

To control infectious disease, use hand sanitizers available to passengers near dining areas and throughout the ship. If you do get sick, tell a crew member right away.

● Schedule your wake-up call to allow time for breakfast. An early morning meal is, after all, a smart way to start an effective work or vacation day. Some hotels include light breakfast service in the room rate. Or if your hotel provides room service, order breakfast the night before.

● When work continues through a meal or a cocktail hour, tune into your food and drinks, and your body's hunger and satiety signals, as well as your business issues. A second round of drinks or another basket of chips can appear without much notice.

Drinking is often part of the social side of business travel, or is viewed by travelers as a way to relax. Yet calories in a cocktail or two, and perhaps wine with dinner, add up fast. Depending on the size, a single drink can supply 10 percent or more of your day's calorie needs! Be careful, too, that cocktails and salty snacks don't replace a nourishing meal.

● As a leisure or business traveler, make time to move: explore museums, historic spots, parks, and shops on foot. Use athletic facilities at the hotel or a local park. Get up early enough for a walk or a work-out. Too often people complain that travel upsets their workout routine. *For tips on fitting physical activity into your travel schedule, see "When You're on the Road" in chapter 20.*

Breakfast on the Road

A 2-egg omelet, 3 strips of bacon, ½ cup of hash browns, 1 slice of toast with 2 teaspoons of butter or margarine, ¾ cup of fruit juice, and coffee: This hearty restaurant breakfast can total up to 685 calories and 40 fat grams. For a quick, nutritious start, order one of the following breakfasts instead for fewer calories, and perhaps more overall nutrition:

● Fresh fruit, small bagel with jam, low-fat or fat-free milk

● Ready-to-eat dry cereal (preferably low in added sugar), grits, or oatmeal with low-fat or fat-free milk, fresh or dried fruit, a handful of nuts, coffee or tea

● Low-fat yogurt, whole-wheat English muffin with spread served on the side, fruit juice or fresh fruit, coffee or tea

● Whole-wheat pancakes or waffles topped with fruit; hot cocoa made with milk

● One poached egg, whole-wheat toast with jam, ½ grapefruit, fat-free milk

● Vegetable omelet to fit veggies in. Have it made with egg whites or an egg substitute for less solid fat and cholesterol. Consider a side of Canadian bacon, whole wheat toast, and coffee latte.

Ordering a Continental breakfast (bread, juice, and coffee)? For breads with less fat, ask for a bagel, toast (perhaps whole-wheat or rye), or an English muffin with jam or with butter or margarine served on the side. Skip doughnuts, sweet rolls, croissants, and other pastries to cut down on calories, solid fats, and added sugars.

For more breakfast advice see "Break-FAST" in this chapter.

Have Food, Will Travel

If your job, vacation, or weekend outings take you on a road trip, train, or bus trip, brown-bag it or fill a cooler. Then you don't need to rely on vending machines, convenience stores, or snack bars.

● Fill sealable plastic bags with vegetable finger foods: raw vegetables (broccoli and cauliflower florets, jicama and carrot sticks, zucchini and bell pepper circles, or snow peas). Take seasonal fruit. Besides taking the edge off hunger, fruit can be a thirst quencher.

TRAVELING ABROAD? EATING FOR SAFETY'S SAKE

BE CAUTIOUS—SKIP THESE FOODS . . .	EAT THESE FOODS INSTEAD . . .
Salads, fruit with peels, raw vegetables (in uncertain areas)	Fruit peeled by you, cooked vegetables
Raw, rare, or partly cooked meat, poultry, and fish	Well-cooked meat, poultry, or fish
Softly scrambled or sunny-side-up eggs (unless the egg is well cooked)	Well-cooked scrambled eggs or hard-cooked eggs
Unpasteurized milk	Canned or ultrapasteurized (UHT) boxed milk, or pasteurized milk from a large commercial dairy (ask to be sure)
Juice or juice drink with added "local" water	Canned or boxed juice or juice drink from a commercial processor (ask to be sure.)
Cheese made from unpasteurized milk	Cheese made from pasteurized milk
Food and drinks sold by street vendors	Only commercially bottled drinks and commercially packaged foods from vendors
Local water, ice made with local water	Commercially bottled water and drinks without ice

● Tuck in single-portion beverages: canned or boxed 100 percent fruit juice, canned tomato juice, boxed low-fat or fat-free milk, and bottled water. Take other portable, nonperishable foods—for example, crackers, peanut butter, raisins, small boxes of ready-to-eat cereal, single-serving cans of tuna or fruit, other dried fruit, pretzels, or plain popcorn. Tuck in packages of instant oatmeal and perhaps dry milk powder to make a quick, easy, hot breakfast in your hotel.

● Stock an insulated cooler with perishable foods: deli sandwiches, yogurt, and cheese, among others. Keep fresh fruit and raw vegetables in the cooler, too, to keep them crisp. *For more tips see "Carry It for Safety" in chapter 13.*

● When you're hungry, stop to eat. Get out of the car. Stretch. Take a short walk, too. You'll enjoy your meal more—and feel more relaxed as you continue driving. To help prevent constipation—a frequent complaint on long-distance car trips—stop every hour or two for a brisk walk and drink of water.

Food Safety in Faraway Places

From cozy cafés, open-air markets, and food stalls to seeing rice paddies, tropical fruit plantations, and fishermen haul in their nets, new foods and flavors, as well as local farming and markets, offer unique cultural experiences for curious travelers. Americans' growing enjoyment of ethnic foods comes in part from their travel experiences, including culinary and agriculture travel.

Today more business and pleasure travelers (adults and youth) venture to places where sanitation standards are less strict than in the United States. In some environments, bacteria, parasites, and viruses can transfer to food from poor sanitation or agricultural practices. To help control the spread of disease, immigration forms to enter the United States ask if the traveler has visited a farm; travelers and their baggage also go through an agricultural inspection.

An Ounce of Precaution

No matter what you call it—Montezuma's Revenge, turista, or something else—travelers' diarrhea most often is caused by contaminated food and/or water. Typically, it lasts no more than three to four days. However, that's enough to upset or even ruin an other-wise wonderful vacation—and certainly puts a business trip into a tailspin.

The first bout won't "immunize" you from the next. But you can reduce your risk by being cautious and careful with everything you eat and drink.

Like other types of foodborne illness, travelers' diarrhea is most commonly caused by bacteria—probably 80 percent of all cases. Improperly handled and contaminated food and drink also can cause *E. coli* infections, hepatitis, giardiasis, shigellosis, and other contagious diseases.

To avoid foodborne illness, guidelines in "Eating Out Safely" in this chapter apply, no matter where you eat away from home. In less developed places of the world, you need to take added precautions: "Boil it, cook it, peel it, or forget it." *For more about foodborne illness see chapter 13.*

● If you will travel to developing or rural areas, ask your physician and county health department about immunizations and preventive medication suggested for your destination. The Centers for Disease Control and Prevention (CDC) (wwwnc.cdc.gov/travel) provides food, water, and immunization alerts and advice for travelers in some regions of the world. Even if you will stay with friends and relatives abroad, take pretravel preventive care. For an infant, child, or someone at high risk (*see chapter 13*) who travels, immunizations are a must, as are pretravel precautions for foodborne and other infectious illness.

● Check travel guides and talk to staff in the better hotels, or to your tour guide, to find restaurants with high sanitation standards. Restaurants in better hotels usually have high standards. Food and drinks eaten from street vendors increase the chance of illness.

● When you aren't sure what you may encounter, carry packable, nonperishable foods. Single-serve foods, sold for lunch boxes, are great for travelers.

● As at home, always wash your hands with warm, soapy water, and dry them before eating! *Remember:* Your hands can transfer diarrhea-causing bacteria to your mouth. Carry an antibacterial hand wash, wet wipes, and maybe a small bar of soap.

● Like anywhere, avoid buffets if food is just rewarmed after sitting for a while, or if it's been kept at room temperature for longer than 1 to 2 hours.

● *Be aware:* Fresh dairy products in developing countries may not be pasteurized. They also may be diluted with untreated water.

● If you travel with a baby, breast milk guarantees food safety. If your infant takes formula, prepare it from commercial powder, and boiled or commercially bottled water. Wash pacifiers, teething rings, and toys that fall to the floor, too. *For more about infant formula see "A Healthful Option: Formula-Feeding" in chapter 16.*

● Be cautious about different types of fish and shellfish when you travel abroad, especially from tropical waters of the West Indies and the Pacific and Indian Oceans. Avoid barracuda, morey eel, and puffer fish. Other tropical reef fish also can carry toxins (ciguatera fish poisoning): grouper, amberjack, sea bass, sturgeon, parrot fish, and red snapper.

The CDC advises travelers to avoid or limit ingestion of these reef fish, particularly if they weigh 6 pounds or more, and to avoid parts of the fish where the toxin may be concentrated (such as liver, intestines, roe, and head). Some fish contain toxins even when they're cooked. Ciguatera toxins do not affect the texture, taste, or smell of fish, and they aren't destroyed by cooking, smoking, freezing, canning, salting, or pickling, or during digestion.

For other issues related to seafood safety if fishing is part of your travel, see the website: wwwnc.cdc .gov/travel.

What's Safe to Drink?

You're always smart to play it safe. In developed countries, tap water generally is fine. Still, be cautious.

Better hotels in less-developed areas also may filter and chlorinate their tap water for safety. Before you use water from the faucet, find out if the hotel has a water purification system. When you're not sure, don't drink or brush your teeth with tap water. Instead, use commercially bottled or canned water with the seal or cap intact. Keep a bottle or can of water in your carry bag.

● Be aware that in some places bottled water may not be superior to tap water. Knowing how to disinfect water may be important, especially for long-term travelers. Check with the CDC, Traveler's Health to learn how: http://wwwnc.cdc.gov/travel/yellowbook/2010.

Soft drinks, canned or bottled juices, beer, and wine are safe to drink. Coffee, tea, and other hot beverages usually are safe; the long heating time destroys most and perhaps all bacteria, viruses, and parasites that might be present in the water. You also can boil or chemically treat water you drink. In addition, the CDC advises you to dry any wet cans or bottles before opening them, then wiping clean any surfaces where your mouth contacts the can or the bottle. *For guidelines on treating water see "Safe Enough to Drink" in chapter 8.*

In less-developed areas avoid beverages made with water or ice cubes unless you know that commercially bottled water was used. Also avoid bottled water without an intact seal or cap; it may have been refilled with local tap water. Be cautious of locally bottled water; the standards may not be high for bottling. Even crystal-clear water in wilderness areas anywhere, including the United States and Canada, should be treated before drinking it.

If You Do Get Sick . . .

● For most cases of travelers' diarrhea, dehydration is the biggest concern. If it strikes you, increase your fluid intake—with plenty of safe water, canned juice, and soup. Canned or bottled soft drinks (preferably without caffeine) are okay, too.

● If the problem persists (for more than three or four days) or if your symptoms are severe, seek qualified medical care. Your hotel or tour guide should be able to suggest a physician.

● Prepare before you travel. Talk with your physician at home; take recommended precautionary medication with you. Check the CDC website to learn more (wwwnc.cdc.gov/travel). *For more about dealing with diarrhea, see "Gastrointestinal Conditions" in chapter 22.*

Need more tips on eating out? Check here for how-tos:

● Eating out with kids and dealing with their fussy restaurant eating—*see chapter 17.*

● Handling allergies when eating out—*see chapter 21.*

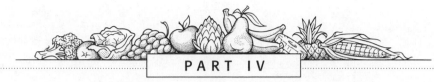

Food for Health
Every Age, Every Stage of Life

Off to a Healthy Start
Feeding Baby

Should our baby be breast-fed or bottle-fed?" "Can solid foods be given too soon?" "How do I know if my baby has eaten enough?" "Do I give my baby juice from a cup or a bottle?" "Should solid foods be warmed?"

New and experienced parents ask so many questions! Wouldn't it be great for parents and other caregivers if newborns were delivered into their parents' arms with a "how-to" manual filled with feeding instructions? Still, it's amazing how fast infant feeding becomes routine. However, as soon as babies and parents master one feeding stage, they're both ready to move on and learn the next.

As you feed your baby, keep two main goals in mind: Offer the right amount of food energy (or calories) and nutrients at the right time to support your baby's optimal growth and development . . . and nourish the emotional bonds between you and your baby.

Breast-Feed or Formula-Feed?

If you're a new parent, either approach—*breast- or formula-feeding*—can provide adequate nourishment and the strong emotional bond that your growing baby needs. Whenever possible, though, breast milk is best for baby during the first year. If you're not sure which approach to use, start with breast-feeding. If it isn't right for you, switch to formula-feeding. Starting with a bottle, then trying later to breast-feed is difficult. *Either way— or both ways—you'll find guidance in this chapter.*

Consider this: A baby's birth weight doubles by about five months of age and triples by one year. He or she grows about 30 percent longer by five months of age, and about 50 percent longer by 12 months. At birth a baby's brain is about 25 percent of its adult size and grows to 75 percent of its adult size by 12 months.

Good feeding practices are not only essential for proper growth; they set the stage for food patterns and a healthy weight throughout life. From the very start, help your baby develop a positive relationship with food and eating. That includes learning and trusting his or her hunger and fullness signals.

Learning baby feeding basics takes the guesswork out. Practical guidance from your pediatrician, pediatric nurse, registered dietitian, and other parents is a blessing. Your own patience, time—and creativity— build warm, memorable feeding experiences for your baby, your family, and you.

Your feeding relationship and how you shift from breast milk or formula, to solid foods, and then to family foods may have long-term health outcomes for you and your baby. Feeding practices in this first year will affect your baby's food choices, their nutrient and diet quality, and your baby's weight status in childhood and beyond.

Breast-Feeding Your Baby

Nature provides ideal nourishment for babies: breast milk. Medical and nutrition experts highly recommend breast-feeding at least for an infant's first year of life. Breast milk alone can provide optimal nutrition and health protection to support most babies' growth and development during the first six months of life. Then when solid foods are introduced, they complement breast milk as the ideal feeding pattern. Breast milk continues to be important for your baby for the first year—and even longer.

The decision to breast-feed is a personal one. It takes into account the family's lifestyle, economic situation, and cultural beliefs, along with the mother's and the infant's physical ability to do so.

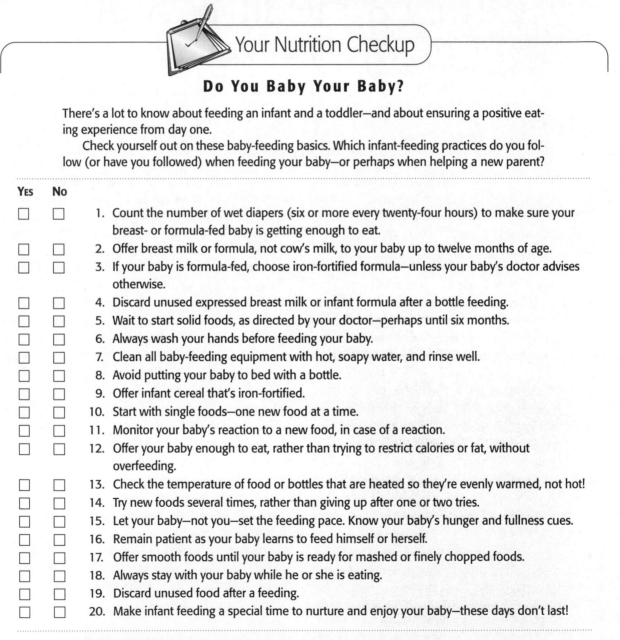

Your Nutrition Checkup

Do You Baby Your Baby?

There's a lot to know about feeding an infant and a toddler—and about ensuring a positive eating experience from day one.

Check yourself out on these baby-feeding basics. Which infant-feeding practices do you follow (or have you followed) when feeding your baby—or perhaps when helping a new parent?

YES	No	
☐	☐	1. Count the number of wet diapers (six or more every twenty-four hours) to make sure your breast- or formula-fed baby is getting enough to eat.
☐	☐	2. Offer breast milk or formula, not cow's milk, to your baby up to twelve months of age.
☐	☐	3. If your baby is formula-fed, choose iron-fortified formula—unless your baby's doctor advises otherwise.
☐	☐	4. Discard unused expressed breast milk or infant formula after a bottle feeding.
☐	☐	5. Wait to start solid foods, as directed by your doctor—perhaps until six months.
☐	☐	6. Always wash your hands before feeding your baby.
☐	☐	7. Clean all baby-feeding equipment with hot, soapy water, and rinse well.
☐	☐	8. Avoid putting your baby to bed with a bottle.
☐	☐	9. Offer infant cereal that's iron-fortified.
☐	☐	10. Start with single foods—one new food at a time.
☐	☐	11. Monitor your baby's reaction to a new food, in case of a reaction.
☐	☐	12. Offer your baby enough to eat, rather than trying to restrict calories or fat, without overfeeding.
☐	☐	13. Check the temperature of food or bottles that are heated so they're evenly warmed, not hot!
☐	☐	14. Try new foods several times, rather than giving up after one or two tries.
☐	☐	15. Let your baby—not you—set the feeding pace. Know your baby's hunger and fullness cues.
☐	☐	16. Remain patient as your baby learns to feed himself or herself.
☐	☐	17. Offer smooth foods until your baby is ready for mashed or finely chopped foods.
☐	☐	18. Always stay with your baby while he or she is eating.
☐	☐	19. Discard unused food after a feeding.
☐	☐	20. Make infant feeding a special time to nurture and enjoy your baby—these days don't last!

Now Score Yourself:
Give yourself—and your baby—a big hug if you said "yes" to all twenty items. If you said "no" to any item, read on. Then practice what you learn. Your baby's health depends on it!

For Good Reasons . . .

Breast-feeding offers a host of physical, emotional, and practical benefits for both baby and mother. The benefits are greatest when mother's milk is baby's exclusive source of nourishment for at least the first four, and preferably six, months, and continues when solids are introduced at about six months. The longer a baby breast-feeds, the greater the benefits. However, your baby benefits even when breast-feeding lasts for only a short time, perhaps only during a six- to eight-week maternity leave.

Human milk provides optimal nutrition! It has the right amount and balance of carbohydrates (lactose), protein (casein and whey), fat, water, and other nutrients to meet the growth, development, and energy needs of infants. It's easily digested; its nutrients, easily absorbed and used. As a baby matures and grows, the composition and amount of breast milk that a mother produces naturally changes.

For most nutrients, what a mother eats has little if any effect on the nutrient content of breast milk. If her nutrient intake is low, her body's own stored nutrients may be used for breast milk, putting her at potential nutritional risk. That's especially true for calcium and folate. For overall health, a nutritious diet during breast-feeding is important, as it was during pregnancy. *See "For Those Who Breast-Feed" in chapter 18.*

Breast-fed babies get protection from allergies, intolerances, and common illnesses. Unlike formula, breast milk is rich in antibodies and other substances that build the immune system and help protect an infant from illnesses such as ear infections, diarrhea, respiratory illnesses, allergies, intestinal infections, and perhaps sudden infant death syndrome (SIDS). Breast-fed babies aren't sick as often and have fewer doctor's visits. In fact, human milk contains at least a hundred ingredients that infant formula doesn't have!

Colostrum, the clear or yellow fluid secreted for two to four days after delivery, is rich in protein and vitamin A, with more antibodies than the mature milk that follows. It helps protect a newborn's intestines from infection during the first few months. Think

Have You Ever Wondered **?**

. . . if breast size affects breast-feeding success? No; it doesn't affect the volume of milk production, either. When a woman isn't breast-feeding, glands that produce milk are very small, regardless of breast size. The amounts of fat and fibrous tissue a woman has, not the glands that produce breast milk, determine breast size.

. . . if premature babies can breast-feed successfully? Many premature babies can. But if your baby is born prematurely, get help from a lactation counselor, pediatric nurse, or your doctor. You may need to express milk at first; you'll still feed your milk to your baby, perhaps mixed with a nutrient supplement for preterm infants. For premature babies, breast milk offers benefits that help them grow and stay free from illness. There's another reason to start right away: You need to establish your milk supply if you plan to nurse.

. . . if the foods you eat during pregnancy or breast-feeding increase your baby's risk for food allergies? Plenty of research indicates that breast-feeding reduces the risk for food allergies, particularly if there's a fam-ily history of allergies. Food allergies are less common in breast-fed babies than in formula-fed babies.

For pregnant and nursing mothers? The American Academy of Pediatrics in 2008 noted: Avoiding known food allergens hasn't been shown to protect against food allergies. As a precaution, if a parent or sibling has a food allergy, such as for peanuts, then the woman is advised to avoid that food allergen. Avoiding certain foods during nursing possibly may prevent eczema; talk to your doctor. Exclusive breast-feeding doesn't appear to protect a child from allergic asthma that starts after early childhood (after age six years).

. . . what to do if your baby reacts to something you eat? Be watchful. If your baby seems to react poorly after you eat certain foods, including those with known allergens, stop eating them for a while. Any allergic reaction usually comes from a protein in a food that a mother consumes, not from breast milk itself. If your pediatrician identifies an allergy, eliminate that food or ingredient in your diet until your baby is weaned. *See "Food Allergies: A Growing Concern" in chapter 21.*

of colostrum as a newborn's first immunization. Colostrum also helps a baby pass his or her first stool.

Breast milk changes with baby's changing needs. From about the third to the tenth day after delivery, the body produces transition milk—a mix of colostrum and mature milk. Then mature milk, bluish in color and thinner in consistency, comes in. As a baby needs to eat more often, a mother's breasts produce more milk.

Breast milk is easy for babies to digest. It's clean and safe. Babies may react to something their mothers eat, but they're rarely allergic to their mother's milk. Breast-feeding requires more sucking than bottle-feeding. This helps strengthen and develop the baby's jaw and so helps teeth and speech patterns. Despite the benefits of sucking, don't overuse a pacifier!

Later on, those who were breast-fed may be less likely to develop certain chronic diseases, including heart disease, high blood pressure, type 1 and 2 diabetes, asthma, lower respiratory infections, childhood leukemia, and certain stomach and intestinal diseases. Research in this area is not conclusive, but it is promising.

Breast-fed babies are less likely to become obese later, with potentially more benefits each added month of nursing—a wise strategy for reducing childhood obesity! Breast-feeding may also increase mental function; breast-fed babies score higher on childhood IQ tests, especially those born prematurely. They also have lower risk of sudden infant death syndrome (SIDS) and infant disease and death.

How about Mom?

Besides knowing that your baby is well fed, you as a nursing mom get many benefits from breast-feeding,

Do Babies Need Extra Water?

Newborns need little or no extra water. In fact, water before a feeding may interfere with a baby's interest in eating. Except for periods of hot weather when your baby perspires, breast milk or infant formula usually supply enough fluid. If water is needed, offer 1 to 2 ounces of plain water after a feeding; water shouldn't take the place of breast milk or formula. For safety's sake when your baby is less than four months of age, boil water first, then chill it, or offer sterilized bottled water. When babies begin eating solid food, offer plain water.

Your child needs water in addition to breast milk or formula to replace fluids lost through diarrhea or vomiting. Diarrhea and vomiting can lead to dehydration—and its complications—if fluids aren't replaced. Rather than water or juice, your doctor or pediatric nurse may recommend an oral electrolyte maintenance solution, sold near baby foods in your grocery store, to prevent dehydration. Besides fluid, the solution contains glucose (a form of sugar) and minerals (sodium, chloride, potassium) called electrolytes. Electrolytes help maintain fluid balance in your baby's body cells. These minerals are lost through body fluids.

Consult your doctor or pediatric nurse before feeding an oral electrolyte maintenance solution to children under two years of age (or older children, too). Besides the risk of dehydration, diarrhea and vomiting signal possible illness that may require medical attention! If diarrhea, vomiting, or fever persist longer than twenty-four hours, consult your doctor or pediatric nurse. An electrolyte maintenance solution won't stop diarrhea or vomiting, but it does prevent dehydration.

Click Here! Websites to Know . . .

- Bright Futures, www.brightfutures.org
- American Academy of Pediatrics, www.healthychildren.org
- Food and Nutrition Service, USDA, www.fns.usda.gov/tn/resources/feeding infants-ch7.pdf

See "Resources You Can Use" for more websites.

too. The longer a woman breast-feeds, the greater the benefits to both baby and mother.

Breast-feeding nurtures a close bond between mother and baby. Skin-to-skin contact is often a gratifying, emotionally fulfilling extension of pregnancy and a chance to build self-esteem as a parent. In addition, breast-feeding helps decrease the chance of postpartum depression.

Always ready-to-feed, breast milk doesn't need measuring, mixing, or warming. So it's easy, especially in the wee hours of the night. With no bottles to prepare or wash and no infant formula to shop for, nursing moms have more time to relax with the baby, or to catch a nap as baby sleeps.

Breast-feeding also may help a new mother regain her prepregnancy figure and reduce postpartum bleeding. Because nursing stimulates the release of oxytocin, a hormone that helps the uterus to contract and shrink, a mother's abdomen trims down more quickly. Nursing burns calories. Her body also uses the fat pad that was deposited on her hips and thighs during pregnancy as some fuel for milk production. Gradual weight loss during breast-feeding doesn't affect milk production.

Breast-feeding is economical, too—even when you account for the extra food a mother eats and the cost of breast-feeding supplies, such as nursing bras and a breast pump. And since breast-fed babies often aren't sick as much, there's less cost for doctor visits and lost work income when babies are breast-fed. Women who breast-feed do need to add about 330 to 400 calories a day to their normal meals and snacks to cover the energy required for milk production. These calories are best added with nutrient-rich food-group foods. *See "Planning to Eat Smart," chapter 10.*

There's less odor involved with breast-feeding. Diaper-changing odor is less offensive, and if a breast-fed infant spits up, there's very little smell, and it doesn't stain clothing.

An added benefit: With nursing, a mother takes time to relax every few hours. That's often a welcome and needed change of pace from the added demands of being a new parent.

What about long-term benefits? Women who have breast-fed have a lower risk of developing premenopausal breast cancer, ovarian cancer, type 2 diabetes, and osteoporosis and hip fractures. Breast-feeding also helps with blood glucose levels for women with gestational diabetes.

See "For Those Who Breast-Feed" in chapter 18.

Perfecting the Breast-Feeding Technique

While breast-feeding is nature's way of providing ideal nutrition for infants, the "art" of breast-feeding might not come as naturally! Like learning any new skill, the keys to success are knowledge, practice, and the support of family, friends, and perhaps coworkers and employers. Discuss your decision to breast-feed with your doctor before delivery, and remind hospital staff when you arrive at the hospital. Most hospitals provide assistance and instruction.

Getting Started

● To build confidence and to help ensure an adequate milk supply, start nursing as soon after delivery as possible. The best time to start is within twenty to thirty minutes after your baby is born, perhaps right in the delivery room. The first feeding will be short, about ten minutes. "Rooming in" at the hospital may make your first days with nursing more successful.

● Relax and make yourself comfortable. Find a comfortable chair with good arm and back support. Or lie down with pillows strategically positioned to help you support your baby. If you are comfortable and well supported, it's easy to hold your baby, and you won't feel much tension in your neck, back, and shoulders.

● Plan to nurse on demand—that is, whenever your baby says it's time to eat. Increased alertness or activity, rooting toward your breast, hand-to-mouth activity, and mouthing are all signs that your baby is hungry. Typically, crying is a late signal of hunger. Trying to establish a schedule early on may frustrate you both. As reassurance, you can't "spoil" your baby by feeding on demand. Most babies fall into a schedule with time.

● Be prepared to nurse very frequently during the first months—about eight to twelve times every twenty-four hours. That's because a newborn's stomach is small and because nutrient needs are exceptional now during rapid growth and development. Good news: After about three months, babies feed less often, and some start to sleep through the night.

Frequent nursing helps establish your milk supply and keeps your breasts from becoming hard and swollen. Full, heavy breasts signal that it's time to nurse. As milk "lets down," or moves from the inner breast to the nipple, you may get a tingling feeling.

Latching On

Some newborns instinctively suck when they're first put to their mother's breast. (Maybe they practiced sucking their thumb before birth.) Others nuzzle first, just to get used to the warmth, security, and softness from their mother. Either way is normal.

● Help your baby by stroking baby's cheek nearest your breast. As your baby turns toward your nipple, guide your baby's mouth to take in as much of the areola (dark area of the nipple) as possible, not just the nipple. Newborns have a "rooting reflex" at the breast; they open their mouths naturally.

● Try to offer both breasts at each feeding. Let your baby nurse as long as he or she wants (about ten to twenty minutes on each breast). The last portion from each breast is "hind milk." This milk is higher in fat and helps the baby feel full and satisfied after feeding.

● Release your baby from the breast by gently putting your finger into the corner of his or her mouth. (Wash your hands before nursing.) This will ease the baby's grip and break the suction without discomfort. Wait until you feel the suction release before pulling away.

Latching on correctly helps your baby get enough milk and protects you from sore nipples. Ask about breast compression as a way to create and maintain a natural flow of milk and to stimulate a natural letdown reflex if your baby is no longer drinking on his or her own.

Breast-Feeding: About Your Baby

● Burp your baby when you change breasts and at the end of the feeding. This relieves any discomfort from air swallowed while nursing. Hold him or her upright, chin on your shoulder, or lay your baby "tummy-side down" across your lap. Then gently rub or pat your baby's back. It's normal for a baby to spit up a bit of milk.

● Trust your baby to let you know when he or she has had enough to eat. When your baby feels full, he or she may close his or her lips, turn away, or even fall asleep. Sometimes babies rest during a feeding, too, making it hard to know when one feeding stops and the next begins! Is your baby getting enough milk? *See "Nursing: Reassuring Signs of Success" in this chapter.*

● Don't worry about your baby's loose stools. It's normal for a breast-fed baby to have loose, yellowish stools, which may resemble watery "mustard seeds."

● Try to skip a pacifier or bottle nipple between feedings. It can interfere with your baby's ability to learn to breast-feed. Although a between-meal pacifier may help quiet your baby, crying is okay if your baby is hungry, tired, or sick. Excessive use of pacifiers can interfere with normal development of oral motor skills, such as rotary chewing and up-and-down munching.

Some Steps in Breast-Feeding

1. *Snuggle "tummy to tummy."* Cradle baby in your arms with his or her tummy against your tummy. Baby's head should rest in the bend of your elbow. Your forearm should support the baby's back, with your hand on his bottom.

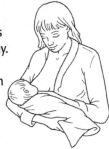

2. *Place nipple directly in front of your baby's mouth.* Your baby's head should be in a straight line with his or her body. If his or her head is tilted back or your baby has to turn to reach your nipple, your baby is in the wrong position.

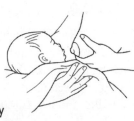

3. *Keep a good position.* Keep your baby well supported. Make sure your baby is facing straight on to the nipple and does not have his or her head back or neck turned. Make sure your back is straight and you are not leaning over your baby.

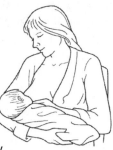

4. *Nurse as long as your baby wants.* Try to use both breasts at each feeding. To take your baby off the breast, release the suction by putting your little finger in the corner of his or her mouth. Wait until you feel the suction release before removing your baby.

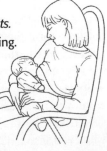

Breast-Feeding: About You

● Because babies nurse more vigorously when they start feeding, alternate the breast you offer first. Clip a safety pin to your bra as a reminder. Alternating ensures that both breasts are emptied regularly, and helps prevent breast tenderness. Vary the nursing position, and allow your nipples to "air dry" after feedings to avoid breast tenderness and cracking.

● If your breasts are tender or reddened, or if you feel achy and feverish, contact your doctor. You may have a plugged duct or breast infection (mastitis). An antibiotic might be prescribed. Usually you can keep on nursing while an infection clears up.

● If your breasts feel tight and full, soften them with a warm shower, or express a small amount of milk. To express milk means to stimulate milk flow by hand or with a breast pump. Fullness and discomfort are signs of engorgement and may happen when your milk supply first comes in or if you've gone too long between feedings. Feed your baby often. Wearing undergarments with proper support helps, too. When breasts become too full, your baby won't be able to latch on correctly, which can cause nipple soreness.

● Don't be surprised if your milk "lets down" and leaks a bit when you hear your baby cry, or even when you think about him or her. It's natural. You might wear pads (without plastic liners) for protection.

● Pour yourself some water or juice before nursing.

Breast-Feeding Cautions

Smoking, drinking alcoholic beverages, using some herbal supplements, and taking medication may affect milk production and the let-down reflex. Some of these substances pass into the mother's milk, too, at the same levels as in her bloodstream.

When you're nursing, avoid smoking and drinking alcoholic beverages. Dietary Guidelines advises: Breast-feeding women should be very cautious about drinking alcoholic beverages, if they drink at all. Alcohol concentrates in breast milk; drinking alcoholic beverages can inhibit milk production. An occasional single drink to celebrate is okay—consumed at least four hours before nursing and if nursing is well established, consistent, and predictable (no earlier than an infant's third month). When mothers smoke, babies are more likely to get sinus infections, colic, or become fussy. Even secondhand smoke is harmful, so dads and other caregivers are wise to avoid smoking, too. Smoking around babies increases the risk for Sudden Infant Death Syndrome (SIDS). *The bottom line:* Now's a great time to quit smoking! That said, breast-feeding is still best, even when the mother is exposed to smoke.

Talk to your doctor about taking medications, including over-the-counter medications, and herbal supplements during breast-feeding. Take your own medications, even if they're safe for babies, after nursing, not before.

In a few circumstances, breast-feeding isn't advised. Mothers who test positive for HIV can pass the virus on through breast milk. Women with untreated tuberculosis or on chemotherapy should not breast-feed. And babies born with galactosemia, who can't tolerate breast milk, need a special diet free of lactose and galactose. Recreational drugs are never advisable; they can also pass to the baby and cause serious, perhaps lasting, side effects.

Getting Help for Breast-Feeding

You and your baby are learning about breast-feeding together. It's okay to ask for help. Besides the delivery

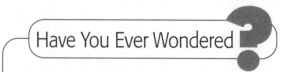

Have You Ever Wondered

. . . if you can breast-feed if you're sick? Yes—usually it's safe to continue breast-feeding. It even offers added protection for your baby, who already has been exposed to any "bug" before you experienced any symptoms. In breast milk you pass on some immunity through the antibodies your own body produces to fight the infection. If you're taking any medications to treat an illness, talk to your pediatrician to make sure they're compatible with breast-feeding. Severe illness may require weaning; again consult your doctor.

. . . if a baby can be sensitive to lactose in mother's milk? That's highly unlikely. A baby's body makes lactase, so he or she can digest lactose in breast milk. If a child does become lactose sensitive, that usually starts later. *See "Lactose Intolerance: A Matter of Degree" in chapter 21.*

Breast-Feeding Positions

If you're a nursing mom, you may want to experiment with these positions as you feed your baby:

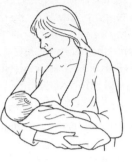

Cradle position. Sit up straight with your baby cradled in your arm. His or her head should be slightly elevated and resting in the crux of your elbow. You and your baby should be comfortably positioned "tummy to tummy," with baby's mouth level with your nipple. Be sure that your baby is facing straight toward you, without having his or her head, back, or neck turned.

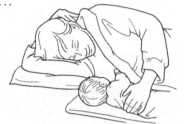

Lying down. Lie on your side with the baby on his or her side, too. Place pillows under your head and behind your back for comfort. Position your baby "tummy to tummy" so his or her mouth is next to your nipple. Use a folded towel or a pillow to elevate your baby to the correct height. This position is especially comfortable for women who've had a cesarean delivery. You can feed your baby from both breasts on one side, or turn onto your other side to nurse from your second breast.

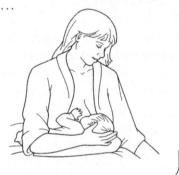

"Football" position. Hold your baby with the head facing your breast, and his or her body tucked under your arm at your side. Your forearm supports the baby's back, and his or her legs and feet should point toward your back. Rest the baby on a pillow near your elbow to give support and slightly raise his or her head.

Whatever the position, enjoy eye contact with your baby. (Put your cell phone away!) This helps build the mother-baby bond and helps your baby feel secure.

---

room nurse, certified lactation consultants in many hospitals teach breast-feeding techniques and answer parents' questions. Some may visit at home later to help you perfect your skills. Some nursing support groups offer peer dad support, too.

Within the first week or two, nursing mothers and their newborns should see their pediatrician or health-care professional. That's a chance to check feeding techniques. If you're discharged from the hospital less than forty-eight hours after delivery, your first checkup should be within two to four days after birth.

You can also seek help and get support and reassurance from the La Leche League, a registered dietitian (RD), a nurse midwife, or another health professional with experience in lactation counseling. Women who have been successful at breast-feeding, such as La Leche League volunteers, offer great support and practical advice to new mothers. The government's National Women's Health Information can also help: 800-994-9662. *To find sound, reliable advice on infant feeding and breast-feeding, see "How to Find Nutrition Help . . ." in chapter 24.*

Nursing: Reassuring Signs of Success

Not knowing how much milk their infant consumes, some parents feel uncomfortable about breast-feeding. You probably don't need to worry about having enough milk. Your body is miraculous. If your baby needs and demands more, your body probably will make more milk to satisfy the demands of nursing—even when you try to lose extra pounds gained during pregnancy. Even mothers of twins and triplets can produce enough milk to nurse successfully.

Look for these signs that nursing is going well:

● Following the third or fourth day after birth, your baby has six or more wet diapers, soiled with light-colored urine, every twenty-four hours. Most newborns wet fewer diapers with only colostrum.

● Your baby nurses at least eight times every twenty-four hours, and maybe up to twelve times daily, in the first month. If your baby sleeps longer than a four-hour stretch, you may need to awaken him or her for a feeding. While nursing, you should feel sucking and hear the infant swallowing.

● The baby's weight steadily increases. Make certain your baby is weighed at the doctor's office within a week or two after delivery to monitor weight gain, and regularly thereafter. During checkups, your baby's weight and length will be assessed. Doctors check a baby's measurements against reference growth curves. If your child doesn't gain weight properly, there may be a feeding or a medical problem.

Initially babies may lose a little weight right after their birth. That's normal. However, if your baby doesn't regain his or her birth weight by three weeks of age, your doctor or pediatric nurse will need to monitor him or her frequently. From birth to six months, babies typically gain 4 to 8 ounces per week.

Other signs of breast-feeding success: Your baby's urine will be pale yellow urine, not deep yellow or orange, and he or she will sleep well, yet be alert and healthy when awake.

A Few Words for Dad . . .

A father can play a very important role in the success of breast-feeding. He can offer support, encouragement, and confidence to a new mother. Fathers can attend prenatal breast-feeding classes with an expectant mother, read a book on breast-feeding, arrange pillows, and bring a snack or a beverage for mom when breast-feeding. A father also can burp the baby, change diapers, massage mom's neck and shoulders to encourage relaxation, and give baby a supplemental bottle. By sharing household responsibilities, caring for other children, shopping, and doing other tasks, he takes other pressures and interruptions away from mom.

What about Supplemental Bottles?

Breast-feeding abides by the law of supply and demand. Nursing stimulates the flow of milk—and increases its production as baby demands more to meet his or her needs. So supplemental bottles usually aren't needed—unless your pediatrician advises it, perhaps if your baby loses weight and doesn't regain it.

Although nursing may temporarily limit your independence, offering a supplemental bottle too soon may discourage your baby from nursing. Until your milk supply is established, stay close for feeding.

If you choose to offer a supplemental bottle or a pacifier, wait about four weeks after birth, or until breast-feeding is well established. Because the nipple on a bottle or a pacifier is different from the breast, it can confuse a baby who is just learning to breast-feed.

Once the milk supply is constant—and both you and your baby are comfortable with nursing—a supplemental bottle lets dad, siblings, and other caregivers share in feeding. Expressed breast milk or commercially prepared infant formula may be offered in a supplemental bottle. *Note:* When nursing sessions are replaced regularly with supplemental bottles—without expressing milk—a mother's breasts will compensate by producing less milk.

For tips on storing breast milk, see "Breast Milk: Safe Handling and Storage" in this chapter. For more about infant formula and bottle feeding, see "A Healthful Option: Formula-Feeding," in this chapter.

Breast-Feeding for a Back-to-Work Schedule

To continue breast-feeding, changing from maternity leave to a back-to-work schedule takes adjustment. Some moms express milk during their workday. In that way, their baby can have bottles of mother's milk when mom's away. Other moms breast-feed when they can be with their baby; caregivers offer infant formula when mom can't. Some babies take both—bottles of expressed breast milk and of formula. Choose the option that works best for you and your baby.

If you're a back-to-work nursing mom (or need to be away from home regularly), consider these guidelines for breast-feeding success:

● Before your maternity leave, make a plan with your employer. Perhaps work at home for a while, or plan your schedule for short days, flextime, or longer breaks. Check your state law for breast-feeding at work.

● Select a caregiver for your baby who is supportive of breast-feeding.

● Plan to nurse before you leave for work, soon after you return from work, and during the evening to keep your milk supply strong. A routine helps.

● If you plan to express (pump) milk during the workday, try to make your plans before your maternity leave. If necessary, arrange for a private area to relax, free from interruptions. (You'll need fifteen to thirty minutes, usually twice a day.) Unoccupied offices or women's lounges may be options. And you'll need access to a refrigerator, or a small cooler with ice packs, to store breast milk, and an outlet if you use an electric pump. By 2010 federal law, a nursing mother must have a reasonable break time and a clean place (not a bathroom) to express breast milk for one year after an infant's birth. An employer doesn't need to pay you during that time; small workplaces (fewer than 50 workers) are exempt. Since state laws may be stricter, check. *For tips on safe handing of expressed milk, see "Breast Milk: Safe Handling and Storage" in this chapter.*

● Before you go back to work, help your baby learn to take expressed breast milk or infant formula from a bottle. Wait at least four weeks after delivery so your own milk supply is well established. If you wait too long, your baby may be less willing to take a bottle. Experiment with different types of bottle nipples to find one your baby likes. This may be the perfect chance to involve dad in feeding! *For more about different types of bottle nipples, see "Bottles and Nipples: Baby Feeding Supplies" in this chapter.*

● If your work schedule and the travel distance from work allow, schedule feeding visits with your baby during your breaks. Let the caregiver know when you'll arrive. In that way, your baby won't be fed too soon before your visits. To make it easier, choose a caregiver near your workplace.

● For the same reason, let the caregiver know when you'll pick up your baby after work. Together, schedule feedings so your baby won't eat too close to the end of your workday.

Have You Ever Wondered

...if a human milk bank is an option if you can't breast-feed? Perhaps—but generally only as a medical emergency. Human milk banks require a prescription. Currently supplies are limited, and the cost is high.

. . . if breast-feeding affects fertility? Ovaries may stop releasing eggs, but it's still possible to get pregnant. While you're nursing, talk to your doctor about a birth control method that's right for you.

. . . how to successfully breast-feed twins? Wonder if you'll produce enough milk? *Remember:* Your milk supply operates on the principle of supply and demand; with more breast-feeding, your body produces more breast milk. In the early weeks, you may be able to feed both infants simultaneously—an efficient use of time.

Talk to your pediatrician about the need for a supplemental bottle. If your babies are growing normally, it's probably not needed unless you need help from other caregivers. Seek help from a lactation counselor for any special guidance for successfully nursing "multiples," such as help with positioning for two infants.

Vitamin and Mineral Supplements for Breast-Fed Babies

Until solid foods are introduced—preferably at about six months—breast milk can be a complete source of nutrition for infants. However, three nutrients may warrant additional consideration. Ask your doctor for advice.

Vitamin D. This vitamin helps your baby use calcium from breast milk (and infant formula) to help bones grow and develop. When skin is exposed to sunlight, the body can make vitamin D; always protect a baby's skin from sunlight with sunscreen or clothing.

Unlike infant formula and fortified cow's milk, breast milk doesn't contain much vitamin D. That's why the American Academy of Pediatrics advises at least 400 IU of vitamin D daily for breast-fed infants, starting within the first few days after birth, even if the baby consumes supplemental formula. For most children, a vitamin D supplement should continue through childhood.

Iron. Iron is important for the manufacture of hemoglobin, the part of red blood cells that carries oxygen throughout the body. Iron also is essential for a baby's brain development and growth.

In the last trimester before birth, babies accumulate enough iron stores to last through their first four to six months of life. Breast milk also contains easily absorbed iron for the first six months. Then an iron-rich cereal can provide the additional iron babies need.

Premature infants who breast-feed may need iron supplementation earlier. They had less time to build adequate iron reserves before birth. Low-birth-weight babies may need an iron supplement, too. Talk to your dietitian or health professional about what is best for your baby.

Fluoride. Your baby's teeth started to develop even before you could see them. Fluoride, a mineral often found in tap water, helps develop strong teeth and prevent cavities later.

Breast milk contains little fluoride—even if the mother's drinking water is fluoridated. If your breast-fed infant takes supplemental formula made with fluoridated water—at least 0.3 ppm (parts per million) of fluoride—your baby may get enough fluoride. If your child is breast-fed only or drinks formula made with well water, distilled water, unfluoridated bottled water, or city unfluoridated water, your doctor may advise a fluoride supplement starting at about six months. Breast-fed infants who take supplemental ready-to-use formula also may need a fluoride supplement; these formulas usually are prepared with water low in fluoride.

At your baby's six-month checkup, ask your doctor if fluoride supplementation is needed. A fluoride supplement may be prescribed.

Other vitamins. Babies of strict vegetarian mothers may need a vitamin B_{12} supplement. *See "The Vegetarian Mom" in chapter 18 for more advice.*

Always get advice from your baby's healthcare provider or a registered dietitian before giving nutrient supplements to a baby—or a child, or a teen of any age!

Weaning . . . When and How?

Weaning is the slow, gradual process that helps your baby eat and enjoy your family's foods. The time for weaning is an individual matter for mother and baby. Experts encourage moms to breast-feed for at least twelve months. Babies benefit from breast-feeding for as long as it's mutually right for mother and baby. Some older babies naturally wean themselves.

Breast Milk: Safe Handling and Storage

- Wash your hands before expressing milk.
- If you use a breast pump, review the operation and cleaning instructions.
- Refrigerate breast milk in clean collection bottles. Plastic retains the protective properties of refrigerated breast milk better. To avoid BPA (bisphenol A), look for plastic bottles labeled "BPA-free" or use glass bottles. *Refer to "Bottles and Nipples: Baby Feeding Supplies" in this chapter to learn more.* You also can freeze breast milk in either plastic or glass containers.
- Keep expressed breast milk stored in the refrigerator. Use refrigerated breast milk within 24 hours. Otherwise freeze it.
- If you work outside your home, or need to be away, consider stocking a milk supply in your freezer during maternity leave. Breast milk can be frozen:
  - In a freezer compartment inside the refrigerator, not the freezer door, for up to two weeks
  - In a refrigerator-freezer with a separate freezer door for three to four months
  - In a separate freezer at temperatures below 0° F for six months or longer.
  Date expressed milk kept in the refrigerator or freezer. Then rotate the milk—first in, first out.
- Store expressed milk in 2- to 4-ounce portions to avoid wasting unused milk after a feeding. Because bacteria from the baby's mouth can contaminate milk in the bottle, always discard milk that's left in the bottle after feeding.
- Thaw breast milk in the refrigerator; under warm, running water; or in a pan of water on the stove. Do not thaw or heat breast milk in a microwave oven. Before feeding thawed breast milk, gently shake the container to mix layers that may have become separated. Once thawed, use breast milk within 24 hours; avoid refreezing it.

No matter how long you choose to nurse, start complementary foods, too, when your baby's ready. If your baby is exclusively breast-fed, that's about at six months of age. Talk to your pediatrician about timing. When your baby eats other foods, too, you'll probably nurse less often: typically first thing in the morning, naptimes, and bedtime.

When you choose to wean your baby, introduce either infant formula or cow's milk, depending on your baby's age. Start slow. Replace breast milk with formula or cow's milk for just one feeding on one day. A few days later, change another feeding. If your baby is under twelve months of age, wean from breast milk to iron-fortified infant formula. If your baby is twelve months or older, whole cow's milk is appropriate.

Should you wean your baby to a bottle or a cup? That depends on his or her developmental readiness. Between four and six months, most infants will drink or suck small amounts of liquid from a cup or a glass when someone else holds it. Older babies and toddlers usually have the coordination to drink fluids from a cup or a straw. However, for infants under six months of age, a bottle is probably the best choice. After 12 months, most health professionals advise to offer only water in a bottle, and by age 12 to 18 months, to give up the bottle entirely. Some babies develop feeding skills more slowly. Daily practice with a cup help helps develop drinking skills. Be consistent and patient as your baby learns.

A Healthful Option: Formula-Feeding

Breast-feeding may or may not be right for you. In rare cases, a woman may not be able to breast-feed for physical or health reasons. Some may feel uncomfortable. Others may take medications that wouldn't be safe if passed through their breast milk to the baby. Still others have cultural or work-related reasons. In all of these cases, parents can feel reassured that bottle-feeding is a healthful option.

Infant formula also is a good complement to breast milk when a nursing mother chooses to skip a breast-feeding, or when the mother doesn't make enough breast milk for her baby.

If you choose formula-feeding, feel assured: Commercially prepared infant formulas are as similar to mother's milk as currently possible. Infant formulas have enough nutrients and food energy (calories) for your baby until you introduce solid foods—usually at about four to six months of age. And infant formulas supply the right balance of fats, carbohydrates, and proteins. Whether generic or branded, infant formulas must meet the U.S. Food and Drug Administration's

A Healthy Weight Starts Early

Developing eating and physical activity habits that lead to a healthy weight start as early as infancy. Respect your baby's appetite from the beginning; learn hunger and fullness cues, *as described in this chapter*. That helps your baby learn to eat the right amount, not over- or under-eat. Take time to burp and cuddle your baby. Know that your baby's brain needs a little time to signal a sense of fullness. Try to wait 2 to 2½ hours between feedings. For older babies, a little more protein in the last feeding of the day may help with satiety, or feeling full.

Not only can overfeeding make your baby feel uncomfortable, it also sets the stage for weight problems later. Even in the first few months, overfeeding with formula is linked to childhood obesity; some babies drain a bottle fast because they suck so strongly. With breast-feeding overfeeding is less likely; breast-fed babies have less chance of being overweight or obese later. Avoid overfeeding or forcing a baby to finish meals if he or she isn't hungry. And avoid introducing foods without overall nutrition value, just to provide calories. Instead offer nutrient-rich foods—at regular feeding times—even if your baby initially won't eat them.

Too much juice can be an issue. Wait until at least six months old to offer juice. Then if you do introduce juice, start with an ounce or two. The American Academy of Pediatrics suggests no more than 4 to 6 ounces per day for children age one and younger.

On the flip side, restricting food/underfeeding may keep your baby from getting nutrients and food energy (calories) needed to grow and develop, and may cause failure to thrive. Overly restrictive feeding also can keep your baby from learning the hunger and fullness cues that can lead to a healthy weight throughout life.

Talk to your baby's doctor about the right weight for your baby's proper and healthy growth and development. A healthy weight starts early—and helps prevent childhood obesity.

nutrient requirements. Unlike breast milk, formulas lack protective factors such as antibodies to promote immunity.

Even after babies take solids, continue infant formula until your baby's first birthday. Similar to breastfeeding, cuddling a baby while he or she takes formula also builds a close, nurturing relationship with all those who share the responsibility of feeding: dad, siblings, grandparents, and other caregivers.

Formula: What Type?

Commercially prepared infant formulas are powdered, liquid concentrate, or more costly ready-to-feed. Before feeding, dilute powdered and liquid-concentrate formulas with boiled or sterile water. Ready-to-feed formulas don't need to be diluted. They're ready "as is"—packaged in cans or in bottles.

What's in a name? Regardless of which formula you use, commercially prepared infant formulas are usually cow's milk–based or soy-based. Formulas based on modified cow's milk are appropriate for most babies. A soy-based or specialty formula might be best

---

Cow's Milk: When? What Type?

As a great source of calcium and other nutrients, cow's milk is an ideal food for toddlers, children, and adults. However, it isn't appropriate for infants younger than twelve months of age. Some infant formulas are made from cow's milk, but modified for infants.

Unmodified cow's milk isn't the best food for young infants for several reasons. Its high protein content is hard for a baby's immature system to digest and process. The potassium and sodium contents also are higher than recommended for babies. Cow's milk is low in iron, vitamin E, and linoleic acid; the iron it does contain isn't absorbed well. And it doesn't provide enough zinc, vitamins C and E, copper, and essential fatty acids—nutrients that babies need to grow and develop.

Goat's milk isn't a suitable alternative either, for many of the same reasons. If you choose to offer goat's milk after age one, make sure it's vitamin D fortified. To clear up a misconception, babies who are allergic to the protein in cow's milk are probably allergic to the protein in goat's milk, too. And about one in five babies who are allergic to cow's milk are also allergic to soy milk.

With Baby . . . That's More Than One!

Are you an experienced parent—with one or more other children? If so, feeding a newborn isn't new to you. Yet, every baby is different—so be prepared to learn new parenting skills. One child may be a fussy eater; another, ready and eager to eat. One may be ready for solid foods at five months; another, at six months. Observe, respect, and enjoy their unique differences.

Do you wish that you had handled feeding differently with your first child? That's normal, too, especially after being a first-time parent. You were learning! It's okay to change your feeding approach with your next child.

Perhaps the biggest change is trying to do several things at once: trying to feed a baby, older children, and others in your family—including you. Enlist help from your preschooler or school-age child, without expecting too much. An older child can be your helper, but shouldn't be responsible for your baby. Tasks as simple as wiping baby's sticky hands, getting a bib, or picking up a bottle that falls to the floor make your older child feel helpful, "grown up," and important. A younger child can listen to music or a story as you are nursing.

A new baby competes for your attention, which may lead to fussy eating from another child. Give your older child personal time at the table, too; include him or her in table talk. And try to keep mealtime calm and pleasant—despite all that's happening around the table.

---

for the small number of babies who are sensitive to protein in cow's milk. Vegetarian moms who don't choose to breast-feed may prefer a soy-based formula, too. As an aside, soy-based formulas do not seem to prevent allergies. For premature or low-birth-weight babies, a soy-based formula probably won't be recommended. Ask your baby's healthcare provider about choosing the right formula.

Old-fashioned homemade formulas from canned evaporated milk and corn syrup may have nourished you or your mother, but they're nutritionally inferior to today's commercial formulas. And corn syrup and honey may contain botulinum spores, which can produce a deadly toxin. *The bottom line:* Homemade infant formulas generally aren't recommended and may be harmful. Recreating the nutrient balance babies need and get from commercial formulas is nearly impossible with a homemade formula.

Consider this when choosing a formula:

Iron. Many infant formulas are iron-fortified. Iron is a key mineral in forming hemoglobin, the part of red blood cells that carries oxygen to cells to make energy. Your baby also needs iron for brain development; an

Have You Ever Wondered

. . . if your baby needs formula fortified with DHA and ARA? Infant formulas with two fatty acids—docosa-hexaenoic acid (DHA) and arachidonic acid (ARA)—now are sold in the United States.

Found naturally in breast milk, DHA and ARA are important components of cell membranes in the brain and the retina. Infants also produce these fatty acids inside the body when adequate amounts of essential fatty acids—alpha-linolenic acid and linoleic acid—are present in infant formula. Inconclusive evidence suggests some benefits from directly consuming DHA. *See chapter 5, "Fat Facts."*

DHA and ARA, added to almost all infant formula, may provide developmental benefits (brain and vision), especially for premature infants. These nutrients are generally recognized as safe (GRAS) for full-term infants by the U.S. Food and Drug Administration (FDA), but not yet for preterm infants. The benefits of these formulas are still inconclusive. For more current information, check www.FDA.gov. Ask your physician before choosing these formulas for your infant. The formula label will indicate the presence of DHA and ARA.

. . . why carrageenan and mono- and diglycerides are added to some liquid formulas? They pose no health risks and are added to ensure that the formula doesn't separate during its shelf-life.

. . . if formula fortified with probiotics helps build immunity? Perhaps. Probiotics are friendly bacteria that may help protect against unhealthy bacteria in the intestines that cause infections and may provide other health benefits while the baby consumes them. Breast-fed babies already have friendly bacteria. Adding probiotics to formula may have similar benefit; however, there's not enough conclusive research yet to know. These formulas appear safe, but before offering formula with probiotics, ask your baby's doctor.

iron deficiency may cause irreversible developmental delays. Full-term babies are born with enough iron stores to last four to six months. An iron-fortified formula right from the start helps keep a baby's iron stores adequate.

Choose an iron-fortified formula, or ask your baby's doctor, pediatric nurse, or a registered dietitian to recommend one. If your baby starts on a formula without iron, switch to an iron-fortified formula by four months. To clear up a common misperception, iron added to infant formula won't cause constipation or other feeding problems. Continue an iron-fortified formula until twelve months, when your baby is already eating a variety of foods and starts cow's milk.

Fluoride. This mineral helps your baby develop strong teeth and protects teeth from cavities. Use fluoridated water if available, but don't overdo it since too much fluoride can stain baby and permanent teeth. Talk to your baby's doctor about the water you use. When you mix powdered or liquid concentrate formulas with water, you add fluoride, too—if your water supply is fluoridated. Ready-to-feed formulas aren't prepared with fluoridated water. If you regularly offer ready-to-feed formula or if your water supply isn't fluoridated, ask your baby's doctor about fluoride supplementation. After six months a fluoride supplement may be advised.

Recipe for Success

For mixing infant formula, careful measurement, cleanliness, and refrigeration constitute the "recipe for success." When properly mixed, powdered, concentrated, and ready-to-feed infant formulas are identical in their nutritional composition. The primary differences are price and how much time you need to prepare formula. Pay attention to the "use by" date on the label. If it's expired, don't use it.

Whatever formula chosen, follow these guidelines:

● Wash your hands first, and clean the preparation surface. With an immature immune system, your baby is highly susceptible to foodborne illness.

● Pay careful attention to mixing instructions on the formula label. Adding too much water dilutes it. Then your baby may not get enough nutrients or calories (food energy). Conversely, adding too little water concentrates the formula too much. Then it's hard for a baby to digest, and it supplies too much food energy at one feeding and not enough fluid to prevent dehydration.

Powdered and concentrated formulas should be mixed with water that's pathogen-free and low in minerals. One option is to bring tap or bottled water to a rolling boil for one minute, then cool it. Longer boiling may concentrate the minerals too much. Cooling the water before mixing the formula lessens both clumping and the loss of heat-labile vitamins. Bottled water that's labeled "sterile" is another option, unless your baby's doctor advises otherwise. If the label on bottled water says it's meant for infants, the water must meet Environmental Protection Agency (EPA) standards for tap water, and it must say "sterile." *See "What about Bottled Water?" in chapter 8.*

Shake ready-to-feed formula and concentrated formula before pouring it into a bottle since some solids may have settled to the bottom.

● If your baby does well with one type and brand of infant formula, stick with it unless your baby's doctor advises otherwise. If you switch, check the label. The "recipe" for mixing the new formula may differ from the brand you used first.

● Always use clean bottles and baby-bottle nipples. *See the following "Bottles and Nipples: Baby Feeding Supplies" for cleaning tips.*

● For convenience, prepare a supply of bottles— enough for the day ahead. Date and refrigerate the prepared infant formula as soon as you make it; use it within forty-eight hours. Once opened, ready-to-feed formula and liquid concentrates must be covered and refrigerated and used within forty-eight hours. Cover

How Much Formula?

Your baby's appetite is a good guide to the amount of infant formula he or she needs—and how often. That depends in part on the stage of development. In addition, some babies drink a little more or less depending on body weight and when solid food is introduced. Use this chart *only* as a guide. On average, babies need about 2½ ounces of formula per day for each pound of body weight.

Age	Number of Bottle Feedings per Day	Total Amount of Formula per Day (oz.)
Birth to 4 months	6–8	18–32
4 to 6 months	4–6	28–45
6 to 9 months	3–5	24–32
9 to 12 months	2–4	24–32

a powdered formula container that's been opened; use it within one month.

● Infant formula can be fed to a baby at a cold temperature, room temperature, or slightly warm. Always test the temperature of the formula to make sure it's not too hot. *Caution:* Avoid feeding cold formula to a newborn. Doing so may lower his or her body's core temperature. *To bring chilled bottles to room temperature or to slightly warm, see "Play It Safe: Warming Baby's Bottle and Food" later in this chapter.*

● Make only as much as your baby needs. Discard formula left in the bottle within one hour after feeding. Bacteria from your baby's mouth can contaminate formula and cause spoilage. To avoid too much leftover, fill the bottle with less. Make more as your baby's appetite dictates.

Bottles and Nipples: Baby Feeding Supplies

Baby bottles. Plastic or glass bottles, or disposable bottle bags? The choice is yours. Some parents keep a variety of baby-bottle sizes and styles on hand for different purposes. For example, disposable bottle bags are handy when you're on the go and when washing facilities are limited. For convenience, bottles with disposable liners let you toss away the used liner when the feeding is done. Small-size bottles are perfect for holding 2- or 3-ounce feedings during the first weeks

Knowing When Your Baby's Had Enough

There's no exact science to formula-feeding. These signs suggest that your baby's had enough formula:

● Your baby may close his or her mouth and turn away from the nipple.

● Your baby may fall asleep.

● Your baby may get interested in other things.

● Your baby may bite, spit out, or play with the nipple.

● Your baby's sucking may slow or stop.

after delivery. Be cautious of bottles with cute shapes; they're often hard to clean.

Try to use plastic baby bottles that are free of bisphenol A (BPA). Although there's no scientific proof linking health risks to BPA in hard plastics, you can take reasonable steps to reduce exposure to them. Switch to glass baby bottles or to plastic baby bottles and sippy cups labeled BPA-free. *Refer to chapter 9 for more guidance.*

Baby-bottle nipples. They come in many shapes and sizes. Choose nipples that match your baby's mouth size and developmental needs. A baby's comfort and ease of sucking are the criteria to use when choosing a nipple.

There are four basic baby-bottle nipple types: regular nipple with slow, medium, or fast flow (the number and size of the holes will determine flow); nipple for very small or premature babies; orthodontic nipple, which imitates the shape of a human nipple during breast-feeding; and cleft-palate nipple. A cleft-palate nipple is meant for babies with a lip or palate problem that keeps them from sucking properly.

Keep bottle-feeding equipment in good condition:

● Discard cracked or chipped bottles that could break and spill formula onto your baby. Toss scratched plastic bottles.

● Replace nipples regularly, as they can become "gummy" or cracked with age. Check them by pulling the tip before each use.

● Check the size of the opening on new nipples and then periodically as you use them. Formula should flow from the nipple in even drops—not a steady stream. If the milk flows too quickly, your baby could choke, so discard the nipple. If the milk flows too slowly for your baby, consider trying a nipple with more holes, designed for older babies.

When it comes to preparing infant formula and washing bottles, cleanliness is essential! Your baby's immune system isn't fully developed, so he or she is very susceptible to foodborne illness from improperly cleaned feeding equipment.

● Use hot, soapy water to wash your hands, work area, measuring utensils, bottles, and nipples. If possible, wash bottles right away when they're easier to clean.

● Thoroughly clean reusable bottles, caps, and nipples by washing them with hot, soapy water and rinsing them well before each use. Sanitize nipples and bottles in boiling water for two minutes. Then let them air-dry. Or wash bottles, rings, and caps in the top dishwasher rack. Look for dishwasher baskets designed to hold bottle parts and to keep them from falling to the dishwasher bottom.

● *Remember:* The outer "shell" of bottles with disposable bottle bags needs regular washing to destroy bacteria.

● Opening a new can of formula? First, wash the can opener and the can's lid with soap and water; rinse well.

Bottle-Feeding Techniques: All in the Family!

Bottle-feeding gives the whole family warm, cozy moments with the baby. Nestled in the arms of a parent, sibling, grandparent, or other caregiver, babies feel safe and comfortable. Consider these tips for your bottle-feeding techniques:

● Find a comfortable place, perhaps a chair for you with an armrest. Hold your baby across your lap with his or her head slightly raised, resting on your elbow. That allows a baby to suck from the bottle and to swallow easily. Keep eye contact.

● Avoid propping your baby in bed or in an infant seat with a bottle, even if your baby can hold a bottle. Babies can choke! Propping a baby on a pillow can also cause eating discomfort and ear infections. And if he or she falls asleep with a bottle in the mouth, formula that bathes the teeth can promote baby-bottle tooth

---

Need more parenting tips for feeding your baby? Check here for "how-tos":

● Look ahead to toddler and preschool feeding—see chapter 17.

● Eat smart during pregnancy and breast-feeding—see chapter 18.

● Know signs of food allergies or intolerances—see chapter 21.

● Find a nutrition expert experienced in infant feeding—see chapter 24.

decay. Remove the bottle promptly if your baby falls asleep while eating.

● Angle the bottle to help prevent your baby from swallowing too much air. The nipple should stay full with formula when your baby is eating.

● To ease discomfort from air bubbles swallowed during feeding, burp your baby in the middle and at the end of feedings. Hold him or her upright, chin resting on your shoulder, or lie your baby tummy down across your lap. Then gently pat or rub your baby's back.

● Keep a clean, damp washcloth handy. It's normal for babies to spit up some formula during burping.

● When your baby's done, take the nipple out of his or her mouth. Sucking on an empty bottle causes air bubbles in your baby's tummy.

● If your baby doesn't finish a bottle, don't refrigerate it for later. Don't keep formula at room temperature for more than one hour, either.

Baby's Bottle-Feeding Routine

Newborns eat frequently in the first months after birth—perhaps every two hours! Since their stomachs are small, just about 2 ounces, or as many as 4 ounces of infant formula, may be enough for the early feedings. *See "How Much Formula?" in this chapter for guidelines during the first twelve months.*

Formula-fed babies usually need twenty to thirty minutes to finish a bottle. If it takes less than fifteen minutes for a newborn to finish a bottle, use a nipple with smaller holes. If it takes longer and if the baby is sucking actively, make sure the holes aren't clogged. Or try a nipple with more holes.

As with a breast-fed baby, plan to formula-feed on demand—when a baby signals hunger: fussy sounds, hand-to-mouth activity, pre-cry facial grimaces, and waking and tossing around. Trying to impose a feeding routine will frustrate you both. You can't spoil your baby by feeding on demand. A formula-fed baby may not eat as often; formula digests more slowly than breast milk.

Should formula be warm, cool, or at room temperature? That's up to you. Your baby will become accustomed to whatever temperature you usually provide. If you warm it, just be careful so your baby

Physical Activity: Guidelines for Infants

Physical activity is important from the beginning of life! Activity can encourage rolling over, crawling, and walking as well as cognitive development, and can lead to a preference for active play. Conversely, inactivity may set the stage for childhood obesity. Rather than confine your baby to a stroller or playpen too much, start a habit of active living now. During this first year of life:

● Spend part of each day with active baby games such as peekaboo and pat-a-cake.

● Find ways to help your infant safely and actively explore his or her surroundings. Floor play is great!

● Avoid restricting your infant's movements for prolonged periods of time.

● Choose activities that encourage your infant to move large muscles (arms, legs, hands, and feet).

● Talk to your child care provider about how much time is spent moving about, too.

● Play when your baby's awake; don't interrupt sleep to play.

● Avoid rough-and-tumble play. Gentle bouncing, rolling, and swaying are good from the start.

● Join a parent-infant play group.

doesn't get burned. *For tips, see "Play It Safe: Warming Baby's Bottle and Food" later in this chapter.*

Let your baby decide how much to drink. Pay attention to his or her appetite; your baby doesn't need to finish a bottle. In fact, forcing your baby to finish it focuses too much on eating—which may lead to over- or underfeeding. To learn good eating habits, babies need to learn hunger and fullness cues.

If your baby has six or more wet diapers a day, seems content between feedings, and his or her weight increases steadily, your baby's probably getting enough. If not, check with your doctor or pediatric nurse. *For more hunger and fullness cues, see "Knowing When Your Baby's Had Enough" in this chapter.*

Solid Advice on Solid Foods

Just when parents master breast-feeding routines or formula mixing, babies show that they're ready to join the high-chair crowd! Starting solid foods is just one more adventure in the journey of child feeding.

Throughout the first year, breast milk or iron-fortified infant formula continues to be your baby's main nutrient and energy source. (Wait until after twelve months for cow's milk.) Around the middle of your baby's first year, he or she will be ready to start solid foods to complement the nutrition from breast milk or formula. Typically they're added in this order:

● Iron-fortified, single-grain infant cereal (mixed with breast milk or formula)—six months or somewhat sooner.

● Strained meats/poultry; single strained fruits and vegetables; unsweetened 100 percent fruit juices (vitamin C fortified) in a cup; toast; and teething biscuits—six to nine months. The order isn't important—as long as solids provide your baby with an iron source and the consistency and texture are developmentally appropriate.

● Chopped soft fruits, vegetables, and meats; unsweetened dry cereals; plain, soft bread; and pasta—ten to twelve months.

For more detailed guidelines, see "Infant Feeding Plan: A Basic Guideline" later in this chapter.

Ready, Willing, and Able

Although most babies are ready to start solid foods about six months of age or perhaps somewhat earlier, don't rely solely on the calendar! Babies must be physically and developmentally ready for solid foods. *Remember:* Each baby is different. Age is just a point of reference. If babies aren't ready to eat solid food, it likely will end up on their laps—not in their tummies. Offering solids too soon only frustrates baby, parents, and other caregivers.

Until about four months, babies are unable to effectively coordinate their tongue to push food to the back of their mouth for swallowing. Instead, they have a tongue-pushing reflex needed for nursing or bottle-feeding. Well-meaning friends and family may tell you to start solid foods earlier to help your baby sleep. However, babies sleep through the night only after their nervous system develops more fully. In fact, solid foods offered too soon stress a baby's immature digestive system, and most passes right through to the diaper.

When is the right time to start solid foods? Usually, around six months of age. Then, if your baby weighs at least 13 pounds and has doubled his or her birth weight, it might be time. Let your baby be the judge. There's no one calendar date that's right for all babies. According to the American Academy of Pediatrics, introducing complementary solid foods before six months generally doesn't increase total calorie intake or growth rate, but may substitute foods that lack the nutrients and protective factors in breast milk (and formulas). Watch for these milestones that suggest that he or she may be ready to eat solid foods:

For Vegetarian Babies . . .

Breast milk is the best first food for babies. Commercial infant formulas, including soy formulas, are also healthful options for vegetarian babies. *Caution:* Vegetarian milk, such as rice beverages, are not! For these beverages, wait until after two years of age; talk to your doctor, pediatric nurse, or registered dietitian first. Rice and almond beverages in particular are often low in protein and other nutrients. They can't adequately substitute for cow's milk or soy beverages.

Give special attention to sources of zinc, iron, vitamin D, and vitamin B_{12}. Vegetarian or not, the American Academy of Pediatrics advises a vitamin D supplement for breast-fed babies, starting within the first few days after birth, even if the baby consumes supplemental formula. Infant formula contains vitamin D. For breast-fed vegan infants, a vitamin B_{12} supplement may be recommended if the mother doesn't consume vitamin B_{12}–fortified foods. Healthcare providers may advise an iron supplement.

Time to introduce protein-rich solid foods? Offer pureed tofu, cottage cheese, cooked egg, soy or dairy yogurt, and *very* pureed or strained beans (legumes). Later start tofu cubes, cheese or soy cheese, and soy-burger pieces. At age one year or older, it's okay to start a full-fat commercial, fortified soy beverage or cow's milk. When infants are weaned, provide energy-rich, nutrient-rich foods, such as mashed avocado, bean spreads, and tofu. Before age two years, babies need enough fat to develop a healthy nervous system; this isn't the time to restrict fat in food!

Most important: If you choose a vegetarian eating style for your infant, consult a registered dietitian, your doctor, or a pediatric nurse for support and nutrition counseling.

● *Baby can sit with little support.* Your baby can control his or her head and may be able to lift up his or her chest, shoulders, and head when lying tummy down. By now your baby can turn away to signal "enough."

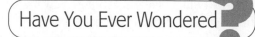
Have You Ever Wondered

... if it's okay to offer solid foods in a bottle? No, not for most babies. One problem: a possible delay in learning feeding skills. Cereal or other foods from a bottle also can cause choking and may encourage your baby to overeat (too many calories). With spoon-feeding, resting between bites gives your baby time to feel full and learn self-regulation. Cereal in a bottle also may replace breast milk or formula, along with the nutrients they supply. To clarify a misconception, offering cereal in a bottle won't help baby sleep or stop crying.

... how you can help relieve the discomfort of teething? Rub your baby's tender gums gently with your clean finger, perhaps with a little teething gel along the gumline. A chilled teething ring—kept in the refrigerator, not the freezer—can help. Chewing on textured solid foods, such as teething biscuits or bagel pieces, helps teething. Offer these foods when your baby is sitting up; stay nearby. Chill baby foods, too; they may feel better on a baby's gums than warm foods.

More drooling and swollen, tender gums signal teething. Be aware that a runny nose, diarrhea, fever, or rash probably are symptoms of illness, not teething.

... if I should comfort my baby with a bottle or food? No, instead just cuddle, rock, or walk your baby. Comforting an infant with food may teach him or her to eat in response to emotions, not hunger. A fussy baby may just need attention. Remember, it's normal for babies to cry, especially if they're hungry, wet, *or* tired!

... if my baby is growing at a healthy rate? Your baby's doctor will assess your baby's growth rate during regular visits. With support from the American Academy of Pediatrics and the National Institutes of Health, the Centers for Disease Control and Prevention (CDC) in 2006 recommended using growth charts from the World Health Organization (WHO) to assess growth for infants and toddlers ages one to twenty-three months. After that CDC growth charts are used. For both WHO and CDC charts, see www.cdc.gov/growthcharts/who_charts.htm.

● *Baby has an appetite for more.* If your baby is hungry after eight to ten breast-feedings or drinks more than 32 ounces of formula, it may be time for solids.

● *Baby shows interest in foods you're eating.* As your baby watches, he or she leans forward and may even open his or her mouth in anticipation, or perhaps grabs things to put in his or her mouth. Take a trial run with appropriate solid foods. If your baby doesn't seem interested, wait a few weeks, then try again. Avoid forcing a child to eat solid foods.

● *Baby can move foods from the front to the back of the mouth.* Up to about four months of age, babies will try to push food out with their tongue. As they develop, the tongue becomes more coordinated and moves back and forth. This allows babies to swallow foods from a spoon. When a baby is ready, eating solids helps with motor development, such as swallowing and using facial muscles.

Something New: Eating from a Spoon!

Learning to eat the first solid food—usually iron-fortified cereal—from a spoon is a big transition in infant feeding. It's a step toward independence. And it encourages chewing and swallowing skills.

Spoon feeding has challenges. It's messier. At first, more food may end up on the bib and face than in the mouth. Try this to make the transition pleasant:

● Relax. This is a new eating adventure for both of you! Pick a time when your baby is relaxed and not ravenously hungry. Smile, and talk as you feed your baby. Your soothing voice will make new food experiences more pleasant—and talking helps with language development, too.

● Of course, wash your hands first. And keep baby food safe and clean.

● Use a small spoon with a long handle—and just a little bit of food on the tip of the spoon.

● Start with a teaspoon or two of food. Then work up to one to two tablespoons, two to three times a day.

● Let your baby set the pace for feeding. Don't try to go faster or slower.

● Seat your baby straight or propped upright, facing forward. This makes swallowing easier and helps prevent choking. Position the feeder in front of your baby.

Use the seat belt in a high chair. Have direct eye contact with your baby.

● Introduce new foods at the start of the meal. Once satisfied, your baby may be less willing to try a new taste. If he or she refuses a new food, that's okay; try it again in a few days or weeks.

Infant Cereal: Timing Is Everything

By tradition, single-grain cereal is typically introduced as the first solid food. Make it a source of iron, such as iron-fortified infant cereal, which is often the most convenient iron source. Whether they are dry or premixed, opt for cereals developed for babies. They digest more easily than varieties for older children and adults. Iron-fortified infant cereals help babies maintain their iron stores.

● Although there's no strict order, you might start with rice cereal. It's often best as the first cereal because it's least likely to cause allergic reactions. *To determine if a food may be causing a reaction, see "Food Sensitivities and Your Baby" on this page.* Hold off on wheat cereal until after your baby's first birthday. Some infants are sensitive to wheat before one year of age.

● When it comes to your baby's first cereal feedings, keep the cereal mixture thin. Start with just one part dry cereal to four parts of breast milk or infant formula. Once your baby develops eating skills—and a taste for cereal—mix in less liquid so it's thicker. Don't mix in honey or corn syrup, which may contain small amounts of bacteria *(Clostridium botulinum)* spores that can cause severe foodborne illness.

● Be prepared if your baby refuses cereal at first. Try again in a few days. Infant cereal tastes different from the familiar breast milk or formula. The texture is different, too—not to mention the difference between a nipple and a spoon!

● Once your baby starts eating more cereal, he or she will take less breast milk or infant formula. Breast milk or iron-fortified formula still should be the mainstay of the diet during the first year.

Solid Foods: What Comes Next?

Once your baby accepts cereal, try strained meats and beans (legumes), which are good sources of vitamin B_6, phosphorus, iron, and zinc. Especially for breast-fed babies, these nutrients are likely to be limited. Offer strained vegetables or fruits, too. It doesn't matter which you offer first: vegetables or fruits. Some pediatricians advise vegetables first.

Even if your baby refuses a food three to four times, don't give up! Babies often need twelve or even fifteen different tries before finally accepting a new food. Just be patient and persistent as your baby learns.

● One by one, offer a variety of foods. This lays the

Food Sensitivities and Your Baby

Some babies are sensitive to certain foods. You know by their reaction—perhaps a rash, wheezing, diarrhea, or vomiting. Most babies outgrow these reactions once their digestive and immune systems mature. (To reassure you . . . a baby's stool often changes color and consistency when new foods are eaten. These changes don't necessarily indicate a food sensitivity.) To best monitor your baby for food-induced reactions:

● Keep track of foods your baby eats. Choose single-grain infant cereals and plain fruits, vegetables, and meats instead of mixed varieties or "dinners" until you know what your baby can handle. If your baby has a reaction, stop that food for a while.

● Offer one new food at a time. Wait three to five days before offering the next new food. If your baby has trouble with a certain food, you'll more likely know what food causes the reaction.

● Be watchful of foods with common allergens: peanuts, tree nuts, soy, eggs, fish, shellfish, wheat, and milk. Use the ingredient list and allergen labeling on food labels to identify these ingredients.

● If any food causes a significant or ongoing reaction stop giving it. Talk to your baby's doctor, pediatric nurse, or registered dietitian about it. Together, you can establish an eating plan that's best for your baby.

Whether a baby has a family history of food allergies or not, delaying or avoiding foods with common allergens, such as wheat, peanuts, fish, or eggs, after six months of age doesn't appear to reduce the risk of food allergies. From an allergy prevention standpoint, neither does delaying solid foods beyond four to six months.

For more about food intolerances and allergies, see chapter 21, "Sensitive to Food."

groundwork for healthful eating throughout life. *See "Variety: Good for You, Good for Baby!" in this chapter.*

● Try single foods first: for example, meat—beef, chicken, turkey, ham; beans or tofu (for vegetarian infants); fruits—applesauce, pears, peaches, prunes (dried plums), bananas; vegetables—sweet potato, carrots, squash, peas, green beans; and eggs.

● Start with smooth foods that are easy to swallow. Babies can eat mashed or finely chopped foods when their teeth start to appear and when they start to make chewing motions.

● If you offer juice, offer it from a cup, not a bottle. Sucking juice too long from a bottle exposes a baby's teeth to natural sugars in fruit juice. Prolonged contact with sugars can promote tooth decay. Offer mashed or pureed fruit first.

● At about six to nine months of age, most babies enjoy drinking from a cup—or at least trying to! Offer formula, breast milk, or water in a child-size unbreakable cup. A cup without handles may be easier for a young child to hold. Covered cups with a spout are helpful at this stage. Babies are clumsy with a cup at first but usually catch on quickly.

● As your baby gets more teeth and gets interested in self-feeding—at about nine to twelve months of age—introduce finger foods. Soft, ripe fruit without peels or seeds and cooked vegetables are good for tiny fingers. Avoid foods a baby can choke on. *See "For Babies, Toddlers, and Preschoolers: How to Avoid Choking" in this chapter.*

● Teething biscuits, breadsticks, and rice cakes are good natural "teethers." Chewing on them eases a baby's sore gums while offering a healthful snack—eaten "all by myself"! *See "'Feeding Myself'" in this chapter.*

● Babies need the opportunity to develop a taste for the natural flavor of foods without added sugars, salt, or other flavorings. Seasonings are not added to many varieties of commercially prepared baby foods. Read the product label to find out.

● Gradually expose your baby to foods with herbs and spices, including flavors of your family's food culture. There's no need to keep food plain.

● As you choose foods for your baby, don't restrict fat for the first two years. Growing babies need the calories and essential fatty acids that fat provides for brain development.

● As your baby grows and develops a bigger appetite, offer more solid foods. *The chart "Infant Feeding*

Caring for Baby Teeth

Good dental care begins at birth—even before baby teeth appear! Healthy teeth let children chew food more easily, learn to talk clearly, and smile with self-assurance.

Make cleaning your baby's teeth and gums part of the daily bathtub routine. Starting at birth, clean your baby's gums with a soft infant toothbrush and water, or use a clean, wet washcloth or gauze pad. Do this after every feeding. Skip toothpaste, which babies often swallow.

Schedule your baby's first visit to a pediatric dentist after the first tooth appears (at about six to twelve months).

Fluoride is a mineral that helps teeth develop and resist decay. In many places, fluoride is naturally present in local water supplies at various levels. If you live in an area that doesn't have fluoridated water, ask your baby's doctor if your baby or child needs a fluoride supplement. Unless your child's dentist advises otherwise, wait until after age two or three years to start with fluoridated toothpaste. *For more information on fluoride, see "Vitamin and Mineral Supplements for Breast-Fed Babies" and "Formula: What Type?" earlier in this chapter. For more about fluoridated water, see "The Fluoride Connection" in chapter 8.*

To avoid tooth decay, do not put your infant, toddler, or young child to bed with a bottle of juice, formula, or milk. The liquid that bathes the teeth and gums from sucking on the bottle stays on teeth and can cause tooth decay. That happens even if a baby's teeth haven't yet erupted through the gums. If your child won't nap or go to bed without a bottle, fill it with plain water instead.

For more about dental care, see "Your Smile: Carbohydrates and Oral Health" in chapter 3.

Have You Ever Wondered ?

. . . if it's okay to sweeten baby foods with honey or to dip a pacifier in honey? No. Until after a baby's first birthday, avoid giving honey in any form. Very occasionally, honey can harbor spores of a toxic bacterium called *Clostridium botulinum.* For adults and older children, these spores are harmless. But for babies younger than twelve months, they can cause botulism, a severe foodborne illness that can be fatal. *Note:* Sucking on a sweetened pacifier promotes cavities.

. . . when your baby can have fruit juice? Before six months fruit juice offers no nutritional benefits, advises the American Academy of Pediatrics. After six months pasteurized 100 percent fruit juice (not fruit drinks) is an option, as long as your baby doesn't drink too much of it. Four ounces of vitamin C–fortified juice a day are enough.

Offer juice in a small cup at mealtime or snacktime—not from a bottle, covered cup, or juice box, which promotes sipping juice throughout the day. Juice shouldn't be given in a bedtime bottle, or to manage diarrhea. Except that fruit has more fiber, fruit juice and fruit offer the same nutritional benefits for older babies.

. . . if your baby needs a vitamin supplement when he or she starts solid foods? Ask your pediatrician. A specially formulated infant supplement may be recommended if you're not sure if foods supply enough, if your family is vegetarian, or if your baby needs to restrict food for any reason.

Plan: A Basic Guideline" in this chapter suggests when.

To refute a myth, feeding your baby cereal before bedtime doesn't lead to sleeping through the night.

Variety: Good for You, Good for Baby!

Variety certainly is the spice of life—especially when it comes to forming good eating habits for your baby. Offering your baby a wide variety of foods with different flavors, colors, shapes, and textures helps ensure that his or her nutrition needs are met. Variety makes mealtime more fun, too! As an aside, babies perceive sweet tastes first; both amniotic fluid and breast milk are sweet. Other taste perceptions develop during a baby's first year.

Like you, your baby may like some foods better than others. That's normal. Likes and dislikes may change from week to week. Continue to offer food variety. Don't let your own food biases limit your baby's preferences. Your baby or toddler may like those foods!

Skip foods with added sugars or salt. Consuming them now just enhances a baby's preference for them later, and the added sugars only provide added calories.

If your baby has little or no interest in solids and continues to struggle with spoon feeding or more textured foods, talk to your baby's healthcare provider. Your baby may need help from a health professional who specializes in infant feeding issues.

Learning to enjoy a variety of nutrient-rich solid foods helps establish a lifetime of good eating habits. This is why variety is so important, even in the early years.

Breads, Cereals, and Other Grain Foods

Offer iron-fortified cereal to babies and toddlers. To enhance iron absorption, serve iron-containing foods with vitamin C–rich foods, such as fruits and fortified infant juices. Other grain products include soft, cooked pasta or rice, soft breads, dry cereals, crackers, and teething biscuits.

Caution with high-fiber foods: Some high-fiber cereals, such as bran, are low in calories yet high in bulk. Avoid offering large amounts to infants; they fill a small stomach without providing many nutrients or calories. Infants and young children can get enough fiber from a variety of foods.

Meats, Milk Products, and Other Protein Sources

These foods are valuable sources of protein, calcium, iron, zinc, and other minerals that your baby needs to develop bones and muscles, as well as for his or her blood supply and brain development.

Offer a variety of soft, pureed, or finely chopped meats such as chicken, turkey, or beef.

Feeding Myself

As babies master spoon feeding, they're gradually ready to feed themselves. Watch for signals that suggest your baby is ready, at about eight to nine months: perhaps trying to help you, or taking a cup away, or putting his or her hand on yours.

● Start with finger foods. It's easy because eating by hand is utensil-free.

● Give your baby a spoon to hold in one hand while you use another for feeding. This gives your baby practice grasping a utensil.

● Offer baby-friendly utensils: a small, rounded spoon with a straight, wide handle, and a dish with high, straight sides.

● Use the two-spoon approach. Give an empty one to your baby, and fill the other with baby food. Then switch so baby has a filled spoon for self-feeding.

● Be patient—and relaxed. Food will end up on the floor. Your baby will need lots of practice before being able to eat a whole meal without your help.

● Always stay with your baby when he or she is self-feeding. In that way you'll be around if he or she starts to choke.

Tip: Start a lifelong habit of family mealtime. Bring your baby's high chair to the family table, even if you need to feed your baby first.

By age seven to eight months, well-cooked, pureed beans (legumes) (perhaps strained) or mashed tofu are options for vegetarian infants; since tofu is made of soy, be watchful for potential food allergies. (Wait until after one year of age to offer smooth nut and seed butters, spread on bread or crackers.)

Offer only cooked eggs; before age one, your doctor may advise only egg yolks in case your baby has a reaction to egg whites.

After twelve months, if children no longer take breast milk or infant formula, whole cow's milk is an important source of calories, calcium, vitamin D, proteins, essential fatty acids, and some other nutrients. Growing bones need an adequate supply of calcium and vitamin D. Good calcium sources include cheese, milk, and calcium-fortified cottage cheese. Health experts don't advise feeding lower-fat dairy foods, such as low-fat or fat-free milk, for children under two years of age. *(See chapter 17.)* If you offer yogurt (often sold as low-fat), offer whole-milk dairy foods, too, for vitamin D and essential fatty acids, as well as calcium.

Fruits and Vegetables

They're good sources of vitamin C, beta carotene, other nutrients, and phytonutrients. By offering these foods frequently at mealtime, children become familiar with fruit and vegetable flavors. That helps set the stage for accepting and enjoying them throughout life.

Introduce vegetables and fruits in any order. If you want to start with applesauce, bananas, and carrots, that's fine. Offer new flavors along with familiar vegetables and fruit. Respect what your baby likes and

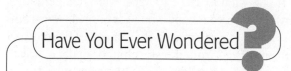

Have You Ever Wondered

. . . what foods help your baby avoid constipation? Offer a combination of foods to keep stools a consistency that's easier to pass. Some foods produce softer stools: for example, apricots, peas, peaches, pears, and prunes (dried plums). Drinking enough fluid helps soften stools.

If your baby gets constipated, offer apple or pear juice twice a day, or prune juice for something stronger. Get advice from your pediatrician if this doesn't work.

. . . how to tell if your older baby is hungry or full? Older babies might signal hunger by opening and moving their mouth toward a spoon, by trying to swipe food toward their mouth, or by pointing, nodding, or grabbing a spoon. Fullness signals might be turning their head away from the spoon, spitting out or pushing familiar foods away, or being distracted. Learn your baby's hunger and fullness cues, as you help him or her learn to avoid overeating later in life.

. . . whether lead poisoning is an issue for your infant? You need to check! The American Academy of Pediatrics and the Centers for Disease Control and Prevention advise lead screening at ages one and two. Talk to your doctor. *Refer to chapter 8 for more about lead poisoning.*

. . . if organic baby food is worth the extra price? That's your choice. The American Academy of Pediatrics advises that organic baby foods are no more nutritious or safer than traditional options—but usually cost more. Organic or not, nutrient-rich foods from the start are the key to a lifetime of healthy eating.

may not like. No one fruit or vegetable is essential for health, so relax. Encourage a rainbow of colorful vegetables and fruits. The goal? Learning to like as many vegetables and fruits as possible.

No evidence indicates that introducing fruit before vegetables makes a baby prefer fruit.

Play It Safe: Warming Baby's Bottle and Food

Babies enjoy breast milk, infant formula, and baby foods either warm or cool. Unlike most adults, babies have no physical or emotional need for warmed liquids and warmed foods. That said, cold formula fed to a newborn can lower his or her core body temperature.

● If you want to serve foods at warm temperatures, play it safe so your baby won't get burned. Warm bottles of formula or breast milk in a pan of warm water that's removed from the stovetop, or under a stream of warm tap water. You can do the same with frozen breast milk, or defrost it overnight in the refrigerator.

● Avoid heating milk to a boiling temperature. Boiling temperatures destroy some nutrients, and for breast milk, some protective properties.

● Shake the bottle during and after warming to evenly distribute the heat. And always test a few drops on the back of your hand, not your wrist; the back of your hand is more sensitive. The formula or milk should be tepid, or just slightly warm to the touch.

Microwave Warming: Be Very Cautious

Be very cautious if you heat baby food in a microwave oven. Avoid using the microwave oven to warm breast milk or infant formula. Microwaving creates uneven heating, or "hot spots," that can burn a baby's mouth, throat, and skin. Food may feel cool on the outside while the inner contents reach scorching temperatures. And since food doesn't heat evenly, microwaving may not destroy bacteria that cause foodborne illness.

Besides the chance of burning your baby, microwave heating produces high temperatures quickly; some vitamins and protective factors in breast milk may be destroyed. Another problem: Sometimes plastic bottle liners explode if their contents become too hot.

For solid foods . . . warm foods in the microwave oven until only just lukewarm.

● Warm food in a microwave-safe dish. As in baby bottles, food heated in jars can develop hot spots.

● Heat only the amount you'll need. Less food heats faster than more food, and some ovens heat faster than others. Fifteen seconds on high (100 percent power) for 4 ounces of baby food are enough. Heat higher-fat foods such as meat and eggs on the stove, not in the microwave oven. They heat faster and splatter or overheat more.

● Read warming guidelines on baby food labels. And remember that baby foods can be served cold, at room temperature, or slightly warm.

● After microwaving, allow food to "rest"; food will continue to heat through. Stir the food to distribute the heat. Let it stand for at least 30 seconds.

● Test the temperature of the food before feeding it to your baby; the food should be just lukewarm. Use a clean spoon to feed the baby.

For more about the safe use of a microwave oven, see "Play It Microwave-Safe" in chapter 13.

Baby Food—Make It Yourself?

In spite of the added work, some parents get satisfaction from preparing baby food themselves. However, that requires extra care to keep baby's food safe and to retain the nutrients from fresh foods.

Commercial baby foods are nutritious options for feeding baby, too. Today's commercial baby foods provide balance and variety with carefully controlled and consistent nutrient content.

If you choose to prepare homemade baby food:

● Wash your hands before preparing baby food.

● Always use clean cutting boards, utensils, and containers to cook, puree, and store homemade baby food.

● Wash, peel, and remove seeds or pits from produce. Take special care with fruits and vegetables that are grown close to the ground; they may contain spores for *Clostridium botulinum* or contain other harmful bacteria that can cause foodborne illness.

● Start with fresh or frozen vegetables. Cook them until tender by steaming or microwaving, then puree or mash. There's no need to add salt, other seasonings, or sweeteners. A baby's tastes aren't the same as yours.

INFANT FEEDING PLAN: A BASIC GUIDELINE

Babies differ in their size, appetite, and readiness for solid food. This guide offers a general time frame for introducing baby foods and table foods into an infant's eating pattern.

However, some babies may be ready for certain foods a little sooner; others, somewhat later. Your baby's doctor, pediatric nurse, or a registered dietitian will recommend an eating pattern to meet your baby's individual needs.

What Are Your Baby's Developmental Signs?

	NEWBORN/HEAD UP	SUPPORTED SITTER	INDEPENDENT SITTER
Physical Skills	—*Newborn:* need head support —*Head Up:* has more skillful head control	—Sits with help or support —On tummy, pushes up on arms with straight elbow	—Sits independently —Can pick up and hold small objects in hand —Leans toward food or spoon
Eating Skills	—*Newborn:* establishes a suck-swallow breathing pattern —*Head Up:* tongue moves forward and back to suck	—May push food out of mouth with tongue —Moves pureed food forward with tongue to swallow —Recognizes spoon and holds mouth open as spoon approaches	—Able to keep thick purees in mouth —Pulls head downward and presses upper lip to draw food from spoon —Rakes food toward self in fist —Can transfer food from one hand to another —Can drink from a cup with help
Appropriate Foods and Textures	—*Newborn & Head Up:* breast milk or formula	—Breast milk or formula —Infant cereals —Thin pureed foods, such as single-ingredient baby foods	—Breast milk or formula —Infant cereals —Thin pureed foods, such as single-ingredient baby foods —Thicker pureed foods, such as more advanced pureed baby foods —Soft, mashed foods without lumps, such as cooked potatoes and carrots, 100% juice
What You Do to Help	—If breast-feeding, eat a wide variety of healthy foods to teach your baby flavors, tastes, and aromas through your breast milk	—Enhance baby's acceptance of cereal by mixing it with breast milk or formula —Respect baby's hunger and fullness cues—stop feeding when he/she indicates he/she is full	—Introduce one new food 2 to 4 days in a row before starting a new one —Give baby a variety of thin and thick textures to help develop the skills needed

Source: Copyright 2005 Gerber Products Company. Reprinted with permission.

● Puree or mash fresh fruit or fruit canned in its own juice. Never add honey, sugar, or corn syrup.

● Offer cooked eggs only, whether they're whites and/or yolks.

● Cook meats, poultry, and eggs until well done. Babies are especially susceptible to foodborne illnesses caused by eating undercooked meats, poultry, and eggs. Again, there's no need for added flavorings.

● Prepare foods with a texture appropriate for the baby's feeding stage. Puree foods in a food processor, blender, or baby food grinder; mash them with a fork; or chop them well, so your baby won't choke.

● Cover, and refrigerate or freeze homemade baby food immediately after it's prepared. Homemade baby food keeps in a covered container for one to two days in the refrigerator or three to four months in the freezer. Label and date homemade baby food.

Avoid Feeding from the Baby Food Jar

Feeding directly from the jar introduces bacteria from your baby's mouth to the spoon and into the food. If you save the uneaten food, bacteria in leftovers can grow and may cause diarrhea, vomiting, and other symptoms of foodborne illness if used at a later feeding.

● Instead, spoon small amounts of baby food from the jar into a feeding dish, and feed from there. Toss what's uneaten from the dish. If your baby needs a second helping, just take more from the jar with a clean spoon.

● As soon as you finish feeding your baby, cap opened jars of baby food that haven't come in contact with your baby's saliva. You may then safely refrigerate them: opened strained fruits for two to three days; strained meats and eggs, one day; and meat and vegetable combinations, one to two days.

Unopened jars of baby food have the same shelf life as other canned foods. Check the product dating on the label or lid, then use the baby food while it's still at its peak quality. *To learn how to read product dating, see "More Reading on the Food Label" in chapter 12.* Most jars of baby food have a safety button on top. If the button's down, the food should be safe. As the vacuum seal releases, you'll hear a "pop" when you open the jar. Discard jars with chipped glass or rusty lids.

Tips for Travel and Day Care

● Pack unopened jars of commercial baby food. Even cereal comes in jars. Ready-to-feed formula in a prepackaged bottle is handy, especially since it doesn't require refrigeration. Or use powdered formula. Just premeasure water and powder into separate containers, then mix when it's needed.

● Keep perishable food, such as bottles of prepared infant formula or breast milk, well chilled. Pack them in an insulated container with frozen cold packs or buried in ice in a plastic bag. When you arrive at your destination, refrigerate.

Bottles, already cold from your refrigerator, can stay safe for up to eight hours in sterile sealed bottles in an insulated bottle bag with cold packs or for about four hours if they're stored in ice cubes in a plastic bag.

● Have everything handy: food, utensils, bib, and baby wipes or a clean, damp washcloth. If someone else is feeding your baby, provide feeding instructions, too, including the time and approximate amount.

● Keep food separate from soiled diapers. And don't put food and bottles in a diaper bag that's frequently exposed to soiled diapers.

● For convenience, freeze prepared baby food for later use. Freeze it in small portions in a clean ice cube tray. Once frozen, put the cubes into clean, airtight, plastic bags for single-serve portions. As another method, use the "plop and freeze" technique: Plop meal-size spoonfuls of pureed food onto a clean cookie sheet, freeze, then transfer the frozen baby food to clean plastic bags for continued freezing.

For Babies, Toddlers, and Preschoolers: How to Avoid Choking

Having teeth doesn't mean children can handle all foods. Small, hard foods . . . slippery foods . . . and sticky foods can block the air passage, cutting off a child's supply of oxygen.

● Don't offer these foods to children younger than four years of age:

● *Small, hard foods*—nuts, seeds, popcorn, dry

flake cereal, snack chips, pretzels, raw carrots, raw celery, raw peas, whole olives, cherry tomatoes, whole kernel corn. For toddlers and preschoolers, cut or break these foods into ½-inch pieces or smaller to bite and chew, but not to put whole into their mouths.

● *Slippery foods*—whole grapes; large pieces of meats, poultry, and frankfurter; and hard candy, lollipops, and cough drops, which may be swallowed before they're adequately chewed. Chop grapes, meat, poultry, hot dogs, and other foods in small pieces.

Food Labels: For Children under Four Years

The Dietary Guidelines for Americans doesn't apply to children under age two—and neither do the Nutrition Facts on food labels, which are for adults and children ages four years and above.

Although they use the Nutrition Facts format, infant and toddler food labels differ from adult food labels—and supply different information. *This page shows two typical Nutrition Facts panels: for a toddler food (less than two years) and for food for children ages two to four years.* The label gives information that helps parents choose food with the kinds and amounts of nutrients that infants, toddlers, and young children need.

Serving size. For infant foods, serving sizes are based on average amounts that infants and toddlers under four or under two years of age usually eat at one time. For example, for oatmeal, that's ¼ cup. On adult food labels, serving sizes are based on average amounts adults typically eat at one time; again for oatmeal, that may be given as ½ cup or 1 ounce of uncooked oatmeal.

Total fat. Infant food labels (foods for children under two years and four years) list the total fat and *trans* fat content in a single serving of food. But unlike adult food labels, they don't give the calories from fat or from saturated fat. The saturated fat and cholesterol content are listed only on labels for foods for children ages two to under four years. These details aren't included on foods for babies and toddlers under two years of age, who need fat as a concentrated energy source to fuel their rapid growth. Parents and other caregivers shouldn't try to limit an infant's fat intake.

% Daily Values (DVs). The % Daily Values for protein and some vitamins and minerals are listed on food labels for infants and children under four years of age. You won't find % DVs for fat, cholesterol, sodium, potassium, carbohydrates, and fiber, however; no Daily Values for them are set for children under age four.

For more about food labels, see *"Today's Food Labels"* in chapter 12, which includes more detail on the Nutrition Facts panel on adult food labels.

Check the required use-by date on a food label for infant formula and baby food, too, so you don't offer baby food with an off-flavor or texture. That date is for quality, as well as for nutrient retention.

Fruit dessert for children less than 2 years old

Nutrition Facts	
Serving Size 1 jar (140g)	
Amount Per Serving	
Calories 110	
Total Fat	0g
Trans Fat	0g
Sodium	10mg
Total Carbohydrate	27g
Dietary Fiber	4g
Sugars	0g
Protein	0g
% Daily Value	
Protein 0% • Vitamin A 6%	
Vitamin C 45% • Calcium 2%	
Iron 2%	

Fruit dessert for children ages 2 years to 4 years

Nutrition Facts	
Serving Size 1 jar (140g)	
Amount Per Serving	
Calories 110	Calories from Fat 0
Total Fat	0g
Saturated Fat	0g
Trans Fat	0g
Cholesterol	0mg
Sodium	10mg
Total Carbohydrate	27g
Dietary Fiber	4g
Sugars	0g
Protein	0g
% Daily Value	
Protein 0% • Vitamin A 6%	
Vitamin C 45% • Calcium 2%	
Iron 2%	

Source: Food and Drug Administration 2009.

● Be careful with sticky foods, too, such as peanut butter. Spread only a thin layer on bread. Avoid giving your baby peanut butter from a spoon or finger. Avoid chewing gum. If these foods get stuck in your baby's throat, he or she may have trouble breathing.

● Watch out for these foods: taffy, soft candies with a firm texture such as gel or gummi candies, caramels, marshmallows, jelly beans, raw peeled apple and pear slices, cherries with pits, dried fruits, and fruit leather.

When an Infant Is Choking . . .

If the infant is choking and is unable to breathe, cough, cry, or talk: Call 911 immediately! Then alternate and repeat these steps until the object is expelled:

● *Back slaps:*
  ● Lay the infant along your forearm, facing down on your lap or thigh, and with the head lower than the torso.
  ● Give five quick, forceful back slaps between the shoulder blades with the heel of your hand.

● *Chest thrusts* (if the object doesn't come out of the airway after five blows):
  ● Turn the baby face up on your lap, head supported.
  ● Please two or three fingers on the middle of the breastbone just below the nipples.
  ● Give up to five quick chest compressions.

Remove any object blocking the airway, only if you can see it.

Do not perform these steps if the infant has strong coughs and strong cries. These can push the object away.

If your baby isn't breathing: Clear any obstructions from the mouth. If there is no pulse, start infant CPR (two breaths followed by five gentle chest thrusts). Continue CPR until baby starts breathing or help arrives.

Source: Medline Plus, National Institutes of Health. Accessed October 26, 2011.

● Avoid propping your baby's bottle. Refrain from feeding your baby in the car, too; helping a choking baby is harder when the car's moving.

● Offer appropriate foods. Finger foods for older babies and toddlers are pieces of banana, graham crackers, strips of cheese, or bagels.

● Watch young children while they eat. That includes watching older brothers and sisters who may offer foods that younger children can't handle yet.

● Insist that children sit to eat or drink, not when they're lying down, walking, or running. As they develop eating skills, encourage them to take time to chew well.

● Look for warning labels on foods with a high choking risk.

● Be prepared to do first aid for choking quickly to dislodge solid foods that obstruct the air passage. Do this when a child is choking and can't breathe, cough, talk, or cry. The technique for infants and toddlers differs somewhat from that for adults. *See the illustrated description. For first-aid for choking, see chapters 13 and 17.*

● Always have your doctor see your child after a serious choking incident to be sure that the lungs and airway are clear.

Another Food Safety Reminder for Feeding Infants

Infants and young children are very vulnerable to foodborne illness! Their immune systems aren't developed enough to fend off foodborne infections. Safe food handling and preparation are essential. For feeding infants: *Avoid raw (unpasteurized) milk or any products made from unpasteurized milk, raw or partially cooked eggs or foods containing raw eggs, raw or undercooked meat and poultry, raw or undercooked fish or shellfish, unpasteurized juices, and raw sprouts. Refer to chapter 13 for advice on food safety.*

CHAPTER 17

Food to Grow On
Toddlers to Teens

Food nourishes at every age and stage in a child's life: infancy, the toddler and preschool years, school-age years, and adolescence. Careful food choices not only help ensure the physical nourishment of a child's growing body but also nourish his or her social, mental, and psychological development. Childhood is also a time to establish patterns of healthful eating and active living that lead to lifelong health and wellness. The implications can extend even further, when children someday role model these food behaviors to their own children.

Whatever the age, children and teens need the same nutrients as adults. Only the amounts differ. Like you, they need energy from food—in fact, more than you do relative to their body weight. They enjoy many of the same foods you like, but the form and combinations may differ.

Your challenge as a parent or a caregiver? First, be a good role model for healthful eating and active living for kids. After all, parents and other caregivers are a child's first and most influential teachers. Second, support your child's chances to make wise food choices and enjoy food. It's up to you to recognize and respect his or her unique needs, to provide a variety of nourishing, appropriate foods, and to set a routine (time and place) for eating. Your child has responsibilities: learning skills to make sound food choices, listening to body cues to learn to eat the right amount, and making active play a part of daily life!

You influence your child's or teen's well-being in ways beyond role modeling. When you take care of yourself (eat smart and move more), you have better health and are better able to care for your child and your family!

Toddlers and Preschoolers: Food and Active Play for the Early Years

Young children can seem like sponges, absorbing all the sights, sounds, and tastes around them. They are impressionable, and ready and eager to learn. That makes the preschool years a great time to nurture positive attitudes as children learn to eat and enjoy a variety of foods. Establishing good eating habits and active lifestyles now starts a lifelong pattern.

Compared to infants, toddlers and preschoolers grow at a slower rate. However, they continue to require the right amount of food and nutrients for energy, active play, learning, and the next stages of growth. Providing your child with good nutrition and promoting an active lifestyle can reduce the risks of overweight and obesity, type 2 diabetes, heart disease, cancer, and other chronic diseases later in life.

The 2006 World Health Organization International growth charts are used to assess the growth of children ages 0 to 23 months. *The Centers for Disease Control and Prevention (CDC) growth charts for children and teens ages 2 to 19 years appear in the appendices.* All these growth charts can be accessed on the CDC website: www.cdc.gov/growthcharts.

Your Nutrition Checkup

Eating and Physical Activity: Family Matters

Family styles influence a child's eating and physical activity patterns and attitudes for life. What children eat and how much they move—and their attitude toward both—have lifelong implications.

Take a moment to assess your own family's eating and physical activity practices. As a parent, family member, or caregiver:

Do You . . .	ALWAYS	USUALLY	SOMETIMES	NEVER
Eat your meals together as a family on most days of the week?	____	____	____	____
Serve meals and snacks on a regular schedule?	____	____	____	____
Give your youngster freedom to choose how much he or she eats from the foods offered?	____	____	____	____
Respect a child's appetite and offer child-size portions?	____	____	____	____
Involve children in planning and preparing family food?	____	____	____	____
Make an effort to keep mealtimes pleasant?	____	____	____	____
Include nutrient-rich snacks as part of the day's eating plan?	____	____	____	____
Attempt to keep eating to the kitchen, dining room, or another designated place?	____	____	____	____
Set a good role model with your food choices?	____	____	____	____
Avoid rewarding or punishing a child with food?	____	____	____	____
Give kids enough time to eat—make meals last at least fifteen minutes?	____	____	____	____
Turn off the TV whenever you and/or your child eat? Limit cell phone use during meals?	____	____	____	____
Make breakfast a family habit?	____	____	____	____
Serve a variety of nutrient-rich foods for meals and snacks?	____	____	____	____
Expand food experiences by offering new foods and new food combinations?	____	____	____	____
Avoid forcing a clean plate? Let your child stop eating when he or she feels full?	____	____	____	____
Set a good role model by being physically active?	____	____	____	____
Limit screen time (TV and computer and use of handheld device) to one to two hours daily?	____	____	____	____
Encourage children to play actively?	____	____	____	____
Enjoy physical activity regularly as a family (at least once or twice weekly)?	____	____	____	____
Subtotal	____	____	____	____

Now score yourself:

Count the number of check marks in each column. Then multiply by these scores.

What's your total?

"Always":	3 points
"Usually":	2 points
"Sometimes":	1 points
"Never":	0 point

Your total score _____

What does your score suggest?

If you scored 40 to 60 points, you already apply what you know about nurturing positive eating and physical activity patterns. *Read on for more ideas.*

A score of 20 to 39 suggests you're on the right track for feeding and exercising with kids. But you still have room to make positive changes in your family's lifestyle. *Check this chapter for more practical tips.*

Less than 20, try to incorporate a few changes in your family's approach to food and physical activity. *Read on for some steps to get you started.*

Food for Hungry Tummies

A variety of foods with different textures, tastes, and colors—in adequate amounts (but not too much)—provides the nutrients and the calories (food energy) children need to thrive.

What is a healthful eating pattern for young children? Their meals and snacks should have many of the same attributes as yours: a variety of nutrient-rich food and beverages in the right amounts, reasonably sized portions, and limits on added sugars and solid fats (saturated and *trans* fats).

Variety for young children is defined this way: enough calcium-rich dairy foods and iron-rich protein foods (lean meat, lean poultry, fish, and beans), as well as enough vegetables, fruits, and grain products, including whole grains. Offered in child-size portions and at the calorie level that's right for them, a variety of nutrient-rich foods:

● Provides the vitamins and minerals that young children need to thrive. Calcium, vitamin D, potassium, and iron are among the nutrients that may need special attention.

● Should provide most of your child's calories (food energy).

Click Here! Websites to Know . . .
● Action for Healthy Kids, www.actionforhealthykids.org
● Families, Food and Fitness, Cooperative Extension, www.extension.org/families_food_fitness
● Kids Eat Right, Academy of Nutrition and Dietetics, www.eatright.org/kids
● MyPlate (resources for children), www.ChooseMyPlate.gov/kids
● Let's Move!, www.letsmove.gov
● Team Nutrition, www.fns.usda.gov/TN
● We Can!, National Heart, Lung, and Blood Institute, USHHS, www.nhlbi.nih.gov/health/public/heart/obesity/wecan

See "Resources You Can Use" for more websites.

Preschoolers: Behavioral Milestones

The preschool years are an important time for developing healthful habits for life. During this time children grow and develop in ways that affect behavior in all areas, including eating. The timing of these milestones may vary with each child.

Two years
● Can use a spoon and drink from a cup
● Can be easily distracted
● Growth slows and appetite drops
● Can be very messy
● May suddenly refuse certain foods

Three years
● Makes simple either/or food choices, such as a choice of apple or orange slices
● Pours liquid with some spills
● Comfortable using fork and spoon
● Can follow simple requests such as "Please use your napkin"
● Likes to imitate cooking
● May suddenly refuse certain foods

Four years
● Influenced by TV, media, and peers
● May dislike many mixed dishes
● Rarely spills with spoon or cup
● Knows what table manners are expected
● Can be easily sidetracked
● May suddenly refuse certain foods

Five years
● Has fewer demands
● Will usually accept the food that's available
● Dresses and eats with minor supervision

Source: USDA.

● Provides alternatives with similar nutrient content. If sweet potatoes are rejected with some initial fussiness, carrots and cantaloupe are good vitamin A sources, too. If plain milk is rejected, try low-fat fruit yogurt or low-fat cheese.

● Helps children learn to enjoy them —and so reap their benefits throughout life.

For toddlers, age twelve to twenty-four months, whole milk (rather than low-fat) is advised. Toddlers need the fat and food energy (calories) that whole milk provides. After age two years, low-fat (1 percent) or fat-free milk is advised. In 2008 the American Academy of Pediatrics advised that reduced-fat milk (2 percent) is appropriate for children ages twelve to twenty-four months if overweight or obesity is a concern or if they have a family history of obesity, high cholesterol, or heart disease. The Daily Reference Intakes advise 30 to 40 percent of calories from fat for those ages one to three years, and 25 to 35 percent of calories from fat, mostly unsaturated, for those ages four to eighteen years.

A low-fat eating plan isn't advised for children less than two years of age—and cutting way back on fat for older children isn't recommended, either. Fat is a concentrated energy source that supports a young child's rapid growth, learning, and play. In fact, two fatty acids—linoleic and alpha-linolenic acid—are essen-

tial for growth and brain development. Food must supply them because the body can't make them. Kids also need some fat from food to help their bodies use vitamins A, D, E, and K and to add flavor to food. After age two years, the advice for children's fat intake matches that for their parents; *see chapter 5*.

Carbohydrates—in the form of starches and naturally occurring sugars—should be young children's main energy source. How much? Their calorie needs depend on their age, growth rate, body size, and level of physical activity. Most moderately active to active children ages three to five need 1,200 to 1,600 calories a day. Younger children likely need somewhat less. Fiber, another form of carbohydrate, is important, too; many kids don't consume enough fiber. For children ages one to three years, the Institute of Medicine advises 19 grams of total fiber a day; for children ages four to eight years, the advice is 25 grams a day. Access to foods with added sugars, such as soda, fruit drinks, cookies, and candy, should be limited.

Protein? Children need enough for growth and for the body substances (hormones and enzymes) that stimulate body processes. Five to 20 percent of total calories should come from protein. *See chapter 4 to learn more about protein.*

Can your child eat French fries, chicken nuggets, cheese, and ice cream? Yes, an occasional child-size portion is fine if the child's overall choices are moderate in fat, are low in solid fats and added sugars, and match calorie needs.

The USDA Food Patterns are useful daily food guides for planning healthful meals and snacks for young children ages two to five years; *see chapter 10 to learn about food group amounts for children ages two and above. "For Starters: Meal and Snack Patterns for Preschoolers" in this chapter shows how much from each food group for them.* Remember it's not what your child eats at a single meal, or even one day, that counts. Instead your child's overall eating plan for several days is important for now—and for lifelong health.

For helping your child eat wisely for his or her healthy weight, refer to "Weighty Issues for Children—Teens, Too!" in this chapter.

Enough to Eat, without Overfeeding

You can lead a young child to the table, but you can't make a child eat—nor should you! Let your child's

---

Have You Ever Wondered?

. . . what to do if your preschooler seems overweight? First discuss your concerns with your child's doctor, who is trained to assess a child's weight. Your child's size may be normal. A growth chart, recorded in regular health exams, will track your child's height and weight and show how he or she fits within a healthy range. Some kids gain a little extra weight to support an upcoming growth spurt.

Healthful eating habits, combined with plenty of active play, can help most overweight kids grow into their healthy weight—without a special diet. *See "Weighty Issues for Children—Teens, Too!" in this chapter.*

. . . how to find out if your child is getting enough iron? For young children, iron deficiency anemia is a common nutrition problem. That's why children are screened for anemia in regular checkups. Children need enough iron to support growth, replace normal iron loss, and produce energy for learning and play. The best iron source is food, including red meats and certain vegetables such as beans (legumes). Fruits with vitamin C, such as orange juice, enhance absorption of iron from eggs, grain products, beans, and other vegetables. A healthcare provider may advise liquid iron supplements or chewable multivitamins for some children. *See chapter 6 for ways to include iron-rich foods in family meals.*

appetite guide how much food is enough. A pattern of overeating can lead to overweight, starting in these early years. *Of concern:* Even among two- to five-year-olds, more than 10 percent are considered overweight, according to 2007–2008 data from the CDC. Underfeeding can cause feelings of deprivation and can even lead to weight gain if your child sneaks food to satisfy hunger when you're not looking.

How much do toddlers and preschoolers need to eat? Although they're no longer babies, young children aren't ready for adult-size portions. Adult servings can overwhelm small appetites and lead to overeating and too many calories. Judge how much your child needs to eat:

● Serve a toddler or a preschooler small helpings—smaller than yours. Let the child ask for more if he or she is still hungry. As a guide, some experts advise one tablespoon of every food served for every year in age.

● Respect your child's hunger and fullness (satiety) cues. When he or she starts to play with food, becomes restless, or sends signals of "no more," remove the food. Knowing what fullness feels like—and when to stop—helps children learn to eat enough, but not too much.

● Do away with the "clean plate" club. This practice may encourage overeating or a food aversion—habits

"Do as I Do": Are You a Good Role Model?

Did *you* eat *your* vegetables today? Did *you* drink milk? Did *you* take a walk or do something physically active, not just sit by the TV or the computer? Did *you* eat just a handful of chips, or the whole bagful?

Children learn their habits, attitudes, and beliefs about eating and physical activity by watching and interacting with you: parent, older sibling, other caregiver. By mimicking, they explore their world, try "grown-up" behavior, and hope to please you. Whether you intend to or not, role-modeling probably is the most powerful, effective way to help your child eat smart and move more.

Most young kids want to do what others do! So the next time you order a drink to go with a fast-food meal, eat when you're stressed or bored, or decide how you'll spend a leisurely afternoon, think about the messages you send. The best way to help your child eat healthier and be physically active is for you to do so!

Have You Ever Wondered

... how to make sure food is safe for your young child? Infants and young children are at greater risk for food-borne illness; *chapter 13 offers plenty of advice.* Among the many lessons: Teach kids about proper handwashing and skip the raw cookie dough! Another food safety issue: Avoid offering foods your child could choke on. Hard, smooth foods and round, firm foods, as well as chewing gum, can get lodged in a child's windpipe. Because children don't master chewing with a grinding motion until about age four years, choking is a significant danger until about age five years. The American Academy of Pediatrics (AAP) advises against whole peanuts until age seven years or older. *Refer to chapter 16 for more advice.*

... what to do if your child is choking? Know what to do in advance! You might save his or her life, or the life of another child.

For children ages one to four years, the AAP advises: If your child has breathing difficulties but can still speak and has a strong cough, let the coughing itself dislodge the object. However, if the child can't breathe or speak and has just a weak cough, have someone call 911 immediately, then give quick inward and upward abdominal thrusts just above the navel and well below the bottom tip of the breastbone and rib cage until the object is coughed up; *see chapter 13.* If the child becomes unconscious, use the tongue-jaw lift to remove the object and begin CPR; refer to the AAP's website, www.healthychildren.org, for instructions.

that could set up a child for weight or eating problems later. If your child always leaves food on his or her plate, serve less; you may be offering too much!

Day-to-day and meal-to-meal appetite fluctuations are normal. Children's appetites often decrease after their first birthday as their growth slows. In fact, expect a child to pick at meals occasionally. Chances are, he or she will make up for it later. If your child is growing normally, seems healthy, and has energy to play, he or she probably is eating enough. Unsure? Talk to your child's doctor.

How often should young children eat? Most children do best with a routine—when meals and snacks are served at about the same time each day. Younger children may need to eat five to six times a day because their small stomachs don't hold much. *See "Snacks Equal Good Nutrition" in this chapter.*

For daily amounts that meet the nutrient and energy needs of most young children, see "For Starters: Meal and Snack Patterns for Preschoolers" in this chapter.

Feeding Choosy Eaters

Does your child refuse green foods? Does he or she suddenly react to an all-time favorite food with "I don't like this," or just "no"? Are you concerned because your youngster won't eat vegetables?

Bouts of independence are part of being a toddler or a young child. "Choosy" eating may be your child's early attempts to make decisions and be assertive—a natural part of growing up. It may reflect a smaller appetite as his or her growth rate slows a bit, too. Or "no" may really mean "I want your attention."

Relax; be patient. Arm yourself with practical

Mealtime Tactics: For Young and School-Age Kids!

Parents and caregivers supply the three *w*'s of meals and snacks: *what* foods are offered, and *when* and *where* they're eaten. The child fills in the other *w* and *h*: *which* offered foods to eat and *how* much.

- Wash hands before eating.
- Remember that your child learns by watching you and older siblings. Eat as a family. Set a good example by eating a variety of foods—including vegetables—yourself.
- Even if you can't eat together, be there! Young children need supervision in case they start to choke. Someone who's choking may not be able to make sounds you can hear easily. *For foods that may cause choking, see chapter 16 and earlier in this chapter; for ways to safely handle a choking incident, see "Have You Ever Wondered . . ." earlier in this chapter.*
- Encourage kids to sit while they eat. Provide a booster seat so they can reach their food easily. Discourage eating while standing, walking, or lying down.
- Reward children with affection and attention—not food. Using food as a reward or a punishment only promotes unhealthy attitudes about food and perhaps emotional overeating.
- Respect food preferences. Give young children the freedom to choose and reject foods, just as older children and adults do. Just encourage young children to politely say "No, thank you." Making food choices is a competency children need to master.
- Stay positive! Avoid the notion of "forbidden" foods. That may cause your child to want them more. In the right amounts, any foods can be part of your child's healthful eating plan.
- Bring into the house only the foods you want your child to eat.

- Experiment with "designer dinners," featuring a variety of colors and textures. Cut food into interesting shapes, and arrange it attractively on the plate. Kids react to inviting foods just as you do!
- Involve kids in meal preparation. Even young children can tear apart lettuce leaves for a salad or break green beans into smaller pieces. Children are more likely to try foods that they have helped prepare.
- Encourage children to practice serving themselves—for example, pouring milk from a small pitcher, spreading peanut butter on bread, or spooning food from a serving bowl to their plate. Even though spills are messy, they're part of becoming independent.
- Make eating and family time the focus of meal and snack time—not TV watching or texting. Use this chance to talk together and reinforce their good eating habits.
- Focus on the whole meal, not just on desserts. Avoid making desserts a reward.
- Stock your kitchen with child-size dishes and utensils that children can use with ease: cups they can get their hands around; broad, straight, short-handled utensils; spoons with a wide mouth; forks with blunt tines; and plates with a curved lip.
- Even in this fast-paced world, give kids enough time to eat. *Remember:* They're just learning to feed themselves. Time pressure puts stress on eating and takes the pleasure away.
- Encourage a sense of fun and adventure by making family meals pleasant. Recall the day's events, share each other's company, and talk about the food: its colors, flavors, and textures.
- Eating together is a good chance to talk and practice appropriate table manners.

Also see "Eating Out with Kids" later in this chapter.

For Starters: Meal and Snack Patterns for Preschoolers

A healthy meal and snack pattern for preschoolers can be planned in different ways to get enough daily from each of the five food groups, with many different menus. Here's an example for 1,000 calories a day.

Check USDA's MyPlate (*described in chapter 10*) for more 1,000-, 1,200-, 1,400-, and 1,600-calorie meal and snack patterns, and sample menus, for preschoolers.

Breakfast

1 ounce Grains
½ cup Fruit
½ cup Dairy*

Breakfast Ideas

Cereal and Banana
1 cup crispy rice cereal
½ sliced banana
½ cup milk*

Yogurt and Strawberries
½ cup plain yogurt*
4 sliced strawberries
1 slice whole-wheat toast

Applesauce Topped Pancake
1 small pancake
¼ cup applesauce
¼ cup blueberries
½ cup milk*

Morning Snack

½ ounce Grains
½ cup Fruit

Morning Snack Ideas

½ slice cinnamon bread
½ large orange

½ cup toasted oat cereal
½ cup diced pineapple

Frozen Graham Cracker Sandwich
1 graham cracker
(2 squares)
¼ cup mashed banana
¼ cup apple juice

Lunch

1 ounce Grains
¼ cup Vegetables
½ cup Dairy*
1 ounce Protein Foods

Lunch Ideas

Open-faced Chicken Sandwich and Salad
1 slice whole-wheat bread
1 slice American cheese
1 ounce sliced chicken
¼ cup baby spinach (raw)
2 Tbsp. grated carrots

Soft Taco (meat or veggie)
1 small tortilla
¼ cup salad greens
2 Tbsp. chopped tomatoes
2 Tbsp. shredded cheese*
1 ounce cooked ground beef or ¼ cup refried beans

Bagel Sandwich
1 mini whole-grain bagel
¼ cup sliced cherry tomatoes
¼ cup diced celery
1 ounce tuna
½ cup milk*

Afternoon snack

¼ cup Vegetables
½ cup Dairy*

Afternoon Snack Ideas

¼ cup sugar snap peas
½ cup yogurt*

¼ cup carrot "matchsticks"
½ cup milk

¼ cup tomato juice
1 string cheese*

Dinner

½ ounce Grains
½ cup Vegetables
½ cup Dairy*
1 ounce Protein Foods

Dinner Ideas

Chicken and Potatoes
1 ounce chicken breast
¼ cup mashed potato
¼ cup green peas
½ small whole-wheat roll
½ cup milk

Spaghetti and Meatballs
¼ cup cooked pasta
2 Tbsp. tomato sauce
1 meatball (1 ounce)
½ medium ear corn on the cob
½ cup milk*

Rice & Beans
¼ cup cooked brown rice
¼ cup black beans
¼ cup bell pepper
¼ cup broccoli
½ cup milk

*Offer your child fat-free or low-fat milk, yogurt, and cheese.

Source: USDA.

USDA Food Patterns Plan (1000 calories)	Total amount for the day
Grain Group	3 oz.
Vegetable Group	1 cup
Fruit Group	1 cup
Dairy* Group	2 cups
Protein Foods Group	2 oz.

Have You Ever Wondered?

. . . what to do if you think your child is lactose intolerant? Milk sensitivity is often a matter of degree. Lactose intolerance, or difficulty digesting the sugar in milk, is more common than a milk allergy. And it's easy to manage—often by giving the child smaller, more frequent portions of milk. Also easier to digest: yogurt or cheese, which has milk's nutrients without the lactose.

If you suspect a lactose sensitivity, seek advice from your child's doctor, pediatric nurse, or a registered dietitian. Don't simply give up milk! Your child depends on you for calcium and other nutrients that milk provides for proper growth. Find alternative foods with comparable nutrition. For more tips, *see "Lactose Intolerance: A Matter of Degree" in chapter 21.*

. . . what to do if your child has a fear of trying new foods? Just relax; give your child time to outgrow it. Even kids who resist trying new foods can eat in a healthful way, according to studies of kids' eating behavior. In the meantime, offer a variety of foods, and enjoy them yourself.

solutions to handle the "downs and ups" of child feeding. Your child won't starve if you consistently offer healthy choices with reasonable alternatives. Remember, there's a fine line between encouraging your child to eat well and pressuring him or her too much to eat.

● At mealtime, serve at least one food you know your child likes. But encourage your tot to at least try foods that others in your family enjoy. Avoid being a "short-order cook." At first, trying a new food may mean touching, smelling, licking, and even spitting it out into a napkin.

● Offer choices, but not too many, rather than asking open-ended questions such as, "What do you want to eat?" Deciding between or among two or three foods gives your child a feeling of control. It's also good practice for learning to make food decisions.

● Make food simple and recognizable. "Unmix" the food if it's an issue; put aside some ingredients for mixed dishes before assembling the recipe, even a salad or a sandwich. Then let your child put food together as he or she likes.

● Involve kids. Even choosy eaters eat foods they help plan, buy, or make. Together, plan a meal around

foods your child likes. When you shop, ask your child to pick a new food for the family to try. Ask for a kitchen helper; even small children can wash fresh fruit or put meat between bread slices for a sandwich.

● If your child won't eat certain foods, perhaps spinach, don't worry. Just offer a similar food-group food, maybe broccoli. Or try carrots. Foods from the same food group supply similar nutrients.

● Moisten dry foods such as meat if they're hard to chew. A little cheese sauce or fruit or vegetable juice might help. Serve drier foods alongside naturally moist foods such as mashed potatoes or cottage cheese. Or offer "dipping" sauces, such as ranch dressing, with finger foods—kids love to dip!

● Ensure that your child is seated high enough on the chair to easily see and reach the food, which makes trying new foods more pleasant.

● Trust your child's appetite. Forcing children to eat can start a lifelong habit of overeating. Instead, following hunger and fullness cues helps a child learn to eat the right amount.

● Allow ample time for your child to eat and try new foods; however, excuse your child after a reasonable time, say 20 to 30 minutes.

● Most of all, relax. And be a good role model (eat your veggies, drink your milk).

● Avoid conflict and criticism at mealtime; otherwise your child may use food for "table control." Focus your attention on the positives in your child's eating behavior, not on your child's food. And unless you're pre-

Food Jags

What do you do when youngsters get "stuck" on a food? If he or she keeps asking for the same food meal after meal, the child is on a "food jag." Food jags are common in the toddler years. More frustrating for you than harmful for kids, you're smart to stay low-key. The more you focus on this behavior, the longer it lasts.

Actually, it's okay to offer the food they want again and again and again! Just include other foods alongside to encourage variety. Most "monotonous diners" soon tire of eating the same food so often.

If your child rejects whole categories of food for more than two weeks, talk to your child's doctor or a registered dietitian.

pared for a self-fulfilling prophecy, skip labeling your child as a "picky eater."

● *Remember:* What your child eats over several days—not just one meal—is what really counts!

Tasting Something New!

Babies try one new food after another as they start solids, each time adding more food variety to their diet. The tasting adventure continues throughout childhood—and on into adulthood. More variety increases the chance for good nutrition and adds interest and fun to eating.

Help children be willing food "tryers." It's part of the challenge and pleasure of learning about food. Sometimes, at about age two, children start avoiding bitter-tasting vegetables; this may be nature's way of protecting them from poisonous plants, which are typically bitter, too. Young children also typically have

---

Child-Friendly Snacks

For children under age four, avoid popcorn, nuts, seeds, and other hard, small, whole foods to avoid choking. Chop raw carrots and grapes and cooked hot dogs in small pieces.

Grain Group
Animal crackers; unsweetened cereal (dry or with milk); bagel; English muffin; graham crackers; pita (pocket) bread; rice cake; toast; tortilla; crackers; pretzels. Go for whole-grain varieties whenever possible.

Dairy Group
Cheese stick; pudding; low-fat or fat-free milk; string cheese; yogurt; frozen yogurt

Vegetable Group
Any raw vegetable (cut in strips or circles); vegetable soup; salsa

Fruit Group
Any fresh fruit (sliced for finger food); canned or frozen fruit (in juice or water); fruit juice*; fruit leather; dried fruit; applesauce

Protein Foods Group
Bean soup; peanut butter; hard-cooked egg; turkey or meat cubes; tuna salad; hummus

* See advice about fruit juice in "Have You Ever Wondered . . . are fruit juices and fruit drinks good choices for kids?" in this chapter.

---

more tastebuds and may be more sensitive to flavors than you are.

● Offer new foods at the start of meals. That's when children are the most hungry. Make the rest of the meal familiar.

● Keep quiet about foods you don't like. Your food dislikes may keep your child from trying new foods.

● Before offering the new food, talk about it: color, texture, size, shape, aroma, sweet, bitter, salty, or tart, not if they like it. Let kids help you prepare it. They'll be more willing to taste!

● Serve the same food in different forms—for example, raw carrot sticks and cooked carrot coins.

● Just be matter-of-fact and perhaps say, "Maybe you'll like it next time," or "Maybe you'll like it when you get your grown-up tastes." Don't force a child to taste a food.

● Keep trying! Kids may need to taste a food at least eight to ten times before they learn to like it. Accept a fact of life: It's okay to not like every food.

Snacks Equal Good Nutrition

Young children like to snack. That's good news! With their small stomachs, they may not meet their nutrition needs with just three meals a day. Snacks can fill in the nutrient and food-energy gaps from their meals.

If snacks conjure up images of high-calorie, low-nutrient foods—think again! Wise snack foods for young children come *mostly* from a variety of nutrient-rich foods. Low-fat or fat-free milk is a good snack drink; go easy on fruit juice. Make snacks a healthful part of your child's day:

● Let snacks supplement regular meals, not replace them. Plan for two to three food-group snacks plus three meals a day. Children age two to five usually need to eat every two to three hours. Younger children may need to eat more often.

● Plan ahead by keeping food-group snacks handy. *Check "Child-Friendly Snacks" on this page.* An occasional piece of candy is okay, but avoid labeling it as a "special treat" to avoid undue emphasis. Just be matter-of-fact about it.

● Offer snacks two hours or more before meals. In that way youngsters are hungry at mealtime. "Pacifier snacks" eaten while standing in line at the supermarket—or snacks just a half hour before a meal—may interfere with a child's eating routine.

● Offer snacks when kids are hungry, not to calm tears or reward behavior. Otherwise you teach a pattern of emotional overeating. Maybe your child just needs attention, not food.

● Offer vegetables, fruit, or whole-grain foods at snacktime if your child's meals come up short on them.

● Offer small snack portions. Let your child ask for more if he or she is still hungry.

● Think "fun" at snacktime: brightly colored fruits and vegetables; the aroma of baking bread or freshly cut watermelon; the texture differences of soft, creamy cheese with crisp, crunchy crackers.

● Encourage toothbrushing after snacks of any kind, not only after sweets. *See chapter 3 for more about dental care.*

Exploring More about Food

Food offers a world of learning experiences. Because buying and preparing food are "hands-on" activities, everyday tasks can involve kids in food—and so promote healthful eating. To explore food with young children:

● As you walk the store aisles, encourage children to name the fruits and vegetables in the produce aisle or the canned food aisle, or to say the colors of foods they know. Find foods that are new to them; talk about their color, shape, size, and feel.

● Take your child to a farmers' market.

● At home, as you take vegetables out of grocery bags, talk about the part of the plant each one grows on: leaf (cabbage, lettuce, greens), roots (carrot, potato), stalk (celery, asparagus), flower (broccoli, cauliflower, artichoke), and seed (peas, corn).

● Grow foods from seed or a small starter plant in your backyard garden or in plant pots. Perhaps start the seeds in paper cups on your windowsill. Pick produce together. And gather garden waste together for the compost pile. Kids enjoy eating foods they grow themselves—and it's a great science lesson!

● Have children help decide what foods to serve. Perhaps show them pictures of vegetables and fruits. Have them pick the ones to make together for family meals.

● As preschoolers are ready, give them simple tasks to help with family meals. Most children like to help. They feel good about themselves when they can say, for example, "I poured it!" Working together in the kitchen

---

"I Can Help": Preschoolers in the Kitchen

Helping in the kitchen encourages children to try new foods. You know your child best, so simply use this as a guide since children develop these skills at different ages:

At 2 years:
● Wipe tables.
● Hand items to adult to put away (such as grocery shopping).
● Place things in trash.
● Tear lettuce or greens.
● Help "read" a cookbook by turning the pages.
● Make "faces" out of pieces of fruits and vegetables.
● Rinse vegetables or fruits.
● Snap green beans.

At 3 years:
All that a 2-year-old can do plus:
● Add ingredients.
● Talk about cooking.
● Scoop or mash potatoes.
● Squeeze citrus fruits.
● Stir pancake batter.
● Knead and shape dough.
● Name and count foods.
● Help assemble a pizza.

At 4 years:
All that a 3-year-old can do plus:
● Peel eggs and some fruits, such as oranges and bananas.
● Set the table.
● Crack eggs.
● Help measure dry ingredients.
● Help make sandwiches and tossed salads.

At 5 years:
All that a 4-year-old can do plus:
● Measure liquids.
● Cut soft fruits with a dull knife.
● Use a manual egg beater.

Source: USDA.

Need more practical, easy ways to help your kids eat healthy? Check here for "how-tos":

● Help your child with proper dental care—see chapter 3.

● Help your child or teenager eat smart for sports—see chapter 20.

● Deal with food allergies or intolerances at home, at day care, in school, or in a restaurant—see chapter 21.

● Find a nutrition expert experienced in issues for feeding kids—see chapter 24.

offers many chances to nurture children. *See "'I Can Help': Preschoolers in the Kitchen" in this chapter.*

● Expand their world by reading books about food to children. Ask a librarian, preschool teacher, or head of the children's book department in a store to suggest titles. Prepare some foods from the stories.

For more about cooking with kids, including kitchen safety tips, see "Kids in the Kitchen" later in this chapter.

Food in Child Care: Check It Out!

Warm and caring staff, a safe environment, opportunities for development and self-expression—that's what most parents look for when they choose child care. The nutrient quality of meals and snacks—as well as the eating environment—needs consideration. That's especially important for children who eat two or more meals and snacks in a child-care center. Eating skills and food attitudes learned and reinforced in child care can have long-lasting impact on food behavior, health, and body weight. If your child has a food allergy or needs to avoid any food for religious or other reasons, find out how that's handled.

Food safety is a top priority, too! Child-care settings offer many opportunities for spreading illness: food service, diapering, toileting, and close contact with others. That's why cleanliness and safe food handling are "musts." Infants and young children with immature immune systems are more vulnerable to catching a cold, flu, or other illness from others.

Active play and active learning? To help establish a

lifelong habit of active living, children regularly involved in child care need a program with safe, fun, and developmentally appropriate ways to move more and sit less. Besides health, active play teaches social skills and helps develop muscle and body skills.

As you choose child care, look for high standards of cleanliness, nutrition, and active play:

Food preparation and storage areas . . .

● Neat and very clean

● Properly labeled and well-covered foods

● Adequate refrigeration and heating equipment

● Perishable foods stored in the refrigerator or freezer

Hand-washing area . . .

● Child-size sinks, or safe stepping stools for adult-size sinks

● Soap and paper towels

Mealtimes and snacktimes . . .

● Meals and snacks with a variety of nutrient-rich foods. Many child-care settings have specific menu guidelines for food types and amounts from each

Hand-Washing Basics

Kids can't see them—but germs that cause illness are everywhere! For children, who have less immunity, proper hand washing and food safety are especially important.

Teach children good hand-washing habits—always before and after handling food and eating, and after using the bathroom, touching a pet, combing hair, blowing their nose, or coughing or sneezing into their hands:

● Wash hands with soap and warm water, rubbing hands for twenty seconds. (It's good counting practice, too.) Sing "The Alphabet Song" while handwashing, which takes about twenty seconds, too. And dry hands well.

● Get a safe stool so your child can reach the sink, the faucet, the soap, and a towel.

● Practice with your child. Rub a little cinnamon and oil on your child's hands. Watch what happens if he or she doesn't wash hands well. Cinnamon that stays on hands represents germs.

● Be a good role model. *Always* wash and dry your hands properly, too.

food group vegetables, fruit, grain, dairy, and protein foods. They're matched to the nutrient and calorie needs of children. Ask to see the menus.

● Tables and chairs appropriately sized for children's comfort, or high chairs, or booster seats

● Child-size utensils and cups to help young children master their feeding skills

● Adult supervision at snacktimes and mealtimes and adequate staffing for feeding infants and children with special needs

Diaper-changing and toilet areas . . .

● Very clean

● Located away from food, eating, and play areas

● Closed containers for soiled diapers, tissues, and wipes

● Daily removal of soiled items

Active Play for Toddlers and Preschoolers

Run, jump, throw, and kick! Active play helps your child develop and learn a variety of body skills, mental skills, and social skills, and begins a habit of lifelong active living and a healthy weight. And it's fun! Those skills develop with maturity when structured play develops physical (motor) skills and when children have opportunities to move in their daily life. As a parent, it's up to you to encourage free and structured play that's physically active:

● Balance quiet play (such as reading together) with plenty of active play. Limit sitting time to no longer than 30 to 60 minutes at a stretch.

● Choose child care that makes safe, active play a priority.

● Set aside time each day to play together, perhaps tossing a ball, playing tag, or taking a family walk.

● Designate an inside and an outside area that's safe, where your child can freely jump, roll, and tumble.

● Pick toys that "move"—perhaps a ball or a tricycle.

● Join a play group together.

Inactive TV watching is discouraged for kids under two years. For children over age two years, the American Academy of Pediatrics (AAP) recommends no more than one to two hours of quality entertainment media per day. Videos and computer games that encourage active "follow me" games can encourage moving for older children.

Other areas . . .

● Separate storage for each child's toothbrush, comb, and clothing

● Ample space between cots, nap rugs, or cribs

Observe what goes on in the child-care setting. You should be able to answer "yes" to these questions:

● Do children, staff, and volunteers wash and dry their hands before and after eating or participating in food activities?

● Do children wash and dry their hands after outdoor play, toileting, touching animals, sneezing, or wiping their nose?

● Does each child have his or her own washcloth?

● Do child-care providers and parents wash their hands thoroughly after every diaper check and change?

● Are child-care providers practicing appropriate sanitation and food-handling techniques?

● Are bottles and foods brought from home refrigerated, and if necessary, heated safely? (*Hint:* When you send food, always label it with your child's name. Transport perishable foods in an insulated sack with a cold pack.)

● For infant care, is space provided for moms to breast-feed?

● Is food that's left on a child's plate discarded properly?

● Do children each have their own dish, cup, and utensils, rather than share?

● Does an adult eat with the children, helping them learn table skills and serving as a good role model? Can you volunteer or drop in for a visit from time to time?

● Are menus posted online or on a bulletin board, or are they sent home with the children?

● Are the foods appropriate for the age of the children (e.g., no foods that may be choking hazards)?

● Are plates, cups, and utensils washed and sanitized after each use?

● Can you visit during the day, including meal and snack times?

● Are the program's policies on meals, active play, and other issues consistent with yours?

● Are toys that go into a child's mouth sanitized regularly?

● Are food activities such as tasting parties, food preparation, growing food from seed, field trips, and circle time activities part of the child-care program? Can you be a parent volunteer?

● Is safe, physically active indoor and outdoor play part of the daily routine? Is it well supervised? Does it match the abilities of children? Do adults direct some of the activities?

● Can you talk to the staff regularly and comfortably, especially about sensitive issues?

For more guidance on choosing a child-care center, check the American Academy of Pediatrics website: www.HealthyChildren.org.

Parents as Partners

For the many children in child care, feeding is a shared responsibility. Together, parents and child-care providers offer foods that nourish kids. And together they help children develop skills and a positive attitude about eating. Here's what you can do:

● If your child has a feeding issue—perhaps a food allergy—make a plan with your child and the caregivers.

● Ask for a meal and snack menu. Identify new foods. Talk about and prepare them at home. Reinforce tasting by serving foods your child tries first in child care.

● Practice hand washing before kids start child care.

● If schedules and policies allow, volunteer in a child-care setting to support the center's nutrition program. Offer to help with meal planning. Occasionally eat with children or help chaperone a food-related field trip. Or gather empty food packages and other kitchen supplies for play areas or for food activities. Early childhood educators appreciate this help!

School-Age Kids: Eat Smart, Move More

School-age youngsters—no longer preschoolers, not yet teens—are establishing habits that last a lifetime. For their good health and healthy weight, nutrition *and* physical activity should rank as high priorities.

During these years, children gain control of the world around them. They push for independence, associate more with their peers, and make more choices of their own. Because they're away from home more often, people other than family have a growing role in shaping their food decisions.

Parents, teachers, and schools provide much of kids' nutrition education. Advertising in all kinds of media, as well as websites and even phone apps, also influence kids' food decisions. Parents' challenge: to help their children access youth-focused websites, apps, and games that provide sound nutrition information. *Hint:* Access many reliable sites through www.kids.gov.

Nutrition for Active, Growing Kids!

Help your school-age child develop healthful eating and active living habits that last a lifetime!

Growth. Children ages six to twelve years grow about 2 inches and about 5 pounds yearly. To look at it another way, children grow 1 to 2 feet and almost double their weight during these years.

Before you compare your child with another, remember that children's body sizes, shapes, and growth patterns vary. Most children grow in a pattern that's more like a parent than an unrelated friend. (Get out your family photo album for a visual memory.) *"For Kids: Tracking Their Growth" in this chapter helps you look at your child's growth pattern.*

A school-age child's appetite gradually increases; most eat more just before a growth spurt. During childhood, growth is gradual, accelerating most just prior to and during early adolescence: generally for girls this is from ages ten through fourteen, and for boys, from ages twelve through sixteen. As long as a child is growing normally, he or she is getting enough calories. By tracking a child's weight and height, your child's healthcare professional will advise if your child is consuming adequate calories for healthy growth or if he or she is consuming too much or too little.

Nutrients and Calories. Children don't need any special foods for their growth, energy, and health, just enough calories, or food energy (but not too much) and nutrients. In fact, they need the same nutrients as their parents do, only in different amounts.

For children, what nutrients may need special attention? The 2010 Dietary Guidelines identifies calcium, potassium, vitamin D, and fiber as nutrients that may be low among children. Zinc, important for growth, and iron may be issues for some children, as well.

With a day's worth of meals and snacks that follow food group guidelines, they can consume enough of these nutrients, except perhaps for vitamin D. For example, consuming two to three cups of milk or an equivalent supplies enough calcium, and eating more

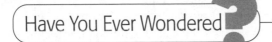

Have You Ever Wondered

... are fruit juices and fruit drinks good choices for kids? Actually, that takes a two-part answer.

Fruit juices: You know that kids are urged to eat fruit every day; 100% fruit juice is one option, but be aware that too much juice can add up to a lot of calories, or crowd out other nourishing foods and beverages such as milk, and can spoil appetites. An excessive amount also can lead to diarrhea and intestinal discomfort. Sipping a lot of juice even promotes tooth decay. For children and teens, the American Academy of Pediatrics advises:

- *ages 1 to 6 years:* ½ to ¾ cup (4 to 6 ounces) of fruit juice daily, maximum

- *ages 7 to 18 years:* 1 to 1½ cup (8 to 12 ounces) of fruit juice daily, maximum

For food safety sake, avoid unpasteurized juice.

Juice drinks: They have some juice and perhaps added vitamin C or calcium, but offer fewer nutrients than 100% fruit juice or milk. Juice drinks and fruit drinks cannot replace 100 percent fruit juice. Read the Nutrition Facts and ingredient list to compare. *See "Fruit Juice, Juice Drink, Fruit Drink?" in chapter 8.*

... about iron poisoning—how does it happen? Iron poisoning from adult iron capsules or tablets—or from vitamin pills with iron—occurs when children accidentally swallow them. This can happen, too, if iron tablets meant for children aren't taken as directed, but instead at a higher dosage in a short period. If your doctor prescribes extra iron for your child, give it *only* as directed.

Iron poisoning can cause serious injury, even death. Call your doctor or a poison control center immediately if your child accidentally swallows an adult supplement with iron. Keep all pills in child-safe containers where your child can't reach them. *Note:* A healthful diet with iron-fortified foods won't cause iron poisoning!

whole fruit, vegetables, and whole-grain foods helps kids eat more fiber. And for potassium: fruits, many vegetables, and beans. *See "A Healthy Eating Plan for Kids" in this chapter.*

For vitamin D, the Dietary Reference Intakes advise 600 IU (15 micrograms) per day for children and teens. Low-fat and fat-free milk are your child's best food source, providing 100 IU of vitamin D per 8 ounces of milk. Kids benefit from outdoor time since the body makes vitamin D from sun exposure, except during winter months in northern latitudes. Encourage outdoor play, caring for a small garden, reading together outside, or taking messy activities such as painting outdoors—with sunscreen! With these strategies, a vitamin D supplement likely isn't needed.

How many calories? Energy (calorie) balance is key to your child's healthy weight. Age, gender, and activity level determine your child's calorie needs. Talk to your child's doctor about the right amount, without overdoing on calories; *see "Estimated Calorie Needs per Day" in the appendices.* Calorie estimates help you plan, but your child's internal hunger cues are the best gauge. Most calories should come from grain products, fruits, vegetables, low-fat or fat-free dairy foods, and other protein foods (lean meat, poultry, fish, eggs, beans, and nuts) and not from foods high in solid fats and added sugars.

Many children consume more calories than their bodies use—especially inactive kids. What foods deliver their excess calories? Perhaps too many energy-dense foods, "too big" portions, or poorly chosen snack and snack drinks. *See "Weighty Issues for Children—Teens, Too!" in this chapter.*

Calorie sources are an issue, too. For carbohydrates, offer foods such as whole fruit, vegetables, and mostly whole grains. Limit those with added sugars, such as most cookies and candy as well as juice drinks and all sugar-sweetened drinks, including regular sodas. If kids fill up on these foods and drinks, they may miss out on the nutrient-rich foods they need; too many sugary drinks increase the chance of unhealthy weight gain, too. Another carb issue: preventing cavities. *Refer to "Your Smile: Carbohydrates and Oral Health" in chapter 3.*

Regarding fat, another other calorie source, the Institute of Medicine advises between 25 to 35 percent calories from fat for youth ages four to eighteen years, with most fats coming from sources of polyun-saturated and monounsaturated fatty acids, such as fish, nuts, and vegetable oils. Like adults, kids need to limit solid fats in foods such as cakes and cookies. *For more about dietary fat and Dietary Guidelines for fat intake, refer to chapter 5.*

Protein isn't an issue for kids who consume enough from the dairy group and protein foods group. *The advice:* Make most of these choices low-fat, fat-free, or lean. *See chapter 4 for more about protein.*

Food Preferences and Habits. Children's appetites and food preferences are changeable. Eating small amounts or not eating certain foods simply may mean that your child is testing his or her tastes, or perhaps exerting independence.

Children learn their food habits by watching others—not just parents, but also siblings, friends, teachers, and media. How big are your portions? Do you eat a variety of foods including vegetables? Try new foods? Skip the urge to eat to relieve stress? Fit in phys-

For Kids: Tracking Their Growth

Growth charts—using the body mass index (BMI) designed for children ages two and over, and teens—track growth, and a child's or a teen's weight in relation to height. These charts are used to assess whether a child *may be* underweight, overweight, or obese. As important, the growth charts assure parents and kids that there's a wide range of "normal." A muscular kid isn't necessarily fat, and a slim kid isn't necessarily underweight. They're simply different.

As children mature, it's normal for their body fat to change. Each child's growth clock, body size, and shape are individual; girls differ from boys, too. Some kids plump up before puberty to prepare for their next rapid growth spurt. *Remember:* Your child will likely grow as one of his or her parents did at a similar age.

As a parent, you, with your healthcare provider, can use these charts to help track your child's growth. Be aware that even the extremes—5th percentile or 95th percentile—don't necessarily mean your child is at an unhealthy weight. Children can be fit at any size. Let your healthcare provider make that determination, using additional measures. *See the appendices for the CDC Growth Charts with Body Mass Index-for-Age Percentiles for Boys and for Girls, 2 to 20 Years.*

Empower Your Kids: Seven How-tos for Smart Snacking

Here's the key to healthful food choices: very visible, convenient, effortless—great taste.

1. Ask your kids what foods from each food group they like and buy some to have on hand. Buy them!
2. "Walk" your kids through the kitchen so they know where these foods are kept.
3. Keep fresh fruit on the counter where kids see it.
4. Wash and cut veggies ahead, so they're ready to eat.
5. Use see-through containers, clear plastic bags, or containers covered with plastic wrap so kids can see what's inside.
6. Put nutrient-rich foods where kids can reach them, perhaps on lower shelves in your refrigerator, pantry, or cabinet. Keep "sometimes" foods such as cookies and chips away in cabinets where they're less convenient to reach, especially for impulse eaters.
7. Buy food in "single-serve containers" for grab-and-go eating—for example, milk, raisins, juice, fruit cups, pudding, baby carrots. Or prepare "single-serve" portions yourself (with your child's help) to save money and packaging.

ical activity each day? Early influence from all of you help determine how children relate to food later in life.

Healthy Eating for Growing Up

School-age children love to measure their progress from year to year on a growth chart. They want energy to run and play—and the energy to do well in school. Parents, teachers, and other caregivers have the same priorities: helping children grow up healthy—and have the energy to experience their world.

A Healthy Eating Plan for Kids

The USDA Food Patterns are healthy eating guides for all members of the family. *The advice:* "Eat Right. Exercise. Have Fun." Among its goals: to help combat obesity, starting at a young age. *The advice:*

● *Be physically active every day.* Reminds kids to be physically active every day: 60 minutes of moderate activity on most days! *Read "Get Up and Move!" in this chapter.*

Grow a Family Garden!

Gardening offers family fun. In a garden, you can be active, relax, and spend time together. Growing vegetables or herbs teaches children that plants, like people, need tender loving care to grow and stay healthy: soil (food), water, sunshine (smiles), and nurturing. Caring for plants helps develop responsibility. It also builds self-esteem when kids see what they can grow. A garden can teach your child about new foods. Kids usually taste what they grow.

Tip: Call your county Extension Agent for help.

What you need:

- Containers for city gardens: milk and juice carton, empty cans, empty bleach bottle, dishpan, plastic bucket, fish bowl, bushel basket
- Garden plot: a two-foot plot is big enough. *Hint:* Preparing soil is hard for young children.
- Child-size tools: watering can, hose, shovel, old spoon and fork, rake, digging stick, hoe and spade, sticks to label plants
- Seeds or seedlings (young plants)
- Water for your hose or watering can
- Soil for container gardens
- Fertilizer: compost, manure, chemical types

Tip: In the city, vegetables and herbs can grow in a sunny place on the roof, fire escape, or balcony. No garden? Volunteer as a family to help plant and care for a community garden, or visit local farmers' markets.

Easy foods for kids to grow:

- Beets,* carrots,* cherry tomatoes,* collard greens, cucumbers,* green beans, herbs,* lettuce,* okra, onion,* peppers,* spinach, tomatoes, zucchini
- In windowsill pot: herbs, seeds to germinate and replant as young plants in the garden

* These grow easily in a container.

"I Can Grow Things!"

Most kids are proud of what they grow. Even when gardening is messy, your child is learning. He or she can help with almost any gardening task. It's okay if the garden isn't planted perfectly.

Source: Written by R. Duyff for *Nibbles for Health*, Food and Nutrition Service,

---

- *Eat a variety of foods each day from all five food groups—grain, vegetables, fruit, dairy, and protein foods—plus oils.* For example, encourage many colorful vegetables, not just fries; fruit as a sweet snack, not just ice cream; and milk, not sugary soda.

- *Choose healthier foods from each food group.* Every food group has foods that kids should eat more often—more nutrient-rich foods. Offer mostly whole-grain crackers instead of cookies; yogurt rather than ice cream; broiled chicken fingers, not fried chicken nuggets; raw veggies instead of chips; fruit in place of fruit pies. *See "Foods to 'Chews'" in this chapter for more ideas.*

- *Eat more from some food groups than others.* Most children need more vegetables and fruits than they eat now. *"Vegetables for Kids: The Challenge" in this chapter offers tips.* Most children need more whole-grain foods, too; choose whole grains for crackers, breakfast cereals, and sandwich bread. And they need milk group foods for bone-building calcium and vitamin D.

- *Make the right choices.* For help in making personal choices for eating better and moving, check the website (www.ChooseMyPlate.gov).

- *Take it one step at a time.* To eat smart and move more is sensible; start with one new, good thing a day. Add another new one every day.

The Dietary Guidelines, *discussed in chapter 1*, provides healthy eating advice for those ages two and over. *See chapter 10 to learn about the nutrients, foods, and amounts from the food groups and oils.* You'll also learn about the food group amounts recommended, based on your child's calorie needs.

Sweet Ideas for Your Kids... and Less Added Sugars

- Shopping with your kids? Use the checkout line without the candy display.
- Snack beverage? Offer smoothies with fruit juice and yogurt, not soda and fruit drink.
- Dessert? Offer fruit or frozen 100% juice bars.
- Sweets? Provide only small portions, occasionally, in small plates or bowls.
- Kids don't eat a meal? Skip "extras" (cookies, candy) as replacements.

Vegetables for Kids: The Challenge

Most kids come up short on vegetables! But what's a parent to do when vegetables are greeted with a chorus of "yuck"?

● Add veggies to kid favorites. Mix peas into macaroni and cheese. Add carrot shreds to spaghetti sauce, chili, lasagna, even peanut butter. Put zucchini shreds into burgers or mashed potatoes.

● "Fortify" ready-to-eat soup with extra vegetables or canned beans.

● Offer raw finger-food veggies. Kids may prefer uncooked vegetables. They like to "dip," too. So offer salsa, bean dip, or herb-flavored plain yogurt.

● Kids like the bright colors and crisp textures of vegetables. To keep them appealing, steam or microwave veggies in small amounts of water, or stir-fry.

● Start a "veggie club." Try to taste vegetables from A to Z, and check off letters of the alphabet as you go! As you shop, let kids pick a new vegetable as a family "adventure." Post a tasting chart on the refrigerator door to recognize family tasters.

● Grow veggies together. If you don't have a backyard garden, plant in a container for a porch or windowsill. Most kids eat vegetables they grow!

● From your library, check out children's books about vegetables. Read the story, then taste the veggies together!

● Nothing works? Offer more fruit or other sources of vitamins A and C, and phytonutrients.

● Encourage them to choose a vegetable when you shop together at the supermarket or farmers' market.

Check chapter 14 for more ways to add vegetables and fruits to your child's meals and snacks.

Source: "Healthy Start: Food to Grow On," volume IV (Food Marketing Institute, American Dietetic Association, and American Academy of Pediatrics, 1995). Reprinted with permission of the Food Marketing Institute, ©1995.

Learning to Eat Healthy

In school most children learn the basics about healthful eating: what eating smart is and why it matters. They learn why physical activity is important, too. But acting on what they know doesn't just happen. Your support and reinforcement can help your child practice healthful eating and active living until these become everyday habits.

Foods to "Chews"

Chances are that some of your child's favorite foods may be higher in food energy and lower in nutrients. To get the most nutrition:

MORE OFTEN . . .	LESS OFTEN . . .
Baked potato, baked sweet potato, colorful veggies	French fries, deep-fat fried veggies
Baked or grilled chicken	Fried chicken strips and nuggets
Bagels or English muffins	Doughnuts and breakfast pastries
Graham crackers, animal crackers, fig bars	Chocolate-chip cookies, cupcakes
Pretzels, plain popcorn	Most potato chips, cheese puffs
Low-fat or fat-free milk, 100% fruit juice*	Soft drinks, fruit drinks
Raw vegetable snacks, fruit	Candy
Frozen yogurt	Ice cream

See earlier in this chapter for amount per day.

Reinforce what your child is learning at school. For example, help your child use advice represented by MyPlate (*see chapter 10*) and the food groups to plan a family meal or snacks; count how many colorful vegetables he or she eats each day; prepare foods (perhaps with fruit or vegetables) at home that he or she learned about at school; and track physical activities.

Encourage healthful snacks and physical activity in your child's after-school program or activities, too. Some programs and clubs offer "junior chef" or gardening activities. Pick one that gives your child experiences with healthful food choices.

What about Nutrient Supplements?

Does your child eat a variety of foods? Do his or her meals and snacks have enough nutrient-rich foods from each food group? If so, your child probably doesn't need a nutrient supplement. Meals and snacks likely supply enough vitamins and other nutrients for growth and health. Food is the best nutrient source, anyway.

If your child has a feeding problem that lasts for several weeks or if you're unsure about your child's nutrient intake, get expert advice. If your child is short on vitamin D, perhaps due to a milk allergy, a vitamin

D supplement may be advised. Before you give your child a supplement, talk to your child's doctor or a registered dietitian.

Beware of claims for supplements targeted to help children get over colds, depression, or attention deficit disorder, among others. These claims aren't supported by sound science; such supplements may be harmful. An appropriate supplement may be recommended if your child avoids an entire food group due to a food dislike, allergy, or intolerance, or if your child is a strict vegetarian. If your water supply isn't fluoridated, a fluoride supplement may be advised by your dentist.

If your health provider recommends a nutrient supplement for your child:

● Buy what's advised, perhaps a children's supplement. Check with the pharmacist if you need help. It should have no more than 100 percent of the Daily Values (DV). Unless stated otherwise, the % Daily Values stated on the Supplement Facts panel are meant for children age four or older, as well as for adults. On supplements for younger children, look for the % DV for children under age four. *Beware:* An adult iron supplement can be dangerous for children!

● Choose a supplement with a childproof cap. Store it out of your child's reach.

● Give a supplement only in the safe, advised dose.

● *Remember:* Supplements are just that—supplements—not an excuse to forgo smart eating.

● Remind children: supplements aren't candy, even if they come in fun names, colors, shapes, and packages.

● Remember that enriched and fortified foods may have the same added nutrients that the supplement has. Read labels so your child doesn't get too much.

For more about supplements, see chapter 23.

Eating Strategies for Children

How can you help your school-age child eat well? Many feeding strategies you used during the preschool years apply now, too. *See "Mealtime Tactics" earlier in this chapter.* Keep these ideas top-of-mind, too:

Regular meal schedule. Most school-age children do best with a regular meal schedule. When meals aren't regular or when meals are missed, children tend to snack more heavily throughout the day, so they're less hungry at mealtime. Space snacks at least one hour before a meal. Two to three snacks per day are enough for most children; make their calories count for good nutrition!

Breakfast-skipping is a concern. Breakfast is a healthful, important start for a day of learning and active play. *See "Nutrition and Learning" and "Breakfast: Ready to Learn, Healthier Weight!" in this chapter.*

The family table. According to recent research, kids who eat frequent and regular family dinners also consume more calcium, iron, fiber, and several vitamins, and less saturated fat and *trans* fats. They also eat more fruit or vegetables daily. Family mealtime offers more than nutrition to school-aged kids: Studies link frequent family meals to healthier weight, better school performance, and language development from family "talk time" at the table—and for teens, less risk for substance abuse. So the family table matters!

Telling kids to eat nutritious foods and have good table manners is one thing; showing them is better! The family table promotes family bonding—a time to talk, listen, and create family memories.

● Eat as a family—if possible, at least once a day. If it's breakfast, set the table the night before for less effort in the morning.

● If your family is always "on the go," designate family dinner nights. Mark them on your calendar. Planning ahead makes it easier to fit family meals in.

● Turn off the TV, cell phone, and other electronic devices if you can to make food and family important.

● Eat around a table, not side by side at the counter. That's better for conversation and eye contact.

● Keep family mealtime positive: pleasant talk, a chance for everyone (including your child) to share and get attention, a mealtime that's neither rushed nor prolonged.

Making food decisions. Children usually eat better when they feel in control of their choices. As the adult, provide a variety of nutrient-rich foods—new and familiar—from which your child can choose.

● Let your child choose what and how much to eat from what you offer. Respect his or her food preferences and appetite. Help your child learn to eat slowly and pay attention to feeling full. By learning hunger and fullness cues, your child will learn to eat enough, but not overeat. Give your child the freedom to politely refuse foods he or she doesn't want.

● Involve kids in planning meals and snacks. It's a chance to practice making food decisions. Children often eat foods that they help plan and prepare.

● Encourage your child to try new foods—without forcing or bribing them. Trying new foods is like a new hobby; it expands his or her food knowledge, experience, and skills. Include foods from cultures other than your own. Acknowledge that your child will like some, but not all, of those foods. That's okay.

Kids learn to like foods they are exposed to often. If you offer fruits and vegetables regularly—and if they see you eating them—your child likely will learn to like them.

● Keep nutrient-rich snacks such as fruit, baby carrots, and yogurt dip on hand for kids. If you buy empty-calorie foods such as regular soda, candy, and cookies, then restrict them, it creates the chance for confrontation.

Snacks for health. Chosen carefully, they supply nutrient-dense food-group foods—and nutrients—that

---

Have You Ever Wondered

… how you know if your child is eating right, but not too much? Start by asking: Is my child growing well? Does he or she have energy to play and learn? If so, he or she probably is eating enough. Your child's doctor, pediatric nurse, or a registered dietitian can help you monitor your child's growth and development by plotting his or her progress on a growth chart. The other question to ask: Is your child eating a variety of foods and the recommended amount of nutrient-rich foods from the five food groups of the USDA Food Patterns? If so, he or she probably is getting enough nutrients to grow well.

… if your child gets enough to drink? Active children need eight or more cups of water during the day, as you do. Children perspire with active play, even outside in cold weather when they're bundled up. Just plain water is great for replenishing fluids; bring some along if you plan to be out for longer than an hour or on an extended car trip. Kids may drink more water if it's offered in appealing reusable "sports bottles." *Check chapter 20 if your child is involved in sports.*

---

may be missing from the day's meals. Snacks can help supply the calories, or food energy, that growing, active children need. Kids who use more energy in active play, organized sports, or after-school activities need more calories—and more snacks—than kids who watch a lot of TV, play electronic games, spend time on a computer, or have a sedentary after-school routine. *For snacks kids can make, see "Kitchen Nutrition: Healthful, No-Cook Snacks for Kids" later in this chapter. See "Snacks Count!" in chapter 11.*

Overall eating pattern. What children eat over several days counts—not what they eat for one meal or one day. There's no need for concern if your child occasionally skips food-group foods or doesn't eat much at a meal.

Pleasant mealtimes. Mealtime stress can lead to emotional overeating or undereating, so try to avoid fussing, nagging, arguing, or complaining at the table.

Nutrition and Learning

A well-nourished child is ready to learn. Fit kids more likely have the energy, stamina, and self-esteem that enhance their ability to learn. Healthful eating, along with regular physical activity, helps kids get and stay fit.

Eating breakfast is linked to learning. A morning meal may help children succeed with learning and provide energy to learn. Studies show that breakfast eaters tend to have higher school attendance, less tardiness, and fewer hunger-induced stomachaches in the morning. Their overall test scores tend to be better. And they may have better short-term memory, may concentrate better, solve problems more easily, and have better muscle coordination. Conversely, regular breakfast-skipping is linked to lower school achievement and performance. Kids who eat breakfast are less likely to be overweight and more likely to get enough bone-building calcium. Nutrients kids miss with breakfast-skipping, such as calcium, iron, B vitamins, and vitamin D, typically aren't made up during the day. For more about breakfast and solutions to breakfast skipping, see *"Breakfast Matters" in chapter 11 and "Breakfast: Ready to Learn, Healthier Weight!" in this chapter.*

Mild undernutrition isn't easily recognized. But it may affect how children learn; for example, a mild iron deficiency can affect brain function. Meal-skipping

Have You Ever Wondered

... if a bag lunch would be a better option than school lunch? Not necessarily. In a study comparing lunches from home with USDA-funded School Lunch, the school meal provided significantly more dairy foods, fruit, and vegetables, and had less fat and more food variety. If you decide to send a packed lunch, provide variety (lean-protein foods, whole-grain bread, plenty of fruit and veggies, and milk money), and, if you pack them, include only a small portion of cookies, sweets, or chips.

... if children outgrow weight problems? Sometimes, with good food habits and regular physical activity! However, don't count on growth alone to compensate. Poor eating habits and inactivity often lead to more weight gain as children grow. *This chapter offers guidance to help you.*

... if your child is really just "big boned," not overweight? If the BMI for children indicates that your child is overweight or obese (when looking at weight in relation to height), take heed—even if your family is big. Your healthcare provider should work with you to make the judgment.

and poor food choices can lead to mild undernutrition. Reasons are many, not just family economics.

Nutrition experts, other health professionals, and educators recognize that severe nutrient deficiencies—which may be linked to improper growth, retarded mental development, and very low energy levels—hinder learning. Iron deficiency among children leads to poor behavior, difficulty concentrating, and poor performance.

For Kids Only—Today's School Meals

What's for school lunch? What's for school breakfast? For parents, school meals offer an inexpensive, convenient, and nutritious solution for one or two meals daily for their kids. For many students, school meals contribute significantly to their overall nutrient and energy intake. For kids who aren't hungry first thing in the morning, school breakfast, if available, may offer the perfect solution.

Despite stereotypes, school meals are nourishing—and designed to promote kids' healthy weight. In most public school districts, school menus must follow national nutrition standards from the National School

Food Service Program (NSFSP) of the U.S. Department of Agriculture (USDA). Meal patterns must support advice from the Daily Reference Intakes and the Dietary Guidelines for Americans, 2010, *both discussed in chapter 1.*

As part of the NSFSP program, School Breakfast supplies about one-quarter of a child's or teen's need for key nutrients and energy. School Lunch provides about one-third of energy and nutrient needs for the day. For both, no more than 30 percent of calories can come from fat and less than 10 percent from saturated fat. Portions are age-appropriate portions (no supersizing) for different age or grade groups. Schools that meet these patterns receive federal reimbursement for each meal served.

Many school menus have expanded the variety of nutrient-rich foods kids can choose: more fruits, vegetables, and whole grains. Most school districts offer fresh fruits and vegetables, according to a 2009 study from the School Nutrition Association, and more than 90 percent offer salad bars or packaged salads. Lean beef, oven-baked fries, baked (not fried) chicken nuggets, low-fat and fat-free milk, whole-wheat bread, and whole-wheat pizza crusts also promote good nutrition on today's school menus.

Increasingly, schools engage in farm-to-school initiatives with local "farmers' market" salad bars and may provide foods such as baked sweet potato fries and low-fat and fat-free cheese. Cafeteria staff often offer tastings of new foods. Local chefs may help with food and nutrition education. Many schools include parent and student input in planning school meal initiatives.

Because most school meals have federal financial support, children and teens of all income levels have access to nutritious meals during school at a low cost. Some kids qualify for free or reduced-price meals.

If your child buys school meals, he or she may have choices on the cafeteria line, perhaps more than one vegetable or several types of milk including fat-free flavored milk. In many schools, students can select three to five items from the school lunch menu for the same price. Other schools provide up to seven items, including more fruits and vegetables. Having choices helps students build smart eating skills—and it helps ensure that children eat healthful meals. It's part of "eating right" education!

Breakfast: Ready to Learn, Healthier Weight!

Breakfast—with a variety of nutrient-rich foods—improves school performance, provides important nutrients, and puts kids on a path to a healthy weight. What's for breakfast? Even if kids are on their own in the morning, most can make these easy breakfasts. And they go down even "healthier" with juice or milk!

G = Grain, **V** = Vegetable, **F** = Fruit, **D** = Dairy, **PF** = Protein Foods

- Low-fat cheese slices served with—or melted on—whole-wheat toast, fruit juice **D G F**
- Iron-fortified cereal and low-fat or fat-free milk, with banana slices **G D F**
- Peanut butter spread on toasted whole-grain bread or a waffle, or rolled inside a wheat tortilla, tangerine **PF G F**
- Fruit—bananas, strawberries, raisins—and milk on instant oatmeal **F D G**
- Cold meat and veggie pizza **G D V PF**
- Leftover spaghetti or macaroni and cheese, banana **G D F**
- Apple and low-fat cheese slices between whole-wheat or graham crackers **F D G**
- Breakfast cereal topped with fresh fruit and a scoop of frozen yogurt **G F D**
- Toasted frozen waffle, topped with low-fat yogurt and berries **G F D**

To learn more, see "Breakfast and Learning" in chapter 11.

Competitive foods. Foods and drinks sold in the school cafeteria that compete with the USDA-regulated School Breakfast and School Lunch are "competitive foods." That includes the à la carte and vending machine foods. By federal law those defined as "foods of minimal nutritional value" can't be sold during meal periods, wherever meals are served or consumed at school, unless the USDA's Food and Nutrition Service grants an exemption as an à la carte item. These include soda water (carbonated and aerated drinks), water ices, chewing gum, and certain candies. Many school districts, counties, and states have additional policies about selling competitive foods before, during, and after school meals in the cafeteria and on the school campus. Ask at the administration about your Local School Wellness Policy.

Parent Involvement. You can be involved in and support school meals in your community—and help your child or teen choose healthful meals at school:

- Get familiar with the menu. Keep a current school lunch menu and perhaps a breakfast menu in your kitchen. Find menus in school mailings or on your school's website. You can ask for nutrition information about the menus from the school food service director.

- Go over the menu with your child. Talk about making choices on the cafeteria line; practice at home.

- If your child has a food allergy, restricts food for any reason (perhaps for religious, cultural, or health reasons), or chooses to be a vegetarian, talk to a school administrator and school food service staff. Most schools can prepare meals that match your child's unique needs—if they know ahead. *For dealing with food allergies, refer to chapter 21.*

- Join or set up a parent advisory committee for the school food service program. Schools involved in the NSFSP must have Local School Wellness Policies set by each school or school district. Parents can be involved!

- Have lunch—or breakfast—with kids occasionally to become familiar with the school food service program, the foods served, and the atmosphere in the cafeteria.

- Get to know the school food service staff. Volunteer to help with meal events, with tastings, or at regular meal hours. Help in a school garden. Express support. As you build relationships, share constructive suggestions.

● Support school nutrition education. Help children practice at home what they learn at school. Find sound, often interactive, nutrition education for kids and families on websites. See www.kids.gov. *Refer to chapter 24 for judging "Nutrition in Cyberspace."*

● Encourage school clubs and parent associations to serve nutrient-rich snacks and drinks at athletic and fund-raising events and school parties. Advocate for school policies that promote healthful competitive foods.

Another school-related tip: Advocate for physical education (PE) as part of the school curriculum—to the school board, administration, and other parents. Recess before lunch encourages more physical activity, too. Encourage your child to play actively during recess. Balancing stringent academic standards with physical activity during the school day is challenging for schools; however, being physically active helps children stay healthy and ready to learn.

Brown-Bagging It!

If your child prefers a bag lunch, pack easy-to-prepare and fun meals that are healthful, safe, and nutritious.

● What tote: brown bag, insulated bag, or lunch box? Ask what your child prefers. For some kids, having the "right" tote is important. A lunch box is easier to clean; it may keep food cool longer. Wash it after every use! Always use a clean, new paper bag.

● For perishable foods, such as a meat sandwich, include a small, frozen cold pack. Remind the child to bring it home! An insulated bag or frozen pouch or juice box also keeps helps keep food cool.

● Plan easy-to-eat foods—for example, sandwiches, raw vegetable pieces (carrots, red or green bell peppers, cucumbers, cherry tomatoes), crackers, low-fat cheese slices or cubes, string cheese, whole fruit, individual containers of pudding, or an oatmeal cookie. If you pack an orange, score the rind so it's easy to peel—or tuck in a tangerine instead! It's okay to pack a brownie or a small bag of chips as part of a healthful bag lunch. Kids may need the extra calories these foods supply.

● Are foods traded between kids? Ask what food was traded at lunchtime to get an idea of what foods your child prefers.

● At the store or farmers' market, ask your child to choose foods to enjoy in a packed lunch for school.

● Expect children to help plan and prepare their school lunches. When involved, they'll probably eat every morsel—rather than trade their raw veggies for someone else's cookie.

● Remind kids to store their carried meals at school in a clean, safe place—away from sunlight and the heat vent in the classroom and not in a dirty gym bag!

● *Hint:* Add extra pleasure to a carried meal with an occasional surprise tucked inside—a riddle, a comic, or a note that says, "You're somebody special!" Knowing that someone cares is "nourishing" in its own way.

See "Carry It for Safety" in chapter 13.

Weighty Issues for Children—Teens, Too!

Over the past thirty years, the number of overweight or obese children in the United States has risen dramatically; about one-third of children and adolescents are obese or overweight today, according to government statistics. Over 10 percent of children ages two to five years of age, nearly 20 percent of six- to eleven-year-olds, and about 18 percent of youth ages twelve to nineteen years are considered obese, according to data from the 2007–2008 National Health and Nutrition Examination Survey (NHANES). In fact, overweight and obesity have been described as the most common health problem among American youth today.

The 2010 Dietary Guidelines encourages children and teens to maintain calorie balance to support their normal growth and development without promoting excess weight gain.

Weighing the Risks

Excess body weight during these early years can have physical and psychological consequences, both immediate and later in life.

Even during youth, obese children and teens more likely have risk factors related to heart disease (such as high blood pressure and high blood cholesterol levels). In a population sample of five- to seventeen-year-olds, 70 percent of the obese children had at least one risk factor for cardiovascular disease (CVD), while 39 percent of obese children had two or more CVD risk factors.

Obese kids may have sleep apnea (short cessation of breathing while sleeping), problems with balance or ease of moving, and early puberty. With early puberty girls have more estrogen over a lifetime, and perhaps greater risk for breast and ovarian cancer later on. Childhood obesity is also linked to asthma and orthopedic problems. When coupled with low calcium intake and weakened bones, overweight children have more forearm fractures when they try to catch themselves during a fall.

Of concern, too, children who are overweight or obese are more likely to develop insulin resistance, which often precedes adult-onset type 2 diabetes. Type 2 diabetes, usually seen in overweight adults, now is being seen in children and teens as well! Complications from diabetes are appearing sooner, too. *See "Children and Diabetes" in chapter 22.*

There are psychological costs, too: overweight children may lose their self-esteem, have a poor body image, or feel emotionally stressed. Another consequence: Overweight children may be teased or bullied, feel stigmatized, or isolate themselves from their peers, teachers, and family. A bullied child may feel reluctant to go to school; absences can result in low grades, which further lower self-esteem. *See "Dangers of Bullying" later in this chapter.*

Compared with their normal-weight peers, overweight and obese children are more likely to become obese adults, who in turn are more prone to health problems such as diabetes, heart disease, high blood pressure, stroke, osteoarthritis, gallbladder disease, and some forms of cancer.

Childhood Overweight and Obesity: Why?

The easy answer is that overweight and obesity result from a child consuming more calories than his or her body uses. However, the underlying reasons—genetic, behavioral, and environmental—are complex and interrelated.

Do genetics play a role? Yes, they factor in as much as food choices. A child with one or two overweight parents has a higher risk. Certain genetic factors increase the chance of extra body weight, but a hormone imbalance probably isn't the cause.

How "nature" impacts "nurture" depends on what a child's body is exposed to. The family environment and interaction can affect how genetic make-up influences a child's weight. Children often mimic the food and lifestyle habits they see at home. Heavy snacking, irregular meals, and having high-calorie foods easily available are factors, as is a lot of sit-down time, such as screen time, that make it easier for genetics to affect body weight. However, parents can control the environment and hence the genetic propensity for overweight and obesity.

Although rare, obesity is a clinical feature of some genetic and metabolic disorders such as Prader-Willi or Cushing syndrome. Talk to your child's healthcare provider if these are concerns.

Factors influencing childhood overweight and obesity extend well beyond family issues. For example, many communities aren't designed for physical activity. Lacking sidewalks, bike paths, and parks, many kids don't have places for safe, active play. Physical education at school may be limited. Young people may spend free time watching TV and DVDs, playing electronic games, or being online with social media. Screen time often fosters snacking; media itself may encourage less healthful food choices. Large portions (often fast food), frequent snacking on high-calorie foods, and too many sugary beverages are factors, too.

A child with a family history of overweight and obesity isn't destined to become an overweight adult. A physically active lifestyle and healthful food choices are essential for reducing the chances. The risk goes up as children get older if they still carry excess weight. Increased physical activity and balanced, healthful eating are keys to helping prevent a child from becoming overweight. Addressing weight problems early is important.

Is My Child Overweight?

Children grow at different rates and have different body heights and shapes at the same age, so you may not be able to easily detect when a child is obese or overweight.

Never assess a child's body weight by adult standards. BMI charts for adults aren't meant for kids! *Instead "For Kids: Tracking Their Growth" earlier in this chapter presents an indicator.* Your child's doctor should make the assessment.

To Help Your Child or Teen Get to a Healthy Weight . . .

Because their bodies are growing and developing, weight loss isn't the best approach for most children. Instead, for most kids, slowing or stopping weight gain

Feeding Vegetarian Children and Teens

Not surprisingly, vegetarian parents often raise vegetarian kids. Today, an awareness of and concern for animals may prompt kids' interest in becoming a vegetarian. Some teens opt for an eating style to be independent or reflect their emerging beliefs. Whatever the reason, a vegetarian eating pattern for growing, active children and teens can be healthful—if well planned and carefully followed. Even a vegan plan, with no animal-based foods, can supply enough nourishment, but the planning takes effort from kids, parents, and other caregivers.

The potential benefit is that vegetarian diets generally encourage nutrient-rich foods that many children and teens need more of: fruit, vegetables, beans (legumes), low-fat and fat-free dairy foods, and whole grains. That can mean meals and snacks have more fiber and polyunsaturated fat, and less solid fats and calories.

Vegetarian diets differ; so do the nutrition concerns for vegetarian kids. Your healthcare provider may advise a nutrient supplement, especially if your child or teen is a vegan.

● *Lacto-ovo-vegetarian kids:* eating dairy foods and eggs makes it easier to get enough nutrients. However, with no meat, iron, zinc, and some other minerals may come up short, which may delay kids' normal growth and healthy weight gain. Milk, yogurt, cheese, and eggs each provide all the essential amino acids (proteins) for normal growth.

● *Vegan kids:* calcium, vitamin B_{12}, and vitamin D, as well as iron and zinc, need special attention. Although some vegetables provide calcium, it's generally not enough for bone growth. Without milk, children also need another vitamin D source for bone growth, too, often advised in supplement form. Check the calcium and vitamin D content of fortified soy beverages, a potential milk alternative. (*See chapter 8.*) For vitamin B_{12}, many fortified breakfast cereals are options. To support growth, vegan kids need the right balance of essential amino acids from several sources, such as from beans (legumes), soybeans, nuts, and seeds. A vegan diet, if poorly planned, may not supply all the nutrients children and teens need to grow properly.

Ensuring that a vegetarian child or teen gets enough food energy (calories) for proper growth and health is another concern. Because vegetarian meals can be low in fat and high in fiber ("bulky"), they may fill kids up without supplying enough calories. To meet the nutrient and calorie demands of growth, offer frequent meals and snacks. Provide some foods with more unsaturated fats such as nuts, seeds, avocadoes, and nut butters. Foods with some added sugars, such as oatmeal cookies and ice cream, may provide calories, or food energy, but go easy. These nutrient-rich snacks provide calories, too: a peanut butter sandwich and milk, raw vegetables with hummus or tofu dip, ready-to-eat breakfast cereal, fruit, finger-food veggies, nuts, and dried fruit.

Is it okay for your teenager to control weight with a vegetarian diet? Yes, if your teen's food choices are varied and balanced as he or she maintains a healthy weight. However, vegetarian eating isn't always lower-calorie eating! The calorie content of food depends on a teen's overall food choices. Feel assured that vegetarian eating doesn't lead to eating disorders; however, it may be used to camouflage one. If a vegetarian teen loses too much weight or shows other signs of disordered eating, be concerned. Eating disorders can be harmful, even life-threatening. If that happens, seek professional help. *See "Disordered Eating: Problems, Signs, and Help" in chapter 2.*

School Meals for Vegetarian Kids

If your school-age child or teen is a vegetarian, help him or her make smart choices from the array of foods that fit in vegetarian diets.

● Review school menus together, and practice what he or she might order. If the school doesn't provide menus to parents, ask the school staff.

● Suggest the salad bar as a nutritious option—if it's available. A salad bar can be a good place to go for fresh vegetables and possibly for other nutrient-packed choices, including fruits, beans (legumes), sunflower seeds, cheese, or hard-cooked eggs.

● When the school menu doesn't offer a vegetarian option, a packed lunch is an option. A peanut butter sandwich is always popular (if your child doesn't have a peanut allergy)!

Advice for Family Meals

If your child or teen decides to be a vegetarian, support the decision with food options that continue to promote growth, health, and a healthy weight. A vegetarian eating plan can supply enough of the nutrients and

Feeding Vegetarian Children and Teens *(continued)*

food energy needed—without overdoing on calories—if kids know how to make smart choices. Most of all, be supportive and learn how to make healthful vegetarian choices together.

- Together make a shopping list of food-group foods that fit your child's or teen's vegetarian "style"—and keep those foods on hand: perhaps hummus, cheese, and crackers; cow's milk; calcium-fortified soy beverage; trail mix with nuts; fruit; raw veggies; yogurt; and other quick, portable vegetarian snacks. Filling up on mostly cookies, chips, sugary drinks, ramen noodles, and fries may be vegetarian, but not healthful.
- Plan vegetarian dishes that your whole family can enjoy, such as chili with beans, vegetarian pizza, or bean tacos, so you aren't a short-order cook.

- For some dishes, prepare them two ways with just a simple substitution: a veggie burger for your teen and beef burgers for the rest of the family.
- Prepare vegetarian foods that can be the main dish for your teen and a side dish for others—for example, rice and beans, or pasta primavera. Offer low-fat or fat-free milk.
- Encourage your child or teen to help prepare food to practice the basics of healthful vegetarian eating.
- Talk about eating-out options so your teen is prepared to make wise choices with peers.
- As a parent, whether you're a vegetarian or not, be a role model for healthful eating and healthful living.

For more guidance on vegetarian eating, refer to chapter 10.

with good food habits and physical activity, so a child grows into his or her weight, is usually best. In other words, let a child's height catch up with his or her weight. A diet that's too restrictive—with too few calories—may not supply the calories, or food energy, and nutrients a child needs for normal growth and development and can trigger unhealthy binge eating if the child feels too deprived.

For overweight or obese children or adolescents, the Dietary Guidelines advises: Change eating and physical activity behaviors so that their BMI-for-age percentile (*see the appendices*) doesn't increase over time. A healthcare provider should be consulted to determine appropriate weight management for the child or adolescent. The guidelines recognize the important roles that families, schools, and communities play in supporting changes in eating and physical activity behaviors for children and teens.

Weight problems aren't just about food. Many factors, such as emotions, family problems, lifestyle, and self-image, intertwine with eating behavior. Address the whole child—emotionally, socially, mentally, and physically—as you address weight management.

Lifestyle changes—often for the whole family— offer a good approach for helping an overweight child manage his or her weight. *"Eating Strategies for Children" earlier in this chapter apply to every child—overweight, normal weight, or underweight.*

- Seek professional advice with a medical evaluation first. A registered dietitian, your doctor, or the school nurse can help you find an approach that's right for the nutritional and developmental needs of your child. Weight loss approaches for adults aren't necessarily right for children. *See "How to Find Nutrition Help . . ." in chapter 24.*
- Encourage physical activities your child enjoys, but not excessive exercise. Besides burning calories, physical activity indirectly affects eating—for example, appetite control, stress release, and mental diversion from eating. Make physical activity a family affair. When parents are physically active, their kids are often active, too.

Overweight children are often self-conscious in organized or competitive games. Instead of forcing a child to join a team, encourage activities such as walking the dog or biking, where skill and an audience are less important. *For more about physical activity, see "Get Up and Move!" in this chapter.*

- Give your child more control over how much to eat. That may seem counterintuitive; however, when parents pressure or restrict food choices too much, kids don't learn self-regulation. They may overeat if they can't read their body signals for hunger and satiety.
- *Be aware:* An overly restricted eating approach may keep your child from getting nutrients he or she

needs. Restrictions also may lead to sneaking food elsewhere, then to feeling guilty or bad about himself or herself or even to overeating later.

● Be a role model. Involve your whole family in healthful eating so your overweight child won't feel singled out.

● Tailor portion sizes for your child. Large portions encourage overeating. Use smaller plates so less looks like more. A hungry child can ask for more.

● Avoid undue attention to eating. For example, forget rewarding or punishing a child with food. In that way you won't reinforce an emotional link to eating.

● Stock your kitchen with lower-calorie snack choices such as raw vegetables, fruit, low-fat or fat-free milk, or

vanilla wafers. Instead of heavy snacking, meals should provide most of your child's nutrients and calories.

● Avoid labeling food as "good" or "bad." Instead, help your child see how any food can fit in a healthful eating pattern. Even kids who need to reduce body fat can have an occasional cookie or a piece of candy. In fact, they probably need a high-calorie snack from time to time to meet their energy needs. Anyway, the body doesn't see food in black-and-white terms. It's the whole eating plan that counts.

● Be careful about bringing higher-calorie foods into the house. Hiding restricted foods or forbidding access to certain foods makes them more attractive.

● Set time limits on watching television—no more

Should You Have Your Child's Cholesterol Level Checked?

Until recently, cholesterol screening was only advised for children considered at higher risk (family history) of heart disease. In late 2011 new recommendations from the National Heart, Lung and Blood Institute/National Institutes of Health, with AAP endorsement, also advised cholesterol screening for every child between the ages 9 and 11 years, and again between ages 17 and 21 years. The growing obesity epidemic among youth is one reason for the new advice; another, children with high cholesterol haven't been identified. The report also advised diabetes screening every two years starting at age 9 years for children who are overweight and have other risk for type 2 diabetes.

If your child has a higher than normal blood cholesterol level, don't panic. High cholesterol levels among children don't necessarily predict high levels in adulthood. When children come from high-risk families, it's prudent to check with a doctor and work with a registered dietitian to bring the levels down: good advice for the whole family!

For cardiovascular health, young people, ages two through nineteen years, should maintain acceptable blood cholesterol levels, established by the National Cholesterol Education Program's Expert Panel on Blood Cholesterol in Children and Adolescents:

HDL levels should be greater than or equal to 35 mg/dL; triglycerides should be less than or equal to 150 mg/dL.

Compelling evidence shows that fatty buildup in arteries begins in childhood and is more likely with higher blood cholesterol levels. It slowly progresses into adulthood, often resulting in heart disease. For that reason, the American Heart Association offers advice for children and teens to reduce cholesterol levels and fatty buildup in arteries:

● Cigarette smoking: discourage it.

● High blood pressure: identify and treat it.

● Overweight and obesity: prevent them or reduce weight.

● Diabetes: diagnose and treat it.

● Inactivity: encourage regular aerobic exercise (30 to 60 minutes) on most days of the week.

● Kids also need to eat enough fruits and vegetables each day, and choose a variety of foods that are low in saturated fats, *trans* fats, and cholesterol.

Refer to "Your Healthy Heart" in chapter 22. For more about cardiovascular health for infants, children, and adolescents, go to the American Heart Association's website: www.americanheart.org.

LEVELS	TOTAL CHOLESTEROL (MG/DL)	LDL CHOLESTEROL (MG/DL)
High:	200 or greater	130 or greater
Borderline:	170 to 199	110 to 129
Acceptable:	Less than 170	Less than 110

than one or two hours daily of total media time, advises the American Academy of Pediatrics (AAP). Limit video games and computer time, too. Screen time keeps kids away from active play. Children who watch four or more hours of television a day are twice as likely to be overweight as youngsters who don't.

● Eat only in the kitchen or dining room. Refrain from eating meals in front of the TV or computer screen. It's easy to eat more when attention is shifted away from the meal and satiety cues to the screen.

● Talk to your child about his or her feelings. Observe emotions and subsequent behavior. Together look for ways other than eating to address emotions. Help your child understand: Even though eating may feel good for a while, food can't solve problems!

● *Be aware:* Kids may say they're hungry when they're bored or want attention. Probe a little. Offer a snack, perhaps a cracker or an apple. If neither appeals, the child is probably bored, not hungry.

● Help your child get enough sleep. Besides being a health essential, adequate sleep may lower a child's risk for overweight and obesity, notes some research. The American Academy of Pediatrics offers this advice for daily sleep: Ages three to ten need ten to twelve hours; ages eleven to twelve years, about ten hours; and teenagers, about nine hours.

Consider this advice about childhood weight issues, even if your child's weight seems healthy: *See "Obesity and Kids: A Heavy Burden" in chapter 2.*

Fear of Weight Gain

A desire to be overly thin, prompted by media messages and by what parents say and do, is reaching down to children as young as age three. Children,

mostly girls, as young as age six express concerns about their body image and gaining weight. Inappropriate weight loss can interfere with growth—and may lead to eating disorders down the road.

Parents may play an even bigger role than media in shaping a child's body image. Even before your child hits adolescence:

● Focus on your child's inner qualities, not your child's looks or weight. Instead, strive for a positive eating relationship with your child. Avoid pressuring your child to conform to any body size or shape. Teach healthful eating habits.

● Refrain from negative comments about your own weight or anyone else's weight.

● Set a good example in the way you manage your own weight and feel about your own body image. Skip the lure of fad dieting yourself.

● Encourage physical activity to build muscles and coordination. And work to develop your child's social skills, self-confidence, and self-esteem.

See "Disordered Eating: Problems, Signs, and Help" in chapter 2 and "Pressure to Be Thin" later in this chapter.

Dangers of Bullying

Overweight and obese kids are more likely to be bullied, teased, and harassed. Skinny kids can be the brunt of bullying, too. Whether physical or verbal, this abuse can have a tremendous, even dangerous, effect on a child's or a teen's self-esteem and well-being.

While bullying behavior often comes from peers, parental and sibling bullying is equally damaging. With concerns about childhood obesity, parents may nag, tease, or pressure kids, trying to inspire weight loss. That strategy usually backfires and may reinforce poor food habits. A sibling may tease or exclude an overweight or obese brother. Food may instead become an emotional tool to replace the comfort or support so needed from the family. Rather than taking blame or feeling shame, kids with weight issues need empathy, open and supportive communication, inclusion, and support for healthful food choices and physical activity. Get professional help from a registered dietitian or a specialist who addresses self-esteem, body image, and food, if needed. Make the school counselor aware of ongoing bullying behavior.

Have You Ever Wondered

... if lead is harmful to children? Infants and children are at higher risk for lead poisoning than others. Among other problems, lead that builds up in the body over time can cause brain damage. Health experts advise that children get screened at ages one and two, perhaps more often if there's a risk. *For more about screening and addressing lead in drinking water, see "Get the Lead Out!" in chapter 8.*

On another note: Whether or not your child has a weight problem, he or she can be a thoughtful classmate, friend, or sibling to those who are overweight or underweight. Remind your child that dealing with weight problems isn't easy. Yet all children have the same basic needs and lots to offer, no matter what their body size. Teasing or bullying isn't caring, respectful, or fair and can lead to dangerous consequences.

Eating Out with Kids

Whether eating out is a necessity in your busy lifestyle or a special treat for your family, make it an opportunity to teach kids how to make healthful food choices and to behave away from home. To make restaurant meals a healthful and pleasant experience for the whole family:

● Choose a restaurant that caters to children, perhaps with healthy options on its children's menus. Many restaurants now serve children's meals with 600 calories or less and more fruits and vegetables.

A place that serves food quickly is best; waiting too long at the table is hard for kids. If you have a young child, ask for a high chair or a booster seat. Save upscale table service for older children, teens, and adults.

● Match your eating-out schedule to a child's needs. When meals are delayed, kids can't compensate for hunger pangs as adults can. You'll only end up with a cranky meal companion! Offer a small snack ahead.

Go early before the rush, call ahead for reservations to avoid waiting, and provide the full order the first time you're asked so the waiting time for food is shorter.

● Discuss your expectations before you eat out—and the consequences if your child doesn't behave politely in the restaurant. Then follow through if need be, even if it means leaving the restaurant and opting for take-out.

● Look beyond the children's menu—even though it makes ordering easier. Instead of fried chicken nuggets and fries, expose them to new foods. Or give your child a bite or two of new foods from your plate.

● Before ordering, ask about the preparation. If children like plain foods, ask for sauce or the dressing on the side. That way kids have a choice. Substitute "sides": perhaps carrot sticks in place of fries. Order milk instead of soda.

What If . . . Your Child Gets Fussy in a Restaurant?

● Excuse yourselves from the table. Take a short walk.
● Talk in a calm, quiet, and positive way.
● Avoid forcing your child to eat. Instead, have the meal packed to take home.
● Ask if the restaurant has a paper placemat to color or draw on. Bring your own crayons—just in case.
● Bring along a stuffed animal to "share" the fun.

Source: Duyff, R. L. *Nibbles for Health* (Washington, D.C.: U.S. Department of Agriculture, 2002).

● Choose two or three suitable menu items. Then let your child pick—and even place the order if he or she wants to. (Avoid pressuring your child.) Making choices encourages independence and gives kids control over their eating.

● If regular portions are too big, ask for appetizer-size portions. Or share an order . . . perhaps between two kids or with you. Kids shouldn't be urged or expected to "polish" their plate. Instead, bring leftovers home safely.

● Curb your child's appetite while you wait. Ask for a small portion of raw vegetables or bread—just enough to take the edge off hunger, not enough to interfere with a meal. Ask for drinks *with* the meal, not before, so your child doesn't fill up on liquids.

● Make eating out a pleasant experience for kids. Engage them in table talk as you wait for your meal.

● As you're seated, childproof your table if needed.

● Have kids help with clean up in quick-service restaurants.

● Remain patient and positive as your child learns. Mastering table and eating-out manners, including sitting still and being quiet takes skill and practice—and your gentle guidance and role modeling.

For more about restaurant ordering, see chapter 15.

Get Up and Move!

Smart eating is just part of a healthy start on life. Kids need to be physically active, too. Inactivity is linked to the dramatic rise in childhood overweight!

Today's children often watch TV or play computer games during their "prime time" for active play. In fact, by first grade, many kids have clocked five thousand hours of screen time. According to health experts, children who watch too much TV may not get enough physical exercise or time for creative activity. Besides spending too much leisure time at the computer, TV, or video games, there's concern about safe outdoor play. Kids often ride instead of walk to school and have less chance at school for noncompetitive play. To prevent your "tater tots" from becoming the next generation of "couch potatoes," make physical activity fun and part of your family's routine.

When family, school, and community provide opportunities for active play or sports, kids are more likely to participate.

Why Active Play?

Good physical health and a healthy body weight are two good reasons for active play, appropriate sports, and other physical activities. Children can develop social skills, build a positive self-image, enhance their ability to learn, and even help protect themselves from danger. An active child is also more likely be an active adult! Regular physical activity that includes both free play and structured play, meant to develop a variety of motor skills:

● *Helps with a child's physical development.* It builds muscular strength, including a strong heart muscle. Strong muscles promote good posture, which, in turn, affects a child's health and self-image. Weight-bearing activities such as running and skating help strengthen

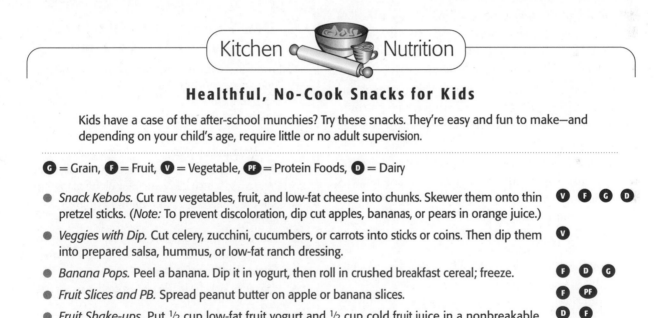

Kitchen Nutrition

Healthful, No-Cook Snacks for Kids

Kids have a case of the after-school munchies? Try these snacks. They're easy and fun to make—and depending on your child's age, require little or no adult supervision.

G = Grain, **F** = Fruit, **V** = Vegetable, **PF** = Protein Foods, **D** = Dairy

● *Snack Kebobs.* Cut raw vegetables, fruit, and low-fat cheese into chunks. Skewer them onto thin pretzel sticks. (*Note:* To prevent discoloration, dip cut apples, bananas, or pears in orange juice.)   **V F G D**

● *Veggies with Dip.* Cut celery, zucchini, cucumbers, or carrots into sticks or coins. Then dip them into prepared salsa, hummus, or low-fat ranch dressing.   **V**

● *Banana Pops.* Peel a banana. Dip it in yogurt, then roll in crushed breakfast cereal; freeze.   **F D G**

● *Fruit Slices and PB.* Spread peanut butter on apple or banana slices.   **F PF**

● *Fruit Shake-ups.* Put ½ cup low-fat fruit yogurt and ½ cup cold fruit juice in a nonbreakable, covered container. Make sure the lid is tight. Then shake it up, and pour into a cup.   **D F**

● *Sandwich Cutouts.* Using cookie cutters with fun shapes like dinosaurs, stars, and hearts, cut slices of low-fat cheese, lean meat, and whole-grain bread. Then put them together to make fun sandwiches. Eat the edges, too.   **D PF G**

● *Peanut Butter Balls.* Mix peanut butter and bran or cornflakes in a bowl. Shape the mixture into balls with clean hands. Then roll them in crushed graham crackers.   **PF G**

● *Salsa Quesadillas.* Fill a soft tortilla with low-fat cheese and salsa, fold over, and grill.   **G D V**

● *Ice Cream–Wiches.* Put a small scoop of ice cream or frozen yogurt between two oatmeal cookies or frozen whole-wheat waffles. Make a batch of these sandwiches ahead, and freeze them.   **D G**

● *Ants on a Log.* Fill celery with peanut butter. Arrange raisins along the top.   **V PF F**

growing bones. Being active also helps build stamina, a quality that promotes learning and play. Once children master basic physical skills they feel self-confident moving, which leads to enjoying physically activities more and being more active.

● *Promotes a healthy body weight.* Increased physical activity is one of the best ways for kids to trim extra body fat.

● *Supports learning.* Many activities develop coordination. Playing catch develops eye-hand coordination. Jumping rope or hopscotch help teach spatial relationships, while soccer helps develop manipulative skills.

● *Develops social skills.* As children play actively with others, they share, cooperate, communicate, support each other, and act as a team.

● *Builds self-esteem.* Succeeding at any physical activity (not just team sports)—riding a bike, swimming a lap, or catching a ball—helps build self-confidence and a positive self-image.

● *Keeps kids fit to handle danger.* Although each circumstance has different physical demands, strong, physically fit children deal better with many possibly harmful emergencies.

● *Comes with the joy of childhood!* Physical activity that's pleasant more likely becomes a lifelong habit. A lifestyle that includes regular physical activity lowers the risk of many chronic diseases.

Kids, Move More!

For good health, children need to move! The Centers for Disease Control and Prevention's Physical Activity Guidelines for Americans advise at least 60 minutes of physical activity every day for kids. It doesn't have to occur at once. While most of the activity should be of moderate intensity, doing activities that are vigorous (running), that build strength (climbing), and that build bones (jumping rope)—at least three times a week—is important, too. Kids need structured play to develop large and small motor skills. Competitive sports aren't needed and may not be appropriate for some kids; they can create unnecessary pressure and take the fun away.

Active play—biking, in-line skating, playing tag, jump-roping, swimming, or tossing a Frisbee, among others—can offer enough exercise for most children. Even household chores count—sweeping can be fun!

Hint: Be sure that children have appropriate safety gear such as helmets, knee pads, or life jackets, as well as sunscreen (even in cold weather) and appropriate clothing.

Next time your kids say they don't know what to do, suggest something active. *See "Ten Things for Kids to Do Instead of Screen Time" on this page.*

To help your child to an active lifestyle you need to make your moves, too. Be a role model. Join kids in active play—perhaps hike together as a weekend outing, ride bikes after dinner, play a quick game of catch or hopscotch after work, clean up a local nature trail, knead a loaf of bread, try a rock-climbing gym, or take an active vacation (perhaps with hiking, swimming, or skiing). Plan for family activities, perhaps after dinner or every Saturday morning so that exercise happens!

Ten Things for Kids to Do Instead of Screen Time

1. Encourage kids to jump rope. If they're older, go "double dutch" with two ropes. (A Hula Hoop contest is fun, too.)
2. Take the dog for a brisk walk or play fetch. No dog? Have kids take their teddy bears for a walk instead. Walking as a family is good talking time!
3. Give kids colored chalk to create a sidewalk mural. Draw a hopscotch game—to play alone or together.
4. Don't let rainy days put a damper on fun! Dance inside.
5. Start a "hundred" walking club. Who's first in your family to walk a hundred times up and down the sidewalk or the stairs in your house?
6. Play tag or kickball in the playground, park, or backyard.
7. If there's snow, make a snowman or go sledding. Or take the family skating at an ice rink—even in July!
8. On warm days, go in-line skating, roller skating, or ride bikes (remember the helmet and pads), or run through sprinkler "rain."
9. Hike together in a nearby park. Have kids find ten points of natural interest to enjoy as you hike.
10. Host a neighborhood bicycle or scooter wash outside—or a dog wash instead!

Source: Adapted from *"Healthy Start: Food to Grow On,"* vol. IV (Food Marketing Institute, American Dietetic Association, and American Academy of Pediatrics, 1995). Reprinted with permission by the Food Marketing Institute, ©1995.

Party time? Make fun activities the main event: swimming, bowling, or skating. Going to a party? Give gifts that encourage physical activity, such as sporting equipment, kites, balls, or physically active games. A walk together in the park or neighborhood provides more than exercise. It's a time to talk, requires no equipment or planning, and it's free!

A few more tips:

● Limit screen time; keep the television, digital devices, and video games out of your child's bedroom. (They don't need a fridge in their room, either.) Give your child enough free time for active play.

● Until your child is a teen, avoid the urge to compete with him or her in organized games such as tennis; usually a child is no match for adult strength and skill. Physical activity needs to feel good to the body and the mind. Encourage "personal best."

● Encourage active play so exercise doesn't seem like punishment. If your child is uninterested or feels embarrassed about not being good enough in a sport, find something active your child likes or feels good about. It doesn't need to be a team or group activity. Do it together to build confidence.

● Do you need after-school care for your kids? Look for programs that include physical activity: perhaps in Scout groups, outdoor centers, recreational and community centers, or your child's school. Or sign them up for gymnastics, dance, karate, or swim classes.

● If your child has a disability, talk to your healthcare provider about the appropriate amount and types of physical activities.

For more ideas, see "Twenty Everyday Ways to Get Moving" in chapter 2.

Kids in the Kitchen

Your kitchen is a learning laboratory! Just like learning to read and write, becoming self-sufficient with food preparation is a life skill. Knowing how to cook is a strategy for healthful meals that also promotes a healthy weight! Your child also may share responsibility for healthful family meals and be expected to feed himself or herself sometimes. Depending on age, your child may help with food shopping, preparation, and

---

Microwave Oven Safety for Kids

Because burns are a common hazard related to microwave oven use, make sure children know how to use a microwave oven safely.

● Make sure the microwave oven is on a sturdy stand—one that's low enough for kids. If children need to reach too high, they may pull a hot dish down on themselves.

● Teach children to read the controls on the microwave oven—the time, the power level, and the "start" and "stop" controls. If kids can't read them, they're too young to operate a microwave oven alone.

● Keep microwave-safe containers in one place—within a child's reach.

● Always have a child use child-size kitchen mitts to remove heated food from the microwave oven—whether the food is hot or not. In that way it becomes a habit. Keep potholders handy for kids.

● Teach children to stir heated food before tasting. That distributes the heat and avoids hot spots that can cause burns.

● Show them how to open containers so that steam escapes away from their face. That includes packages of popped microwave popcorn.

● Until you're sure that children have mastered the art of microwaving, provide supervision.

For more tips on using a microwave oven safely, see "Play It Microwave-Safe" in chapter 13.

---

cleanup. Kitchen skills are more than fun. They may be a necessity! Shop, cook, and eat together!

For more ideas, see "Exploring More about Food" earlier in this chapter.

Let's Cook!

Prepare food with your child—and explore a wide variety of foods. When kids "cook," they practice many skills—not just how to handle and prepare foods to nourish themselves and keep food safe to eat. By reading a recipe, children learn new words and practice reading. They identify foods and learn their qualities as they gather ingredients. By preparing a recipe, they practice measuring, counting, timing, sequencing, and following directions. Slicing, pouring, rolling dough, and shaping meat patties are among the food preparation activities that develop small-muscle movement and eye-hand coordination. Food preparation is practical science. Children might watch dough rise, see eggs coagulate, or observe how sugar dissolves in water.

Preparing food also promotes your child's social and emotional development. Children feel good about themselves when they successfully prepare foods to eat—and share with others. It's an opportunity to explore foods of other cultures and respect the similarities and the differences. Most important, preparing food together is a chance to be together.

● Choose foods and recipes that match your child's abilities. With foods a child might prepare alone, first make them together.

● For young cooks, choose illustrated children's cookbooks that show the foods, measurements, and steps along the way. Go over the safety and sanitation tips at the front of a child's cookbook.

● Ask your child to suggest foods he or she would like to make. Make it a total experience by shopping for ingredients together, too.

● Besides cooking together, have your child help you store food properly. Use this chance to show your child how to handle food to keep it clean and safe from spoilage and foodborne illness.

● Sign up for a cooking class where kids and parents cook together. Volunteer to help with food activities in after-school programs. Suggest a summer cooking camp for your child.

● As you prepare food, help children learn to be "green" in the kitchen. *See "The 'Eco' Kitchen" in chapter 14.*

For easy recipes that children can prepare for snacks—or any meal of the day—see "Kitchen Nutrition: Healthful, No-Cook Snacks for Kids" in this chapter.

Kitchen Safety Alert

With all that goes on in a kitchen, food preparation sends some "red flags" for kids' safety. Cooking is safe—if your child learns to be careful.

● Remind children to always wash their hands with soap and water before and after they handle food, and dry them well. Follow good cleanliness habits. Review safety precautions. *See "Hand-Washing Basics" earlier in this chapter.*

● Supervise your child in the kitchen. As your child is ready, teach kitchen safety tips. *See kitchen safety rules in chapter 13 and "Microwave Oven Safety for Kids" in this chapter.*

● Set limits on what your child can—and can't—do without proper supervision. For example, your child can't use the oven if he or she is home alone.

● Remind your child to be aware of his or her hair and clothes before using the stove. Large, loose-fitting garments and long hair can catch fire.

● Be a good kitchen role model. Your child will take his or her kitchen-safety cues from you. Among the things to learn and practice: using clean utensils for different foods and using a food thermometer. *For more guidance on food safety, see chapter 13.*

● Practice what to do in case of fire. That includes "drop and roll" to smother the flames in case his or her clothes catch fire. Keep a fire extinguisher in view, and teach your child how to use it.

● Try to keep food and utensils your child will use within easy reach. Keep a sturdy stool handy if he or she needs to reach higher. Remind your child not to climb on the counters or on a wobbling stool!

● Teach kids—even preschoolers—to call 911 (or emergency numbers such as those for the fire department, poison control center, or police in your area). Post the phone numbers in your kitchen where children can see them easily.

● Know first aid for choking. *See "If You or Someone Else Is Choking" in chapter 13.*

● Keep a first-aid kit handy and stocked. Teach your child how to use it for a minor cooking injury.

For more on preventing injuries, see "Quick Tips for Injury Prevention" in chapter 13.

Feeding the Teen Machine

Seeing teenagers make wise food choices is your reward for providing healthful food and teaching good nutrition in their younger years. By adolescence, many kids make most of their own decisions about food. Other than filling the refrigerator and kitchen shelves with food and preparing family meals, parents have far less control over what their adolescent child eats.

Teenagers themselves exert stronger influence over family eating than before, perhaps sharing the shopping and food preparation. Compared with their childhood years, they probably consume more food and beverages away from home.

Chances are that teenagers know the basics of nutrition and healthful eating. However, peer pressure; busy school, after-school activity, and work schedules; a sense of independence; unrealistic notions about body weight; and a poor self-image are among the barriers to healthful eating. Food choices may not reflect what teens know about eating for fitness.

The same holds true for physical activity. Kids know why they should move more and be physically active, but doing so has barriers, too.

Sound familiar? In a nutshell, adolescents often don't connect their immediate food and physical activity patterns to their long- or short-term health. Many teens live in a wonderful world of invulnerability. Others follow misguided advice: supplements for muscle building, unsafe dieting for weight loss, energy drinks—for energy! Read on for a few "teen-friendly" fitness strategies.

Teens, Did You Know

... unhealthy dieting can stop you from growing to your full height? Your body needs calories and other nutrients to grow and develop fully. Most teens shouldn't "diet."

... your bones take in the most calcium during your teen years? The best sources are milk, yogurt, and low-fat cheese, and most teens need the equivalent of three to four cups of milk daily.

... if you don't eat breakfast, your body is like a computer without power?

... eating cookies, candy, or other sweet foods before an athletic event won't give you an energy boost?

... for girls, when you have a menstrual period you lose iron? If you don't eat iron-rich foods to replace this loss, you may feel weak and tired.

... pizza and hamburgers can be healthful food choices, especially if you know which toppings to choose (veggies, fruit, beans, lean meat or chicken)—and you eat sensible amounts?

... eating smart and moving more help you feel good, look good, and do your best!

Many nutrition issues for adults also apply to your teenager: for example, calorie-dense snacking, meal-skipping, mindless eating, too-big portions, fad diets, eating too few fruits and vegetables, vegetarian eating, fast-food choices, sports nutrition. *Throughout the book, you'll find strategies your teen can use to address these issues.*

Food, Nutrients, and the Teen Years

Second only to infancy, adolescence is the fastest growth stage in life! Even when teens reach their adult height (for girls sooner than for boys), their bodies are still growing and developing.

Puberty marks the start of the teenage growth spurt. That time differs for each child. For girls, puberty typically begins at about age twelve, about two years younger than for boys. From the school-age years through the teens, the average youngster grows to be 20 percent taller and 50 percent heavier. Body changes that happen as children mature are stressful for some, and may affect their self-image and perhaps the choices they make about eating and physical activity.

How your teenager grows—when, how, and how much—has more to do with genes than with food choices. However, smart eating does help determine if your teen grows to his or her maximum height potential—with strong bones, a fit body, and a healthy weight. Teens need understanding parents who appreciate that their adolescent's growth pattern, although different from a friend's, is perfectly normal.

All teens need enough calcium and vitamin D for bone growth and strength, protein for every body cell including muscles, carbohydrates and fats for energy, vitamins and minerals for the "sparks" that make it all happen, and enough water. Calorie and nutrient needs increase to meet the growth demands of adolescence.

Food Energy: How Much?

Teens need somewhat more calories than when they were a bit younger. Teenage boys on average need 1,800 to 2,600 calories a day if they're eleven to thirteen years, and 2,200 to 3,200 calories a day if they're fourteen to eighteen years of age. Teenage girls need on average 1,800 to 2,200 calories a day if they're ages eleven to thirteen, and 1,800 to 2,400 calories a day if they're age fourteen to eighteen. Their gender, body size, growth rate, and physical activity level determine how many calories they need. Those who do a lot of strenuous physical activity such as soccer, basketball, football, or other sports may need 3,500 calories daily. Let internal hunger cues, rather than charts and tables, be the guide. *Refer to "Weighty Issues for Children—Teens, Too!" earlier in this chapter.*

Nutrients: For Some, An All-Time High

Many nutrient recommendations go up during adolescence. *Check the Dietary Reference Intakes in the appendices to see how much.* As teens consume more food-group foods, they also need a nutrient and calorie boost to meet the demands of growth and perhaps more physical activity.

Several nutrients may need attention in a teenager's food choices: calcium, iron, potassium, vitamin D, and perhaps zinc. That's usually due to poor food choices, or for girls especially, simply not eating enough. Dairy foods provide some of these nutrients; protein foods provide some, too, but not the same ones. Potassium and fiber likely need attention; eating enough fruit, vegetables, and whole-grain foods can provide enough of these. And saturated fat, *trans* fat, added sugars, and sodium are likely too high. Read on to learn more.

Pregnancy affects a teenage girl's nutrition needs. Like any pregnancy, the need for nutrients and calories goes up; for teens, the recommendations are higher than for adult women, for their own growth and development, and for the developing fetus. *For more on the nutrition needs of a teenage pregnancy, see "For Pregnant Teens: Good Nutrition" in chapter 18.*

Calcium and Vitamin D: Growing Issues. "I'm sixteen, and I've stopped growing. So why do I need milk?" Actually, bones keep on developing into the adult years. Even when teenagers reach their adult height, bones continue to strengthen as they become more dense. In fact, almost half of an adult's bone mass forms during the teen years. The stronger bones become during adolescence, the lower the risk of osteoporosis later on. Yet in the United States, only 10 percent of girls and 42 percent of boys ages fourteen to eighteen consume the recommended amount of calcium daily. And many are short-changed on vitamin D!

Osteoporosis is an adolescent health problem that manifests itself in later years. Teenagers—children, too—who don't consume enough calcium put their bones at risk for the long term. They may start their

Have You Ever Wondered

. . . besides drinking milk, how can teens keep their bones healthy? Like milk, yogurt, cheese, and pudding are all calcium-rich, bone-building foods. In addition, calcium-fortified soy beverage and tofu, as well as calcium-fortified juice and dark-green vegetables, provide calcium, too. Regular weight-bearing activities such as dancing, soccer, running, weight lifting, tennis, and volleyball are important since they trigger bone tissue to form. Going easy on soft drinks if they edge out calcium-rich milk is smart advice. Smoking also may have a negative effect on bone formation; teens who smoke are smart to kick the habit for many reasons!

adult years with a calcium deficit in their bones. With bone loss that comes as a natural part of aging, they have less to draw on, and their risk for osteoporosis, or brittle bone disease, goes up. Poor bone health, perhaps related to low intake of calcium and vitamin D, can also result in stress fractures. These are tiny cracks in the bone, usually from overuse. They're among the most common sport injuries, especially for those who are involved in basketball, dance, gymnastics, tennis, and track and field.

Teens are advised to consume enough calcium- and vitamin D-rich foods so their bones become as strong as they can be. For teens, the Recommended Dietary Allowance for calcium is 1,300 milligrams daily and 600 IU (15 micrograms) daily for vitamin D. An 8-ounce glass of milk has about 300 milligrams of calcium and 100 IU of vitamin D.

What foods are teens' best calcium sources? Dairy group foods including milk, yogurt, and cheese (preferably low-fat or fat-free)—although a variety of foods have smaller amounts of calcium. Milk also contains other nutrients essential to healthy bone: vitamins A, D, and B_{12}, potassium, magnesium, and protein. Canned salmon and sardines with bones, as well as some vegetables (such as mustard greens, collard greens, okra, broccoli, and bok choy), supply calcium. And some prepared foods are calcium- and vitamin D-fortified, including some juice, fortified soy beverages, breads, and breakfast cereal. *For more on calcium, vitamin D, and bone health, see chapter 6.*

Why don't many teens consume enough calcium-rich dairy foods? Perhaps there's no milk on hand at home, or perhaps they say they don't like it. Maybe kids haven't made a habit of drinking milk with meals. Or perhaps soft drinks or other sugar-sweetened drinks compete. If milk is cold, convenient, and "cool," your teen more likely will drink it. *Tip:* Fill the fridge with flavored milk or yogurt drinks. Look for low-fat and fat-free options.

Many teenage girls misguidedly link milk drinking to their fear of getting fat, including teens on fad diets or those with eating disorders. Yet those who watch calories could consume low-fat or fat-free dairy foods or maybe a latte or flavored milk when they eat out. Eight ounces of fat-free milk supply fewer calories than 8 ounces of a soft drink or juice: only 86 calories and almost no fat, yet fat-free milk has as much calcium and vitamin D as whole milk!

Vegan eating patterns and lactose intolerance may be barriers, too. In either case, teens have plenty of practical ways to get enough calcium and vitamin D. *See chapter 21 for more about lactose intolerance.*

For more about bone health during adulthood, see "Osteoporosis: Reduce the Risks" in chapter 22.

Iron: The Fatigue Connection. Does your teenager seem chronically tired? Fatigue may come from too little sleep, an exhausting schedule, strenuous activity (a good kind of fatigue), or the emotional ups and downs of adolescence. Feeling tired also may be a symptom of a health problem due to low iron levels in blood.

Iron is part of blood's hemoglobin, which carries oxygen to body cells. Once there, oxygen helps cells produce energy. When iron is in short supply, there's less oxygen available to produce energy—hence fatigue.

Iron needs go up dramatically in the teen years. During childhood (ages nine to thirteen) both boys and girls need about 8 milligrams of iron daily, according to the Dietary Reference Intakes. For adolescence, more muscle mass and a greater blood supply demand more iron, so the recommendation jumps to 15 milligrams of iron daily for girls ages fourteen to eighteen to replace iron losses from their menstrual flow. For boys that age the advice is 11 milligrams daily. *See "Menstrual Cycle: More Iron for Women" in chapter 18.*

Many teens—girls especially—don't consume enough iron. Poor food choices or restricting food to lose weight are two common reasons. Kids who don't eat protein foods regularly may not consume enough either.

Iron comes from a variety of foods: meat, poultry, and seafood as well as beans (legumes), enriched grain products, and some vegetables.

Teens who drink orange juice with their morning toast or iron-fortified cereal get an iron boost, too. Its vitamin C content makes iron from plant sources and eggs more usable by the body. Kids who just grab toast to eat at the bus stop, but skip the juice, don't get the full benefit of the iron in bread. Some teens don't consume enough vitamin C, either.

For more on iron in a healthful diet, see chapter 6.

Many nutrition issues faced by teens are also adult nutrition issues, discussed elsewhere in this book.

Food Guide for Teens

USDA's MyPlate, which represents advice from the five food groups and oils, is meant for teens, too! How much from the food groups? That depends on how many calories they need. The more active they are, the more calories they need—and the more they can eat. *Check the appendices to estimate calorie needs and find a food-group pattern that matches.*

Here's top-line food group advice to share with teens. *For more guidance, refer to chapter 10, "Planning to Eat Smart," and refer to the Dietary Guidelines, discussed on chapter 1.*

● Grain group—*make calories count.* Carbs should provide most food energy for teens. The best choices

Have You Ever Wondered

... if you should be concerned if your teenager skips meals? That depends. If your teen skips meals regularly, nutrients needed for growth, development, and health may come up short. Some teenage girls often skip breakfast or lunch to save on calories, then perhaps miss out on nutrient-rich foods of special concern: high-calcium, high-vitamin-D foods such as milk, iron-fortified cereals, fiber-rich whole grains, and fruits and vegetables. Later teens may satisfy their hunger with high-calorie, high-fat snack foods. The net result: more calories, fewer nutrients, and perhaps a potential for weight issues.

have more fiber and less solid fats and added sugars; for example, replace donuts with whole-grain bagels. Order pizza on whole-grain crust, sandwiches on whole-wheat bread, plain popcorn, or whole-wheat crackers.

● Vegetable and fruit groups—*eat more* fruits and veggies than you're used to. They deliver vitamins, minerals, fiber, and more, generally with fewer calories. Choose with variety in mind, less fat, and without added sugars. Go for color! Ease up on fries!

● Dairy group—*eat enough* low-fat or fat-free dairy foods for calcium and vitamin D and their nutrient partners for a lifetime of healthy bones.

● Protein foods group—*eat enough* lean meat and beans to get the iron your body needs. These foods, along with poultry, fish, eggs, and nuts, provide protein, too. Go easy on fried chicken and fried fish.

● Oils—*choose an amount within your calorie budget* from vegetable oils, oily fish such as salmon, avocado, and nuts, in place of foods with more saturated and *trans* fats.

Healthy eating at school makes a difference. For school lunch, encourage teens to choose from the full variety of foods on the menu—preferably not a burger, pizza, or fries every day—and to make lunch a chance to drink milk. *For more about school meals, see "For Kids Only—Today's School Meals" earlier in this chapter.*

Great Snacking!

With their high energy and nutrient needs, especially during their growth spurt, teens often need snacks as a "refueling stop." Boys especially may need snacks to fill their bottomless pit. Snacks help to fill in nutrient gaps that meal choices miss: yogurt as a snack, for example, if a teen doesn't drink milk for lunch, and hummus and baby carrots as another way to fit veggies in. Snacking is part of a social pattern and something to do when teenagers get together!

The real issue with teen snacking isn't whether they do—or don't. Instead it's about what and how much. These are among the nutrition issues: (1) high-calorie snacks replacing nutrient-rich foods; (2) mindless or emotional snacking that adds to excess calories; (3) large, even oversized, portions that add up on calories;

and (4) overdoing on drinks and snacks that are high in total fat, including solid fats, or high in sodium or added sugars; for example, regular soft drinks, sweetened tea, candy, chips, cookies, and fruit pies.

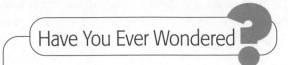

Have You Ever Wondered

. . . what to eat to control acne? Although all kinds of foods get blamed, teenage acne is linked to hormonal changes, rarely to food choices. The best approach to healthy skin is to eat an overall varied and balanced diet, keep skin clean, get enough rest—and wait. After the body matures, most acne clears up. If problems are severe or persist, talk to a dermatologist. Sometimes a skin application that contains a derivative of vitamin A is prescribed; simply taking a vitamin A tablet won't clear the skin.

Caution: If the doctor prescribes Accutane (isotretinoin) to treat severe acne, avoid supplements with vitamin A. Together, Accutane and vitamin A have toxic effects. Taking Accutane can also raise cholesterol and blood lipid (fat) levels until the treatment stops. Because of the many potential psychological (depression, lack of concentration, irritability, and suicidal thoughts, among others) and physical (including unusual fatigue and appetite loss) side effects of Accutane, make sure your teen follows dosage directions carefully, *under close supervision of a physician.* Accutane can cause birth defects.

. . . if chocolate causes acne? No, chocolate doesn't cause acne or make acne worse. Hormones and hygiene, rather than a chocolate allergy, are more likely the culprits. A true food allergy to chocolate is rare. Instead, a reaction to a chocolate bar may come from other ingredients mixed in, such as nuts or milk.

. . . if kids who wear braces should avoid eating raw vegetables and fruits? No! It's true that hard, crunchy, or sticky foods can damage braces. But kids don't need to give up vegetables and fruits. Instead they might choose softer types: perhaps a ripe peach or a banana rather than a crisp apple; or cucumber sticks rather than a whole, raw carrot; or soften sliced carrots or broccoli in a microwave oven. Or they might cut these foods into bite-size pieces instead of eating them whole. Consult your child's orthodontist for a list of foods that might damage braces.

Teens snack! Support their ability to snack smart: water, milk, or juice from a vending machine; a small burger with milk at a fast-food restaurant; or fruit, raw vegetables, yogurt, or cereal with fat-free or low-fat milk from the kitchen at home. Have healthful snacks on hand when teens bring friends home. *For easy, nutritious snack ideas, see chapter 11.*

Your Teen's Food Choices: What You Can Do

Bigger appetites, busy lifestyles, emotional swings, struggles for independence, peer pressure: they challenge how and what teens eat. As a parent you can influence your teen's eating habits—subtly, of course!

● Stock the kitchen with easy-to-grab nutrition. Foods that take little or no effort—for example, whole fruit, yogurt, hummus, cut-up veggie sticks, string cheese, and bagels—are most likely eaten. (Ease is one reason why kids reach for chips.) *See "Empower Your Kids: Seven How-tos for Smart Snacking" earlier in this chapter for more ideas.*

● Still . . . make time for family meals, even if you need to schedule around after-school activities and jobs, and put family meals on the calendar days in advance. It's a good time to get connected. (Save stressful conversations for later.) What's more, research suggests nutritional benefits! For teens, eating family meals is linked to consuming more fruit, vegetables, and milk and fewer soft drinks and fried, high-fat, and sugar-laden foods. Another link: Some research also links family meals with better emotional health; fewer risk-taking behaviors, such as alcohol and drug abuse; and better school performance.

● Encourage an elective class in foods (cooking), nutrition and wellness, or consumer health. That's a great way for teens to learn practical basics of sound nutrition and healthful eating. These classes are also full of applied science, math, and social studies!

● Help teens build skills. Your teen can plan, shop for, and cook family meals. The kitchen is a place to practice what's learned in a foods class. *Some tips in "Kids in the Kitchen" in this chapter might help younger teens.*

● Check out the options together at fast-food restaurants, vending machines, and convenience stores. Your teen may not be aware of all the choices out there. There's more than burgers, fries, chips, and soft drinks.

Alert: Teenage Drinking!

"It's just beer; it's not like I'm using drugs!" That's common logic for some teens. But scientific evidence, the Dietary Guidelines, and the law are clear: for teens, do not drink! What may start as social drinking with a seemingly "safe" sweet wine cooler or beer can turn high risk. The alcohol in wine coolers, which are wine plus carbonated fruit drink, and beer quickly adds up to dangerous levels of blood alcohol. The effects are faster and stronger for some than others; there's no way to predict how a teen will be affected.

Besides being illegal, alcohol use by young people can have serious outcomes. For one, it can contribute to alcohol-related problems later on. Driving accidents, with potentially life-altering and fatal consequences, are among the obvious risks of drunkenness *for anyone*, not just for confirmed alcoholics. In addition, alcohol use is highly linked to sexual assaults and potentially to alcohol-induced blackouts. Under the influence of alcohol, sexually active youth are less likely to use precautions for pregnancy and sexually transmitted disease (STD); because heavy drinking lowers immunity, risks for STDs are higher.

As a parent, talk openly about the risks. For weight-conscious girls, just knowing the calories in beer and wine coolers may be a deterrent. Practice ways your teen can refuse alcoholic drinks and leave drinking situations. Be mindful of alcohol use among your child's peers and within the community, so you can help your child avoid them. Show by example your responsible use of alcoholic beverages, if you choose to drink them. *For more about alcoholic drinks, including the risks, see chapter 8.*

● Help kids tune into portion size. A small bag of chips can be as much fun to eat as a bigger bag, with far fewer calories! The same goes for soft drinks. *See "Portion Distortion?" in chapter 11.*

● Set a good example for wellness and lifestyle—for example, with regular physical activity, lower-fat eating, sensible portions, and not smoking. Kids notice when adults "walk their talk." Not surprisingly, research suggests that boys tend to follow their dad's lifestyles; girls, their mother's.

● Help your teen deal with peer pressure. In that way he or she will have strategies to follow personal goals for smart eating, rather than going with the crowd.

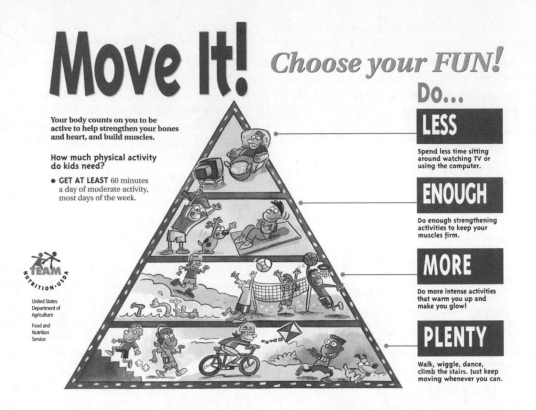

Move It!

Choose your FUN!

Your body counts on you to be active to help strengthen your bones and heart, and build muscles.

How much physical activity do kids need?

● **GET AT LEAST** 60 minutes a day of moderate activity, most days of the week.

United States
Department of Agriculture

Food and Nutrition Service

Do...

LESS
Spend less time sitting around watching TV or using the computer.

ENOUGH
Do enough strengthening activities to keep your muscles firm.

MORE
Do more intense activities that warm you up and make you glow!

PLENTY
Walk, wiggle, dance, climb the stairs. Just keep moving whenever you can.

● In your talk, tie smart eating and active living to what matters to your teen—growing normally; feeling good; looking good; and doing well in school, sports, or a personal interest (music, drama, art, whatever). Even when teens seem to disregard what you suggest, they likely "hear" your encouragement, concern, and example.

Refer to "Feeding Vegetarian Children and Teens" earlier in this chapter.

Move It!

Does your teen move in high gear on a "24/7" schedule—school to after-school activities and perhaps to a job? Do homework, time with friends, and hours on the phone or online fit in between? Research shows that unless they are involved in sports, kids' physical activity drops dramatically when they hit the teen years. *Remember:* A busy schedule may not be an active lifestyle!

Moving more promotes benefits that are dear to teenage hearts: looking good, being in shape, being strong, feeling energetic, being self-confident, doing well in school, and having a good outlook on life.

There's more. Being active now helps them keep a healthy weight and helps reduce the risk for some chronic health problems later, including diabetes, heart disease, obesity, and osteoporosis. That's especially true if teens make active living a lifelong habit.

The physical activity guideline for teens? For teens, the Physical Activity Guidelines for Americans advises 60 minutes or more of physical activity each day. Divide it up. Do mostly aerobic activity (moderate or vigorous). At least three days a week fit in vigorous activity, muscle-strengthening activities, and bone-strengthening activities. Get a good balance of activities that stretch, strengthen, and give your heart a workout. *For more about guidelines and benefits of physical activity, see "Get Physical!" in chapter 2.*

Kids on the Move: Overcoming the Barriers

Why are more and more teenagers less and less active? Perhaps it's the family pattern they "inherited." But for every reason teens give, there's an easy, often fun solution.

Reason: Video games, social media, computer time, and TV take precedent. According to the American Academy of Pediatrics, children and teens spend on average about seven hours daily with screen time and media. While the mental exercise of computer games is great, one's eyes, brain, and body need an active break from sitting. In fact, brain synapses may work faster with some physical activity.

Tactic: Encourage kids to balance social media and online time with physically active time, either with friends and family or on their own.

● Do something active while watching TV: perhaps lift weights, do push-ups or sit-ups, or dance!

● Find video games that make your body move, not just sit.

● Surf the Internet to find ways to have active fun.

● As a parent, set limits on screen time. Have a "landing place" for computers and digital devices that are within adult control.

Reason: Kids say, "It's too far to walk there." So they ride in or drive cars nearly everywhere: to school, the store, friends' homes, the library, or work.

Tactic: Encourage the independence and physical activity benefits of getting to close places by foot or bike.

● Get a foot scooter, in-line skates, or bike. (Remember a helmet and perhaps knee pads for safety.)

● For a parent, encourage kids to walk or bike when possible rather than to be the family chauffer.

Reason: Kids say they don't have time, especially if they work after school or if they're involved in sports or other after-school activities.

Tactic: Fit physical activity into what kids do anyway.

● Read a book while on a stationary bike. Balance on a large balance ball while doing homework at a desk or table.

● Pick household chores that take more movement, such as washing the car, raking leaves, or sweeping sidewalks.

Reason: School doesn't require much physical education.

Tactic: Make personal health the priority, not just school requirements.

● Sign up for PE at school anyway, and not just as a summer course.

● Take a community aerobics, dance, or martial arts class.

● As a parent, support efforts to include physical education at school.

Reason: Some kids feel self-conscious about sports, especially if they aren't athletic or they're overweight.

Tactic: Put the emphasis on fun, not performance.

● Try individual physical activities, such as biking, walking, and in-line skating.

● Download music for your kids to listen to as they walk to keep up a quick pace.

Reason: Kids (especially girls) say, "I don't want to sweat or mess up my hair."

Tactic: Shift mind-set. Even if your teen sweats, fitness is more important.

● Do everyday activities such as walking to school or household tasks that don't work up a sweat.

● Come up with an active day "look."

Weight: Right-Sized?

Body image is a big issue for most teens, who are eager for acceptance, yet self-conscious about body

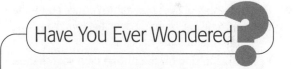

Have You Ever Wondered

. . . if kids can turn computer time into physically active fun? Sure, on the right website! BAM (Body and Mind) at www.BAM.gov from the Centers for Disease Control and Prevention and the U.S. Department of Health and Human Services website, www.smallstep.gov/kids/flash/games_and_activities.html, get kids moving while they're online.

. . . how to help my teen avoid the "freshman fifteen"? That number refers to the belief that many teens gain fifteen pounds during their first year at college. However, poor food habits may be promoted by academic pressure, the stress of being away from home, and perhaps unlimited food access. Encourage your teen to eat smart and take time for physical activity, perhaps a study break. You might send a "care package" with healthier and lower-calorie snack foods, too. After college, in fact, that amount is likely overstated, and some weight gain results from adolescent development.

changes. Despite different body sizes, shapes, and growth stages, many weigh in within a healthy range. In growing numbers, overweight and obesity are concerns, however. Some use misguided approaches for trying to achieve an unrealistic weight or body size. Still others are victims of disordered eating. *Remember:* The right weight is a range, not a single number; and it's about health and a healthy weight for the individual teen, not just looks.

If Your Teen Is Overweight or Obese

Teens who truly are overweight or obese—or at risk for it—need a healthful, realistic, safe way to manage their weight. That includes both physical activity and smart eating, not "dieting." Adult weight-loss diets aren't meant for teens. Unless a doctor advises it, the teen years aren't a time for a weight-loss diet. For many, growing into an appropriate weight is healthier—if the teen eats sensibly and gets enough physical activity. Otherwise a growth spurt won't resolve a weight prob-

lem. Dieting may deprive a growing teen of needed nutrients.

Weight is a sensitive issue for everyone, especially kids. The best approach is positive—no nagging, forbidden foods, or criticism; a negative approach is surefire defeat. Instead, understanding, love, and support go a long way in helping teens and children cope with and address weight issues.

- Help eliminate eating triggers, such as the sight of high-calorie snacks on the kitchen counter.

- Reassess the family's eating style. Make gradual improvements together. Gradual changes often become permanent ones.

- Do fun, active things together. You both benefit!

- Talk, listen, and offer support and alternatives for emotional issues that trigger eating.

- Gather the resources your teen needs. Keep nutritious, lower-calorie foods, including vegetables and fruits, on hand. Prepare family meals that support your teen's strategies for managing weight.

- Make this book, the *American Dietetic Association Complete Food and Nutrition Guide*, available for your teen to read.

- Most of all, be accepting. Your love doesn't depend on your teen's weight loss. Unconditional acceptance goes a long way in promoting a positive self-image, which helps promote a healthy weight.

For more about weight issues, see "Weighty Issues for Children—Teens, Too!" earlier in this chapter.

Pressure to Be Thin

To many teens, looks are almost everything! As their bodies develop and take on adult shapes, it's normal to focus on body image. Often, however, teens have unrealistic notions about their own weight. Many girls, especially those ages nine to fifteen years, view themselves as overweight when they really aren't. Although less common, many boys in that age group do, too.

Pressure to be thin is closely linked to pressure to fit in and to be accepted by peers. Thin people are viewed as successful, popular, and attractive. This message gets reinforced by media images and celebrities—and often by parents and friends. However, even celebrities they try to emulate may not have a "perfect look" in reality; computers can manipulate photo images.

Get Fit with a Friend

Is your teenager looking for something to do? Suggest these active ways to get fit with a friend—and have fun!

- Do something active: play table tennis, go in-line skating, go hiking, or enjoy dancing. *Hint:* You don't need a partner for line dancing.

- Walk while talking on the phone with your friends.

- Sign up for a school or community sports team. You don't need to "play varsity" to get health benefits.

- Join the marching band if you play a musical instrument. Try out for cheerleading, majorettes, or the pom-pom squad.

- Volunteer as a stagehand for school plays. You'll get plenty of activity doing stage chores.

- Do community service—perhaps at a community garden, home-building project, children's day camp, community clean-up, or animal center.

- Baby-sit! Play actively with children.

- Get a neighborhood job: mow lawns, shovel snow, wash cars, do yardwork, walk a neighbor's dog.

- Enjoy interactive computer and video games that promote physical activity.

  For more physical activity ideas for teens, see "Twenty Everyday Ways to Get Moving" in chapter 2.

Teenage girls tend to diet, often poorly, as their main approach to having an attractive body, while boys often put more emphasis on exercise and body building. For girls, the pursuit of thinness often leads to fad dieting—usually ineffective, often dangerous. These diets are especially risky during adolescence, when teenagers' nutrient needs for growth and energy are high. Trying to lose weight fast to "look good" for a dance or a swim party is neither realistic nor healthful. *For more on fad diets, see "'Diets That Don't Work!" in chapter 2.*

Teens who truly are overweight—or at risk for overweight—need a realistic, safe, and healthful way to manage their weight. That includes both physical activity and a healthful eating plan, not "dieting."

Disordered Eating. Sometimes a teen's pursuit of thinness leads to obsession, perhaps caused by a traumatic event or a life change. Although not overweight, and perhaps even underweight, some teenagers see themselves as fat. Sometimes a distorted body image begins as teens develop sexual characteristics.

A distorted body image may lead to disordered eating. Teens, whose nutrient needs are high, instead may eat very little, or purge with self-induced vomiting or laxative abuse. Disordered eating can result in extreme undernourishment and weight loss—even death. Because eating disorders are linked to psychological problems, attention from a mental health professional, as well as your child's physician, is essential.

Most victims of eating disorders are teenage girls and young women. For example, 1 percent of girls age twelve to eighteen have anorexia nervosa. Although less common, teenage boys, in increasing numbers, have eating disorders, too. Other eating disorders, such as bulimia and binge eating disorder, also afflict adolescents. Binge-eating is a common eating disorder of obese people. *To learn more, see "Disordered Eating: Problems, Signs, and Help" in chapter 2.*

Also refer to "Dangers of Bullying," which addresses weight issues, earlier in this chapter.

Bodybuilding

Most teenage boys want to build muscle (have great "abs"), not lose weight, to look good. Many know the value of weight training for bodybuilding. But for some, the size and shape of their muscles become obsessions that lead to seemingly constant weight lifting and workouts. They may also have the misguided notion that eating more protein builds muscle mass, too. Some opt for more meat portions, perhaps at the expense of whole-grain starchy foods; others take protein supplements and "bulk-up" drugs such as steroids. Muscle-building steroids are dangerous; *see "Ergogenic Aids: No Substitute for Training" in chapter 20.*

Although protein needs go up from childhood, an extra amount has no bodybuilding benefits. Following the food-group recommendations supplies the protein that most teens need—whether they're involved in weight training or not. Like extra carbohydrate or dietary fat, extra calories from protein are deposited in the body as fat, not muscle. *See chapter 20 for advice about the variety and amount of food for sports.*

A high-protein diet may contribute a high percentage of calories from fat. That's especially true when teens opt for fewer foods high in carbohydrates, such as bread, pasta, rice, and cereal. The best advice for teenage bodybuilders? *Follow the USDA Food Patterns guidelines in chapter 10,* and be sensible with a weight-training program.

The key to building muscle is a good exercise program and enough nutrient-rich foods to fuel longer workouts. Through exercise, which creates a demand for more muscle, protein enters the muscles and makes them larger. *See "Muscle Myths" in chapter 20.*

What about making weight for wrestling or football—or for a lean strong body for gymnastics, figure skating, or cheerleading? Unhealthy weight management—either to gain or to lose weight—can be dangerous for anyone, including young athletes. Cutting down on food and beverages, along with overexercising and sweating off water weight, can lead to dehydration, heat stress, and other health problems—and certainly does not enhance performance. Instead, muscles may get weaker and smaller, even for those who consume protein. Without enough calories, the body burns some protein in muscles for energy. Crash dieting for sports and body image, along with a poor self-image, are factors that can lead to disordered eating and decreased performance.

For more on food for sports and making weight, see "Making Weight" in chapter 20.

CHAPTER 18

For Women Only

Women—this chapter is meant especially for you and your unique nutrition needs! Until recent years, women's health needs were projected in studies done mostly with men. Except for a focus on reproductive health, women's health concerns were largely ignored. Today medical research, health promotion, and healthcare address gender differences. And nutrition often is center stage in initiatives for women's health.

Women need the same nutrients that men do—perhaps more of some, depending on their age. Yet, if physically smaller, they likely need fewer calories to deliver those nutrients.

Unless men shift their physical activity level, the nutrition needs of healthy males don't change much over a lifetime. That's not true for women. Complexities of the reproductive system, the ups and downs of female hormones, and the physical demands of childbearing affect nutrition needs and healthcare. Menstruation, pregnancy, breast-feeding, and menopause all have nutrition implications.

- *If you're in your reproductive years, check the beginning of the chapter for healthful eating advice.*
- *For nutrition advice during pregnancy and breast-feeding, go to the middle of the chapter.*
- *If you're near to or dealing with menopause or post-menopause, turn to the end of the chapter, where you'll find nutrition guidance for your continued health and well-being.*

Healthy eating fuels women's busy lifestyles and provides nourishment or overall health at every stage in a woman's life. For the right food variety and amounts, check the food guides—and learn the advice represented by the visual cue for healthy eating known as MyPlate—*discussed in chapter 10.*

Childbearing Years: Nutrition, Menstruation, Prepregnancy

The choice is yours! Healthful eating, active living, and hormones are intertwined in the unique and complex issues of women's health. Whether or not you choose to have children, the choices you make now, during your childbearing years, affect the quality and length of your life for the long run. That includes keeping a healthy prepregnancy body weight. Many of those choices are uniquely female.

Menstrual Cycle: More Iron for Women

In your childbearing years you need more iron than men do. Why? To replace iron loss from menstrual flow. On average, women lose about ¼ cup of blood with each menstrual period. Those with a heavy flow may lose more. For women who don't replace that iron, menstrual loss—combined with low iron intake, frequent dieting, and a low vitamin C intake—can contribute to iron deficiency and even to anemia.

The Dietary Guidelines advises women of child-bearing age: *Choose foods that supply heme iron, which is more readily absorbed by the body; additional iron sources; and enhancers of iron absorption, such as vitamin C-rich foods.* For women ages nineteen to fifty, the Recommended Dietary Allowance (RDA) for iron is 18 milligrams daily. During pregnancy, the recommendation increases to 27 milligrams daily. To compare, adult men need 8 milligrams of iron daily. With menopause, a woman's need for iron drops to that of men.

To get enough iron from food, eat iron-rich foods such as lean meat, poultry, fortified cereal, enriched rice, and beans (legumes). Iron from grain products, beans, and eggs isn't absorbed as well. So to help absorption, enjoy these foods with vitamin C-rich foods: perhaps citrus fruit with your morning cereal or scrambled egg. Consult your healthcare provider about an iron supplement, too. *For more about iron*

and food sources, see chapter 6. See chapter 22 for "Anemia: 'Tired Blood'" and chapter 23 for "Iron Supplements: Enhancing the Benefit."

Food Choices: Control for PMS?

Do you experience uncomfortable symptoms of premenstrual syndrome (PMS)? Women describe as many as two hundred symptoms: physical, such as acne, backaches, bloating, tender breasts, and headaches; food cravings; and psychological, such as anxiety, irritability, and insomnia.

PMS—a condition, not a disease—starts as early as fourteen days before a woman's period, then stops when menstrual flow starts. Shifts in hormone levels are the likely cause. Because body water fluctuates during the menstrual cycle, the body may retain fluids prior to a period that disappear soon after it's over.

PMS gets plenty of attention in women's media, yet there's little consensus on its causes or treatment, and little conclusive research on links between nutrition and its symptoms. Despite claims, no evidence links PMS and nutritional deficiencies. Here's what's known—and unknown—about PMS "headlines."

- *Calcium* may help reduce fluid retention and regulate mood-related brain chemicals, but research isn't conclusive. Regardless, there's good reason to boost your calcium intake. Calcium is essential for lifelong bone health, yet most women don't get enough!

- *Phytoestrogens* are weak, naturally occurring plant estrogens that may help relieve some PMS symptoms. Science hasn't yet determined how much is adequate,

---

Girl Friends: A Great Support Network for Health!

Whether you're age 25, 50, or 75, most women value the support and social interaction that comes from being together. Yet getting together doesn't need to involve food. If it does, it's a great chance for a healthful fitness and food adventure.

- Set workout dates together, or walk the neighborhood as you talk. It's easier to stick to an exercise plan when you don't want to let someone else down.

- Share healthful recipes. You or your friends may have a great makeover recipe—with more vegetables and whole grains (and fewer calories)—that are already family-tested!

- When friend time is also food time, snack on baby carrots, bell peppers, berries, or grapes. Quench your thirst with ice-cold water instead of sugary drinks.

- Be each other's best cheerleader. Surround yourself with those who make positive food and lifestyle choices. Encourage one another to eat healthier and stay active.

- If you use social media, tweet, text, or e-mail a healthful meal idea, a great value at a farmers' market, or an active play-day idea for your kids, grandkids, nieces, or nephews.

Click Here! Websites to Know . . .

- The American College of Obstetrics and Gynecology, www.acog.org/publications/patient_education
- Women's Health: Medline Plus, www.nlm.nih.gov/medlineplus/womenshealth.html
- U.S. Department of Health and Human Services, www.womenshealth.gov

See "Resources You Can Use" for more websites.

Have You Ever Wondered

. . . if you need extra vitamins if you use oral contraceptives? No. An overall eating plan that's varied and balanced can supply enough nutrients if you're on the pill. However, taking an oral contraceptive over a period of time may exacerbate symptoms of a nutrient deficiency. For example, vitamin B_6—found in whole grains, legumes, meat, poultry, and fish—helps the body produce serotonin, which helps regulate mood and pain. Vitamin B_6 deficiency may trigger mood-related side effects related to oral contraceptives.

. . . if drinking cranberry juice helps protect you from urinary tract infections? Maybe. It appears that substances in cranberries and blueberries (same berry family) may help prevent certain bacteria that cause infection from sticking to the urinary tract wall. Many women suffer from urinary tract infections sometime in their lives. Although urine is normally bacteria-free, bacteria can travel from the rectum, across the skin surface, and into the bladder and cause infection. Studies are investigating the role of drinking cranberry juice in reducing urinary tract bacteria.

If you feel the symptoms—frequent and urgent need to urinate, painful urination, cloudy or bloody urine, or lower back or abdominal pain—seek advice for proper treatment from your doctor. Drink water.

. . . can food choices reduce symptoms of fibromyalgia? A syndrome more common in women in their twenties and thirties than in men, fibromyalgia results in chronic pain in fibrous tissues, muscles, tendons, and other connective tissues, and often sleeplessness. Although there's no known cure, a healthy weight helps keep pain in check by putting less pressure on muscles and tissues around joints. Relieving stress, staying physically active, and avoiding caffeine six to eight hours before sleeptime helps. *For more tips, see "Drink Smart—and Get Your Zzzzzzzs!" in chapter 8.* Some herbal supplements are touted for relief, but research isn't conclusive; some may be harmful.

. . . why an eating disorder or missed periods can affect bone health? Estrogen levels may drop from overexercising, eating so little that a woman gets very thin, or from disorders of the ovaries or the pituitary gland, which directs hormone production by the ovaries. Low estrogen levels can result in missed periods and lowers the body's ability to form new bone in the ongoing process of bone turnover. That, in turn, promotes bone loss.

---

or the interaction between phytoestrogens and other hormones. Still, foods with phytoestrogens such as tofu, tempeh, soy beverage, and many other soy foods are worth enjoying for their potential health benefits.

● *Salt.* If you retain a lot of water (five pounds or more) before your period, try cutting down on salt for a week to ten days before your period, or ask your doctor about a diuretic. Research suggests that higher progesterone levels before a period cause the body to excrete sodium naturally. Limit sodium intake to less than 2,300 milligrams per day; *refer to chapter 7 to see if further limits apply to you.* Do not limit fluids!

● *Dietary supplements?* Despite anecdotal claims, no conclusive research indicates that vitamin B_6, vitamin E, or magnesium alleviate PMS symptoms—and megadoses of vitamin B_6 can cause nerve damage. Except for any psychological effect, large doses of other vitamins, herbals, or botanicals such as evening primrose oil don't alleviate the symptoms either, and they may be harmful. *For more about supplements, see*

chapter 23 and the "Have You Ever Wondered . . . ?" at the end of this chapter.

Until more is known, general guidelines for good health may help you cope with PMS, if it's a problem. Live an active lifestyle. Relax, learn to alleviate stress, and cope with mood swings. Get plenty of rest. Eat an overall healthful diet.

The American College of Obstetricians and Gynecologists (ACOG) suggests simple dietary changes for relief as long as you keep calorie intake within your calorie need. Eat foods rich in complex carbohydrates and calcium; eat less fat, salt, and added sugars, and no caffeine or alcohol. Learn smart strategies to overcome any food cravings, especially if they lead to excess calories; *see chapter 2.*

Physical activity may offer benefits! First, a good workout stimulates the release of brain endorphins, which can help relieve PMS moodiness. Just before your period, endorphin levels are low. Second, if you tend to eat more before your period or experience food cravings, exercise can help you keep your weight stable. And third, sweating may help reduce bloating if you retain less fluid.

Consult your doctor if PMS symptoms incapacitate you. Before you attribute ongoing symptoms to PMS, talk to your healthcare provider. Diabetes, pelvic infections, depression, and other health problems may be misdiagnosed as PMS.

Other Health Issues: A Nutrition Link?

Vaginal Yeast Infections

Do food choices either promote or prevent vaginal "yeast infections," or *Candida vulvovaginitis*? ("Vulvo" means the external female genitals.) *Candida* is a fungus that commonly lives in the mouth, intestinal tract, vagina, and other moist, warm, and dark body areas. For teenage girls and women, *Candida* may cause vaginal "yeast infections" with several symptoms: vaginal itching, redness, or pain; a thick, white, "cheesy" vaginal discharge; discomfort during urination; and perhaps white or yellow skin patches around the vaginal area. Recent use of antibiotics, uncontrolled diabetes, pregnancy, high-estrogen contraceptives, immunosuppression, thyroid or endocrine disorders, and corticosteroid therapy are among the risk factors linked to yeast infections.

Does eating yogurt prevent it? Eating a cup of yogurt with *active cultures* each day may offer some protection from vaginal "yeast infections." However, the evidence isn't conclusive. Regardless, that same 8-ounce cup of yogurt does supply 300 to 450 milligrams of calcium, which is good for bone health!

To refute a common myth, no scientific evidence shows that eating sugary foods contributes to "yeast infections." Neither do processed foods, fruit, or milk. Avoiding these foods or taking certain dietary supplements or antifungal drugs doesn't appear to prevent it.

Candida isn't the only cause of vaginitis. Other health conditions, such as diabetes and overweight, are among contributing factors. The best way to proper diagnosis and treatment is accurate diagnosis from your healthcare provider. If you're prone to "yeast infections," lower your risk with good hygiene, avoiding vaginal sprays and douches, and wearing cotton undergarments that don't hold in moisture and heat.

Fibrocystic Breast Disease

Between 10 and 20 percent of women experience fibrocystic breast disease (FBD), benign but often painful breast lumps. Despite anecdotal claims, no carefully controlled research evidence links noncancerous breast lumps to caffeine intake. In fact, both the National Cancer Institute and the American Medical Association's Council on Scientific Affairs report that FBD isn't associated with caffeine intake. While not harmful, the use of vitamin E as a treatment is controversial.

Because FBD is linked to hormone levels, it usually subsides with menopause—unless a woman receives hormone replacement therapy.

As a safety check for breast health, examine your breasts carefully each month. Get recommended mammograms and professional examinations every one to two years after age forty. And consult your doctor immediately about any breast lumps.

Polycystic Ovary Syndrome

Polycystic ovary syndrome (PCOS) is an often undiagnosed hormonal problem with a cluster of symptoms, including obesity (common clue), ovarian cysts, irregular menstrual cycles, acne, excess facial hair, fertility problems, and male pattern hair thinning. The concerns extend farther. PCOS increases other health risks: diabetes, heart disease, high blood pressure, and uterine and breast cancers.

Although the causes of PCOS aren't known, it's a lifelong problem that may run in families and begin in adolescence. Insulin resistance (which affects the way the body uses blood glucose), obesity, and a high level of male hormones such as testosterone may explain some symptoms. PCOS isn't easy to diagnose; however, blood tests for hormone levels and ultrasound exams for ovarian cysts reveal clues.

Because of the short- and long-term health implications, talk to your healthcare provider if you suspect PCOS. Some women with PCOS have no signs. Treatment may include weight loss, hormone therapy, and regular physical activity. Some women also need treatment for diabetes or high blood pressure.

Body Image

For some young women, the links among unrealistic goals about body weight, self-image, and self-esteem

Your Nutrition Checkup

Screening Tests: Do You Keep Up?

Screening is key to health promotion and disease prevention! Many chronic health problems are linked to food choices or nutrition in one way or another. Find your age on the chart below, then talk to your healthcare provider about getting the tests you need. For the complete chart and other important tests, refer to "Screening Tests for Women," www.womenshealth.gov/prevention/general/part4.cfm.

Screening Tests*	Ages 18–39	Ages 40–49	Ages 50–64	Ages 65 and older
Blood pressure test	Get tested at least every 2 years if you have normal blood pressure (lower than 120/80). Get tested once a year if you have blood pressure between 120/80 and 139/89. Discuss treatment with your doctor or nurse if you have blood pressure 140/90 or higher.	Get tested at least every 2 years if you have normal blood pressure (lower than 120/80). Get tested once a year if you have blood pressure between 120/80 and 139/89. Discuss treatment with your doctor or nurse if you have blood pressure 140/90 or higher.	Get tested at least every 2 years if you have normal blood pressure (lower than 120/80). Get tested once a year if you have blood pressure between 120/80 and 139/89. Discuss treatment with your doctor or nurse if you have blood pressure 140/90 or higher.	Get tested at least every 2 years if you have normal blood pressure (lower than 120/80). Get tested once a year if you have blood pressure between 120/80 and 139/89. Discuss treatment with your doctor or nurse if you have blood pressure 140/90 or higher.
Bone mineral density test (osteoporosis screening)			Discuss with your doctor or nurse if you are at risk of osteoporosis. Get this test at least once at age 65 or older.	Talk to your doctor or nurse about repeat testing.
Breast cancer screening (mammogram) **		Discuss with your doctor or nurse.	Starting at age 50, get screened every 2 years.	Get screened every 2 years through age 74. Age 75 and older, ask your doctor or nurse if you need to be screened.
Cervical cancer screening (Pap test)	Get a Pap test at least every 3 years if you are 21 or older or are younger than 21 and have been sexually active for at least 3 years.	Get a Pap test at least every 3 years.	Get a Pap test at least every 3 years.	Ask your doctor or nurse if you need to get a Pap test.
Cholesterol test	Starting at age 20, get a cholesterol test regularly if you are at increased risk for heart disease. Ask your doctor or nurse how often you need your cholesterol tested.	Get a cholesterol test regularly if you are at increased risk for heart disease. Ask your doctor or nurse how often you need your cholesterol tested.	Get a cholesterol test regularly if you are at increased risk for heart disease. Ask your doctor or nurse how often you need your cholesterol tested.	Get a cholesterol test regularly if you are at increased risk for heart disease. Ask your doctor or nurse how often you need your cholesterol tested.
Colorectal cancer screening (using fecal occult blood testing, sigmoidoscopy, or colonoscopy)			Starting at age 50, get screened for colorectal cancer. Talk to your doctor or nurse about which screening test is best for you and how often you need it.	Get screened for colorectal cancer through age 75. Talk to your doctor or nurse about which screening test is best for you and how often you need it.

Screening Tests*	Ages 18–39	Ages 40–49	Ages 50–64	Ages 65 and older
Diabetes screening	Get screened for diabetes if your blood pressure is higher than 135/80 or if you take medicine for high blood pressure.	Get screened for diabetes if your blood pressure is higher than 135/80 or if you take medicine for high blood pressure.	Get screened for diabetes if your blood pressure is higher than 135/80 or if you take medicine for high blood pressure.	Get screened for diabetes if your blood pressure is higher than 135/80 or if you take medicine for high blood pressure.

Refer to the website for screening tests for sexually transmitted diseases.

Source: U.S. Department of Health and Human Services, Office on Women's Health, www.womenshealth.gov. Accessed January 1, 2012.

* In your regular check-ups, ask about overweight and obesity, alcohol use, thryoid testing, among others.

** The American Cancer Society/National Cancer Institute (2010) recommends yearly mammograms starting at age 40 and continuing for as long as a woman is in good health.

result in poor eating behavior. Healthful eating, managing weight, and being physically active can lead to overall health and better body image. Conversely, disordered eating, linked to poor body image, is more common among young women than young men. *See chapter 2 to learn more about disordered eating.*

Before Pregnancy

Thinking about pregnancy? Be fit and ready! Inventory your health and nutrition habits now. Initiating good health and nutrition habits before pregnancy—or simply nudging healthful eating and active living back into your lifestyle—promotes your health and normal weight and establishes the healthy environment your baby needs to develop normally during pregnancy. Your baby develops rapidly during the first weeks of pregnancy, perhaps before you even know you're expecting!

Preparing for pregnancy or not, advice for all healthy women is the same: Get enough of the forty or so nutrients essential for your good health—and your baby's health, too. *Customize a healthy food pattern explained in chapter 10, as your "before, during, and after" pregnancy guide to healthful eating.*

Healthy Prepregnancy Weight

Reaching a healthy weight in a healthful way *before* conceiving is important—and not just for you! A healthy weight reduces obstetric risks; it also increases your chances of a normal infant birth weight, and lowers the risk of obesity for you and your offspring later in life. Especially for overweight and obese women, preconception counseling on nutrition and physical activity is important, along with access to contracep-

tion, to allow time to reach a healthy weight before conceiving. *See "Every Age and State of Life: Why a Healthy Weight?" in this chapter, as well as chapter 2.*

If You Have Diabetes or Prediabetes . . .

You can have a healthy baby—but talk to your doctor now to learn how to keep your blood glucose level under control before and during pregnancy. Uncontrolled diabetes, starting in the first few weeks of pregnancy, increases the chances of miscarriage, premature delivery, stillbirth, or having a baby with a serious birth defect. Work with your healthcare provider on how to get your blood glucose under control before you get pregnant; you might need to adjust medication for diabetes and delay pregnancy. S*ee "Pregnancy and Diabetes" later in this chapter.*

Fertility: Nutrition Links

Healthful eating not only prepares your body for pregnancy but also can affect fertility in ways that aren't yet clear. If you're trying to get pregnant:

● Aim for your healthy weight. Either extreme underweight or extreme overweight may affect the menstrual cycle and ovulation and so reduce fertility. How? The body produces estrogen in the ovaries and in fat cells. If very thin, the body won't produce as much estrogen in fat cells. With obesity, the body's fat cells produce too much. Either way throws off the delicate hormonal balance that promotes fertility.

● Take caution with dietary supplements touted to enhance fertility. Not enough is known about the risks of extra vitamins, minerals, or herbals and how they might affect the unborn baby.

● If you're having difficulty getting pregnant, explore

the reasons and a sound approach to addressing infertility with your doctor. You'll also rule out any health problems that you or your spouse may have. *See "Polycystic Ovary Syndrome" in this chapter.*

Fertility is a couple's issue; one-third of infertility cases are related to the male partner. For men, overall healthful eating and lifestyle choices have a positive effect on fertility and sperm count. Among the advice for men to promote conception: follow healthy eating guidelines (*see chapter 10*), limit alcoholic beverages, avoid smoking, keep a healthy weight, and be physically active without overexercising.

Bottom line: You both benefit from healthful eating and active living. Get advice from your doctor if you have concerns about fertility.

Folic Acid: Take Note!

To prepare for pregnancy, all nutrients are essential. One merits special consideration: folate, or folic acid (a B vitamin). Folic acid is the form of folate in fortified foods and supplements. Folate is essential to good health, and your body needs it to manufacture new cells and genetic material. Soon after conception, folate helps develop the neural tube, which becomes your baby's spinal cord and brain.

Women who consume enough folate, particularly in the weeks prior to conception and during the first three months of pregnancy, may reduce the risk of neural tube defects, which occur when the neural tube does not close completely. As many as 75 percent of serious birth defects in the spine and neural tube (spina

---

EVERY AGE AND STAGE OF LIFE: WHY A HEALTHY WEIGHT?

For girls . . . A healthy weight—not overweight—during childhood offers protection for the long term: protecting them from adult obesity and type 2 diabetes, and helping blood cholesterol and triglyceride levels stay at healthy levels. During the growing-up years, a healthy weight boosts self-esteem, important for emotional, mental, and social development. Overweight increases the chance of early puberty. A healthy weight now helps ensure a healthy weight by the time they become pregnant for the first time!

For teen and young-adult women . . . As with girls, a healthy weight—not overweight—reduces the chances of adult obesity later and helps ensure a healthy pregnancy and nursing. Beyond that, maintaining a healthy weight promotes physical health in other ways: lower risk for high blood cholesterol levels, for type 2 diabetes, and for high blood pressure; less arthritis risk in later life; and perhaps easier breast cancer detection. On the flip side, a healthy weight—not underweight—helps teens and young women develop and maintain strong bones for peak bone mass. For emotional health, a healthy weight feels good and boosts self-esteem.

For women in their child-bearing years . . . The benefits of a healthy weight mirror those of the teen and young-adult years. In addition, a healthy weight promotes fertility and helps reduce the risk for gallbladder disease. For babies, there's increased risk of congenital (conditions at birth) abnormalities and macrosomia (when the fetus grows very large), with possible birth injury.

For pregnant and breast-feeding women . . . Most important, healthy weight gain (not dieting) helps ensure a healthy pregnancy: promotes normal fetal development and improves the chances of a healthy, full-term birth. When maternal weight is healthy, childbirth is easier and safer. Obesity increases the risk for high blood pressure, gestational diabetes, caesarean sections, premature delivery, birth defects, and stillbirth. Maternal overweight and obesity may also affect a child's health in other ways, including increased risk of obesity during childhood and later in life. During breast-feeding, a healthy weight helps maintain the quality and volume of breast milk. For all these reasons, returning to a healthy weight after delivery (postpartum) and between pregnancies is important.

For women after menopause . . . As before, a healthy weight protects against some health problems, including breast cancer, some other cancers, heart disease, and diabetes. That includes preventing risky abdominal weight gain, as weight shifts after menopause. As always, a healthy weight feels good!

For older women . . . A healthy weight continues to protect against some cancers, heart disease, and type 2 diabetes. A healthy weight—not underweight—helps bones remain strong, cushions bones and organs from fracture and other injury (in case of a fall), and protects against wasting related to serious illness.

See "Weighing the Risks" in chapter 2 for more reasons!

bifida) and brain (anencephaly) might be prevented if women consumed enough folic acid at this critical time. Since 1998, when it became law for many grain products to be fortified with folic acid (a form of folate), the incidence has gone down significantly.

Even a varied, well-balanced eating plan may not supply enough folate to protect against birth defects. So nutrition experts advise that all women of child-bearing age consume 400 micrograms of folic acid daily from fortified foods, vitamin supplements, or both, in addition to the folate naturally found in food.

● Eat a variety of foods with naturally occurring folate—for example, citrus fruits and juices, dark-green leafy vegetables, nuts, beans (legumes), and liver.

● Read food labels to identify foods fortified with folic acid—for example, in most refined grains, such as breads, flour, crackers, cornmeal, farina, pasta and rice. If folic acid is added to breakfast cereals, it's listed on the Nutrition Facts. For fortified foods, the label may carry a health claim—that adequate folate intake may decrease the risk for neural tube defects. *Caution:* If you're cutting carbs or eating gluten-free, make sure you're getting enough folic-acid-fortified foods! In addition, whole-grain products, such as brown rice, may not be folic-acid fortified. If most of your grains are "whole," your food choices may not provide much folate.

● Consult your doctor or a registered dietitian (RD) about appropriate levels of supplements with folic acid. Taking too much folate (more than 1,000 micrograms a day) can mask the symptoms of pernicious anemia, which can cause nerve damage. (Pernicious anemia may result from a vitamin B_{12} deficiency.) Taking large doses from vitamin pills, not food sources, is the usual reason why symptoms are masked.

Even if pregnant women do consume enough folate, obesity increases the chance of neural tube defects. *For more on folate, see chapter 6.*

More Prepregnancy Advice

Consume enough iron-rich foods. If you're iron deficient before pregnancy, it's harder to make it up during pregnancy. *See chapter 6 for more about iron.*

● Even before pregnancy, refrain from practices that may harm your developing baby: cigarette smoking, drinking alcoholic beverages, and inappropriate drug use. Important stages in your baby's development start right after conception. Before you know you're pregnant, potentially harmful substances may have effects.

● Discuss over-the-counter and prescription medications you take with your doctor. They may be harmful to your unborn baby.

● Stay physically active or initiate moderate physical activity in your daily life. That will help prepare you to be "fit" and at your healthy weight for pregnancy.

● Two foodborne risks can affect your baby, even before you conceive: methylmercury and toxoplasmosis. *Refer to chapter 13 to know how to protect yourself now!*

You're Expecting!

Being a nurturing parent begins even before conception. Although you can't change your age or genetic

---

HOW MUCH WEIGHT GAIN IS ADVISED?

BMI before Pregnancy: If You're . . .	WITH ONE BABY		WITH TWINS
	TOTAL PREGNANCY WEIGHT GAIN (POUNDS)	2ND/3RD TRIMESTER AVERAGE WEIGHT GAIN PER WEEK (POUNDS)	TOTAL PREGNANCY WEIGHT GAIN (POUNDS)
Underweight (BMI <18.5)	28–40	1	(Insufficient data for guidelines)
Normal weight (BMI 18.5–24.9)	25–35	1	37–54
Overweight (BMI 25.0–29.9)	15–25	0.6	31–50
Obese (BMI ≥30.0)	11–20	0.5	25–42

Source: Institute of Medicine, 2009.

traits, there's plenty you can do during the nine months of pregnancy to ensure your well-being and that of your unborn baby: eat wisely, maintain a healthy pregnancy weight, stay physically active, get plenty of rest. More good advice: See your doctor regularly, stop smoking (if that's a habit), and avoid alcoholic drinks and inappropriate recreational drugs. The likely outcome: fewer complications during pregnancy, labor, and delivery, and a healthier baby.

"Weighting" for Your New Arrival

"How much weight should I gain?" That's one of the top questions expectant mothers ask. In the last twenty-six weeks of pregnancy, your baby will grow fast, gaining about 1 ounce every day. Besides "baby weight," the weight you gain supports changes in your body and helps prepare you for breast-feeding. Appropriate weight gain helps ensure a healthy outcome.

If you don't gain enough, your chance for delivering a low-birth-weight infant goes up. Babies who weigh less than 5½ pounds at birth are at greater risk for developmental difficulties and health problems.

Gain too much? Excessive weight gain during pregnancy can be risky. Both delivery and returning to a prepregnancy weight may be harder with too much weight gain. As research reveals, health professionals share these concerns for the health of both mother and baby. For mom, excess weight gain during pregnancy contributes to the rising obesity risk for adult women; too much weight gained often isn't lost. Extra pounds also can lead to back and joint problems, gestational diabetes, and a difficult delivery (including a baby born too large, which can result in birth injury) or a cesarean section. And babies? They tend to be heavier at and after birth and at greater risk for obesity and type 2 diabetes later in life.

If you were dieting for weight loss before pregnancy, put that regimen aside for these nine months. Pregnancy is *not* a good time to skimp on calories, follow a weight-loss diet, or restrict weight gain! A doctor may advise modest weight loss during pregnancy for a woman with a BMI of 40 or higher, but that should *only* happen under a doctor's care.

How much should you expect to gain during pregnancy? Because every woman is unique, your doctor will advise you about the weight-gain range that's right for you. That advice depends on:

● *Your weight before pregnancy.* For a healthy pregnancy outcome, the Institute of Medicine provides general guidelines for weight gain based on pre-pregnancy BMI. *See "How Much Weight Gain Is Advised?" in this chapter.* A healthcare professional can help calculate your body mass index.

● *Your height.* Because women differ, weight gain is recommended as a range—not one targeted weight. For instance, very short women (62 inches or less) should aim for the lower end of the weight-gain range.

● *Your age.* Young, normal-weight teens (until age eighteen), who are at greater risk for delivering low-birth-weight babies, are encouraged to gain at the higher end of the weight-gain range. Pregnancy puts greater demands on their own growing, developing bodies. *For more on teenage pregnancy, see "For Pregnant Teens: Good Nutrition" in this chapter.*

● *Expecting multiples? For twins, see "How Much Weight Gain Is Advised?" in this chapter.*

Weight Gain and Loss: Slow and Steady

Your rate of weight gain during pregnancy is as important as the amount. Expect 2 to 4 pounds of weight

Where Does Weight Gain Go?

Your baby may weigh about 7 to 8 pounds at birth—but you'll gain more. Why? Many parts of your body support pregnancy. Your blood volume expands by about 50 percent. Your breasts increase in size. Your body stores fat to sustain the baby's rapid growth and to provide energy for labor, delivery, and breast-feeding.

	Average Weight Gain
Baby	7½ pounds
Placenta	1½ pounds
Amniotic fluid (water around the baby)	2 pounds
Mother	
Breast growth	2 pounds
Uterus growth	2 pounds
Maternal stores (body's protein and fat)	7 pounds
Increased blood volume	4 pounds
Body fluids	4 pounds

Source: American College of Obstetricians and Gynecologists, 2010.

gain during your first three months; for teens, 4 to 6 pounds. (More weight than that is likely body fat without added benefit to mother or baby.) After that, you'll probably gain somewhat faster; *see "How Much Weight Gain Is Advised?" in this chapter*. From month to month, you may gain a little more or a little less.

If your healthcare provider advises you to cut calories without depriving yourself or your baby of nutrients:

● Substitute fat-free or lower-fat milk, yogurt, and cheese for whole-milk products. And choose lean meats, poultry, and fish.

● Broil, bake, grill, or stir-fry foods instead of frying them.

● Eat smaller portions. *See chapter 10 for advice and tips on portion sizes.*

● Cut down on foods high in fat, added sugars, and calories and low in nutrients, such as candy, cake, pastries, and rich desserts. Eat more nutrient-rich foods such as fruit and vegetables instead.

● Increase your physical activity within your doctor's guidelines.

Delivering your baby may be the fastest weight you ever lose! Between the baby and fluid loss, some moms lose up to 10 pounds right after delivery, and another 5 pounds within the first month or so. For others, weight comes off gradually, over a longer period. Most women continue to lose weight slowly and steadily for six to twelve months after delivery. How fast you shed "baby weight" depends on how physically active you are, your calorie intake, and, if you breast-feed, for how long.

Returning to your prepregnancy weight is very important for your ongoing health—and, if you choose, to prepare for another pregnancy! *See "After Pregnancy" later in this chapter.*

Nutrients: For You and Baby, Too!

During pregnancy, your need for most nutrients and calories goes up somewhat. Eating the right amounts from a variety of nutrient-dense foods is the best way to get what you need. An inadequate diet may impair your baby's development, and he or she may be underweight at birth.

For an eating plan that's right for your individual pregnancy, refer to www.ChooseMyPlate.gov. These resources are meant to help you determine your calorie needs before and throughout pregnancy, then to create an eating plan to meet your calorie and nutrient needs. (That may include cutting back on sugar-sweetened drinks and drinking low-fat milk instead. Even by following the food guidance for pregnancy and breast-feeding, it may be hard to get enough iron.)

Caution: If you've been pregnant recently, or if you've breast-fed within the past year, your body's nutritional reserves may be low. Problems during a previous pregnancy are another reason to make a special effort to eat wisely for a healthy pregnancy.

For specific nutrient recommendations during pregnancy, see the appendices. If you're vegetarian, see "The Vegetarian Mom" in this chapter.

Baby-Building Protein

The structural components of body cells—your baby's and yours—are mostly protein. Changes in your own body, particularly the placenta, also require protein. An eating plan that matches advice from the USDA Food Patterns provides enough protein for a healthy pregnancy.

Pregnancy requires somewhat more protein. The Institute of Medicine advises 71 grams of protein daily for pregnant teens and adult pregnant women compared with 46 grams before. Most nonpregnant women easily consume that much. To put the extra in perspective, a 3-ounce meat patty has about 20 grams of protein; 8 ounces of milk have about 8 grams of protein.

Refer to chapter 4 for more about protein.

Fueling Your Pregnancy

Did you know it takes about 75,000 calories for a healthy pregnancy (for the fetus and changes in the mother's body) for a single birth? Your baby needs a constant supply of energy—every minute for about 280 days—to grow! For protein to build body cells, your body also needs an adequate energy supply. Otherwise your body uses protein for energy instead of cell building.

Eating for two (or more!) doesn't mean your calorie need doubles. In fact it's not that different from eating for one. So stop eating when you're full so you don't overeat! Just a few more nutrient-rich food group foods can supply the relatively small increase in extra calories needed for pregnancy. Nutrient-rich foods provide a healthful dose of nutrients, too.

Most pregnant women need 2,200 to 2,900 calories a day, with the amount increasing within this range during the course of pregnancy. For the first trimester you don't need more than before. However, the Dietary Reference Intakes advises an additional 340 calories a day during the second trimester and 450 calories more than when you're not pregnant during the third trimester.

How many calories for you? That's an individual matter. You healthcare provider's advice will depend on your prepregnancy body mass index, your rate of weight gain, your age, your physical activity level, and your appetite. Carrying more than one baby is a factor, too. If you're overweight or obese, your healthcare provider may advise somewhat fewer calories.

Most of your calories, or food energy, should come

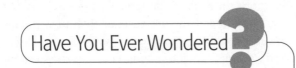

Have You Ever Wondered

. . . if low-calorie sweeteners are safe to consume during pregnancy? Current research shows no reason to avoid foods and beverages with low-calorie sweeteners, such as aspartame, saccharin, acesulfame potassium, sucralose, tagatose, neotame, or stevia.

Exception: Women with the rare genetic disorder called phenylketonuria (PKU) should avoid foods sweetened with aspartame starting before pregnancy. People with PKU cannot break down phenylalanine, which is an amino acid in aspartame. When that happens, phenylalanine can reach high levels in the mother's blood and may affect the developing baby. Studies show that women with the PKU gene, but not the disease, metabolize aspartame well enough to protect their unborn baby from abnormal phenylalanine levels. If you have PKU or carry the gene, talk to your doctor.

Low-calorie sweeteners in moderation can be useful to pregnant women with diabetes, or to pregnant women who enjoy sweet flavors without adding calories. Instead of calorie-free soft drinks and candies, more nutritious foods and beverages may be better choices. Drink low-fat milk, juice, and water. *For more about low-calorie sweeteners and about aspartame and PKU, see "Low-calorie Sweeteners: Flavor without Calories" in chapter 3.*

from carbohydrates. How much? The RDA advises at least 175 grams of carbohydrate a day, just for enough glucose for both mother and baby. For overall nourishment during pregnancy, you need more: 45 to 65 percent of total calories from carbohydrates. Let carbs come from nutrient-rich fruits, vegetables, beans (legumes), and grain products (including whole grains).

Dietary fat? The percentage of calories advised from fat doesn't change during pregnancy. Restricting fat too much isn't advised. For your baby's central nervous system, including brain cells, you need enough essential fatty acids. During pregnancy, the Institute of Medicine advises an Adequate Intake of 13 grams of omega-6 fatty acids and 1.4 grams of omega-3s daily.

DHA, one form of omega-3s, is especially important for your baby's brain and eye development and function; that's why you're advised to consume at least 8 and up to 12 ounces of a variety of seafood per week while you're pregnant, including those high in omega-3s, yet low in methyl mercury. *See "Pregnancy: More Reasons for Food Safety" for types of seafood to avoid for safety reasons later in this chapter. Refer to chapter 5 for more about fat, including essential fatty acids.*

How do 340 calories additional daily translate into "real food"? Try these nutrient-rich "combos" for about that amount:

- 1 ounce of cold cereal, 1 banana, and 1 cup of fat-free milk, *or*

- 1 baked potato with skin, topped with ½ cup each of broccoli and cauliflower, and 1 ounce of low-fat cheese, *or*

- 2 ounces of turkey on 2 slices of whole-grain or enriched bread, topped with lettuce and tomato

A nutrient-rich snack, such as low-fat yogurt or fruit, during the day might be your best strategy for getting those extra calories or nutrients. *See chapter 10 for more guidelines for healthy eating.*

Vital Vitamins

If carbohydrates are the fuel of human life, vitamins are sparks that make body processes happen! Although all vitamins are important during pregnancy, some need special attention, including those important for cell division and the formation of new life.

A varied and balanced approach to eating is the best

way to get the vitamins you and your unborn baby need. Your doctor may prescribe a prenatal vitamin/mineral supplement, too. *See "Vitamin/Mineral Supplements: Benefits and Risks" in chapter 23.*

Vitamin A. Vitamin A promotes the growth and the health of cells and tissues throughout the body—yours and your baby's. Your everyday food choices can provide enough vitamin A for pregnancy.

Supplements? Not advised. Too much vitamin A from supplements—10,000 IU of vitamin A or 3,000 micrograms preformed vitamin A daily—during pregnancy can increase the risk of birth defects. Only with your healthcare provider's advice, take low levels of vitamin A in a supplement. Use the Supplement Facts on the label; choose one with no more than 100 percent of the Daily Value for vitamin A.

Eating plenty of fruits and vegetables high in beta carotene (which forms vitamin A) isn't a problem. Beta carotene does not convert to vitamin A when blood levels of vitamin A are normal.

Folate and Other B Vitamins. By consuming an extra 340 to 450 calories a day, you'll likely consume enough extra of most B vitamins. During pregnancy you need more thiamin, riboflavin, and niacin to use the extra energy from food. And you need more vitamin B_6 to help protein make new body cells.

The 2010 Dietary Guidelines for women of childbearing age who may become pregnant and those in the first trimester of pregnancy: *Consume 400 micrograms per day of synthetic folic acid (from fortified foods and/or supplements) in addition to food forms of folate from a varied diet.* The Recommended Dietary Allowance increases from 400 micrograms before pregnancy to 600 micrograms daily. Get 400 micrograms from fortified foods or supplements and the remaining 200 micrograms from foods with naturally occurring folate. For women who have had a child with a neural tube defect or who are taking certain drugs, a healthcare provider may advise more. Consuming enough during the first three months is especially critical for lowering a newborn's risk for neural tube, or brain and spinal cord, damage. *For more about folate prior to and during pregnancy, see "Before Pregnancy" in this chapter.*

Caution: Pregnant women who avoid products with wheat, perhaps to eat gluten-free or low-carb, or who eat only whole-wheat products may get short changed on folic acid. If you need to eat gluten-free, talk to your doctor about a folic acid supplement, even before pregnancy.

The need for vitamin B_{12} also goes up during pregnancy. This vitamin is found in foods of animal origin such as milk, eggs, cheese, and meats.

Choline. The recommendation for choline, a nutrient for normal cell functioning, also goes up during pregnancy and breast-feeding, yet it's often low in the eating patterns of women. Although this nutrient isn't fully understood, it appears that choline is important for an infant's development. It works with folic acid during pregnancy to develop the nervous system. Egg yolks are an excellent source; *see chapter 6 to learn more about choline.*

Vitamin C. The need for vitamin C goes up a bit, too. But ¾ cup of orange juice still supplies enough for a day! Besides its other functions, vitamin C helps your body absorb iron from plant sources of food. Your iron needs increase by about 50 percent during pregnancy.

Vitamin D. To help your body absorb the calcium needed for pregnancy, consume enough vitamin D, a nutrient that often comes up short because many

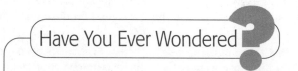

Have You Ever Wondered

... if you need a multivitamin/mineral supplement during pregnancy? Check with your doctor. A balanced diet with a variety of foods can provide healthy women with enough nutrients for pregnancy. Your doctor or registered dietitian may recommend a prenatal multivitamin/mineral supplement to help ensure that you get enough iron, folic acid, and other nutrients.

A multivitamin/mineral supplement is advised during pregnancy if: you have iron-deficiency anemia, follow a poor-quality diet, eat little or no foods from animal sources; smoke, or abuse drugs or alcohol. When pregnant with multiples (such as twins), you may also need a "multi." Talk to your doctor. *See chapter 23, "Dietary Supplements: Use and Misuse," and "The Vegetarian Mom" in this chapter.*

women don't drink enough milk. Vitamin D-fortified milk is a good source. Calcium-fortified foods with vitamin D, too, are other options.

See "Vitamins: The Basics" in chapter 6.

Minerals: Giving Body Structure

Minerals are part of a baby's bones and teeth. Along with protein and vitamins, minerals help make blood cells and other body tissues, too. Minerals also take

---

The Vegetarian Mom

Can a vegetarian eating plan promote a healthy pregnancy? What about breast-feeding?

Yes, if you plan your food choices carefully, *as noted in this chapter.* Either a lacto-ovo-vegetarian or a vegan eating plan can supply the nutrients and the calories, or food energy, needed to support the increased needs of both mother and baby. Adjusting for pregnancy and breast-feeding is easier if you've already mastered vegetarian eating skills. If, however, you decide to become a vegetarian during pregnancy, *first* consult a registered dietitian.

For a vegetarian approach to eating during pregnancy or nursing, keep this additional advice in mind:

● Keep tabs on your weight gain during pregnancy. Research shows that babies born to vegetarian moms are similar in birth weight to babies born to nonvegetarian women—as long as the mother is well nourished during pregnancy. *Caution:* If your vegetarian eating plan doesn't provide enough calories during pregnancy, you may not gain enough weight to sustain normal fetal development; that may result in a low birth weight. If your calorie intake is too low while nursing, your body may not produce enough breast milk.

● Get enough high-quality protein. Eggs and dairy foods can provide enough protein for lacto-ovo-vegetarians. With proper planning vegans who consume plenty of beans (legumes), grain products, seeds, and nuts can get enough high-quality protein, too. *See chapter 4.*

● Consume enough calcium. Doing so is easier if you consume dairy products, and perhaps more challenging if you're a vegan. Either way, a calcium supplement may be advised; check with your healthcare provider.

● Consume enough vitamin D. Among other reasons, you need enough to help absorb calcium. Milk fortified with vitamin D is great for lacto-ovo-vegetarians. Vegans likely need a vitamin D supplement, especially if exposure to sunlight is limited. Other sources: vitamin D–fortified juice, cereal, and other food products.

● As for nonvegetarians, take an iron supplement as advised by your healthcare provider. Follow the rec-

ommended dosage. Too much iron can interfere with zinc absorption, putting your newborn at risk for a zinc deficiency.

● Consume a reliable vitamin B_{12} source—perhaps fortified breakfast cereals or a vitamin B_{12} supplement—especially if you're a vegan. Vitamin B_{12} is found naturally only in foods of animal origin. Pregnancy requires more vitamin B_{12} for the developing fetus and mother's own increased blood supply. Without enough vitamin B_{12} during pregnancy and nursing, a baby is put at greater risk for anemia and nerve damage.

● Get enough folate prior to and during pregnancy to avoid neural tube (spinal cord) defects in the fetus. A vegetarian diet likely provides enough folate since many plant-based foods are good sources: leafy vegetables, beans, some fruits, wheat germ, and grain products fortified with folic acid. Be aware that whole-grain foods may not be folic-acid fortified. As a precaution a folic acid supplement or folic-acid-fortified foods may be advised.

● Take a zinc supplement if your food choices come up short. The need for zinc increases by 50 percent during pregnancy.

● If you're a vegan or avoid fish, consume sources of alpha-linolenic acid (ALA), an essential omega-3 fatty acid and a vegetarian source of DHA, perhaps in fortified foods. Only small amounts of ALA—found in foods such as walnuts, ground flaxseed, and flaxseed, canola, or soy oils—convert to DHA. That's why your doctor may advise a supplement with DHA. During pregnancy and breast-feeding, consuming enough essential fatty acids is not only healthful for the mother, but may also promote baby's brain and visual development. *For more about omega-3s, see chapter 5.*

For more about feeding vegetarian babies, see chapter 17. Before you take any dietary supplement, talk to your healthcare provider; *for more on supplements refer to chapter 23. Chapter 6 addresses vitamins and minerals in more depth.*

part in many body processes that support pregnancy. A few minerals require special attention during pregnancy: calcium, iron, and sometimes zinc.

Calcium. You need enough calcium now for two reasons: developing your baby's bones and preserving your own bone mass. Without enough calcium, your body will withdraw calcium from your bones to build your baby's bones. You can't afford the loss! Research suggests that you also may reduce the chances of developing toxemia and high blood pressure if you consume enough calcium.

The calcium recommendation doesn't change for pregnancy. The body absorbs calcium more efficiently during pregnancy: 1,000 milligrams of calcium daily for adult women; 1,300 milligrams daily for pregnant teens. Yet before, during, and after pregnancy, many women don't get enough calcium to protect against osteoporosis later in life. *See "Osteoporosis: Reduce the Risks" in chapter 22.*

The equivalent of three cups of milk from the dairy group supply nearly all the calcium adult women need daily. An 8-ounce serving of milk or yogurt provides about 300 milligrams of calcium. *Refer to chapter 6 for more about calcium, and to "Calcium Supplements: A Bone-Builder" in chapter 23.*

Doctors may prescribe a supplement for women who don't consume enough calcium-rich foods. But the advice is calcium-rich food and calcium-fortified food first, *then* a calcium supplement.

Iron. Why do you need so much more iron during pregnancy—up from 18 to 27 milligrams daily for adult women? Iron is essential for making hemoglobin, a component of blood. During pregnancy your blood volume increases by about 50 percent. Hemoglobin carries oxygen throughout your body, including to the placenta for your unborn baby.

For enough iron, consume good iron sources every day: lean meat, poultry, beans, eggs, iron-fortified grain products, and green, leafy vegetables. Eat good sources of vitamin C, such as citrus fruits and juices, broccoli, tomatoes, and kiwifruit, with iron-rich foods since vitamin C helps your body absorb iron from eggs and plant-based foods.

Besides an iron-rich diet your doctor probably will prescribe a low-dose (30 milligrams per day) iron supplement or a prenatal vitamin supplement with iron. Why? Iron deficiency, the most common nutritional deficiency during pregnancy, increases the risk for low birth weight and possibly premature delivery or perinatal death; fatigue that may come with a deficiency may impair the interaction between mother and baby. (Perinatal is the period shortly before and after birth.)

Although widely available in food, iron isn't always well absorbed. Many women start pregnancy with marginal iron stores, which increases the chance for anemia. If you have iron-deficiency anemia, your doctor may prescribe a higher dosage.

Your body absorbs iron from a supplement best on an empty stomach or with vitamin C-rich juice, but not with meals. Taking an iron supplement with coffee or tea may decrease its absorption.

Iron can interfere with the absorption of some other minerals. An iron supplement with 15 milligrams of zinc and 2 milligrams of copper is recommended.

Iron supplements during pregnancy may cause side effects such as nausea, constipation, and appetite loss. If that happens, try taking the supplement with meals even though the iron may not be absorbed as well. Then make sure you eat more food sources of iron. A lower dosage might help, too; talk to your doctor.

For more about iron, see chapter 6, and refer to "Iron Supplements: Enhancing the Benefit" in chapter 23.

Zinc. The need for zinc, essential for cell growth and brain development, increases by 50 percent during pregnancy. Zinc comes in a variety of foods, but it's most available from meat, seafood, and poultry. Whole-grain products have zinc, too, but it's not absorbed as well. Most women, except some vegetarian women, get enough zinc during pregnancy from their everyday food choices. *Caution:* Take an iron supplement according to the recommended dosage; too much iron can interfere with zinc absorption.

Sodium. Pregnant or not, choosing and preparing food with little salt (and less sodium)—and more potassium-rich fruits and vegetables—is good advice. You don't need to further restrict sodium during pregnancy—unless your doctor advises you to do so. And if you limited your sodium intake before pregnancy, continue to do so as your doctor recommends. *See chapter 7, "Sodium and Potassium: A Salty Subject."*

For more about minerals in a healthful eating plan, see "Minerals—Not 'Heavy Metal'" in chapter 6.

Fiber

Hormone changes during pregnancy may cause digestive problems, such as constipation and hemorrhoids. Getting enough fiber—from whole-grain foods, bran, vegetables, beans, fruits, nuts, and seeds—may help lower the chance during pregnancy. The Adequate Intake for total fiber for pregnant women, regardless of age, is 28 grams per day—likely more than normally consumed.

And Water, Too

Remember: Water is a nutrient. As part of your body's transportation system, it carries nutrients to body cells and carries waste products away. That includes nourishment that passes through the placenta to your baby. You need fluids—about 12 cups (3 liters) daily—for your own and your baby's increased blood volume. When you feel thirsty, drink more!

For Pregnant Teens: Good Nutrition

Most teenagers don't plan to get pregnant; when it happens, it's high risk for both mother and baby. A teen

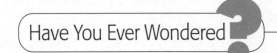

Have You Ever Wondered

. . . if caffeinated drinks are okay during pregnancy? There's no conclusive evidence about the effects of caffeine on fetal development.

Prudent advice: Most research notes that up to 300 milligrams of caffeine daily is safe during pregnancy and nursing. That's about two to three 8-ounce cups of medium strength coffee, or about six cups of tea. The March of Dimes is more conservative: limit caffeine intake to about 200 milligrams a day. The American College of Obstetricians and Gynecologists states that moderate caffeine intake (less than 200 milligrams, or one cup of coffee, daily) doesn't increase the risk of miscarriage or preterm birth. Still, it's wise for pregnant women to monitor their caffeine consumption, listen to body cues, and talk to their healthcare provider about consuming caffeine; individual sensitivities vary.

For more about caffeine and caffeinated drinks, see chapter 8.

more likely delivers a low-birth-weight baby. The chances of anemia, premature delivery, and pre-eclampsia (or toxemia) are higher. Untreated, pre-eclampsia is potentially life-threatening to mother and baby. *See page 504 for symptoms of pre-eclampsia.*

Why high risk? Teens often don't get timely prenatal care. Their bodies are still growing, perhaps competing with the unborn baby for calories and nutrients. Their needs for calories, protein, and some vitamins and minerals are higher than those of an adult pregnant woman. School, activities, social schedules, and emotional ups-and-downs often take good nutrition off a teen's "top ten" list. Teen eating patterns of meal skipping and high-calorie/low-nutrient foods and drinks often don't provide the ongoing nutrient supply that the teen and her unborn baby need. With potentially poor food choices and inadequate nutrient intake, her body isn't prepared for a healthy pregnancy—and she may not get the right nourishment, at least in the first few weeks before knowing she's pregnant.

Figure-conscious teens may be reluctant to gain weight during pregnancy. However, teens need to understand that pregnancy isn't the time to restrict calories or follow a weight-control diet! Pregnancy is just a temporary body change, and extra pounds aren't just the fetus or the mother's body fat.

Until age eighteen, pregnant teens need to gain more weight than adult women do. Most healthy, normal weight young mothers gain 25 to 35 pounds by the end of their pregnancy. Gaining at the upper end of the suggested range helps the teen mother deliver a healthier, normal-birth-weight baby.

A varied, balanced eating plan that's developed with the teenage girl can provide enough calories (food energy) and nutrients during her pregnancy. Use the "Daily Food Plan for Moms" at www.choosemyplate.gov and *refer to chapter 10 to learn more.* A multivitamin/mineral supplement for pregnant teens may be prescribed to supplement, not replace, meals or snacks. Regular physical activity, enough sleep, and prenatal care are essential!

For more about nutrition during adolescence, see "Feeding the Teen Machine" in chapter 17.

Discomforts of Pregnancy

With so many changes taking place in your body, occasional discomforts during pregnancy really aren't surprising, but are common, especially during the first trimester. A few changes in what—and how—you eat may relieve vomiting and nausea, constipation, heartburn, and swelling.

Dealing with Nausea and Vomiting

Often referred to as "morning sickness," nausea or vomiting is experienced by many moms-to-be. Hormonal changes, particularly rising estrogen levels, are likely responsible. Somewhat of a misnomer, "morning sickness" may occur at any time—day or night—and usually goes away after the first three months of pregnancy.

Mild queasiness isn't harmful to you or your baby. However, persistent, severe nausea with spells of vomiting can leave pregnant women at risk for dehydration and weight loss. If these discomforts continue beyond the first trimester, get advice and support from your healthcare provider. These suggestions might keep nausea at bay:

● Avoid foods with strong flavors (perhaps spicy foods) or aromas if they trigger nausea. Pregnant women often have an exaggerated sense of smell, making a common aroma seem unappealing.

● Before getting out of bed, eat starchy foods such as crackers, plain toast, or dry cereal to help remove stomach acid. Get out of bed slowly.

● Enjoy small meals every two to three hours to prevent an empty stomach. Drink beverages between meals, and stay well hydrated!

● Eat easy-to-digest carbohydrate foods, such as plain pasta, crackers, potatoes, rice, fruits, and vegetables, and low-fat protein foods such as lean meat, fish, poultry, and eggs. Limit fried and other high-fat foods if they cause discomfort.

● Savor every bite! Eat meals slowly. In fact, try to make your surroundings stress-free.

● Before bedtime eat a small snack such as peanut butter on crackers and milk, or cereal and milk.

● Experiment with beverages that may calm a queasy stomach: lemon or ginger tea, lemonade, ginger ale, or water flavored with lemon or ginger.

● Choose those foods that appeal and that "stay down." Even if your food choices aren't "nutritionally perfect," that's okay if queasiness doesn't last longer than a few days. If the problem persists, talk to your doctor or a registered dietitian.

● Skip the urge to take a supplement, unless advised by your doctor. No evidence shows that taking vitamin B_6 or other herbal products effectively

Pregnancy and Alcoholic Beverages Don't Mix!

Your blood passes through every organ in your body, through the placenta, and into the circulatory system of your unborn baby. Your baby will be exposed to any alcohol or drugs in your blood.

The Dietary Guidelines advises that women who are pregnant or who may be pregnant should not drink alcoholic beverages. Especially in the first few months of pregnancy, there may be negative behaviorial or neurological consequences for the baby.

Drinking during pregnancy is linked to serious birth defects. Even moderate levels (one drink a day) during pregnancy may lead to behavioral or development problems for your baby. The risks are greater for older moms and binge drinkers. Fetal alcohol syndrome (FAS) is associated with excessive drinking. Infants with FAS may be born with birth defects: retarded growth, mental impairment, or physical malformations.

If you're trying to conceive or you're already pregnant, health experts advise to avoid beer, wine, and other alcoholic beverages completely. There is no known safe level for alcohol intake during pregnancy. Health experts don't know if babies differ in their sensitivity to alcohol. As a reminder, alcoholic beverages carry a label warning about the dangers of drinking during pregnancy and its relation to birth defects.

Once you know you're pregnant, it's time to stop alcohol consumption. If you've had a glass of wine or two before you knew, you likely don't need to worry, but stop as soon as you find out.

GOVERNMENT WARNING:

(1) ACCORDING TO THE SURGEON GENERAL, WOMEN SHOULD NOT DRINK ALCOHOLIC BEVERAGES DURING PREGNANCY BECAUSE OF THE RISK OF BIRTH DEFECTS. (2) CONSUMPTION OF ALCOHOLIC BEVERAGES IMPAIRS YOUR ABILITY TO DRIVE A CAR OR OPERATE MACHINERY, AND MAY CAUSE HEALTH PROBLEMS.

treats morning sickness. Some herbals may have harmful side effects.

● Get enough rest!

● Consult your doctor, especially if severe nausea and vomiting continue after fourteen weeks, or if you have any of these problems: a small amount of dark-colored urine, inability to keep liquids down, dizziness when standing up, a racing or pounding heart, or bloody vomit.

Constipation during Pregnancy

Since becoming pregnant, do you occasionally feel constipated? Many women do. Hormonal changes relax muscles to accommodate your expanding uterus, and that slows the action in your intestines. Taking an iron supplement can aggravate constipation, too.

For some women, constipation, along with pressure from the baby, leads to hemorrhoids. Hemorrhoids are large, swollen veins in the rectum.

Try these ways to prevent or ease constipation and the discomfort of hemorrhoids:

● Consume about 12 cups of fluid daily. Besides water, include milk, fruit juice, and perhaps broth in your fluid allowance. *For more about fluids in a healthful eating plan, including food sources of water, see chapter 8.*

● Eat high-fiber foods: whole-grain foods, bran, vegetables, fruits, and beans.

● Enjoy the natural laxative effect of dried plums (prunes), prune juice, and figs.

● Be physically active every day. Like swimming and prenatal exercise classes, walking is good exercise during pregnancy. Regular activity stimulates normal bowel function.

● Unless your doctor prescribes them, don't take laxatives. For hemorrhoids, ask your doctor to recommend a safe suppository or ointment.

Heartburn

Especially during the last three months, you may complain about heartburn. That may happen as a result of hormonal changes that slow the movement of food through the digestive tract. To relieve your discomfort:

● Eat small meals often, every two to three hours.

● Cut down on caffeinated and carbonated beverages, chocolate, and highly seasoned food.

● Eat slowly in relaxed surroundings.

● Walk after you eat to help gastric, or stomach, juices go down, not up. Or at least remain sitting up for an hour or two after eating, rather than lie down.

● Avoid large meals before bedtime.

● Sleep with your head elevated to avoid acid reflux.

● Wear comfortable, loose-fitting clothes.

● Consult your doctor before taking antacids. Some contain sodium bicarbonate (baking soda), which can interfere with nutrient absorption.

Swelling: Part of Pregnancy

Swelling is normal, especially in the last trimester. Water retained in your ankles, hands, and wrists is a reservoir for your expanded blood volume. It offsets the water lost during delivery, and it's used later for breast milk. Even with swelling, drink plenty of water!

Unless your doctor advises otherwise, avoid diuretics that increase water loss through urination. There's no need to limit salt to prevent swelling; use iodized salt—just enough to match your taste. Iodine is a mineral essential for you and your baby.

To relieve the discomfort of moderate swelling:

● Put your feet up. When you sit, get up to stretch to improve your circulation. Try not to stand for a long time. Rest on your left side to aid circulation.

● Wear comfortable shoes, perhaps a larger size. Avoid tight clothes, tight stockings, tight-fitting rings, and anything else that restricts circulation.

Excessive swelling may signal pre-eclampsia, or toxemia. Other signs include high blood pressure, a sudden weight gain, headaches, and abdominal pain. Advise your doctor right away if you develop these symptoms. Untreated, pre-eclampsia can be dangerous later in pregnancy, even life-threatening for mother and baby. Pre-eclampsia is linked to low calcium and low protein intake during pregnancy. Cutting back on sodium won't prevent toxemia, as was once believed.

Pregnancy and Diabetes

Gestational diabetes—which may start around the middle of pregnancy and end after delivery—is a health problem for some pregnant women. Who's at risk? Women with a family history of diabetes, overweight and obese women, those with previous gestational diabetes or who have delivered a baby who was large for gestational age, and those with poly-cystic ovary syndrome are among those at risk. Most women are routinely tested for gestational diabetes at about twenty-four to twenty-eight weeks.

Whether it's preexisting or gestational, diabetes during pregnancy increases the risk for high blood pressure, pre-eclampsia, and toxemia. Toxemia, accompanied by swelling, high blood pressure, and excess protein in urine, is dangerous. Women with gestational diabetes often have big babies, who may be difficult to deliver, and these women may need a cesarean delivery. The risk for getting diabetes later in life is higher among women who develop gesta-tional diabetes—and their babies may be more prone to overweight or obesity during childhood or adoles-cence, too.

If you have diabetes, you can deliver a healthy baby. However, it's important for your doctor to monitor carefully and prescribe treatment, typically a combination of diet and physical activity. A regis-tered dietitian can help you develop an eating plan to control your blood glucose levels. *See "Dia-betes: A Growing Concern" in chapter 22.* Control-ling existing diabetes before pregnancy is important.

High Blood Pressure during Pregnancy

Gestational hypertension, or high blood pressure—another health risk—happens in 12 to 22 percent of pregnancies in the United States. A significant num-ber of these women develop pre-eclampsia, a serious health risk for mother and baby. Obesity, a multiples pregnancy, being African American, and being age thirty-five years or older are some risk factors for ges-tational hypertension. Healthful eating and healthy weight can reduce the risk. Your doctor will monitor your blood pressure and treat hypertension if it devel-ops. *See "Blood Pressure: Under Control?" in chap-ter 22.*

Pregnancy: More Reasons for Food Safety

Handling food properly to avoid foodborne illness is always essential. For the safety of you and your baby,

pregnancy is no exception. Besides general cautions, some issues are of special concern:

● *Listeria,* bacteria that may contaminate soft cheese, unpasteurized milk, hot dogs, and deli meats, can cause miscarriage in the first trimester and serious ill-ness, premature birth, or stillbirth later.

● *Toxoplasmosis,* a parasite linked to undercooked meat or poultry, can pass from mother to unborn baby, causing severe symptoms including infant death or mental retardation. Because cat feces carry this para-site, avoid cat litter, always wash your hands with soap and water after handling a cat, and keep your cat indoors.

● *Salmonella*, bacteria that can contaminate un-cooked meat, poultry, eggs, seafood, and unpasteur-ized milk, are as risky during pregnancy as before. Although rare in the United States one type—*Sal-monella typhi*—may be passed to the developing baby and can cause abortion, stillbirth, or premature labor.

● *E. coli O157:H7*, a bacterium associated with raw and undercooked meat and unpasteurized milk, is highly toxic. This life-threatening strain, which can

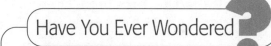

Have You Ever Wondered

. . . if herbal supplements or botanicals are safe during pregnancy and nursing? There's not enough scientific evidence yet to recommend safe levels for herbal sup-plements for pregnant or nursing moms. Some are known to be harmful to a baby—for example, comfrey may cause liver damage, blue cohosh may cause heart defects, and pennyroyal may cause spontaneous abor-tions. Other herbs identified as potentially harmful include aloe, buckthorn, burdock, cascara, chamomile, coltsfoot, cornsilk, devil's claw root, Dong Quai, ephedra, feverfew, ginseng, goldenseal, hawthorne, horseradish, licorice, lobelia, mate, rue, sassafras, senna, St. John's wort, uva ursi, and yarrow. *See chapter 23, "Dietary Sup-plements: Use and Misuse."*

. . . if herbal teas are okay to drink during pregnancy? Some, but not all, are considered safe if you enjoy no more than two to three cups a day. Blackberry, citrus peel, ginger, lemon balm, orange peel, and rosehip teas are among those considered safe if they've been processed according to government safety standards.

cause severe kidney, intestinal, and brain damage, can pass to your unborn baby.

● *Lead* exposure during pregnancy is linked to miscarriage and stillbirth, low-birth-weight babies, and damage to a baby's nervous system. Among the sources of lead: water from lead pipes or pipes with lead solder, food served on ceramic plates with improperly applied lead glaze, and beverages kept and served in lead crystal decanters or glasses. *See chapter 13 for more about lead poisoning.*

● *Methyl mercury and PCBs (polychlorinated biphenyls)*, chemical pollutants found in some fish, are especially harmful to unborn babies and young children, whose bodies are just developing. Mercury poisoning, for example, may damage the nervous system. No matter how you prepare or cook fish, you can't get rid of the methyl mercury!

That said, seafood is a good source of protein, omega-3 fatty acids, and other essential nutrients. However, since you may pass contaminants in some fish on to your baby, avoid large, long-lived fish (shark, swordfish, king mackerel, and tilefish) during pregnancy and breast-feeding. They contain the highest levels of methyl mercury. During pregnancy and breast-feeding limit white (albacore) tuna to 6 ounces per week; it has more methyl mercury than light canned tuna.

Especially during pregnancy and breast-feeding, avoid raw fish and seafood to reduce viral and bacterial infection risks. For locally caught fish, check advisories; limit to 6 ounces if an advisory isn't posted.

During pregnancy the Dietary Guidelines for Americans offers special precautions: not to consume unpasteurized (raw) juice or milk or foods made from unpasteurized milk, like some soft chesses (Feta, queso blanco, queso fresco, Brie, Camembert cheeses, blue-veined cheeses, and Panela). Reheat deli and luncheon meats and hot dogs to steaming hot to kill *Listeria*, the bacteria which causes listeriosis, and do not eat raw sprouts, which also can carry harmful bacteria.

See chapter 13 for specific precautions for food-borne illnesses and for general food safety guidance. Chapter 8 addresses safe water supplies.

Pass the Pickles: Cravings and Food Aversions

Whether it's pickles and ice cream or other foods, cravings, as well as food aversions, are common during pregnancy. Although the exact cause is unknown, taste perceptions may change with hormonal changes.

If you avoid an entire food group, food aversions are harmless unless foods you crave replace more nutritious foods. Instead substitute nutritionally similar foods. For instance, if broccoli loses its appeal, substitute another vegetable that you enjoy and tolerate.

Caution: Cravings for nonfood substances, a condition called pica, can be dangerous. The cultural practice of craving cornstarch, ashes, laundry starch, clay, or other odd substances comes from folklore that started hundreds of years ago. It was believed that eating a particular substance might decrease nausea, promote a healthy baby, or ease delivery. There's no evidence that this practice works—and it can be harmful for you and your baby. Some substances contain lead or other toxicants.

As an aside, craving ice may indicate an iron deficiency. Usually, once the iron-deficiency anemia is corrected, the craving for ice goes away.

Stay Active!

For most pregnancies, mild to moderate physical activity benefits mom—and won't affect an unborn child. If you're healthy, physical activity will not increase your chances of low birth weight, early delivery, or miscarriage. Being active offers relief for some normal discomforts of pregnancy. Consider the unique benefits! Regular physical activity:

● Helps you look and feel good as your body changes

● May lower the risks for gestational diabetes and pre-eclampsia

● Promotes muscle tone, stamina, and strength

● Helps reduce leg and back pain, constipation, swelling, and bloating

● Promotes blood circulation and may help prevent varicose veins, and helps keep your lungs healthy

● Helps your posture and balance—important as your center of gravity shifts

● Helps you sleep better

- Prepares your body for labor and childbirth
- After delivery, helps your body get in shape!

For healthy women, the 2008 Physical Activity Guidelines for Americans advises at least 150 minutes per week of moderate-intensity aerobic activity during and after their pregnancy. Spread it out over the week.

- Talk with your doctor about physical activity during pregnancy—including the type of sport or activities you plan to do. Doctors may advise against exercise for a high-risk pregnancy: high blood pressure induced by pregnancy, symptoms or a history of early contractions (preterm labor), vaginal bleeding, or early rupture of membranes. Other health conditions, such as heart or lung disease or high blood pressure, may limit physical activity.

- With your doctor, choose an activity plan that keeps you fit, matches your health needs and lifestyle, and prepares you for delivery. Your hospital, clinic, or health club may offer an exercise program for pregnant women with exercises to help with labor.

- Choose physical activities that are safe and comfortable. With minor changes you may be able to continue your regular physical activity routine.

With moderate intensity, most pregnant women— even beginners—can do the following activities: walking, swimming, low-impact and water aerobics, or cycling. Include strength-building and endurance activities; stretch before and afterward. The right intensity depends on your health and how active you were before pregnancy. (Later in pregnancy, stationary or recumbent biking might be best since you'll be more prone to falling.)

If you're healthy and already do vigorous-intensity aerobic activity, such as running, you likely can continue during and after pregnancy—if you stay healthy. Talk to your healthcare provider about how and when to modify your routine during pregnancy. For example, as your balance shifts, your risk of falling with some racquet sports may increase.

Avoid activities that increase your risk of falling or abdominal injury, such as horseback riding, downhill and water skiing, gymnastics, and contact sports such as soccer or basketball. Scuba diving is also risky; the water pressure can put your unborn baby at risk for decompression sickness.

For your routine, start slowly and work up. If you haven't been physically active, start with low-intensity activity as your doctor advises. Work up to a daily routine of about thirty minutes on most days. Now isn't the time to stop and start with bursts of heavy exercise. Remember to start with a five-to-ten-minute warm-up of light activity and stretching and to end with five to ten minutes of a slower activity and stretching to cool down.

- Drink plenty of water—before, during, and after physical activity—and wear appropriate clothing to avoid getting overheated and dehydrated. Avoid brisk exercise in hot, humid temperatures.

- Wear a supportive bra to protect your breasts.

- If you feel tired, stop before you feel exhausted. If you can talk as you move, your level of physical activity is right. Talk with your doctor about the right target heart rate for you. *See "Your Physical Activity: How Intense?" in chapter 20.*

A few words of caution:

- As your body shape changes and you gain weight, your center of gravity shifts. That puts more stress on your muscles and joints, particularly in your lower back and pelvis. Your balance changes, too. Some activities get harder to do, especially during the last three months. Injury is more likely as your hormones cause ligaments in your joints to stretch. Exercise with care. Avoid jerky, bouncy movements—and don't overdo it.

- With the added weight of pregnancy, your body must work harder as you exercise. Overexertion isn't healthy for you or your unborn baby. If your unborn baby becomes overheated at a critical time of development, the risk for birth defects goes up.

- After the first trimester, avoid exercises you do while lying on your back. In that position it may be harder for your blood to circulate.

- Pregnancy isn't the time to exercise to lose or keep from gaining weight!

- If you experience any problems, stop your activity; consult your doctor right away. These are warning signs from the American College of Obstetricians and Gynecologists: chest pain, headaches, pain (in general, or in your back or pubic area), dizziness or feeling faint, vaginal bleeding, increased shortness of breath, uterine contractions, fluid leaking from your vagina, calf pain or swelling, muscle weakness, or decreased fetal movement.

After Pregnancy

If you made some lifestyle changes for a healthy pregnancy, keep them up! Perhaps you stopped smoking, or ate more vegetables, fruit, or whole grains, or drank more milk.

For your continued health, returning to your pre-pregnancy weight—slowly and steadily—is very important. That's often easier after a first pregnancy—and harder after later pregnancies. Moreover, accumulated weight gain from one pregnancy to the next isn't healthy—for your long-term health or a future pregnancy. *For more guidance on healthy weight loss, see "Weight Management: Strategies That Work!" in chapter 2.*

Losing "baby weight" may require a shift in your lifestyle, not just in your eating pattern. New demands of parenthood can make that difficult.

Physical activity is part of the strategy! Resume a prepregnancy routine—or start one—when you recover from delivery and get your strength back; check with your healthcare provider first. Then make physical activity a family affair. Start with walking, then work up to more strenuous activity; use a stroller or a front/back carrier so your baby can go on walks with you. Play actively together. Check in your community for a postpartum exercise class. *See "Stay Active!" in this chapter.*

If you had gestational diabetes, get a blood glucose screening at six weeks after delivery and perhaps at your regular medical check-ups later—even if the symptoms disappear. You're at higher risk for type 2 diabetes later in life.

Have You Ever Wondered

... if your food choices affect the flavor of breast milk? Yes, eating strongly flavored foods such as onions, garlic, broccoli, cabbage, cauliflower, garlic, "hot" spicy food, or beans may give breast milk an unfamiliar flavor. These flavors make some babies fussy; other babies don't notice. If some foods seem to upset your baby, eat less of them, less often. What you eat may cause a harmless color change. Breast milk usually is white or bluish-white.

For Those Who Breast-Feed

The decision to breast-feed is personal. If you decide it's right for you and your baby, make smart eating a priority. Your needs for calories and some nutrients are higher now than during pregnancy.

If you're able, breast-feeding is good for your baby—and for you. Besides the physical benefits to your baby and the emotional nurturing you share, breast-feeding may help you return to your prepregnancy shape and weight faster than if you were formula-feeding. Breast-feeding releases the hormone oxytocin, which helps your uterus return to its normal size faster and also helps reduce blood loss after delivery. The impact of nursing alone on weight loss is likely small and short-term—and depends on how much and how long you breast-feed. While inconclusive, research suggests that breast-feeding may offer other health benefits later: reduced risks of breast cancer, ovarian cancer, and osteoporosis. *See "Breast-Feeding Your Baby" in chapter 16.*

In some cases, it's better not to breast-feed. If you have HIV or active tuberculosis, breast-feeding could pass the infection to the baby.

Your Energy Sources

Your fuel supply for milk production comes from two sources: energy stored as body fat during pregnancy, and extra energy from food choices. To produce breast milk, your body uses about 100 to 150 calories a day from the fat you stored during pregnancy. That's why breast-feeding may help many new mothers lose pregnancy weight—for the short term!

While you're nursing, you'll also need somewhat more calories: an extra 330 calories daily for the first six months, an extra 400 calories daily if you nurse for the second six months. Small amounts of nutrient-rich foods provide enough extra food energy (calories) and nutrients needed to support breast-feeding. *See "A Food Guide for You?" in chapter 10.*

After you've established your breast-feeding routine, evaluate your calorie intake. Consider your physical activity level and your weight gain during pregnancy. Ask your lactation counselor or a registered dietitian for guidance.

While nursing, steer away from restrictive weight-loss regimens. Dipping below 1,800 calories daily may decrease your milk volume and compromise your nutritional status. Losing 2 to 4 pounds a month probably won't affect your milk supply; gradual weight loss is healthier anyway. Losing more than 4 to 5 pounds a month after the first month isn't advised. Conversely, overweight and obesity may decrease milk production. To help you return to prepregnancy weight and maintain a healthy weight, work out a plan with your healthcare provider.

Now about Nutrients

The need for most nutrients increases during breast-feeding. A few need special attention, especially if you breast-feed longer than two or three months. *Also see "The Vegetarian Mom" in this chapter.*

Macronutrients. When you breast-feed, the advice for protein, essential fatty acids, and carbohydrates is higher than if you didn't breast-feed. Everyday food choices can supply enough if chosen wisely. Consuming at least 8 and up to 12 ounces of a variety of seafood weekly, including fish high in omega-3 fatty acids (in particular DHA) and low in methyl mercury, may increase the DHA in breast milk, and so promote your baby's brain and visual development. In fact, this is the reason DHA is now added to formula. Breast milk is best, but scientific advances in formula research have brought formula closer to the composition of breast milk. *For guidance on safe seafood intake during pregnancy and breast-feeding, see "Pregnancy: More Reasons for Food Safety" in this chapter. Refer to the USDA Food Patterns in the appendices for amounts of seafood to consume.*

Calcium. Your calcium needs don't change when you're breast-feeding. Still, make sure you consume enough. If you come up short, your body may draw from calcium in your bones so the calcium content in breast milk remains adequate. Bone loss puts you at greater risk for osteoporosis later in life. Periodontal problems also may crop up after pregnancy and nursing, perhaps related to calcium drain. Enjoy the equivalent of 3 cups of milk daily. Eat leafy-green vegetables and fish with edible bones; they're both good calcium sources. *See "Osteoporosis: Reduce the Risks" in chapter 22.*

Zinc. Nursing increases the need for zinc. Zinc easily comes from foods of animal origin.

Vitamin B_{12} and Vitamin D. Consume enough to ensure an optimal amount of these vitamins in breast milk. If you eat meat, poultry, fish, eggs, and dairy products, you're likely getting enough vitamin B_{12}.

Breast milk doesn't have much vitamin D. If your meals and snacks are low in vitamin D or if you aren't exposed to sunlight, your breast milk may have less. Milk is fortified with vitamin D; sunlight helps your body produce it.

Folate. Especially if you're considering another pregnancy soon, consume the recommended 500 micrograms daily of folate—from fortified grain products and supplements as well as from fruits and vegetables—while breast-feeding. *For more about folate, see "Before Pregnancy" earlier in this chapter.*

Vitamin B_6. The need for this B vitamin goes up, yet nursing mothers often don't consume enough.

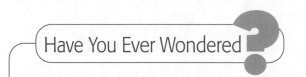

Have You Ever Wondered

. . . if you can drink caffeinated beverages while you're nursing? Yes, enjoy your morning coffee, or a soft drink for a snack, in moderation. Caffeine does pass into breast milk and may affect baby's sleep or feeding. However, caffeine in 1 or 2 cups a day probably won't bother your baby.

. . . if you can pass food allergens through breast milk to your baby? For starters, it's highly unlikely that your baby can't tolerate breast milk; allergic reactions from human milk are extremely rare. No current convincing evidence shows that avoiding known food allergens during pregnancy or while breast-feeding prevents allergies—although limited research says avoiding certain foods while nursing may prevent eczema. In 2008 the American Academy of Pediatrics (AAP) updated its advice: Pregnant and nursing women don't need to avoid eating peanut and other potential allergens. If a baby has a natural parent or sibling with allergies, or if a baby already has a known allergy, then a doctor may advise a nursing mom to avoid certain food allergens. If you suspect an allergy, never make the diagnosis yourself! Talk to your doctor. Then get help from a registered dietitian to help you manage any allergy and continue breast-feeding. *See "Food Allergies: A Common Concern" in chapter 21.*

Chicken, fish, and pork are the best sources, followed by whole-grain products and beans.

Multivitamin/Mineral Supplement. If you took a prenatal vitamin/mineral supplement during pregnancy, your doctor may recommend that you continue. You probably can get enough nutrients from food—if you choose wisely. If your own food choices come up short on nutrients, in most cases your breast milk still will be sufficient to support your baby's growth and development—but at the expense of your own nutrient reserves! *See "Vitamin/Mineral Supplements: Benefits and Risks" in chapter 23.*

For more about vitamins and minerals, see chapter 6; for specific Dietary Reference Intakes during breast-feeding, see the appendices.

Remember Fluids!

To ensure an adequate milk supply and to prevent dehydration, drink enough fluids to satisfy your thirst. That's the amount to keep your urine pale yellow or nearly colorless. During breast-feeding, you need about 15 cups of fluids daily—more if you're thirsty. That includes water from food sources. If you're constipated or if your urine is concentrated (dark-yellow), drink more! *Tip:* Keep water, milk, or 100% juice handy to sip as you nurse. Milk and juice supply other nutrients you need in extra amounts for nursing: calcium from milk, and vitamin C from most fruit juices.

Nonfoods: Effect on Breast Milk?

While breast-feeding, take the same precautions you did during pregnancy: what you consume may be passed to your baby.

Alcoholic Beverages

Alcohol passes into breast milk; drinking alcoholic beverages can decrease milk production. Steer away from wine or beer for relaxation. Contrary to popular belief, no scientific evidence suggests that an alcoholic drink promotes the "letdown" reflex.

An occasional alcoholic drink doesn't mean you should stop nursing, but heavy drinking may inhibit your "letdown" reflex. Alcohol that passes into breast milk may cause your baby to be less alert. In excess, it may affect brain development.

The Dietary Guidelines advises breast-feeding women to be very cautious about drinking alcoholic beverages. If breast-feeding behavior is well-established, consistent, and predictable (not before the baby is three months of age), a nursing mom may consume a single drink if she waits at least four hours before breast-feeding. Another option: express breast milk before drinking an alcoholic beverage so your baby has expressed milk later. For a celebration drink, do so *after* breast-feeding.

Smoking

Nicotine passes into breast milk. If you're a smoker and quit during pregnancy, breast-feeding isn't the time to start again. Nicotine can reduce your milk supply and increase your baby's chance for colic, a sinus infection, or fussiness. Too close to a nursing session, smoking may inhibit your "letdown" reflex. Smoking is also linked to the increased rate of lung cancer.

Smoking near your baby exposes him or her to the risks of secondhand smoke and possibly to getting burned. If you choose to smoke, don't smoke near your baby—not even in the same room. Try to avoid smoking for 2½ hours before nursing: never smoke as you nurse!

Food Safety Issues

As during pregnancy, food safety precautions are advised during nursing. That includes prevention of foodborne illness and exposure to contaminants such as methyl mercury. *See food safety advice earlier in this chapter.*

Medications

Consult your doctor about any prescription and over-the-counter medication you're taking, even an aspirin! Most pass into breast milk in concentrations that pose no harm to your infant. There are some exceptions.

Recreational drugs—which pass into breast milk—are never considered safe for you or your baby!

See "Breast-Feeding Your Baby" in chapter 16.

Stay Active!

Being physically active now helps shed "baby weight," when combined with eating fewer calories. It's good for your health and postpartum mood.

Being active likely won't affect the amount or the composition of breast milk, or your baby's growth. If you're highly active, your milk may have more lactic acid right after exercise, which may affect flavor, but doesn't appear harmful to infants.

For more about physical activity, refer to "After Pregnancy" in this chapter.

Midlife and Beyond . . .

Menopause, when hormone levels slowly drop, is a natural passage in a woman's life cycle. So relax. Accept the changes as normal and very individual. Make healthy lifestyle choices: eat well, be physically active, and reduce calories if pounds start to creep on. *See chapter 10 for a guide to healthful eating, and*

chapters 1 and 2 for guidance on physical activity.

Being proactive by eating smart and being active promotes a healthy weight, heart and bone health, and lowers risks for heart disease, diabetes, and cancer. An active lifestyle also can reduce the discomforts of menopause. Taking care of yourself makes this normal midlife transition easier.

The menopausal years are gradual, and the transition, called perimenopause, starts earlier. Menopausal changes are linked closely to hormone levels, most specifically to estrogen. As reproductive hormones diminish, every body cell—particularly in the cardiovascular, skeletal, and reproductive systems—is affected. Perimenopause typically starts in a woman's

---

Breast Cancer: Do Food Choices Make a Difference?

Breast cancer: it's a common fear for good reason. Breast cancer is the most common cancer among North American women, striking nearly two hundred thousand women annually. It's the second most common cause of cancer death for women, killing nearly fifty thousand women a year.

All women are vulnerable to breast cancer—although some have more risk than others. What's your risk? Among risk factors: a family history of breast cancer (although most women diagnosed with breast cancer don't have a family history of the disease); early menstruation (before age twelve); late menopause (after age fifty-five); inherited gene mutations (most commonly BRCA1 and BRCA2); older-age pregnancy (after age thirty-five) of first child; overweight or obesity; radiation treatment to the chest when young; and simply getting older. While you need to be "breast cancer aware," having these risk factors doesn't make cancer inevitable. A healthful eating pattern and regular physical activity have been shown to help reduce the risk.

Are you a "pear" or an "apple"? The place where extra pounds of body fat settle on your body may make a difference. Early research suggests that women who carry excess body fat around the abdomen (apple shape) may have an increased breast cancer risk. After menopause, more excess weight accumulates there. After menopause, weight gain is linked with increased cancer risk, perhaps related to estrogens formed in the body's fat tissues. Being physically active helps you keep your healthy weight and have less body fat and more muscle, so move more, too!

Another possible link: excessive alcoholic beverage consumption may increase breast cancer risk. A daily limit of 5 ounces of wine, 12 ounces of beer, or 1½ ounces of 80-proof distilled spirits is recommended. If you're at high risk for breast cancer, you may be better off enjoying non-alcoholic drinks instead.

Are foods with phytoestrogens—for example, soy with the isoflavone genistein—an appropriate alternative to hormone therapy if you're at high risk for breast cancer? New research also suggests that phytoestrogens in soy are selective and don't have much effect on breast tissue. Talk to your physician before adding soy to your meals and snacks if you have breast cancer, if you're at high risk for breast cancer, or if you're taking tamoxifen, a hormone-blocking drug related to estrogen. Dietary soy supplements aren't advised, either. Research is under way to explore flaxseed, which contains a type of phytoestrogen called lignan that may protect against hormone-sensitive cancers.

The causes of breast cancer aren't understood. Yet, healthful eating and lifestyles, maintaining healthy weight throughout life, being physically active, and reducing alcoholic-beverage consumption may help protect you from breast lesions and cancer. Breast-feeding for at least several months also may help you keep from increasing your breast cancer risk. Make early detection a habit: monthly self-examination, mammograms every one to two years, and routine breast examination. *See chapter 22 for more about nutrition and cancer.*

Have You Ever Wondered ?

. . . if foods designed for women are worth it? "Feminine foods," or those nutritionally designed for women's needs, may offer health benefits—for example, soy beverage products, cereals fully fortified with folic acid, and juice with added calcium and vitamin D. Read food labels, then decide if you need what they provide. These foods often cost more. If you already consume enough from other foods, you may not need them.

. . . if feeling tired could be a thyroid problem? Perhaps. Symptoms of hypothyroidism include fatigue and mood swings. However, with mild hypothyroidism, you may feel fine. Cold intolerance; dry, brittle hair and skin; hoarseness; difficulty swallowing; and forgetfulness are other symptoms, usually associated with more severe hypothyroidism. Of the eleven million people in the United States with hypothyroidism, most are women and elderly people. *For more about a thyroid problem and its potential consequences, see chapter 22.*

you cope: sleep in a cool room, wear clothes that don't make you too warm, reduce stress, and stay physically active. Hot flashes generally go away, or at least become less severe, in time.

Trouble sleeping? Try consuming milk or yogurt (low-fat or fat-free) at bedtime and perhaps taking a relaxing shower. Keep physical activity, preferably early in the day, in your daily routine; done later, it may keep you awake at night.

Many women experience mood swings and memory problems. Getting enough sleep, eating in a healthful way, and staying physically active help!

Can eating foods with phytoestrogens, such as isoflavones, make a difference? Foods with isoflavones (genistein and daidzein) in many soy protein foods (such as tofu, tempeh, soy beverages) are getting research attention. Similar to the hormone estrogen, these substances may help offset the effects of reduced estrogen production—but there's no solid evidence to know for sure. *See "Soy Good?" in chapter 4.*

midforties and lasts for four to six years as the ovaries gradually produce less estrogen and progesterone. Periods may become irregular, unusually heavy or light, perhaps with more time in between. Menopause is twelve months after the last period, on average—at age fifty-one; postmenopause follows.

Once symptoms such as hot flashes, mood swings, and sleeplessness disappear, postmenopausal women are free of discomforts from a monthly menstrual cycle.

Hot Flashes, Insomnia, and Other Symptoms

Many women deal with uncomfortable symptoms during perimenopause and menopause. Nutrition and lifestyle strategies—rather than hormone therapy—may help. Talk to your healthcare provider about the best approach for you. Nonhormonal medications may be prescribed.

Hot flashes, or a short-term feeling of heat, perhaps accompanied by sweating (perhaps night sweats) and a flushed face and neck, are common symptoms of perimenopause and menopause. Hot flashes probably can't be prevented entirely. But you might avoid or manage some common triggers: caffeine, spicy foods, stress, alcoholic drinks, heat, cigarette smoke, and tight clothing. Some lifestyle changes may help

Iron Needs Drop

Your iron need drops with menopause—from 18 to 8 milligrams of iron a day. Since you no longer have menstrual loss, your risk for iron deficiency goes down. Unless your doctor advises otherwise, stop taking iron supplements. Consuming too much iron, typically from a supplement, can be harmful—especially if you have a genetic disorder called hemochromatosis.

Weight Gain

Some menopausal women gain weight—perhaps for the first time in their life! The reasons: partly lifestyle shifts, partly physical aging. In midlife, lifestyles often get more sedentary, demanding less food energy (calories). With age, metabolic rate, or the speed at which the body uses energy, also slows as hormone levels change. Both contribute to weight gain and to muscle mass being replaced by body fat. Why more belly fat and a thicker midsection? Hormone shifts—and perhaps more stress and less sleep—promote more visceral fat that accumulates under the abdominal wall. As an aside, research doesn't show that hormone therapy causes weight gain.

Being overweight increases the chances for many

Have You Ever Wondered

. . . if hormone therapy may ease menopausal discomforts? Perhaps so for some women bothered by moderate or severe symptoms; it may also help reduce osteoporosis risk. However, although low for many women, there's an increased risk for heart disease, stroke, or breast cancer with the use of hormone therapy medications that combine estrogen and progesterone. Since there has been a change of thinking on this issue, discuss with your doctor whether hormone therapy outweighs your personal risks. If you choose to use it, see your healthcare professional regularly. If you already use hormone therapy, reconsider your options.

health problems that start to appear after menopause. Abdominal or visceral body fat appears to be riskier for heart disease, higher cholesterol levels, high blood pressure, and insulin resistance (which can lead to diabetes) than lower body fat. The greater the abdominal fat, the greater the waist size and the greater the health risks.

You don't need be resigned to weight gain after menopause! To maintain your weight or to drop a few pounds if you need to, adjust your food choices. Follow healthful eating guidelines; *see chapter 10*. Balance the calories you take in with those you burn. Move more, too—that includes strength training to maintain muscle and to keep your bones healthy! *See chapter 2, "Your Healthy Weight."*

Bone Health: Calcium and Vitamin D Needs Go Up

Bone loss is part of aging. With a drop in estrogen levels during menopause, women lose bone faster, so calcium needs increase. In the first years after menopause women lose 3 to 5 percent of bone mass per year and 1 percent bone loss per year after age sixty-five. Since ovaries produce most of the estrogen, that's also true for those who go through early menopause.

Boosting your calcium and vitamin D intake and regular weight-bearing exercise helps slow bone loss and reduce risks for osteopenia/osteoporosis and fractures. For women age fifty-one and over, the Recommended Dietary Allowance, set by the Institute of Medicine, is 1,200 milligrams of calcium daily, and for vitamin D, 15 micrograms (or 600 IU) a day. As a reference, 8 ounces of milk supply about 300 milligrams of calcium and 2.5 micrograms (or 100 IU) of vitamin D. *For more about calcium, vitamin D, and bone health, see chapter 6.* Taking a calcium supplement does make a difference in bone health.

For bone health, phytoestrogens (*see chapter 6*)

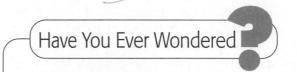

Have You Ever Wondered

. . . if supplements are safe, effective treatments for menopause symptoms? Even though they're "natural," herbal and botanical supplements may not be safe or effective. The American College of Obstetricians and Gynecologists advises:

- *Soy foods and their isoflavones* in amounts in food are safe and perhaps helpful. Because soy products have some estrogenlike qualities they may have some risks.

- *Black cohosh* may act like estrogen. It may offer some relief from hot flashes, sleep disorder, and depression. But side effects may include nausea and low blood pressure. For safety's sake, products with black cohosh may offer this label warning: "Discontinue use and consult a healthcare practitioner if you have a liver disorder or develop symptoms of liver trouble, such as abdominal pain, dark urine, or jaundice."

- *Dong quai* doesn't appear effective when used alone. Of concern, it may increase sensitivity to sunlight and perhaps affect blood clotting time, which can be risky.

- *Wild or Mexican yam* doesn't appear to reduce menopause symptoms, unless perhaps large amounts are consumed.

- Other products without proof of effectiveness: *evening primrose, valerian root, ginseng, and chasteberry.* Again, probably not worth the money.

Before you take supplements to reduce menopause symptoms, talk to your doctor. They may interfere with other medications you're taking. Some of these dietary supplements may affect hormone levels and shouldn't be taken by women on birth control pills or those with a hormone-sensitive condition such as breast cancer. *Refer to chapter 23 for more about dietary supplements.*

haven't been shown to prevent osteopenia/osteoporosis, or lower fracture risk. While hormone therapy may reduce bone loss, any benefit—from estrogen only—must be balanced against increased heart disease risk. *Refer to "Osteoporosis: Reduce the Risks" in chapter 22.*

Heart Disease: A Woman's Issue, Too!

As estrogen levels drop with menopause, women no longer have the same protection from heart disease and high blood pressure that estrogen gives. HDL ("good") cholesterol levels drop; triglyceride levels increase. That's true whether menopause is natural or surgical. Studies show from age fifty-five on, women's blood cholesterol levels are higher than those of men the same age. As a result, women's heart-disease risks parallel those of men—seven to ten years later in life! Their death rate goes up, perhaps due to increased age or more risk factors. In fact, heart disease (not breast cancer) is the top killer and disabler of American women; a woman is three times more likely to get cardiovascular disease than breast cancer. About two-thirds of women who die of heart disease had no previous symptoms.

The signs of heart disease for women often differ from those of men—and may go unrecognized or ignored. Women often have angina first, rather than a heart attack , and a lower HDL cholesterol level. When their HDL drops, they're twice as likely to have a heart attack than men. A woman's symptoms may be intermittent: unexplained heartburn, profound fatigue, nausea, shortness of breath, and pain that comes and goes. Treadmill stress tests for diagnosis are less reliable for women than for men, too. Also less reliable: taking a lose-dose aspirin.

Women—if you haven't done so already, make heart-healthy choices. Start with small steps, then work up. This book is full of practical advice.

In 2011, the American Heart Association suggested the following for women:

● Eat a diet rich in fruits and vegetables; choose whole-grain, high-fiber foods; eat oily fish at least twice a week; limit saturated fat, cholesterol, and sugar; avoid *trans*-fatty acids. *See chapter 10.*

● Consume omega-3 fatty acids by eating fish, or in capsule form if they have high cholesterol. *See chapter 5.*

● Achieve a healthy body weight. *See chapter 2. Note:* Heart disease risk is higher if most fat is around the abdomen.

● Be physically active, getting 150 minutes a week of moderate exercise or 75 minutes a week of vigorous exercise. *See chapter 1.*

● Establish a comprehensive risk-reduction regime if diagnosed with heart disease or have had a heart event. *See chapter 22.*

● Avoid smoking and exposure to environmental smoke.

Other advice:

● Control diabetes if you have it. A healthy weight lowers your risk of type 2 diabetes. Diabetes increases heart disease risk, for women even more than for men. Aim for a normal blood glucose level.

● Prevent high blood pressure, or lower your blood pressure to optimal levels. Choose and prepare foods with little salt; consume potassium-rich foods to blunt sodium's effects on blood pressure.

● Control everyday stress, especially if it leads to overeating, smoking, or other risky behaviors.

● Know your risk factors. Know your heart health numbers.

Need more tips specific to women's health? Check here for "how-tos":

● Help an adolescent girl address some nutrition issues that start during puberty—see chapter 16.

● Follow a safe, effective strategy for reaching and keeping your healthy weight after pregnancy, menopause, or at any other time of life—see chapter 2.

● Protect yourself from—or deal with—chronic health problems that afflict women: heart disease, diabetes, cancer (including breast cancer), osteoporosis, and anemia—see chapter 22.

● Choose a supplement ("multi," calcium, iron) if you need it—see chapter 23.

● Find a nutrition expert experienced in women's health issues—see chapter 24.

CHAPTER 19

For Mature Adults
Age Fifty Plus!

Are you age fifty plus—or do you have an older relative or a friend? Are you in the "sandwich generation"—in between caring for kids and older parents?

Due to better healthcare, longer life expectancy, and the aging of the baby boom generation, the number of Americans ages fifty plus is on the rise. By 2015 more than 45 million American adults are projected to be sixty-five years or older. By 2030 that number will rise to 76 million Americans. Compare that to a decade or so ago in 2000, when 35 million were age sixty-five or older. The group expected to grow the fastest? Eighty-five plus!

There's no single way to describe adults whose ages span a half century—from their fifties into their hundreds. In fact, today's sixty is often described as the new forty—with a different mind-set than past generations. Many live a full, active lifestyle that differs little from life in their thirties or forties. Others are limited by health and lifestyle challenges that began at a younger age. Except for a few shifts in nutrient needs, overall health and attitude define aging more than calendar age does.

So, with what you know now, do you wish you were sixteen again? If so, would you make smarter food choices? Fit more physical activity into your life? Deal with stress better? Try to sleep more?

You can't change the past—or stop the clock. "Anti-aging" is impossible, but the choices made now, or at any age and health condition, can slow the changes and the challenges that come with getting older, and may even extend your youth. Start now—to eat smarter and move more!

Aged to Perfection!

It's no secret: How you eat—and how active you are—have plenty to do with your biological age. Smart food choices and active living today not only keep your mind sharp, but may also help you feel younger, stay healthier, more productive and self-sufficient, and enjoy a healthier, higher quality of life. You may even spend less on health care. *See "How 'Old' Are You?: Biomarkers of Age" in this chapter.*

Of course, life and health change gradually as the years go by. Yet for each of us, getting older differs. And diversity describes every decade of the mature years: "fifty plus," "seventy plus," even "ninety plus"!

Eating for Healthy Aging

Whether you're over fifty or seventy, you (or an older relative or friend) need the same nutrients—proteins, carbohydrates, fats, vitamins, minerals, and water—but perhaps in slightly different amounts. When health or lifestyles limit food choices, or when meals and medications need careful coordination, consuming enough may be a challenge!

After age fifty, a few nutrients may need special

How "Old" Are You?: Biomarkers of Age

Eager to slow the physical changes of aging? Want to feel as young as you are? Rather than wait until you notice signs of aging, a fitness routine—healthful eating and regular physical activity—can help slow or reverse "biomarkers," or changes, that can come with getting older.

● *Your muscle mass and strength.* Stamina, ease of movement, ability to handle heavy objects, feeling energetic, even physical appearance depend on muscle strength and flexibility. Yet, with age, muscle size and strength decrease naturally; for each decade of adult life, people lose about six to seven pounds of muscle. That rate hastens after age forty-five. This natural loss of lean muscle is called sarcopenia. Regular physical activity helps maintain muscle size, strength, and other qualities of youth.

● *The rate your body uses energy.* The rate your body uses energy (metabolic rate) declines with age: about 2 percent for every decade. Loss of lean body tissue (muscle mass), along with hormone changes, is part of the reason. If you're physically active and keep your muscle mass, your body burns energy a little faster; muscle burns more energy than body fat.

● *Your percentage of body fat.* With age, body fat gradually replaces muscle—even if your eating and activity patterns stay the same. Besides losing that firm, muscular shape of youth, extra body fat increases your risk for high blood pressure, heart disease, stroke, some cancers, diabetes, arthritis, and breathing problems. "Midriff bulge" is a sure sign that you're probably not twenty-five anymore! *The bottom line:* Try to keep lean.

● *Your bone density.* Healthy bones let you enjoy physical activity as you age with less risk of fractures. Yet bone loss is a natural part of aging. If you keep your bones strong, you also may avoid a "dowager's hump," which often appears with osteoporosis and compression fractures along your spine, which can affect your breathing and displace your organs. *See "Osteoporosis: Reduce the Risks" in chapter 22 for ways to slow bone loss.*

● *Your cholesterol/HDL levels.* Age is one reason why total and LDL cholesterol rise. As a heart-healthy strategy, losing weight, regular physical activity, and smart eating can help bring down your total and your LDL blood cholesterol levels, lower your triglycerides, and raise your HDL ("good") blood cholesterol levels. *See "Heart Disease: The Blood Lipid Connection" in chapter 22.*

● *Your blood glucose tolerance.* With age, blood glucose levels may rise for several reasons. In part, your body may not produce as much insulin with age. Physical activity, along with keeping a healthy weight, can help keep blood glucose levels within normal range and help you avoid type 2 diabetes.

● *Your body's "thermostat."* Fluids are your body's natural cooling system. As you get older, your sense of thirst may diminish, putting you at greater risk for dehydration. Still, your body needs at least 9 to 12½ cups of water daily. Total water comes from food, beverages, and drinking water. Physical activity helps your body regulate its internal temperature.

● *Your aerobic capacity.* With age, your body's ability to use the oxygen you breathe efficiently declines. With continued vigorous physical activity, your body pumps more oxygen to your muscles.

attention, *as discussed in this chapter*. Among the reasons? Physical changes that can accompany aging affect how your body digests food, absorbs its nutrients, and excretes wastes. And if you take medication, it may affect the way your body uses some nutrients.

For nutrients, the DRIs provide guidance for two groups of healthy older adults: those age fifty-one or over and those age seventy-one or over. *For specific amounts, see the charts in the appendices.* Advice may differ with health problems; *see chapter 22.*

Nutrient-Rich: Spend Calories Wisely

As people get older, most use less energy, or calories, than they did in their younger years. In fact, calorie needs may decrease by as much as 25 percent for two reasons. First, basic body processes use energy at a slower rate. Most adults lose about 2 to 3 percent of their lean body mass, or muscle, each decade of their adult life; the body uses less energy to maintain body fat than to maintain muscle. Second, many older adults need fewer calories for their less physically active lifestyles. Yet nutrient needs don't change much; in some cases they're somewhat higher.

How many calories? Although calorie needs vary for activity level, gender, health status, and age, as well as height and weight, many women over age fifty need 1,600 to 1,800 calories daily. Many older men need about 2,000 calories each day. Doesn't seem like many calories? Chosen carefully, those calories can—*and should*—be nutrient-rich! Another concern for many older adults: As calorie intake declines, vitamin and mineral intake often does, too. That's why nutrient-dense foods are so important! *Use "Estimated Calorie Needs per Day by Age, Gender, and Physical Activity Level" in the appendices to estimate your calorie needs.*

As for younger adults, a healthy weight is important, too, when you're fifty plus! The benefits? Better quality of life, ease of handling any disabilities if they arise, and less risk for many chronic health problems, such as type 2 diabetes and heart disease. In later adult years, however, some evidence suggests that a high BMI is less predictive of mortality, or death, than it is among younger adults. In fact, being underweight, with a BMI that's too low, was more predictive of mortality than having a high BMI.

The challenge for healthy, older adults: getting about the same amount of nutrients as before, but likely with fewer calories!

● Know your calorie goal; make your calories count. Choose mostly nutrient-packed foods that are lower in calories: fruits; dark-colored vegetables; low-fat and fat-free milk and milk products; lean meat, poultry, seafood, eggs, and beans and peas; whole-grain and enriched breads and cereals. Use Nutrition Facts on food labels to check calorie amounts.

● Focus on variety. Get the nutrients your body needs with the right amounts from and variety within five food groups; *see chapter 10.* That includes nutrients of special concern for older adults: potassium, calcium, vitamin B_{12}, vitamin D, and fiber.

Click Here! Website to Know . . .

● NIH Senior Health, nihseniorhealth.gov/eatingwellasyouget older/toc.html

See "Resources You Can Use" for more websites.

Eat Your Fruits and Vegetables!

The advice you've likely given kids applies to you, too: Eat your fruits and vegetables! Colorful and nourishing, they're mostly nutrient-rich and provide plenty of phytonutrients. Along with their many health-promoting benefits, their fiber can help overcome constipation. Their potassium may help counter the effects of sodium on blood pressure, and their antioxidants may provide anti-aging properties that may reduce disease risk.

Chewing problems? That's no reason to give up fruits or vegetables. Make "softer" choices: perhaps ripe bananas, baked or steamed squash, cooked peas, sliced peaches, baked sweet or baking potatoes, cooked spinach, stewed tomatoes, or steamed cauliflower.

Concerned that fresh produce might take a bite out of your pocketbook? Buy seasonal fruits and vegetables, when they typically cost less. And stock up on canned and frozen fruits and vegetables, and dried fruits, when they're specially priced. Canned and frozen fruits and vegetables offer convenience, especially for housebound adults. If you or someone you're caring for needs a special diet, talk to a registered dietitian about buying these foods. Use the Nutrition Facts on food labels, too. Some canned vegetables and frozen vegetables with sauces contain added salt and added sugars. Plain, frozen vegetables and no-salt-added canned vegetables may be better choices. Canned fruit in natural juices and frozen fruit without added sugars may be better choices, too.

● Know your fats. Replace solid fats (saturated and *trans* fats) with healthful oils such as canola, olive, corn, and soybean oils. Check Nutrition Facts on food labels to keep your overall food choices low in saturated and *trans* fats and cholesterol; that helps manage risk factors for heart disease and other chronic health problems, too. Most fats should be poly- and monounsaturated fats.

Remember: One gram of fat supplies more than twice the calories that a gram of either carbohydrate or protein does. Watching your total fat intake is a healthy way to ease up on your calorie intake for weight control.

● Limit added sugars—from sugar-sweetened drinks, sugary desserts, candy, and more.

● Balance calories in and out. Pay attention to your food and drink portions, perhaps with smaller portions.

And stay physically active in ways that match your lifestyle and health.

Use MyPlate (www.ChooseMyPlate.gov), *described in chapter 10,* as a visual cue to healthful eating. *Chapter 10 also provides food guides* for planning a day's worth of healthful meals and snacks. If you have diabetes, high blood pressure, or other health problems (or if you're at risk for them), your food and nutrient needs may differ. Get advice from a registered dietitian or your doctor. *Refer to chapter 22*, "*Smart Eating to Prevent and Manage Disease*."

Protein: An Issue for Some

Protein: You need enough! If you follow advice from the protein foods group in the food guide (*see chapter 10*), you're likely consuming enough protein. So what's the issue?

Besides its other roles, consuming enough protein, along with regular strength building exercise, may help you retain muscle mass, or lower your risk of sarcopenia, as you age. Consuming enough protein also may be linked to bone health. Emerging research suggests that older adults may need somewhat more protein than advised in the Recommended Dietary Allowances (RDAs). Many older adults don't meet the RDA for protein.

Why might protein intake come up short? Meat and poultry may be hard to chew and swallow, so they may be left on the plate. Those with limited finances might avoid meat, poultry, or fish because they are often costly. Other people may have trouble digesting milk, another good protein source. To avoid these challenges:

● Combine lean meat, poultry, and fish with other ingredients in casserole dishes so a small amount goes

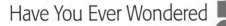

Have You Ever Wondered

. . . why milk doesn't seem to agree with you anymore? Some older adults have trouble digesting milk, even though they had no problem in younger years. The reason? The small intestine may no longer produce as much lactase. Lactase, an enzyme, digests the natural sugar, called lactose, in milk and some milk products.

To enjoy milk and reap its nutrient benefits, try this. Drink milk in small amounts; usually your body can handle a little at a time. Try buttermilk, yogurt, cheese, or lactose-reduced milk. Custard, pudding, and cream soup may be tolerated better. Calcium- and vitamin D-fortified soy milk, yogurt, and cheese can be alternatives. Try other foods that supply calcium, including some dark-green leafy vegetables and canned fish (sardines, salmon) with bones. *For more tips, see "Lactose Intolerance: A Matter of Degree" in chapter 21.*

. . . if you should avoid animal-based foods (meat, eggs, milk, cheese), which contain fat and cholesterol, to protect yourself from heart disease? There's no reason for "fat phobia." Thinking that you need to avoid meat, dairy foods, and eggs to protect against heart disease is unfounded—especially if that means missing out on these nutrient-rich foods. They supply other nutrients that often end up short in the eating patterns of older adults: calcium, iron, zinc, and vitamins B_6 and B_{12}.

If you don't have heart disease, and if your blood cholesterol levels are within a healthful range, be sensible—and enjoy these foods in moderation.

. . . if extra vitamin E will keep you young? We all dream of the fountain of youth. Many claims made for vitamin E are really distortions of research done with animals not humans. Taking vitamin E supplements won't stop or reverse the aging process. And research doesn't show that older adults lower their chances of heart disease, cancer, or mental decline by taking vitamin E.

That said, research is exploring the potential benefits of taking extra amounts of vitamin E. As an antioxidant it may play a protective role against some health problems including building immunity and cataract formation. It's too soon to advise levels higher than the Recommended Dietary Allowance of 15 milligrams of alpha-tocopherol a day; *see chapter 6 for more about vitamin E.*

Until more is known, choose foods that supply enough vitamin E such as nuts and wheat germ; switch to sunflower or safflower oil. If you take a supplement, choose one with no more than 100 percent of the Daily Value for vitamin E. And talk to a registered dietitian to help you sort through the current research about vitamin E.

farther. Consider less-expensive protein sources, such as eggs, beans (legumes), and peanut butter.

● Trouble chewing? Have your teeth and gums (perhaps dentures) checked. *See "Chewing Problems?" in this chapter.* Chop your meat or poultry well if you need to.

● Include dairy products, an economical protein source: milk, cheese, and yogurt—and foods made with these ingredients. If milk disagrees with you, try cheese, yogurt, or a soy-based alternative. *See chapter 21 if you're lactose-sensitive.*

● Consult a registered dietitian for other ways to ensure enough high-quality protein in your food choices.

See chapter 4, "Protein Power."

Calcium: As Important as Ever

Why does calcium remain so important? Its benefits go well beyond bone health and reducing the risks of osteopenia and osteoporosis, or brittle-bone disease. That's true for both men and women! As you age, calcium may promote cardiovascular health and help lower the risk for breast cancer.

After age fifty, calcium needs are higher. To help maintain bone mass, calcium recommendations increase by 20 percent. For both men and women over age fifty, the Adequate Intake level is 1,200 milligrams of calcium daily. That's almost as much as growing children and teens need daily.

The risk for osteoporosis goes up with age. By age seventy, between 30 and 40 percent of all women have had at least one fracture linked to osteoporosis. Even before that, many are diagnosed with osteopenia, or bone loss. The percent continues to climb, even for men, who may develop bone disease later in life. *See "Osteoporosis: Reduce the Risks" in chapter 22.*

Age is only one reason why older adults have a higher risk for bone disease. Many don't consume enough calcium-rich foods, especially if dairy foods or calcium-fortified alternatives aren't a regular part of meals or snacks. With age, the body doesn't absorb calcium from food as well. In addition, many older adults don't get enough weight-bearing exercise, which helps to keep bones stronger. Vitamin D, which helps the body use calcium, may be limited in food choices, too, and it isn't absorbed as well as it once was.

There's good news if you're an older adult: even if you haven't been consuming enough calcium all along, it's not too late to consume more now. You still can reduce your risk of bone fractures. At the same time, consume enough vitamin D and do some weight-bearing exercise, such as walking. *See "Never Too Late for Exercise" in this chapter.*

Which foods supply calcium? Milk, yogurt, and cheese have the highest amount along with some calcium-fortified foods. *See chapter 6.*

Hint: Calcium in food is more bioavailable than from a supplement. But if you do take a calcium supplement, choose one with vitamin D, too. Check to see if the supplement should be taken with or between meals. *See "Calcium Supplements: A Bone Builder" in chapter 23.*

Vitamin D: Often Shortchanged!

To keep bones strong as you age, your body needs enough vitamin D, along with enough calcium. Together they help protect you from fractures and bone loss: osteopenia and osteoporosis. But that's not vitamin D's only health benefit. Emerging research suggests that adequate vitamin D also promotes health and may reduce the risks for some cancers, heart disease, infectious diseases, and autoimmune diseases, among other possible benefits. Of concern, the majority of adults over age fifty don't consume enough!

Vitamin D is unique. Known as the sunshine vitamin, your body makes it after sunlight or ultraviolet light hits your skin. With age, the body doesn't make vitamin D from sunlight as easily; by age seventy, 50 to 75 percent less vitamin D is made than for someone age twenty. The body doesn't absorb vitamin D from food as well as it once did either. Adding to the risk, some older adults are housebound or covered when they go outside, especially in northern climates, so sun exposure is limited. And if they don't drink milk or another beverage that is vitamin D-fortified, they likely don't consume enough either.

Like calcium, the need for vitamin D goes up after age seventy. In fact, it goes up to 800 International Units (IUs), or 20 micrograms, daily.

Even if you drink milk regularly and eat vitamin D-fortified cereal, you may need a vitamin D supplement; consult your doctor or registered dietitian about the dosage. Taking high doses from a dietary supplement can be harmful. Kidney damage, weak bones or muscles, and excessive bleeding are all associated with taking too much over time.

The Dietary Guidelines advises: *Choose foods that provide more vitamin D*. Vitamin D-fortified dairy foods and soy beverages provide it.

Calcium and vitamin D aren't the only nutrients important for bone health. Others, including protein, vitamins A and K, magnesium, as well as phytoestrogens, play a role—another reason why overall healthful eating is so important to reducing osteoporosis risk!

The Iron–Vitamin C Connection

Most people who follow guidelines of the USDA Food Patterns or the DASH Eating Plan (*see chapter 10*) consume enough iron and vitamin C. Yet, for some

---

Vegetarian Fare for Older Adults

Are you a fifty-plus vegetarian? If so, your overall nutrition needs and concerns are similar to those of other adults your age, and the nutrition issues are like those of other vegetarians.

Now vitamin D and vitamin B$_{12}$ need special attention. If you're confined to the house without sunlight exposure, you may be vitamin-D deficient unless you consume enough vitamin D-fortified foods, such as milk and some cereals; you likely need a vitamin D supplement, too. With age, the body may not absorb vitamin B$_{12}$ efficiently either; what's more, vitamin B$_{12}$ isn't found naturally in foods from plant sources such as grain products, vegetables, fruits, nuts, and seeds. Eating foods fortified with vitamin B$_{12}$ or taking a supplement can prevent a deficiency.

Protein? Though controversial, it probably isn't a problem, except for those on very-low-calorie diets. For vegans, eating a variety of protein-rich plant-based foods, such as beans (legumes), tofu, and soy beverages, each day likely can provide enough; dairy foods and eggs—both good product sources—fit in some vegetarian diets.

Good news: Fiber in a vegetarian eating plan may help older adults avoid constipation.

In later years, people are at greater risk for some health problems if they don't get the variety of nutrients they need, especially when recovering from illness. A healthy approach to vegetarian eating is an essential—and a unique challenge for those needing medical nutrition therapy. *Refer to chapter 10 for a healthful eating guide for vegetarians.*

---

older adults, a poor diet may lead to low intake of one or both. Iron deficiency causes anemia, which can make you feel weak, tired, and irritable, or lose concentration. *See "Anemia: 'Tired Blood'" in chapter 22.* Iron deficiency may have other causes: reduced iron absorption as the body secretes less digestive juices or when antacids interfere; blood loss from ulcers, hemorrhoids, or other health problems; and medications (perhaps too many aspirins) that cause blood loss.

That said, for older adults too much iron—taken in supplement form—is usually more of a concern than too little.

For iron, the advice for adults ages fifty-one on is 8 milligrams a day; that's less than half of what women need before menopause. Consult with your doctor before taking an iron supplement. A supplement with too much iron can be harmful for older adults. For some people with a genetic illness called hemochromatosis, iron is absorbed more readily and can build up in body organs, causing irreparable damage.

Although iron and vitamin C come from very different foods, their health roles are connected. Vitamin C helps your body absorb iron from eggs and plant sources of food. Vitamin C is especially important if you rely heavily on beans, whole-grain foods, and iron-enriched cereals as iron sources. *Refer to chapter 6 for more about iron and vitamin C.*

As an antioxidant, vitamin C (in citrus, fruit, melon, and berries) may help lower the risk for cataracts and some cancers.

For any nutrient, including vitamin C, try to get enough from food first, not a supplement. Besides, vitamin C-rich foods have other nutrients, such as potassium, and phytonutrients that promote health. Insufficient intake of vitamin C is linked to memory loss. Excessively high amounts from supplements can be harmful, especially if you have hemochromatosis, recurring kidney stones, or kidney disease.

Vitamin A and Carotenoids

Vitamin A helps your eyes adjust to darkness, a safety precaution. Carotenoids (forms vitamin A) also may help reduce the risk of age-related macular degeneration and cataracts. Colorful vegetables and fruits are good food sources. Consult with a registered dietitian or your healthcare provider before taking a vitamin A supplement regularly. With age, the liver can't handle excess vitamin A as well; too much from supplements can be especially harmful.

Folate

Folate, a B vitamin, helps your body make red blood cells. Not consuming enough over time may lead to anemia and age-related hearing loss. Along with other B vitamins, folate from food may play a role in heart health, by removing homocysteine from the bloodstream; high homocysteine levels are a potential risk factor for heart disease. Since refined flour and uncooked cereals are fortified with folic acid, you likely get enough.

If you also take a supplement with folic acid, you may consume too much, over the Tolerable Upper Intake Level (UL) of 1,000 micrograms per day. *Advice for those age fifty years and over:* So you don't exceed the UL, choose a supplement that delivers no more than 400 micrograms of folic acid per day. Why the limit? While folic acid fortification may promote cardiovascular health, limited evidence suggests that too much folate could trigger nerve damage in people with a vitamin B_{12} deficiency. On both counts, more research is needed. If you're over age fifty years and take a folic acid supplement, talk to your doctor about a need for additional vitamin B_{12}.

Enriched grain products are fortified with folic acid by law; that's not required for whole-grain products. If you eat mostly whole grains such as whole-wheat bread, choose some whole-grain foods that are folic acid-fortified. Check nutrition information on the label to find out. Leafy green vegetables, some fruits, beans (legumes), and liver also contain folate.

Vitamin B_6

Vitamin B_6 may come up short for some older adults. The recommendation for vitamin B_6 goes up slightly after age fifty, from 1.3 milligrams per day for men and women to 1.5 milligrams daily for women and 1.7 milligrams daily for men. Among the good sources: chicken, fish, and pork, and to a lesser degree, whole grains, nuts, and beans (legumes).

Vitamin B_{12}

Vitamin B_{12}, or cobalamin, works with folate to make red blood cells. Not getting enough vitamin B_{12} also can lead to anemia and high levels of homocysteine.

Miracles? Dream On!

Charlatans prey on older adults with promises of easy cures or "anti-aging"! Many products they peddle are foods, substances from food, or supplements. No substantial evidence is provided for many claims that their products help treat arthritis, cancer, Alzheimer's disease, or other maladies—or help people live longer.

Many "miracle" products are costly. Money used to buy them is better spent on healthful, flavorful foods or proper medical care.

Their harm may go farther than the pocketbook. These remedies may mask symptoms, offer false hope, or worse yet, keep people from seeking reliable healthcare. These products also may interfere with the action of prescribed medications—or perhaps with the absorption of nutrients in food.

Always be cautious of promises that seem too good to be true. *To learn how to judge what you read and hear about nutrition and health, see chapter 24.* Always consult your doctor or a registered dietitian before trying these products—or any alternative healthcare. *Chapter 23 explores what's known and unknown about many supplements, some promoted as "anti-aging."* Many people claim to be nutrition experts; some aren't qualified. *To find a registered dietitian, other qualified health expert, or community resource, see chapter 24.*

Among older adults, low levels of vitamins B_{12} and B_6 (pyrodoxine) are linked to memory loss, and low levels of B_{12}, to age-related hearing loss. With coexisting conditions, other symptoms of vitamin B_{12} deficiency may go unrecognized.

Meat, poultry, fish, eggs, and dairy foods are all good sources. To avoid a deficiency, the 2010 Dietary Guidelines advises that individuals age fifty years and older *consume foods fortified with vitamin B_{12} such as fortified cereals, or dietary supplements.* Many adults this age have a reduced ability to absorb naturally occurring vitamin B_{12}; the crystalline form of the vitamin is well absorbed. The recommendation is 2.4 micrograms per day.

Sodium and Potassium

As people get older, the risk for prehypertension and hypertension (high blood pressure) goes up. At the same time, blood pressure becomes more salt- (sodium-) sensitive. (Salt is sodium chloride.) Of concern, most adults consume much more sodium than they need. Yet, among many adults, as sodium intake goes down, so does blood pressure. To reduce the risk of hypertension, the 2010 Dietary Guidelines advises adults age fifty-one and older to *reduce intake of sodium to 1,500 milligrams daily.* Two ways to do that: Read labels to choose lower-sodium foods, and replace salt with herbs and spices in food preparation.

Because potassium blunts sodium's effects on blood pressure, people of all ages, including older adults, are urged to consume more potassium-rich foods—fruits, many vegetables, beans (legumes), milk, and yogurt. Most Americans—including most older adults—don't consume enough potassium.

To learn more, see chapter 7, "Sodium and Potassium: A Salty Subject."

Zinc

Zinc from foods such as beef, whole grains, and milk helps your body fight infections and repair body tissue. Yet absorption decreases with age. Even a marginal deficiency may affect the ability to taste, heal wounds, and provide immunity.

Two other nutrients may also be of concern: vitamin E and vitamin K. *For more about vitamins and minerals, see chapter 6.*

Fiber

Fiber-rich foods aid digestion and help prevent the discomfort of constipation—two nutrition concerns that arise with aging. Beyond that, fiber plays a role in heart health, blood glucose control, weight management, lower colorectal cancer risk, and more. Adequate Intake for total fiber intake is slightly less after age fifty: 30 grams for men and 21 grams for women daily. Even though you need somewhat less fiber, you might come up short, especially if you don't eat enough vegetables, fruit, and whole grains. Many people don't consume enough fiber. *For more about fiber, see chapter 3.*

Thirst Quenchers: Drink Fluids

Thirsty? The average healthy adult loses about 3 quarts or more of fluid daily by urinating, perspiring, breathing, and eliminating other body wastes. To keep from getting dehydrated, your body needs these fluids replaced. Thirst is a signal to drink more.

With age come changes that may affect fluid intake. The sense of thirst often diminishes, so some older adults may not be able to count on thirst as their primary reminder to drink fluids. Kidneys may not conserve fluids as well as they once did either, so the body holds on to less water. Those who have trouble getting around may deliberately limit fluid intake to avoid bathroom trips. Fear of incontinence also keeps some older people from drinking enough.

Dehydration is a health concern especially for the elderly in hot weather and among those who don't drink enough fluid. Other health issues:

A Day of Good Nutrition

Here's an easy-to-make, easy-to-digest, low-cost menu for a whole day of good nutrition. Count up the servings. You'll see it supplies enough from all five food groups. It's a menu that adds up to about 1,700 to 1,800 calories. *Note:* Choose mostly foods with little added salt.

Breakfast:

½ medium grapefruit
½ cup fortified oat flakes with ½ cup low-fat or fat-free milk
Coffee, tea, or water

Snack:

2 squares graham crackers
1 cup low-fat fruit yogurt
½ cup orange juice (perhaps calcium fortified)

Lunch:

1 cup split-pea or lentil soup, low sodium
½ cup coleslaw
1 small corn muffin
½ cup canned, juice-packed peaches
½ cup low-sodium tomato juice

Dinner:

3 ounces skinless chicken breast, baked with Italian seasoning
1 medium baked sweet potato
½ cup green beans, frozen or canned, no-salt-added
1 small dinner roll
½ cup low-fat ice cream
Coffee, tea, or water

Snack:

½ whole-wheat English muffin with 1 tablespoon apple butter
1 cup low-fat or fat-free milk

● Everyone needs enough water to help rid the body of wastes. With less fluid, the chances of constipation rise.

● Many older adults have less saliva to help with chewing and swallowing. Drinking water or other liquids at meals makes eating easier.

● Some medications need to be taken with water. Some, such as diuretics, cause the body to lose water. Understand how medications affect fluid status!

● While fluid helps keep kidneys healthy, dehydration can cause kidney problems.

● In older adults, dehydration may cause symptoms that seem like dementia, or impaired mental function, or might worsen existing dementia.

● In extreme cases dehydration can lead to death.

Day to day, the amount of water you need varies, depending on your physical activity level, the weather, how much you perspire, and other factors. Food provides some water, but drinking at least 9 to 12½ cups daily, depending on your gender, is a good guideline. Any beverage—juice, milk, soup, tea, coffee, soft drinks—supplies water. Plain water is great! Juice, milk, and soup offer other nutrients as well.

Caffeinated beverages? Consume regular coffee, tea, and colas in moderation. Caffeine can have a mild diuretic effect, perhaps increasing the need to urinate. The beverage itself usually cancels out any fluid loss.

The 2010 Dietary Guidelines advises: *If alcohol is consumed, it should be consumed in moderation—up to one drink per day for women and two drinks per day for men.* Don't consume alcoholic beverages if you take medications that can interact with alcohol or have certain medical problems. *See chapter 8 to learn more about alcoholic beverages.*

If you can't recall how much water you drank, try this: Fill a jug (or two) or a jar with at least 9 cups (72 ounces) of water each morning. Place it in your refrigerator. Use that water for drinking and for making juice, lemonade, soup, tea, and coffee. When the water is gone, you've probably met your day's fluid goal. Another option: Carry a water bottle with calibrated measurements with you.

For more about water as a nutrient and the risks of dehydration, see "A Fluid Asset" in chapter 8.

Never Too Late for Exercise

No matter what your age, it's never too late to get moving! Whether you're fifty, or pushing sixty, seventy, eighty, or perhaps even ninety, regular physical activity strengthens your muscles, improves agility and balance, and provides other benefits, even if you haven't been physically active for a while. Regardless of overall health, most people can participate in some form of enjoyable physical activity.

For people of all ages, the 2010 Dietary Guidelines advises: *Increase physical activity and reduce time spent in sedentary behaviors. See "Physical Activity: How Much?" in this chapter for advice on how much if you're over age fifty.*

The Reasons Are Many

Regular physical activity just may be one of the most important health-promoting things you can do—and may prevent many health problems that seem to come with age. Regular physical activity:

● Burns calories. By helping you balance energy out with energy in, active living helps you keep your healthy weight. Beyond that, it helps speed up your metabolism, especially if you build up more muscle mass.

● Helps reduce your bone disease risk. Activities that put weight on your bones, such as walking, help preserve bone density.

● Helps keep your heart and lungs healthier. Do some aerobic activity if you can; ask your doctor first.

● Helps keep your blood pressure, blood cholesterol, and blood glucose levels normal. That reduces the risks related to health problems, such as high blood pressure, heart disease, and diabetes.

● Minimizes muscle loss, improves balance, and keeps muscles strong. Strength helps reduce your risk of falling and helps you remain independent.

● May aid digestion and stimulate appetite—a benefit if food loses its appeal.

● Helps promote sleep. Trouble sleeping often comes with getting older.

● Boosts your mental outlook and energy levels, and may promote a better memory. Being active can be an antidote for depression and perhaps "senior moments."

Physical Activity: How Much?

Any physical activity is better than none. Being inactive isn't healthful, no matter what your age or health condition. The more active you are, the more benefits you get.

If you're generally fit with no limiting health conditions, the 2008 Physical Activity Guidelines for Americans for older adults advises:

Ages fifty to sixty-four:

● For substantial health benefits, do 150 minutes of moderate-intensity aerobic activity (such as brisk walking) every week . . . *or* 75 minutes of vigorous-intensity aerobic activity (such as jogging or running) every week . . . *or* an equivalent mix of moderate- and vigorous-intensity aerobic activity. *Bonus:* If you do more, you get more health benefits!

● Do muscle-strengthening activities on two or more days a week that work all major muscle groups (legs, hips, back, abdomen, chest, shoulders, and arms).

If 150 minutes seem like a lot, remember: You don't need to do them all at once. Break them up; spread them out during the day and week. As long as you're moderately or vigorously active for at least ten min-utes at a time, you get the benefits! An activity that's of moderate intensity for one person may be vigorous for another. Talk to your doctor.

Ages sixty-five or over:

Follow the adult guidelines above, but if you can't meet these adult guidelines, be as physically active as your abilities and health allow. If you're at risk of falling, do exercises to maintain or improve your balance. And understand if and how any chronic health conditions affect your ability to do regular physical activity safely. *The bottom line:* It's all about you, how fit you are, what you feel comfortable doing, and your overall health.

For more about these guidelines from the Centers for Disease Control and Prevention and about activities defined as of moderate and vigorous intensity, refer to chapter 1.

You Can Do It!

The key to fitting physical activity into your everyday routine is to make it fun and matched to your abilities! Even low-intensity activity can make a difference. Choose a variety of activities that improve endurance, strength, and flexibility.

Health Alert: Foodborne Illness

Keep food safe! Older adults are at greater risk for foodborne illness. The reason? The immune system can't always fight back as easily with age, especially the frail elderly and those battling other health problems, such as an organ transplant or liver disease, or those dealing with some cancer treatments. With age, stomach acids, which help reduce intestinal bacteria, decrease, and your kidneys are less able to filter bacteria from your blood. Even mild foodborne illness can have a serious health effect, and once contracted, foodborne illnesses can be hard to treat and may recur. Keep yourself and food preparation areas clean; wash your hands often!

Although the kitchen seems clean, poor eyesight or inadequate lighting may keep people from noticing food spills or visual signs of food spoilage. For those with less energy, proper cleaning may be hard to do.

● If you need glasses, wear them as you handle food.

● Turn up the lights. Mature adults may have more trouble with glare from one light source.

● Label perishable food with a date. Use a dark marker that's easy to read. Don't count on memory alone to know your own "use by" date.

● Don't rely on your sight, smell, or taste to determine if food is safe to eat. Contaminated food may not have an off-flavor or off-smell. With impaired vision, cross-contamination of salad vegetables and raw meat juices may not be obvious.

● Cook simply to save energy for cleanup. Frozen and canned foods are quick, nutritious, and easy to cook.

● Feeling short on energy? Feel comfortable about asking a younger family member or a friend to help occasionally with kitchen tasks.

● Portions too big when you eat out? If you bring food home in a "doggie bag," refrigerate it right away, and reheat it to steaming or boiling before you eat it.

Follow the general steps for food safety, and check a list of foods that have greater health risks; see chapter 13.

- Walk—around the block or around the mall. Walk a dog or invite a friend if you'd like companionship. If you don't have a sidewalk, mall walking is safe—especially in bad weather.

- Do some gardening without electric tools.

- Go swimming. Or try aqua exercises, such as stretching, walking, dancing, or water aerobics. These are great activities, especially if you're not steady on your feet. They may help relieve some joint pain that accompanies arthritis.

- If you golf, "go the course"—without the cart.

- Go dancing. Even a moderate two-step is good exercise—and a great way to be with other people.

- Take a class in Tai Chi, a series of slow, controlled movements, or balance training that may include backward walking, sideways walking, heel walking, and toe walking.

- To keep your arms strong, do strength exercises. Use canned foods from your kitchen shelves, bean bags, or 1- to 5-pound hand or ankle weights.

- Learn some chair exercises—good for people who aren't steady on their feet or who have degenerative joint disease. You can "sit and be fit" even if you're confined to a wheelchair or need a walker.

- Want to keep up with everyday tasks such as bending for a newspaper, reaching an upper shelf, or making a bed? Fit in some stretching activities that increase the range of motion in your ankles, knees, hips, shoulders, neck, and back.

- Sign up for an exercise class or an individual fitness program especially designed for older adults. If needed, check with your community center or area hospital for special classes.

For more ideas, see "Twenty Everyday Ways to Get Moving" in chapter 2.

If you haven't been physically active, or if you have a health condition such as heart disease, arthritis, or diabetes, or a physical disability, talk to your doctor before getting started. Together plan activities and a sensible approach that's safe, effective, and right for you. Even if you have a health condition like these, you can be physically active—and doing so can improve your quality of life and even reduce your risk of other health problems. Most important, start slowly, work toward your goal gradually, and enjoy!

Tip: No matter what activity you're involved in, drink plenty of water before, during, and afterward.

When Lifestyles Change

Lifestyle changes accompany each stage in life. Think about the independence that came with becoming an adult, the responsibility with parenthood, or the freedom of having kids finally leave the "nest." At some point the mature years also bring new lifestyles and health conditions that impact what, where, when, and even with whom you eat. And losing a spouse, moving away from a lifelong community, even retiring can change social interaction that includes food.

Eating Alone: Special, Too!

For many, eating provides a time to enjoy others. That's especially true for those who've spent their time cooking for a family. However, the pleasure of preparing food, even eating, may diminish when eating alone. Eating alone can feel boring or depressing. If you're in that position, or know someone who is, you can help spark a tired appetite and nutrition!

Making Meals Special: Solo or Not

If you're a "single," you don't need to always dine alone. Eat with friends occasionally:

- Set a standing date with a friend or relative (perhaps a grandchild) for lunch or dinner at your home.

- If you're "into cooking" but need someone to cook for, organize a dining club of like-minded friends.

- Cut down on the effort. Get together with other older adults for weekly or monthly potluck suppers. Take turns acting as host.

- Take advantage of meals offered at senior and community centers. Many serve full midday meals on weekdays. Usually the price is right. In some communities, religious centers and schools serve meals for older adults.

Added benefits: These meals offer a place to meet old and new friends. You can enjoy a meal that takes more work to prepare than you may do for yourself. Take advantage of an exercise class when you go!

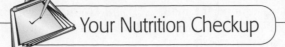

Your Nutrition Checkup

Older Adults: Nutritionally Healthy?

If you're an older adult, use this checklist for insight into your nutritional health. If you care for an older adult, use it to be a better caregiver.

Read each statement. If it applies to you or someone you know, circle the number in the "yes" column. Then tally up the nutritional score of "yes" answers.

	Yes
I have an illness or a condition that made me change the kind and/or amount of food I eat.	2 points
I eat fewer than two meals per day.	3 points
I eat few fruits or vegetables, or milk products.	2 points
I have three or more drinks of beer, wine, or spirits almost every day.	2 points
I have tooth or mouth problems that make it hard for me to eat.	2 points
I don't always have enough money to buy the food I need.	4 points
I eat alone most of the time.	1 point
I take three or more different prescribed or over-the-counter drugs a day.	1 point
Without wanting to, I have lost or gained 10 pounds in the past six months.	2 points
I am not always physically able to shop, cook, and/or feed myself.	2 points
Total	_____ points

What's your nutritional score? If it's . . .

0–2 . . . Good! But check again in six months.

3–5 . . . You're at moderate nutritional risk. Try to make some changes—suggested here—that improve your eating habits and lifestyle. Get advice from a registered dietitian or another qualified nutrition professional . . . or from an office on aging, a senior citizens' center, health department, or senior nutrition program. And check again in three months.

6 or more . . . You're at high nutritional risk. The next time you see your doctor, registered dietitian, or other qualified health or social service professional, bring this checklist. Talk about any problems, and ask for help to improve your nutritional health. Read on for practical ways to follow their advice.

Source: Reprinted with permission by the Nutrition Screening Initiative, a project of the American Academy of Family Physicians, the American Dietetic Association, and the National Council on Aging, Inc., and funded in part by a grant from Ross Products Division, Abbott Laboratories Inc. Go to *www.aafp.org/nsi.xml* for a print or interactive copy of this checklist.

● When eating out, enjoy lunch and early-bird specials. Portions are usually smaller; prices are lower. Go to restaurants with senior-citizen discounts. Consider splitting an order or take home half for another meal if restaurant portions seem too large. *For more tips on eating out, see chapter 15.*

When you dine solo, make eating a special event. Looking forward to mealtime can offer a boost to both your appetite and your morale!

● Set your place at the table, perhaps with a place mat, napkin, your best dishes, and a centerpiece. You'll feel more like you've had a meal—with more enjoyment—than if you had eaten from the cooking pot!

● For a change of pace, enjoy eating in different places: the kitchen, patio or deck, dining room, or perhaps on a tray by the fireplace or a window.

● Create some atmosphere or interest. Turn on the radio or your favorite music.

● Take your meal to a park. Treat yourself to lunch out.

See "Have You Ever Wondered . . . how to feel comfortable when you dine alone?" in chapter 15.

Meals: Fast, Simple, Nutritious

Some older adults say they have no time to cook. They're too busy living life to its fullest. For others, lack of inclination or energy or perhaps less mobility require quick and easy solutions for nutritious eating. And some get bored eating the same foods over and over; so variety of nutrient-rich foods is often lacking.

Whatever the reason, make food preparation easy, varied—and healthful! *See "A Day of Good Nutrition" in this chapter for a day's worth of easy-to-prepare, healthful meals and snacks.*

● For a quick breakfast, add milk to instant hot cereal. It's as fast to prepare as ready-to-eat cereals.

● Keep frozen dinners and entrées (perhaps a low-calorie version) on hand for quick cooking and easy cleanup. Buy frozen meals (but check the sodium content) with meat, poultry, or fish; a starchy food (such as rice, pasta, or potato); and a vegetable. Team them with a salad, a roll, a piece of fruit, and milk for a hearty meal that takes little effort.

DETERMINE the Warning Signs of Poor Nutrition

If you're an older adult, or if you care for someone older, be alert for these warning signs of poor nutrition. They spell the word "determine." Anyone with three or more of these risk factors should consult a doctor, a registered dietitian (RD), or other healthcare professional:

Disease

Eating poorly

Tooth loss or mouth pain

Economic hardship

Reduced social contact

Multiple medicines

Involuntary weight loss or gain

Needs assistance in self-care

Elder years above age eighty

Source: Reprinted with permission by the Nutrition Screening Initiative, a project of the American Academy of Family Physicians, the American Dietetic Association, and the National Council on Aging, Inc., and funded in part by a grant from Ross Products Division, Abbott Laboratories Inc.

These warning signs suggest risk but don't diagnose any health condition.

● Prepare food ahead, or to freeze as plan-overs. Perhaps make lower-fat meatballs with lean, ground turkey or beef. Brown, drain any grease, then combine with tomato sauce. Serve over pasta on one day, over rice the next, and freeze the rest for later. For a lower-sodium version use salt-free tomato sauce and flavor with herbs.

● Freeze homemade soups, stews, lasagna, and other casserole dishes in single-serving containers. Then thaw enough for one or two meals at a time. Label and date your packages to track what's in the freezer.

● For easy-to-prepare salads, wash, tear, and dry salad greens. Then store them in a plastic container for three or four days. Or purchase pre-washed and cut salad greens in a bag. So when you want a salad, just top greens with sliced tomatoes, grated carrots, sliced deli meat, cheese, or canned kidney beans. Serve with milk, whole-wheat bread, and canned fruit.

● Visit the supermarket salad bar for single servings of washed and chopped fruits and vegetables.

"Maxing Out" Your Food Dollar

Another adjustment may affect food decisions: learning to live and eat on a fixed income. If medical and prescription costs go up at the same time, there may not be much money to spare. Economic challenges can get in the way of healthful eating. By shopping wisely, you can maximize your food dollar for the most nutrition. *See "Nutrition $ense" in chapter 12 for more ways to maximize your food dollar.*

Depending on income, many older adults qualify for SNAP food benefits (formerly the Food Stamp Program), handled by the U.S. Department of Agriculture. Provided through an electronic benefits card, it works like cash at most grocery stores, giving people access to a healthful diet and nutrient-rich foods. If you're helping an older adult who's never used or qualified for SNAP, be sensitive; he or she may feel there's a social stigma with signing up or accepting SNAP benefits. Usually SNAP benefits aren't for dining out, although for older adults, some restaurants are authorized to accept them in exchange for low-cost meals; check before you order. SNAP at farmers' markets also gives qualified adults ages sixty years and older more access to fresh fruits and vegetables. Other government programs also provide food and nutrition assistance for older adults who qualify. *Refer to chapter 24 for more information about these programs.*

To find out if you—or someone you know—qualifies for SNAP (food stamps) or other food assistance, talk to a registered dietitian, social worker, or your local senior center. Or check the government pages in your phone book for your local SNAP office.

Hassle-Free Shopping

As people get older, popping in and out of the store may take more effort. Shop with fewer hassles:

● Start your shopping trip before you get to the store. Plan ahead. Make a grocery list, then you won't need to repeat your steps through the store.

● Shop at quiet times, such as weekday mornings, when stores aren't crowded. Daytime shopping, when it's easier to see curbs and potholes, is safer anyway, especially if you have trouble with night vision. If you must shop at night, pick a store with a well-lit parking lot, or ask someone to go with you.

● Ask for help with your groceries. It's also extra security for you in the parking lot. Or hire a home health aide to shop and cook for you.

● Feeling less stable? Use the shopping cart for balance—even to buy just a few items.

● If you have trouble reading food labels and unit price codes on shelves, take a magnifying glass.

● If you're less mobile, shop in stores with a battery-powered, sit-down grocery cart. It's a courtesy service that your supermarket may offer.

● Don't drive or use public transportation? Check with your local area Agency on Aging or Community Action Center for shopping assistance. Your community may offer shopping transportation for adults.

● Keep an emergency supply of nonperishable foods: nonfat dry milk or boxed milk, dried fruit, canned foods (fruit, vegetables, juice, tuna, soup, stew, beans), peanut butter, and cereal. Then you won't need to shop when it's raining or snowing.

● If you have ideas to make shopping more convenient for older shoppers, talk with the store manager. With the growing numbers of older customers, they'll likely listen.

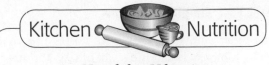

Meal in Minutes

Check the clock. Prepare this nutritious, flavorful supper without much effort!

● Place a sliced red or white potato and sliced carrots into a small baking dish with vegetable oil spray. Toss with 2 teaspoons of olive oil and ½ teaspoon of crushed rosemary or basil, or your favorite herbs. Bake at 350° F for about thirty minutes, until tender.

● In another small baking dish, place a chicken breast or two smaller pieces of chicken. Sprinkle with lemon juice or Italian salad dressing before placing it into the oven. Check the internal temperature; the chicken's done when it reaches 170° F.

● Set the table. Relax with a book or television for about twenty minutes.

● Spoon canned apricot halves into a dish.

● Take out a whole-wheat dinner roll.

● Pour a tall glass of refreshing milk.

● Enjoy your dinner!

● If you qualify, get a sticker for your car that lets you park in handicapped spots.

● Ask about special services from your supermarket: home delivery or phone orders. If you're computer savvy, you might order online.

When Cooking Is Too Much

Can't cook anymore? That doesn't necessarily mean giving up living on your own. Many communities offer services for older adults to assure access to nutritious meals. In fact, the Older Americans Act, first funded nearly fifty years ago, supports many home and community services for adults age sixty and over. Look for these services in your community:

● Meals on Wheels brings food to housebound people. You can ask for vegetarian menus and for menus for special dietary needs such as low sodium.

● Home healthcare aides help by shopping and preparing meals for older disabled people.

● Community centers offer hot meals. Some are part of adult day programs. Minivans may be available to transfer people to the center. *See "Food in Adult Day and Residential Care: Questions to Ask!" below.*

● Many churches, synagogues, mosques, and other community groups provide volunteers who help older adults with shopping and food preparation.

For assistance, talk to a registered dietitian or a social worker, or call your local Agency on Aging. *See "How to Find Nutrition Help . . ." in chapter 24.*

Food in Adult Day and Residential Care: Questions to Ask!

Meals offer more than nourishment to daily life. That's especially true for many older adults, who look forward to meals as a time to be with others.

As you look for adult day or residential care for yourself, or for a friend or family member, ask about the food service. Look for "yes" answers:

Facilities:

● Is the dining area clean, safe, comfortable, and attractive?

● Are menus printed with lettering that's big enough for older people to read?

Have You Ever Wondered

. . . if taking lecithin or ginkgo biloba can help prevent memory loss? No, but it's a common wish, especially for those who constantly misplace eyeglasses or shoes! In fact, no conclusive studies show that taking lecithin (a type of fat) or ginkgo biloba improves memory, thinking, or learning. Under a doctor's supervision, ginkgo biloba may be used to help treat the symptoms of age-related memory loss and dementia.

. . . if taking a multivitamin/mineral supplement is a good idea? Consuming a wide variety of food, in sufficient amounts, is the best approach to adequate nutrition, no matter what your age, if you're healthy. However, your physician may suggest a multivitamin/mineral supplement meant for older adults, especially if you limit your food choices. For older adults, supplements with vitamin B_{12}, vitamin D, and perhaps calcium are recommended. Talk to your doctor about any supplement before you take it.

● Is the dining area well lit throughout, not just "mood" lighting or single lights that cause glare?

● Does the dining area encourage socializing?

● Can the resident decide where, when, and what he or she wants to eat—and with whom?

● Is the table at a height appropriate for proper and comfortable seating?

Food:

● Are people given a variety of food choices and given a voice in meal planning if desired?

● Are beverages and snacks available throughout the day?

● Is the menu changed often, so the menu cycle doesn't get monotonous?

● Are fresh fruits and vegetables served often?

● Is food served attractively and at the right temperature?

● Are portion sizes acceptable? Are second helpings available if allowed?

● Are religious and cultural food restrictions honored and respected? How about food preferences?

● Are holidays and special events celebrated with special menus or appropriate foods?

● Are special meals, such as low-sodium, diabetic, or soft-textured meals, provided to those who need them?

● Are food and nutrition needs given individual attention? Are special utensils offered if needed?

Staff:

● Is mealtime viewed as important to daily life?

● Is a registered dietitian on staff?

● Are people encouraged to eat in a common dining room? Are they offered assistance to get there?

● Do staff or volunteers help those needing assistance, perhaps cutting food or helping them eat?

● Do staff or volunteers wear sanitary gloves when helping people eat so they don't spread infection?

● Are people given enough time to eat, and not rushed?

● For those who can't leave their rooms, is food brought to them on attractive trays and properly set up for ease of in-room dining?

Sandwiched In?

Are you among the many adults who fit in the "sandwich generation," with children or teens yet to raise and an elderly parent to care for? If so, learn to cope without becoming overly stressed:

- Start by taking care of you: Eat smart, fit regular physical activity in, and try to stay rested. Overcome stress or lack of time so they don't become barriers! You'll be more effective in all your family roles as parent, son or daughter, or perhaps spouse—and perhaps in the workforce or your volunteer work.

- Plan openly with your family, including kids and an elder parent(s), so that goals, responsibilities, and expectations are clear. That includes activities that surround eating: shopping, food preparation, cleanup, eating schedules, and family meals.

- Share responsibilities as a family rather than attempt to do everything yourself. Try to avoid neglecting one family member to care for another.

- Gather a support network that may include adult day programs, home-delivered meals if you work all day, and other senior citizen services for your parent. Ask for help, and accept when it's offered.

- Accept the fact that you'll be tired and perhaps angry sometimes. That's okay, so discard any feelings of guilt. Instead, get help so you can have a break, even if it's just for a few hours. Maybe it's a good time to do something physically active. If negative feelings trigger eating, find another emotional outlet.

- Respect privacy, dignity, and independence.

● If residents need assistance, is it given promptly so food doesn't get cold? Are trays removed promptly?

● For a long-term care facility, does the staff track each person's weight and how much he or she eats and drinks?

Changes That Challenge

What's changed? That depends. If you've inherited a great set of genes, and taken care of yourself throughout life, you have a better chance of living a long, vital life. You may feel "fit as a fiddle" without many apparent physical signs of aging. Wrinkles and gray hairs hardly seem to count. In fact, they make you look wise and distinguished.

In the long run, some physical changes are inevitable. The reasons that the human body ages—and the rate of change—are still scientific speculation. But genetics, nutrition, lifestyle, disease, and environment are among the reasons. Many physical and lifestyle changes affect food choices and nutrition.

Medications may have side effects related to food or nutrition. *To learn about interactions, see "Food and Medicine" in chapter 22.*

Aging with "Taste"

"That recipe just doesn't taste the way I remember!" You might hear that from an older adult. Maybe you've said it yourself! The truth is, the senses of smell, taste, and touch decline gradually, with acuity loss starting at about age sixty; some people notice the effects more than others. Fortunately, you can boost the flavor and the appeal of food.

Less Sense-Able

You've probably given it little thought, but throughout your life, smell and taste have affected the quality of your life, your overall health, and your personal safety. Think about simple pleasures: the variety of flavors in a holiday meal, the aromas of bread baking or turkey roasting in the oven, the sounds of popping popcorn, or the sizzle of food on the grill. Food's wonderful flavors encourage a healthy appetite and help stimulate digestion. On the flip side, if nutrient-rich foods don't smell or taste appetizing, they will not be eaten.

Your senses also provide clues to the off-flavor or appearance of deteriorating food, or perhaps to a kitchen fire or a gas leak in the kitchen stove. All these sensory experiences may change with age and health problems, posing potential health risks.

Flavor is really several perceptions: the senses of smell and taste, as well as touch (temperature and mouth feel). With aging, taste buds and smell receptors may not be quite as sensitive or as numerous. Loss of smell is often greater than loss of taste. When flavors seem to change, people often mistakenly think they can't taste as well; instead, loss of smell may be the issue. Appealing foods may be less appealing. That's why some older people reach for the salt shaker or the sugar bowl. Differences in saliva—composition and amount—may affect flavor, too. *See "What Is Flavor?" in chapter 14.*

Age isn't the only reason why foods may taste different. Reducing the salt, added sugars, or fat in your foods also may alter familiar flavors. Medications and health problems may interfere. Some medicines leave a bitter flavor that affects saliva and, as a result, flavor. Some cause nausea, resulting in appetite loss, or dry mouth. Medicines may suppress taste and smell. And health problems such as diabetes, high blood pressure, cancer, and liver disease, common among older people, may alter taste and smell. Loss of smell also can be an indicator of other health problems such as Parkinson's and Alzheimer's diseases.

You can overcome, or at least accommodate to, many sensory changes that gradually affect your food experiences and thus your personal nutrition.

● Can't easily read food labels, recipes, an oven thermometer, or medication instructions? Get glasses for the first time, change your eyeglasses or contact lens prescription, or keep a magnifying glass handy. Large-print cookbooks are useful, too.

● Have trouble hearing a kitchen timer, food bubbling over on the stove, or a faucet you forgot to turn off? How about hearing the answers to your questions in a restaurant or supermarket? Find out from a doctor if you need a hearing aid.

● Pay attention to smell and taste losses—and their effects on nutrition and the pleasure of eating. When food "just doesn't taste as good as it used to," some older adults lose interest in eating. Small appetites and skipped meals can result in poor nutrition and the "anorexia" of aging.

"Sage" Advice for a Flavor Boost

Compensating for diminished taste or smell is within your control—so perhaps is making special, restricted diets more appealing. One approach: Intensify the taste and the aroma of food. Vary the temperature and the texture—and make food more visually appealing. And consider: Sensory loss may not be the issue; soft, colorless, and bland food and mushy vegetables don't appeal to most people.

● Perk up flavors with more herbs, spices, and lemon juice—not with more salt or sugar! To compensate for age-related taste loss, you might need two or three times as much herb or spice and twice the flavor extract. *For ideas, see "A Pinch of Flavor: Cooking*

with Herbs and Spices" in chapter 14. Despite a common myth, older adults can tolerate spicy foods. *Hint:* If any spices cause stomach irritation, stick with herbs.

● Unless you're sensitive to it, use MSG, not salt. It has one-third of the sodium than the same amount of salt. One-half teaspoon can season a pound of meat or two to three cups of cooked vegetables.

● Add crunch! Texture adds to food's mouth feel and flavor. A variety of textures helps make up for a loss of taste and smell. Add whole-grain breads, whole-grain cereals, and cooked beans for more texture. What else is easy? Crushed crackers on soup, chopped nuts on vegetables or in rice dishes, and crushed cornflakes on pudding.

● Use strong-flavored ingredients: garlic, onion, sharp cheese, flavored vinegars and oils, concentrated fruit sauce, and jam.

● For less fat, impart flavor with herb rubs instead of gravy or sauces. Fat carries flavor, too. Use small amounts of flavorful oils such as olive and peanut oils for health benefits, too. A little dribble will do!

● Include foods of different temperatures. Serve hot foods hot, not lukewarm, to enhance flavor. Extreme hot or cold temperatures, however, tend to lessen flavors.

● Serve colorful, attractive food. A simple lemon or tomato slice on the plate adds appeal.

● Chew well to enjoy the foods' full flavors.

● If you smoke, stop. Smoking reduces the ability to perceive flavors.

● Avoid overexposing your taste buds to strong or bitter flavors, such as coffee, which can temporarily deaden sensitivity to other flavors.

● If you've lost interest in eating, talk to your doctor, and consult a registered dietitian about other ways to make food more appealing. *Be aware:* Sensory loss may signal serious health problems; tell your doctor!

For more about flavor, see "Flavor and Health" in chapter 14.

A Few Words about Constipation

Constipation is a persistent problem for many people as they get older. The reason? The digestive system may get a little sluggish. Not getting enough fluid or

Have You Ever Wondered ?

. . . if taking mineral oil helps keep you regular? Taking mineral oil isn't recommended. It can promote the loss of fat-soluble vitamins (A, D, E, and K).

fiber and being inactive may compound the problem. With constipation, stools get hard and can't be passed out of the body without straining. And the body's normal elimination schedule may change.

Being physically active, drinking enough fluids, and eating enough fiber are ways to stay regular and avoid constipation—and a better approach than using more laxatives! If these remedies don't work, ask a registered dietitian or your doctor for more advice.

● Drink enough water or other fluids. Fluids help your stools stay softer, bulkier, and easier to eliminate.

● Consume plenty of fiber-rich foods: beans (legumes), whole-grain breads and cereals, vegetables, and fruits. Fiber gives bulk to stools, making them easier to pass through the colon, and won't interfere with the digestion and absorption of nutrients as laxatives might. *For more about fiber, including fiber pills and powders, see chapter 3.*

● Listen to nature's call! The longer waste remains in your large intestine, the more difficult it is to eliminate. The body continues to draw out water, so stools get harder.

● Keep physically active and get enough rest. Both help keep your body regular.

● Avoid taking laxatives, as well as fiber pills and powders, unless your doctor recommends them. Food may pass through your intestinal tract faster than vitamins and minerals can be absorbed. And some may cause your body to lose fluids and potassium. A cup of tea or warm water with lemon, taken first thing in the morning, can act as a gentle, natural laxative.

For more about dealing with constipation, see "Gastrointestinal Conditions" in chapter 22.

Not Hungry?

While many older adults say they just don't have an appetite, there's no single cause for that complaint. As

noted, sensory loss plays a role. Some have digestive problems that cause appetite loss. And medication or health problems also may be a cause. For some, the problem is psychological: loneliness, depression, or anxiety, among others.

Regardless, people who don't eat adequately increase their chances for poor nutrition and its negative consequences. If you're not hungry, skipping meals actually may suppress appetite—especially if you already have appetite loss. And skipping meals may cause your blood glucose level to drop too low, then surge too high later with a big meal. To perk up a tired appetite:

● Try to identify the problem. If certain foods cause heartburn or gas, find alternatives. Talk to your doctor about your medication; if it's the cause, something else might be prescribed.

● Start the day with breakfast, when your appetite is likely at its best. Then try to eat something at every meal.

● Eat four to six smaller meals; keep portions small. You may take seconds if you're hungry for more. And smaller meals may be easier to digest.

● Give yourself enough time to eat. Rushing through a meal can cause discomfort.

● To get your digestive juices flowing, serve foods hot. Heat brings out the aroma of food, usually making it more enticing.

● Make your overall meal look appealing. Food that's attractively arranged and served may help bring your appetite back!

● If possible, increase your physical activity. That may promote a healthier appetite.

● If you're confined to bed, ask for help to keep your room pleasant. Remove bedpans and other unpleasant things. Enjoy a plant; turn on music!

Chewing Problems?

For many mature adults, poor appetite isn't much of a nutrition problem. Instead, tooth loss or mouth pain may be. An astounding number lose all their teeth by age sixty-five. Many also have poorly fitting dentures that cause chewing problems and mouth sores.

What's at the root of oral health problems? Cavities may come to mind first. Yet gum, or periodontal, disease is the most common cause of tooth loss among older adults. As a result, many have missing, loose, or diseased teeth and sore, diseased gums. People with dentures may be able to eat all the foods they've always enjoyed if dentures fit right. If not, the resulting discomfort and mouth pain may keep them from eating a well-balanced diet. Osteoarthritis also can hinder chewing if it affects the lower jaw.

A dry mouth is another problem that may cause chewing and swallowing difficulties, especially if food is dry and hard to chew. As people get older, they may not have as much saliva flow to help soften food and wash it down. Medications, some health problems, and treatment such as chemotherapy also may decrease saliva flow or cause chewing and swallowing problems. *See "Cancer Treatment: Handling Some Side Effects" in chapter 22.*

If you have chewing problems, make sure oral problems don't become a barrier to good nutrition.

● See your dentist, or go to a dentist who specializes in care for older adults. Many oral health problems can be treated. Have poorly fitted dentures adjusted.

● Choose softer foods that are easier to chew. Chop, grate, grind, puree, or cook hard vegetables or fruit to reduce your risk of choking. These nutrient-rich foods are softer and easier to eat.

  ● *Grain group:* cooked cereal, cooked rice, cooked pasta, soft bread or rolls, softer crackers
  ● *Fruit group:* fruit juice, cooked or canned fruit, avocados, bananas, soft fruit
  ● *Vegetable group:* vegetable juice, cooked vegetables, mashed potatoes, salads with soft vegetables, chopped lettuce
  ● *Dairy group:* milk, cheese, yogurt, pudding, ice cream, milk shakes
  ● *Protein foods group:* chopped lean meat, chopped chicken or turkey, canned fish, tender cooked fish, eggs, tofu, hummus, peanut butter

● Drink water or other fluids with meals and snacks to make swallowing easier.

● Consult a registered dietitian. Together you can plan for foods that you can eat comfortably without compromising your nutrient intake.

There's good news! Tooth loss and chewing difficulty aren't inevitable parts of aging. Good oral care— starting now, whatever your age—can help you keep the teeth you were born with. *See "Your Smile: Carbohydrates and Oral Health" in chapter 3.*

Gum disease is highly preventable. Proper brushing, daily flossing, and regular cleaning by a dentist or a hygienist can keep gum disease at bay. If you can, have your teeth cleaned twice a year, and perhaps more often if you have gum disease. *See "Keep Smiling: Prevent Gum Disease" in chapter 22.*

Weight Loss—or Gain?

Does clothing fit as it did before? Too loose? Have you lost weight as a result of a poor appetite or health problems? Or have extra pounds crept on? Maintaining or improving your weight may be a health step you need to take. Talk to your doctor or a registered dietitian about the weight that's healthy for you.

Weight Loss: A Concern

Weight loss may signal a health problem, especially if losing weight isn't your intention. If that happens, first and foremost, find out why! Perhaps the reason is poor oral health, appetite loss, or immobility that makes grocery shopping or food preparation difficult, or it's eating smaller meals and fewer snacks to lower food expense. Weight loss may signal an emotional problem, perhaps depression and/or bereavement, or social isolation. Unexpected weight loss also is a symptom for some serious health problems, including cancer. Talk to your doctor! Besides weight loss, talk about chewing or digestive problems, depression, and medications. Ask for screenings to detect nutrition-related problems.

Weight loss may be linked to physical weakness when muscle mass, not just body fat, is lost. Loss of physical strength and frailty increase the risk for falls, and as a result, bone fractures and other health problems that affect quality of life and health. Being underweight also may slow recovery from sickness or surgery. Severe weight loss may be life-threatening.

Note: Intentional weight loss among overweight and obese older adults is advised and is linked to lower risk of type 2 diabetes and to improved cardiovascular health.

To gain or to maintain weight:

● Eat enough. *See chapter 10 for your guide for consuming enough among and within the five food groups.*

● Eat five or six small meals a day if you fill up quickly at three bigger meals.

● Stick to a regular meal schedule so you don't forget to eat.

● Keep healthful, easy snack foods handy: cheese milk, yogurt, fruit, vegetables, crackers, whole-wheat bread, cereal, peanut butter, even ice cream.

● Eat with someone else to spark your appetite.

● Instead of coffee or tea, which supplies few calories, drink cocoa, milk, soup, or juice.

● Make casseroles, soups, stews, and side dishes heartier. Add whole milk, cheese, beans, rice, or pasta.

● Talk to a registered dietitian (RD) or your doctor about ways to boost calories and nutrients in your meals and snacks. An RD can provide ideas for high-calorie meals and drinks, and if necessary, can help you select the right canned nutrition supplement drink or dietary supplement. Find an appropriate way to stay physically active so you maintain your body's muscle mass—and your strength. Talk to your doctor, and perhaps a trained physical therapist.

Be aware that some medications, including low-dose antidepressant drugs, may enhance appetite; others may interfere with appetite, digestion, or nutrient absorption.

Weight Gain: An Issue, Too

As you get older, you need fewer calories to maintain your weight. It's not surprising, then, to gain a few pounds—especially if you're more sedentary and still eat as you always have. The concern is that being overweight or obese increases the risks for high blood pressure, heart disease, diabetes, and certain cancers. If you have one of these problems already, or if you're carrying extra weight, dropping just a few pounds may lower your blood pressure, total blood cholesterol level, or blood glucose level. Extra body weight affects how easily you move and intensifies the discomfort of arthritis. It also can contribute to disabilities, which may lead to an earlier death. As older adults lose muscle mass they often gain body fat.

Before you start trying to lose weight, talk to your physician about an effective, safe approach that matches your health needs.

To lose weight:

● Know your calorie target; *refer to chapter 10 for a*

healthy eating pattern to match your calorie needs. Choose mostly lean and low-fat or fat-free foods and those without much solid fats and added sugars. Eat the recommended amount of nutrient-rich foods from the five food groups and healthy oils, based on your calorie target. That may mean smaller portions.

● Eat regular meals. Meal-skipping often leads to snacking and possibly overeating.

● Choose snacks carefully: fruits, vegetables, low-fat yogurt, fat-free or low-fat milk, breakfast cereal, and frozen yogurt.

● Trim fat and added sugars from food choices to cut calories. Remove skin from turkey or chicken before eating it. Choose lean meats and trim visible fat. Bake, broil, microwave, or steam foods instead of frying them. Use low-fat or fat-free milk, yogurt, and cheese. Go easy on butter, margarine, cream, and sour cream and sugary desserts. *For more ways to trim fat and added sugars in food preparation, see chapter 14.*

● Eat smaller portions—and still meet food group guidelines for your calorie needs. *See chapter 10.*

● If you drink alcoholic beverages, do so in moderation: no more than one drink a day for women, and two for men. If you take medication, you might need to avoid alcoholic drinks altogether.

● Keep physically active and busy to prevent eating from boredom or loneliness. And learn to recognize signals for hunger and satiety (fullness).

● Find safe and appropriate ways to move more and sit less. You'll get more health-promoting benefits than weight control alone!

● Beware of weight-loss plans with unrealistic promises. *See "'Diets' That Don't Work!" in chapter 2.*

"Moving Ideas" for Physical Limitations

Some older adults move with the same grace, stamina, and dexterity of their earlier years. For others, health problems limit physical abilities: for example, arthritis, diabetes, osteoporosis, Parkinson's disease, respiratory diseases, and strokes. Even healthy, mature adults may become gradually less active, so they have less strength and stamina for everyday tasks.

For those who enjoy independent living, these tips can make food preparation and eating easier:

● Does your tile or wooden floor seem slippery? Wear flat, rubber-soled shoes in the kitchen. And wipe up spills immediately so you don't slip!

● Be careful of loose rugs by the sink or other places in your kitchen. They may feel good underfoot, but they're easy to trip or slip on.

● If you're unsteady or need a cane, use a rolling tea cart to move food, dishes, and kitchen equipment from place to place.

● A wheelchair or a walker with a flat seat can be used to move things, too; check with a medical supply store.

● Sit while you work. Use the kitchen table for food preparation, or get a stable chair or stool that's high enough for working at the counter or the stove.

● Give yourself time. Things may take a little longer to do as you get older.

● Get a loud kitchen timer if you have trouble hearing. Especially if you're forgetful, using a timer when you cook can avoid burned food and kitchen fires.

● Cooking for just one? Use a microwave or toaster oven rather than the conventional oven.

● Organize your kitchen for efficiency—everything within easy reach. Keep mixers, blenders, and other heavy, small appliances on the counter. Keep heavy pots and pans on lower shelves, too.

● If you have vision problems, keep a magnifying glass handy, and have your eyes checked and fitted for glasses. That makes it easier to read expiration dates and small type on food labels.

● Use a cutting board with contrasting colors if you have trouble with vision; for example, it may be hard to safely cut an onion on a white plastic cutting board.

● Have trouble with manual tasks such as opening jars and cans, or perhaps cutting? Kitchen devices are sold to make food preparation easier for people with arthritis or other problems, and for those partly paralyzed by a stroke. Again, check a medical supply store. Place a wet paper towel under the cutting board so it doesn't move around. *See "Have You Ever Wondered . . . if you can eat anything to relieve arthritis?" in chapter 22.*

● Keep your cordless or cell phone handy and charged. You won't need to dash to the phone while you're cooking. It's a good safety measure, too, in case you fall.

● If you use a walker or a wheelchair, talk to a registered dietitian or a physical therapist about ways to change your kitchen for independent living.

● *Another kitchen safety tip:* Avoid using your oven as a room heater. It can be dangerous! If heating is a problem where you live, let someone know—a relative, landlord, building manager, or social worker, among others. *For other kitchen safety tips, see "Quick Tips for Injury Prevention" in chapter 13.*

● Use an all-in-one fork and spoon if you have trouble with one hand. Check with a medical supply store or catalog to find one.

● Drink soup from a mug. It's easier than using a soup spoon—and there's one less utensil to wash.

● Get dishes with a high rim and a rubber, no-slip back. The rim helps you push food onto your spoon or fork.

● Set your table with plastic placemats. They're easy to clean. And dishes won't slide on them, as they might on the table surface.

Need more practical, easy ways to eat smart as the years go by? Check here for "how-tos":

● Boost your appetite if you don't feel hungry—see chapter 2.

● Find smart ways to lose, gain, or maintain your weight—see chapter 2.

● Make a personal plan for healthful eating—see chapter 10.

● Make quick, simple meals if you don't have a lot of energy—see chapter 11.

● Get more for your food dollar on a fixed income—see chapter 12.

● Protect yourself from foodborne illness—see chapter 13.

● Prepare food to get more nutrition for fewer calories—see chapter 14.

● Perk up food's flavor with herbs and spices if food no longer tastes as good. Improve food's look, too—see chapter 14.

● Eat out, yet still match your health needs—see chapter 15.

● Eat to manage health problems—see chapter 22.

● Get easy, personalized tips from a nutrition expert—see chapter 24.

● Shaky with a cup? Get a covered cup with a drinking spout or place for a straw.

● If you use a wheelchair, buy an oven with front controls and a side-hinged door. Install it next to the sink or your work area, not across the kitchen. Put in low countertops and "pull-outs," such as cutting boards, in your kitchen. Talk to a physical therapist or a registered dietitian about other kitchen solutions.

● Rather than avoid certain categories of foods, accept food preparation help if you need it. You need nourishment from a variety of foods.

Meals and Snacks: When You Need a Special Diet

Many health problems—physical and emotional— that arise with aging require major changes in what and how people eat. Discuss that with your doctor during your regular checkups—annually or more often as your doctor advises. Never self-diagnose an ongoing disease or prescribe your own special diet or dietary supplement to treat it. And be careful of so-called miracle cures. *See "Miracles? Dream On!" earlier in this chapter.*

For any health condition, there's no one recommended diet. Each person needs individual nutrition advice because needs differ so much. And sometimes more than one health problem needs to be treated at the same time. If a special (therapeutic) diet is prescribed for you, consult your doctor or a registered dietitian for guidance. Have your progress monitored, as advised. *For more tips, see "If Your Doctor Prescribes a Special Eating Plan . . . " in chapter 22.*

To manage your health, your food choices may need as much of your attention as following directions for medications. It's all for your good health! To find a registered dietitian, ask your doctor. *See "How to Find Nutrition Help . . ." in chapter 24.*

Give a Helping Hand!

To people who are sick, weak, or injured, good nutrition is often the best medicine! Visit during mealtime or invite someone you care about to your home for a meal. Regardless of age, those with difficulty feeding themselves may need a caring, helping hand. If you offer help, make mealtime pleasant:

● Help with hand washing before and after eating. Use a wet, soapy washcloth or premoistened towels or a hand sanitizer if the person can't get to the sink. Offer a towel for drying.

● Make sure that the food is the right consistency. Chop, grind, or puree it if chewing is difficult.

● Let the person decide what foods to eat first, next, and so on. Even when people can't feed themselves, most want to feel in control.

● For dignity's sake, provide a napkin or an apron to help him or her keep clean.

● Offer some finger foods to eat independently. For example, try banana slices, orange sections, bread (cut in quarters), a soft roll, cheese sticks, or meat (sliced in strips).

● Offer a drink between bites to help with chewing and swallowing. Provide a straw and a cup that's not too big. You can always pour more.

● Consider how far the person can reach for a cup or a dish. Arrange the place setting for easy reach.

● Sit together at the same level as you offer food. Share pleasant conversation in a normal tone, even if you need to do all the talking. To be sure you understand a response, repeat or rephrase it.

● Relax; be patient. Encourage self-expression of any kind. Meals should not feel rushed, especially if the person has trouble chewing or swallowing.

● Offer small bites, and suggest a spoon rather than a fork. It's easier for holding food and less likely to jab his or her mouth.

● If you can, eat your meal at the same time to continue the normalcy of social interaction at mealtime.

● Clean spills right away. Keep a clean cloth handy.

● Most important, respect the person's needs and desires. Expect frustration, and handle it without a negative reaction. Counting on others for personal care can be emotionally difficult.

● Let the nurse or other caregivers know what and how much the person has eaten. In that way other meals and snacks can be adjusted accordingly.

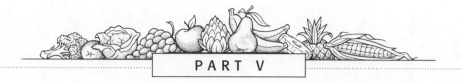

PART V

Healthful Eating
Special Issues

CHAPTER 20

Athlete's Guide
Winning Nutrition

O n your mark . . . get set . . . go! Whether you train for competitive sports, or work out for your own good health or just for fun, what you eat and drink—and when—is part of your formula for athletic success. Good nutrition can't replace training, effort, talent, and personal drive. But what you eat and drink over time makes a difference for peak performance or your personal best.

Whether competitive or recreational, physical activity puts extra demands on your body. You use more energy, lose more body fluids, and put extra stress on your muscles, joints, and bones. Fortunately, your "training table" can increase your endurance and help prevent dehydration and injury. Most important, healthful eating helps you feel good and stay fit overall—the positive "mental edge!"

For more about the benefits of regular physical activity and physical activity guidelines for the general public, see chapters 1 and 2.

Nutrients for Active Living

Good nutrition truly is fundamental to peak physical performance. No matter what your level of physical activity, your nutrient needs are similar to others of the same age and gender. If you're highly active, you may need slightly more of some nutrients: more water to replace fluid loss during high activity and more energy-supplying nutrients, especially carbohydrates.

Thirst for Success!

Do you drink plenty of water, but not to excess? Your physical endurance and strength depend on it!

When you're physically active, even with recreational activity, you lose fluids as sweat evaporates from your skin. As you breathe, often heavily, you exhale moisture, too. A 150-pound athlete can lose 1½ quarts, or 3 pounds, of fluid in just one hour. That equals six 8-ounce glasses of water. With heavy training, fluid loss can be higher. To avoid dehydration you must replace the fluids you lose.

Fluids for Peak Performance

What's the risk if you begin physical activity even slightly dehydrated, or lose too much fluid while you're active? Even small losses of 1 percent of your body weight may hinder your physical performance, particularly during warm weather. Losing more than

> ### Did You Know
>
> . . . heat stroke, caused by severe dehydration, ranks second among the reported cases of death among high school athletes?
>
> . . . taking extra vitamins or minerals (beyond the Recommended Dietary Allowances) offers no added advantage to athletic performance?
>
> . . . a high-carbohydrate diet can boost your endurance?

1 percent is a known detriment. (That's about 2 or 3 pounds for a 150-pound person.) Dehydration can affect strength, endurance, and aerobic capacity. How?

For energy production. Fluids are part of the energy-production cycle. As part of blood, water helps carry oxygen and glucose to muscle cells. There, oxygen and glucose help produce energy. Blood removes waste by-products as muscle cells generate energy and passes them to urine. Fluid losses decrease blood volume; your heart must work harder to deliver enough oxygen to cells.

For cooling down. Exercise generates heat as a by-product of energy production. Evaporation of sweat helps cool you down. As you move, your overall temperature goes up, and you sweat. As sweat evaporates,

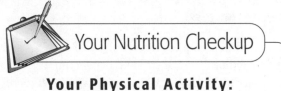

Your Nutrition Checkup

Your Physical Activity: How Intense?

Light, moderate, or intense? Estimate your activity level: Determine if your heart rate is within your target zone.

1. *Decide on your goal:*
   ● *Moderate intensity:* Your target heart rate should be 50 to 70 percent of your maximum heart rate.
   ● *Vigorous intensity:* Your target heart rate should be 70 to 85 percent of your maximum heart rate.

2. *Figure your maximum heart rate.* It's 220 minus your age. So, if you're 50 years old, your maximum heart rate is 220 minus 50 to equal 170 beats per minute (bpm).

3. *Determine your target zone.* Multiply your maximum heart rate by your workout intensity. For example, for moderate intensity, multiply 170 bpm by 50 percent to equal 85 bpm, or by 70 percent to equal 119 bpm.

4. *Take your heart rate.* Stop exercising. With your index and middle fingers, take your pulse at your neck, wrist, or chest. Count the beats for 60 seconds; the first beat is zero. (Or count for 30 seconds, then double it for bpm.) In this example, between 85 and 119 beats is moderate activity.

   The talk-sing test, *described in chapter 1,* is another quick way to assess your workout intensity.

Click Here! Websites to Know . . .
● American College of Sports Medicine, www.acsm.org
● Sports, Cardiovascular, and Wellness Nutrition Dietetic Practice Group, Academy of Nutrition and Dietetics, www.scandpg.org
See "Resources You Can Use" for more websites.

your skin and the blood just under your skin cool. Cooler blood that flows throughout your body helps protect you from overheating. If you don't replace this fluid loss, your body's fluid balance is thrown off—a bigger problem as working muscles continue to generate more heat.

For transporting nutrients. Water in your bloodstream carries other nutrients for performance, including electrolytes, which help maintain body fluid balance.

As a cushion. The water around your body's tissues and organs offers protection from all the jostles and jolts that go along with exercise.

Protection from dehydration. Fluid loss—beyond the early stages of dehydration—increases your chances of heat injury, such as heat cramps, heat exhaustion, and heat stroke. *Severe dehydration can be life-threatening. See "Dehydration Alert!" in this chapter. See "A Fluid Asset" in chapter 8.*

Fluids: Tips to Drink Enough

No matter what your sport—running, bicycling, swimming, tennis, even walking and golfing—or rigorous activity, drink enough fluid to avoid dehydration. Getting enough isn't always easy.

● Drink adequate amounts of fluids—before, during, and after physical activity. Carry a water bottle in a bottle belt or fluid pack, especially if you have no available water source. Or find out where you can get fluids: store (bring money), water fountain. Rehydrating after activity helps you recover faster, physically and mentally.

● Drink early and often—not too much. Drink fluids every fifteen minutes during activity—even when you don't feel thirsty. Your thirst mechanism may not send thirst signals when you're exercising. Thirst signals

When You're on the Road

Planes, trains, and automobiles get you where you're going. But to keep physically active—or perhaps keep up a training regimen—when you travel, plan ahead!

- Pack comfortable workout clothes and footwear. Take a jump rope, running or walking shoes, or plastic dumbbells to fill with water.

- Choose a hotel with exercise equipment, then make time to use it. Before you make your reservation, ask about the facilities: an indoor or outdoor pool; tennis courts; bicycle rentals; and gym equipment such as a treadmill, step machine, or rowing machine.

- If you belong to a health club at home, check ahead for membership benefits elsewhere.

- At the airport, wait for your flight by walking the concourse; skip people movers. On a long train or plane trip, walk up and down the aisle several times if allowed. Ask for an aisle seat so you won't have to climb over your fellow passengers. Do simple stretching exercises to avoid feeling stiff.

- Ask for an early wake-up call so you can get a jump start on your day with a thirty-minute walk or jog. Get a guidebook to map out your way—or the hotel's front desk may have a walking map.

- Skip the taxicab. If it's a safe, reasonable distance, walk to your business meeting, museums, shops, or restaurants in comfortable walking shoes.

- If you're driving, take regular breaks. You'll ride more comfortably after some physical activity.

- Check the television guide for a workout or yoga program. Or bring an exercise DVD for your laptop.

dehydration; drink fluids before that happens. *Follow the schedule in this chapter, "For Physical Activity: How Much Fluid?"*

- Stop to drink if you need fluids. You'll more than make up for any lost time with better performance.

- Wear lightweight, loose-fitting clothing that wicks moisture, especially in warm weather. Fabrics that hold heat—such as tights, body suits, heavy gear—as well as helmets and other protective gear, won't let sweat evaporate.

- Replace water weight. Weigh yourself before and after a physical workout. (Your nude weight is best.) Wear the same clothing when you weigh yourself—

before and after. Replace each pound of weight loss with 3 cups of water, carbohydrate drink, or other fluid to bring your fluid balance back to normal. Perhaps plan to drink more before your active workout next time. If you weigh more after exercise, you drank too much during activity; drink less while exercising next time.

- Check the color of your urine. Dark-colored urine indicates dehydration. Drink more fluids, so your urine is pale and nearly colorless before exercising again.

- Be especially careful if you exercise intensely in warm, humid weather. Consider how much hotter you feel on humid days. Sweat doesn't evaporate from your skin quickly, so you don't get the cooling benefits. That's why on humid days it's easier to get hyperthermia, or overheated, as you exercise. Hyperthermia can lead to heat stroke, which can be fatal!

- Know the signs of dehydration. Some early signs are flushed skin, fatigue, increased body temperature, and faster breathing and pulse rate. Later signs are dizziness, weakness, and labored breathing with exercise. Replace fluids before symptoms get serious. *See "Dehydration: Body Signals!" in chapter 8.*

- Drink, rather than simply pour water over your head. Drinking is the *only* way to rehydrate and cool your body from the inside out.

For more about fluids and active children, see "Fluids: Caution for Kids" later in this chapter.

Be cautious about overdrinking, which can lead to hyponatremia, or abnormally low blood sodium levels. This occurs when extra water moves into body cells, including brain cells. The extra pressure affects vital functions, with potentially fatal outcomes.

Which Fluids?

For workouts of less than thirty minutes of continuous activity and recreational walking, sports drinks, juices, and water are good choices. For fluid replacers for other sports, read on.

Water: A good choice. Water helps lower and normalize your body's core (inside) temperature when you're hot. Water moves quickly from your digestive tract to your tissues.

Cold water is fine. Contrary to myth, drinking cold water during physical activity doesn't cause stomach

For Physical Activity: How Much Fluid?

Make a point of drinking fluids at all times during the day—not just after your workout or competition. How much fluid is enough? Here's a schedule that can keep you from becoming dehydrated:

WHEN TO DRINK	ABOUT HOW MUCH (One medium mouthful of fluid = about 1 ounce; 1 cup = 8 ounces.)
2 to 3 hours before activity	2 cups (and drink plenty with meals)
15 minutes before activity	1 to 1½ cups
Every 15 minutes during activity	½ to 1½ cups, enough to minimize body weight loss, without overdrinking
After activity	3 cups for each pound of body weight lost

Adapted from: Christine Rosenbloom, ed., *Sports Nutrition: A Practice Manual for Professionals* (Chicago: Academy of Nutrition and Dietetics, 2012).

cramps. For outside activity in cold weather, drink water that's warm or at room temperature to help protect you from hypothermia, or low body temperature. Cool water, preferred by many exercisers, can enhance performance.

Sports drinks. Sports drinks can benefit athletes who exercise hard for more than ninety minutes. Sports drinks with 6 to 8 percent carbohydrate (14 to 19 grams of carbohydrate per 8 ounces) may be better than water or diluted fruit juice for fluid replacement. More than 8 percent carbohydrate solution may decrease the rate of fluid absorption and gastric (stomach) emptying.

If you're a long-distance runner or long-distance bicyclist, or involved in other endurance events (longer than ninety minutes), sports drinks offer performance benefits. Research also shows a benefit for high-intensity activity (perhaps sprinting or playing hockey) lasting thirty minutes or more.

Glucose (simple form of carbohydrate) in sports drinks is a more immediate fuel, or energy, source for working muscles. It may help prevent muscle glycogen from depleting too fast and so help lengthen per-

formance time. (Muscle glycogen is carbohydrate stored in muscle.) Glucose in sports drinks also helps fluid get out of the gut and into the bloodstream.

Compared to juice or soft drinks, sports drinks are more diluted, so their fluid and glucose can be absorbed and used faster by the body.

Besides fluid and calories, sports drinks supply electrolytes. As you perspire, your body loses very small amounts of sodium and other electrolytes. For most athletes, normal meals and snacks replace what's lost. The amount of sodium and other electrolytes in sport drinks is low compared to what you get from typical foods. During exercise that's longer than 60 minutes, or for exercise performed in high heat or humidity, drinks with electrolytes help to enhance fluid absorption. *See "Electrolytes: Sweat 'Em!" later in this chapter.*

You don't lose vitamins when you sweat, so you don't need sports drinks with extra vitamins. The extra food you eat for more calories also provides any extra B vitamins you need for energy production.

For endurance sports, experiment with sports drinks and other fluids during practices and low-key competition. If the flavor encourages you to drink more fluids—or if they give you a psychological boost—enjoy them, but don't overdo. Watching your weight? *Remember:* They supply calories.

Energy drinks? They typically contain more carbohydrates than commercial sport drinks. They're also usually higher in caffeine. Since these aren't formulated for athletes' needs, they aren't advised for use during exercise. *See chapter 8.*

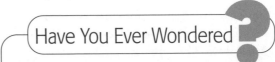

Have You Ever Wondered

. . . if swimmers need to worry about dehydration? Like any athlete, swimmers perspire to keep from overheating. However, they may not notice their sweat—at least not while they're in the water. They too need to drink plenty of fluids before, during, and after rigorous swimming.

. . . if dehydration is a concern with cold-weather sports such as ice skating or skiing? Even in a cool or cold environment, you sweat. Attire for cold weather sports such as downhill skiing, snowmobiling, and ice hockey doesn't "breathe" or allow the body to cool down either.

Some energy drinks are designed for athletes and may delay the onset of fatigue; their caffeine may enhance athletic performance. The American Academy of Pediatrics (AAP) advises against energy drinks for children and teens; the advice also applies to young athletes. AAP notes these reasons: (1) health risks of stimulants in energy drinks for young people and (2) increased risk of overweight and obesity and dental caries with routine intake of carbohydrate-containing sports drinks by children and teens. In addition, high school and college athletes should check the rules for consuming caffeinated energy drinks.

For adult athletes, energy drinks are generally okay if used in moderation and if the athlete has no underlying heart condition or high blood pressure. If you're an athlete, be aware of any caffeine sensitivity, and check with your doctor before consuming energy drinks.

Have You Ever Wondered ?

. . . if caffeine can boost your physical performance? Maybe—and maybe not. People react to caffeine in different ways. Caffeine stimulates the central nervous system, so it may help you feel more alert and attentive. And there's some evidence that caffeine, consumed before physical activity, may improve performance and endurance.

For caffeine-sensitive athletes, caffeine may exacerbate pre-event anxiety and its symptoms. If you enjoy coffee, tea, or soft drinks with caffeine, experiment during training, not competition. A single cup may help—or at least not hinder—your performance. But avoid caffeine tablets or several cups of caffeinated drinks. The National Collegiate Athletic Association (NCAA) limits caffeine concentration to no more than 15 micrograms per milliliter of urine. You likely won't reach this level from caffeine in food (equivalent to seventeen caffeinated, 12-ounce sodas). But athletes who consume three 200-mg caffeine tablets may exceed this limit. Beginning in 2004 the International Olympic Committee no longer prohibited caffeine but monitors caffeine content in urine instead.

Caffeine doesn't cause dehydration or electrolyte imbalance. *For more about caffeine, see "Drinks: With or without Caffeine?" in chapter 8.*

Dehydration Alert!

As you exercise, be alert for conditions that increase your fluid loss through sweat. With more perspiration, your body dehydrates faster.

● *Temperature.* The higher the temperature, the greater your sweat loss.

● *Intensity.* The harder you work out, the greater your sweat loss.

● *Body size.* The larger the athlete, the greater the sweat loss. Males generally sweat more than females.

● *Duration.* The longer the workout, the greater your fluid loss.

● *Fitness.* Well-trained athletes sweat more, starting at a lower body temperature. With training, the body cools more efficiently.

Source: Debbi Sowell Jennings and Suzanne Nelson Steen, *Play Hard, Eat Right* (Minneapolis: American Dietetic Association, Chronimed Publishing, 1995).

Fruit juice or soft drinks? Compared with sports drinks, sugars in soft drinks and fruit juice are more concentrated: 10 to 15 percent carbohydrate. They aren't recommended during exercise because of their high sugar content and, for soft drinks, their carbonation. Drinks with a lot of sugar take longer to be absorbed, and they may cause cramps, diarrhea, or nausea. Carbonation can make you feel full and make your throat burn, so you drink less fluid.

You can dilute fruit juice with water—if you like the flavor. Add a dash of salt, and you'll have a homemade sports drink at a low cost!

Alcoholic drinks: Not now! They can impair, not enhance, your physical performance. Skip alcoholic drinks—at least until *after* you replenish the fluids lost in your workout:

● If you're looking for a carbohydrate source, look elsewhere. A 12-ounce can of beer has less than a third of the carbs provided by a 12-ounce serving of orange juice. Calories from alcohol don't fuel muscles.

● Alcohol may have a short-term diuretic effect. It works as a depressant, affecting your brain's ability to reason and make judgments and perhaps your reaction time. And it may impair your coordination, balance, muscle reflexes, and visual perception.

● For endurance sports there's another effect. When you drink a beer, wine, or mixed drink, your liver works to detoxify and metabolize the alcohol. That can interfere with the liver's job of forming extra blood glucose for prolonged physical activity. Possible result? Early fatigue.

Energy to Burn

To have enough energy for physical activity you need to consume enough energy. How much energy, or calories, per day? That's an individual matter. A 200-pound body builder has very different needs than an 80-pound gymnast or a 130-pound jogger, walker, or bicyclist. Physical training may use 500 to 3,000 or more calories daily—a huge range!

● The amount of energy for sports depends partly on your body composition, body weight, and level of fitness. Body size (consider a male football player and a female gymnast) also makes a big difference. When two people ski together at the same intensity, the person weighing more likely burns more calories.

● The harder, the longer, and the more often you work out, the more energy required for muscle work. Any activity such as cycling, power walking, or swimming is a bigger energy burner if done more vigorously.

● Not surprisingly, some sports burn more energy than others. That's simply because they're more intense or their duration is longer. Both a golf game and downhill skiing may last several hours. But skiing uses more energy since it's more physically demanding for larger muscle groups.

Have You Ever Wondered

. . . how you can avoid "hitting the wall"? When endurance athletes run out of their source of glucose, they're too tired to continue exerting themselves. To maintain your supply for as long as possible for endurance sports, follow a pre-exercise eating regimen that's high in carbohydrates. Have a sports drink if your workout lasts an hour or more. Eat a carbohydrate-rich snack right afterward when your body can store glycogen at a faster rate. Regular physical training also helps; your muscles adapt, gradually storing more glycogen for intense workouts.

YOUR DAILY CARBOHYDRATE GOAL IS ABOUT . . .*			
IF YOU WEIGH . . .	5 GRAMS	7 GRAMS	10 GRAMS
	PER KILOGRAM OF YOUR BODY WEIGHT		
100 pounds (45 kg)	225	320	455
125 pounds (56 kg)	280	400	570
150 pounds (68 kg)	340	475	680
175 pounds (80 kg)	400	560	800
200 pounds (91 kg)	455	640	910
225 pounds (102 kg)	510	715	1,020
250 pounds (114 kg)	570	800	1,140

Energy needs vary among athletes. For your target amount check with a registered dietitian.

*Amounts are rounded.

How does that translate to food? *See the chart "Carbohydrates in Food: Quick Rule of Thumb" in this chapter.*

Carbohydrates supply energy for activities that take high-intensity, short bursts of energy, and both carbohydrates and fats supply energy for longer activity.

For the energy costs of several sports, see chapter 2. To estimate your energy needs, see "Your 'Weigh': Figuring Your Energy Needs" in chapter 2. Or have a registered dietitian help you.

Carbohydrate Power

For sports and everyday living, carbohydrates are your body's foremost energy source—and the main fuel for working muscles. Nutrition experts advise athletes to consume 3 to 12 grams of carbohydrate a day for every kilogram of body weight depending on their sport. For an athlete who weighs 120 pounds (55 kilograms), that's 165 to 660 grams of carbohydrate; for a 175-pound (80-kilogram) athlete, that's 240 to 960 grams of carbs. While 5 to 7 grams of carbohydrate per kilogram of weight daily is right for general training, some athletes, especially endurance athletes, need 6 to 10 grams per kilogram body weight daily. Some ultraendurance athletes may need more. (One pound equals 2.2 kilograms.) Recreational athletes who participate in low-intensity or fuel-based activities with light training need 3 to 5 grams of carbohydrates daily.

Along with training, a high-carbohydrate eating

plan promotes overall fitness and offers a competitive edge. With carbs (not fats or proteins) as the main fuel, you can maintain rigorous activity longer. Training helps your body use carbohydrates efficiently and store more as muscle glycogen. Stored in muscles, glycogen is fuel ready to power your physical activity.

For Working Muscles

To power working muscles, stored energy comes mostly from glycogen in muscle or the liver, and from blood sugar (or blood glucose). Glycogen is your body's storage form of carbohydrate. Depending on the intensity and the duration of exercise, fat and, for endurance athletes, even a small amount of protein supplies energy.

Carbohydrates are broken down during digestion and changed to blood sugar, or glucose. Some blood sugar, which is circulated in your bloodstream, is used immediately for energy. The rest is stored as muscle and liver glycogen, or it's converted to fat if excess calories are consumed. The more muscle glycogen you can store, the more you have to power physical activity.

Your body's glycogen stores are continually used and replenished. For more energy, your body fuels muscles with a mix of both carbohydrate (glycogen) and fat. The higher the immediate intensity of an activity, the more glycogen used. Lower-intensity and longer activities use more fat and less glycogen.

● For sports that require short, intense energy spurts (anaerobic activities), muscle glycogen is the main energy source used. That includes tennis, volleyball, baseball, weight lifting, sprinting, and even bowling.

● Sports requiring intensity and endurance use mostly muscle glycogen. Basketball and football are examples.

● For endurance activities (aerobic activities) such as long-distance running or bicycling, your body uses glucose, glycogen, and fat for fuel; the proportion depends mainly on the activity's intensity and duration.

See chapter 3 for more about carbohydrates.

Fuel Up!

Carbs are an athlete's best energy source. (Eat enough every day to keep your muscle and liver glycogen stores up.) Both starches and sugars supply energy and replenish your muscle glycogen.

"CARBOHYDRATES" IN FOOD: QUICK RULE OF THUMB

FOOD	CARBOHYDRATES
Breads and cereals: 1 slice bread, or ½ cup rice or pasta, or 1 ounce dry cereal	About 15 grams
Starchy vegetables: ½ cup	About 15 grams
Fruits: ½ cup, or 1 small to medium whole fruit	About 10 to 15 grams
Vegetables: ½ cup cooked or raw	About 5 grams
Milk: 1 cup	About 12 grams

Starches come from cereals, breads, rice, pasta, vegetables, and beans and peas (legumes). Sugars (naturally occurring and added) are in fruit, fruit juice, milk, cookies, cakes, candy, and soft drinks, among other foods.

Get carbs from mixed dishes, too:

● *Made with breads, grains, cereals, and pastas:* wild rice pilaf; pasta salads; whole-wheat or buckwheat pancakes; sandwiches made with bread, including a bagel or pita bread; animal crackers, gingersnaps, graham crackers, or oatmeal-raisin cookies; homemade fruit and nut breads.

● *Made with fruits or vegetables:* dried fruit; stuffed spuds such as a baked potato with broccoli; fresh fruit salad; and raw vegetables with yogurt dip.

● *Made with beans and peas (chickpeas, kidney or black beans, lentils, and other dried peas and beans):* bean enchiladas, split pea soup, baked beans, and chili.

Carbohydrate Loading

Your muscles and liver store glycogen—only a limited amount—which must be replaced after each bout of exercise. Endurance athletes worry that they may "hit the wall," or feel extremely fatigued, before finishing. When this happens, they're out of glycogen.

The more glycogen you store, the longer it lasts. Carbohydrate loading (or glycogen loading) may help you "stockpile" two to three times more glycogen in your muscles for extended activity. Carbohydrate loading won't make you pedal harder or run faster. But it may help you perform longer before getting tired.

To "load up" your muscles for endurance sports, combine training, rest, and eating extra carbohydrates.

Starting a week before the endurance event, taper off on training to rest your muscles so they can "restock" muscle glycogen. Consume a carbohydrate-based diet, with at least 5 to 8 grams of carbohydrate per kilogram of your weight. (2.2 lb. = 1 kg)

The biggest pre-event change is in your training, not in what you eat. All along, eat a carbohydrate-based diet to support your training. Now rest your muscles so they have the time to refuel.

Recent research has tried to simulate carbohydrate loading with a short bout of high-intensity exercise, then one to two days of 'high-carb" eating. More research is needed to see if this helps store extra muscle glycogen.

Reminders: In your normal training diet, most of your calories should come from carbohydrates. Whole grains, cereal, beans (legumes), and starchy vegetables are good sources of starches (complex carbs).

What sports should you "carb load" for? If you're a trained athlete, try it for either endurance events such as marathons and triathlons that last longer than ninety minutes, or for all-day events such as swim meets, a series of tennis matches, distance bicycling, or soccer games. For shorter events, a normal, carbohydrate-rich approach to eating supplies enough glycogen.

Caution: If you have diabetes or high blood triglycerides, talk to your doctor and a registered dietitian before trying this regimen.

Smart about Fat, Still Best!

Fat also fuels working muscles. In fact, it's a more concentrated energy source. And it performs other body functions, such as transporting fat-soluble vitamins and providing essential fatty acids. For good health, consume fat as one source of fuel. Rather than try to eat almost "fat-free," be smart: low in saturated fat and *trans* fat, and moderate in your total fat intake.

Fat as Fuel

For energy, fat helps power activities of longer duration such as hiking or marathon running. Because fat doesn't convert to energy as fast as carbohydrates, fat doesn't power quick energy spurts such as returning a tennis serve or running a 100-yard dash.

Unlike glycogen, fat needs oxygen for energy metabolism. That's why endurance sports, fueled in part by fat, are called aerobic activities. "Aerobic" means with oxygen, and aerobic activities require a continuous intake of oxygen. The more you train, the more easily you breathe during longer activity; the oxygen you take in helps convert fat to energy.

No matter its source—carbohydrates, proteins, or fats—your body stores extra energy as body fat. Fat stores supply energy for aerobic activity. Even if you're lean, you likely have enough fat stores to fuel prolonged or endurance activity. You don't need to eat more fat!

For Athletes: How Much Fat?

Advice for athletes is the same as that for all healthy people: Eat a diet low in saturated fat, *trans* fat, and cholesterol and moderate in total fat. To get enough calories for sports, yet not too much fat, 20 to 35 percent of your total calories from fat is a good guideline. Most of your calories should come from carbohydrates. With a high-fat diet your carbohydrate or protein intake may come up short. Less than 15 percent of calories from fat doesn't provide enough calories or enough fat for other health roles, especially for those involved in endurance sports. Getting enough essential fatty acids is also important for health and peak performance.

Athletes who consume too little fat, often to keep weight and body fat down, may risk a calorie shortfall; young athletes on a very low-fat diet may not consume enough essential fatty acids for normal growth and development. For female athletes—often dancers, gymnasts, and skaters—a low-calorie, low-fat diet may interfere with menstrual cycles, with lifelong health implications.

If your calorie needs are higher, your total fat intake is probably higher, too. That's often true for football linemen and weight lifters, who may use 4,000 calories or more a day. Still, fats shouldn't contribute more than 35 percent of total energy.

Action plan. Do you need to eat less fat? If so, get more calories from carbohydrates. Remember that fat isn't stored as muscle glycogen; carbs are. Here's one strategy for cutting fat and boosting carbohydrates: Eat a baked potato more often than fries. Replace the fat calories from fries with carb calories from a slice of whole-grain bread.

See chapter 5, "Fat Facts: Cholesterol, Too."

. . . if eating a candy bar right before rigorous activity supercharges your body? For endurance activities of ninety minutes or longer, a sugary snack food (energy) bar or drink before exercise (or even during an event) may enhance your stamina. Fig bars, graham crackers, bananas, and raisins work, too. Drink water along with these snacks.

Keep your snack or drink small: no more than 200 to 300 calories. Too much sugar may slow the time it takes water to leave your stomach, so your body won't replace fluids as quickly. Your best approach? Enjoy a sports drink. You'll consume a little sugar to fuel your muscles—but not too much to impair rehydration.

Protein: More Is Not Necessarily Better

Athlete or not, you need protein. But what's enough? Is consuming more protein better if you're an athlete? This nutrient needs no special attention just because you're physically active or building muscle. For overall fitness or strength building, extra protein—beyond the amount recommended—offers no added performance benefits.

Your body uses protein for many purposes: to build and repair tissues; to make enzymes, hormones, and other body chemicals; to transport nutrients; to make your muscles contract; and to regulate body processes such as water balance. If you don't consume enough carbohydrates for your high-energy demands, your body uses protein for energy instead. That's counterproductive to your physical goals!

Although protein supplies energy, extra amounts aren't your best fuel. Extra calories from excess protein are stored as fat, not used for energy—if you already consume enough calories. For anyone, protein should supply 10 to 35 percent of overall calorie intake.

Most athletes need just slightly more protein than nonathletes do. Because athletes usually eat more, they easily get what they need.

How Much Protein?

Interestingly, you may think of muscles as all protein. Actually 15 to 20 percent is protein; 70 to 75 percent

is water; and 5 to 7 percent is fat, glycogen, and minerals. How much protein do you need for sports? Base the amount on body weight, not calorie need.

● For most recreational exercisers, 0.5 to 0.75 gram of protein per pound of body weight is enough. (The upper end of the range is recommended for athletes involved in strength training or for those who must restrict calories.) For a 150-pound athlete that's about 75 to 115 grams of protein each day . . . and just 2 to 4 ounces more meat, chicken, or fish a day than recommended for nonathletes. For reference, 3 ounces of lean beef supply about 30 grams of protein, 8 ounces of milk supply 8 grams of protein, and a slice of bread has 2 grams of protein or more.

● Adult endurance athletes need 0.6 to 0.7 gram of protein per pound of body weight. Adults building muscle mass, including weight lifters and football players, may need 0.7 to 0.8 gram of protein daily per pound. Teen athletes need enough for growth and muscle building: 0.7 to 0.9 gram of protein per pound.

Source for protein needs: N. Clark, *Nancy Clark's Sport Nutrition Guidebook,* 4th ed. (Champaign, Ill.: Human Kinetics, 2008).

Muscle Myths

You've likely heard the myth: Extra protein builds more muscle. In truth, only athletic training builds muscle strength and size. Consuming more protein—from food or dietary supplements—won't make a difference. You've got to work your muscles!

Can amino acid supplements build muscle? Despite claims, they won't increase muscle size or strength. Amino acids are building blocks of protein. Twenty different amino acids link to make proteins in food and in body tissue. Food supplies amino acids in proportions your body needs. To your body, amino acids in supplements are no different from those in foods. In food they "taste" better and likely cost much less.

Most athletes get enough protein—and enough amino acids—from food. Protein-rich foods supply other nutrients, too; amino acid supplements supply only amino acids. So an extra protein shake? Save your money!

Caution about excess protein: Extra protein is *not* stored in your body for future use as protein. Instead, it's either used as energy or stored as body fat. A high-protein diet also may be high in fat.

Excessive protein or amino acids can be harmful. Side effects include metabolic imbalance, toxicity, nervous system disorders, and perhaps kidney problems.

When you consume excess protein, you need more water to excrete the urea, a waste product formed when protein is broken down. So excess protein increases the chances of dehydration—and increases the need to urinate. That's an inconvenience during a workout.

The bottom line: To build muscle, consume enough calories from carbs, follow advice for protein from food (no need for extra), and train regularly.

See "Ergogenic Aids: No Substitute for Training" later in this chapter.

Protein-Rich Foods: How Much?

The average American diet supplies more than enough protein. Just 6 to 7 ounces total of lean meat, poultry, or seafood, or the equivalent from eggs, beans, nuts, or seeds daily, along with protein from dairy foods and grain products, supply enough for most athletes. Athletes involved in endurance sports and weight lifters need somewhat more. Timing is important, too. A high-protein snack within the first hour or two after strength training helps stimulate muscle protein synthesis.

Good protein sources include lean meat, poultry, and fish; low-fat and fat-free milk, cheese, and yogurt; eggs; beans and tofu; and nuts, seeds, and peanut butter. Cereal, breads, and vegetables contain smaller amounts of protein. If you're a vegetarian, choose a variety of protein-containing foods carefully.

For more about protein and amino acids, see chapter 4, "Protein Power."

Vitamins and Minerals: Sense, Nonsense

Vitamins and minerals trigger body processes for physical performance. They don't supply energy, but some help produce energy from carbohydrates, fats, and proteins. Some help muscles relax and contract. Others are part of hemoglobin in blood that carries oxygen to cells to power aerobic activity. *See chapter 6 to learn more about vitamins and minerals.*

If you burn more energy, you need more of some vitamins and minerals. By eating enough from each of the five food groups, you likely consume enough vitamins and minerals. For those who might need slightly more, eating more food probably provides the extra. In fact, an athlete with a hearty appetite has a better chance of consuming enough vitamins and minerals than someone who's less active and eats less. However, athletes who try to lose weight by consuming too few calories or eliminating whole food groups are at greater risk for vitamin and mineral deficiencies.

For enough vitamins and minerals, eat recommended amounts from food group foods; *see chapter 10.*

Electrolytes? Sweat 'Em!

Sweat is made of water along with electrolyte minerals, including sodium, chloride, and potassium. Among their functions, electrolytes help maintain your body's water balance—crucial for athletes. They help your muscles, including your heart muscle, contract and relax. And they help transmit nerve impulses.

Taste the sweat on your upper lip. How salty it can be! As you perspire during a physical workout, your body loses small amounts of electrolytes, mostly sodium. Most athletes replace sodium and other electrolytes through foods they normally eat. Since you probably consume more than enough sodium to

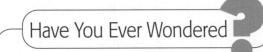

Have You Ever Wondered

. . . if athletes benefit from extra chromium? No, but misleading claims about chromium picolinate, which is a dietary supplement, have raised the question. No scientific evidence shows that taking a chromium supplement improves physical performance, builds muscle, burns body fat, or prolongs youth. For that matter, the role of chromium in your overall health isn't well understood, although early research suggests benefits to some people with diabetes or glucose intolerance.

Whole-grain foods, ready-to-eat cereals, beans, apples, and peanuts are some sources of chromium; most people get enough from their normal diet. Supplements aren't advised; chromium supplements may interfere with the work of iron in the blood.

. . . if taking salt tablets prevents muscle cramps? Sodium loss is only one factor that contributes to muscle cramping during exercise, especially during hot weather. Muscle fatigue and dehydration also increase the chance. Athletes who sweat heavily and whose skin becomes encrusted with a salt residue should consume salty foods, such as soup, ham-cheese-mustard sandwiches, or pasta with tomato sauce.

replace losses—no need for extra sodium. When you perspire heavily, focus on extra fluids instead.

Endurance athletes, who sweat heavily for long periods, may need to replace sodium and other electrolytes. A sports drink with electrolytes, plus salty foods such as crackers and cheese, probably offer enough. Sodium from those sources helps speed rehydration. *See "Sports Drinks?" earlier in this chapter.*

For more about electrolytes, chapters 6 and 7.

About Iron

Athletes: Your muscle cells need iron to produce energy! Iron is part of hemoglobin, the part of red blood cells that carries oxygen to your body cells. Oxygen is used in energy metabolism, specifically for aerobic activities where fat converts to energy. An iron shortfall, even if it's small, can affect your physical performance. Women who engage in vigorous, prolonged activity may be at special risk for iron depletion. Getting enough iron may be an issue—especially if you're female, or if most of your iron comes from foods of plant origin such as beans (legumes) and grains.

Even if you consume enough iron, you may be iron-depleted if you're involved in endurance sports. Prolonged exercise such as marathon running and long-distance bicycling promotes iron loss. With more exercise you sweat more, losing some iron through perspiration. Endurance athletes may lose iron through urine, feces, and intestinal bleeding. If you're an endurance athlete, have your iron status checked periodically by your doctor.

Unless prescribed by your doctor, don't take an iron supplement. Be aware that iron supplementation is harmful to those with a genetic disorder called hemochromatosis.

For more about iron, its recommended amounts, and food sources, see chapter 6; also see "Menstrual Cycle: More Iron for Women" in chapter 18.

Calcium, Vitamin D, and Weight-Bearing Exercise: Bone-Building Trio

Calcium, vitamin D, and weight-bearing exercise: They're a winning combination for building and maintaining strong, healthy bones. Your goal? To maximize your calcium stores early in life, then maintain that level to later minimize the loss that comes with age.

Consuming enough calcium, at least 1,000 to 1,300

Have You Ever Wondered

. . . if heavy training causes "sports anemia"? Perhaps, early in training. "Sports anemia" isn't really anemia. Because blood volume increases in the early weeks of endurance training, iron concentration in blood dilutes slightly as the body adapts to more physical activity.

If you develop sports anemia, that's normal. It will disappear once your training program is off and running. With endurance training your blood's capacity to carry oxygen and your athletic performance will improve. Taking iron supplements isn't helpful or advised.

Feeling tired may result from other aspects of training. If fatigue persists, or if you think you're at risk for other types of anemia, check with your doctor. *See "Anemia: 'Tired Blood'" in chapter 22.*

milligrams a day, depending on your age, and enough vitamin D offers protection against bone loss. Outdoor athletes likely get enough vitamin D because their skin is exposed to sunlight; indoor athletes may not. *See chapter 6 for more about vitamin D.*

Weight-bearing activity such as running, cross-country skiing, tennis, and soccer promotes the deposit of calcium into the matrix, or structure, of bones. While swimming and cycling offer many benefits of physical activity, they aren't weight-bearing, so they don't help to build bone.

Calcium and female athletes. Calcium is an issue. Why? To start with, many (including teens) don't consume enough calcium and vitamin D for bone health.

Active women who repeatedly consume too few calories—perhaps due to disordered eating—to meet their training needs risk having their menstrual periods stop. For teens and young women this hinders the deposit of calcium into bones at a time when bones should be developing at their maximum rate. Female athletes who've stopped menstruating are at special risk for developing stress fractures, decreased bone mineral density, and other bone problems.

When these three issues—low calorie intake, disrupted menstrual function, and poor bone health—come together, it's called the female athlete triad. Female athletes involved in sports that focus on leanness and aesthetics, such as cheerleading, diving, distance running, figure skating, and gymnastics, are at greater risk.

Women: For your bones' sake, pay attention if your periods stop. Talk to your doctor. This is *not* a normal outcome of physical activity. Stress fractures caused by weakened bones may seriously affect your physical performance. The long-range impact on bone health: increased osteoporosis risk. For bone health, your doctor may recommend a higher calcium intake, or perhaps a calcium supplement. *See "Osteoporosis: Reduce the Risks" in chapter 22.*

Supplements: Not "Energy-Charged"

Contrary to unscientific claims, there's likely no need for vitamin or mineral supplements for sports if you're already well nourished. The "extra" won't offer an energy boost or added physical benefits—immediately or over the long run. Even if you're deficient in one or more nutrients, popping a supplement pill right before physical activity has no immediate effect.

Although B vitamins help your body use energy from food, no vitamin supplies energy. Since you likely eat more when you're physically active, you'll get the extra B vitamins you need from food—if your food choices are varied and nutrient-rich.

If you decide to take a supplement, choose a "multi" with no more than 100 percent of the Daily Values (DVs) for vitamins and minerals—unless your doctor prescribes more for special health reasons. *See "Dietary Supplements: Defined" in chapter 23.*

A High-Performance Diet

Healthful eating prepares you to achieve and maintain your strength, flexibility, and endurance. What's the best training diet? One that's varied, moderate, and balanced. Sound familiar? It's high in carbohydrates, with enough proteins, vitamins, minerals, and it's moderate in fat. High-performance eating is appropriate for all physically active people, not just those training for sports.

Food Guide for Athletes

Except for calories, healthful eating for athletics and for rigorous active living doesn't differ much from advice for nonathletes. Both on- and off-season, the USDA Food Patterns offer healthful eating guidelines. Because they're flexible, they work—no matter how many calories you need or what sport you choose. There's no single eating plan for sports. You can customize!

For many athletes, energy needs are high—as many as 6,000 calories a day, for example, for some football players. To meet higher energy demands, choose more servings of nutrient-rich, carbohydrate-rich foods, mostly from the grain group and the vegetable and fruit groups of the food guide. In contrast, although a high-fat diet offers plenty of concentrated energy (from fat), it carries risks for heart disease—even for highly active people. *For more about food guides, see chapter 10.*

The "USDA Food Patterns" in the appendices can help you determine how much to eat from each food group based on your calorie needs.

An added reminder: Drink enough fluids during training. It's a good time to practice drinking "on schedule," not just for thirst.

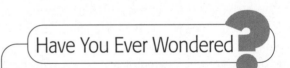

Have You Ever Wondered

. . . if vegetarians have other sports nutrition concerns? Vegetarian eating styles can provide enough fuel and nutrients for peak athletic performance—if chosen wisely. *See "The Vegetarian Way," in chapter 10.* As with any high-performance diet, carbohydrate-rich foods should provide the most calories, or food energy—usually not an issue for vegetarians. Consuming enough calories from an eating plan of bulky, plant-based foods may be challenging for some vegetarian athletes. Eating six to eight meals or snacks of nutrient-rich foods a day is one practical solution.

. . . how to eat after you're no longer in training? Many athletes never address that! Whether you're a college athlete who stops training or an elite athlete who retires, "retrain" for healthful eating. Less physical activity; loss of muscle mass; and for some, increased food intake can contribute to weight gain. You'll likely need fewer calories, even though your nutrient needs remain about the same. *For guidance see chapter 10, "Planning to Eat Smart."* A registered dietitian can help you, too. See *"How to Find Nutrition Help . . ." in chapter 24.*

Especially for Children and Teens

You've heard that today's kids don't move enough. Yet many do enjoy vigorous play or competitive sports. And their food and beverage choices power all they do: first and foremost, for growth and development, and second, for the added demands of physical activity.

Many situations, often unplanned, affect what kids eat and, as a result, their physical performance: early lunch hours and after-school competition; practice that goes into family meal hours; two-sport athletes with little time to recover before competing again; sports fatigue that preempts homework and meals; and nervousness so kids don't eat planned precompetition carried food. These challenges need smart, practical snack and meal solutions.

Nutrients for Active Kids. Healthy eating guidelines apply to young athletes. Except for calories and fluids, the nutrients for young athletes and nonathletes are about the same. For serious young athletes who train intensely, talk to your doctor or a registered dietitian for guidance; getting enough iron, calcium, and vitamin D, for example, may be issues. Also be aware that growing bones are more susceptible to sports injury from impact and excessive use.

Food Energy for Active Kids. Energy needs depend on age, growth stage, body size, and sport. *Check "Estimated Calorie Needs Per Day by Age, Gender, and Physical Activity Level" in the appendices.* Some very active kids may need more calories to fuel activity.

Does your highly active child consume enough calories? Here's a clue: Watch his or her performance. Children who tire easily may not be eating enough. Another clue: Monitor your child's growth with your physician. If your child is growing normally, his or her energy (caloric) intake is likely okay. If you're still unsure, ask your doctor to refer you to a registered dietitian who can help you create an eating plan that matches your child's calorie needs.

Fluids: Caution for Kids. Children are more likely to get overheated from strenuous activity. As a result, they're at greater risk for dehydration. Even when they play actively in the backyard, they need plenty of fluids.

Why is the risk for dehydration higher? Because kids perspire less than teens and adults, their body's "air conditioning" system is less effective. Kids generate more body heat with exercise, too. A child's "thermostat" doesn't adjust as quickly during exercise in hot weather. Protective gear for many sports, such as hockey and football, hinders the ability to cool off, too.

To protect children from becoming dehydrated:

● Encourage them to drink plenty of cool fluids before, during, and after physical activities.

● Offer regular fluid breaks (every fifteen minutes) and ensure that fluids are readily available. Perhaps give them each a water bottle. Once they're thirsty, they're already on the way to dehydration.

● Weigh them before and after exercise, then replace fluids: 3 cups per pound of weight loss.

● Supervise them carefully, especially on hot days, when fluid needs are even greater.

See chapter 17 for more about food for active kids.

Weight: For Young Athletes

For all children, normal growth and development should be the top priority. Their weight should never be manipulated to meet goals required for sports!

Child athletes aren't the same as teen and adult athletes. Because they're growing and because their growth spurts aren't always predictable, their body composition can't be judged in the same way. At certain times—for example, before puberty—a child's body naturally stores more body fat to prepare for the next growth spurt. Each child matures at his or her own time and rate.

An eating approach for sports can't change the genetic "body clock" and so speed up physical changes that enhance athletic performance. Supplements and ergogenic aids that are promoted to build muscle, prevent fat gain, or improve performance are never appropriate for children and teens! *For more about healthful eating during childhood and adolescence, see chapter 17.*

For young athletes, weight goals should be healthy ones. A distorted body image that drives overexercising and undereating can lead to serious developmental and health problems. That includes the "female athlete triad": a problem of disordered eating, low bone density, and amenorrhea (cessation of menstruation).

Always talk to your doctor about the best weight for your child. An inaccurate assessment may result in a weight goal that isn't healthy.

For more information about body weight, see "Compete in a Weight Category?" later in this chapter.

During Pregnancy and Breast-feeding

Pregnancy. With their doctor's approval, active women may continue their sport. Less active women may start low-level activities gradually—again with their doctor's approval. Being physically active during pregnancy offers many benefits, among them a psychological lift, optimal weight gain, better aerobic fitness, and an easier labor and delivery

If you're pregnant, or planning to be, ask your doctor about precautions. Overheating your body from exercise, a sauna, or a steam room early in pregnancy can affect the development of your unborn baby. If you have anemia, hypertension, diabetes, or other health problems, rigorous activity during pregnancy may not be advised.

All the nutritional issues that relate to a healthy pregnancy apply to female athletes, too. Eat a varied and balanced diet—with enough calories to support your pregnancy, your own needs, and the demands of physical activity. If your calorie intake is too low, you may not gain enough weight and your baby may not grow adequately.

Fluid replacement, always important, has even more health implications now. During pregnancy you need more fluids as your own and your baby's blood volumes increase. If you don't drink enough, you're at greater risk for dehydration and overheating.

Breast-feeding. With a doctor's guidance, most women can engage in sports or some other form of regular physically activity if they're breast-feeding.

Breast-feeding requires an additional 330 to 400 calories a day for milk production. With more physical activity, you need more; the actual amount depends on the duration and the intensity of your workout.

For athletes and nonathletes alike, the USDA Food Patterns offer guidance for planning a varied, balanced, and moderate eating plan during breast-feeding. Your fluid needs increase during breast-feeding, too. Without exercise, you need about 4 cups more, or at least 15 cups daily from food, beverages, and drinking water. When you work out, drink even more.

For more about healthful eating and physical activity during pregnancy and breast-feeding, see "You're Expecting!" and "For Those Who Breast-feed" in chapter 18.

Different Sports, Different Eating Approaches

No matter what the sport, the USDA Food Patterns are basic guides for high-performance eating: enough nutrient-rich food-group foods for the calories you need.

Calorie, or energy, need is the most significant nutrition difference from sport to sport. The duration and intensity of activity, as well as body size, make the difference.

● A 200-pound football player uses more energy than a 90-pound gymnast.

● A baseball player uses less energy than a soccer player, who's almost constantly in motion.

● An endurance cross-country skier or a long-distance runner likely uses more energy overall than a tennis player or a golfer, who uses spurts of energy for a shorter time.

Every sport demands adequate fluids to replace perspiration and breathing losses, too. In sports with prolonged, intense activity, athletes may perspire more—especially during hot weather.

Endurance Sports

Both in training and in competition, endurance sports—cross-country and marathon running, cross-country skiing, distance bicycling, field hockey, long-distance swimming, and soccer—require more energy. Activity that lasts longer than several hours depletes glycogen stores. Carbohydrate consumed during exercise helps endurance athletes maintain a fast pace; fat is used more efficiently for fuel as exercise continues. Also, protein is a minor fuel source during endurance exercise. Endurance athletes do not need to consume more protein than strength-training athletes; adult endurance athletes should aim for 0.6 to 0.7 gram of protein per pound of body weight.

Energy needed for endurance sports depends on body size, duration of activity, and overall effort. An elite athlete may need 4,000 to 6,000 calories daily, chosen from a high-carbohydrate diet. *Best sources:* nutrient-rich foods from all food groups of the USDA Food Patterns.

Nonendurance Sports

Nonendurance sports—baseball, bowling, golf, martial arts, softball, speed skating, sprint swimming, tennis, track and field, volleyball, and weight lifting—are fueled by short bursts of energy, perhaps just for two or three minutes or even several seconds. While these sports take an intense, all-out effort, they don't use as much energy overall.

Still, nonendurance sports might be of high or moderate intensity. The overall energy demand depends not only on the duration but also on the intensity and the athlete's body size.

Except for calories, nutrient needs for athletes involved in endurance and nonendurance sports are about the same. Again, the USDA Food Patterns represented by MyPlate offer a healthful eating guideline, with an emphasis on nutrient-rich, carbohydrate-rich foods. *See chapter 10 for more information.*

Making Weight

Most athletes are concerned about their weight. For football, extra weight may be an advantage for a defensive lineman. For swimmers, some body fat may offer buoyancy. For gymnasts and skaters, a slim body may add to the aesthetics of performance.

For some athletes, weight cycling is an issue. Those who weigh more during their off-season may need to drop a few pounds for training and competition. Others need to "bulk up," perhaps to train and compete in contact sports. Either way, what's the healthful, most effective approach to your best competitive weight?

Whatever your sport, for your peak performance, enter the competitive season at your best weight. Instead of trying to "make weight" quickly to train and compete, stay at your best weight year-'round.

Body Composition: Fit, Not Fat

For athletic performance (strength, speed, endurance), your body composition is more important than your weight—even if you compete in a weight category. (That's true for nonathletes, too.) Health risks go up as the proportion of body fat increases beyond "healthy." A lean, muscular body has benefits beyond athletics and good looks: overall fitness for life!

What's healthy for athletes? There's no single body fat percentage to aim for, even for the same sport. For your own best performance, the percent body fat for you depends on the body type you were born with. *Refer to "Body Fat for Adults: Leaner with Physical*

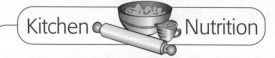

Food for Your Training Table

For meals that are high in carbohydrates, adequate in protein, and moderate in fat, try these meal combos:

- Chili made with kidney beans and lean beef.
- Stir-fry with vegetables and lean pork, chicken, shrimp, or tofu served over rice (easy on the oil).
- Soft corn tortillas filled with vegetarian refried beans and topped with tomato sauce or salsa, and cheese. (On a can of refried beans, check the fat content on the label's Nutrition Facts.)
- Grilled fish kebobs (chunks of fresh fish alternating with cherry tomatoes, green peppers, and pineapple on a skewer) served on brown rice.
- Lentils (alone or mixed with lean ground beef) in spaghetti sauce on whole-wheat pasta.
- Green peppers stuffed with a lean ground turkey–brown rice mixture. Add a mixed green salad. Finish the meal with angel food cake topped with strawberries.
- Lean roast sirloin strips with a baked potato, steamed carrots, cauliflower, and whole-wheat rolls.
- Chicken salad (with reduced-calorie mayonnaise, grated lemon peel, and tarragon) on rye bread with tomato slices and sprouts. Serve with vegetable soup, whole-wheat crackers, and cantaloupe.

Training" in this chapter. Calorie restriction associated with too little body fat not only jeopardizes athletic performance but also health. In general, less than 5 percent body fat for men and less than 12 percent body fat for women have been defined as risky; the percent body fat that's considered risky for you may differ.

You can't measure your body fat or composition accurately. Instead, seek a trained health expert who uses professional methods for measurement, such as skinfold measurements, air displacement, and bioelectrical impedance (done with a computer). A registered dietitian or an exercise physiologist can help you target goals for a healthy weight and body composition for your best physical performance. *See "How to Find Nutrition Help . . ." in chapter 24. For more about body composition, see "Body Weight, Body Fat?" in chapter 2.*

Lose Fat, Not Muscle

Do you need to lose weight? Choose an approach that helps you lose fat, not muscle. Start your weight loss strategies ahead—well before training and competition. Then maintain your healthy weight so you have energy and strength when you need them most.

Getting the Lean Advantage

Most important, set a weight goal that's realistic and healthy for you—one that considers your body composition and that offers the best competitive edge for your sport. If you need to drop a few pounds, make your weight loss gradual: ½ to 1 pound a week. To lose about 1 pound a week, cut back on your day's energy intake by about 250 calories and boost your training to burn 250 calories more. (*Hint:* 1 pound of body fat equals 3,500 calories.) To cut back on calories, follow guidelines of the USDA Food Patterns at a calorie level that's lower for you than usual, and somewhat lower in calories than what your body uses. *See "Food Guide for Athletes" earlier in this chapter.*

Carbohydrates are the fuel that your working muscles need. Get most of your calories from starches (complex carbohydrates): grain products, including whole grains, beans (legumes), vegetables, and fruits. Cut back on higher-fat foods.

For weight loss, physical activity does more than burn calories. Exercise boosts your metabolic rate, or the rate at which your body uses energy. Muscles use more energy than body fat does.

A quick weight-loss regimen that's low in calories may interfere with your physical performance, first by shorting your energy supply. With many quick regimens you may lose muscle, along with body fat, and deplete your stores of muscle glycogen. Weight loss may be partly water loss—a problem for athletes, who need to keep adequately hydrated.

In your off-season training program, learn to maintain weight so you stay at the best weight for your sport. *To lose weight in a healthful way, see "Weight Management: Strategies That Work!" in chapter 2.*

"Leanest" Isn't Always Better!

The notion that you can never be too thin or too lean may compromise your physical performance. Athletes obsessed with a lean, thin body risk eating disorders and all the dangers (some life-threatening) that accom-

---

Body Fat for Adults: Leaner with Physical Training

Optimal body fat ranges vary from athlete to athlete, sport to sport, and even for a specific position or event on a team. If you're a serious or perhaps an elite athlete, talk to your physician, qualified trainer, or registered dietitian to set your goal for body fat composition.* It's usually lower than that for most active healthy people.

| | **Percent Body Fat** | | |
	Age (years)	Women	Men
For overall health	<55	20–35	8–22
	>55	25–38	10–25
For people in substantial	<55	16–28	5–15
physical training	>55	20–33	7–18

Source: Marie Dunford, editor, *Sports Nutrition: A Practice Manual for Professionals* (Chicago: American Dietetic Association, 2006).

*Specific goals vary among sports.

---

pany severe weight loss. Among other concerns, a poorly fueled body that's too lean may not sweat and cool down properly. The chance for dehydration goes up. Some body fat has other functions: Fat cushions body organs, providing protection from injury. During endurance sports, both carbohydrate and fat provide energy for working muscles. If you're too lean, you may tire quickly. Restricting calorie intake too much to avoid body fat may result in a nutrient deficiency.

If you, someone you train with, or your child or teen show signs of an eating disorder, seek help. Talk to the person about your concern, as well as the family, friends, or the coach. *See "Disordered Eating: Problems, Signs, and Help" in chapter 2.*

Compete in a Weight Category?

If you're a wrestler, weight lifter, oarsman, boxer, or body builder who competes in a weight category, body weight may be critically important. Being the heaviest competitor in a lower weight class often is believed to provide a competitive edge. Even an extra pound or two may affect weight class or performance.

For good health, endurance, strength, and best performance, the better advice is to compete in a weight class that's realistic for your body composition and to maintain your optimal weight throughout the competitive season, rather than cycle to "make weight" in unhealthful ways for competition.

Water weight is *not* unnecessary body weight, so sweating off pounds to make weight for wrestling—or any other sport—can potentially hinder performance. Because it leads to dehydration, losing as little as 2 to 3 percent of body weight from sweat (e.g., 3 or 4 pounds, or 6 to 8 cups of fluid, in a 150-pound athlete) can be very dangerous.

Fasting, or drastically cutting back on food, isn't healthy or performance-enhancing, either! Feeling hungry is distracting. Never advised, with fasting your body won't store muscle glycogen as energy for training and competition. Fasting often causes fatigue, the potential for muscle loss, dehydration, and decreased performance. A careful healthful eating plan—that starts well before "weigh in"—is the smartest way to reach and stay in your weight class. Without ongoing, sensible weight management you might continue with the same weight dilemma and "weight cycle" for the next competition—and the next and the next!

Gain Muscle, Not Fat

Hockey and football are among the sports where extra body weight aids performance. Trying to "bulk up" too fast, however, may put on more fat than muscle—especially if you eat extra calories without enough exercise. If you're already in strenuous training, gaining weight may not be as easy as it sounds. You may use energy faster than you consume it!

To build muscle, engage in strength-building activity and consume enough calories. Contrary to myth, you need only a little extra protein to help build muscle. *See "Muscle Myths" earlier in this chapter.*

As with weight loss, the key to weight gain is "gradual and steady": about ½ to 1 pound a week. To get the extra energy to fuel exercise and build muscle:

● Increase portions at mealtime.

● Snack between meals.

● Drink extra 100 percent juice, low-fat chocolate milk, or fruit smoothies.

● Get most of your extra calories from nutrient-rich, high-carbohydrate foods—for example, granola or muesli topped with nuts or dried fruit. *For guidance on healthy weight gain, see chapter 2.*

The Game Plan

It's the day of the big event. You're excited and perhaps a bit anxious. You've trained hard. What should you eat to maximize your performance? Your game plan now—what you eat before, during, and after competition or a heavy workout—makes a difference.

For endurance events, think further ahead—before your pre-event meal. Several days beforehand, you might eat more carbohydrates and gradually rest your muscles. In that way, you'll store extra muscle glycogen and won't tire as quickly during the event. *See "Carbohydrate Loading" earlier in this chapter.*

For any sport, eat well ahead for peak performance. Most energy for competition comes from foods you ate earlier, not from your pre-event meal. For training, eat plenty of carbohydrates, moderate amounts of protein, and not much fat, and drink plenty of fluids. On competition day, even carefully planned meals can't make up for a poor training diet. Eat for fitness all along. Read on for general advice.

Before You Compete

Choose a pre-event meal or snack—light, easy to digest, high-carbohydrate—that matches your physical performance goals. In that way you can perform to your ability without tiring too soon. Eating helps prevent the distraction of hunger pangs and supplies energy for exercise that lasts an hour or more. Drink enough, too, to fully hydrate your body before strenuous exercise.

The "right" pre-event meal or snack differs from athlete to athlete, event to event, and time of day. During your training, experiment with different foods, food combinations, amounts, and timing.

Timing. Finish eating one to four hours before your workout or competition. That allows enough time for food to digest so you don't feel full or uncomfortable.

Morning competition? Eat a hearty, high-carbohydrate dinner and bedtime snack the night before. In the morning, eat a light, high-carbohydrate meal or snack. Eating two hours before exercise helps replenish your liver glycogen and satisfy hunger.

Small meals. Choose a small meal or snack. The amount depends on what makes you feel comfortable.

High "carbs." Enjoy a high-carb meal or snack that's moderate in protein and low in fat. It gets digested and absorbed faster. (About 1/2 gram to 2 grams of carbohydrate per pound of body weight is about right.)

Make pasta, rice, potatoes, or bread the "center" of your plate. A high-fat meal may cause indigestion or nausea with heavy exercise. *See "Pre-Event Meals . . . For Starters."*

Contrary to common belief, eating small amounts of fat won't keep your body from storing muscle glycogen. A little fat adds flavor and helps you meet your overall energy needs.

A steak dinner? The fats and proteins in steak take longer to digest than carbohydrates do. If steak gives you a "mental edge," enjoy a small portion, along with carbohydrate-rich foods: perhaps a baked potato, pasta, or rice; carrots; a dinner roll; a fruit salad; and frozen yogurt for dessert. Allow several hours for the meal to digest.

No discomfort. Skip foods that may cause intestinal discomfort during competition: gas-causing foods such as beans, cabbage, onions, cauliflower, and turnips, and bulky, high-fiber foods such as raw fruits and vegetables with seeds and tough skin, bran, nuts, and seeds.

Familiar foods. Enjoy familiar foods and beverages. This isn't the time to try something new that may disagree with you.

Enough fluids. About two to three hours ahead, drink at least 2 cups of fluids. Then about fifteen minutes ahead, drink another 1 to 1 1/2 cups of fluids. Milk's okay. Stress and loss of body fluids—not milk—often slow saliva flow, causing "cotton mouth," or a dry mouth.

"Feel-good" foods. If a certain food or meal seems to enhance your performance, enjoy it—if you can fit it into your pre-event eating strategy.

During Competition

Nourishment now depends on your sport.

● *During most activities,* drinking plenty of fluids is the only real issue. Every fifteen or so minutes, drink enough to minimize loss of body weight, without over-drinking: 1/2 to 1 1/2 cups every 15 minutes.

● *During endurance sports of sixty minutes or more,* a slightly sweetened carbohydrate drink (sports drink) or snack may help maintain your blood glucose levels, boost your stamina, and enhance your performance. Figure about 0.5 gram of carbohydrate per pound of your body weight per hour.

Sports drinks are easy to digest, especially during intense activity. And they count as fluids. Their flavor may encourage their consumption, especially among children. Drink fluids every fifteen or so minutes!

● *During day-long events or regional tournaments,* snack on high-carbohydrate, low-fat foods. Between matches, sets, or other competitive events, crackers, bagels, rice cakes, orange slices, apples, bananas, and fruit bars are good choices. Bring snacks so you don't need to rely on a concession stand. Consuming fluids all day long remains important.

After You Compete

Your cool-down routine is as important as your warm-up. What you eat and drink for recovery after a work-

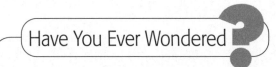

Have You Ever Wondered

. . . about competing on an empty stomach? You're better off eating. Food consumed within four hours of physical activity is fuel for working muscles. For morning events, eating is especially important for endurance. It replenishes liver glycogen and helps maintain your blood sugar level. Don't skip breakfast; eat something light!

. . . what to eat before competition if you feel too nervous to eat? Drinking a liquid meal supplement or a fruit milk shake might help. It provides nutrients and fluids needed for competition. And it might be more easily digested and absorbed than a full meal.

. . . if a "complete nutrition supplement," perhaps an energy bar or drink, or a power gel, aids performance? Not "complete nutrition," energy bars and drinks may be an energy source, but not a meal replacement. Power gels supply "carbs," too, but usually few vitamins or minerals. A quick check of the Nutrition Facts reveals their calorie and nutrient contribution. Energy bars, drinks, or gels may be convenient during an endurance event; enjoy a carbohydrate-protein combination food afterward, such as low-fat chocolate milk or a fruity yogurt.

out is as important as your pre-event eating routine. Start with a snack or meal within fifteen to sixty minutes after practice or competition.

Make fluids your first priority! After competition or a heavy workout, replace your fluid loss. The amount depends on how much weight you lose through exercise. Simply weigh yourself before and afterward; the difference is your water weight. Replenish the loss: For every pound you lose, drink 3 cups of fluid. Continue to drink fluids throughout the day or several days until you return to your pre-exercise weight if you lost weight.

What fluids are best? Drink fluids with carbohydrates, such as juice or sports drinks. They replace fluids and electrolytes and help your body replenish muscle glycogen. Plain water and watery foods, such as soup, watermelon, and grapes, are good fluid recovery foods, too. *See chapter 8.*

Refuel your muscles with carbohydrates. Within the first several hours after competition or a heavy workout, eat a carbohydrate-rich meal or snack. For muscle recovery, the sooner, the better. For strength training and muscle recovery, include a high-quality protein source, such as milk, lean meat, fish, or poultry.

For every pound of body weight, strive for about 0.5 gram of carbohydrates. For example, if you weigh 150 pounds, eat at least 75 grams of carbohydrates. That's easy to do with a high-carbohydrate snack or meal. For strenuous exercise that lasts ninety minutes or longer,

consume that much in carbohydrates within thirty minutes after exercise, then again about two hours later. A little protein eaten with carbohydrate foods, perhaps milk with cereal, aids recovery.

If you aren't hungry right after a training session, drink juice or a sports drink for fluids and carbs.

Have You Ever Wondered ?

… where to get sports-specific nutrition advice—or to find out if your food choices help or hinder your training? Talk to a sports dietitian, a registered dietitian with a specialty in sports nutrition, or other qualified expert for help in determining your energy needs, evaluating your eating plan, and strategizing ways to eat for peak performance. *Be aware:* "Personal trainer" isn't a regulated professional specialty. Some trainers are highly qualified exercise specialists; others aren't. To find a local sports dietitian, use the referral network from the Academy of Nutrition and Dietetics: www.SCANdpg.org.

… if drinking milk before a heavy workout causes stomach cramps? Contrary to myth, drinking milk before physical exertion doesn't cause stomach discomfort or digestive problems. If you have any discomfort after drinking milk, you may be sensitive to lactose, the naturally occurring sugar in milk. *See chapter 21 to learn about lactose maldigestion and intolerance.* Besides its role in bone health, calcium in milk is needed for muscle contraction.

Pre-Event Meals: For Starters

There's no single menu prescribed for pre-event eating, but these three high-carbohydrate menus show what you might eat before you compete:

MEAL 1	MEAL 2	MEAL 3
● 1 cup cornflakes	● 2 cups beef noodle soup	● 2 6-inch pancakes with 2 tbsp. syrup
● 1 small banana	● 6 whole wheat crackers	● 1 large scrambled egg
● 8 oz. fat-free milk	● 1 medium baked potato	● ½ cup sliced strawberries
● 1 3-inch bagel with 1 tbsp. jelly and 1 tbsp. peanut butter	● 8 oz. low-fat fruit yogurt	● 1 cup apple juice
● ¾ cup cranberry juice drink		
Calories 715	*Calories* 670	*Calories* 685
Carbohydrates 139 g	*Carbohydrates* 115 g	*Carbohydrates* 106 g

Because sports drinks are a diluted source of "carbs," double the amount of sports drink to get the same amount of carbohydrates—for example, 32 ounces of a sports drink and 16 ounces of juice each supply about 50 grams of carbohydrates. When your hunger returns, enjoy a high-carbohydrate meal or snack.

How about electrolytes? Through perspiration, you lose electrolytes such as sodium. Your meal—and perhaps a sports drink—after endurance sports will undoubtedly provide enough sodium and other electrolytes to replace your losses.

Protein for recovery. Eat foods that provide protein to help repair damaged muscle tissue and stimulate the development of new tissue. That's especially important if you're involved in high-intensity training that may damage muscle tissue (e.g., resistance training, interval sessions).

Ergogenic Aids:
No Substitute for Training

"Blast your body with energy!" "Best muscle volumizers!" "Guaranteed for muscle growth!" "For faster muscle recovery and longer endurance!"

Of course, you want to make the most of every workout and increase your competitive edge. But do you take supplements without questioning their merits? It's easy to be lured by advertising claims that dietary and hormonal supplements improve strength, endurance, or recovery time, especially when anatomical graphics and charts make claims appear well-researched. Yet, valid and invalid advice often appear side by side in fitness magazines.

"Ergogenic" means the potential to increase work output. Only proper training and nutrition can do that.

What about "proven results"? Perceived performance benefits of ergogenic aids often come from individual reports, a misunderstanding of physiology, or from claims taken out of scientific context. Benefits may be more psychological than physical. It's well documented that the side effects of taking many ergogenic aids may hinder performance and may cause harm, especially in the long run!

Dietary Supplements

Many dietary supplements—amino acid supplements, bee pollen, carnitine, chromium picolinate, ephedra, glutamine, and HMB (beta-hydroxy beta methylbutyrate), among others, as well as many herbs—are promoted for better physical performance. Yet, their effectiveness and safety are undetermined. (*Note:* Ephedra is now banned by the U.S. FDA for sale as a supplement although the ruling has been challenged; some over-the-counter medications may contain ephedrine.) And they're costly!

● *Amino acids.* Amino acid supplements such as arginine, branched-chain amino acids (BCAAs), and ornithine are promoted to build muscle and increase fat loss. Most athletes consume more than enough amino acids from food; these products are an unnecessary expense. *See "Muscle Myths" in this chapter.*

● *Carnitine.* Promoted for more energy, aerobic power, and body fat reduction, carnitine is composed of two essential amino acids, lysine and methionine. However, the human body produces adequate amounts; foods of animal origin are good sources. There's no need for extra. For improved athletic performance, it's ineffective.

● *Creatine monohydrate.* This ergogenic aid is promoted to increase muscle mass and strength, enhance energy, and delay fatigue. In fact, creatine is

---

Snacks and Meals—For Recovery

Snack Ideas

● Smoothie made with yogurt and frozen berries
● Sports drink (carbohydrate, electrolyte fluid) + sport bar (carbohydrate, protein)
● Graham crackers with peanut butter + low-fat chocolate milk + banana

Meal Ideas

● Whole wheat pita sandwich with turkey and veggies + pretzels + low-fat milk
● Rice bowl with beans, cheese, salsa, avocado + whole-grain tortilla chips or whole-wheat tortilla
● Stir-fry with lean steak, broccoli, bell peppers, carrots + brown rice

Source: Sports, Cardiovascular and Wellness Nutrition (SCAN) Dietary Practice Group, Academy of Nutrition and Dietetics.

a nitrogen-containing compound that's found naturally in meat and fish, in the human brain, and in muscle. Research suggests that creatine supplements may promote muscle strength, help increase body weight, and aid recovery after strength training or short bouts of high-intensity activity. Creatine supplements aren't advised for teenage athletes, who need to learn what their bodies can do with hard training.

● *Spirulina.* Spirulina, a blue-green algae, is marketed as a high-energy food. It's high in protein with small amounts of vitamin B_{12}, but has no unique energy-producing qualities. Much of its vitamin B_{12} is inactive and cannot be absorbed by humans.

● *Wheat germ and wheat germ oil.* Both products are promoted as ergogenic aids. Although no proven benefits exist, there are no known side effects or adverse reactions from ingesting them. Wheat germ supplies nutrients such as proteins, B vitamins, and vitamin E.

The NCAA advises school athletes to check with the athletics staff before using dietary supplements, as some may contain banned substances not listed on the supplement label. *See chapter 23 for more about dietary supplements.*

Hormone Supplements

Hormone supplements, or steroids, are another type of supplement that may increase muscle mass—but at a price to health. An ergogenic aid, they're powerful yet dangerous drugs!

Teens should *never* use steroids. Contrary to many a young adolescent boy's wish, steroids won't bulk up muscles before puberty. Adolescents who use them may not grow to their normal height.

● *Androstenedione*, or "andro," is an anabolic steroid that acts like testosterone, a male sex hormone. "Anabolic" refers to the metabolic processes of synthesizing body tissue. Steroids can help build bigger muscles, as well as increase strength, alter mood, and decrease body fat. However, they don't ensure better physical performance.

Of concern, their use can have dangerous and often permanent side effects. For example, in men, steroids may cause acne, testicular damage, enlarged breasts, and a lower sperm count. Used by women, steroids may cause masculine qualities: a lower voice, facial hair, smaller breasts, and loss of (or an irregular) menstrual cycle. Other potential risks: increased risk for injury, blood clots, and gastrointestinal problems as well as liver damage, heart disease, and cancer. Steroid use is banned by the International Olympic Committee (IOC) and most other sports governing bodies and condemned by the American Academy of Pediatrics and the American College of Sports Medicine. In the Anabolic Steroid Control Act androstenedione is a controlled substance, listed as a banned anabolic steroid and an illegal performance-enhancing drug.

● *Dehydroepiandrosterone (DHEA)*, sold as a safe alternative to anabolic steroids, is an androgenic steroid, banned by the IOC and the National Collegiate Athletic Association. "Androgenic" refers to the development of male characteristics. Evidence doesn't back up claims to increase energy, decrease body fat, counteract stress, and slow aging. In the short run, DHEA can have unpleasant side effects, including facial hair growth, acne, enlarged liver, rapid heartbeat, and testicular damage. With its potential effect on testosterone and estradiol (a female steroid produced in the ovaries) levels, its use may be risky for people with a family history of prostate or breast cancer.

Building muscle gradually through physical activity is the healthful, time-honored, most effective, and fair approach! *See "Muscle Myths" in this chapter.*

Need more tips specific to eating for active living? Check here for "how-tos":

● Manage weight for sports sensibly—see chapter 2.

● Spot the signs of eating disorders in athletes—see chapter 2.

● Exercise safely during pregnancy—see chapter 18.

● Sort through claims for ergogenic dietary supplements—see chapter 23.

● Seek advice from a sports dietitian, especially if you're an athlete who aspires to peak performance, an elite or professional athlete, or a physically active person with a health condition—see chapter 24.

CHAPTER 21

Sensitive to Food

A queasy stomach, itchy skin, or diarrhea—must be a reaction to something you ate, right? Maybe. But it may not be what you think. Before blaming food, take time to explore the cause.

Any food sensitivity—allergy, intolerance, or other adverse reaction—can be a health concern. Some reactions cause discomfort. Others can seriously affect and disrupt the quality of life. And unfortunately for some people, some reactions can be life-threatening. Causes of these reactions are more numerous, and perhaps more complex, than you may think.

● *Food intolerances.* Different food intolerances have different causes. For metabolic reasons, people may not be able to digest a component of certain foods, perhaps because a digestive enzyme such as lactase is deficient. Naturally occurring substances such as theobromine in coffee or tea, or serotonin in bananas or tomatoes, may cause reactions, but they aren't life-threatening. Since food intolerances may prompt some similar symptoms (nausea, diarrhea, abdominal cramps), they're often mislabeled as food allergies.

● *Food allergies.* A food allergy rallies the body's disease-fighting (immune) system to action, creating unpleasant, sometimes serious, symptoms in response to a food component, usually a protein. The immune system starts to work even though the person isn't sick. That's why symptoms appear.

● *Other adverse reactions to food.* Infectious organisms such as bacteria, parasites, or viruses, which cause foodborne illness, or waterborne contaminants where seafood is harvested, can cause adverse body reactions. *See chapter 13, "The Safe Kitchen," to learn about foodborne illnesses.*

● *Psychological reasons.* Feelings of discomfort after eating also can be wrapped up with emotions. Even with no physiological reason, just thinking about, smelling, or tasting a certain food that someone associates with an unpleasant experience can make him or her feel sick. Even misperceiving a food as harmful may trigger discomfort!

Managing various adverse reactions differs. People with food allergies must eliminate certain foods from their diet. In contrast, with a food intolerance small servings of a problem food usually provide few, if any, unpleasant side effects. There are exceptions; those with celiac disease or a sulfite sensitivity must eliminate certain foods.

If a certain food seems to bother you, skip the temptation to self-diagnose. For example, a reaction to milk could be a digestive problem, not a food allergy. This chapter can help familiarize you with possible causes, health risks, and ways to handle food allergies and food intolerances. Your doctor should diagnose your symptoms!

Lactose Intolerance: A Matter of Degree

Do you like milk but think that milk doesn't like you? Then you may be lactose-intolerant—not allergic to milk. The good news is that milk may be "friendlier" than you think!

Lactose is a natural sugar in milk and milk products. During digestion, an intestinal enzyme called lactase breaks down lactose into smaller, more easily digested sugars. Not fully digested, lactose instead is fermented by "healthy" bacteria in the intestinal tract. This fermentation may produce uncomfortable symptoms—for example, nausea, cramping, bloating, abdominal pain, gas, and diarrhea.

Lactose maldigestion or intolerance? They aren't the same. With *lactose maldigestion*, the body may not produce enough lactase to completely digest lactose—but the person may have no symptoms. In fact, lactose maldigestion is normal for many people. In varying degrees after about age two years, lactase activity may gradually decline. It's in the genes!

In contrast, those with *lactose intolerance* have symptoms of gastrointestinal discomfort when they can't completely digest or absorb the amount of lactose they consume. Symptoms may begin from fifteen minutes to several hours after consuming foods or drinks containing lactose. The severity varies from person to person—and how much and when lactose is consumed in relation to other foods.

Because lactase insufficiency varies, most people with lactose intolerance or with lactose maldigestion can eat dairy products in varying amounts.

If you suspect a lactose intolerance, avoid self-diagnosis. Instead, see your doctor for a medical diagnosis; discomfort in your gut might be caused by another condition, such as irritable bowel syndrome or celiac disease, which can cause lactose intolerance. Lactose intolerance is diagnosed with several tests: lactose tolerance test, hydrogen breath test, or stool acidity test for infants and young children.

To clarify a misconception, lactose intolerance differs from a milk allergy. Lactose intolerance results from an inability to adequately digest lactose, a milk sugar. A milk allergy is an immune response to milk protein; it happens when the body's disease-fighting (immune) system reacts to a protein, such as casein, in milk. With a milk allergy usually people must avoid all milk products unless they outgrow the allergy. A physician's diagnosis, management, and treatment of a milk allergy is imperative. *See "Food Allergies: A Growing Concern" in this chapter.*

Who's Likely to Be Lactose-Intolerant?

Anyone may have some degree of lactose maldigestion, or perhaps intolerance. From birth, most infants produce the lactase enzyme, so it's rare in young children, at least until they're weaned. With age, however, the body gradually may produce less lactase. For those with a genetic tendency, lactose maldigestion or intolerance often starts in the late teens or early adulthood.

Not enough evidence exists to really know how many people have low levels of lactase, but lactose intolerance appears to be less common than originally thought. Past estimates, which were higher, were based on studies of people consuming unrealistic

HOW MUCH LACTOSE?

Current research notes that those with lactose intolerance likely can handle the amount of lactose in about one cup of milk without any, or with just minor, symptoms.

LACTOSE IN COMMON DAIRY FOODS

PRODUCT	PORTION	GRAMS
Milk, whole, 2%, 1%, fat-free	1 cup	12
Lactaid milk, low-fat, lactose-free	1 cup	0
Goat milk	1 cup	9
Nonfat dry milk	⅓ cup	12
Evaporated milk	1 cup	24
Cottage cheese: low-fat, 2%	½ cup	3
Aged cheese: Cheddar, Swiss, mozzarella	1 oz.	<0.1
American processed cheese	1 oz.	1
Yogurt, low-fat	1 cup	5–19
Ice cream	½ cup	2–6

Sources: U.S. Department of Agriculture, National Nutrient Database for Standard Reference, Release 24, 2011. N. S. Scrimshaw et al., *American Journal of Clinical Nutrition Supplement* 48 (4), 1988; http:www.lactaid.com.

Lactose-free foods include:
- Broth-based soups
- Plain meat, fish, poultry
- Fruits and vegetables (plain)
- Tofu and tofu products
- Soy, rice, potato, nut, and hempseed beverages; coconut milk
- Bread, cereal, crackers, and desserts made without milk, dry milk, or whey

amounts of lactose; today's estimates reflect real-life intake. On average, as few as 12 percent of the U.S. population have this condition. Many people who think they're lactose-intolerant really aren't; some have lactose maldigestion instead, with few if any symptoms.

Certain ethnic and racial populations are more widely affected than others: African Americans, Native Americans, Asian Americans, and Hispanics. The condition is least common among persons of northern European descent, who tend to maintain adequate lactose levels throughout their lives.

Lactose intolerance is sometimes linked to other health issues. For example, some medications may lower lactase production in the body. Lactose maldigestion or intolerance can be a side effect of certain medical issues such as intestinal disease, gastric (stomach) surgery, Crohn's disease, celiac disease, or chemotherapy. Depending on the cause, this type of lactose intolerance may be short-term.

Lactose in Food: Which "Whey"?

Lactose usually comes from foods containing milk or milk solids. *The chart "How Much Lactose?" in this chapter suggests how much.* Prepared foods, even those labeled "nondairy," may contain lactose. If you're very lactose-intolerant, check labels carefully.

● Check labels for ingredients that suggest lactose: milk, dry milk solids (including nonfat milk solids), buttermilk, lactose, malted milk, sour or sweet cream, margarine, whey, whey protein concentrate, and cheese.

● Be aware that baked and processed foods often contain small amounts of lactose: bread, pancake or baking mixes, candy and cookies, cold cuts and hot dogs, drink mixes, commercial sauces and gravies, cream soups, dry cereals, prepared foods (such as frozen pizza, lasagna, waffles), salad dressings made with milk or cheese, margarine, sugar substitutes, and powdered meal-replacement supplements.

> #### Click Here! Websites to Know . . .
>
> *See "Resources You Can Use" later in this book for website links to information on specific food sensitivities.*

> ### For Those with Lactose Intolerance: Another Option
>
> Food products have been developed for people with lactose intolerance. Some are lactose-reduced. Others contain lactase, the enzyme that digests milk sugar. If you're lactose-intolerant and if *"Lactose: Tips for Tolerance" in this chapter* aren't enough:
>
> ● Buy lactose-free milk and other dairy foods. Lactose-free milk is regular milk, with less or no lactose.
>
> ● Add lactase enzyme, available in drops, to fluid milk before drinking it. You'll find instructions on the package. Your milk will taste slightly sweeter because added lactase breaks down the lactose in milk into simpler, sweeter sugars.
>
> ● Before eating lactose-rich foods, take lactase, often in capsule or tablet form. With a supplemental supply of lactase, you can eat without discomfort. Read the timing and dosage instructions on the label.

● Know that some medications contain lactose. If you're lactose-intolerant, consult your doctor or pharmacist about appropriate medications.

Dairy Foods: Don't Give 'Em Up!

Even if your doctor has diagnosed you with lactose intolerance, there's no reason to give up dairy foods—or to miss out on the nutrient package they provide. Lactose intolerance isn't an "all or nothing" condition. Instead, it's a matter of degree. Whether you have lactose intolerance or maldigestion, learn to manage the amount of lactose you consume; know your own tolerance level.

Needlessly avoiding milk and other dairy foods may lead to nutrient shortfalls and, as a result, possible health risks. Dairy foods are important sources of calcium, protein, riboflavin, vitamins A and D, magnesium, potassium, phosphorus, and other nutrients essential for bone health and more health benefits.

Without milk and other dairy foods, meeting calcium and vitamin D recommendations can be challenging. Calcium and vitamin D are especially important for bone health. Adequate amounts help children and teens grow strong, healthy bones and help prevent the bone-thinning conditions called osteopenia and osteoporosis later in life. For children, adequate vitamin D helps prevent bone-softening rickets. *For more about nutrients in dairy foods, refer to chapter 6.*

For children and teens with lactose intolerance, the American Academy of Pediatrics advises that dairy foods can provide nutrients essential for growth. Lower-lactose dairy foods are options. The Special Supplemental Nutrition Program for Women, Infants, and Children (WIC) advises lactose-reduced and lactose-free dairy options first, before non-dairy alternatives. Many heath organizations agree.

If you're lactose-intolerant, consult a registered dietitian (RD) to help you plan meals and snacks adequate in calcium and vitamin D, while controlling the lactose. In extreme cases or for children or pregnant women with lactose intolerance, a physician or a registered dietitian also may recommend a calcium supplement with vitamin D.

Lactose: Tips for Tolerance

Lactose intolerance, or any discomfort from lactose maldigestion, is easy to manage. Most people with lower lactase levels can include some dairy and other lactose-containing foods in their meals and snacks. In fact, most can drink a cup of milk without discomfort.

If you or someone in your family has one of these conditions, try these tips to comfortably enjoy lactose-containing foods:

● Experiment! Start with small amounts of lactose-containing foods. Gradually increase the portion to your tolerance level.

● Enjoy lactose-containing foods as part of a meal or a snack, not alone. Try a milk-fruit smoothie, or milk and fruit on your cereal. The mix of foods slows the release of lactose into the digestive system, making it easier to digest. Think of this as "diluting" the lactose.

● Eat smaller, more frequent portions of lactose-rich foods. For example, drink ½- or ¾-cup servings of milk several times throughout the day instead of a 1-cup serving one, two, or three times daily.

● Choose dairy foods that are naturally lower in lactose, such as natural cheeses. When cheese is made, curds (or solids) separate from the whey (or watery liquid); most lactose is in the whey, which is drained away. Natural cheeses such as Swiss, Colby, Parmesan, and Cheddar lose most of their lactose during processing and aging.

● Try yogurt, kefir, and buttermilk with active cultures. Their "friendly" bacteria help digest lactose. Not all cultured dairy foods contain live cultures. Look for the National Yogurt Association's seal "Live and Active Cultures" on the carton.

● Opt for whole-milk dairy products. Their higher fat content may help to slow the rate of digestion, allowing a gradual release of lactose. Then in your overall food choices, choose other foods with less fat.

● Enjoy a variety of other calcium-rich foods in your diet daily. Nondairy sources of calcium include dark-green leafy vegetables; calcium-fortified products such as juice, bread, and cereal; and canned sardines and salmon with bones. For canned fish, eat the bones to get the calcium!

● Check labels for ingredients that indicate lactose. *See "Lactose in Food: Which 'Whey'?" in this chapter.*

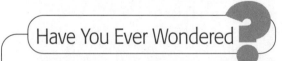

Have You Ever Wondered

. . . if goat's milk is a good substitute for cow's milk for someone with lactose intolerance or a milk allergy? Goat's milk has slightly less lactose: 9 grams of lactose per cup, compared with about 13 grams of lactose in one cup of cow's milk. For a milk allergy, the protein in goat's milk is similar to that of cow's milk; it's not a suitable alternative.

. . . if a nondairy creamer can replace milk for someone who's lactose-intolerant? How about nonfat dry milk? No for both. Nondairy creamers may contain lactose. Check the ingredient list on the label. The nutrient content of creamer and milk differs; in a nondairy creamer, the protein quality and the amounts of calcium and vitamins A and D are lower than in milk. Regarding nonfat dry milk, remember that fat, not lactose, has been removed.

. . . if a/B milk offers unique health benefits? Milk with added a/B cultures (acidophilus and bifidobacteria cultures) is similar to the milk it's made from. Although research isn't conclusive, these cultures may help improve lactose digestion, promote healthy bacteria in the GI tract, and help lower blood pressure, but it isn't acceptable for a milk allergy.

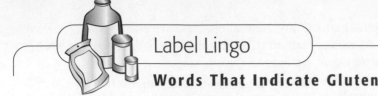

Label Lingo

Words That Indicate Gluten

For people with gluten intolerance (celiac disease and nonceliac gluten sensitivity) label reading is very important! These are among the ingredients to watch out for, but it's not a complete list:

Grains and grain-derived ingredients with gluten:
- Barley
- Rye
- Triticale
- Wheat (durum, einkorn, graham, semolina, kamut, spelt, emmer, farro, germ)
- Malt, malt flavoring (made from barley)
- Malt vinegar (made from barley)

Ingredients/foods/products that may or often do contain gluten:
- Batter-dipped foods
- Beer
- Breading, coating mixes, Panko*
- Brewer's yeasts
- Broth, soup bases
- Brown rice syrup
- Candy—e.g., licorice, some chocolates
- Croutons
- Egg substitutes such as liquid egg products
- Flour or cereal products
- French fries
- Some herbal teas
- Imitation bacon and seafood
- Marinades and salad dressings
- Modified food starch, dextrin (usually made from corn, but may be made from wheat)
- Pastas, instant rice mixes
- Processed luncheon meats
- Pudding and pudding mix
- Sauces and gravies
- Seasoning mixes
- Self-basting poultry
- Soy sauce, Worcestershire sauce, or soy sauce solids
- Stuffing, dressing
- Thickeners (roux)
- Communion wafers
- Matzoh (matzah, matzo)
- Herbal and nutrient supplements
- Some medications
- Some mouthwash, personal care products
- Play-Doh—a potential problem if hands are put on or in the mouth while playing with Play-Doh or are not washed after use

*Bread crumbs used in Japanese cooking.

● Kefir *without* active cultures, sweet acidophilus milk, and other fermented dairy foods? *Be aware:* Most are no lower in lactose than other dairy foods; they're tolerated at least as well as milk.

Gluten Intolerance: Often a Lifelong Condition

Pasta, tortillas, bagels, and whole-wheat bread are great sources of starches, other nutrients, and perhaps fiber. Yet those who react to gluten need to get their nutrients from other grain products that are gluten-free.

Gluten intolerance is an overriding term for a spectrum of gluten-related disorders. Whether it's nonceliac gluten sensitivity or celiac disease, it's an intestinal disorder, not a true food intolerance.

For those who have either of these conditions, the body can't tolerate gluten. "Gluten" refers to proteins in certain grains (wheat, rye, barley) and foods made from them. Oats are considered naturally gluten-free, although may contain gluten from cross-contamination. To clarify, gluten is a protein comprised of the prolamin *gliadin* and the glutelin *glutenin*. Many grains contain prolamins, including oats, rice, and corn. Prolamins aren't harmful to those with celiac disease.

How do these conditions differ?

Nonceliac gluten sensitivity is currently thought to be an immune-system response to gluten but not an autoimmune condition. Intestinal symptoms are uncomfortable and often worsen over time; a gluten-free diet relieves them. This condition probably won't damage the intestine. That said, there's scant research on gluten sensitivity.

Celiac disease, an autoimmune digestive disorder, is much more serious. With an autoimmune disease, the immune system attacks itself; it causes damage to the body when it contacts something perceived as harmful. Unmanaged celiac disease damages the villi that line the small intestine. Villi—small, hairlike projections—shorten and flatten. As a result, the damaged intestine can't absorb nutrients properly into the bloodstream.

Without healthy villi, someone with celiac disease becomes malnourished, even when eating enough nourishing foods. Malabsorption causes gasintrointestinal symptoms such as diarrhea, gas, and stomach pain. Over time, damage from unmanaged celiac disease increases many health risks, including premature osteoporosis, gastrointestinal cancers, anemia, delayed puberty, arthritis, miscarriage, and birth defects. Celiac disease also is called celiac sprue, nontropical sprue, and gluten-sensitive enteropathy.

Who's at Risk? What are the Symptoms?

Nonceliac gluten sensitivity doesn't appear to be genetic. Celiac disease is. It's more common among people with European roots, but Asian, Hispanic, African, and Middle Eastern populations may have it, too. The actual incidence of celiac disease in the United States is unknown but may run as high as 3 percent of Americans; the Centers for Disease Control and Prevention report 1 in 133 people.

The challenges: Celiac disease often is misdiagnosed or underdiagnosed. Its varying symptoms may imitate other health problems such as irritable bowel syndrome, anemia, inflammatory bowel disease, diverticulitis, intestinal infections, and chronic fatigue syndrome. Some people may have no symptoms yet still can develop complications over time. Often celiac disease goes undetected until triggered by other body stresses: perhaps surgery, a viral infection, pregnancy, or severe emotional stress.

What are the symptoms of celiac disease? They vary from person to person: abdominal cramps, bloating, appetite loss, chronic diarrhea or constipation, fatigue, vomiting, and weight loss are classic symptoms. Some people experience a painful rash, muscle cramps, joint pain, and other symptoms. For women, celiac disease may affect the menstrual cycle.

For children, chronic irritability could be a warning sign. For growth and development, a child's high energy and nutrient needs require adequate nourishment; unmanaged celiac disease can affect a child's behavior and ability to grow and learn. Malabsorption of nutrients can lead to failure to thrive in infancy, delayed growth and short stature, delayed puberty, and dental enamel defects of the permanent teeth.

Celiac disease can occur at any age. Symptoms may appear first during infancy after cereal is started. Most cases are diagnosed in adulthood, often four to five years after the first symptoms. The longer celiac disease goes undiagnosed and untreated, the greater the chance of long-term complications. Temporary lactose maldigestion may accompany celiac disease, at least until the condition is under control and the small intestine heals. Healing may take months or years.

If you think you have nonceliac gluten sensitivity or celiac disease, ask your doctor for a diagnosis *before* starting a gluten-free diet. That allows testing for biomarkers of celiac disease—and an accurate test result. Celiac disease is diagnosed with blood, intestinal biopsy, and other tests. No medical tests can confirm nonceliac gluten sensitivity; instead, an elimination diet or a challenge test, done by reintroducing foods with gluten, is done. If celiac disease runs in your family, you may wish to be tested.

What's the Treatment?

For celiac disease the only treatment is a lifelong, strict eating regimen. A gluten-free diet is a must. Once gluten is eliminated, the small intestine in people with celiac disease can start to heal. Nutrient absorption then improves, and symptoms gradually disappear. Currently the treatment for nonceliac gluten sensitivity is also a gluten-free diet. Those with either condition can live a long, healthy life—and enjoy nourishing, flavorful foods, too.

Which Foods Are Gluten-Free?

Gluten-free means no wheat, rye, or barley. These grains and their hybrids are harmful for those with celiac disease. To manage any gluten intolerance, these grains, and any food or food component made from them, must be avoided. For those with celiac disease, even trace amounts of gluten in the diet can damage the small intestine. While gluten is mostly in food

Have You Ever Wondered?

... if a wheat allergy is the same as gluten intolerance? No; they're different conditions: different physiological responses, treated in somewhat different ways. With both a wheat allergy and gluten intolerance, wheat products and foods made with wheat products must be avoided. Wheat substitutes, including rye and barley, are okay with a wheat allergy but not with gluten intolerance. *See "Gluten Intolerance: Often a Lifelong Condition" in this chapter.*

... if glutathione in an ingredient list is gluten? No; glutathione is a common, safe protein sometimes used in gluten-free products. It can enhance the texture and volume of gluten-free bread.

including many processed foods, products such as medicines and supplements may contain it, too.

Avoiding gluten, wheat especially, is challenging. That's because wheat is the main ingredient in baked foods such as bread, breakfast cereals, breaded foods, crackers, pretzels, and pasta, among others. Gluten-containing ingredients can show up as additives (thickeners, fillers, malt) in other products as well.

Gluten-containing ingredients on food labels may appear under different names or as part of other ingredients. *See "Label Lingo: Words That Indicate Gluten" in this chapter.* The U.S. Food and Drug Administration (FDA) is working on voluntary labeling regulations to help consumers more easily identify gluten-free products. Until then, "gluten- free" can appear on food labels if the claim is truthful and not misleading.

Caution: Avoiding all grain foods isn't a smart option! Without fortified breads and cereals you miss out on their folate and iron; *see chapter 6.* Avoiding whole grains may shortchange you on fiber; *see chapter 3.* Instead, check labels and choose gluten-free grain products that are folate- and iron-fortified; try naturally gluten-free whole grains such as amaranth, buckwheat, and quinoa.

Eating Gluten-Free!

Coping with either nonceliac gluten sensitivity or celiac disease requires a strict eating regimen. While a gluten-free diet is hard to follow at first, these conditions are managed with food choices, not medication. In time this becomes second nature.

If you—or someone you know—must eat gluten-free, follow these guidelines:

● Consult a registered dietitian to learn to eat gluten-free—and enjoy eating! Ask about a supplement if you must make up for nutrients missed in a gluten-free diet. *See "How to Find Nutrition Help . . ." in chapter 24 to find a qualified nutrition expert.*

● Gluten-free doesn't mean no grain. Choose grain products and other starchy foods without gluten: amaranth, arrowroot, beans (legumes), buckwheat, cassava, corn, flax, garfava, millet, Montina, nut flours, potato, quinoa, rice, sago, seeds, sorghum, soy, tapioca, teff, wild rice, and yucca.

● Ask your doctor and/or registered dietitian about oats. Eat them only with medical supervision. In the past, people with celiac disease were advised to avoid oats. Evidence indicates that gluten-free oats in small amounts ($\frac{1}{2}$ cup dry oats or $\frac{1}{4}$ cup dry steel cut oats) not contaminated with wheat, barley, or rye during processing are usually safe. If allowed, use only "gluten-free"-labeled oats. A small percentage of people with celiac disease can't tolerate gluten-free oats.

● Choose plain foods. Plain meat, fish, rice, fruits, and vegetables (no added ingredients) don't contain gluten.

● Learn about ingredients and how to read an ingredient list on a food label. Examples: flavored chips may be dusted with an ingredient made with wheat; malt flavoring, made from barley, is used in many dry cereals.

If an ingredient such as modified food starch is made from wheat starch and contains wheat protein, allergen labeling on FDA-regulated food labels requires that "wheat" be declared. Malt (made with barley) would be on the ingredient list only; it's not included in allergen labeling. For USDA-regulated foods (meat, poultry, egg products) allergen labeling is voluntary, so the allergen "wheat" may not be shown. Only common or usual names, such as modified food starch or malt, are required.

● Check the label's ingredient list *every time* before consuming any product. Many commercially prepared foods—baked, frozen, and canned—have gluten-containing ingredients, but the ingredients may change. Contact the food manufacturer with ingredient questions. The company name, address, and perhaps the toll-free information number or website will appear on the food label. *Remember:* "Wheat-free" does not mean gluten-free.

● Try gluten-free products. Today gluten-free flour, baking mixes, pasta, pizza, snack foods, soups, and bakery items are widely available in most grocery stores. Or check specialty and health food stores, and online and mail order outlets.

● Cook with care. Use separate cooking and serving equipment for gluten-free foods. Keep food preparation surfaces crumb-free. Store gluten-free ingredients away from and above gluten-containing ingredients. Use good dishwashing skills to remove any gluten ingredient.

● Substitute gluten-free flour for wheat flour in food prep. Try corn, rice, brown rice, soy, arrowroot, tapioca, potato, or quinoa flours. Mix different flours. Because they give a different flavor and texture to baked foods, using these flours takes practice and experimentation. (Gluten gives dough its elasticity, and bread, its structure.)

● Skip alcoholic and nonalcoholic beer unless labeled "gluten-free." Beer, including ale, lager, and stout, usually is made with barley or wheat.

● Eating away from home? Pack gluten-free bread to take. Read restaurant menus carefully; ask questions. See if the restaurant has a gluten-free menu or if it participates in the Gluten-Free Restaurant Awareness Program. *See "Dining Out Tip List" in chapter 15 for the gluten-free symbol.*

● If you're a guest in someone's home, share your special food needs ahead. Offer to bring food.

● Ask your pharmacist if prescribed medications contain wheat. Gluten may be an unexpected additive in some products. Read labels and ask the manufacturer questions. Individuals with celiac disease probably don't need to worry about toothpaste, lipstick, and lip balm.

● Find local and national support groups to share information and gluten-free recipes. Many support groups publish lists of acceptable food products by

Have You Ever Wondered

. . . if you can be gluten-sensitive without having celiac disease? Yes, you may have nonceliac glucose sensitivity. Regularly check with your physician. Research doesn't yet know if a gluten sensitivity could progress to celiac disease.

. . . what wheat gluten is, and how it's used in cooking? Wheat gluten, also known as seitan, is wheat protein. Sold in specialty stores, it has a chewy, meaty texture, making it a good, protein-rich ingredient in casseroles, soups, pasta sauces, and other recipes calling for chopped or ground meat or poultry. *Caution:* People with celiac disease, nonceliac gluten sensitivity, and wheat allergy should avoid wheat gluten.

brand name, which can serve as a guide. A registered dietitian can help you find a support group, a trustworthy blog, or online support.

Sensitive to Additives? Maybe, Maybe Not

Do you wonder what less familiar ingredients on food labels do? Additives serve important functions in food. Some improve the nutritional value. Some, such as spices and colors, enhance a food's taste and appearance. Others prevent spoilage or give foods the consistency you expect. Without them our food supply likely would be far more limited. *See "Additives: Safe at the Plate" in chapter 9.*

Consuming food additives rarely causes adverse reactions. When it does, the response is commonly an intolerance—not a true allergy—to the additive.

The U.S. FDA, which regulates food additives, considers food intolerances and allergies in the approval process. Certain food additives—preservatives, colors, and flavors—are linked more commonly to food sensitivities than others.

For the Sulfite-Sensitive

Have you ever wondered why dried apricots and dehydrated potatoes list "sulfites" on a label's ingredient list? Sulfites help prevent certain foods, such as light-colored fruits, dried fruits, and vegetables, from browning. In beer, wine, and other fermented foods, sulfites slow bacterial growth.

The term "sulfites" is a catchall, referring to several common food additives. Usually they have "sulf" in their names. Sulfites may be listed on food labels as sulfur dioxide, sodium sulfite, sodium or potassium bisulfite, sodium or potassium metabisulfite, sulfurous acid, and sodium dithionite.

Sulfites in a varied diet pose no risk of side effects for most people. However, the U.S. FDA estimates that one in a hundred people is sulfite-sensitive. Asthmatics react more often to sulfites than the general population; the reaction may be severe.

For those who are sulfite-sensitive, reactions may include wheezing, diarrhea, stomach ache, hives, or swelling. Fortunately, side effects are mild for most people. However, reactions may become life-threatening for those who are very sensitive to sulfite. In rare cases they may experience anaphylactic shock and require immediate medical care; *anaphylaxis is discussed later in this chapter*. Consult your doctor if you think you're sulfite-sensitive. Don't self-diagnose or self-impose dietary restrictions; that may lead to nutrient deficiencies.

Because sulfites can trigger intense reactions in sulfite-sensitive asthmatics, the FDA prohibits using sulfites on fruits and vegetables (except potatoes) intended to be served or sold raw. In the past, sulfites sometimes were used to keep fruits and vegetables fresh longer on restaurant salad bars; that's no longer allowed.

Sulfites also can destroy the B vitamin thiamin. That's why they're not allowed in foods such as enriched bread and flour, which are major thiamin sources in the U.S. diet. Among other functions, thiamin is needed to produce energy; *see chapter 6*.

If you're among those rare individuals who are sulfite-sensitive:

● Check food labels. Choose foods without sulfite-containing additives. Be aware that they're used in varying amounts in many packaged foods, not just dried fruit, dehydrated potatoes, and fruit juices. By law, when sulfites are present in detectable amounts, the label must say so. *See "Where Might You Find Sulfites?" in this chapter.*

Where Might You Find Sulfites?

● Baked goods

● Beverages (beer, wine, hard cider, fruit and vegetable juices, tea)

● Bottled lemon and lime juices, grape juice (white, pink, and red sparkling)

● Condiments, pickled cocktail onions

● Dried fruits, fruit toppings, maraschino cherries, dried potatoes, sauerkraut

● Sauces, sauerkraut juice, wine vinegar, molasses, gravies

Source: Nutrition Care Manual, Academy of Nutrition and Dietetics. Accessed January 1, 2012.

● Check alcoholic beverages. Labels on beer and wine must state "Contains Sulfites" if applicable. Dealcoholized beer and wine still may contain sulfites.

● Ask in restaurants before ordering. For example, ask if dried or canned foods, vegetables, or potato products contain—or were treated with—sulfites.

● Make a plan with your doctor if you consume sulfites accidentally. Carry a rescue inhaler with you always!

● Be aware that some asthma medications contain sulfites. If you're sulfite-sensitive, ask for another medication.

● People sensitive to *sulfites* can consume foods with *sulfates*. Sulfates such as calcium sulfate (an additive used to fortify food with calcium) don't cause the same adverse reaction in sulfite-sensitive people.

Coloring by Any Other Name!

Although the incidence is rare, a very small number of people are sensitive to a coloring added to food. FD&C Yellow No. 5, also called tartrazine, is a dye used to color foods, beverages, and medications. Research indicates that FD&C Yellow No. 5 may trigger hives, itching, and nasal congestion but not asthma attacks. The incidence is limited: just one or two of every ten thousand people. This is the only food coloring known to cause such reactions.

When added to a food or a medication, FD&C Yellow No. 5 must be listed on the label or package insert. If you're sensitive to it, read labels carefully. Foods and beverages likely to contain tartrazine include soft drinks; ice cream; sherbets; gelatins; salad dressings; cheese dishes; seasoned salts; candies; flavor extracts; and pudding, cake, and frosting mixes.

Aspartame: PKU Warning

Since their discovery, low-calorie or non-nutritive sweeteners—aspartame, saccharin, acesulfame K, sucralose, and tagatose—have been investigated thoroughly by regulatory agencies worldwide and by leading scientific organizations. Evidence indicates that their long-term intake is safe and not associated with adverse health effects. *See "Non-Nutritive Sweeteners: Flavor without Calories" in chapter 3.* With one exception, they don't cause symptoms of food sensitivity. However, people with the rare genetic disorder

phenylketonuria (PKU) should avoid foods sweetened with aspartame.

Aspartame is made from two amino acids (aspartic acid and phenylalanine) and methanol. (The same amino acids are found naturally in meat, milk, fruit, and vegetables.) Regardless of the source, people with PKU cannot metabolize phenylalanine properly, so they can consume only limited amounts. Unmanaged, PKU can cause tissue damage, and in infants, brain damage. As a precaution, all babies are screened for PKU at birth; that is when a diagnosis is made.

For those who suffer from this disorder, foods and beverages containing aspartame carry a label warning stating "Phenylketonurics: Contains Phenylalanine." Aspartame, one of the most widely accepted food additives, is used in many products, including carbonated and powdered soft drinks, yogurt, pudding and gelatins, frozen desserts, hot beverage mixes, and candy. You'll find aspartame in the label's ingredient list. The PKU warning is a signal, too.

Does Food Cause Hyperactivity?

The commonly held notion linking sugar or other food additives to hyperactive behavior or attention deficit hyperactivity disorder (ADHD) in children never has been scientifically proven. Although the exact cause of ADHD isn't known, factors such as genetics and environmental influences have been suggested.

The Feingold diet, popularized for its claimed ability to manage ADHD, has been touted for treating hyperactive children. The eating plan restricts foods containing salicylates, present in almonds, certain fruits and vegetables, artificial flavors and colors, and preservatives. However, the reported success is based on anecdotal data, not scientific research methods. Extra attention given to children on the Feingold diet—not the change in food choices—may explain why a child's behavior changes. Although many other studies have been conducted attempting to link eating with hyperactivity, a clear cause-and-effect link between food colors and hyperactivity hasn't been shown.

Until researchers learn more, the best management of ADHD includes behavioral modification and medication, if warranted by a doctor. If you choose to avoid food colorings, check the ingredient list on food labels.

For more about the misconceptions between sugar and behavior see "Dispelling Carbohydrate Confusion" in chapter 3.

Food Allergies: A Growing Concern

Have you ever heard parents say that their child is allergic to milk, then remark that he or she has no adverse reactions to chocolate milk? Or maybe you avoid a particular food yourself, believing you're allergic to it?

People often use the term "allergy" loosely to describe almost any physical reaction to food—even if it's psychological! Why? Because the symptoms of food allergies can mimic other food-induced ailments such as foodborne illness and food intolerances.

Because reactions may be severe, even life-threatening, food allergies can't be taken lightly. Although the reasons are unclear, food allergies—and related severe reactions—appear to be on the rise; the true incidence is hard to determine.

Who is likely to develop a food allergy? Anyone, at any age. A family history of allergies is a contributing factor. Almost all are identified early in life. Young children are much more likely to have food allergies than adults; many allergies are outgrown. However, food allergies can occur in adulthood without a prior history of allergies. Studies are under way to determine if strictly avoiding a specific allergen from an early age increases the chance of outgrowing that allergy. Nonfood allergies are more common than food allergies.

Food Allergies: What Are They?

A true food allergy is an adverse physical response that happens when the body's disease-fighting (immune) system reacts to a component, usually a protein, in the offending food. Sometimes called food hypersensitivity, it causes the body's immune system to react even though the person isn't sick. The body reacts to a normally harmless food substance, thinking it's harmful. An allergen sets off a chain of immune system reactions.

When an allergy-prone person eats a food that causes an allergic reaction, his or her body scrambles to protect itself by making immunoglubulin E (IgE) antibodies. These antibodies trigger the release of body chemicals, including histamine. In turn, these body chemicals cause uncomfortable symptoms associated with allergies, such as a runny nose, itchy skin, nausea, even a rapid heartbeat, or in severe cases anaphylaxis.

Something You Ate?

It's lunchtime. You make your toddler his or her first peanut butter and jelly sandwich. An hour later the child has broken out with an itchy rash. You've heard that peanuts can be allergenic. Is your child allergic to peanut butter? Maybe, or maybe not! In any case, a call to the child's doctor is certainly in order.

Have You Ever Wondered

. . . if you can be sensitive to MSG? Perhaps, but not likely. Some people describe varying symptoms, including body tingling or warmth after eating foods containing monosodium glutamate (MSG). The symptoms, usually mild, commonly last less than an hour. Collectively the symptoms have been called "Chinese restaurant syndrome" because MSG was once common in Chinese cuisine.

Actually, research hasn't found a definitive link between MSG or Chinese food, and any adverse side effects. Other food components, perhaps a common allergen such as soy, could cause an adverse reaction.

If you want to moderate your MSG intake—or seem sensitive to it—ask to order food without added MSG in Asian restaurants. If the menu says "No MSG," it likely means no *added* MSG. MSG is likely in other ingredients, such as soy sauce. Glutamate, a component of MSG, is naturally in most protein-containing foods. Check food labels. Glutamate-containing ingredients such as MSG, hydrolyzed protein, and autolyzed yeast extract appear on the ingredient list. Glutamate that naturally occurs in food won't be listed. Consult a registered dietitian for guidance. *To learn more see "MSG—Another Flavor Enhancer" in chapter 7.*

. . . why some people get a reaction from fresh fruit and vegetables? Not a true food allergy, oral allergy syndrome (OAS) causes some people with pollen allergies and hay fever to react to certain raw fruits and vegetables such as apples, cherries, kiwis, celery, tomatoes, and green peppers. Just touching them can cause a reaction. Mild symptoms (such as itchy or swelling mouth and lips, runny nose, watery eyes, sneezing, or rash) are like other reactions to pollen; rarely, symptoms may be more severe.

To help manage reactions, cook these foods to break down the protein, remove their skin (perhaps with kitchen gloves), or choose canned forms. *Note:* An OAS reaction is not caused by pesticides, chemicals, or wax on fruit. If you think you or a family member has OAS, talk to your doctor.

. . . what fructose malabsorption is? It's a condition that may cause abdominal pain, gas, bloating, and diarrhea caused by difficulty digesting fructose, but it doesn't cause organ damage. Fructose is a sugar found naturally in fruit, honey, and some syrups.

Fructose malabsorption may be mislabeled by consumers as a more serious and rare genetic disorder called hereditary fructose intolerance, whereby a person lacks the enzyme that breaks down fructose. This condition can result in kidney and liver damage.

If you suspect either of these conditions, talk to your physician for a diagnosis and a list of foods to avoid. For hereditary fructose intolerance, foods with fructose, sucrose, and sorbitol (a sugar alcohol) should be avoided.

More than 170 foods are known to cause allergic reactions in susceptible people. However, some foods are more likely to set off a reaction than others. Milk, eggs, wheat, and soy as well as fish, crustacean shellfish (such as shrimp), peanuts, and tree nuts (such as pecans or walnuts) are the most common foods with allergens, causing about 90 percent of allergic reactions in the United States.

By age ten years—and often by age five—most kids outgrow milk, egg, soy, and wheat allergies. However, allergies to shellfish, fish, peanuts, and tree nuts are often lifelong. Only about 20 percent outgrow a peanut allergy; only about 10 percent outgrow a tree nut allergy. A board-certified allergist should determine whether a person has outgrown an allergy with a food challenge test.

Symptoms? Something to Sneeze About

Different people react to the same allergen in different ways. Even if a food contains a common allergen, you can't predict whether you may have an allergic reaction.

My Aching Head

Two to 20 percent of Americans suffer migraines (severe head pain plus a range of other symptoms such as nausea, vomiting, or increased sensitivity to light, sound, and smells). Migraine headaches can affect anyone, but women are three times more likely than men to suffer. Certain foods are blamed, but there's little agreement about the link between foods and headaches.

The causes of migraine headaches are complicated and not well understood. Certain food components—natural or added—have been suspected, not proven, to cause headaches in some people. Tyrosine (in cheese and chocolate), histamine (in red wine), caffeine (in coffee and cola), benzoic acid (a preservative), and alcohol may be food-related triggers. Susceptible individuals may be affected by several factors, not just food.

If you experience chronic headaches, check with your doctor for a medical diagnosis. To determine which foods or drinks, if any, trigger migraine attacks, keep a journal, often for several weeks, of what you eat and drink.

If you're diagnosed with migraine headaches and feel you're susceptible to food triggers, a registered dietitian can recommend substitutes for suspected triggers and ensure adequate nutrition.

Symptoms typically appear within minutes or up to several hours after eating the food that triggers the reaction. In exceptionally sensitive people, just skin contact or inhaling the allergen (perhaps from steam cooking or flour dust) can provoke a reaction!

What Are the Signs?

The most common symptoms include swelling, sneezing, and nausea. Most symptoms affect the skin, respiratory system, stomach, or intestines. A severe allergic reaction also may cause anaphylaxis, with a drop in blood pressure, loss of consciousness, and even death.

Skin reactions:
- Swelling of the lips, tongue, and face
- Itchy eyes
- Hives
- Rash (eczema)

Respiratory tract reactions:
- Swelling, itching, and/or tightness in the throat
- Shortness of breath
- Dry or raspy cough
- Runny nose
- Wheezing (asthma)

Digestive tract reactions:
- Abdominal cramps
- Nausea
- Vomiting
- Diarrhea

Keep in mind that these symptoms may be caused by other food- or nonfood-related conditions. *See "Itching for a Cause?" later in this chapter.*

To date there's no known scientific link between food allergies and arthritis, migraine headaches, behavioral problems, ear infections, or urinary tract infections, although research is under way. Recent studies show a link between food allergies and severe asthma in children.

Food Allergies: The Dangerous Side

For most people with food allergies, the reactions are more unsettling and inconvenient than life-threatening. In rare cases, however, an anaphylactic reaction can occur. When many different body systems react at the same time, the allergic response to food can be severe. Just a tiny bite of a food—and in rare instances, a touch or a whiff—can be harmful.

With an anaphylactic reaction, symptoms often develop quickly—within seconds or minutes after eating—and progress quickly from mild to severe, even fatal. Symptoms may start with itching, tingling, or a metallic taste in the mouth, then progress to extreme itching, a swollen throat that makes breathing difficult, sweating, rapid or irregular heartbeat, low blood pressure, nausea, diarrhea, loss of consciousness, cardiac arrest, and shock. Without immediate medical attention the affected person may die.

What foods may cause a severe reaction? Although rare, any food can cause anaphylactic reactions; most are caused by proteins in tree nuts, eggs, peanuts, or shellfish (crustacea). Those with asthma and a food allergy, especially peanut and tree nut allergies, are at highest risk.

Is the reaction the same every time? Perhaps not. Severity depends on two things: how allergic a person is and how much allergen is consumed.

Warning! If you—or a family member—experience true food allergies, plan ahead how to handle accidental ingestion of the trigger allergen. The person should wear an identification bracelet or necklace to alert others, and should carry epinephrine (Adrenalin) to inject quickly to counter the allergen and open the airway and blood vessels. A healthcare professional will provide a prescription. Because the body's responses can be life-threatening, call 911 or an ambulance immediately if someone has severe allergic reactions.

Itching for a Cause?

If you have symptoms, never try to self-diagnose. For an accurate diagnosis you need a complete medical evaluation by a board-certified allergist (certified by the American Academy of Allergy, Asthma, and Immunology). Someone with a food allergy should be under a doctor's care.

True food allergies can be measured and evaluated clinically—with no need for guessing. In that way unrelated medical conditions are eliminated. Typically the diagnosis includes a medical history, a physical exam, a food journal, elimination diet, and laboratory

Have You Ever Wondered?

... if avoiding certain foods during pregnancy can prevent food allergies in the baby? There's no conclusive evidence that restricting foods during pregnancy makes a difference. In fact, it's not recommended. Babies born to mothers who have restricted their diets during pregnancy often have lower birth weights. Eating a known food allergen during pregnancy won't cause a food allergy in the infant either. *See "Food Sensitivities and Your Baby" in chapter 16 for more guidance.*

... if breast-feeding can prevent food allergies in the baby? For those with a family history of allergies, there's no strong evidence that breast-fed babies are less likely to have food allergies. In addition, research doesn't show that eating peanuts while breast-feeding causes a baby to have a peanut allergy. A doctor can make an individual determination about whether a woman should avoid peanuts while breast-feeding.

tests. As an initial screening the doctor may use a skin test; an allergist will confirm a food allergy with more definitive tests.

Pass the Test?

Various medical tests help diagnose a food allergy but not its possible severity.

● A *skin-prick* test uses small amounts of diluted food extracts "pricked" into the skin. If skin reacts with a mosquito-bite-like bump (wheal) within about 15 minutes, you may have a food allergy.

● *Blood tests* check for IgE antibodies. *Remember:* The presence of antibodies, released by the immune system, signals a reaction to an allergen. For example, a radioallergosorbent test (RAST) uses a sample of blood to determine the presence of IgE antibodies from response to a specific food.

● In a *food challenge test*, likely given in a doctor's office, the patient gets a sample that's either the suspected food allergen or a placebo. The placebo won't produce an allergic reaction. The response is watched carefully. With no symptoms, the challenge gets repeated with higher doses. This test must be done under a doctor's supervision—never on your own.

Tests using a food extract are unreliable and costly.

Even with a positive test, many people can eat the problem food without symptoms. Conversely, negative results may not tell the whole story; the test won't detect allergies that don't involve IgE antibodies, according to the *NIAID Food Allergy Clinical Guide 2010*.

Keeping track of physical reactions to a specific food one time after another may help you detect a possible food allergy or intolerance. Still, avoid self-diagnosis. The cause may be a more serious medical problem. Eliminating groups of foods from your eating pattern based only on a hunch may limit nutrients and other food substances needed for overall good health!

For the Record

Suspect a food allergy? During a medical exam you'll need to describe your symptoms and give some medical history. Prepare to answer such questions as:

● What are your symptoms?

● How long does it take for symptoms to appear after eating the food in question?

● How much of the food must you eat before you get a reaction?

● Do symptoms occur whenever you eat the food?

● What else, such as physical activity or drinking alcoholic beverages, brings on symptoms?

Helping Kids Deal with Food Allergies

Whether your child—or his or her pal—has a food allergy, kids need to learn how to deal with it. Use the same basic advice if your child has celiac disease or any food sensitivity.

To help your child cope:

● Get a letter from your child's healthcare provider for school. It should include your child's name, diagnosis, the effect of the allergy on your child, the treatment (with suitable ingredient substitutions), and what to do if the child accidentally consumes it. Provide emergency contact information.

● Make a written plan for your child with the school personnel. Include the administration, nurse, food service staff, teacher, and perhaps coach and bus driver. Together develop an approach for avoiding allergens without making your child feel "different" or isolated. Include food-related events: parties, birthday treats, in-class and after-school food activities, recess, field trips, and food that children bring from home.

● With your healthcare provider, other responsible adults, and your child, make a plan for epinephrine administration (for severe reactions) or antihistamine (for milder reactions) if needed. Come up with a way your child can signal for help—fast!

● Help your child know symptoms of allergic reactions, and how and when to tell an adult when having an allergy-related problem.

● Visit the cafeteria before school starts so your child can meet staff who can help. Choose a place for him or her to sit, perhaps an allergy-free table, to avoid cross-contact with allergen-containing foods. Arrange for a responsible lunch buddy to help.

● Go over the menu with your child to identify safe and unsafe foods. Plan for food substitutes—with the food service staff—or for home-prepared food.

● Teach your child why and how to avoid "food swapping" and pressure to try new foods. Talk about strategies to avoid exposure to unsafe food. Role-play scenarios so your child will know how to react in these situations.

For more parenting tips, see chapter 17.

● Equip your child. When old enough to be responsible, children and teens who have severe reactions should carry an EpiPen or other form of epinephrine (and know how to use it), a personal emergency card (perhaps in a fun card holder), a medical-alert necklace or bracelet, and a parent's phone number. Antihistamine may be enough for milder reactions.

Even if your child doesn't have a food allergy, help him or her be a friend to a food-allergic friend:

● Take friends seriously if they say they have a food allergy. Ask questions. Help them at school, with foods you offer at home, and with party foods.

● Don't swap or share food—even if you think it's safe.

● When you're nearby, avoid eating a food that's allergenic to a friend.

● Wash your hands after you eat so you don't transfer food to other things your friend may touch.

● Get immediate help if your friend gets sick.

Have You Ever Wondered

. . . if peanut, soy, or nut oils can cause an allergic response? Most peanut and soy oils are highly refined, making them free of the protein allergen. Research shows that people with peanut or soy allergies don't have reactions to these commonly used oils; extremely sensitive people are still wise to be cautious. Cold-pressed peanut and tree nut oils are processed differently and may contain small amounts of protein allergens that can trigger a reaction.

. . . if foods modified by biotechnology contain allergens? It's possible. But no biotech foods to date have protein from known allergenic foods. The U.S. FDA policy states that any protein taken from a food causing a known allergic reaction should be considered allergenic, too. It also must be listed on the label of a food produced by biotechnology. *See "Food Biotechnology: Enhanced Farming" in chapter 9.*

. . . if food allergies trigger asthma? Only in very rare cases. The usual triggers are allergens in dust, molds, pollen, and animals; pollutants in the air; respiratory infections; some medications; physical activity; and perhaps weather changes. If food appears to be a trigger, consult your doctor.

. . . if foods labeled as "nondairy" are okay for people with milk allergies? Carefully read the label to find out. For most people with a milk allergy, a key protein in milk called casein causes a reaction. Casein or caseinates are common additives.

. . . if there's a cure for food allergies? At this time, no. Research is under way to find a vaccine that may reduce or eliminate the symptoms of severe food allergies. Avoiding foods with allergens is the only protective approach.

. . . if soy is a good substitute for people with other allergies? Yes, if the person isn't allergic to soy, too. Calcium- and vitamin D-fortified soy beverages can substitute for cow's milk—if you get enough of milk's other nutrients elsewhere. Soy nuts can substitute for peanuts or tree nuts.

. . . if a flu shot or an MMR vaccine is safe for someone with an egg allergy? Flu vaccines may contain a small amount of egg protein, since they're grown on egg embryos. If you have an egg allergy, talk to your doctor before getting a flu shot. The American Academy of Pediatrics acknowledges the safety of—and recommends—a one-dose administration of MMR vaccine for children with egg allergies.

. . . if calcium carbonate in fortified foods is safe for someone with milk allergy? Calcium carbonate adds calcium, not milk protein, to food.

. . . if a kiss can result in an allergic reaction? Yes, if it causes cross-contact with a food allergen. If you have a food allergy, wait at least four hours before kissing someone who's eaten the problem food.

● Does a family member have allergies? Food allergies?

You may need to keep a food journal, with all the foods, beverages (including alcoholic beverages), and medications you consume over a determined period. That includes brand names of commercially prepared foods. Also keep track of physical reactions and how soon after eating they appear. By itself, a journal can't confirm a cause-and-effect relationship between a food and symptoms, but the information can suggest a connection to investigate.

An elimination diet also may help uncover a cause. Your doctor may instruct you to completely avoid the suspicious food for a while. If the symptoms go away, then reappear when you eat the food again, you may be allergic to it. If your symptoms aren't life-threatening, your doctor may recommend a rechallenge where the suspected allergen or allergens are reintroduced, one at a time.

Keeping a food journal or following an elimination diet may seem easy. However, detecting ingredients in prepared foods that cause allergic reactions may not be. A registered dietitian has the expertise to help you.

"How-tos" for Coping with Food Allergies

If you're diagnosed with a true food allergy, what's next? There's no cure—and no pill to avoid a reaction. Instead, managing food allergies is life-altering and requires constant attention, often by family and friends, too.

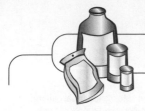

Label Lingo

How to Read a Label for Food Allergies

HOW TO READ A LABEL FOR A PEANUT-FREE DIET

All FDA-regulated manufactured food products that contain peanut as an ingredient
are required by U.S. law to list the word "peanut" on the product label.

Avoid foods that contain peanuts or any of these ingredients:

artificial nuts	goobers	nutmeat
beer nuts	ground nuts	peanut butter
cold pressed, expeller	mixed nuts	peanut flour
pressed, or extruded	monkey nuts	peanut protein
peanut oil	nut pieces	hydrolysate

Peanut is sometimes found in the following:

African, Asian	baked goods	chili
(especially Chinese,	*(e.g., pastries,*	egg rolls
Indian, Indonesian,	*cookies)*	enchilada sauce
Thai, and	candy *(including*	marzipan
Vietnamese), and	*chocolate*	mole sauce
Mexican dishes	*candy)*	nougat

Keep the following in mind:

● Mandelonas are peanuts soaked in almond flavoring.

● *The FDA exempts highly refined peanut oil from being labeled as an allergen.* Studies show that most allergic individuals can safely eat peanut oil that has been highly refined (not cold pressed, expeller pressed, or extruded peanut oil). Follow your doctor's advice.

● A study showed that unlike other legumes, there is a strong possibility of cross-reaction between peanuts and lupine.

● Arachis oil is peanut oil.

● Many experts advise patients allergic to peanuts to avoid tree nuts as well.

● Sunflower seeds are often produced on equipment shared with peanuts.

HOW TO READ A LABEL FOR A TREE NUT-FREE DIET

All FDA-regulated manufactured food products that contain a tree nut as an ingredient
are required by U.S. law to list the specific tree nut on the product label.

Avoid foods that contain nuts or any of these ingredients:

almond	litchi/lichee/lychee	nut pieces
artificial nuts	nut	pecan
beechnut	macadamia nut	pesto
Brazil nut	marzipan/almond	pili nut
butternut	paste	pine nut *(also referred*
cashew	Nangai nut	*to as Indian, pignoli,*
chestnut	natural nut extract	*pigñolia, pignon,*
chinquapin	*(e.g., almond, walnut)*	*piñon, and pinyon*
coconut	nut butters *(e.g.,*	*nut)*
filbert/hazelnut	*cashew butter)*	pistachio
gianduja *(a chocolate-*	nut meal	praline
nut mixture)	nut meat	shea nut
ginkgo nut	nut paste *(e.g.,*	walnut
hickory nut	*almond paste)*	

Tree nuts are sometimes found in the following:

black walnut hull extract *(flavoring)*
natural nut extract
nut distillates/alcoholic extracts
nut oils *(e.g., walnut oil, almond oil)*
walnut hull extract *(flavoring)*

Keep the following in mind:

● Mortadella may contain pistachios.

● There is no evidence that coconut oil and shea nut oil/butter are allergenic.

● Many experts advise patients allergic to tree nuts to avoid peanuts as well.

● Talk to your doctor if you find other nuts not listed here.

HOW TO READ A LABEL FOR A MILK-FREE DIET

All FDA-regulated manufactured food products that contain milk as an ingredient
are required by U.S. law to list the word "milk" on the product label.

Avoid foods that contain milk or any of these ingredients:

butter, butter fat,	cheese	lactalbumin, lactalbumin	*milk and milk from*	rennet casein
butter oil, butter	cottage cheese	phosphate	*other animals, low-fat,*	sour cream, sour
acid, butter ester(s)	cream	lactoferrin	*malted, milkfat, nonfat,*	cream solids
buttermilk	curds	lactose	*powder, protein,*	sour milk solids
casein	custard	lactulose	*skimmed, solids, whole)*	tagatose
casein hydrolysate	diacetyl	milk *(in all forms, including*	milk protein hydrolysate	whey *(in all forms)*
caseinates *(in all*	ghee	*condensed, derivative,*	pudding	whey protein hydrolysate
forms)	half-and-half	*dry, evaporated, goat's*	Recaldent®	yogurt

Milk is sometimes found in the following:

artificial butter	caramel candies	lactic acid starter	luncheon meat, hot	nisin
flavor	chocolate	culture and other	dogs, sausages	nondairy products
baked goods		bacterial cultures	margarine	nougat

(continued)

How to Read a Label for Food Allergies *(continued)*

HOW TO READ A LABEL FOR A SOY-FREE DIET

All FDA-regulated manufactured food products that contain soy as an ingredient
are required by U.S. law to list the word "soy" on the product label.

Avoid foods that contain soy or any of these ingredients:

edamame
miso
natto
shoyu
soy *(soy albumin, soy cheese, soy fiber, soy flour, soy grits, soy ice cream, soy milk, soy nuts, soy sprouts, soy yogurt)*

soya
soybean *(curd, granules)*
soy protein *(concentrate, hydrolyzed, isolate)*

Soy is sometimes found in the following:

Asian cuisine
vegetable broth

soy sauce
tamari
tempeh
textured vegetable protein *(TVP)*
tofu

vegetable gum
vegetable starch

Keep the following in mind:

● *The FDA exempts highly refined soybean oil from being labeled as an allergen.* Studies show most allergic individuals can safely eat soy oil that has been highly refined (not cold pressed, expeller pressed, or extruded soybean oil).

● Most individuals allergic to soy can safely eat soy lecithin.
● Follow your doctor's advice regarding these ingredients.

HOW TO READ A LABEL FOR A WHEAT-FREE DIET

All FDA-regulated manufactured food products that contain wheat as an ingredient are required by U.S. law
to list the word "wheat" on the product label. The law defines any species in the genus *Triticum* as wheat.

Avoid foods that contain wheat or any of these ingredients:

bread crumbs
bulgur
cereal extract
club wheat
couscous
cracker meal
durum
einkorn
emmer
farina

flour *(all purpose, bread, cake, durum, enriched, graham, high gluten, high protein, instant, pastry, self-rising, soft wheat, steel ground, stone ground, whole wheat)*
hydrolyzed wheat protein

Kamut©
matzoh, matzoh meal *(also spelled as matzo, matzah, or matza)*
pasta
seitan
semolina
spelt
sprouted wheat

triticale
vital wheat gluten
wheat *(bran, durum, germ, gluten, grass, malt, sprouts, starch)*
wheat bran hydrolysate
wheat germ oil
wheat grass
wheat protein isolate
whole wheat berries

Wheat is sometimes found in the following:

glucose syrup
soy sauce
starch *(gelatinized starch, modified starch, modified food starch, vegetable starch)*
surimi

HOW TO READ A LABEL FOR AN EGG-FREE DIET

All FDA-regulated manufactured food products that contain egg as an ingredient
are required by U.S. law to list the word "egg" on the product label.

Avoid foods that contain eggs or any of these ingredients:

albumin *(also spelled albumen)*
egg *(dried, powdered, solids, white, yolk)*
eggnog
lysozyme

mayonnaise
meringue *(meringue powder)*
ovalbumin
surimi

Egg is sometimes found in the following:

baked goods
egg substitutes
lecithin
macaroni

marzipan
marshmallows
nougat
pasta

Keep the following in mind:

● Individuals with egg allergy should also avoid eggs from duck, turkey, goose, quail, etc., as these are known to be cross-reactive with chicken egg.

HOW TO READ A LABEL FOR AN SHELLFISH-FREE DIET

All FDA-regulated manufactured food products that contain a crustacean shellfish as an ingredient
are required by U.S. law to list the specific crustacean shellfish on the product label.

Avoid foods that contain shellfish or any of these ingredients:

barnacle
crab
crawfish *(crawdad, crayfish, ecrevisse)*
krill
lobster *(langouste,*

langoustine, Moreton bay bugs, scampi, tomalley)
prawns
shrimp *(crevette, scampi)*

● *Mollusks are not considered major allergens under food labeling laws and may not be fully disclosed on a product label.*

Your doctor may advise you to avoid mollusks or these ingredients:

abalone
clams *(cherrystone, geoduck, littleneck, pismo, quahog)*
cockle
cuttlefish

limpet *(lapas, opihi)*
mussels
octopus
oysters
periwinkle
scallops

sea cucumber
sea urchin
snails *(escargot)*
squid *(calamari)*
whelk *(Turban shell)*

Shellfish are sometimes found in the following:

bouillabaisse
cuttlefish ink
fish stock
glucosamine
seafood flavoring *(e.g., crab or clam extract)*
surimi

Keep the following in mind:

● Any food served in a seafood restaurant may contain shellfish protein due to cross-contact.
● For some individuals, a reaction may occur from inhaling cooking vapors or from handling fish or shellfish.

Source: © Food Allergy and Anaphylaxis Network, 2011.
Used with permission

The only way to prevent an allergic reaction is to avoid the troublesome food. Prepare and choose meals and snacks with care!

● Seek professional help. Get a written plan for any medication from your doctor. Ask a registered dietitian to help you identify safe foods, avoid problem foods, and still eat for good nutrition. Learn about making food substitutions, reading food labels, and dining away from home. Ask about a supplement in case you need to make up for any nutrients missed in an allergen-free diet. *See chapter 23 for more on supplements.*

● Prepare for emergencies! Always carry injectable epinephrine (Epi-Pens) once a food allergy has been diagnosed. Keeping an antihistamine and a bronchodilator handy, in case you accidentally consume a food allergen, is a good backup plan. Prepare to use it as directed. Get immediate medical help if needed. Wear an identification necklace or bracelet that identifies your allergy. *Be aware:* An antihistamine addresses symptoms but won't help with anaphylaxis.

● Tell others: family, coworkers, friends. Let them know how they can help keep your risk for exposure to allergens low—and what to do if you do have a reaction.

Eating Allergen-Free at Home

Simply cooking a food or scraping the allergenic food (e.g., peanuts) off the plate won't make it safe for food allergy sufferers. Whether for yourself or a family member, buy, prepare, and serve food to cope with a food allergy.

Allergen-Free: Sharpen Your Cooking Skills

Preparing dishes without allergenic foods seems obvious. Just leave the ingredient out of the recipe or off the plate! A few other "how-tos" can help ensure a reaction-free meal or snack:

● Wash your hands with warm, soapy water before handling and serving allergen-free foods.

● Cook the allergen-free meal first. Set it aside; cover it to avoid cross-contact with other foods before serving it.

● Use different and clean (washed well in warm, soapy water) utensils (including knives and spatulas), containers, cutting boards, and serving utensils for foods prepared without the food allergen.

　● For example, for a peanut allergy: just wiping off a knife used to spread peanut butter isn't enough. Use a clean, separate knife for the next ingredient, perhaps jelly. The same holds true for another utensil, such as cleaning a blender after making an ice cream shake with peanut ingredients.

● Use different oils to cook allergenic and nonallergenic foods. Frying doesn't destroy allergens.

　● For example, for a seafood allergy: use different cooking oil in a clean frying pan to deep-fry shrimp rather than what you used to make French fries or other foods. Serve them on a separate plate with different utensils, too.

● Be careful to note allergenic ingredients.

　● *For example, for a tree nut allergy:* ground-up nuts added to a muffin batter or a breading mix may go unnoticed. Even a bottle of barbecue sauce, pasta, or meat-free burgers may have nuts!

　● *For a fish allergy:* bottled fish sauce in a stir-fry, Worcestershire sauce, or salad dressing could be an undetected problem. Anchovies flavor some Italian foods such as caponata.

　● *For an egg allergy:* sometimes eggs are used to hold meatballs and fish croquettes together. They may be used in the foam for specialty coffee drinks, as an egg wash on pretzels, in some dry pasta, or in egg substitutes that contain egg whites.

　● *For a soy allergy:* soy flours and soy protein are used in increasingly more baked goods and other prepared foods.

　● *For a milk allergy:* milk protein is in many brands of tuna. Currently many foods labeled as "nondairy" have casein, a milk derivative. Meat may have casein as a binder.

　For a peanut allergy: peanuts are sometimes an unexpected substitute for tree nuts and may be found in some sauces, vegetarian foods, and other prepared foods.

● Read the ingredient list on food labels carefully to uncover allergens every time you buy or use even familiar foods. If, for example, you're allergic to eggs, remember that eggs are common ingredients in mayonnaise, many salad dressings, and ice cream. No package label? Make a different choice. *"Label Lingo: How to Read a Label for Food Allergies" in this chapter gives some ingredients to watch for.*

Since 2006 the Food Allergen Labeling and Consumer Protection Act (FALCPA) has required allergen labeling of U.S. FDA-regulated packaged foods sold in the United States. The top eight food allergens, or ingredients with a protein derived from them, must be labeled in common language: milk, egg, fish (such as salmon and flounder), crustacean shellfish, tree nuts, wheat, peanuts, and soybeans. For tree nuts, fish, and shellfish, the specific types must be stated. Major food allergens used in spices, flavorings, additives, and colorings must be listed, too. When in doubt, contact the manufacturer.

For food allergen labeling, the package will be labeled in one of two ways: (1) a "Contains" statement, for example, "Contains milk, egg, peanuts," at the end of the ingredient list, or (2) the common name of the allergen from which the ingredient is derived, for example, "albumin (egg)," listed in parentheses after the ingredient within the ingredient list. The law doesn't apply to restaurants. Alcoholic beverages such as beer may be labeled voluntarily.

● Check labels on medications and on body care and oral care products. They also may contain food allergens such as milk, egg, wheat, and tree nuts; FALCPA doesn't apply to them.

● Keep up-to-date on ingredients in food products. Periodically, food manufacturers change ingredients. Also the same food from different manufacturers likely has a different "recipe." Even if you're a long-time consumer of a certain food, check the label's ingredient list every time you buy it.

● If you have a milk or casein allergy, be cautious about kosher foods labeled as "pareve" or "parve." For religious purposes these foods are milk-free, or perhaps have only a very small amount of milk. Although appropriate for those with lactose intolerance, the food may not be milk-free from a food science perspective or for those with food allergies. If, however, a "D" appears next to the kosher symbol, it does have an ingredient derived from milk or was produced in equipment shared with a dairy. "F" printed near the kosher symbol indicates that it contains fish ingredients. *See chapter 12 for kosher symbols.*

● Contact food companies with your questions about allergens in their products. The company name, address, and perhaps a toll-free consumer information number or website are on the food label.

● Practice new ways to cook. In time, substituting one food for another will become second nature. Find a

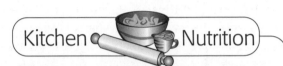

Kitchen Nutrition

Handy Substitutions for Allergen-Free Cooking

Egg-free recipes—substitute for 1 egg:

● 1 teaspoon baking powder, 1 tablespoon liquid, 1 tablespoon vinegar
● 1 teaspoon yeast dissolved in ¼ cup warm water
● 1½ tablespoons water, 1½ tablespoons oil, 1 teaspoon baking powder
● 1 packet plain gelatin, 2 tablespoons warm water (Don't mix until ready to use.)

Wheat-free recipes—substitute for 1 cup wheat flour:

● ¾ cup rice flour plus ¼ cup cornstarch
● 1 cup fine cornmeal or corn flour
● ⅔ cup brown rice flour and ⅓ cup potato flour
● 1 cup soy flour plus ¼ cup potato starch flour
● 1 cup of any of the following flours: amaranth, garbanzo/fava, quinoa, sorghum
● *1 tablespoon wheat flour equals:*

    1½ teaspoons cornstarch, arrowroot, white rice flour, *or* potato starch

    2 teaspoons tapioca *or* uncooked rice

Milk-free recipes—substitute for an equal amount of milk:

● Fruit juice
● Rice, soy, potato, nut, hempseed beverages, and coconut milk
● Water

* Experiment, as cooking or baking characteristics of the end result may differ with ingredient substitutions.

cookbook or online source of allergen-free recipes. Experiment to find substitutions that work.

● Be careful with cooking and serving to avoid cross-contact so a food allergen won't creep into an allergy-safe food. Even invisible traces on a utensil or a splatter can cause a reaction! *See "Allergen-Free: Sharpen Your Cooking Skills" in this chapter.* The same rule applies elsewhere—for example, for a milk allergy, avoid deli-sliced meats since cheese and meat may be cut with the same slicer.

Eating Allergen-Free away from Home

If you suffer from a food allergy, eating away from home can be challenging! You're not in control of the ingredients or the food preparation. So be ingredient-savvy:

● Review the restaurant menu ahead when possible. Menus are often online, or try to get a menu from the restaurant.

● Choose restaurants where you can special-order.

● Make a chef card to explain your food allergy or sensitivity. Share it with your server and the chef

---

To the Chef:

WARNING! I am allergic to _____ .
In order to avoid a life-threatening reaction, I must avoid all foods that might contain _____, including these ingredients:

_____

_____

_____

_____

_____

_____

Please ensure that my food does not contain any of these ingredients and that all utensils and equipment used to prepare my meal, as well as to prep surfaces, are thoroughly cleaned prior to use. Thanks for your cooperation.

Reprinted with permission from the Food Allergy & Anaphylaxis Network.

---

as you order. If you travel to places that don't speak or read English, get a translation of the chef card as you prepare for your trip.

● Explain your needs to your food server. Ask about the menu—ingredients and preparation—before ordering. The same dish prepared in different restaurants may not have the same ingredients. To play safe, order plain foods such as grilled meats, steamed vegetables, and fresh fruits—but still ask questions!

● Ask for the chef or manager if your server seems unsure about the ingredients or preparation. It's okay to leave the restaurant if your request isn't understood.

● Skip sauces and condiments. They may contain allergens.

Caution! Avoid these situations:

● Buffet-style or family-style service—the same serving utensils may be used for different dishes.

● Steak—since butter, which melts into meat, is often added to grilled meat for flavor, an issue if you have a milk allergy.

● Coffee drinks with foam or milk topping (may contain eggs) if you have an egg allergy.

● Fried foods—since the same oil may be used for different foods.

● Seafood restaurants if you have a fish allergy—since cooking utensils may contact fish protein.

● Many Chinese, Indonesian, Malaysian, Thai, Vietnamese, Mexican, and African foods if you have a tree nut, peanut, or fish allergy—since peanuts, nuts, and fish sauce are common in some of these ethnic cuisines. Soy sauce contains wheat.

What Food Allergies Are Most Common?

● *Adults:* peanuts, crustacean shellfish (crab, crawfish, lobster, shrimp), tree nuts (almonds, Brazil nuts, cashews, hazelnuts, macadamias, pecans, pine nuts, pistachios, walnuts, others), fish

● *Children:* milk, eggs, peanuts, soy, tree nuts, wheat

● Breaded foods—for a wheat, milk, or egg allergy. The problem protein may transfer if the same breading mix is used for different foods. Breaded foods may have an egg wash.

● Scooped ice cream—since the scooper for several flavors may be kept in the same tub of water.

● Baked goods if you're allergic to soy or wheat. Today more breads, pizza crusts, and other doughs are made with soy flour; wheat is often added to rye bread. Tongs and other utensils are reused.

Have You Ever Wondered ?

. . . what is an exercise-induced food allergy? It's a very infrequent reaction from eating a certain food before exercising. Crustacean shellfish, alcohol, tomatoes, cheese, and celery are common causes. Allergic reactions may appear once exercising starts and the body temperature starts to rise. Anaphylaxis may even develop. Managing it is easy: avoid eating that food for a couple of hours before exercising. Evidence isn't clear whether this can happen only to those with a food allergy.

. . . if you should avoid coconut and water chestnuts if you have a tree nut allergy? Ask your doctor; a coconut is actually a fruit (a drupe), not a true nut. Any reaction is not from a nut allergy. Some people do react to coconut. Regarding water chestnuts, they're from a plant root, not a nut—so enjoy them!

. . . if carrageenan is a problem if you're allergic to fish or shellfish? No; it's a seaweed extract, not a fish. An additive in many foods, it appears safe for most people with allergies to fish and seafood.

Refer to chapter 15, "Your Food Away from Home," for restaurant tips.

● Carry your own food on airlines. Ask for the peanut-free snack if you have a peanut allergy.

● If you're not sure about the food, brown-bag your own. If you're a guest in someone's home, offer to bring your own food or to help with food preparation.

● Be a sensitive host. With your invitation, ask about special food needs—in case guests feel uncomfortable telling you. Adjust the menu or prepare some foods differently if needed to address their needs.

For more about managing specific food allergies, and a cookbook, newsletters, and other support, contact the Food Allergy and Anaphylaxis Network. *See "Resources You Can Use" for contact information.*

Need more strategies for handling food sensitivities? Check here:

● Sharpen up on ingredient detection as you shop—*see chapter 12.*

● Ask the right menu questions when you eat out—*see chapter 15.*

● Monitor an infant's food-induced reactions—*see chapter 16.*

● Get more help from a registered dietitian—*see chapter 24.*

● Find organizations that offer additional help—*see "Resources You Can Use."*

CHAPTER 22

Smart Eating to Prevent and Manage Disease

A healthful eating pattern and lifestyle from the start are your best approaches for staying healthy and preventing disease, or at least slowing its course. Most health problems don't start with a single event in your life. Instead, they're a combination of factors. Some you can't control, such as your family history, gender, or age; many you can.

This chapter addresses several common health problems that concern Americans: (1) their prevention and risk reduction and (2) the management of health problems or their symptoms. This overview may or may not apply to your unique needs. For advice specific to you or to someone you care for, consult with your doctor, a registered dietitian, and other members of your personal healthcare team. For detailed information on the diet-related health conditions discussed in this chapter, check the websites of the health organizations *noted on page 583 and in the appendices.*

Your Healthy Heart

We've all heard the statistics. Heart disease is America's number one killer. Although its onset is slightly postponed for women, it's a disease that affects both genders. About 81 million people in the United States have some form of cardiovascular disease, about 37 percent of the U.S. population (2010 data, American Heart Association). The truth is, many deaths from

---

DAMAGE CONTROL

Of the thirteen leading causes of death in the United States, six are associated directly with diet, and six with excessive intake of alcoholic beverages. Paying attention to what you eat and drink can pay off in good health and longevity.

RANK AND CAUSE*	RISK FACTORS	
	DIET-RELATED	ALCOHOL-RELATED
1. Heart disease	X	X
2. Cancers	X	X
3. Chronic lower respiratory diseases		
4. Strokes	X	
5. Accidents		X
6. Alzheimer's disease		
7. Diabetes	X	
8. Influenza and pneumonia		
9. Kidney diseases	X	X
10. Suicide		X
11. Septicemia (bacterial infection in the blood)		
12. Chronic liver disease and cirrhosis		X
13. Hypertension and hypertensive renal disease	X	

Source: National Vital Statistics Reports (reflecting preliminary data for 2009).

Your Nutrition Checkup

Do It for You!

Take care of you for you—and all those in your life! You can't control your age, gender, or family history, but there's plenty you can do to stay fit. For many health problems, the risk factors are the same, so the same smart living patterns may protect you from several chronic diseases.

How well are you protecting your health? If you can answer "yes" to the following questions, great! Then check to the left; fill in your own numbers in the blanks on the right.

Your Body's "Maintenance" Program . . . Your Markers of Health!

_____ Have you had a recent physical exam?

_____ Does your body mass index (BMI) fit within a range with fewer health risks?   _____ BMI*

_____ Is your waist circumference 35 inches or less for women, or 40 inches or less for men?

Do you know your numbers? Are they within a normal/optimal range?

_____ Total blood cholesterol (below 200 mg/dL)   _____ mg/dL

_____ LDL blood cholesterol (below 100 mg/dL)   _____ mg/dL

_____ HDL blood cholesterol (60 mg/dL or more)   _____ mg/dL

_____ Triglycerides (below 150 mg/dL)   _____ mg/dL

_____ Blood pressure (below 120/below 80 mm Hg)   ___/___ mm Hg

_____ Fasting blood glucose (sugar) (below 100 mg/dL)   _____ mg/dL

_____ Bone mass density (BMD) (T-score at −1.0 and above)   _____ mg/dL

Eat—for the Health of It!

_____ Do you know about how many calories you need a day to maintain or lose weight?

_____ Do you watch your portion sizes?

_____ Do you try to consume the equivalent of about 6 ounces of breads, cereals, rice, pasta, and other grain products daily?** (One ounce is about 1 regular slice of bread, ½ cup of cooked rice or pasta, or 1 cup of ready-to-eat cereal.)

_____ Of these grain products, do you eat at least half as whole grain?†**

_____ Do you try to eat at least 4½ cups or more of fruits and vegetables with a colorful variety each day?**

_____ Do you consume enough calcium-rich dairy foods daily: three cups of low-fat or fat-free milk or an equivalent?**

_____ Do you try to eat lean protein foods that add up to about 5½ ounces daily (e.g., lean meat, poultry, seafood, eggs, beans and peas, and nuts)?

_____ Do you choose foods low in solid fats, saturated fat, *trans* fat, and cholesterol most of the time (e.g., lean meat, skinless poultry, fish, low-fat or fat-free dairy foods)?

_____ Do you try to eat beans and peas several times a week? (Besides being low in fat, they're high in protein, iron, and fiber.)

_____ Eat a variety of seafood in place of some meat and poultry?

_____ Do you go easy on foods with solid fats and added sugars?

_____ Do you choose and prepare food with little sodium and salt?

*See "Body Mass Index: Fit or Fat?" in chapter 2 to figure your BMI.
**For a 2,000-calorie daily diet. Check chapter 10 for more about a healthful eating pattern.
†See "What Is a Whole Grain? in chapter 3.

Do It for You! (continued)

Now . . . Your Lifestyle

_____ Do you get at least 150 minutes a week of moderate, or at least 75 minutes of vigorous, physical activity a week, or a combination?

_____ Are some of your physical activities weight-bearing (e.g., walking, dancing, tennis, basketball)?

_____ If you drink alcoholic beverages, do you do so in moderation (no more than one drink daily for women, or two for men)?

Now count up all your "yes" answers:

For each checkmark, give yourself four points. What's your total score? _____

Of course, these eating and active living strategies aren't the only ways to promote your good health. But the more often you said "yes," the better your chances are for a long, healthy life.

What does your score suggest? It only indicates how many different ways you already may be protecting yourself from health problems. And it suggests where you might improve.

Having a score of 50 compared with a perfect 100 doesn't mean you're twice as likely to develop heart disease, cancer, diabetes, or some other health problem. And this quick checkup is not meant for diagnosis, either. That's the role of your doctor in your regular physical checkups. However, your responses might point to risk factors that may contribute to health problems later. Read on to explore the role of nutrition and regular physical activity in common health conditions.

---

heart attacks or strokes are preventable. The higher your blood cholesterol level, the greater your risk for developing heart disease or having a heart attack. High blood pressure is also a risk factor.

What Is Heart Disease?

"Heart disease," or cardiovascular disease, describes several health problems that relate to the heart and blood vessels. Heart attacks and strokes may come to your mind first. However, high blood pressure, angina (chest pain), poor circulation, and abnormal heartbeats are among the other forms of heart disease.

Heart Disease: The Risks

What increases your risk? Knowing your risks for heart disease is the first step in creating a personal plan for prevention. Two risk factors aren't within your control: age and genetic tendency. Yet many other risk factors are. Do any apply to you?

Risk factors you can't control:

● Heredity. Family history of early heart disease (father or brother with heart disease before age fifty-five; mother or sister, before age sixty-five). African Americans, who are more likely to have high blood pressure, are at higher risk. So are Mexican Ameri-

cans, Native Americans, Native Hawaiians, and some Asian Americans.

● Age and gender. Getting older (men over age forty-five; women over age fifty-five). Before menopause, women usually have lower cholesterol levels than men their age; after menopause, women's LDL cholesterol often rises.

Click Here! Websites to Know . . .

● American Diabetes Association, www.diabetes.org
● Academy of Nutrition and Dietetics, www.eatright.org
● American Heart Association, www.heart.org
● American Cancer Society, www.cancer.org
● Health Check Tools, National Institute of Health, www.nlm.nih.gov/medlineplus/health checktools.html
● National Osteoporosis Foundation, www.nof.org

See "Resources You Can Use" for more websites.

Risk factors within your control:

- Smoking. That includes cigarette, cigar, and pipe smoking, as well as exposure to secondhand smoke.

- High blood pressure. This condition causes the heart to work harder and so enlarge and weaken. *See "Blood Pressure Levels: For Adults" later in this chapter.*

- High total blood cholesterol (240 mg/dL and above) and low HDL cholesterol levels (less than 40 mg/dL). *See "Strive for Desirable Blood Lipid Levels" in this chapter.*

- Diabetes, even if under control. People with diabetes have a higher risk of dying from a heart attack. *Learn more about diabetes control later in this chapter.*

- Being overweight or obese, especially with excess abdominal fat. The excess puts strain on the heart, raises blood pressure, raises total cholesterol and triglyceride levels, and lowers HDL cholesterol level. *Refer to chapter 2 for more about healthy weight.*

- Physical inactivity, or living a sedentary lifestyle. *Refer to chapter 1 for physical activity guidelines.*

Lifestyle issues and poor nutrition contribute to the risks, too. Too much alcohol intake can raise blood pressure, which can cause heart failure and lead to a stroke. And it can contribute to high triglycerides and irregular heartbeat. Stress can be a risk, too, as it often leads to overeating, smoking, and other factors that aren't heart healthy.

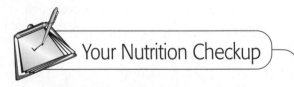

Your Nutrition Checkup

Heart Disease: Your Risk?

Use these interactive calculators for your heart attack risk assessment:

- My Life Check, American Heart Association, www.heart.org/mylifecheck

- National Cholesterol Education Program, hp2010.nhlbihin.net/atpiii/calculator.asp?usertype=pub

Metabolic Syndrome

Metabolic syndrome, sometimes referred to as insulin resistance syndrome, is defined by a large waist circumference (> 40 inches for men, > 35 inches for women), raised blood pressure, a high fasting blood glucose level, and abnormal blood lipid levels (high triglycerides and/or low HDL ["good"] cholesterol). When these conditions exist together, the risks for heart disease (heart attack and stroke) and diabetes are higher. Several factors are among those that play a key role in the development of insulin resistance syndrome: inactivity, overeating, and insulin resistance itself.

With insulin resistance, body cells don't respond normally to insulin. The pancreas produces more insulin to overcome this insensitivity; however, insulin instead builds up in blood, contributing to high blood pressure, glucose intolerance, and abnormal levels of cholesterol and triglycerides. Upper body obesity (abdominal) adds to the problem.

The treatment? Address all conditions at the same time; the recommendations for dealing with them are consistent. This includes increased physical activity, achieving a healthy weight, and eating a healthful diet that's *low* in saturated fat (less than 10 percent of total calories), *moderate* in total fat content (20 to 35 percent of total calories), and *moderate* in carbohydrates. For advice on amounts, talk to your healthcare provider.

To the contrary, a high-carbohydrate, low-fat diet may aggravate the effects of this syndrome. Along with diet therapy, medications also may be prescribed to help control blood glucose, hypertension, and high blood lipids (cholesterol and triglycerides). Stop smoking if you smoke. *See "Diabetes: A Growing Concern" in this chapter.*

Having a high risk doesn't mean you're sure to have a heart attack or a stroke. That's good news! However, the more risks for heart disease you have, and the greater their level, the greater your statistical chances. A total cholesterol level that's 300 mg/dL is riskier than one that's 250 mg/dL, although both are high risk (240 mg/dL and above). Changes in your food choices and lifestyle, and perhaps weight reduction and medication, can lower your risk score.

See "Heart Disease: A Woman's Issue, Too!" in chapter 18.

Heart Disease: The Blood Lipid Connection

High total and LDL cholesterol levels, and high triglyceride levels are major risk factors for heart disease. Conversely, lowering these cholesterol numbers and raising HDL cholesterol levels reduce the risk. What's the link?

Cholesterol, a fatlike substance produced in your liver, is found in everyone's bloodstream. As part of every body cell, it's essential to human health and cell-building. There's no Recommended Dietary Allowance for dietary cholesterol because your body makes it, too. The Dietary Guidelines advise eating less than 300 milligrams of cholesterol a day for adults if their LDL cholesterol is less than 130 mg/dL. As part of a therapeutic diet for adults with elevated LDL blood cholesterol (≥ 130 mg/dL), less than 200 mg cholesterol per day—and less than 7 percent calories from saturated fat—are advised.

Blood cholesterol is a problem if your total or LDL blood cholesterol gets too high and your HDL gets too low. When total and LDL blood cholesterol levels are elevated, deposits of cholesterol, called plaque, collect on arterial and other blood vessel walls. This condition is called atherosclerosis, or hardening of the arteries. As fatty plaques build up, arteries gradually become more narrow and may slow or block the flow of oxygen-rich blood. Chest pain may result without enough oxygen to the heart.

Plaque buildup happens silently, usually without symptoms. Warnings in the form of chest pains may not occur until vessels are about 75 percent blocked. Often a heart attack or a stroke strikes with no warning at all. A clot in a narrowed artery blocks blood flow to the heart, causing a heart attack. With a stroke, blood can't flow to the brain. The higher the blood cholesterol level, the greater the risk. When abnormally high total and LDL blood cholesterol levels go down, so does the risk for heart attack and stroke.

Arteries

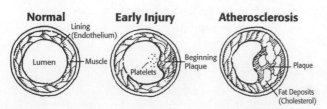

Normal **Early Injury** **Atherosclerosis**
Lining (Endothelium)
Lumen — Muscle
Platelets
Beginning Plaque
Plaque
Fat Deposits (Cholesterol)

…what medical nutrition therapy is? Often abbreviated as MNT, it's essential to comprehensive health care. For Medicare reimbursement, MNT is defined by the government as nutrition diagnoses, therapy, and counseling for the purpose of managing disease. Appropriate for many different health conditions and diseases, these services must be provided by a registered dietitian or other nutrition professional often referred by a physician, as part of safe, effective, overall care. Medical nutrition therapy is always individualized, in-depth care that's provided over time, not in a single visit, to meet very specific needs.

Most important, many people receiving care for health problems and illness can improve their health and well-being with medical nutrition therapy, and perhaps reduce their doctor visits, hospitalizations, and medication use.

For good health, aim to fit your blood cholesterol level within a desirable range. *Check "Strive for Desirable Blood Lipid Levels" in this chapter.* High total blood cholesterol isn't the only risk factor for heart disease. Even a total of 200 or less won't automatically keep you safe.

Why Do Blood Cholesterol Levels Rise and Fall?

Usually there's no single reason. For some people, high or low blood cholesterol is an inherited tendency; in part, genetics affects how much cholesterol your body makes. Families with heart disease share more than their genetic makeup. People also grow up with similar lifestyle habits that may raise cholesterol levels—perhaps high-fat eating, excessive calories, inactivity, excessive alcohol intake, or smoking (or exposure to tobacco products).

Age and gender are other factors you can't control. Even if you inherited the risk or if you're older, you can follow strategies to bring your total and LDL cholesterol levels down.

From a nutrition standpoint, a diet high in fat, especially saturated fats and *trans* fats, is a risk factor for high blood cholesterol levels. In fact, compared to other dietary components, "sat fats" and *trans* fats have the most significant cholesterol-raising effect for most of us.

Overweight and obesity are other key factors. They not only raise total and LDL cholesterol, but also raise triglycerides and lower HDLs. Physical inactivity not only contributes to overweight and high blood pressure, but also can contribute to high total and LDL cholesterol levels and lower HDLs.

HDLs and LDLs: The ups and the downs. Lipoproteins—both HDLs and LDLs—transport "packages" of cholesterol through your blood. Here's how:

● High-density lipoproteins (HDLs), or "good" blood cholesterol, act like waste removal vehicles. They take cholesterol from blood and artery walls to your liver for removal from the body. According to the National Heart, Lung, and Blood Institute, an HDL level of 60 mg/dL or more protects against heart disease. *Tip:* "H" stands for HDLs and "healthy."

To increase HDL blood cholesterol: Stay physically active and trim any extra pounds of body fat if you're not at your healthy weight. Reduce fat intake to no more than 20 to 35 percent calories from fat in your overall diet. Replace some saturated fats with monounsaturated fats. Keep *trans* fats as low as you can. If you smoke, quit.

● Low-density lipoproteins (LDLs), or "bad" blood cholesterol, work like delivery vehicles. Produced naturally in the body, they keep blood cholesterol circulating in your bloodstream, depositing plaque on artery walls along the way. As plaque builds up, atherosclerosis risk goes up. For optimal health, keep LDLs at less than 100 mg/dL. *Tip:* "L" stands for LDLs and "lousy."

To decrease LDL blood cholesterol: Substitute unsaturated fats for saturated fats, while keeping total fat and dietary cholesterol low; cut back on *trans* fatty acids (which can be found in partly hydrogenated vegetable oils). Soluble fiber and soy protein may help lower LDL cholesterol. Keeping excess body weight off also may help.

American Heart Association

LIFE'S SIMPLE 7

● Get active.
● Eat better.
● Lose weight.
● Stop smoking.
● Control cholesterol.
● Manage blood pressure.
● Reduce blood sugar.

To assess your heart health and get a heart health plan, refer to the AHA website: mylifecheck.heart.org.

DIETARY GOALS FOR CARDIOVASCULAR HEALTH*

● Balance calorie intake and physical activity to maintain a healthy body weight.
● Consume a diet rich in vegetables and fruit: ≥ 4½ cups/day.
● Choose fiber-rich whole-grain foods (≥1.1 g fiber/10 g carbohydrate: three 1-oz. equivalent servings).
● Limit intake of saturated fat to <7% of energy (calories), *trans* fat to <1% of energy (calories), and cholesterol to <300 mg/day.
● Limit processed meats: ≤ 2 servings/week.
● Include nuts, legumes, and seeds: ≥ 4 servings per week.
● Consume fish, especially oily fish at least twice a week: ≥ two 3½-oz. servings/week.
● Minimize intake of beverages and food with added sugars: Limit sugar sweetened beverages to ≤450 calories (36 oz.)/week.
● Limit sodium to <1500 mg per day.
● If consuming alcohol, do so in moderation.
● When eating food prepared away from home, follow these recommendations.

*Intake goals are expressed for a 2,000-calorie-a-day eating plan.
Source: Circulation, 2010; 121: 586–613.

The AHA's advice parallels the Dietary Guidelines for Americans, 2010, from the U.S. Department of Health and Human Services and the U.S. Department of Agriculture *(see chapter 1).*

Immunity . . . Protecting against Infections

A strong immune system doesn't guarantee that your body can fight off every cold, sniffle, flu bug, or infectious disease. But it is your best defense! Immunity is the body's ability to use its highly complex, natural defense with highly specialized cells, organs, and a lymphatic system (a circulatory system separate from blood vessels). Even your first line of defense—your skin, hair, mucous membranes, and tears and saliva—helps protect your body from potentially harmful substances. Together they protect, defend, and clear your body from "attacks" by infectious bacteria, viruses, fungi, and parasites. A normal immune response ultimately offers protection from other health problems, too, including arthritis, allergies, abnormal cell development, and cancers.

Good nutrition, which includes handling food safely to avoid foodborne illness, is essential to a strong immune response that develops gradually from infancy on. A relatively mild deficiency of even one nutrient can make a difference in your body's ability to fight infection. Among the nutrients well recognized for their many roles in building immunity and immune response: protein, vitamins A, C, and E, and zinc. Others, including vitamin B_6, folate, selenium, iron, and copper, as well as prebiotics and probiotics, may influence immune response also.

Research is under way to investigate other nutrition-related issues that may play a role in immunity, including diabetes and hypoglycemia (low blood glucose), obesity and overnutrition, and the role of lipids (fats).

To promote your own immunity, follow a healthful eating plan. Guidelines from the USDA Food Patterns can supply plenty of immune-boosting nutrients.

"Strive for Desirable Blood Lipid Levels" in this chapter shows target levels for HDLs and LDLs. To learn more, see chapter 5.

Triglycerides: Another Health Issue

High blood triglycerides get much less attention than cholesterol, yet they're significantly linked to heart disease. As with cholesterol, high blood triglyceride levels don't mean you'll develop heart disease, but the chance goes up if you have other risk factors.

Triglycerides are the main form of fat in your body and in foods, whether they're saturated, polyunsaturated, or monounsaturated. Once consumed, your liver processes them. Excess calories from any source—carbohydrates, proteins, or fats—change to triglycerides for storage as body fat. Alcohol also can boost the liver's production of triglycerides.

Your blood triglyceride level normally goes up after eating. The health risk comes from excess. Things that can increase triglyceride levels include: overweight, physical inactivity, cigarette smoking, excessive alcohol use, a very-high-carbohydrate diet, certain diseases and drugs, and genetic disorders.

Because of the risk for heart disease, the National Heart, Lung, and Blood Institute recommends treating people with borderline-high and high triglyceride levels. If your blood triglyceride level consistently exceeds normal, then a healthier weight, regular physical activity, and perhaps medication may bring it down. (Normal is below 150mg/dL.) In fact, the advice for lowering total blood cholesterol levels also applies to reducing triglyceride levels. Of importance:

● Maintain or improve your weight. Weight loss alone may significantly lower triglyceride levels.

● Reduce the solid fats (saturated and *trans* fats), and cholesterol in your meals and snacks. If you have high triglycerides, switching from saturated fats to monounsaturated and polyunsaturated fats in foods such as canola oil, olive oil, or liquid margarine may help. Eating less fat and more carbohydrate may not be effective; in some people this tactic may raise triglyceride levels and decrease HDL cholesterol levels.

● Eat fruits, vegetables, and fat-free or low-fat dairy products often.

● Get regular physical activity. *See chapter 1 for guidelines.*

● If you drink alcoholic beverages, consume less or skip them entirely. Even small amounts of alcoholic drinks can have a significant effect on blood triglyceride levels.

● Eat oily fish, such as salmon and albacore tuna, since their omega-3 fatty acids may help lower triglycerides. *Refer to chapter 5 for more about omega-3s.*

Be aware: High blood pressure multiplies the risk.

Testing, Testing: Know Your Numbers!

Numbers don't tell the whole story of heart health, but they're good predictors. Know your blood lipid numbers—total cholesterol, LDL, HDL, and triglyceride levels—whether or not you're at risk for heart disease and no matter what your adult age or gender.

Unless you're screened regularly, high lipid levels usually go unnoticed because high blood cholesterol has no symptoms. If you're age twenty or older, have your cholesterol level checked at least every five years—and more often if you're considerably older or at risk for heart disease. If you have a father or brother with heart disease before age 55, or a mother or sister before age 65, health experts advise screening before age twenty years. If your first results are high, your doctor may advise another test soon. Rather than self-diagnose, let your physician or a registered dietitian interpret your test results—and guide you to achieve and maintain your cholesterol numbers at healthy levels. *For children, see "Should You Have Your Child's Cholesterol Level Checked?" in chapter 17.*

Blood lipid levels are measured from a blood sample. What about cholesterol screenings at a mall or a health fair? As an initial screening, these finger stick tests for cholesterol may be good indicators. If your cholesterol number is borderline high or high—or if you have other risk factors for heart disease—have it rechecked with your healthcare provider. A finger stick screening may be less accurate than a blood test done in your doctor's office or a health center.

For a complete picture, you need a blood test called a lipoprotein profile: LDL, total, and HDL cholesterol levels as well as blood triglycerides. Triglyceride levels are especially important if you have other risk factors—for example, high total blood cholesterol; two or more risk factors for heart disease, such as smoking and obesity; or health problems related to triglycerides, such as diabetes, high blood pressure, obesity, chronic kidney disease, or circulatory disease. Before you're tested, follow the directions care-

---

STRIVE FOR DESIRABLE BLOOD LIPID LEVELS

To lower your heart disease risk, strive to keep your blood lipid levels at desirable levels for life. If you don't know your blood cholesterol and triglyceride numbers, check soon. Then act on the results!

LEVEL	CATEGORY
Total Cholesterol	
● Less than 200 mg/dL	Desirable
● 200-239 mg/dL	Borderline high
● 240 mg/dL and above	High
LDL Cholesterol	
● Less than 100 mg/dL	Optimal
● 100-129 mg/dL	Near optimal/above optimal
● 130-159 mg/dL	Borderline high
● 160-189 mg/dL	High
● 190 mg/dL and above	Very high
Triglyceride	
● Less than 150 mg/dL	Normal
● 150-199 mg/dL	Borderline high
● 200 or more	High
HDL Cholesterol	
● Less than 40 mg/dL	A major risk factor for heart disease
● 40-59 mg/dL	The higher, the better
● 60 mg/dL or more	Considered protective against heart disease

Source: National Heart, Lung, and Blood Institute, National Institutes of Health: www.nhlbi.nih.gov/health/health-topics/topics/hbc/diagnosis.html. Accessed January 1, 2012.

---

fully from your doctor's office for accurate results.

If you're at greater risk for heart disease, your doctor might order another test: a type of C-reactive protein (CPR) test. This test assesses arteries for inflammation. Inflammation, a protective immune reaction from an injury or infection, can damage the inner lining of arteries. That can cause clots to break off and block blood flow, making a heart attack or a stroke more likely. Many factors may cause CPR levels to rise and fluctuate, including high blood pressure, insulin resistance, high triglyceride levels, and cigarette smoking. Regular physical activity, a healthy weight, and a heart-healthy diet with omega-3 fatty acids may help reduce inflammation. That said, the connection between high CPR levels and heart attack risk is not very well-understood. Studies are being done to see if CPR testing can assess the risk for other health conditions such as diabetes.

What about over-the-counter cholesterol tests? Done properly, they can be relatively accurate. However, home tests measure only total blood cholesterol levels, not HDLs, LDLs, and triglycerides. Like finger stick tests, verify the results with your healthcare provider—especially if your results are 200 mg/dL or more for total blood cholesterol and if you have other risk factors, such as a family history of heart disease. That said, you need blood tests from your healthcare provider to track your blood lipid levels!

If You Need to Improve Your Lipid Levels

Bringing your cholesterol numbers down takes effort and commitment, changes in your eating and lifestyle, and perhaps medication. Here's what you need to do. If you have diabetes and risk factors that affect LDLs, you may need more aggressive treatment for high LDL and total cholesterol levels. Other heart-disease-related problems may require other dietary changes; get advice from your doctor or a registered dietitian.

Eat for Heart Health

If you're among the many Americans with high or borderline high total blood cholesterol or LDL cholesterol levels, a few changes in your food choices and lifestyle may bring your numbers down . . . and even boost your HDLs. Even if your levels are normal, or you take cholesterol-lowering medication, these guidelines make sense.

● Limit saturated fat (solid fats) to less than 7 percent of calories,* ** according to the American Heart Association and the National Cholesterol Education Program of the National Heart, Lung, and Blood Institute, and keep *trans* fats as low as possible. Saturated and *trans* fats boost blood cholesterol levels more than anything else you consume. Substitute foods high in unsaturated fats for those higher in solid fats—saturated fats (fatty meat, poultry skin, bacon, butter, cheese, whole milk) and *trans* fat (stick margarine, packaged foods with partially hydrogenated oils)—without increasing your total fat intake.

● Limit dietary cholesterol to less than 200 mg per day** if you have high blood cholesterol, advises the National Cholesterol Education Program. Although less significant than cutting back on saturated fat, this can make a difference. You don't need to eliminate foods with cholesterol, just be prudent. Foods high in cholesterol include egg yolks (one yolk has about 185 mg of cholesterol), fatty meat, shrimp, lobster, crab, cheese, and whole milk. These same foods have other health benefits.

● Keep the total amount of fat you consume (including heart-healthy fats) to 20 to 35 percent of your calories.* You need fat to stay healthy so don't attempt to cut fat out of your diet entirely. Some fats are heart healthy. Many foods with fat also contain other nutrients your body needs.

● Consume foods with enough dietary fiber. The National Cholesterol Education suggests 10 to 25 grams of viscous fiber daily to enhance LDL cholesterol lowering. In the intestines, fiber binds to cholesterol-rich bile acids, passing them out of the body as waste rather than reabsorbing them. Fiber also may help improve the LDL-HDL ratio. Among the sources of fiber: oatmeal, brown rice, whole-wheat bread, beans (such as kidney and pinto beans), and many fruits and vegetables. *See chapter 3 for more about fiber.* No long-term studies show heart-healthy benefits from fiber supplements; they are not currently advised for reducing heart disease risk.

● Eat a variety of fruits and vegetables daily. Besides their fiber content, most are low in calories and fat. Emerging research also suggests potential benefits from their antioxidant nutrients and phytonutrients.

● Consider plant stanols and sterols (2 grams per day) as therapeutic options to enhance LDL lowering. *See chapter 5 to learn more.*

● Make some of your meals plant-based. In other words, feature beans (legumes) and foods with soy protein as your key protein source.

● Eat only enough calories to reach and/or maintain your healthy weight. Ask your doctor or a registered dietitian what a reasonable calorie level is for you.

*See chapter 5 for figuring percent calories from various types of fat.
**Dietary Guidelines for Americans differ somewhat.

Refer to other chapters in this book for practical eating strategies to achieve these dietary goals.

Manage Your Weight

Maintain or improve your weight. The more excess body fat you have, the greater your risk for heart disease. If you're overweight, losing weight—even ten pounds—can help you lower LDL cholesterol. That's especially important if you have high triglycerides and/or low HDL cholesterol, and carry excess abdominal fat. Those who carry a "spare tire" around their abdomen have a higher cardiac risk than those with extra padding around their hips and thighs. *See chapter 2, "Your Healthy Weight."*

Keep Moving!

Regular, moderate activity helps keep your blood cholesterol and triglyceride levels normal. It helps boost your HDLs and lower your LDLs and triglycerides, helps reduce blood pressure, helps your body control stress, and helps reduce excess body weight as you burn energy. More vigorous aerobic activity gives your heart muscle a good workout and ultimately helps your whole cardiovascular and respiratory systems stay fit. *See chapters 1 and 2 for more about physical activity.*

Have You Ever Wondered

. . . if high blood cholesterol could be linked to a thyroid problem? Yes, it could. Hypothyroidism—when the thyroid gland doesn't produce enough of the hormone thyroxin—has many symptoms. Among them are a sluggish feeling, poor memory, dry skin and hair, feeling cold, constipation, heavy menstrual flow, weight gain, and muscle cramps. Elevated LDL cholesterol may be another and serious side effect.

Treating hypothyroidism with medication—thyroid hormone—also helps reduce high LDL cholesterol levels associated with this condition. Untreated, hypothyroidism can damage the cardiovascular system permanently.

As part of a routine physical exam, have your physician check for thyroid problems. Hypothyroidism is much more common among women than among men.

Make Other Changes

Diet, weight management, and physical activity aren't the only ways to heart health.

● If you have high blood pressure, get it under control. High blood pressure is a key risk factor for heart attack and stroke. *See "Blood Pressure: Under Control?" in this chapter.*

● If you smoke, give up the habit. It's a key factor in sudden death from cardiovascular disease. Smoking seems to raise blood pressure levels and heart rate. It may lower HDL cholesterol levels, too. And smoking may increase the tendency of blood to clot and so lead to a heart attack. For those who stop smoking, heart disease risk goes down over time, even for longtime smokers.

● If you have diabetes, keep it under control.

Consider Emerging Science

Other substances in food also may be cholesterol-lowering. For some, research evidence is strong; for others, it's preliminary but promising.

● *Soy.* Soybeans and soy products such as soy beverage, tofu, tempeh, and soyburgers (but not soybean oil) contain soy protein and several phytonutrients that may promote heart health; isoflavones are the phytonutrients that get the most consumer attention.

DROP YOUR LDL CHOLESTEROL WITH TLC

The Therapeutic Lifestyle Changes (TLC) Program of the National Heart, Lung, and Blood Institute estimates how much you can lower your LDL cholesterol, based on research. The more you do, the lower your LDL will likely go. And if you take cholesterol-lowering medication, you still benefit and keep your dose down.

	CHANGE	LDL REDUCTION
Saturated Fat	Decrease to less than 7% of calories	8–10%
Dietary cholesterol	Decrease to less than 200 mg/day	3–5%
Weight	Lose 10 pounds if overweight	5–8%
Soluble fiber	Add 5 to 10 grams/day	3–5%
Plant sterols/ stanols	Add 2 grams/day	5–15%
Total		20–30%*

*This compares well with many cholesterol-lowering drugs.
Source: National Heart, Lung, and Blood Institute, 2005.

Have You Ever Wondered

. . . how many eggs you can eat as part of a heart healthy diet? Unless your physician advises less, today's advice is more liberal than in the past—even one egg yolk daily—if you limit your overall cholesterol intake to less than 300 milligrams daily; one large egg yolk has about 185 milligrams of cholesterol. To check the cholesterol in any packaged food, check the Nutrition Facts on the label or displayed near fresh produce, meat, poultry, and seafood.

. . . if eating more olive oil may have a cholesterol-lowering effect? Likely so, but not if you end up eating a diet high in total fat. An eating plan that's low in saturated fats, *trans* fats, and cholesterol and moderate in total fat is recommended for heart health. For heart-healthy eating, substitute in some monounsaturated fats for some saturated fats in your food choices. Olive, canola, and safflower oils are all high in monounsaturated fats.

. . . if garlic is good for your heart? Perhaps, but the research on the heart health benefits of allium (a phytonutrient) in garlic and onions is preliminary. Best advice: Enjoy the flavor of garlic, but don't count on it for heart-healthy benefits. Follow medically sound advice to keep your blood cholesterol under control. Although you can buy garlic pills and extracts,

supplements may lack the phytonutrients that impart potential cholesterol-lowering benefits. Garlic supplements may cause stomach irritation and nausea.

. . . if fish oil supplements can protect your heart? Fish oil supplements are promoted for their omega-3 fatty acids and their potential for lowering the risk for blocked blood vessels and heart attacks. However, proper dosage has not been determined, and they can't cancel out the effects of a diet high in solid fats (saturated and *trans* fats). *Best guideline:* Enjoy oily fish instead, and follow an overall moderate-fat eating plan.

High-quality, contaminant-free fish oil supplements may be advised for people with high triglycerides who may benefit from consuming more omega-3s than their diet alone can provide. Some fish oils supplements are high in vitamin A; check the Supplement Facts to avoid consuming toxic levels.

. . . if fat replacers offer heart-healthy benefits? Perhaps—if you use them to replace full-fat foods and avoid consuming too many calories overall. In part because these products are relatively new, no research shows long-term benefits. Until more is known, use them to give you flexibility with fat control. *See "About Fat Replacers . . ." in chapter 5.*

Although research can't confirm a direct benefit between soy intake and blood cholesterol levels, there may be an indirect benefit if soy replaces foods high in saturated fats. For adults, soy protein may have small effects on total and LDL cholesterol levels; however, research findings are inconsistent. *For more about soy protein, see chapter 4.*

● *Plant stanols and sterols.* Plant stanols and sterols, found naturally in fruits, vegetables, and plant oils, have an LDL-cholesterol-lowering effect. They work by inhibiting the absorption of cholesterol (from food and bile acids) in the intestine; instead, cholesterol passes out of the body through waste.

Some spreads, juices, yogurts, and soft gel capsules are formulated to be high in plant stanols or sterols. These can be effective for lowering cholesterol for those with elevated LDL cholesterol levels. To be effective, you need to consume enough: 2 grams of plant stanols and sterols per day, with meals or other foods—as part

of an eating plan that's low in saturated fat and cholesterol. *See "Functional Nutrition: Plant Stanols and Sterols" in chapter 5.*

● *Omega-3 fatty acids.* "Omega-3s" from oily fish, such as salmon or tuna, may help reduce the risk of heart disease, although the data aren't conclusive. That's why the American Heart Association recommends eating at least two 3½-ounce servings of oily fish a week. Omega-3 fatty acids from other sources—for example canola, soy, and flaxseed oils—may have a similar effect. The American Heart Association advises 1 gram of omega-3 fatty acids from an EPA and DHA combination per day, for those with documented heart disease, preferably from oily fish. Before taking fish oil supplements, talk to your doctor. *See "Functional Nutrition: Eat Your Omega-3s and -6s" in chapter 5.*

● *Folic acid.* The fact that today's grain products are fortified with folic acid (a form of folate) to prevent neural tube defects also may benefit heart health (another reason to enjoy grain products). Here's why: A high level of homocysteine, an amino acid (a protein) in the blood, may indicate a higher risk of heart disease. Although the reasons aren't clear, homocysteine may promote buildup of plaque in the arteries. An area of scientific study and controversy: the role of folic acid (a B vitamin), and perhaps vitamins B_6 and

B_{12}, in lowering an elevated level of homocysteine in blood, and so helping to protect against heart disease. (A doctor can order a lab test to check your homocysteine level.)

Folate comes from fortified grain products, vegetables, and fruits. Folate and B vitamin supplementation aren't advised to reduce heart disease risk.

● *Antioxidants.* Antioxidant nutrients and some phytonutrients in food may benefit the heart. For example, vitamin E may offer protection from blood clots and atherosclerosis, and vitamin C may help keep blood vessels flexible. The evidence is too limited to recommend vitamin supplements; instead, enjoy a variety of nutrient-rich foods that supply antioxidant nutrients. Certain flavonoids in foods such as apples, grapes, tea, and cocoa, and lignans in flaxseed and some vegetables may promote heart health too. *To learn more about food's antioxidant benefits for heart health, refer to chapter 6.*

Cholesterol-Lowering Medication

Depending on your numbers, your risk factors, and if you have diabetes, your doctor may recommend cholesterol-lowering medication, too. The higher your heart disease risk, the lower your LDL cholesterol goal. By reducing your LDL and total cholesterol with eating and lifestyle choices, you may need a lower dose of medication.

For women, hormone therapy isn't an alternative for cholesterol-lowering medication. According to the National Heart, Lung, and Blood Institute, research indicates that hormone therapy doesn't reduce the risk for heart disease, stroke, or death after menopause, and it may increase the chances for gallbladder disease and the blockage of blood vessels (perhaps to the heart or brain) by a blood clot.

Talk to your doctor or healthcare provider about specific heart disease prevention guidelines for women and children.

Blood Pressure: Under Control?

Do you know your blood pressure reading? High blood pressure, or hypertension, often creeps up slowly and quietly. Until it's advanced, there usually are no symptoms. But undetected and uncontrolled, high blood pressure may cause damage to the heart, brain, and

---

Warning Signs: Heart Attack, Stroke, and Cardiac Arrest

Heart Attack*

● Chest discomfort or pain: uncomfortable pressure, squeezing, fullness, or pain, usually in the center of the chest, that lasts more than a few minutes or that goes away and comes back

● Discomfort or pain in other areas of the upper body—for example, one or both arms, the back, neck, jaw, or stomach

● Shortness of breath—with or without chest discomfort

● Other signs: perhaps breaking out in a cold sweat, nausea, or light-headedness

Stroke

● Sudden numbness or weakness of the face, arm, or leg, especially on one side of the body

● Sudden confusion; trouble speaking; trouble understanding

● Sudden trouble seeing in one or both eyes

● Sudden trouble walking; dizziness; loss of balance or coordination

● Severe headache with no known cause

Cardiac Arrest

● Sudden loss of responsiveness; no response to tapping on shoulders

● No normal breathing: the victim does not take a normal breath when you tilt the head up and check for at least five seconds.

*Warning signs for men and women may differ. Women will commonly feel chest pain and discomfort. But they're more likely than men to experience other symptoms, such as jaw ache, back pain, nausea, or vomiting. Have these symptoms checked immediately by a doctor—even if you're unsure. Minutes matter—call 911!

Sources: American Heart Association, American Stroke Association.

kidneys for years without you knowing. Sometimes the first sign is a heart attack or a stroke. More than a million heart attacks and half a million strokes yearly are caused in part by high blood pressure.

About one in three American adults have high blood pressure, yet about 21 percent don't know it (2010 data, American Heart Association). Only 45 percent have their blood pressure under control. And about 30 percent of those with high blood pressure aren't being treated. And many Americans have prehypertension.

Take action to prevent and control high blood pressure. Once it develops, it usually lasts a lifetime.

What Is High Blood Pressure? What Risks?

You've heard the term "high blood pressure" many times. But do you know what it really is? And how does it start? For reasons that aren't yet clear, the body system that regulates blood flow malfunctions.

First, what it's not: Hypertension isn't emotional tension or stress, or being hyperactive, although stress may raise blood pressure temporarily. Even calm, relaxed people can have high blood pressure. For some, stress may be a factor, although the evidence isn't clear-cut.

Blood pressure is the force of blood against artery walls. That pressure helps push blood throughout your arteries, blood vessels, and capillaries so oxygen can reach body cells. A blood pressure reading reflects two forces: one that forces blood from the heart to your arteries, the other force from the heart rests between heart beats. It's normal for blood pressure to rise and fall during the day.

High blood pressure, or hypertension, means consistently higher-than-normal pressure on blood vessel walls, in other words, too much force. It happens over time as blood gets pushed with more tension through arterioles, or small blood vessels, that become stretched, stiff, and constricted. Overstretched blood vessels are more prone to rupture. They can also tear, leaving scar tissue, which can trap plaque, cholesterol, and blood cells, narrowing the passage for blood. As plaque builds up in the arteries and blood flow is restricted, blood pressure goes higher. Eventually arteries or blood vessels may get blocked; plaque might break off and block blood flow to the heart or brain, causing a heart attack or stroke. Other organs might get damaged if they don't get enough oxygen.

High blood pressure causes the heart to work harder; the higher the pressure, the greater the work and the greater the risk of heart attack and stroke. By putting pressure on blood vessels in the eye, it may damage the retina, impair vision, and even cause blindness. High blood pressure can cause other problems: heart failure, kidney disease, paralysis, and brain damage. These problems result from permanent damage to the blood vessels of the heart, kidneys, eyes, and brain.

High Blood Pressure: Are You at Risk?

High blood pressure is a complex problem, and in most cases its causes are still unknown. Only about 5 to 10 percent of cases can be attributed to known health problems, such as kidney disease. Yet health experts can identify people with increased risk. While more common after age 35, high blood pressure can develop in children.

● *Family history of high blood pressure?* There's a genetic tendency for high blood pressure. If your parents or close blood relatives have had high blood pressure, your chances are higher.

● *Race?* African Americans have higher average blood pressure levels and tend to be more sodium-sensitive than European Americans. Typically African Americans develop hypertension earlier. As a result, they're at greater risk for kidney disease as hypertension progresses and for death from strokes and heart disease. Some Asians also are at greater risk.

● *Overweight or obese?* Extra body fat, especially around the waist and midriff, increases the risk for high blood pressure. Excessive weight puts more strain on the heart. Losing ten to twenty pounds can bring blood pressure down.

● *Your age and gender?* For many people, blood pressure goes up as they get older and blood vessels lose their flexibility. For men it's sooner, perhaps starting by ages forty-five to fifty. Women often are protected through menopause; for them, high blood pressure often starts about seven to ten years later. Even if you don't have high blood pressure at age fifty-five, you have a 90 percent chance of developing it during your lifetime! Starting at about age sixty-five, the incidence is higher among women.

LIFESTYLE MODIFICATIONS TO MANAGE HIGH BLOOD PRESSURE

MODIFICATION	RECOMMENDATION	APPROXIMATE SYSTOLIC BLOOD PRESSURE REDUCTION (RANGE) *
Reduce weight	Maintain normal body weight (BMI 18.5–24.9)	5 to 20 mm Hg per 10 kg (22 lb) of weight loss
Adopt DASH eating plan	Consume a diet rich in fruits, vegetables, and low-fat dairy products with a reduced content of saturated and total fat.	8 to 14 mm Hg
Reduce dietary sodium	Reduce dietary sodium intake to no more than 2400 milligrams of sodium** per day or 6 grams of sodium chloride.	2 to 8 mm Hg
Engage in regular aerobic physical activity	Engage in regular aerobic physical activity such as brisk walking (at least 30 minutes per day, most days of the week).	4 to 9 mm Hg
Moderate alcohol consumption	Limit consumption to no more than 2 drinks per day for men and to no more than 1 drink per day for women and light-weight persons. (One drink is 12 ounces beer, 5 ounces wine, or 1½ ounces 80-proof distilled spirits.)	2 to 4 mm Hg

For overall cardiovascular risk reduction, stop smoking.

* Blood pressure reduction is greater for some people and depends on time and dose.

** The Dietary Guidelines for Americans, 2010, advises less than 2,300 milligrams of sodium daily for most people. The American Heart Association advises less than 1,500 milligrams sodium daily for all Americans.

Source: The Seventh Report of the Joint National Committee on Prevention, Detection, Evaluation, and Treatment of High Blood Pressure, U.S. Department of Health and Human Services, National Institutes of Health, National Heart, Lung, and Blood Institute, 2003.

● *Sodium-sensitive?* For many, an eating plan that's high in sodium may contribute to high blood pressure. There's no way to predict whose blood pressure may be sodium-sensitive. The 2010 Dietary Guidelines advises reducing daily sodium intake to less than 2,300 milligrams (mg) and to further reduce intake to 1,500 mg among those who are 51 years and older and those of any age who are African American or have hypertension, diabetes, or chronic kidney disease. The American Heart Association advice is lower: less than 1,500 milligrams sodium daily for all Americans. For everyone, consume more potassium-rich foods to help blunt sodium's effect on blood pressure.

A poor diet overall can be a contributing factor, too; it may result in overweight or obesity, and low potassium and/or high sodium intake.

● *Sedentary lifestyle?* Inactivity can be a factor in overweight and obesity. Conversely, regular physical activity may help lower your blood pressure since it's healthful for your heart and circulatory system.

Stress, smoking, and exposure to secondhand smoke, and sleep apnea may contribute to high blood pressure, but scientific evidence doesn't prove that

Medications: Sodium Alert

Are you on a sodium-modified eating plan? If so, talk to your doctor or pharmacist about medications. Some contain sodium, including some antacids and alkalizers, headache remedies, laxatives, sedatives, and others.

If you're taking medication prescribed for high blood pressure, eating less sodium may let your medication work more effectively. If sodium reduction helps control your blood pressure, you may be able to reduce the dosage of antihypertensive medication.

they're causes. All are linked to other health risks, however.

Several health conditions can contribute to increased risk for hypertension:

● *Too much drinking?* Heavy and regular alcoholic drinking may increase the risk for high blood pressure

A Toast to Heart Health

Does moderate drinking reduce the risk for heart disease? Maybe, although for heart health benefits people who don't drink aren't advised to start. Moderate drinking (red or white wine, beer, or distilled spirits) may offer heart-health benefits for some people. Moderate drinking also may raise HDL levels and keep some LDL cholesterol from forming, according to recent research. Resveratrol, a phytonutrient in the skins and seeds of grapes, may function as an antioxidant, promoting heart health; it also may help keep blood platelets from sticking together. There's a fine line between how much alcohol is protective and how much instead may promote heart disease, high blood pressure, and strokes. Remember, alcohol also can raise triglyceride levels. Stick to moderation.

There's reason for caution. Research linking alcoholic beverages and heart health isn't conclusive. For example, we don't yet know who may benefit. Even if a minor benefit exists, moderate drinking is only one factor related to heart health. Other lifestyle factors may play a role—for example, wine drinkers may be more physically active, and they may drink wine with meals, which may help affect blood lipid (fat) levels. *See "Red Wine: Heart-Healthy?" in chapter 8.*

Excessive and binge drinking is risky. Besides potentially leading to high blood pressure, heart failure, and excess calories, too much drinking can lead to stroke, irregular heartbeat, and sudden cardiac death. For pregnant women, drinking is the leading known cause of birth defects. Even moderate drinking isn't advised.

Alcoholic beverages also supply extra calories, so if you're trying to control weight for heart health, control calories from alcoholic beverages, too.

If you take aspirin regularly for heart health, your doctor may advise you to limit alcoholic beverages. Until we know more, moderation is advised.

For more about alcoholic beverages in a healthful eating plan and a definition of moderate drinking, see "Alcoholic Beverages: In Moderation" in chapter 8.

Have You Ever Wondered

. . . what to do if you have prehypertension? Even high-normal blood pressure appears to increase cardiovascular risk significantly. If you fit into this category, you're smart to monitor your blood pressure regularly—and to make lifestyle and dietary changes now to bring your blood pressure down to a healthier level. That's equally important if you have high cholesterol levels, diabetes, or other cardiovascular risk factors, or if you're an older adult.

and may lead to irregular heartbeat, stroke, and heart attack.

● *Diabetes?* People with diabetes may develop high blood pressure if their condition isn't managed carefully—another reason to control diabetes from its first diagnosis. Up to 65 percent of people with diabetes have it. *See "Diabetes: A Growing Concern" in this chapter.*

● *High blood lipids?* If your blood lipids are high, they contribute to hypertension as well as to atherosclerosis. *See "Strive for Desirable Blood Lipid Levels" earlier in this chapter.*

● *Prehypertension?* Even if your blood pressure is between 120/80 to 139/89 mm Hg, be cautious. With prehypertension you'll likely develop high blood pressure later on. Take steps now to prevent it with healthful food and lifestyle choices.

Testing: Know Your Blood Pressure

A blood pressure measurement is two readings that look like a fraction. For example, an optimal reading is 120/80 mm Hg, expressed as "120 over 80" (mm Hg is millimeters of mercury). If it's less, that's okay.

● The higher number on top is systolic pressure. That's the pressure when your heart (the ventricle) contracts, pumping blood out to your arteries.

● The bottom number, diastolic pressure, is the pressure on your arteries between heartbeats, when your heart is at rest.

Whether you suspect high blood pressure or not, have your blood pressure checked at least every two years. If it's high normal (130–139 mm Hg over 85-89 mm Hg) or high, have it checked more often and take steps to bring it down. Even children should be checked as part of their regular physical exams.

If your systolic, but not diastolic, pressure is high, you can have high blood pressure. With age, systolic blood pressure goes up; diastolic pressure does too until age fifty-five or so, then often goes down. "Isolated systolic hypertension" is the most common type of high blood pressure for older Americans.

Blood pressure may fluctuate a bit during the day. Often the doctor's visit itself makes the number rise slightly; that's sometimes called "white-coat hypertension," which refers to white medical lab coats. To diagnose high blood pressure you need two higher-than-normal readings taken one to several weeks apart.

If either your systolic or your diastolic number, or both, are consistently at or above 140/90 mm Hg, there's cause for concern. Usually high blood pressure is managed by a combination of medication, nutrition, and lifestyle changes. For those with diabetes, a still lower blood pressure goal might be advised.

Your local pharmacist may offer blood pressure readings as a free service. Or buy an electronic blood pressure measuring device to use at home. To check its accuracy, bring it to your next doctor's visit.

Not Too "Pressured"

Having a family history of high blood pressure doesn't necessarily mean you'll get it. And you can take preventive steps to reduce blood pressure, or make your

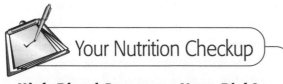

Your Nutrition Checkup

High Blood Pressure: Your Risk?

Use an interactive calculator to assess your high blood pressure risk:

● High Blood Pressure Health Risk Calculator, American Heart Association, www.heart.org/HEARTORG/Conditions/Whats-Your-Risk-Find-out_UCM_306929_Article.jsp

BLOOD PRESSURE LEVELS: FOR ADULTS*

CATEGORY		SYSTOLIC[†]		DIASTOLIC[†]
Normal		<120 mm Hg	and	<80 mm Hg
Prehypertension		120-139 mm Hg	or	80-89 mm Hg
High[‡]	Stage 1	140-159 mm Hg	or	90-99 mm Hg
	Stage 2	≥160 mm Hg	or	≥100 mm Hg

*These categories are for people age eighteen or over. The categories are for those not on a high blood pressure medication and who have no short-term serious illness.

Source: Seventh Report of the Joint National Committee on Prevention, Detection, Evaluation, and Treatment of High Blood Pressure, U.S. Department of Health and human Services, National Institutes of Health/National Heart, Lung, and Blood Institute, National High Blood Pressure Education Program, 2003.

blood pressure medication more effective. In fact, the Dietary Guidelines addresses blood pressure control and protects against hypertension! *See chapter 1.*

● Eat for heart health—with the right amounts of fruit, vegetables, beans, whole-grain and high-fiber foods, fat-free and low-fat dairy foods, lean meat, skinless poultry, and fish (including oily fish with omega-3s). Go low with solid fats (saturated and *trans* fats) and sodium, and limit added sugars.

● Limit sodium to less than 2,300 milligrams daily and 1,500 milligrams daily if you are 51 years and older or of any age if you are African American or have hypertension, diabetes, or chronic kidney disease. And eat more potassium-rich foods, since they blunt the effects of sodium on blood pressure. Use the Nutrition Facts on food labels to make your food choices. *See chapter 7 for more about sodium, potassium, and salt substitutes.*

● Eat plenty of fruits and vegetables. The potassium and magnesium found in many fruits and vegetables may help control your blood pressure. *For more about potassium and magnesium and their food sources, see chapters 6 and 7.*

● Put dairy foods and other calcium-rich foods on the "menu." Three minerals—calcium, magnesium, and potassium—help regulate blood pressure. Calcium, and perhaps magnesium and potassium, which are all found in dairy foods, appear to be protective. *See chapter 6 for more about these minerals.* No conclusive evidence shows that calcium and magnesium supplements offer extra benefits.

The DASH (Dietary Approaches to Stop Hypertension) Eating Plan, established by the National Heart, Lung, and Blood Institute of the National Institutes of Health, emphasizes food rather than nutrients for lowering blood pressure. The DASH plan has been shown to lower blood pressure: down 2 to 8 mm Hg for systolic blood pressure. That's enough to lower hypertension risk significantly. In research studies, the DASH plan worked quickly—lowering blood pressure within two weeks. The benefits of the DASH plan were even better when combined with eating less sodium (down to 1,500 milligrams daily) in the DASH-Sodium study; blood pressure dropped even more, especially for those with hypertension. Lower in fat, abundant in phytonutrients, the DASH plan also may protect against some cancers, heart disease, and other health issues. *See chapter 10.*

● If you have a few pounds to shed, do so. Losing even 10 pounds, through smart eating and physical activity, may bring your blood pressure down and reduce the strain on your heart—perhaps enough to avoid medication. As part of your weight loss plan, reducing solid fats and switching to oil lowers blood lipid levels, too—a benefit to heart health and diabetes management. *See chapter 2, "Your Healthy Weight."*

● Fit in regular moderate to vigorous physical activity, at least 30 minutes a day, on most days. Sedentary living doesn't cause high blood pressure, but regular aerobic activity such as brisk walking, swimming, or biking may help bring it down. Moreover, physical activity can help you maintain a healthy weight. Talk to your doctor about a physical activity plan, including how to pace yourself and your level of exertion.

● Go easy on alcoholic beverages—if you drink. No more than one drink a day for women, and two for men, appear safe. Alcoholic drinks may interfere with medication for hypertension.

● Avoid tobacco smoke, including secondhand smoke. Although evidence doesn't show smoking to cause high blood pressure, each cigarette increases blood pressure temporarily for several minutes.

● Use hot tubs wisely if you have high blood pressure—and not if you're having a hypertensive crisis! Heat causes blood vessels to open, as does taking a brisk walk. If you doctor advises you to avoid moderate physical activity, skip the hot tub, too. Moving back

Have You Ever Wondered

... if caffeine causes high blood pressure? Since caffeine is a mild stimulant, you may think so. However, studies show that caffeine may result in only a very slight, temporary rise in blood pressure level.

and forth between cold water and a hot tub or sauna can raise blood pressure, too. Alcoholic drinks and saunas don't mix either!

● Manage stress. It may lead to overeating, poor eating, smoking, or drinking alcoholic beverages, which may increase your risk. Blood pressure may rise temporarily with the stress of a situation; the effects of chronic stress on blood pressure aren't known.

If You Have High Blood Pressure . . .

Relax. Although it's a lifelong condition, you can control high blood pressure and live a long, healthy life. The key is following your doctor's advice faithfully. Treatment likely will include a shift in your eating approach, weight loss (if you're overweight), more physical activity, smoking cessation (if you smoke), and perhaps blood pressure medication.

● Make a plan of action with your healthcare provider.

● If your doctor prescribes antihypertensive medication, take it faithfully. If other tactics, like weight loss, lower your blood pressure level, taking medication may not be forever. Follow directions for medications carefully. Different blood pressure medications work in different ways; some may interact with other medications—for example, for diabetes or kidney disease.

● If your doctor prescribes a sodium-modified diet, a registered dietitian can help you plan, follow through, and monitor your sodium intake.

Cancer Connection

After heart disease, cancer is the second leading cause of illness and death in the United States, currently accounting for nearly one in four deaths. About 41 percent of the population will be diagnosed with cancer during their lifetime says the National Cancer

Institute. Yet, with early detection and new cancer treatments, the survival rates for all diagnosed cancers have climbed dramatically. The American Cancer Society (ACS) has reported remarkable progress, with a survival rate of 66 percent for all cancers diagnosed between 1999 and 2006. The National Cancer Institute notes that 11.7 million Americans are *living* with a history of cancer.

ACS 2010 data estimates that almost 1.48 million Americans were diagnosed with cancer in 2010. For new cases among men, the incidence of prostate cancer is highest, followed by lung and bronchial cancer, then colorectal cancer. And for women, the prevalence of breast cancer is highest, followed by lung, then colorectal cancer. The overall death rate follows a similar order except that lung cancer for both men and women leaps to the top.

Because of increased survival rates, cancer has become a chronic disease for many, as cancer survivors are living longer. At every stage of this disease—before, during, and after treatment, during remission, during recurrence, and during palliative and hospice care—good nutrition is important.

What Is Cancer?

Cancer is an assortment of more than 100 diseases characterized by abnormal cell growth that can spread and destroy other organs and body tissue. Cancers are classified by the body tissues where the cancer starts, such as the colon, breast, or skin.

Cancer starts with a single cell that divides abnormally. Because the DNA is damaged, the cell does not function as it should. An altered body cell multiplies at an abnormally fast rate to form new abnormal cells, which use the body's resources, including nutrients, to multiply. Unlike normal cells that constantly are repaired or replaced, cancer cells grow out of control. With their damaged DNA, they invade other tissues. In the process, they disrupt and eventually destroy the normal function of the tissue or organ where they grow. These cancerous cells can metastasize, or spread through the bloodstream or the lymphatic system to other parts of the body, invading and destroying healthy body tissues and organs far from the original tumor.

The causes of cancer are varied and not always clear. Some cancers appear to be genetic and run in families. However, most cancers result from environmental and lifestyle factors. In other words, the cell's DNA gets damaged while the normal cell is reproducing or by a carcinogen in the environment, such as cigarette smoke. Cancer promoters, called carcinogens, include viruses, chemicals, and lifestyle and environmental factors.

Reducing Your Cancer Risk

Since some risk factors are controllable, the best prevention is to keep cancer from starting in the first place. Among the risk factors within your control: the use of tobacco; your weight; your physical activity level; your overall food choices; exposure to sunlight (ultraviolet radiation); and exposure to carcinogens, or cancer-causing agents.

In fact, you may reduce your risk of most cancers with lifestyle changes. If you smoke, stop. Limit your skin's exposure to sunlight (ultraviolet radiation). Stay physically active. Eat for good health. And maintain your healthy weight.

Even those with an increased genetic risk for cancer may delay, or perhaps even prevent, its development with these strategies. Based on scientific evidence, the American Cancer Society projects: About one-third of cancer deaths relate to overweight or obesity, physical inactivity, and poor nutrition—and could be pre-

---

Nutrition and Lifestyle Advice for Cancer Prevention

For cancer prevention, the American Cancer Society (ACS) provides specific nutrition and lifestyle recommendations for individual choices. ACS also offers advice for community action—for public, private, and community organizations—to create and support environments that help people follow nutrition and lifestyle recommendations for cancer prevention. For ACS recommendations, check the website www.cancer.org.

The American Institute of Cancer Research (AICR) also provides research-based cancer prevention recommendations related to nutrition, healthy weight, and physical activity as well. Refer to the website: www.aicr.org.

While specifically focused on cancer prevention, the ACS and AICR recommendations parallel advice from the Dietary Guidelines for Americans *(see chapter 1).*

vented. Taking a few small steps may be enough to significantly reduce your cancer risk.

Eat Smart: Reduce Your Cancer Risk

Nutrition guidelines for cancer prevention are similar to those for preventing other health problems, including heart disease, diabetes, and high blood pressure. *Throughout this book you'll find practical tips for eating to prevent cancer.* Keep in mind that no single food or nutrient causes or prevents cancer.

● Maintain a healthy weight throughout your life. Overweight and obesity are linked to cancers of the uterus and breast (among postmenopausal women), esophagus, kidney, colon, and other cancers.

One reason for increased cancer risk: With excess body weight, the body produces and circulates more estrogen and insulin, which may stimulate cancer growth. So, to keep your healthy weight, balance your calorie intake by eating the right amounts of nutrient-rich foods and doing regular physical activity. If you are overweight or obese, reach a healthy weight—and keep it! *For strategies for a healthy weight, see chapter 2.*

● Focus on vegetables, fruits, beans (legumes), and whole grains. These plant-based foods contain a complex mixture of vitamins, minerals, fiber, and phytonutrients, some of which appear to protect against some cancers—from the esophagus through the GI (gastrointestinal) tract to the rectum. These foods also may offer protection from bladder, endometrial (uterine), pancreatic, lung, and larynx cancers. Many of these foods are high in fiber; however, the links between fiber and cancer aren't clearly established. For other health benefits, these foods are mostly low in fat; there's not much evidence to indicate that total fat intake increases cancer risk.

● Choose colorful fruits and vegetables for their potential antioxidant benefits, which may help lower risks for some types of cancer. Antioxidants (vitamins C and E, selenium, and many phytonutrients) may help protect cells from damage, caused by free radicals, *as discussed in chapter 6.* Oxidative damage to cells from normal metabolism and environmental factors is linked to increased cancer risk. What about lycopene, the red-orange pigment in tomatoes, watermelon, and pink grapefruit? It may help reduce risk of some cancers, but the link is uncertain.

● Fit in sources of calcium and vitamin D, too, such as fortified milk and yogurt. Emerging research suggests that calcium may be linked to lower risk of breast cancer; vitamin D, to reduced risk of certain cancers; and both, perhaps to some cancers.

See chapter 10 to learn about an overall healthful eating plan that may lower your cancer risk.

A side note: In cultures where people eat a lot of salt-preserved foods, salt-cured and salt-pickled foods, the risk for stomach, nasopharyngeal, and throat cancers may be higher. No evidence suggests that the amounts of salt used in cooking or in flavoring foods affect cancer risk.

● Go easy on alcoholic beverages, if you drink them. Excessive drinking increases risks for liver, mouth, throat, larynx, and esophagus cancers—even more if you smoke. As with other health problems, moderation is the key—no more than one drink daily for women, two for men. *See chapter 10 for serving sizes of alcoholic drinks.* Some studies suggest: Breast cancer risk may go up even with moderate drinking. Regular consumption of even a few drinks per week is linked to increased risk of breast cancer in women—especially for those who come up short on folate. Drinking also may increase colorectal cancer risk.

Live Smart: Reduce Cancer Risk

● Be physically active. Besides helping you manage your weight, regular physical activity affects hormone levels and keeps your immune system working properly and so aids in protecting against cancer. Regular physical activity is linked to lower risk of colon, prostate, endometrial (uterine), and breast (postmenopause) cancer. *For more benefits of and guidelines for physical activity see chapter 1.*

● Make your life a "nonsmoking" zone. Smoking, chewing tobacco, and secondhand smoke are linked to most cancer deaths in the United States. Although women fear breast cancer, more die annually of lung cancer linked to cigarette smoking. Smoking also lowers blood levels of some protective nutrients. In fact, smoking increases the chances of many other cancers, including oral, throat, esophageal, stomach, pancreatic, cervical, kidney, and bladder cancers, and some types of leukemia. By quitting, the risk gradually declines. For those who don't quit smoking, eat more fruit and vegetables. Many studies show that lung

American Cancer Society's Caution for Early Diagnosis of Cancer

In addition to cancer screening, be alert to these simple visual warning signs and symptoms of cancer.

Change in bowel or bladder habits

A sore that does not heal

Unusual bleeding or discharge

Thickening or lump in breast or elsewhere

Indigestion or difficulty in swallowing or chewing

Obvious change in a wart or mole

Nagging cough or hoarseness

Source: American Cancer Society, www.cancer.org

See your doctor if you observe any of these signs or symptoms. And be aware that these symptoms can indicate other health issues.

---

cancer risk goes down among smokers and nonsmokers when they consumed more fruits and vegetables. *Be aware:* Taking high doses of beta carotene and/or vitamin A supplements *increases* (not decreases) lung cancer risk. Avoid these supplements!

● Preventing skin cancer takes more than the right SPF sunscreen! Limit your exposure to the sun, including midday sun, as well as sunlamps and tanning booths, to reduce your skin cancer risk. As part of your daily routine, wear protective clothing, UV-absorbing sunglasses (blocking 99 to 100% UV rays), wear a hat, and use sunblock to protect your skin.

A sunscreen with an SPF (sun protection factor) of 30 is advised by the American Academy of Dermatology and others. In 2011 the FDA approved new labeling, noting that sunscreens labeled as both "Broad Spectrum" *and* "SPF 15" (or higher), if used regularly, as directed and in combination with other sun protection measures will help reduce the risk of skin cancer, prevent sunburn, and reduce the risk of early skin aging. Many moisturizing creams come with built-in sunscreen. Try to avoid peak sun exposure: 10:00 A.M. to 4:00 P.M. (when your shadow is shorter than you are).

Sunlight that touches unprotected skin is a source of vitamin D, a nutrient often short-changed; *see chapter 6*. To reduce cancer risks, limit sun exposure as a vitamin D source; consume enough from food and beverages and perhaps supplements.

Testing, Testing: Cancer Screening for Early Detection

Cancer develops gradually. *The best cure:* Stop cancer as soon as possible. That's why early detection is so important! On a monthly basis, perform self-exams: breast, testicular, skin. And make sure your regular physical checkups include routine cancer screening, as advised by your doctor. *For women, refer to "Screening Tests: Do You Keep Up?" in chapter 18.* For all ages, check the American Cancer Society's website—www.cancer.org—for "Screening Recommendations

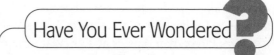

Have You Ever Wondered

... if antioxidant supplements offer cancer-fighting benefits? No scientific evidence shows that supplements—beta-carotene, lycopene, vitamin E, for example—reduce cancer risk. In fact, high-dose beta carotene supplements may increase the risk for some people (current and former smokers). Instead, get your antioxidants from nutrient-rich foods, which provide a full array of substances in a safe and effective mix.

... if cooking methods can increase cancer risk? First and foremost, adequate cooking is essential for cooking meat, poultry, and fish to safe temperatures! (1) High-heat methods such as charbroiling, grilling, broiling, and frying used to cook these foods cause heterocyclic amines (HCAs) to form. Limited research suggests that these substances may contribute to increased cancer risk for some people who eat large amounts of these foods. Braising, steaming, stewing, and microwaving meats produces fewer of these chemicals. (2) Charring creates other substances which are potential carcinogens. When fat from these foods drip onto fire, smoke and flames leave polycyclic aromatic hydrocarbons (PAHs). *The bottom line:* Sensible amounts of meat, poultry, and fish cooked with high heat and occasional darkened or smoked meats are no cause for concern.

... if sugar feeds cancer cells? To refute a misperception, sugar doesn't increase cancer risk directly or speed the growth of cancer cells. Any indirect link to high sugar intake is inconclusive. A food pattern with a lot of sugary foods may, however, be short on the nutrient-rich fruits, vegetables, and whole grains that play unique roles in cancer prevention.

by Age." Cancer screening is done for early detection, to find cancer at an early stage before symptoms appear and when it's easier to treat or cure.

For more specifics on screening, check the American Cancer Society's website at www.cancer.org, and talk to your doctor.

If You're Dealing with a Cancer Diagnosis . . .

Good nutrition is essential if you've been diagnosed with cancer. Your nutrition needs are unique to your cancer, the treatment, and your personal preferences. The goals? To maintain weight and keep up your energy level and strength. To do that, you may need high-calorie foods and more proteins. That may be a change from the way you've been eating and a challenge when you don't feel well. *For tips on boosting calories with a healthful eating pattern, see chapter 2.* Some cancer treatments can cause weight gain. In that case, follow an eating pattern that helps you maintain a healthy weight.

Besides helping you feel stronger and better, good nutrition helps you handle the side effects of cancer treatment, reduce your chance of infection, and assist with your recovery from treatment or surgery.

Safe food handling takes on even more importance since your immune response may not function as well as normal. With a low white blood cell count (common during chemotherapy and radiation therapy) your body may not be able to fight infection or harmful foodborne bacteria effectively. *For guidance on food safety, see chapter 13.*

A registered dietitian can help you make a plan for managing food choices if you're dealing with cancer. Ask your physician or healthcare professional for a referral to a registered dietitian.

Before Treatment or Surgery

Prepare—make good nutrition part of your pretreatment approach to cancer recovery. Start with a positive mind-set. Eat for health; being well nourished is a strategy for building your strength and reserves before surgery or treatment begins. Plan ahead by stocking your kitchen with foods you can eat while you're dealing with the possible side effects of treatment. Have nutrient-rich snacks on hand; you may not have the energy to prepare food, or the appetite to eat. Gather your support team so you'll have help if and

Have You Ever Wondered ?

. . . how to protect against breast cancer? Although there's no certain way to prevent it, you can reduce your risk and boost your odds if you do get breast cancer. Change the risk factors that are within your control: Engage in regular physical activity, avoid or limit intake of alcoholic beverages, and stay at your healthy weight. The risk for many women from hormone therapy after menopause is small; not using hormone therapy may reduce your risk. Follow the American Cancer Society's guidelines (www.cancer.org) for finding breast cancer early. If you are higher risk for breast cancer, perhaps for genetic reasons, talk to your physician. Men can develop breast cancer, too. *See "Breast Cancer: Do Food Choices Make a Difference?" in chapter 18.*

when you need it for food shopping, food preparation, and companionship. A support group can give you psychological support and practical tips. Ask your doctor, nurse, social worker, or other healthcare professional about support groups.

During Chemotherapy and Radiation Therapy

Cancer treatment requires powerful medication or radiation therapy that not only kills cancer cells but may damage healthy body cells, possibly resulting in uncomfortable side effects. Careful food choices can help control some side effects that result from treatment. Most side effects go away once treatment is over.

To deal with side effects of chemotherapy or radiation therapy that affect your ability to eat, try the strategies described here to stay well nourished. *See "Cancer Treatment: Handling Some Side Effects" in this chapter.* Frequent minimeals, for example, might help. If you feel tired, ask your family or a friend to help you with food shoping and meal preparation—or arrange for home-delivered meals to preserve your strength. For more advice, especially if side effects persist, talk to a registered dietitian.

Caution: Talk to your doctor about any alternative or complementary therapies, such as herbal products, antioxidant vitamins, or minerals, before you try them to relieve symptoms or to promote the quality of your life. Although some are safe and harmless, others can interfere with the effects of radiation or chemotherapy,

CANCER TREATMENT: HANDLING SOME SIDE EFFECTS

Treatment and cancer itself often result in uncomfortable side effects that affect the desire and the ability to eat. If you experience these problems, these tips might make eating easier and more appealing. Remember, good nutrition is part of your treatment and your feeling of well-being.

IF YOU . . .	YOU CAN . . .
Have changes in your sense of taste and smell	• Try changing the temperature at which you eat certain foods. Hot foods may smell and taste stronger, so serving at a cool temperature may help. As cold foods get warmer, a sweet taste may get more pronounced, which may or may not be desirable. • Season foods with tart flavors (lemon, other citrus fruit, vinegar) or sweet flavors (sugar, honey, syrup) depending on the taste problem. • Chew sugar-free lemon drops, mints, or gum to remove bitter or metallic taste. (Avoid sugarless gums if you have diarrhea.) Use plastic, not stainless, flatware. • If a food tastes too sweet, add salt or a sour taste to counteract the sweetness. If a food is too salty, bitter, or sour, adding sugar may help. • Rinse your mouth with a water solution—1 quart water, ¾ teaspoon salt, and 1 teaspoon baking soda—before eating to clear your taste buds. Avoid mouth rinse with alcohol if your mouth is sore or irritated. • Rinse your mouth and brush your teeth frequently to help with a bad taste in your mouth.
Have a poor appetite	• Eat small, frequent meals instead of three larger meals. • Make the meal more enjoyable with flowers and nice dishes. Play music or watch your favorite TV show. Eat with family or friends. • Keep nutrient-rich snacks handy to eat when you're hungry: hard-cooked eggs, peanut butter, yogurt, cereal and milk, cheese, ice cream, granola bars, nutritional drinks and puddings, crackers, pretzels, hearty soup. • Eat high-calorie, high-protein foods at meals and snacktime. • Ask your doctor about medications to help relieve constipation, nausea, or pain if these problems are causing your poor appetite. Ask about liquid meal replacements. • Keep commercially prepared, liquid nutritional supplements on hand for times when you don't feel like eating a meal. • Talk to your doctor about an appetite stimulant.
Feel constipated	• Try to stick to regular routines: Eat at the same times each day, and try to be regular with bowel movements. This may include medications such as Metamucil or Senokot. • Drink 8 to 10 cups of liquid daily. Try water, prune juice, warm juice, decaffeinated tea, and hot lemonade. • If you feel gaseous, limit gas-producing foods such as carbonated drinks, broccoli, cabbage, cauliflower, cucumbers, legumes (beans), and onions. To keep from swallowing air, drink through a straw, limit talking while you eat, and avoid chewing gum. To avoid or get rid of gas from gas-promoting food, use a supplement like Beano, or with simethicone. • Eat high-fiber bulky foods, such as whole-grain products, fruits and vegetables (skins on), popcorn, and legumes. Make sure a high-fiber diet is advised. • Talk to your dietitian about a high-calorie, high-protein, fiber-containing liquid supplement. • Use laxatives only with your doctor's advice. Check with your doctor if you haven't had a bowel movement for three days or more.
Have diarrhea	• Drink plenty of mild, clear liquids throughout the day to prevent dehydration. Drink them at room temperature. Fluids without caffeine may be better choices. • Eat small, frequent meals and snacks during the day. • Avoid high-fiber, high-fat (greasy, fried), spicy, or very sweet foods. When diarrhea is over, gradually eat foods with more fiber. • Limit milk products to no more than 2 cups daily if you seem to have problems with milk during the period of diarrhea. • Avoid gas-producing foods. *(See tips for dealing with constipation in this chapter.)* • Drink and eat foods high in sodium and potassium. *(See chapter 7.)* Some sports drinks can help replace electrolytes lost through persistent diarrhea. • Eat foods high in pectin (a type of fiber) such as applesauce and bananas. • Call your doctor if diarrhea persists or increases, or if your stools have an unusual color or odor. • Drink at least one cup of liquid after each loose bowel movement. • Limit sugar-free gums and candies with sorbitol.

If You . . .	You Can . . .
Have mouth sores or throat irritation	• Avoid tart, acidic, or salty beverages and foods (lemon, other citrus, vinegar, pickled foods). • Avoid rough-textured foods such as dry toast, crackers, granola, and raw fruits and vegetables. • Choose cool or lukewarm foods. • Avoid alcoholic and acidic drinks, carbonated beverages, commercial mouthwashes, and tobacco. • Skip irritating seasonings such as chile powder, cloves, hot sauces, nutmeg, pepper, salsa, pepper sauce, and horseradish. Season with herbs instead. • Eat soft, bland, creamy foods such as cream soups, cheese, yogurt, mashed potatoes, cooked cereals, casseroles, milk shakes, and commercial liquid supplements. Suck on fruit ices and ice chips. • Blend and moisten dry or solid foods. • Puree or liquefy foods in a blender to make them easier to swallow. • Tilt your head back and forth to help foods and liquids flow to the back of your throat for easier swallowing. • Drink through a straw to bypass mouth sores. • Eat high-protein, high-calorie foods to speed healing. • Rinse your mouth often with baking soda mouthwash (l quart of water, ¾ teaspoon of salt, and 1 tablespoon of baking soda) to remove food and germs.
Feel nauseous or queasy	• Eat six to eight small meals a day instead of three larger ones. • Eat dry foods such as crackers or dry cereals when you awaken and every few hours. • Stay away from food preparation areas if the aroma makes you nauseous. • Choose foods that don't have a strong odor; eat foods that are cool, not icy cold or hot. • Avoid foods that are very sweet, fatty, greasy, or spicy if they aggravate nausea. • Sit up or recline your head slightly for an hour after eating. • Sip clear fluids—water, juice, flat soda, sports drink—throughout the day. • Talk to your doctor about antinausea medication. • Try bland, easy-to-digest foods: perhaps chicken noodle soup with saltines. • Eat in a cool well-ventilated room without food and cooking odors or other aromas. • Rinse your mouth before and after meals, and after vomiting, with plain water. • Drink adequate fluids daily, and an additional ½ to 1 cup liquid for each vomiting episode. Sip fluids 30 to 60 minutes *after* eating. Try to consume sips of apple and cranberry juice, flat soft drinks, broth, bites of frozen flavored ice.
Have a dry mouth or thick saliva	• Drink adequate fluids daily to loosen mucus. Take a water bottle with you when away from home. • Eat soft, bland foods cold or at room temperature. Try blenderized fruits and vegetables; soft, cooked beef, chicken, or fish; well-thinned cereals; Popsicles; and slushies. • Moisten foods with broth, soup, sauce, gravy, butter, or margarine. Dip or soak food in what you are drinking. • Suck on sour lemon drops. Avoid chewing ice cubes that can damage your teeth. Chew sugarless gum to stimulate saliva flow. • Keep your lips moist and mouth clean with a soft-bristle toothbrush. Rinse your mouth before and after eating with plain water or a mild mouth rinse (made with 1 quart of water, ¾ teaspoon of salt, and 1 teaspoon of baking soda). Floss regularly. • Avoid commercial mouthwashes, alcoholic and acidic beverages, and tobacco. • Limit caffeinated drinks and foods that have a diuretic effect: coffee, tea, cola, chocolate. • Moisten room air with a cool mist humidifier. Keep it clean to avoid the spread of bacteria.
Have trouble swallowing	• Get advice from your healthcare provider on the best diet and fluid consistency for you. • Drink enough liquids daily, thickened to a consistency right for you. • Report any coughing or choking while eating to your doctor right away, especially if you have a fever. • Eat small, frequent meals. • Use liquid nutritional supplements if you can't eat enough food. • Ask a registered dietitian to recommend thickening products and help you know how to use them: gelatin, tapioca, cornstarch, or flour, commercial thickeners, pureed vegetables, instant potatoes, dry infant rice cereal.

Source: Adapted from B. Eldridge and K. K. Hamilton, *Management of Nutrition Impact Symptoms in Cancer and Educational Handouts* (Chicago: American Dietetic Association, 2004) and the *Nutrition Care Manual* (Chicago: Academy of Nutrition and Dietetics). Accessed January 1, 2012.

or with your recovery from surgery. Some may have harmful side effects.

Chemotherapy. Chemotherapy uses oral or injected medications to stop or slow the progress of cancer cell growth. Among its common side effects are fatigue, diarrhea or constipation, nausea and vomiting, mouth tenderness or sores, and changes in the way food tastes and smells. To help you cope with the unpleasant effects of chemotherapy:

● Eat before your treatment. If your treatment takes several hours, bring a light snack along unless a light snack is offered during your treatment.

● When your appetite is good between treatments, nourish yourself well. For may people, breakfast is the best meal.

● Cut yourself some slack. Some people experience changes or loss of taste and smell from chemotherapy. Do your best when it's challenging to eat. Side effects usually go away once treatment is over.

See "Cancer Treatment: Handling Some Side Effects" in this chapter.

Radiation therapy. This form of therapy damages cancer cells with a series of daily treatments of radiation. Side effects depend on the area of the body being treated, the dosage, and the frequency of treatment. These can be nausea, vomiting, sore throat or mouth, loss of taste, dry mouth, difficulty swallowing, diarrhea, or loss of appetite. Many side effects contribute to eating problems, yet good nutrition is important during and after what may be several weeks of treatment. To help you cope with the side effects of radiation:

● Eat before your daily treatment.

● If it takes time to get to a treatment center, bring along food to eat before and afterward. If you need to stay overnight, make plans beforehand for convenient, easy, and nutritious meals and snacks.

● Give your body time to get over any side effects. Often they don't appear right away, but can last two or three weeks after treatments stop.

See "Cancer Treatment: Handling Some Side Effects" in this chapter.

Other cancer treatment options may be recommended, such as biotherapy and anti-angiogenic agents for some patients. They too have nutrition implications.

Your doctor or a registered dietitian experienced with cancer treatment can help with an eating plan that's right for you.

Cancer Survival: After Treatment Ends

No special diet after cancer diagnosis and treatment can prevent the recurrence of cancer. Cancer survivors are at greater risk for other cancers. And obesity is linked to breast cancer recurrence. However, healthful eating, appropriate weight, and a physically active lifestyle can make a difference for overall health, quality of life, and longevity! Being well nourished can help you gradually rebuild your strength.

Try to follow guidance from the USDA Food Patterns; *see chapter 10 to learn more.* Drink alcoholic beverages in moderation, if at all. Prepare and store food safely. Consult with a registered dietitian to help you personalize your healthy eating plan and to manage any side effects that persist. *See "Resources You Can Use" for resources for cancer treatment and cancer survival.*

Diabetes: A Growing Concern

Diabetes has become an epidemic, affecting nearly twenty-six million Americans. Yet about seven million of them—*perhaps you or someone in your family*—don't know they have it! In 2010 the Centers for Disease Control warned: If the current trends continue, one-third of American adults could have diabetes by 2050.

In 2011 the U.S. Department of Health and Human Services and the American Diabetes Association estimated that about 79 million Americans have prediabetes, which sharply raises the risk for developing type 2 diabetes and increases the risk of heart disease and stroke. Because obesity and overweight are predictors of diabetes and insulin resistance, the worldwide rise in obesity parallels a rise in diabetes. Most people with prediabetes are apt to develop diabetes within a decade unless they make modest changes in both their food choices and their physical activity level and lose weight.

If it's not managed properly, diabetes can have serious, even life-threatening, effects on health: eye problems including blindness, circulatory problems, nervous system disease (neuropathy), and kidney disease and failure, among others. In fact, diabetes is the leading cause of blindness, leg and foot amputations, and kidney disease, and the seventh-leading cause of death in the United States. Diabetes also is a major risk factor for heart attacks and stroke; two-thirds of those with diabetes die from these causes. Damage can add up. Even during prediabetes, some long-term damage, especially to the heart and circulatory system, may occur. The best way to reduce the risks for these problems is to keep your blood glucose level near the normal range.

To underscore the seriousness: More deaths result from diabetes each year than from breast cancer and AIDS combined.

On the bright side, you can live a healthier and longer life with diabetes—if you learn how to manage it and follow through. You may lower your risks for prediabetes or diabetes before being diagnosed with improvements in your overall food choices, your weight, and your physical activity.

What Is Diabetes?

Simply defined, diabetes is a physiological condition that affects the way the body converts sugar, starch, and other substances in foods to energy. Carbohydrates (sugars and starches) don't cause diabetes. Instead insulin, a hormone produced by the pancreas, isn't produced or doesn't work correctly in the body and therefore, can't be used properly for energy metabolism.

How does insulin work for healthy people? During digestion, glucose is released from carbohydrates and absorbed to circulate as blood glucose, or blood sugar, to body cells. Among healthy people, insulin regulates blood glucose levels. It lets glucose pass from blood into body cells for energy production. For people without diabetes, their body's insulin helps blood glucose levels stay in a normal range so eating has little effect on blood glucose level.

With diabetes, the body can't control blood glucose levels normally. Too little or no insulin, or the inability to use insulin properly, hinders the body's ability to use energy nutrients—carbohydrates, proteins, and fats. Instead of "feeding" cells, glucose accumulates in blood, causing blood glucose levels to rise. Since it can't be used for energy, blood glucose spills into urine and gets excreted. That makes extra work for the kidneys, causing frequent urination and excessive thirst.

Over time, high blood glucose levels can cause damage to kidneys, eyes, nerves, and the heart. As a key energy source, glucose is lost.

Prediabetes, when a person's blood glucose levels are higher than normal but not high enough for a diagnosis of type 2 diabetes, is a category of increased risk for diabetes. In fact, most people who develop type 2 diabetes had prediabetes first. The heart and circulatory system can be damaged even in these early stages, so being tested is important.

There are several classes of diabetes. Unknown factors trigger the onset of type 1 diabetes. Genetics and lifestyle factors, which are in your control, may trigger type 2 diabetes; being overweight increases the risk.

Type 1 diabetes. Type 1 diabetes, an autoimmune disease, accounts for 5 to 10 percent of diabetes cases. In this form of diabetes, the pancreas can't make insulin. Pancreatic beta cells that produce insulin have been destroyed, perhaps due to heredity or to damage prompted by a virus. The causes aren't clear. Why is it an autoimmune disease? "Auto" refers to "self"; the immune system, which normally protects the body from disease, instead attacks the beta cells that produce insulin.

People of any age can develop type 1 diabetes. Daily insulin injections or a continuous insulin pump, along with a careful eating and physical activity plan, are required to manage type 1 diabetes. Type 1 diabetes requires regular self-monitoring of blood glucose levels.

Type 2 diabetes. Type 2 diabetes, a metabolic disorder, accounts for 90 to 95 percent of diabetes cases, with the incidence rising along with obesity rates, sedentary lifestyles, and an aging population, as well as better and early detection. About 80 percent of those with type 2 diabetes are overweight. With type 2 diabetes, pancreatic cells don't produce enough insulin or the body doesn't respond to insulin normally (insulin resistance), even though the pancreas produces insulin.

Type 2 diabetes often develops slowly with higher risk after age forty; however, obese children are increasingly at risk, too. In type 2 diabetes, blood glucose levels often can be controlled through food choices, weight control, and physical activity alone. Taking glucose-lowering medicines may help the body produce more insulin or better use the insulin the body makes. Insulin injections may be needed, too. Type 2 diabetes also requires regular self-monitoring of blood glucose levels.

Gestational diabetes. Gestational diabetes occurs in about 4 percent of pregnancies, resulting from changes in hormone levels. If diagnosed, it's usually screened for at the first visit and then again 24 to 28 weeks later. The risk is higher among obese and older women.

Although it usually disappears after delivery, gestational diabetes needs careful control during pregnancy. Women with gestational diabetes are at increased risk for type 2 diabetes later in life, and usually in later pregnancies. If you're planning for pregnancy, prepare ahead. Follow your doctor's advice for blood glucose levels. *See "Pregnancy and Diabetes" in chapter 18 for more information on gestational diabetes.*

Early Detection

Early detection of diabetes is important. The longer the body is exposed to high blood glucose levels, the greater the damage to the nervous and circulatory systems and to the blood vessels in the eyes, kidneys, heart, and feet. The early years of diabetes—during prediabetes—offer an opportunity. You can have a significant impact then to prevent or reduce its long-term consequences—and so live a longer life with fewer health problems.

According to the American Diabetes Association, many people don't know they have diabetes—despite the harmful consequences. Some symptoms may seem harmless so diabetes goes undiagnosed. And some people with type 2 diabetes have no symptoms at all.

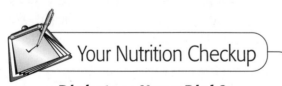

Your Nutrition Checkup

Diabetes: Your Risk?

Use these interactive calculators for your diabetes health risk assessment:

- Diabetes Risk Test, American Diabetes Association, www.diabetes.org/diabetes-basics/prevention/diabetes-risk-test
- My Diabetes Health Assessment, American Heart Association, www.heart.org/HEARTORG/Conditions/Whats-Your-Risk-Find-out_UCM_306929_Article.jsp

How would you know if you have it? These are common symptoms of typical diabetes: extreme fatigue, frequent urination, unusual thirst, extreme hunger, unusual weight loss, and irritability. In addition, those with type 2 diabetes also may experience frequent infections; cuts and bruises that heal slowly; blurred vision; numb or tingling hands or feet; or recurring skin, gum, or bladder infections. Some people with type 2 diabetes have no outward signs associated with high blood glucose levels. Keeping tabs on your blood glucose level is the way to really know.

At Risk for Type 2?

With this growing epidemic, what are the risk factors for type 2 diabetes?

- *Having an impaired glucose tolerance (IGT) and/or impaired fasting glucose (IFG).*

- *Being over age forty-five.* With age, the pancreas is less efficient at producing insulin.

- *Having a close family member with diabetes.* You may have an inherited tendency or share circumstances that increase your risk. To refute a myth, diabetes isn't contagious.

- *Being in certain racial or ethnic groups.* If you're of African American, Hispanic, Latino, Asian American, Hawaiian American, and other Pacific Islander, Native American, or Alaska Native descent, your diabetes risk is higher.

- *Being overweight or obese.* With more body fat, body cells become more insulin-resistant. That's especially true for young people and those who have been obese for a while. That said, many people who are overweight or obese do not develop diabetes and those who do develop it may be normal weight or slightly overweight.

- *Being physically inactive.*

- *Having low HDL cholesterol or high triglycerides levels, and high blood pressure.*

- *Women having had gestational diabetes, or delivering a baby weighing 9 pounds or more.*

Even if you're at risk for type 2 diabetes, there's good news: With healthful eating, regular moderate exercise and weight reduction, if you're overweight, your odds drop.

Testing, Testing: Blood Glucose Checks

Diabetes may be detected first by a urine test, given as a routine part of most physical exams. However, blood glucose readings are much more accurate. Everyone age forty-five or over should have a blood glucose test every three years. If you're at high risk, blood glucose testing should start sooner and be more frequent. Be aware that screening tests, often done at community health events, aren't diagnostic, yet they can identify those at high risk who need further testing.

During a checkup, a blood glucose reading is done after an eight-hour fast. A fasting plasma glucose (blood glucose) of less than 100 milligrams/deciliter (mg/dL) is considered normal. Two readings of 126 mg/dL or higher, taken on different days, are criteria for a diabetes diagnosis. A fasting blood glucose level between 100 and 125 mg/dL signals prediabetes. The Oral Glucose Tolerance Test (OGTT), Fasting Plasma Glucose (FPG), and the Glycated hemoglobin (A1C) tests are used to diagnose diabetes. The A1C, a simple blood test, doesn't require overnight fasting.

If you're diagnosed with diabetes, you may need to self-monitor, or check your own blood glucose level. Without testing you won't know your blood glucose level unless it's very high or very low. Your healthcare team will set realistic target blood glucose levels for you—for example, before meals, after meals, and bedtime. Before meals, a blood glucose level of 90 to 130 mg/dL is considered the target; about 1½ to 2 hours after a meal, it should be less than 180 mg/dl. Your doctor, dietitian, or diabetes educator will show you how to self-monitor. Be aware that target levels for young children and older adults may differ.

Checking your blood glucose level is easy once you get used to pricking your finger or forearm: just a drop of blood on a test strip, read by a blood glucose meter. Record the results, the time, and the date. Or use a blood glucose meter that stores the readings for you. Use the information to see if your diabetes care plan (eating, exercise, and medication) is working. Share your log with your healthcare team.

Once you become adept at self-monitoring, you can use your blood glucose reading to know if you need to make changes in your diabetes treatment plan. If your blood glucose level is too low (perhaps below 70 mg/dL) or too high (perhaps above 240 mg/dL), you'll need to take action. Many factors determine the right blood glucose goals for someone with diabetes. While these levels have been set by the American Diabetes Association, your doctor can help you set your personal targets.

Run every three to six months during your doctor visit, the glycated hemoglobin, or hemoglobin A1C, test measures your average blood glucose levels over the past two to three months, and indicates whether your blood glucose levels are under control over time, not just for a day. There's a new way to report A1C that makes it easier to see how well you are managing overall. Called estimated average glucose (eAG), it correlates with the units of measurement (mg/dl) on your blood glucose meter—so it looks more familiar. If you use it, learn how.

To control blood glucose levels and diabetes-related complications, ongoing monitoring means testing your "ABCs": A for hemoglobin A1C, B for blood pressure, and C for cholesterol (blood lipid) levels.

If you have type 1 diabetes, your doctor also may advise you to take a urine test for ketones, which are acids that may build up in urine to toxic levels. When there is no insulin available, your body cells can't use glucose for energy and so turn to burning fat, not carbohydrates, for energy. Without carbohydrates, or glucose, body cells can't burn fat completely, and ketones form as a by-product of fat burning. When ketones build up, a condition called ketoacidosis can occur and, if left untreated, can lead to a diabetic coma and even death. Talk to your doctor about the early symptoms and an action plan should you experience positive ketones; get immediate medical help if ketoacidosis develops.

If You Have Diabetes . . .

The goal for diabetes management is this: controlling your blood glucose levels so they stay as near to normal as possible. Health problems occur when high blood glucose levels are sustained over time, not from an elevated blood glucose level after a meal.

Like a teeter-totter, blood glucose levels go up (hyperglycemia) and down (hypoglycemia); that's part of dealing with diabetes. Those swings can be dangerous when diet, physical activity, and diabetes medication aren't balanced properly.

● *Too much food or too little insulin?* Your blood glucose level can soar, affecting your health now and very seriously down the road.

● *Too much exercise or too much insulin?* Blood glucose drops, and your body can't use blood glucose to produce enough energy.

To control "the ups and the downs," carefully manage what you eat, how much, and when—*no matter what type of diabetes you have.* Eating raises your blood glucose level; physical activity and medication lower it. For example, in case of low blood glucose (<70), consume a *small amount* (15 grams) of a quick-acting carbohydrate, such as ½ cup juice or three to four glucose tablets.

Your healthcare team likely will advise a regular physical activity plan to help you control your blood glucose levels and prevent weight gain, too—and may advise sensible weight loss if you're overweight. For many people with type 2 diabetes, smart eating, weight loss, and active living are enough to control their blood glucose level and to maintain good health. Others need diabetes medication.

Here's some general advice about managing diabetes and preventing its symptoms. For individualized guidance that matches your needs, consult your doctor and a registered dietitian (RD). Some dietitians, pharmacists, and nurses are certified diabetes educators (CDEs).

If you've just found out that you have diabetes, you may feel healthy. Even if it's hard to remember to stick with your eating and physical activity plan, and if prescribed by your doctor, your medication plan, the long-term benefits are well worth the effort!

Manage Your Meals and Snacks

The game plan for smart eating with diabetes follows this general strategy: *Eat about the same amount of food, in the right balance, at about the same time daily; to avoid weight gain, balance your day's food choices with regular physical activity.* In the big picture, eating with diabetes follows principles of healthful eating for anybody—in fact, for your whole family. *See the Dietary Guidelines in chapter 1.* That can make meal management simpler.

What is the "right balance"? It's *food variety* with a balance of different types of food . . . *portion savvy* to

eat the right amount of food . . . and *control of energy-producing nutrients* (carbohydrates, fats, and proteins).

For diabetes, there's no single eating plan; the guidelines have built-in flexibility. The amount and proportions of carbohydrates, proteins, and fats—the energy nutrients—you consume depend on you and your weight, blood cholesterol levels, and medical needs. Specific food choices are up to you, too, and what foods you enjoy. Your doctor, along with a registered dietitian and your diabetes educator, can help you plan what's right for you—your meal planning approach, portion sizes, types of food, and overall timing.

Carbohydrates: How Much in Food?

Knowing about how many carbohydrate grams a food has or estimating a carbohydrate serving (exchange) takes practice and know-how—especially for mixed foods.

Use Nutrition Facts on food labels: servings per package, serving size, and calories and nutrients per label serving:

● Look at the grams of total carbohydrates per label serving. Divide the total grams of carbohydrate by 15 to determine the number of carbohydrate servings in one label serving. (One carbohydrate serving is the amount of food with 15 grams of carbohydrate.) Sugar isn't counted; it's part of total carbohydrates.

● If the food has significant fiber and sugar alcohols (which have less digestible carbohydrates), you may wish to ask your registered dietitian or diabetes educator to figure the carbohydrate impact. You need to subtract part of these off the total carbohydrates and so lower the carb count. Also ask about "free" foods that have fewer than 20 calories or fewer than 5 carbohydrate grams per serving.

● Use serving sizes to help with exchanges. *For more about reading labels, see chapter 12.*

● As an aside, be wary of label claims, such as "net carbs," "low carb," or "low impact carbs"; these claims aren't approved by the U.S. Food and Drug Administration.

Unpackaged or restaurant foods? Find a book, website source, or app with carbohydrate facts to help you. By law, many restaurant chains provide nutrition information on their websites and at the restaurant. You also will need to learn how to estimate.

FOOD LIST FOR CARBOHYDRATE COUNTING

These portions provide 15 grams of carbohydrate:

Starches
1 slice bread (1 oz.)
1 tortilla (6-inch size)
¼ (1 oz.) large bagel
2 taco shells (5-inch size)
½ (1 oz.) hamburger or
   hot dog bun
¾ cup ready-to-eat cereal
½ cup cooked cereal
1 cup broth-based soup
4 to 6 small crackers
⅓ cup cooked pasta or rice
½ cup cooked beans, peas,
   corn, sweet potatoes,
   winter squash, or mashed
   or boiled potatoes
¼ (3 oz.) large baked potato
¾ ounce pretzels, or potato or
   tortilla chips
3 cups popped popcorn

Fruit
1 small fresh fruit
½ cup canned fruit
¼ cup dried fruit
17 (3 oz.) small grapes
1 cup melon, berries
2 tbsp. raisins
½ cup fruit juice

Milk
1 cup fat-free or reduced-fat
   milk
1 cup soy milk
⅔ cup (6 oz.) fat-free yogurt
   sweetened with sugar-free
   sweetener

Sweets and Desserts
2-inch square cake (unfrosted)
2 (2 oz. or 3 oz.) small cookies
½ cup ice cream or frozen
   yogurt
¼ cup sherbet or sorbet
1 tbsp. syrup, jam, jelly,
   table sugar, or honey
2 tbsp. light syrup

Other Foods
● Count 1 cup raw vegetables
   or ½ cup cooked nonstarchy
   vegetables as zero carbohydrate
   servings or "free" foods.
   If you eat 3 or more servings
   at one meal, count them as
   1 carbohydrate serving.
● Foods that have fewer than 20
   calories in each serving also may
   be counted as zero carbohydrate servings or "free" foods.
● Count 1 cup of casserole or
   other mixed foods as 2 carbohydrate servings.

Source for carbohydrate values: Nutrition Care Manual (Chicago: Academy of Nutrition and Dietetics). Accessed January 1, 2012.

Make a Diabetes Meal and Snack Plan—Follow It!

Your plan should guide the amount and kinds of food for you and help you spread your eating out during the day. Besides controlling blood glucose levels, a smart plan also may help you manage or improve your weight, blood pressure, and cholesterol levels. Consider your food preferences, eating habits, and schedule! Several tools can help:

● *USDA Food Patterns.* The USDA Food Patterns, represented by MyPlate, is a good starting point for planning meals and snacks for managing diabetes—and your healthy weight. Use it to manage carbohydrates and other energy nutrients and to choose a variety of nutrient-rich foods. The good news: It's a healthful guide for your whole family. *See chapter 10.*

● *Exchanges for diabetes.* Exchanges are like food groups in the USDA Food Patterns. They're lists of food, grouped because their carbohydrate, protein, fat, and calorie content is similar. The exchange system

works this way: Meals and snacks are planned with specific amounts from each list. The menu planning goals are: (1) to get enough food variety and (2) to

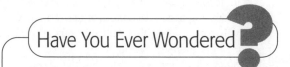

Have You Ever Wondered

. . . if going "low carb" would be a good approach for managing diabetes? Your goal should be to manage the carbohydrates in your food choices, not eliminate them. After all, you need the glucose (blood sugar) from carbohydrates as energy for your brain and other body cells. *Remember:* With diabetes, the issue is how insulin, which may be inadequate or not working properly, handles carbohydrates—not whether you need carbohydrates.

Most women need 45 to 60 grams of carbohydrates per meal; most men, 60 to 75 grams of carbohydrate per meal. They also may need up to two snacks at 15 to 30 grams of carbohydrates each.

manage blood glucose levels by spreading out the carbohydrates, other energy-producing nutrients, and calories throughout the day. Exchange lists are published by the American Diabetic Association and the American Dietetic Association.

Although the exchange system was the most common way to plan meals for diabetes management in the past, today carbohydrate counting is used more often. Still you may see exchanges for recipes. If you want to use the exchange system, ask a registered dietitian or certified diabetes educator to help you.

● *Carbohydrate counting.* Carbs are part of a healthy eating plan for anyone, with diabetes or not. However, because carbohydrates (starches and sugars) affect blood glucose levels more than any other nutrient, they need to be monitored. Starches and sugars have a similar effect on blood glucose levels. That's why you need to consider total carbohydrates, not just sugars.

Counting carbohydrates is a useful meal planning tool. It allows you to more precisely match your food and medication (insulin) intake and so keep your blood glucose levels within your target range. And the

Have You Ever Wondered ?

. . . if people with diabetes should make food choices based on a food's glycemic index(GI)? GI as a tool may help "fine tune" blood glucose response when combined with carbohydrate counting for those already in control—but it's not the first approach for managing food choices. In fact, research shows that the total amount of carbohydrate predicts blood glucose response better than GI does.

Whether there's any health benefit to selecting foods according to their glycemic index is controversial. On one hand, some research suggests that an overall eating plan with a lower glycemic response may reduce insulin response and so help lower the chances of heart disease, diabetes, and obesity. On the other hand, a glycemic index only has been established for single foods, but not for food combinations in meals and snacks or for meal size. Having a low glycemic index doesn't mean a food is high in nutrients, either. And individual responses may differ. Plus, there isn't enough evidence yet to show that using glycemic index actually improves blood glucose levels.

For now, stick to well-accepted approaches for diabetes management. *To learn more, refer to chapter 3, "Hot Topic: Glycemic Index."* For some people with diabetes, glycemic index may be used to "fine tune" glucose response for diabetes management, with the guidance of a healthcare provider.

. . . if eating sugar or a carbohydrate-rich diet causes insulin resistance that results in weight gain? No, it's a common myth. Consuming carbohydrate-rich foods doesn't cause insulin resistance; excessive calories do. People who are overweight and sedentary may have symptoms of insulin resistance, a condition

often diminished with moderate physical activity and weight loss.

. . . if drinking cow's milk during infancy causes type 1 diabetes? There's no scientific evidence that milk protein from cow's milk promotes type 1 diabetes in infants with an inherited tendency for diabetes. Regardless, the American Academy of Pediatrics (AAP) encourages breast-feeding for at least the first year of life, for all babies, including those with a strong family history of type 1 diabetes. Some early research suggests that breast-feeding may reduce a mother's later risk for diabetes. For children age one year or older with diabetes, AAP recommends no restriction for cow's milk.

. . . if you can stop taking insulin if you take chromium supplements? No. Chromium supplements aren't an alternative to insulin. As a nutrient, chromium helps your body use blood glucose properly and helps break down proteins and fats. However, there isn't enough evidence on its safety or effectiveness to recommend routine chromium supplementation for blood glucose control. Its value for those with diabetes is inconclusive and controversial. Talk to your doctor before taking any supplements. Enjoy foods with chromium—meat, eggs, whole-grain products, cheese—to get what you need. *See chapter 6 for more on chromium.*

. . . if herbal products have a glucose-lowering ability? Despite claims, no conclusive evidence shows that herbal products offer benefits for managing diabetes although some may have promise. Some may interact with diabetes medication. Talk to your doctor first, if you choose to try them—and never use them in place of insulin or other prescribed medicine.

more consistent your carbohydrate intake, the more stable your blood glucose level will be. Tight control is getting as close to a normal (nondiabetic) blood glucose level as safely possible. Carbohydrate counting is not a tool that's appropriate for all those with diabetes, including children, elderly adults, and those with some health conditions.

With carb counting, you keep track of—and set limits on—the total carbohydrate grams you eat, trying to eat about the same number of carbohydrates, at the same time, each day. Alternatively, if you take meal-time insulin with an injection or pump, you may learn to adjust your insulin dose to cover the amount of carbohydrate you choose to eat. If you count carbs, work with your healthcare team to set a carbohydrate goal that's right for you. For example, you might set your starting goal at about 45 to 60 grams (or perhaps 60 to 75 grams for men) of carbohydrate per meal, and maybe 20 grams of carbohydrates for a snack. Then match your food and portion sizes to your goal. Try to keep within 5 grams of your target; remember the more carbs consumed, the higher your blood glucose level will be. Take fat and protein into account; they don't impact blood glucose.

For menu planning, one serving of food with carbohydrate has about 15 grams of carbohydrate; *see "Food List for Carbohydrate Counting" in this chapter.* Your carbs can come from any food source. Although bread, pasta, rice, and potatoes are known commonly as carbohydrate foods, remember, that fruit, fruit juice, beans (legumes), corn and other starchy vegetables, milk, yogurt, cake, cookies, sodas, chips, and candy have carbohydrates, too! Meat and oils don't have carbs. For meals and snacks, choose mostly nutrient-rich foods; they also supply vitamins, minerals, and phytonutrients.

● *The plate method.* To make these approaches come together in a quick and easy way, use the plate method to plan a meal. And be portion savvy. The goal: to eat sensible amounts, perhaps less overall, and to shift to bigger amounts of nonstarchy vegetables and smaller amounts of starchy foods and meats. This approach works not only for managing diabetes, but for managing your weight, too!

1. Draw an imaginary line through the middle of your plate. Then divide one half in half again. You'll have three sections.

2. *On half the plate:* Serve nonstarchy vegetables, such as carrots, cucumber, broccoli, tomatoes, spinach, salad greens, okra, peppers, and bok choy.

3. *On one-quarter of the plate:* Serve starchy foods, such as beans (legumes), rice, pasta, grits, whole-grain bread, potatoes, corn, winter squash, low-fat crackers, or pretzels.

4. *On one-quarter of the plate:* Serve lean meat, fish, skinless chicken or turkey, tofu, eggs, or low-fat cheese.

5. *On the side:* Serve 1 cup of low-fat or fat-free milk, 6 ounces of low-fat yogurt, or a small roll.

6. *Also on the side:* Serve ½ cup of fruit in juice, or a small piece of fruit.

With a slight variation, use the plate approach for breakfast, too! For a breakfast plate or bowl, fill half your plate with starchy food, one-quarter with fruit, and one-quarter with meat or a meat substitute. Keep your portions small.

Be portion savvy. No matter what approach—the USDA Food Patterns, the exchange system, carbohydrate counting, or the plate method—amounts are very important! Get out your measuring cups and spoons, and the kitchen scale. Measure your cups, bowls, and dishes, as well as food portions, to get familiar with the right serving sizes. Use your hand for quick estimates: Your fist equals about 1 cup, your palm is about ½ cup (3 to 5 ounces), your thumb is about 1 tablespoon. Learn the serving sizes that match your food plan; for example, ⅓ cup of rice, or one carbohydrate exchange, provides 15 grams of carbohydrate.

Follow This Food-Related Guidance, Too

● Set your carbohydrate target within the guidelines set by the Dietary Reference Intakes; s*ee chapter 3.* Aim for 50 to 60 percent of calories from carbohydrates, based on your metabolic goals. For a 2,000-calorie daily plan, that's 1,000 to 1,200 calories from total carbohydrates, or 250 to 300 carbohydrate grams. (One carbohydrate gram supplies 4 calories.) Your target calorie intake depends on your age, physical activity level, body size, and perhaps a weight-loss plan. *See chapter 3 to learn more about carbohydrates, including fiber.*

● Make the most of your carb choices. Remember that fruits, vegetables, whole grains, and low-fat and fat-free dairy foods are nutrient-rich; their carb content needs to be factored in. *Refer to chapter 10.*

● Choose mostly lean, low-fat, and fat-free foods. They help keep your blood lipid levels within a healthy range and may help with calorie control. *But be aware:* Fat-free foods may have more carbohydrates that their traditional counterparts, so check the Nutrition Facts on food labels. Control salt/sodium in your food choices, too. Remember that people with diabetes often have high blood pressure and risks for heart disease, or they acquire these conditions down the line. *See "Your Healthy Heart" and "Blood Pressure: Under Control?" in this chapter. For ways to limit fat and sodium in your food choices, see chapters 5 and 7.*

● Know how to fit sweetened foods, including desserts and chocolates, into your eating plan. You don't need to give them up. Eat a smaller portion; share with a friend; or learn from a diabetes educator how to prepare them differently. Remember that sugary foods are often low in nutrients, yet high in calories and fat.

● As a sweet flavor option, consider sugar alcohols with fewer calories or carb grams, or low-calorie sweeteners with nearly none; *see chapter 3 to learn about them.*

Foods and drinks with low-calorie sweeteners (such as acesulfame potassium, aspartame, saccharin, and sucralose) may let you fit other foods in. They're much sweeter than the same amount of sugar; for fewer calories you need a very small amount. For example, yogurt sweetened with aspartame instead of sugared fruit lets you spend some of your carbohydrate "budget" on toast or a muffin. Diet soft drinks are sweetened with low-calorie sweeteners, such as aspartame. *Warning:* If you have the disorder phenylketonuria (PKU), avoid foods sweetened with aspartame. *See "Aspartame: PKU Warning" in chapter 21.*

Foods sweetened with sugar alcohols (sorbitol, mannitol, and xylitol, for example) affect blood glucose levels, but not as much as sugar and other nutritive sweeteners do. And they have fewer calories than sugar. *Reminder:* "Sugar-free" doesn't mean "calorie free" or "carb free." *See "Alternatives to Sugar" in chapter 3.* Sugar-free ice cream and candy may have as much carbohydrate as the regular options.

● Eat fiber-rich foods. Among the many health benefits, fiber slows digestion and may control the rise in blood glucose levels after eating. This may reduce the need for medication. Fiber also helps you feel full after eating—an aid to weight control. How much: figure about 14 grams of fiber for every 1,000 calories you consume. You may need more to get a metabolic effect; talk to your healthcare provider for advice. *See chapter 3 for more about fiber's benefits.*

Stick to your "clock." Keep to a regular meal and snack schedule—about the same amount of food, at about the same time daily—to keep your blood glucose level steady. Skipping meals or following an irregular eating pattern puts your blood glucose level out of kilter. To compound the problem, meal skipping may lead to overeating later and to an eating pattern that won't match your plan for managing diabetes.

Advice: Carry an emergency snack in case you must change your regular eating routine. A registered dietitian can help you pick the best food choices for snacking.

If you need insulin or other diabetes medicine, take it on schedule, too.

Go easy: Alcoholic drinks. Can you enjoy alcoholic drinks now and then? Discuss that question with your healthcare team *before* you drink alcoholic beverages. Some people with diabetes are wise not to drink at all.

What are some concerns and risks? The immediate concern is the risk of hypoglycemia soon after drinking and for 8 to 12 hours afterward. Be aware than others may confuse the symptoms of hypoglycemia, such as disorientation and dizziness, with drinking too much; you may not get the right help. That's another reason to wear a necklace or bracelet that identifies you as having diabetes.

Drinking can worsen some diabetes-related health problems such as high blood pressure, nerve damage from diabetes, and high triglyceride levels. Heavy drinking causes liver damage, which makes diabetes control harder. And alcoholic drinks contribute a significant amount of calories when you're trying to keep your weight under control. You need to be cautious, too, if you take diabetes medications that work to lower blood glucose level. With the combination of these medications and alcohol, your blood glucose level may become dangerously low!

If your blood glucose levels are under control and if your doctor indicates that alcoholic beverages in mod-

Children and Diabetes

Type 1 diabetes is the most common form of diabetes among children. With the parallel rise in childhood overweight and obesity, more and more children are at risk for or diagnosed with type 2 diabetes. Dealing with diabetes during the childhood and teenage years adds to the challenges of growing up. Most kids don't want to be different.

The first guideline—help your child maintain or grow into a healthy weight to reduce the chance of type 2 diabetes. If your child is overweight, ask your doctor about testing for diabetes at about age ten or at puberty if your child has other risk factors.

If your child is diagnosed with diabetes, accept and manage it together in a calm, careful, and positive way.

- Work closely with your child's healthcare team to manage diabetes and help your child grow normally—physically, mentally, and emotionally.

- Gradually involve your child in taking responsibility for his or her diabetes. Encourage rather than nag, even when things aren't perfect. Help your child learn when, how, and where to get help. Learning lifelong skills for diabetes management—and making them a habit—is part of growing up. Diabetes won't go away.

- Get advice from your healthcare team about handling special eating events such as birthday parties, sleepovers, field trips, and active play or sports.

- Be matter-of-fact, sensitive, and supportive as you help your child or teen learn about diabetes. A support group or diabetes camp for kids can help. Find a reliable website for kids about diabetes.

- Help teachers, baby-sitters, coaches, school food service staff, the school nurse, and others who supervise your child understand your child's diabetes and how they can support the diabetes healthcare plan. Meet with them. Provide these instructions: how to check your child's blood glucose; how to administer any medication; your child's or teen's ability and willingness to self-monitor and take medication; meal and snack plans; symptoms of hypoglycemia and hyperglycemia and what to do if your child has a reaction; and physical activity requirements. Provide phone numbers for you, your doctor, and other responsible adults. Provide appropriate snacks. Teach a sitter how to do blood glucose checks and give diabetes medication, if needed. Ensure that your child has the time and privacy for diabetes care without discrimination.

- Help your child or teen feel comfortable about asking to leave class or play to monitor blood glucose and take insulin.

- Make diabetes management part of your parenting responsibility, but not the sole focus. Keep the joys of growing up and a healthy family life.

Be aware: The medical needs and fair treatment of children in all public and most private schools and day care centers are protected by law.

For more parenting tips, see chapter 17, "Food to Grow On."

---

eration are okay, a registered dietitian or a certified diabetes educator can help you work them into your meal plan. Keep these guidelines in mind:

- Test your blood glucose level, before you decide if you should have a drink. If your blood glucose level is low or if you haven't eaten for a while, you shouldn't drink. If you do drink, check it again before bedtime; eat something if your blood glucose level is low.

- As always, limit alcoholic drinks: no more than one serving a day for women, and two for men—the same limits as for people without diabetes. A serving of alcohol is 5 ounces of wine, 12 ounces of beer, or $1\frac{1}{2}$ ounces of distilled spirits. Discuss your individual limits with your doctor and registered dietitian.

- *Always* eat when you have an alcoholic drink to reduce the chance for hypoglycemia, or low blood glucose. When your liver is detoxifying alcohol, it doesn't produce as much glucose. Blood glucose that drops too low from drinking can be dangerous.

- As an alternative, choose low-alcohol wine, beer, or distilled spirits. They have fewer calories and less alcohol and carbohydrates than regular beer or sweet wine. Ask how they fit into your eating plan.

- Recognize that some wine coolers and mixed drinks (made with regular soda and juice) contain sugars. Count them as part of your eating plan (as carbohydrate servings/exchanges or as carbohydrate grams). Mix drinks or spritzers with sugar-free mixers such as club soda, diet soft drinks, diet tonic, seltzer, or water.

See "Taking Control: Drinking Responsibly!" in chapter 8.

Get Moving

Get moving! Active living is important for managing diabetes. For one, regular physical activity increases insulin sensitivity, moving glucose out of blood more effectively. Second, being active can lower blood glucose as your muscles use glucose for energy. Third, physical activity burns energy, making weight management easier; your body controls your blood glucose level better at a lower body weight. And fourth, regular physical activity helps reduce your risk for heart disease and high blood pressure, both linked to diabetes.

● Before you start a physical activity plan, talk with your doctor, along with a registered dietitian or a diabetes educator. Balance exercise with eating to keep your blood glucose level within a target range. If you take insulin, planning for physical activity is trickier.

● Before you start your physical activity, check your blood glucose level. If it's low (below 70 mg/dL or less), eat a snack with about 15 carbohydrate grams right away (such as a medium apple or bread slice); wait about 15 minutes, then check again. If it's 70 to 100 mg/dL, enjoy the same 15-carb snack if your next meal is at least an hour away, then get moving. If your blood glucose is 100 to 150, it's okay to start, but eat a light snack if you plan to be active for thirty minutes or more. If your blood glucose is 240 mg/dL or more, wait, and get your blood glucose level down first. This advice is important if you're on glucose-lowering medication. (If your diabetes is managed by lifestyle changes, you don't have these same risks for hypoglycemia.)

● Take a carbohydrate-rich snack along when you're physically active—just in case you start feeling light-headed. If that happens, stop moving and eat it. Too much exercise and not enough food can lead to hypoglycemia, or low blood glucose.

● Get a buddy. Besides being more fun, it's safer. Let your partner know about your diabetes, and what to do if you need help.

● Wear a tag, a necklace, or a bracelet with diabetes identification. And wear proper footwear.

● Keep well hydrated when you're active. Water is a fine choice. Check with your doctor or a registered dietitian about beverage choices if you need a fast-acting carbohydrate source; fruit juice, regular soda, or a sports drink may be advised then.

Control Your Weight

Whether you're overweight or not, manage your body weight as part of your personal approach for diabetes management. If you're overweight, losing 5 to 7 percent of your body weight may make blood glucose easier to control if you have type 2 diabetes. Why? A lower weight helps lower insulin resistance, so you may no longer need as much or any diabetes medication. Other potential benefits of weight loss: lower blood lipid levels and lower blood pressure. Remember, with diabetes your risks for heart disease are higher! (Check with your healthcare team to see if weight loss is right for you.)

Consult a registered dietitian about losing or maintaining weight: how much you need to lose, over what time frame, and how to eat for weight loss and diabetes management. Limiting weight loss to 1 to 2 pounds weekly is generally advised. *See chapter 2 for sensible ways to a healthful weight.*

Team Up for Health!

To manage diabetes properly, seek advice from your healthcare team, whose specialties help you deal with the complexities of diabetes: your physician, a registered dietitian, a diabetes educator, a nurse, an eye doctor, a podiatrist, and a pharmacist, among others. Follow through on your care plan.

Remember: You're the most important team member! For the team to work well:

● Set your target blood glucose levels with your doctor. Be realistic; you can't avoid some "ups and downs." Numbers that are mostly within a safe range reduce your risks for complications.

● Learn to check your own blood glucose level. Self-monitoring, perhaps several times daily, is wise with diabetes, especially if you're taking diabetes medication, if you're pregnant, or if your blood glucose levels are low or out of control. Keep a log of results for your review and to share with your healthcare provider. Use it to see how food, physical activity, and stress affect your blood glucose level.

As an adult, you may choose to use a blood glucose monitor, which is a small, computerized machine that reads your blood glucose level. It's accurate if used correctly and if properly cleaned and maintained. An invasive blood glucose monitor, with a flexible catheter placed under the skin, provides continuous glucose monitoring. You may use it with conventional blood glucose monitoring.

● Learn how to detect and safely treat an insulin reaction (hypoglycemia) and hyperglycemia—before you get into severe danger. "Hypo" means low, or too little, blood glucose; you need glucose. "Hyper" means high, or too much; you need insulin or exercise. Immediate, appropriate treatment, perhaps medical assistance, is essential! Wear a medical alert tag or carry a card to let others know what to do in case you pass out.

● Keep all appointments for checkups, counseling, and laboratory tests. If your blood glucose levels are under control, see your doctor two to four times a year; if not under control, go in more often. Can't make it? Change your appointment—don't skip it!

● Take diabetes medications as directed, even if you're sick. Tell your doctor or pharmacist about all other medicine and supplements (including herbal products) you take, both prescriptions and over-the-counter medications. Also tell your team about any side effects or problems you have with any medicine or supplement. Plan ahead; call for prescription refills well before you run out. If you take insulin, ask about an insulin pump, which gives a constant, small dose, or other newer devices. *Caution:* Diabetes medicines can't substitute for a consistent healthful eating and physical activity for managing diabetes.

● Consult a registered dietitian to create a healthful eating plan (food guide for diabetes, exchange lists, plate method, or carbohydrate counting) specific to you, including a plan for physical activity and managing weight. The dietitian also can offer specific advice on shopping, label reading, eating out, and using alcoholic beverages.

● Get help with stress control if needed. Under stress, it's harder to be diligent about diabetes care: staying active, eating smart, checking your blood glucose level, and perhaps controlling alcoholic beverages. Besides that, stress may raise your blood glucose level.

● Know that you don't need to struggle with diabetes alone. If your medications, eating plan, physical activity, or monitoring program cause problems or concerns, make an appointment to explore new strategies with your healthcare team. Managing diabetes can be complex—but your health now and later depends on it!

Osteoporosis: Reduce the Risks

Keeping your bones healthy is a lifelong process. From childhood on, your eating and lifestyle habits can protect you from osteoporosis, a debilitating disease, later. No matter what your age now, it's not too late to start caring for your bones.

Osteoporosis Is . . .

Osteoporosis is a condition of gradually weakening, brittle bones. As bones lose calcium and other minerals, they become more fragile and porous. They may break under normal use or from just a minor fall, bump, or sudden strain. Because it progresses slowly and silently, people often don't realize they have osteoporosis until they fracture a bone. The spine, hip, and wrist are the most common fracture sites.

A bone mineral density (BMD) test defines osteoporosis, which is a progressive disease. By comparing bone density to that of young healthy adult, test results show bone health as normal or a progression from osteopenia (low bone mass) to osteoporosis.

Osteoporosis is often described as a disease of youth that manifests itself in the senior years. The signs usually don't show up until age 60 years or older.

Among older adults, a "dowager's hump" is an obvious sign of osteoporosis. Vertebrae in the spine collapse as a result of bone loss. Collapse of several vertebrae leads to a loss of height, back pain, and increasing disability.

Osteoporosis affects most Americans over age seventy, especially women. Men get it, too. In fact, if you add up all the cases of heart disease, stroke, and diabetes in a year, osteoporosis is more common. In the United States alone, 1.5 million bone fractures annually are attributed to this bone disease each year. About 10 million Americans have osteoporosis; about 34 million more have low bone density of the hips,

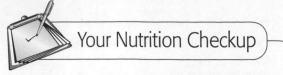

Your Nutrition Checkup

Osteoporosis: Are You at Risk?

While bone loss is a natural part of aging, osteoporosis and fractures don't need to be, according to the National Osteoporosis Foundation. As with any health problem, some women and men are at greater risk than others.

What's your risk? Check all those that apply to you.

Risk factors you can't control. Are you:

_____ **1.** Female?

_____ **2.** Small-boned, with a slight body frame?

_____ **3.** Caucasian or Asian?

_____ **4.** Over age fifty-five?

_____ **5.** From a family with a history of osteoporosis or hip fracture?

Risk factors you can control. Are you:

_____ **6.** Physically inactive?

_____ **7.** Consuming an overall eating plan that's low in calcium and vitamin D?

_____ **8.** Low body mass index?

_____ **9.** Taking high doses of thyroid medication, or high or prolonged doses of cortisonelike medication for asthma, arthritis, or other diseases?

_____ **10.** A current smoker?

_____ **11.** A heavy drinker of alcoholic beverages (three drinks or more per day)?

For the risk factors you can control, make a plan to change!

Adapted from: National Osteoporosis Foundation.

making them at higher risk for osteoporosis. Of those with osteoporosis, most are women. Osteoporosis affects men and women of all races. More people have osteoporosis than report it.

Many fractures, common among older adults, are linked to weakened bones, often overloaded by daily activities or fractures. Besides pain, fractures cause changes in lifestyle and loss of independence. A person may no longer be able to dress alone or walk across a room. Hip fractures also can be fatal. An average of 20 percent of people with hip fractures die from complications within a year after their fracture.

Fractures have emotional consequences. Besides a potential loss of self-esteem and body image, there's the worry of falling or future fractures.

To keep your bones healthy, help them become strong and dense when you're young. After that, help keep them strong by slowing the natural loss that comes with age. *See "Hot Topic: Bone Health" in chapter 6.*

Who's At Risk?

You can't control some risk factors for osteoporosis: genetics, family history, gender, hormonal status, some health conditions, race/ethnic heritage, age, and body frame/weight. You can control other risk factors: what you eat and drink, physical activity, cigarette smoking, alcohol intake, and using medications to help protect against osteoporosis.

Now, how bone-healthy are you?

● *Gender.* If you're female, you're about four times more likely than males to develop osteoporosis: (1) On average, most women have less bone mass to start with—and they lose it faster as they get older. (2) In young women, the hormone estrogen helps deposit calcium in bones. But as estrogen levels drop with menopause, bones are no longer protected. For the first five years after menopause, usually starting at age fifty, women lose bone faster. Estrogen deficiency from early menopause or from a hysterectomy also increases the risk. (3) From the teen years on, women typically eat fewer calcium-rich foods than men do. If you're male, low hormone levels can put your at greater risk, too. Testosterone, as well as estrogen, protect men from bone loss. Drinking too much alcohol or eating too little can lower men's hormone levels; check with your doctor.

● *Low body weight or small body frame.* If you're underweight, you likely have less bone mass than people with a healthy weight. Bone health is one of the benefits of keeping your weight within a healthy range for your height throughout your life.

Women with anorexia or bulimia and those who exercise very strenuously are at higher risk if estrogen levels decrease, causing menstrual periods to become irregular or stop. Women with eating disorders may not consume enough calcium- and vitamin D-rich foods, either. Men also can have eating disorders, which may put them at higher risk for bone loss and osteoporosis, too. *See "Disordered Eating: Problems, Signs, and Help" in chapter 2.*

● *Race/ethnic heritage.* Caucasians and Asians tend to be at higher risk than Latinos and African Americans, although people in these ethnic groups develop osteoporosis, too. Their bones usually are stronger and more dense throughout their lives; all races and ethnic groups need the same amount of calcium.

● *Age.* Bone is dynamic with an ongoing process of bone tissue replacement called remodeling. It's about balance: Older bone is replaced with new bone. Until your early 30s, more bone tissue is re-formed than lost. Call it your bones' preventive maintenance program. Then a few years later that equation flips. With advancing age and menopause for women, more bone is lost than re-formed—up to 1 percent of bone loss per year, depending on individual differences. During the first few years of menopause, there is more rapid bone loss.

● *Family history.* Osteoporosis runs in families. Not only do people inherit a genetic tendency toward bone fractures and osteoporosis, but also families often live similar lifestyles and may follow similar eating patterns that may increase their risk.

● *Physical activity.* Being inactive—perhaps with a desk job, sedentary leisure time, driving—for a long time weakens bones. However, regular weight-bearing activities such as walking, strength training, and dancing trigger your body to deposit calcium in your bones. That makes or keeps them stronger and more dense.

● *Calcium and vitamin D intake.* Throughout life, calcium, along with vitamin D, is a bone builder. If your calcium and vitamin D supplies consistently come up short before ages thirty to thirty-five, your bones may not be as dense as they could be, and less bone gets built. After age thirty-five or so, adults may lose bone faster when their food choices don't supply enough calcium and vitamin D.

● *Some medications.* The use of some medications taken in high doses or for a long time, is linked significantly to increased risk for osteoporosis: ongoing use of steroids, thyroid medicine, and cortisone-like medications. Steroid medications taken for conditions such as rheumatoid arthritis or asthma are especially risky. Some health conditions also may cause or contribute to osteoporosis, such as celiac disease and gastric bypass surgery. Talk to your doctor.

● *Smoking.* For men and women, smoking may lower

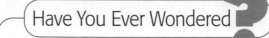

Have You Ever Wondered

. . . if you can get kidney stones by drinking milk? That's a common myth. Research doesn't support this misperception. In fact, drinking milk may reduce the risk. A high-calcium diet may decrease the absorption of oxalate, a substance in some plant-based foods that can form calcium oxalate kidney stones.

. . . if phytoestrogens in soybeans protect your bones? Maybe, since they act much like mild estrogens in the body. After menopause, as natural estrogen declines, phytoestrogens in soy products may help prevent bone some loss.

calcium absorption and so promote bone loss. Among women, smoking lowers estrogen levels, which further contributes to bone loss. If you smoke, that's another good reason to quit.

● *Heavy drinking.* Heavy drinking is linked to weaker bones. But reasons aren't clear—perhaps heavy drinkers don't consume enough food with calcium and vitamin D, or maybe it's a metabolic link.

Protect Your "Support System"

You can't control all factors that keep your "support system," or skeleton, healthy. But regardless of your gender or body build—or your age now—you're still young enough to make a difference in your bone health! You can slow the natural process of bone loss and so reduce your osteoporosis risk. The strategies: wise eating and lifestyle choices.

Ideally, your bone health strategies began in your childhood and have continued throughout adulthood; The denser your bones are before middle age, the better they can withstand bone loss that naturally goes with aging. *For more about bone health see chapters 6 and 19.*

Close the Calcium and Vitamin D Gap

By now you're well aware of the link among calcium, vitamin D, and bone health. So if your food choices come up short, now's the time to close the nutrient gaps!

As an adult you still need calcium; 1,000 milligrams daily is the Recommended Dietary Allowance (RDA) for ages nineteen to fifty; 1,200 milligrams daily for women ages 51 and over and for men over age 70. Remember, an 8-ounce serving of milk or yogurt or 1½ ounces of cheese each supply about 300 milligrams of calcium. Teens need plenty of calcium, too; 1,300 milligrams daily yet during this critical time of bone building, many switch from calcium-rich milk to other beverages.

Vitamin D promotes calcium absorption. If you drink vitamin D-fortified milk, you may consume enough to protect against bone disease. If not, you need other food sources of vitamin D, and perhaps a vitamin D supplement, particularly if you're over age seventy. *See "Vitamins: The Basics" in chapter 6 and "Vitamin D: Often Shortchanged" in chapter 19.*

Consider other links to calcium. Caffeine can increase urinary loss of calcium, but moderate caffeine intake has little influence on bone health. One cup of regular coffee prevents the absorption of the calcium found in one tablespoon of milk. If your caffeine intake is high, you may cut back on caffeinated drinks, since this effect can add up—or enjoy latte (coffee with steamed milk) or tea with milk to make up the difference. Actually, sodium has a greater effect on calcium absorption than caffeine does; however, neither is significant if calcium intake is adequate.

Alcohol and smoking can block calcium absorption. Smoking can speed bone loss; for women, a lifelong habit of smoking a pack of cigarettes a day may lower bone density by menopause an extra 5 to 10 percent. If you smoke, consider the bone-healthy benefits of quitting. Excessive alcohol intake may inhibit some bone remodeling, increase calcium excretion, and increase the chance of falling. If you drink alcoholic beverages, drink only in moderation—for women, no more than one drink a day, and no more than two drinks daily for men.

For many women and men, supplements help ensure an adequate calcium and vitamin D intake and offer protection from osteoporosis. However, the main nourishment for healthy bones should come from food, not pills. If you take calcium and vitamin D pills, use them to supplement, not replace, nourishing foods. *See chapter 23.*

Move Those Bones!

Weight-bearing and resistance training activity—at least three times weekly for adults—helps maintain bone density—if you consume enough calcium and vitamin D. If you're swimming, bicycling, or riding a stationary bike regularly, that's great. But these activities don't promote bone health because they aren't weight-bearing.

Add activities such as these to your "activity repertoire": walking, jogging, aerobic dancing, volleyball, tennis, dancing, or weight lifting—even mowing the grass or shoveling snow. You don't need expensive equipment or a fitness club to lift weights. To build arm and shoulder strength, use things you have around your house, such as canned goods.

Testing, Testing: A Bone Density Scan

Testing for bone mineral density (BMD) isn't recommended for children, teens, or healthy young men or premenopausal women.

If you fit within one of the following groups, the National Osteoporosis Foundation advises testing so osteopenia or osteoporosis can be diagnosed while they can be treated effectively:

Women and men: adults who have had a fracture after age 50 years; all women age 65 years and for older, and men age 70 and older.

Women: those who are at high risk for osteoporosis, especially those who have experienced early menopause, amenorrhea, a fracture from a minor strain, if they have low body weight, or if they have family history of osteoporosis. Not at risk? Still, a BMD test at menopause offers a baseline for later, especially if you're contemplating estrogen or other drug therapy. Consult your doctor.

Men: ages 50 to 69 years who have certain risk factors for osteoporosis.

Your doctor may advise BMD testing if you have other health conditions or if you take high-risk medication, perhaps for arthritis.

BMD tests aren't invasive and take just 5 to 10 minutes. Instead, they scan your spine, hip, and wrist like other X rays do. Your bone density scans are compared to standards of people like you in gender and size: someone age-matched to you and someone younger at peak bone mass. Bone density scanning is now covered by Medicare for many people. The results of a BMD test will be used to help determine if medication is needed.

If You Have Osteoporosis . . .

Prevent and treat osteoporosis with enough calcium and vitamin D, weight-bearing physical activity, and perhaps medication to protect your bones from further deterioration. *Follow the sound advice in "Protect Your 'Support System'" in this chapter.* Also remember this:

● Protect yourself from slips and falls, which might easily fracture a bone, especially if you're over age sixty. Poor lighting, slippery floors and sidewalk, loose rugs, obstacles in walkways, and no assistive devices in bathrooms increase the risk of falling. Check your vision as another precaution.

● Consult with your physician about new medications that may help prevent bone loss or treat osteopenia or osteoporosis. Equally important, talk to your doctor about other medications and supplements you take. Thyroid hormones, oral glucocortoids (steroids), and chemotherapy, among others may promote bone loss.

● Enjoy plenty of calcium- and vitamin D-rich foods. They provide more for bone health—and overall health—than supplements do. A varied, well-balanced eating plan offers other nutrients that appear to promote bone density, including magnesium, phosphorus, potassium, protein, and vitamin K.

● If you cannot meet your calcium and vitamin D recommendations with food and beverages alone, you may need a calcium–vitamin D supplement. Ask a registered dietitian or your doctor about the right dosage and type, and if it should be taken with food to enhance absorption.

Gastrointestinal Conditions

Stomach ache? Diarrhea? Constipation? Heartburn? It's no surprise that discomfort and diseases of the gastrointestinal (GI) tract are linked to nutrition. If you don't feel like eating, or if a health problem interferes with the digestion of food or the absorption of nutrients, GI problems can affect your nutritional status.

For GI problems always see a doctor for a diagnosis if problems persist, and seek guidance from a dietetics professional for eating advice.

Gastric Reflux Disease (GERD)

Is it heartburn—or gastroesophageal reflux disease? Heartburn is a main symptom of GERD; however, gastric reflux disease is a more serious health problem. With GERD, contents of the stomach flow backward into the esophagus. The symptoms? Besides heartburn, symptoms include pain that feels like an ulcer, difficulty swallowing, and regurgitating stomach acid. If you have these ongoing symptoms, check with your doctor.

GERD is associated with several health conditions, such as hiatal hernia, abdominal pressure from obesity, increase of certain hormones (for example, gastrin, estrogen, progesterone), as well as use of some medications and smoking. Caffeine doesn't cause GERD.

Which Bone Is Healthy?

The dense structure of healthy bone depends largely on its calcium stores. As your body withdraws calcium, bone dissolves, leaving a void where calcium was once deposited. Gradually, bones become more porous and fragile. Once the structure of bone disappears, there's no place to redeposit calcium and new bone tissue. Bone loss from osteoporosis appears to be irreversible.

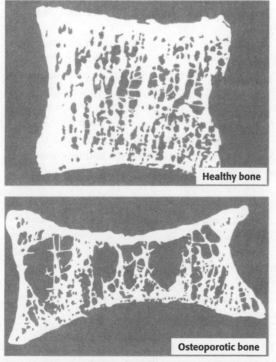

Healthy bone

Osteoporotic bone

Source: Build Better Bone Now. Courtesy of National Dairy Council.

If You Have Gastric Reflux Disease . . .

As part of your treatment, your doctor may recommend an eating plan that eliminates or reduces foods that irritate your esophagus or that cause reflux of stomach acids. Among the common foods and drinks to limit or avoid if they cause discomfort: chocolate, alcoholic drinks, black pepper, any fruit or vegetable that causes symptoms, caffeinated or decaffeinated coffee and tea, high-fat foods, and mint. High-fat foods and large meals may cause problems, too. There's not enough evidence to advise all those with GERD to avoid caffeinated drinks. If other foods, such as tomatoes or oranges, give you trouble, try just small amounts, eaten with other foods. Since obesity increases the risk, your doctor may advise weight loss.

A registered dietitian can provide guidelines for meals and snack planning.

These eating-related tips also can help you treat GERD:

● Eat small, more frequent meals.

● Sit up while you eat, and sit or stand for forty-five to sixty minutes after you eat.

● Eat at least two to three hours before bedtime. Skip late-night meals or bedtime snacks.

Have You Ever Wondered ?

. . . how to relieve hemorrhoids or constipation? Plenty of fiber-rich foods, plenty of fluids, and a physically active lifestyle help prevent constipation and hemorrhoids. As important, pay attention to your body's signals. Delaying a bowel movement can lead to constipation and hard, dry stools, which are difficult to pass. For travelers, lack of access to safe water, sweat loss in a hot climate, or a dry airplane cabin may contribute to fluid loss that leads to constipation.

To help prevent constipation: Eat a variety of fiber-rich foods, drink plenty of fluids, take regular bathroom breaks, and be physically active every day. What's the benefit? Being active helps maintain muscle tone throughout your body, including your intestinal tract.

If constipation is a chronic or a painful problem, talk to your physician. It might signal a more serious problem or an interaction with medication.

See "Fiber and GI Health"" in chapter 3. For tips for easing the problems, see "Constipation during Pregnancy" in chapter 18 and the chart "Cancer Treatment: Handling Some Side Effects" in this chapter.

. . . how you should deal with diarrhea and vomiting? Both are symptoms of other health problems, some more serious than others. In either case, your body loses fluids that need replacing; these conditions can lead to dehydration and electrolyte imbalance.

What causes watery, loose stools, or diarrhea? Perhaps foodborne illness, contaminated water, infection, or medication. With diarrhea, waste passes through the intestine before fluids can be absorbed, or body fluids may pass from the cells into intestinal contents.

For mild diarrhea, drink fluids, but avoid beverages with added sugars, sugar alcohols, caffeine, or alcoholic beverages. Skip high-fiber and gas-producing foods, too, such as nuts, beans, corn, broccoli, cauliflower, and cabbage until you can handle solid food. Prebiotic and probiotic foods such as yogurt, kefir, and cheese may help; *to learn about these foods, see chapter 6.* You might tolerate smaller, more frequent meals better. Rest. For more severe or persistent diarrhea, see your physician.

Vomiting may result from motion imbalance, from a normal reaction to an irritating substance, or it may be symptomatic of many different health problems. When you vomit, the normal rhythmic movements of digestion reverse their direction, expelling your stomach, and perhaps intestinal, contents.

Usually the best "medicine" for vomiting is to drink fluids (in small, frequent amounts) and rest. Start with clear liquids, such as broth, apple juice, or gelatin. About eight hours after you stop vomiting, start to eat solid foods, one at a time in very small amounts. Foods that are odorless, and low in fat and fiber are best for starters. For severe, persistent, or projectile vomiting, check with your physician immediately. You'll need proper rehydration, perhaps with electrolytes, and diagnosis and treatment of the underlying cause. *For more on dealing with diarrhea and vomiting see "Cancer Treatment: Handling Some Side Effects" in this chapter.*

Both diarrhea and vomiting can be especially dangerous for infants and older adults. If they persist, call your healthcare provider immediately!

Have You Ever Wondered **?**

. . . what causes heartburn? The discomfort of heartburn, or indigestion, occurs when digestive juices (hydrochloric acid) and food from your stomach back up into your esophagus. Your stomach lining is protected from acids that form during digestion, but your esophagus lining is sensitive to the burning sensation of stomach acids. That's why you feel discomfort or pain.

Foods themselves don't cause heartburn, but they may aggravate the condition by stimulating acid production. A problem with the esophageal sphincter may be involved, too. Foods high in acids, such as citrus fruit, as well as fatty or highly seasoned foods, may also cause problems for some people.

Heartburn isn't dangerous, just uncomfortable. And it can be treated with antacids. Consult your doctor about the best type for you; antacids can interfere with other medications. The danger can come if you ignore a heart attack, thinking it's simply heartburn. *See "Warning Signs: Heart Attack, Stroke, and Cardiac Arrest" earlier in this chapter.* If the pain continues or if it happens an hour or more after eating, call your doctor immediately!

- Wear loose-fitting clothes that don't put pressure on your abdomen.

- Sleep with your head slightly propped up.

Your doctor also may suggest changes in your lifestyle, medication, and perhaps surgery.

Diverticular Disease

Diverticular disease is really two conditions. *Diverticulosis* is a condition in which pouches, called diverticula, develop in the weakened walls of the intestines, most often the colon. Diverticulosis is linked to an overall eating approach that's low in fiber. Constipation makes the problem worse. These pouches can become inflamed and infected from bacteria in feces that get trapped there—a painful health problem called *diverticulitis*. An estimated 65 to 70 percent of Americans older than eighty-five years have it.

The causes of diverticular disease aren't clear. However, it's likely linked to eating a low-fiber diet. Constipation and lack of exercise also may play a role.

Inflammation may begin when bacteria or feces are caught in the diverticula.

If You Have Diverticular Disease . . .

● For diverticulosis eat plenty of high-fiber foods; keep waste moving through the intestines to avoid constipation. A high-fiber diet is likely the only treatment you need. Nuts and seeds are likely okay to eat. Studies don't support a link between inflammation of the diverticula and eating nuts, seeds, corn, or popcorn. Since people with this condition differ in what and how much they can eat, decide what's best for you if you have diverticulosis. Keep a food journal so you can identity foods that may cause symptoms. *See chapter 3 for more about dietary fiber.*

● For diverticulitis you need to clear up the infection and the inflammation. Treatment often includes antibiotics; perhaps a short-term liquid diet; bed rest; and, if the problem is severe, surgery. Follow the plan from your healthcare provider.

Irritable Bowel Syndrome

Irritable bowel syndrome (IBS), an intestinal problem, doesn't have a clear cause; however, abnormal contractions in the intestines, stress, a low-fiber diet, and a food intolerance all may play a role. Symptoms might be abdominal pain or cramps, as well as diarrhea, constipation, bloating, and gassiness. IBS also is known as colitis and spastic colon.

If you have these symptoms, check with your doctor. They may be a sign of other serious diseases or disorders. Several tests are used to rule out other problems: complete blood count, stool examination, and sigmoidoscopy or colonoscopy.

Irritable bowel syndrome is different from inflammatory bowel disease (IBD)—Crohn's disease and ulcerative colitis—which requires careful medical treatment. With IBD a registered dietitian helps a patient create an individualized approach to eating that not only helps manage gastrointestinal (GI) symptoms but also helps to prevent malnutrition and helps the GI tract function normally.

If You Have Irritable Bowel Syndrome . . .

Many recommendations are good guidance for anyone: a high-fiber, low-fat eating approach. In addition:

● Eat small, frequent meals. Chew your food well to aid digestion. And eat slowly so you don't swallow a lot of air, which may make you feel gassy.

● To prevent constipation, eat plenty of fiber-rich foods. *See chapter 3 for dietary fiber advice.*

● If a food irritates or causes too much gas, avoid it. Beans (legumes), broccoli, Brussels sprouts, cabbage, cucumber, cauliflower, corn, leeks, and onions are some foods that may cause gas.

● Limit any substance or food that makes symptoms worse: perhaps caffeine; alcoholic drinks; high-fat foods; fruit canned in heavy syrup; or sorbitol, a sugar alcohol. Sometimes fructose, the sugar in fruit and fruit drinks, isn't well tolerated; talk to your doctor before avoiding fruit if you suspect a problem.

● Drink more fluids to help prevent constipation. *See chapter 8, "Fluids: Water and More!" for advice about fluids.*

● Learn to manage stress. Anxiety may affect the speed at which food residues pass through your GI tract.

● If you have a food intolerance, learn to manage it.

● Talk to your doctor about your medications. Some, such as antacids, may make symptoms worse. And some dietary supplements can have side effects that affect the GI tract—for example, aloe, black cohosh, garlic, ginkgo biloba, goldenseal, and saw palmetto, among others.

Peptic Ulcers

"Stress is giving me an ulcer!" In truth, it's not, although your body may secrete more stomach acid if you're under emotional strain. Most ulcers in the esophagus, stomach, and small intestine are caused by bacteria called *Heliobactor pylori;* in addition, the use of some anti-inflammatory medications and too much stomach acid, resulting from other health problems, are other causes. When the lining of the gastrointestinal tract is impaired for any number of reasons, the cells underneath can't protect themselves from stomach acids. If the damage goes deep enough, the ulcer may bleed and cause pain.

To refute another common myth, eating spicy foods doesn't cause ulcers either. In fact, no food choices cause or cure ulcers.

Achieve Optimal Digestive Health

● *Consume a balanced diet.* Choose a variety of foods from each food group, especially fiber-rich fruits, vegetables, and grains, as well as certain yogurts and fluids.

● *Establish an eating routine.* Eat regular meals to help promote consistent bowel movements.

● *Eat small, more frequent meals.* Aim for four to five small meals per day versus two to three large meals.

● *Chew more.* Digestion starts in the mouth. Chew thoroughly. Chewing can help with the needed breakdown of some nutrients.

● *Remember a mealtime beverage.* Fluids help move solids through the digestive system.

● *Make half your plate fruits and veggies.* Fiber-rich fruits and vegetables can also provide prebiotics that support the growth of "good" bacteria in the digestive tract.

● *Eat yogurt or kefir daily.* Certain yogurts and kefir contain probiotics that can help promote digestion.

● *Relax after eating.* Give your body time to digest your meal before being active again.

● *Avoid overeating.* Excessive intake can burden the digestive system.

● *Get moving.* Focus on fitting physical activity into your day to help promote digestive health. Even slow activities like stretching and walking will promote good digestive health.

Source: International Food Information Council Foundation, 2011.

If You Have a Peptic Ulcer . . .

Antibiotics or antacids usually are prescribed to treat stomach ulcers: antibiotics to destroy the bacteria, or antacids to suppress stomach acids. In addition, your doctor may recommend dietary treatment. To heal an ulcer, you don't need to eat bland foods, as once thought. Instead, this advice is generally given:

● Follow an overall, well-balanced eating plan. Avoid high-fat foods. Sound familiar?

● Limit foods and seasonings that stimulate the flow of gastric juices: black pepper, chile powder, cloves, garlic, and caffeinated drinks. Decaffeinated coffee or tea may be a problem, too.

Have You Ever Wondered

... if you can eat anything to relieve arthritis? To date, no conclusive research shows that any food or nutrient can relieve the pain that comes with arthritis effectively. Be wary of lures for products, including vitamin supplements, magnets, and copper bracelets, that claim to help, or of taking too many aspirins to relieve pain. Over time aspirin can irritate your stomach, causing bleeding you may not be aware of. That can lead to an iron deficiency. Talk to your doctor about a safe dosage.

Can glucosamine relieve arthritis pain? That's an area of interest and study. Research suggests that, like aspirin and ibuprofen, glucosamine may help dull the pain of stiffening joints. Early findings indicate that it also may help slow the progression of osteoarthritis; however, not enough is known to confirm its safety or effectiveness. Research doesn't show that taking glucosamine and chondroitin sulfate—alone or in combination—reduces pain effectively for most people with osteoarthritis. If you have moderate to severe knee pain, talk to your doctor. Neither supplement is recommended by the Arthritis Foundation for treating arthritis.

People with diabetes, shellfish allergies, and those taking blood-thinning medication or daily aspirin need to be especially cautious about taking glucosamine. Talk to your physician first before trying glucosamine.

The best nutritional advice for arthritis is: Follow a healthful eating plan and maintain a healthy weight. In that way you won't put too much strain on arthritic joints and connective tissue. The medically accepted advice also may include moderate physical activity, prescribed medication, protection of joints, and hot and cold applications.

... if antioxidants can protect your eyes from cataracts or macular degeneration? Maybe. Early research suggests that vitamins A and E, zinc, as well as lutein, zeaxanthin, and some fats may help prevent or slow (not restore) some eye changes that come with aging. Vitamin C may offer protection from cataracts. *See "Functional Nutrition: A Quick Look at Key Phytonutrients" in chapter 6 for lutein and zeaxanthin sources; chapter 6 also gives food sources of nutrients.* Talk to your eye care professional about whether an antioxidant supplement is right for you.

- Eat smaller, more frequent meals.

- Skip alcoholic beverages, smoking, and aspirin.

- Unless a certain food causes repeated discomfort, enjoy any food you choose—as long as it fits within your healthful approach to eating.

- Avoid eating before bedtime.

Anemia: "Tired Blood"

Have that "run-down" feeling? Perhaps you're overworked and underrested. More sleep and relaxation may be what you need to feel energetic again. Or perhaps your fatigue is a symptom of anemia.

Actually, anemia isn't a disease, but instead a symptom of other health problems. With anemia, you may—or may not—feel fatigued. Often there's a nutrition connection.

With anemia, the body doesn't have enough red blood cells, or they're not big enough, to transport oxygen from your lungs to your body cells. Hemoglobin, made with iron, is the part of red blood cells that carries oxygen to other tissues. Without enough oxygen, body cells can't produce enough energy. Then fatigue, pale skin, headache, weakness, lack of concentration, or irritability, among other symptoms, may set in. To produce enough healthy red blood cells, you need enough iron in your diet, as well as enough folate and vitamin B_{12}.

Is It an Iron Deficiency?

Anemia isn't a symptom of just one health problem. A form often described as "iron-poor blood" might come to mind first. In fact, iron deficiency, with its effect on hemoglobin, is the most common form of anemia, more likely affecting adult women of childbearing age, infants and children, and teenage girls. Anemia is a health problem that develops over time. If iron intake comes up short for an extended time, your body can't make enough hemoglobin.

Be aware that having an iron deficiency doesn't necessarily mean you're anemic. For anemia to occur you need a severe depletion of iron stores in your body, with resulting low levels of hemoglobin in your blood.

Before menopause, women need more iron than men do, so women are at higher risk. Why?

● For starters, women need more iron due to monthly blood loss from menstruation. Women with heavy blood loss are at greater risk.

● During pregnancy, women need 50 percent more iron: 27 milligrams a day, compared to 18 milligrams daily prior to pregnancy. The extra is needed for increased blood volume—at least three more pints of blood! Often a woman's stored iron gets used up to meet the demands of pregnancy.

Keep Smiling: Prevent Gum Disease

From an oral health standpoint, a cavity-free mouth doesn't get you home free! Gum, or periodontal, disease, which affects about three-quarters of American adults, is the main cause of tooth loss, which, in turn, can affect food choices. Some chronic health conditions have links to periodontal disease, including diabetes, heart disease, immune deficiency, and osteoporosis, as does poor oral hygiene, tobacco use, and diet. As with tooth decay, bacteria in plaque (the gummy film that forms on teeth) and calculus are at the root of gum disease. In fact, these bacteria may thrive right along the gumline, causing inflammation and infection.

● Help prevent tooth loss by protecting your teeth from gum disease. Brush and floss regularly. By removing plaque along the gumline, bacteria in plaque are less able to irritate your gums. Plaque that isn't removed turns into calculus, or hard deposits, which you can't remove with brushing or flossing.

● Choose an overall eating plan with food variety and balance. Good nutrition affects saliva, making your gums more resistant to infections caused by oral bacteria. And your gums need nutrients to stay healthy.

● Have regular dental checkups. Besides checking for gum problems and oral cancer, the dentist or dental hygienist will remove calculus buildup between teeth and along the gumline.

Have You Ever Wondered

... why fair-skinned people often become pale with anemia? Hemoglobin gives blood its bright red color. With less hemoglobin in circulation, skin is paler. For people with darker skin, check the lining of the eye, which may become pale with anemia.

● Women often don't consume enough iron-rich foods in their everyday food choices, perhaps because they restrict their food intake to their control weight.

● Vegetarian women may come up short on iron. Plant sources of iron aren't absorbed as well as iron from meat, poultry, and fish.

● Like pregnant women, infants and teens need more iron for their increasing blood volume. Infants are at risk if their mothers had low iron status during pregnancy, or, if they bottle-feed, they take formula that's not iron-fortified.

For children, teens, and adults, an iron-rich eating plan can prevent this most common type of anemia. For some, especially pregnant women, iron supplements might be recommended, too.

Some health conditions and medications also cause inadequate iron absorption from food. Iron deficiency anemia in male adults usually results from blood loss.

For more about iron see chapter 6.

Anemia: More than One Cause

Although most common, iron deficiency isn't the only cause of anemia. Deficiencies in vitamin B_{12} or folate are other nutrition-related causes. Anemia also may result from large blood loss, hereditary defects in blood cells (sickle-cell anemia), liver disease that affects body processes that use iron, infections, or congestive heart failure, among other causes. "Sports anemia" isn't really anemia; *see chapter 20.*

Anemia: Linked to Vitamin B_{12}

Anemia from a vitamin B_{12} deficiency doesn't have a single cause; it's not just poor eating, or although uncommon, a low intake of vitamin B_{12}. More often, it's pernicious anemia, caused by poor vitamin B_{12} absorption—perhaps due to lack of intrinsic factor,

Have You Ever Wondered ?

. . . if SAM-e can help someone suffering from osteoarthritis or depression? Derived from the amino acid methionine, SAM-e (S-adenosyl-methionine) is produced in your body and also sold as a dietary supplement in the United States. It may help people suffering from mild depression or joint pain—but shouldn't be used to self-medicate moderate to severe conditions. SAM-e is very costly at the doses used in research studies.

. . . if you can treat chronic fatigue with a special eating plan? Maybe. Studies are under way to determine the best treatment regimen for most sufferers. Of course, an overall healthful eating plan that provides the nutrients and the calories you need to feel energetic, combined with adequate rest, regular physical activity, and stress management, can make a difference. Other ways you might control or relieve your symptoms: improve your sleep habits, adjust your schedule to maximize when you have more energy, and join a support group. Skip unproven remedies, including dietary supplements that haven't shown effectiveness or safety. *(See chapter 23.)* Talk with your doctor about other treatment approaches.

. . . if you should heed the advice "Starve a cold and feed a fever"? Illness is no time to "starve" your body of nutrients. To fight infection, your body needs a supply of nutrients to build and maintain your natural defenses, so you still need balance and variety in your food choices. Extra rest helps, too. With a fever, drink plenty of fluids: juice, milk, soup, or water. If you don't have much appetite, eat bland, simple foods, perhaps more often. How about vitamin C? Well, it won't cure the common cold. No scientific evidence proves that a large dose, perhaps from a vitamin supplement, boosts immunity; however, it may shorten the duration of a cold and decrease the severity of cold symptoms.

. . . if lecithin can keep you healthy? Lecithin is a phospholipid, or a type of fat. Promoters make many claims for lecithin, for example, as a cure for or prevention of arthritis, skin problems, gallstones, and nervous disorders, as well as memory problems and improved endurance. Others claim it dissolves cholesterol that's deposited in arteries. Because your body makes lecithin, taking it as a supplement doesn't appear to offer added benefits. Synthetic lecithin isn't well absorbed.

. . . if other healthcare treatments, such as acupuncture or herbal medicines, are safe and effective? Despite consumer attention to alternative treatments, little research backs up their safety or effectiveness. Although some have been used as traditional medicines for centuries, their success is shared mostly in individual reports, not scientific research. To gather sound research evidence to either support or dissuade their use, the National Center for Complementary and Alternative Medicine recently was established within the National Institutes of Health. Some treatments may offer promise in certain circumstances.

Until more is known, alternative approaches to healthcare shouldn't replace treatment that's known to be safe and effective. If you do choose to try alternative or complementary care, talk to your doctor first. Some alternative approaches may interfere with the effectiveness of your doctor's prescribed treatment.

For other health conditions and problems, see these chapters:

- Breast cancer—chapter 18.
- Celiac disease—chapter 21.
- Choking (Heimlich maneuver)—chapters 13 and 16 (infants) and chapter 17 (children).
- Constipation and hemorrhoids—chapters 3 and 18.
- Dehydration and heat stroke—chapter 8.
- Dental cavities—chapters 3 and 16 (infants).
- Diverticulosis—chapter 3.
- Eating disorders—chapters 2 and 17 (teens).
- Fibrocystic breast disease—chapter 18.

- Fibromyalgia—chapter 18.
- Food allergies—chapters 16 (infants) and 21.
- Foodborne illness—chapter 13.
- Gluten intolerance—chapter 21.
- Lactose intolerance—chapter 21.
- Migraine headaches—chapter 21.
- Overweight and obesity—chapters 2 and 17 (children and teens).
- Polycystic ovary syndrome—chapter 18.
- Reactive hypoglycemia—chapter 3.
- Vaginal yeast infections—chapter 18.

Have You Ever Wondered

... if you need more potassium if you're taking a diuretic medication? That depends on the diuretic that's been prescribed for you. Talk to your doctor or a registered dietitian for advice. You probably don't need to take a potassium supplement, however. Many foods are great sources, including many fruits and vegetables, and milk. *For a list of foods high in potassium, see "Potassium: Another Reason for Fruits and Veggies!" in chapter 7.*

. . . if antacids are okay for ongoing indigestion? Although your body may produce less stomach acid with age, you may suffer from indigestion. Antacids, taken as directed, can help. However, excess amounts can deplete your body's phosphorus reserves, which may lead to softening of the bones, called osteomalacia.

Taking antacids with calcium at mealtime may prevent your body from fully absorbing iron in food. Talk to your doctor about taking antacids. Symptoms that seem like indigestion could be something more serious.

. . . what "medical foods" are? They're a category of functional foods. Medical foods help manage a disease or a health problem. Under a doctor's supervision, they're consumed or given in a tube feeding directly to the stomach.

atrophic gastritis, or the surgical removal of part of the stomach or small intestine.

What's intrinsic factor? It's a body chemical, produced in the stomach, that helps your body absorb vitamin B_{12} in the intestine. If gastric juices lack intrinsic factor, perhaps for genetic reasons, or if the secretion of stomach juices is impaired, vitamin B_{12} can't be properly absorbed. With age (typically over age sixty), atrophic gastritis, a condition that causes the acid content of stomach secretions to decrease, can affect vitamin B_{12} absorption. Injury or surgical removal of part of the stomach also affects gastric juices and nutrient absorption. Your doctor will diagnose these problems and offer advice.

Because vitamin B_{12} comes only from animal sources of food (meat, fish, poultry, eggs, milk, and milk products), strict vegetarians, or vegans, can be at higher risk. They need a reliable source of vitamin B_{12}, perhaps a fortified breakfast cereal or a supplement, to protect against anemia.

Anemia: Short on Folate

A folate deficiency can lead to anemia. Why? Folate is essential for cell growth and development. Without enough folate, red blood cells become enlarged but don't develop normally, so they can't carry oxygen to body cells as efficiently. Today most enriched grain products are folic acid-fortified in the United States, so most people consume enough to avoid anemia. Folate also comes from leafy vegetables, some fruits, beans (legumes), and liver. Some whole-grain foods are folic acid-fortified.

For women, a folate deficiency may show up later in pregnancy when folate needs are high. Early in pregnancy, a shortage of folate may lead to birth defects of the spinal cord. Whether or not you're at risk for anemia caused by folate deficiency, consume enough, especially if you're planning to get pregnant—or if you already are pregnant. *For more about folate and pregnancy, see "Before Pregnancy" in chapter 18.*

Testing, Testing: Do You Have Anemia?

Before you self-diagnose your fatigue as anemia and then pop a pill, consult your doctor about your symptoms. And ask for a blood test.

A hemoglobin test or a hematocrit test is a simple, inexpensive blood test to screen for the possibility of anemia; however, many conditions can affect the results. If the test results are positive, your doctor may conduct more specific tests, for example: *for iron-deficiency anemia*—serum ferritin or total iron-binding capacity (TIBC); *for folate deficiency anemia*—serum folate; or *for vitamin B_{12} deficiency*—serum vitamin B_{12} or a Schilling test.

Proper diagnosis is essential for getting the right treatment for various types of anemia; the wrong treatment may have potentially harmful effects. For example, a folate supplement may "cure" blood-related symptoms of pernicious anemia but mask irreversible, potentially severe damage to the nervous system.

Treatment for sickle cell anemia—a genetic condition that's more common among those of African and Mediterranean descent—differs, too. This condition affects a child's growth patterns. Often a nutritionally adequate eating pattern with more protein and calories is prescribed, but both weight and growth for children must be watched closely by healthcare providers.

If You Have Anemia . . .

● Consult your doctor or a registered dietitian about appropriate treatment for the type of anemia you have. Follow prescribed treatment or professional advice, not self-prescribed supplements.

● Keep any supplements in a safe place, where children can't reach them.

● Enjoy good food sources of all three nutrients: iron, vitamin B$_{12}$, and folate.

● Follow up with your doctor, perhaps with appropriate blood tests to monitor your status.

● For more guidance, check here:

● *Iron—"Menstrual Cycle: More Iron for Women" in chapter 18, "Iron: The Fatigue Connection" for teenage girls in chapter 17, and "Minerals—Not 'Heavy Metal'" in chapter 6.*

● *Vitamin B$_{12}$—"Vitamins: The Basics" in chapter 6.*

● *Folate—"Vitamins: The Basics" in chapter 6.*

Need more tips for preventing or managing health problems? Check here for "how-tos":

● Put more physical activity in your lifestyle —see chapters 1, 2, 17, 19, and 20.

● Manage your weight sensibly and effectively—see chapter 2.

● Manage alcoholic drinks for health—see chapter 8.

● Follow overall eating guidelines for health promotion—see chapter 10.

● Shop smart to match your health needs—see chapter 12.

● Prepare foods to manage your health conditions—see chapter 14.

● Stick to your eating plan when you eat out—see chapter 15.

● Use supplements appropriately to avoid or manage health problems—see chapter 23.

● Find a nutrition expert trained to help with your health problems—see chapter 24.

● Identify resources to help deal with specific health conditions—see "Resources You Can Use."

If Your Doctor Prescribes a Special Eating Plan . . .

Like your medication, a doctor-prescribed eating plan—perhaps sodium-modified, high-fiber, gluten-free, or blenderized liquid—is essential to healthcare and disease management. In the world of medicine, a special meal plan is part of medical nutrition therapy. If your doctor prescribes a special eating plan as part of your treatment for whatever conditions you might have:

● Get enough guidance so you can successfully comply. Ask for a referral to a registered dietitian for help in planning and monitoring your nutrition needs. You need an approach that matches your physical and personal needs and your food preferences. *Caution:* Let your doctor or dietitian know about any supplements you take.

● Follow the special nutrition plan faithfully. Record what you eat, your challenges, and successes to share later with your healthcare provider or dietitian. That's especially important if this is a long-term change in your eating regimen.

● Use Nutrition Facts and ingredient lists on food labels as information aids. A dietitian can help you learn to use label facts effectively—and perhaps direct you to specialized, medically sound resources: websites, phone apps, organizations, or support groups.

● Get family support. Their encouragement and help in food shopping and preparation make any special eating plan easier to follow. Try to dovetail your meal plans; serve the same foods to the whole family whenever you can. For example, if you're on a DASH Eating Plan, almost everyone can benefit from more fruits, vegetables, and low-fat dairy foods.

For more on getting the most from nutrition counseling, see "When You Consult an Expert . . ." in chapter 24.

Food and Medicine

Do you take over-the-counter medications, prescription medications, or both? Their safe, effective use is your responsibility—and an important part of medical treatment. Talk to your doctor, pharmacist, and perhaps a registered dietitian for the guidance you need.

COMMON INTERACTIONS BETWEEN FOOD AND SOME MEDICATIONS: TALK TO YOUR DOCTOR!

MEDICINE CABINET PRESCRIPTION DRUGS AND OVER-THE-COUNTER PRODUCTS	KITCHEN CABINET: COMMON FOOD AND DRUG INTERACTIONS* (FOR SPECIFIC INFORMATION ABOUT YOUR MEDICATIONS, ASK YOUR DOCTOR OR YOUR PHARMACIST.)
Pain relievers ● Aspirin (e.g., Anacin, Bayer) ● Ibuprofen (e.g., Advil, Motrin, Nuprin)	Take these with food to avoid irritating your stomach. Also limit other stomach irritants, such as alcohol and caffeine.
Antibiotics ● Tetracycline (e.g., Achromycin, Sumycin) ● Penicillin (e.g., Pen-Vee K)	The calcium in dairy foods and in calcium and iron supplements can block the absorption of tetracycline-based products. Take these medications one hour or more before or after consuming dairy products or calcium supplements. When taken together, citrus fruits and fruit juices can destroy a type of penicillin.
Blood-thinning medication/anticoagulants ● Warfarin (e.g., Coumadin, Dicoumerol)	Eat in moderation a consistent amount of foods with vitamin K, such as dark-green leafy greens; spinach; kale; turnip greens; green tea; and some soy burgers. Too much vitamin K can make your blood clot faster. Vitamin E supplements can increase the risk of bleeding.
Antidepressants ● MAO inhibitors (e.g., Marplan, Parnate)	When taken with foods high in tyramine (an amino acid found in protein foods), these medications may lead to increased blood pressure, fever, headache, vomiting, and possible death. Ask your doctor or a registered dietitian for a list of foods to avoid, such as beer, cheese, red wine, cured meats, aged cheese, avocados, sour cream, and yeast products.
Antacids containing ● Aluminum (e.g., Maalox, Amphojel) ● Calcium (e.g., Tums) ● Sodium (e.g., Alka-Seltzer)	Wait two to three hours after taking an aluminum-containing antacid before you drink or eat citrus fruits. Citrus fruits can increase the amount of aluminum your body absorbs. Antacids with aluminum also can cause a loss of bone-building calcium. Some antacids can weaken the absorption of heart-regulating medications such as digoxin (e.g., Lanoxin). Some antacids can weaken the effect of antiulcer medication (e.g., Tagamet) or drugs that treat high blood pressure (such as Inderal). Be sure to read all the alerts on the labels. If you have high blood pressure, read the label of antacids for the amount of sodium present.
Garlic pills	It is important for your blood to clot if you suffer a cut or undergo surgery. Substances in garlic appear to thin the blood. If you are already taking aspirin or other blood-thinning medications, taking garlic supplements may thin the blood too much.
Corticosteroids (Prednisone, Solumedrol, Hydrocortisone)	Because these medications increase sodium and water retention, which may lead to edema, go easy on foods high in sodium, such as ham and other cured meats, pickled vegetables (pickled beets, olives, pickles, sauerkraut, others), processed foods, cheese, salty snacks, and salt added in cooking and at the table.
Medications for cancer treatment (Tamoxifen, Methotrexate)	Flavonoids in citrus fruits can help tamoxifen inhibit cancer cell growth. Methotrexate promotes folate deficiency; a folate supplement may be prescribed.

*Many supplements including herbal products may interact with medications, too. *See "Warning: Supplement Interactions!" in chapter 23.*

Adapted from: To Your Health! Food & Activity Tips for Older Adults (National Council on Aging, National Institute on Aging, President's Council on Physical Fitness and Sports, and Food Marketing Institute). Used with permission.

Some Don't Mix

Taking medications may not seem like a nutrition issue. Yet, when food and medicines are taken together, they often interact. That's not surprising since the chemistry of the stomach and the intestine differs before and several hours after eating. Food and the substances released in your body during digestion may either enhance or hinder the effectiveness of some medications. Some medications alter appetite, taste, or smell, and may cause mouth sores or a dry mouth, making swallowing difficult. Others may induce nausea or irritate the GI tract. Medications also can improve or interfere with nutrient absorption or use.

Your goal? To get the full benefits of both food and medicine. To do that, all medications, even aspirin, should be taken as directed:

● Some medications should be taken with meals. With food, they're less likely to irritate the stomach. Aspirin and ibuprofen are two examples.

● Some medications should be taken on an empty stomach, perhaps an hour before or three hours after eating. Food may slow their absorption and action. That's true of some antibiotics, for example.

● Some food and medications shouldn't be consumed within several hours of each other. For example, fruit juice (including grapefruit juice) and other high-acid foods can destroy one type of penicillin. And calcium in dairy foods and calcium supplements binds with tetracycline, so it passes through the body without being absorbed.

● Some medications should be taken with plenty of water. That's true of most cholesterol-lowering medications.

● Many medications shouldn't be taken with alcoholic beverages. Alcohol can block the effects of some medications, and amplify the effects of others to potentially harmful levels. Medication also can intensify the effects of alcohol in your body.

How do you know to take medicine with a meal or on an empty stomach? Read the directions printed on the container or on an accompanying information sheet. You'll find information about when, how much per dose, and how long to take the medication. The directions also may state what to do if you miss a dose. Ask the doctor or the pharmacist if you don't fully understand. You can ask that directions be printed in large type. *Note:* With the long-term use of some medications, your doctor also may prescribe a dietary supplement. *See chapter 23.*

You can't know about the potential interactions between all medicines and food. That's where the advice of your doctor, a pharmacist, or a registered dietitian comes in. *For a quick reference for some medications see "Common Interactions between Food and Some Medications: Talk to Your Doctor!" in this chapter.*

Medication: For Safety's Sake

● Talk to your doctor or pharmacist about all medications you're taking, including over-the-counter medications, dietary supplements such as herbal products, and oral supplements. Some medications and supplements have harmful interactions.

● Always take the medication as prescribed in the directions. If you don't take enough, or stop too soon, the medication may not work. Taking too much, too often can be dangerous. Depending on the medication, excessive amounts also may keep your body from absorbing essential nutrients or deplete your supply.

● Always take medicine in a well-lighted place. Put on your glasses if you wear them! Otherwise you might take the wrong medication or the wrong amount.

● Keep medicines in their original containers with the directions intact. Store them out of a child's reach.

● Only take medicines prescribed for you, even if your symptoms seem similar to someone else's.

● Flush unused or expired medicines down the toilet.

● With each checkup, review your medication plan with your doctor to make sure it's still right for you.

CHAPTER 23

Dietary Supplements
Use and Misuse

Could a supplement replace your dinner? For all those who enjoy the pleasure of eating, there's good news. The answer is unequivocally "no"!

Only food can provide the mixture of vitamins, minerals, phytonutrients, and other substances for health—qualities that can't be duplicated with dietary supplements. Fortunately for most Americans, there's plenty of quality, quantity, and variety in the food marketplace. So most people don't need supplements.

Despite this fact, more than half of Americans take dietary supplements, making it a business of $28.7 billion for 2010, according to the Nutrition Business Journal—and growing! Some people are prudent with their use, limiting the potency of their supplement to 100 percent or less of the Daily Values (DVs) and taking just the recommended dose—at their doctor's advice. For others, supplements, perhaps herbals, are part of or a complement to their medical care—as guided by their healthcare providers. Yet, others self-prescribe, sometimes high, potentially dangerous dosages of supplements, perhaps at the advice of a friend or the media—not their healthcare provider.

Why do many consumers take dietary supplements? The reasons are varied—many times medically valid, sometimes not. In appropriate dosages, *some* supplements offer health benefits under *some* circumstances. Some people use supplements with good intention: perhaps to fill dietary gaps, prevent nutrient deficiencies, or get protection from health problems such as depression, postmenopausal symptoms, aging skin, cancer, or arthritis. Others seek added benefits: perhaps better sleep, athletic performance, or sexual prowess, or more energy. Too often, supplement use is based on scientifically *unfounded* marketing promises.

For many supplements, their use prompts questions with *unknown* answers: *unknown* benefits . . . *unknown* interactions with food, medicines, and other supplements . . . *undetermined* standards . . . *unknown* levels of safety and effectiveness, making dosages on package labels confusing. Yet scientific evidence is being gathered for answers about their safety and effectiveness.

Regardless, no supplements provide a quick, easy road to health. Good nutrition depends on overall healthful eating and active living. Good health requires much more than a supplement or two, or more.

What, then, is appropriate—and inappropriate—use of dietary supplements?

Dietary Supplements: Defined

Dietary supplements are neither food nor drugs. Instead, they're products taken orally that contain a "dietary ingredient" meant to supplement, not substitute for, healthful foods. According to the 1994 Dietary Supplement Health and Education Act (DSHEA), "dietary supplements" refer to a broad range of products: vitamins, minerals, herbs or other botanicals, and

Supplements—Truth or Myth?

Misconceptions about dietary supplements are rampant. What do you think about using them?

FACT OR MYTH?

____	____	**1.**	Nutrient supplements can make up for my poor food choices.
____	____	**2.**	Taking supplements can prevent, treat, or cure disease.
____	____	**3.**	Nutrient supplements boost my energy.
____	____	**4.**	If it's herbal, it's not harmful.
____	____	**5.**	"Stress" vitamins help me cope better with a lot of emotional stress.
____	____	**6.**	A nutrient supplement can help me build muscle or get more from my physical performance.
____	____	**7.**	A vitamin pill could protect my body from the harmful effects of smoking or alcohol.
____	____	**8.**	Supplements make up for foods grown in depleted soil.
____	____	**9.**	Taking the right supplement can help with weight loss.
____	____	**10.**	If I can buy it, it's safe.

Here are the facts: Every statement is false!

1. *Fact:* No supplement can fix an ongoing pattern of poor food choices. Supplements may supply some vitamins and minerals, but not all the substances in food, for optimal health. Only a varied, balanced eating pattern provides enough nutrient variety, phytonutrients, and other substances for health. If you eat smart, you probably don't need a daily supplement.

2. *Fact:* No scientific evidence in humans proves that vitamin and mineral supplements prevent, treat, or cure cancer or other chronic illnesses. Extra vitamin C won't prevent colds and flu but may reduce symptoms. Some antioxidant nutrients may be protective; research is preliminary. *See "Vitamins as Antioxidants" in chapter 6.*

3. *Fact:* Boosting your nutrient intake won't cause your cells to produce extra energy or more brain power. Only three nutrients—carbohydrates, fats, and proteins—supply energy (calories). Vitamins don't. Although B vitamins do *help* body cells produce energy from energy nutrients, they aren't energy sources.

4. *Fact:* Many powerful drugs and toxic chemicals are plant-based. Taking herbal supplements, too—and interactions with medication and allergic reactions—may lead to dangerous side effects.

5. *Fact:* Emotional stress doesn't increase nutrient needs. Claims promoting dietary supplements to "de-stress" your life are misleading, too. The best dietary advice for the physical demands of stress: a healthful eating pattern. More "de-stressing" advice: stay active, get enough rest, and take time to relax.

6. *Fact:* Athletes and other physically active people need about the same amount of nutrients as others do—just more calories for the increased demands of exercise. The extra amount of food that active people eat supplies the small amount of extra vitamins needed for energy production. Although protein needs are somewhat higher for some athletes, especially for those in strength-training sports, food can easily provide the extra. On another note, physical activity, not extra amino acids (protein), builds muscle. *For more on nutrition for athletes and ergogenic aids, see chapter 20.*

7. *Fact:* Dietary supplements won't protect you from the harmful effects of smoking or alcohol abuse. Smoking increases the need for vitamin C; beta carotene supplements may increase lung cancer risk among some smokers. Drinking excessive amounts of alcoholic beverages can interfere with the body's use of most nutrients.

8. *Fact:* If soil can grow crops, the food produced is nutritious. When soil lacks minerals, plants don't grow properly and may not produce their potential yield. Growing area does affect a food's iodine and selenium contents.

9. *Fact:* Weight loss is about calories in, calories out. Weight loss supplements touted to trap fat, block carbs, or boost metabolism typically are no more effective than placebos. Except for some that may temporarily help curb your appetite, no over-the-counter supplement effectively sheds pounds. *For healthy ways to manage your weight, refer to chapter 2.*

10. *Fact:* Unlike medications, supplements don't undergo the same scrutiny. So they may not be as safe as you hope. Marketing claims are related to effectiveness, not safety. Claims on product labels and marketing materials are regulated by the FDA. Most reliable companies don't make unsupported or illegal label claims.

amino acids, as well as substances such as enzymes, hormones, concentrates, extracts, and metabolites. Unlike drugs, dietary supplements aren't intended to treat, diagnose, lessen, prevent, or cure disease.

Supplements are easy to spot. By law, they must be labeled "dietary supplements." Thousands of dietary supplements are marketed in the United States, with new products launched each year. They're sold in many forms—for example, tablets, capsules, softgels, gelcaps, liquids, powders, and energy bars.

Vitamin/Mineral Supplements: Benefits and Risks

Do you take a vitamin and mineral supplement? Maybe you need to, maybe not. A fundamental premise of the 2010 Dietary Guidelines for Americans is: nutrients should come mostly from foods. Food provides not only nutrients often contained in supplements, but also fiber and other naturally occurring substances that promote health. No sufficient evidence supports taking, or not taking, a multivitamin/mineral supplement as the main way to prevent chronic disease for healthy people.

That said, taking certain nutrients in supplements— for some people, under some circumstances—may be appropriate. Conversely, some may be harmful to other subgroups of people. So, is a supplement right for you?

Vitamin/Mineral Supplements: For Whom?

With some exceptions, supplements usually aren't necessary—*if* you're healthy and *if* you're able *and willing* to eat a balanced, varied diet. You probably can get the vitamins and minerals you need from smart food choices. According to national studies, most Americans have enough healthful foods available to do that. *So the advice:* Food first! Under some circumstances, vitamin/mineral supplements offer benefits and are advised.

Many vitamins and minerals are sold as single supplements—for example, vitamins C and E, beta carotene, calcium, and iron. Some are sold in large doses, perhaps more than you need. Others are "combos," sold as multivitamin/mineral supplements. Your doctor or a registered dietitian (RD) may recommend a dietary supplement. Are you . . .

● *A woman with heavy menstrual bleeding?* You may need an iron supplement to replace iron from blood loss. *See "Iron Supplements: Enhancing the Benefit" later in this chapter.*

● *A woman who's pregnant or breast-feeding?* You need more of some nutrients, especially folate and iron—and perhaps calcium (with vitamin D) if you don't consume enough calcium-rich foods. Ask about a prenatal vitamin/mineral supplement. *See "Before Pregnancy" in chapter 18.*

● *A woman capable of becoming pregnant?* Consume 400 micrograms of folic acid (the synthetic form of folate) daily from fortified foods, vitamin supplements, or a combination of the two—*in addition to* folate found naturally in some fruits, vegetables, and beans (legumes). The extra folic acid reduces the risk of spinal cord defects in a developing fetus. Synthetic folic acid is better absorbed than food folate.

Foods fortified with folic acid include enriched grains such as flour, breads, cereals, pasta, and rice. If you take a supplement, choose one with a dosage of no more than 1,000 micrograms of folic acid daily.

● *A menopausal woman?* You may benefit from a calcium supplement with vitamin D, in addition to a calcium-rich diet, to slow calcium loss from bones. *See "Calcium Supplements: A Bone Builder" in this chapter.* For some older men, a calcium supplement is advised.

● *Someone on a restrictive diet (<1,600 calories a day)?* You likely won't consume enough food to meet all your nutrient needs. Your doctor or a registered dietitian may recommend a multivitamin/mineral supplement. *Caution:* Unless under a doctor's supervision, very-low-calorie eating plans aren't advised. *See "'Diets' That Don't Work!" in chapter 2.*

● *A vegetarian?* You may need a supplement with calcium, iron, zinc, and vitamins B_{12} and D—if your regular eating pattern doesn't supply much, if any, meat, dairy, and other animal products or if you don't consume enough from fortified foods.

● *Someone with limited milk intake and sunlight exposure?* If you have lactose intolerance, a milk allergy, or simply don't consume enough dairy foods, you may need a calcium supplement with vitamin D for bone health.

You may be advised to take a vitamin D supplement, too. *See chapter 6 for more about calcium and vitamin D.*

● *Someone with a health condition that affects nutrient use?* Doctors often prescribe supplements for those with health problems that affect appetite or eating, or that affect how nutrients are absorbed, used, or excreted—for example, digestive or liver problems. Surgery or injuries may increase the need for some nutrients. Some medications, such as antacids, antibiotics, laxatives, and diuretics, may interfere with the way the body uses nutrients. If you have a food allergy, gluten intolerance, or other health problems that restrict what you eat, a supplement may be advised.

● *An older adult?* Older adults are often advised to consume a supplement with calcium and vitamin D. *For more about these nutrients for older adults, see chapter 19.*

Ten to 30 percent of adults over age fifty have atrophic gastritis, a condition that causes damage to stomach cells and so reduces the body's ability to absorb vitamin B_{12}. For that reason, adults in this age group are urged to get extra vitamin B_{12} in its crystalline form from a supplement or from fortified food.

● *Some babies* after age six months, children, and teens may need a fluoride supplement—and perhaps iron or vitamin D. *See "Vitamin and Mineral Supplements for Breast-Fed Babies" in chapter 16.*

● *Someone unable—or unwilling—to regularly consume a healthful diet?* You likely need a dietary supplement to fill in the nutrient gaps. However, eating smarter would be better if you don't have food-related health problems! Take a supplement with the advice of a doctor or a registered dietitian. For example, premenopausal women who don't consume enough calcium from food likely need a calcium supplement—unless they're willing to improve their diet.

Except for rare medical conditions, few people need more than 100 percent of their Recommended Dietary Allowances (RDAs) of any nutrient. Large mineral or vitamin doses are prescribed only for certain medically diagnosed health problems. Even then, their use should be monitored carefully by a doctor.

If you have any questions about your own nutrient needs—or think you need a supplement—talk to a registered dietitian or your doctor. *See "How to Find Nutrition Help . . ." in chapter 24.*

More Isn't Always Better!

A little is good, but a lot may *not* be healthier. As with other nutrients, such as fat, added sugars, and sodium, moderation is your smart guideline for vitamins and minerals: enough, but not too much.

Supplements carry labeling, showing the amounts of vitamins and minerals in a single dosage. If you already eat a healthful diet, a low-dose supplement is likely enough. Taking a multivitamin/mineral supplement, with about 100 percent of the Daily Values (DVs) as a safety net, is generally considered safe.

Supplements that boast "high potency"—a much higher dosage than you may need—also are available. Either as single-nutrient supplements or vitamin-mineral combinations, high-potency supplements (significantly in excess of the Daily Values) can be harmful. Be prudent.

Risks. Consuming in amounts that exceed the Tolerable Upper Intake Level (*see appendices*) for nutrients from some supplements can have undesirable side effects such as fatigue, diarrhea, and hair loss. Other side effects may pose more serious risks—for example, kidney stones, liver or nerve damage, birth defects, or even death.

Because fat-soluble vitamins (A, D, E, K) are stored in the body, taking high levels of some for a prolonged time can be toxic. For example, excess amounts of vitamin D in the blood from overuse of supplements can cause kidney damage, and raising blood levels of calcium can cause confusion, disorientation, and problems with heart rhythm. Too much vitamin A, taken over time, can cause bone and liver damage, headaches, diarrhea, and birth defects.

Supplements with water-soluble vitamins or minerals can be risky, too, if taken in excess, over time. For example, taking extra vitamin B_6 may help relieve premenstrual tension. Yet no convincing evidence supports large vitamin B_6 doses for relief of premenstrual syndrome (PMS). Many women have viewed large vitamin B_6 doses as harmless since they are water-soluble. Instead, they may cause irreversible nerve damage when taken in very large doses above the Tolerable Upper Intake Level (UL): 500 to 5,000 mg vitamin B_6 per day.

Other examples: Very high vitamin C doses can cause diarrhea and nausea. Liver damage may be

Have You Ever Wondered

... why a nutrient supplement label may list the percent of vitamin A from beta carotene? The supplement may contain beta carotene but not vitamin A itself. However, the body converts beta carotene to vitamin A.

... if ridges or marks on your fingernails suggest a vitamin deficiency? No, but it's a common misconception. Instead, they're often caused by a slight injury to the nail. A nutrient deficiency isn't a cause.

Appearance-conscious teens often hear that taking gelatin pills strengthens nails, but there's no quick nutritional cure for nails that break and split. Fingernails are mainly dead protein cells that get their strength from amino acids. Gelatin doesn't contain these amino acids.

... if supplements with "phytonutrients" are a good choice? From *phyto,* Greek for plant, these botanical substances are extracted from vegetables and other plant foods. There's not enough scientific evidence to know if supplement manufacturers have picked the right active substance from plant sources for any benefit.

Plants have thousands of phytonutrients. Science hasn't yet revealed which one, if any, or what amount in a supplement might offer any health benefits.

Better advice: Get "phytos" from food. Any health-promoting benefit might come from the interaction of many phytonutrients provided naturally in food.

... how different forms of vitamin C compare? Vitamin C in supplements is usually ascorbic acid. But you might find sodium ascorbate, calcium ascorbate, other mineral ascorbates, and ascorbic acid with bioflavonoids. Research hasn't shown that one is better than another.

... if dietary supplements can protect against biological threats? No, although some supplement promoters may make this claim. According to the Centers for Disease Control and Prevention and the U.S. Food and Drug Administration (FDA), no current and credible scientific evidence suggests that supplements on the market today offer protection from or treatment for biological contaminants such as anthrax, SARS, or bird (avian) flu.

Likewise, FDA advises against taking antibiotics for protection from foodborne illnesses caused by bacteria, unless prescribed by a doctor. Antibiotics can't protect against viruses or chemicals that contaminate food.

---

caused by high niacin doses (as time-released nicotinic acid); sometimes a physician will prescribe high doses of niacin to help lower elevated blood cholesterol. Excessive folic acid can hide symptoms of pernicious anemia, so the disease gets worse without being detected.

Children are more vulnerable to overdoses of vitamins and minerals than adults. In fact, excessive iron—perhaps from iron supplements intended for their mother—can be fatal to children.

The way your body handles large nutrient doses from dietary supplements depends on many factors.

Click Here! Websites to Know . . .

- Dietary Supplement Fact Sheets, ods.od.nih.gov
- National Center for Complementary and Alternative Medicine, nccam.nih.gov

See "Resources You Can Use" for more websites.

Your body size, supplement dose (amount and frequency), and how long you take them influence whether a megadose will be toxic for you.

See the appendices for the Tolerable Upper Intake Level (UL) for many nutrients. The UL is the maximum amount that appears safe for most healthy people. Consuming more may increase some health risks. *See chapter 6 for more about vitamins and minerals that may be sold in supplement form.*

That said, can you overdose on vitamins or minerals naturally occurring in food? That's highly unlikely. The vitamin and mineral content of food is much more balanced than in dietary supplements. In amounts normally consumed, even if you enjoy extra helpings, you won't consume toxic levels of nutrients. *Note:* Nutrient amounts can add up if you consume *a lot* of highly fortified foods; some are classified as supplements because they have as many vitamins and minerals as a multivitamin supplement.

Nutrient-Nutrient Interactions. High doses of some nutrients may result in deficiencies of others. For example, high calcium intake may inhibit the absorption of iron and other trace nutrients. High doses of vitamin E can interfere with the action of vitamin K and make anticoagulant drugs such as Coumadin (warfarin) more powerful.

Even low levels of dietary supplements may contribute to health problems for some people. For example, those at risk for hemochromatosis need to be careful of taking iron in supplements. Folic acid can mask a vitamin B_{12} deficiency, which may cause neurological damage. And zinc supplements in excess of the UL can decrease levels of HDL ("good") cholesterol, impair immunity, and reduce copper status.

What We Know About . . .

Calcium supplements: A bone builder. People of every age need an adequate amount of calcium. As an extra safeguard, many doctors recommend calcium supplements, especially for menopausal and post-menopausal women and for women who simply don't consume enough calcium in their food and beverage choices. The reason? To help stave off bone loss that comes with hormonal changes. If you're advised to take a calcium supplement, consider the following:

● Choose the dosage and the form of calcium that's right for you. Different products have different amounts. Check the serving size on the Nutrition Facts to know how much you need to take to get the amount listed on the label. The calcium amount is generally lower in a multivitamin/mineral supplement than in a product formulated as a calcium supplement.

Calcium supplements are generally compounds, such as calcium carbonate (often found in antacids) and calcium citrate. Calcium carbonate, often less expensive, is best absorbed when taken with food; calcium citrate can be taken any time. Because of lower levels of stomach acids, after age fifty years calcium citrate is absorbed more easily. To aid absorption, chewable and liquid calcium supplements dissolve even before entering the stomach. You might also find calcium gluconate, calcium lactate, or calcium phosphate.

● Choose a calcium supplement or a multivitamin/mineral with vitamin D. Vitamin D is essential for calcium absorption.

● Avoid calcium supplements with dolomite, unrefined oyster shell, or bonemeal without a USP symbol. They might contain small amounts of hazardous contaminants: lead, arsenic, mercury, or cadmium. What's dolomite? A mineral compound found in marble and limestone.

Coral calcium? No evidence shows that it's better. People with shellfish allergies may react since it's from coral reefs. It also may contain lead, which can be dangerous. *Refer to "Get the Lead Out" in chapter 8.*

● Take calcium supplements as intended—as a supplement, not as your only important calcium source. Although calcium supplements may boost calcium intake, they don't provide other nutrients your bones and body need: vitamin D, magnesium, phosphorus, and boron. Milk, for example, provides vitamin D, a nutrient that helps deposit calcium in your bones.

● Take calcium and iron supplements at different times of the day for better absorption.

● If you take two or three low-dose tablets daily, space them throughout the day for better absorption. Calcium in supplements is absorbed best in doses of 500 milligrams or less.

● Follow the dosage advised by your healthcare provider. The Tolerable Upper Intake Level for calcium is 2,500 milligrams daily from food and supplements.

● Drink plenty of fluids with calcium supplements to avoid constipation. The lactose and vitamin D in the milk help to enhance calcium absorption.

● If you take medications or other supplements, ask your doctor or registered dietitian about interactions. For example, calcium and tetracycline bind; neither is adequately absorbed as a result. Calcium also inhibits magnesium, phosphorus, and zinc absorption.

● If you don't drink milk and want an alternative to calcium pills, consider calcium- and vitamin D-fortified juice or soy beverage. One cup of either one can contain about 300 milligrams of calcium, the same amount as in a cup of milk, and juice provides vitamin C, folate, and other nutrients.

Are calcium supplements right for everyone? For people with kidney damage or urinary tract stones, calcium supplements pose risks. If you have a history of kidney stones, take calcium supplements under your doctor's care. *See "Osteoporosis: Reduce the Risks" in chapter 22.*

Iron supplements: Enhancing the benefit. Physicians often advise iron supplements for premenopausal and pregnant women, and for some children and teens. If you're advised to take an iron supplement:

● Pick a better-absorbed form of iron (ferrous, rather than ferric, sulfate).

● Check the dosage when choosing an iron supplement. Dosages of 15 to 30 milligrams per day are likely adequate. Higher amounts should be taken only if prescribed by your healthcare provider; because iron absorption decreases as the dose goes up, your doctor may recommend two or three smaller doses during the day.

● Take an iron supplement on an empty stomach—between meals or before bedtime—to enhance absorption. Absorption may be decreased by as much as 50 percent when taken with a meal or a snack. But if nausea and constipation are problems, take iron supplements with food.

● Take it with water or juice—not milk, coffee, or tea, which can inhibit absorption. As an aside, drinking vitamin C-rich juice with an iron supplement isn't necessary. Unlike nonheme iron in plant-based foods, the iron in supplements is in an absorbable form.

● Drink plenty of water to help avoid constipation, a common side effect from taking an iron supplement.

● Store them where children can't reach them. Adult iron supplements can be extremely toxic to children!

● Adult men and postmenopausal women: be cautious! For you, iron deficiency is uncommon. Taking an iron supplement or a multivitamin/mineral supplement with iron could result in iron overload and lead to hemochromatosis.

Herbals and Other Botanicals: Help or Harm?

Herbs and other botanicals have been used medicinally for thousands of years. They are still commonly used in many cultures and countries, and interest and use for health purposes is growing today in the United States. Among those commonly used: echinacea, flax seed, ginseng, ginkgo, and garlic. Much needs to be learned about the safety and effectiveness of botanicals, as noted in research initiatives from the National Center for Complementary and Alternative Medicine (NCCAM), National Institutes of Health.

Fresh or dried, liquid or solid extracts, tablets, cap-

Have You Ever Wondered?

. . . if antacids are as effective as calcium supplements as an extra calcium source? That depends. Look for an antacid without aluminum hydroxides. Aluminum in antacids increases calcium loss in urine.

. . . if vitamin nasal sprays or patches are effective? No research evidence says so, even though they're promoted for faster, more efficient absorption. In fact, they may not be absorbed at all. Here's the reality check: Fat-soluble vitamins need fat from food to aid absorption. Vitamin C in your intestine aids iron absorption—a problem if vitamin C comes from a spray. Vitamin B_{12} binds with intrinsic factor made in the stomach during digestion. That cannot happen with a spray or a patch!

. . . if zinc lozenges can help people with a cold feel better and recover faster? Different studies have given different results, so the answer isn't clear. *But a caution:* Some people have lost their sense of smell after using nasal sprays and gels with zinc. Talk to your healthcare provider before using them.

. . . if taking a vitamin C supplement will cure or at least protect against the common cold? When taken regularly before getting a cold, a vitamin C supplement might shorten the length of a cold slightly and make its symptoms somewhat milder. For most people, scientific evidence doesn't justify taking large doses of vitamin C regularly to boost immunity and lower the chance of getting a cold. And taking a supplement after getting a cold doesn't appear to be helpful. Research suggests that any benefits from a vitamin C supplement may be the placebo effect.

sules, powders, and tea bags: botanicals are sold in many forms. Consider ginger: fresh gingerroot, dried ginger in tea bags, and liquid ginger extract. Some, such as phytoestrogens from soy, are isolated substances sold as dietary supplements.

Herbal and other botanical supplements may seem safe enough. After all, they're made from natural, fresh herbs or other parts of plants: flowers, leaves, roots, and seeds. And many have been used for centuries.

In reality, there's nothing inherently harmless about botanical supplements, just because they're "natural." Their safety depends on many things, including their chemical makeup, how they work in the body, how they're prepared, and the dose taken.

Their action: mild to potent. The mild action of chamomile and peppermint, for example, often enjoyed in tea, may be gently relaxing and aid digestion. In contrast, kava—*potentially dangerous*—has an immediate, powerful antianxiety action. The form—in a cup of tea, a few teaspoons of tincture, or even less as an herbal extract—makes a difference, too. While peppermint tea is generally safe, concentrated peppermint can be toxic if taken incorrectly.

Many herbals and other botanicals have known medicinal qualities; like many of today's drugs, they come from plants. However, while pharmaceuticals (drugs), meant to cure or prevent disease, are well regulated, government regulations for botanical supplements are less stringent. Many claims have only limited scientific evidence; dosages aren't always standardized and vary among different brands of the same product. *See "Quality and Effectiveness: Who's in Control?" in this chapter.*

That said, use herbals and other botanical supplements with caution. Enough scientific evidence has been collected on only a handful of botanical supplements to support their limited use.

ANTIOXIDANT NUTRIENTS: ENOUGH, OR TOO MUCH?

Antioxidant supplements are "hot" supplements—even though there's no conclusive evidence that taking daily amounts of antioxidant nutrients beyond their Recommended Dietary Allowance (RDA) offers health benefits or protection from cancer or heart disease—whether from food or supplements. That said, research investigating the potential health benefits of antioxidants is ongoing, looking at links to aging, chronic diseases, asthma, allergies, and much more. Listen for science-based updates.

Antioxidants occur naturally in food, but supplements only provide a small number of them. When antioxidants are extracted from food to make supplements, some beneficial qualities may be lost. Excessive amounts from supplements could be harmful.

If you choose to take them for their potential benefits, talk to your doctor first. Then avoid exceeding the Tolerable Upper Intake Level (UL) set for safety. Use Supplement Facts on labels to know how much one dose-serving contains *See "Antioxidants in Supplements" in chapter 6.*

Although Dietary Reference Intakes, with recommended intakes, exist for vitamins and minerals, no recommendation or safe dosage exists for herbals, other botanicals, and other nonnutrient supplements. The National Institutes of Health's Office of Dietary Supplements provides advice on many botanicals.

Herbal Ingredients: Hazardous to Health!

The FDA warns against the use of botanical supplements with these active ingredients, due to their serious, *even deadly,* side effects:

● *Aristolochic acid.* A substance in some traditional Chinese herbal products, aristolochic acid causes kidney damage and is a potent carcinogen. It's known or suspected to be in many products, including those with guan mu tong, ma dou ling, birthwort, Indian ginger, wild ginger, colic root, and snakeroot.

● *Chaparral.* This Native American medicine can cause rapid, potentially irreversible liver damage.

● *Comfrey.* Supplements with comfrey (common, prickly, or Russian) pose serious health risks, notably for liver damage and as a possible carcinogen.

● *Ephedrine, ma huang* (ephedra sinica), *epitonin.* Being medicinal herbs, supplements with these ephedrine alkaloids have been touted as energy enhancers. Ephedrine also has been a component of weight-loss teas and aids. It's a stimulant closely related to methamphetamine, and is especially dangerous when combined with other stimulants. Hazards range from nervousness, dizziness, rapid heartbeat, and changes in blood pressure to muscle injury, seizures, nerve damage, heart attack, hepatitis, psychosis, stroke, and even death. People with health problems, such as high blood pressure, heart disease, or diabetes, are at special risk. Because they are so risky, a 2004 FDA regulation prohibits the sale of dietary supplements containing ephedra; some medications, however, contain a form of it. Bitter orange peel, sometimes used to replace ephedra in weight loss products, contains synephrine, which may be no safer than ephedra; avoid it, too.

● *Kava.* An herbal ingredient promoted for relaxation, and relief of sleeplessness and menopausal symptoms, kava is linked to liver-related injuries. It's especially risky for those with liver disease or liver problems, or persons who are taking drug products that can affect the liver.

HERBALS AND OTHER BOTANICALS (SELECTED): CLAIMS, EFFECTIVENESS

Here's what the symbols mean:

↑ — Evidence comes from several controlled human studies.

↑? — Preliminary evidence comes from only a few controlled human studies or from laboratory studies with cell or tissue samples.

↔ — Evidence is uncertain and based on conflicting, controlled human research.

↓ — Research doesn't support the claim.

↓? — Preliminary evidence from a few controlled trials in humans does *not* support efficacy claims, but more research is needed. (Research that is negative and has only been performed in vitro is so designated in the column.)

NR — Not enough human research has been done yet, or the research quality is poor.

For much more science-based, updated information—*and more warnings*—about many of these and other botanicals, refer to the NCCAM (nccam.nih.gov/health/herbsataglance.htm) and the ODS (ods.od.nih.gov/Health_Information/Botanical_Supplements.aspx).

HERBAL OR OTHER BOTANICAL SUPPLEMENT	MEDIA OR MARKETING CLAIMS	EFFECTIVENESS	ALSO BE AWARE . . . *Caution: Dietary supplements can pose significant and serious health risks,* related to dosage, length of use, health status, age, and interactions with drugs and nutrients. *Before taking them, always* talk to your health-care provider about their safety, risks, and interactions (*not fully listed below*), especially when treating or managing health conditions.
Aloe vera	• Reduces symptoms of gastrointestinal disorders • Helps control blood cholesterol • Helps reduce blood glucose • Reduces constipation	NR NR NR NR	• Consumed as aloe juice • In large doses and excess use, may cause potassium depletion • Prolonged use may lead to nephritis and acute kidney failure
Bitter melon	• Helps reduce blood glucose in people with type 2 diabetes • Reduces blood lipid levels • Prevents cancer • Improved immune response for individuals with HIV	NR NR NR NR	• Avoid during pregnancy. May cause premature contractions, bleeding, miscarriage • Avoid with liver disease • As tea, linked to severe hypoglycemia and hypoglycemic coma in children • For those with diabetes, may have an additive effect when taken with insulin
Echinacea	• Boosts immune function in healthy individuals • Protects against common cold virus, upper respiratory infections	NR ↔	• Do not take if you: — have health problems with reduced immunity (e.g,. lupus, HIV, tuberculosis, multiple sclerosis, scleroderma) — take medications that may be toxic to the liver, such as anabolic steroids • Potential severe allergic reactions if you have asthma or sensitivity to grass pollens
Fenugreek	• Helps control blood glucose in diabetes • Reduces blood cholesterol levels • Prevents cancer	NR ↔ NR	• Those allergic to peanuts may be allergic to fenugreek • May have an additive effect with anticoagulant/antiplatelet or diabetes drugs
Garlic	• Reduces cholesterol levels • Reduces blood pressure • Improves circulation • Reduces cancer risk • Improves immune function	↑? ↑? ↑? ↑? ↑?	• May increase bleeding • Promote undesirable body odor, even from some odor-free varieties • Avoid taking 7 days before surgery • May interfere with the effectiveness of oral contraceptives and certain drugs (e.g., HIV drug saquinavir) • May cause stomach discomfort at high doses • Should be monitored if taken with anticoagulant medications
Ginger	• Treats morning sickness • Treats post-surgery nausea • Treats nausea associated with chemotherapy	↑? ↔ NR	• Conflicting data about safety of ginger before surgery for those on anticoagulation medications • Should monitor closely if also taking glucose-lowering drugs for diabetes management or anticoagulant/antiplatelet drugs
Ginkgo biloba	• Improves memory in individuals with Alzheimer's disease or dementia	↔	• Consuming ginkgo seeds can be fatal; linked to convulsions and repetitive seizures in children • Avoid taking at least 36 hours or longer before surgery

Herbal or Other Botanical Supplement	Media or Marketing Claims	Effectiveness	Also Be Aware ...
Ginkgo biloba (*continued*)	• Improves memory in healthy individuals • Improves symptoms of reduced circulation in individuals with intermittent claudication • Relieves tinnitus (ringing in ears) • Prevents mountain or altitude sickness	↔ ↑? ↓ ↓	• Avoid all fresh ginkgo plant parts • Can cause mild GI upset, headache, dizziness, palpitations, constipation, and allergic skin reactions • Large doses (estimated >600 mg/day) may cause restlessness, diarrhea, nausea, vomiting, lack of muscle tone, weakness • Should be monitored if you take anticoagulant medications • May interfere with diabetes management

Ginseng, American	• Improves exercise performance
	• Improves quality of life, energy mood, cognition
	• Improves sexual function; aphrodisiac
	• Helps control blood glucose levels in diabetes
	• Reduces risk for cancer
		↓
		↔
		
		NR
		
		NR
		
		NR
			• Possible hypertension, nervousness, sleeplessness, acne, edema, headache, and diarrhea linked to > 3g ginseng root/day (about 600 mg ginseng extract)
			• Do not take:
			  – during pregnancy or lactation
			  – if you are at risk or were previously treated for estrogen-related cancer (breast, ovarian, etc.)
			  – before surgery
			• Potential hypoglycemic effect; individuals with diabetes should monitor their blood glucose levels
			• May interfere with phenelzine, corticosteroids, digoxin (digitalis), diabetes medications, and estrogen therapy
			• May increase bleeding time when taken with other blood-thinning drugs or some supplements

Goldenseal (*Hydrastis canadensis*)	• Enhances immune function through antibiotic activity • Reduces risk for infectious diarrhea • Masks drug use in urine drug testing	NR NR ↓	• Safety demonstrated for short-term use • Long-term, high doses linked to cardiac spasms and death. • Oral long-term linked to gastrointestinal upset, hallucinations, delirium • Topical application results in photosensitivity to UVA exposure
Green tea extract (*Camellia sinensis*)	• Acts as an antioxidant • Reduces risk for cancer • Improves heart health • Assists in blood pressure control • Promotes weight control by increasing energy expenditure	↑ ↑? ↔ NR NR	• Moderate doses of green tea extract used for several years have been demonstrated to be safe. • Be aware that caffeine in green tea extract can have side effects • Possible nausea if consumed on an empty stomach • May interfere with iron absorption; may negatively interact with caffeine-containing medications • Discuss with your doctor if on anticoagulant medications • Increases harmful effects of ephedra
Kava (*Piper methysticum*)	• Reduces anxiety • Promotes restful sleep	↑? NR	• Avoid if you have: liver disease; may cause liver damage even death • Potentially dangerous interaction when combined with anti-anxiety medications, such as benzodiazepine, or alcohol • May affect motor reflexes and judgment; do not use while operating heavy machinery • Avoid taking with alcohol, barbiturates, or psychopharmacological agents due to possible sedative effects • Do not use for more than 1 to 3 months without medical advice • May decrease effectiveness of drugs used in Parkinson's disease, other diseases
Ma huang (*Ephedra sinica*)	• Increases metabolism for weight loss	Do *not* use; unsafe; products with with ephedra and ephedrine supplements have been banned by the FDA	• Numerous reports of adverse events, including heart attack, stroke, tremors, insomnia, and death in individuals otherwise in good health • Acts as a heart and central nervous system stimulant • Avoid if you have: hypertension and/or CVD disease, thyroid disease, diabetes, neurological disorders, (men) difficulty urinating due to an enlarged prostate • Do not take with any medications used to treat heart disease, hypertension, depression, Parkinson's disease, asthma, or diabetes or with stimulant herbs

HERBALS AND OTHER BOTANICALS (SELECTED): CLAIMS, EFFECTIVENESS (continued)

HERBAL OR OTHER BOTANICAL SUPPLEMENT	MEDIA OR MARKETING CLAIMS	EFFECTIVENESS	ALSO BE AWARE . . .
Milk thistle	• Improves general liver health • Prevents cancer	NR NR	• Minimal side effects include gastrointestinal upset and allergic skin rash • May alter bioavailability of some medications
Red yeast rice	• Treats high cholesterol	FDA safety alert on some products with red yeast rice	• May increase risk of severe muscle reactions leading to kidney impairment • Risk may be higher when taking lovastain, cholesterol-lowering drugs, some antibiotics, and some drugs to treat depression, and fungal and HIV infections
Saw palmetto (*Seronoa repens*)	• Improves symptoms of enlarged prostate • Prevents prostate cancer • Prevents male-pattern baldness/hair loss	↔ NR NR	• Discontinue at least 2 weeks before surgery due to the herb's anticoagulant effects • May interfere with blood clotting and increase bleeding time if taking anticoagulant medications • May be linked to gastrointestinal discomfort in rare cases • No controlled studies testing the safety of long-term use
St. John's wort	• Alleviates depression • Promotes emotional well-being	↑? NR	• Do not take with antidepressant medications (potentially dangerous combined effects); may limit effectives of some other medications and oral contraceptives • May make skin sensitive to sunlight, especially for fair-skinned people at dosages more than 2 g/day • Discontinue before surgery • Do not take if you have: Alzheimer's disease
Valerian (*Valeriana officinalis*)	• Enhances sleep • Reduces stress and anxiety	↔ NR	• Avoid driving or operating heavy machinery while taking • Do not take if you have: liver disease (due to possible contamination); take barbiturates or other sleep medications • May cause morning drowsiness with high doses (900 mg) • Avoid if taking St John's wort, kava, L-tryptophan, or alcohol due to sedative effects • May experience serious withdrawal symptoms if abruptly discontinued; taper off slowly
Wheat grass, barley grass	• Acts as an antioxidant • Enhances immunity • Reduces cholesterol	NR NR NR	• No studies testing the safety of supplementing the diet with liquid or dried juices of wheat or barley grasses • May cause nausea, appetite loss, and constipation • Gluten content may make celiac disease worse
Yohimbine (*yohimbe*)	• Increases sex drive • Aids in weight loss • Builds muscle	NR NR NR	• Potentially dangerous! • Doses of 4 to 20 mg have been associated with serious harmful effects, such abnormal heartbeat, tremors, and low blood pressure • Toxicity may be enhanced by taking phenothazines (drug used in mental disorders) • Not for people with high or low blood pressure, bipolar disorder, or liver or kidney disease • Should not be used in combination with blood pressure medications, some other drugs

Adapted from Allison Sarubin Fragakis, *The Health Professional's Guide to Popular Dietary Supplements,* Third edition online, http://hpgps.adapocketguide.com/index.cfm. Accessed January 1, 2012.

● *Lobelia.* Also called Indian tobacco, it acts like nicotine; among potential dangers: breathing problems, rapid heartbeat, sweating, low blood pressure, coma, death. It's particularly harmful to children, pregnant women, and people with heart disease.

● *Germander.* Its use may lead to liver disease, possibly to death.

● *Magnolia-stephania preparation.* Its use may lead to kidney disease and permanent kidney failure.

● *Willow bark.* Marketed as an aspirin-free product,

willow bark contains an ingredient that converts to the active ingredient found in aspirin. Potential health hazards include Reye's syndrome, a potentially fatal disease that's linked to aspirin intake in children with chicken pox or flu symptoms. Adults can have an allergic reaction to willow bark.

● *Wormwood.* This herbal ingredient may cause neurological symptoms such as numbness of legs and arms, loss of intellect, delirium, and paralysis.

● *Yohimbe.* Marketed for sexual arousal and derived from tree bark, yohimbe has several active ingredients, including yohimbine, with potentially dangerous side effects: kidney failure, seizures, nervous system disorders, paralysis, fatigue, stomach problems, and death. Because yohimbine is a MAO (monoamine oxidase) inhibitor, it is especially harmful when taken at the same time as tyramine-containing foods such as liver, cheese, or red wine, and with over-the-counter medications with phenylpropanolamine (some nasal decongestants and diet aids).

Other ingredients, often found in herbal supplements, have potential health hazards. For example, germanium (a nonessential mineral) may result in kidney damage, possibly death. Colloidal silver—a nonessential mineral with no known physical benefits when consumed—in supplements may cause permanent grayish or bluish discoloration of the skin, nails, and gums, and conjunctiva (clear membrane covering the white of the eye).

Other Supplements

As supplement categories, nutrient and herbal supplements come to mind. But stores and Internet sites sell others. *Many are addressed in "Selected Other Supplements: Claims, Benefits, Risks" in this chapter.*

For up-to-date, reliable information about safe, effective supplement use, check these websites:

● Office of Dietary Supplements, ods.od.nihs.gov

● U.S. Pharmacopoeia, www.usp.org

● National Center for Complementary and Alternative Medicine, nccam.nih.gov

● Enzymes and hormones—for example, coenzyme Q10, DHEA, melatonin

● Ergogenic aids—for example, chromium picolinate, creatine

● Others—for example, bee pollen, carnitine, conjugated linoleic acid, fish oil, flaxseed, glucosamine, lecithin, royal jelly, shark cartilage

Supplements: Safe? Effective?

Even though dietary supplements are big business, manufacturing standards for their quality, potency, and effectiveness have lagged behind their phenomenal market growth. Product information is often misleading, despite limited government regulations. While scientific claims may be given, well-designed scientific studies for supplements are often limited.

Quality and Effectiveness: Who's in Control?

If you buy a supplement, are you getting what you think you paid for? It may be hard for you to tell from the label. In fact, quality control depends on the production process, likely starting with the supplier of the raw ingredients.

Dietary supplements are regulated differently than food and drugs. Enacted in 1994, the FDA's Dietary Supplement Health and Education Act (DSHEA) requires that supplements be safe, unadulterated, and properly labeled; be produced with good manufacturing practices; and be promoted with label information that's truthful. In 2007, the FDA issued Good Manufacturing Practices for supplements that require manufacturers to guarantee the identity, purity, strength, and composition of their dietary supplements. The aim is to prevent contamination, wrong ingredients, too much or too little of dietary ingredients, and improper packaging and labeling.

The responsibility for proof, however, lies with the manufacturer, not with the FDA. The FDA doesn't analyze the contents of dietary supplements. The manufacturer is expected to ensure that the supplement's label information (Supplement Facts and ingredient list) is accurate, that its ingredients are safe, and that the declared contents match what's in the container.

The FDA doesn't currently require testing—for safety, effectiveness, or interactions—before a supplement is produced or launched into the market-place. If, however, an ingredient is new (marketed after October 1994), manufacturers must provide the FDA with evidence that the supplement is "reason-ably expected to be safe" at the labeled dosage. The FDA can take action if the supplement is either unsafe or mislabeled. Supplements sold in the United States before October 15, 1994, are presumed safe, based on their history of human use.

While some supplements are labeled accurately and completely, some aren't, and what's stated on the label may not be what's in the container. The potency or purity may be misrepresented or inconsistent. Herbs may be misidentified, indicating the wrong part or type of herb. *The bottom line:* It's up to you to be a discrim-inating consumer!

For a growing list of dietary supplements, U.S. Pharmacopeia (USP), an independent, not-for-profit organization, sets quality standards: for strength, quality, purity, and consistency of supplements. If manufacturers voluntarily comply, they may display the USP Verified Mark on product labels, packaging, and promotional materials—and if the products and ingredient meet standards after testing. The mark sig-nals that the supplement:

● Contains the ingredients listed on the label, in the declared potency (or strength) and amounts.

● Doesn't contain harmful levels of specified con-taminants, such as lead and mercury, pesticides, bac-teria, molds, toxins, and others.

● Will break down and release into the body within a specified amount of time, so the person gets its full benefit.

● Is made according to the FDA's Good Manufactur-ing Practices.

This is industry-reported compliance, not outside assessment.

Several other independent organizations—e.g., NSF International, and ConsumerLab.com—have certification programs, too, designed to assess whether a supplement really contains what the manufacturer declares on the label. A fee-based service to industry, each certifying organization sets its own assessment criteria—some more in-depth than others. Some audit manufacturing practices; some do ongoing surveillance.

Have You Ever Wondered

... if any herbal supplement can replace or enhance medication for depression? If your doctor has prescribed medication for depression, follow the guidance; don't mix or change antidepressants. Mixing may result in harmful interactions—for example, St. John's wort inter-acts with antidepressants such as Prozac and amoxa-pine. The combination may be additive. And a herbal treatment may not yield the intended outcome. If you choose to try a herbal, talk to your physician first.

A step in the right direction, it's hard to discern precisely what a specific certification mark on a sup-plement label means and how each mark's criteria differs. Although a certifying mark helps you know if you're getting what you paid for, it does *not* verify a supplement's overall safety or effectiveness. No certifying mark? It could mean several things: the supplement didn't meet certification criteria, the assessment is in progress, or perhaps the supplement hasn't been submitted for review.

What about advertising supplements? The Federal Trade Commission (FTC) regulates supplement advertising, including media infomercials and Inter-net promotion. Like the FDA, its resources for mon-itoring are limited.

Supplements: Marketplace Confusion

Many supplement manufacturers provide reliable product information. By law, supplement labels must bear a Supplement Facts panel: If the label carries one or more claims, they are supposed to be truthful and not misleading.

For well-intentioned consumers—eager to take responsibility for their health—the sea of science and fiction is often confusing and misleading, and ulti-mately may be costly and harmful. Misleading tactics:

● *Borrowed research.* Study results that may or may not apply to the product: perhaps supplements with different potencies or formulations, or derived from different parts of the plant.

● *Distorted data.* Information that's "spun" to match the product claim. Again, the formulation or dosage may differ from the supplement used in the original

For more about supplements . . .

- *Fiber, in chapter 3:* fiber pills and powders
- *Prebiotic and antioxidant benefits, in chapter 6:* acai, fructo-oligosaccharides, inulin
- *Menopausal symptoms, in chapter 18:* black cohosh, chasteberry, dong quai, soy foods and isoflavones, wild or Mexican yam
- *Athletic performance, in chapter 20:* amino acid supplements, androstenedoine ("andro"), carnitine, creatine, dehydroepiandrosterone (DHEA), ergogenic aids, spirulina, wheat germ and wheat germ oil
- *Lactose intolerance, in chapter 21:* lactase
- *Chronic health issues, in chapter 22:* fish oil supplements, garlic supplements, glucosamine, lecithin, SAM-e

study. Less reputable manufacturers may present their "proof" in a format—charts and tables, cited references—that looks like a reliable research study.

- *Claims that research is under way.* In other words, no specific data are available.
- *Unreliable studies.* Poorly designed research that hasn't been published in peer-reviewed publications.
- *Testimonials.* Statements, not based in sound science, from "satisfied" customers or celebrities.

Science behind Supplements: More Needed

To show a supplement's effectiveness and its active ingredients, more good research is needed! Good research provides data from randomized, placebo-controlled, double-blind studies—not just one study, but several that duplicate the results. Manufacturers of supplements are not required to conduct research on their products. *See chapter 24 for defined research terms.*

To further complicate what's known and unknown, many supplements—for example, botanicals—have two or more active ingredients. Yet, all the bioactive substances haven't been identified, nor do we know what they do. Potencies differ when the same herbal supplement derives from different parts of a plant or different varieties. Growing conditions may affect the potency of bioactive substances. Even if sound

Supplements: Questions to Ask an Expert

With so many supplement products and so many unknowns about them, explore these questions with qualified nutrition experts and your doctor—before you take a supplement:

For you . . .

- Do I need a dietary supplement? Can it contribute to my health?
- Are there any dietary supplements I should avoid while taking certain medicines (prescription or over-the-counter) or other supplements?
- If I'm scheduled for elective surgery, should I discontinue use of dietary supplements? If so when?

About the supplement . . .

- What is it for? What are the claims? Who's making them? Why? Are the claims valid?
- Where did the product information come from? Is the manufacturer a trusted, nonbiased source?
- Is the supplement generally safe? Can it cause harm in *any* dosage?
- Does the product come from a company that's known, or highly likely, to follow safe, appropriate manufacturing practices?
- What's known about the supplement's effectiveness for its proposed benefit?
- How do the active ingredients work in the body?
- What plant or plants and part of the plant or plants do the main active ingredients come from?
- How much of the active ingredients does the supplement have? What else does it contain?
- What are its intended potential benefits: for anyone, for you?
- Are there any precautions or warnings I should know about (for example, an amount or "upper limit" that I should not go above)?
- What scientific evidence supports this product formula or brand?
- What side effects might result from taking it?
- How much (dose), how often, and how long is it safe for you to take it?

Adapted from American Dietetic Association/American Pharmaceutical Association, *A Healthcare Professional's Guide to Evaluating Dietary Supplements,* 2002.

Other Supplements (Selected) : Claims, Effectiveness

Here's what the symbols mean:

↑ — Evidence comes from several controlled human studies.

↑? — Preliminary evidence comes from only a few controlled human studies or from laboratory studies with cell or tissue samples.

↔ — Evidence is uncertain and based on conflicting, controlled human research.

↓ — Research doesn't support the claim.

↓? — Preliminary evidence from a few controlled trials in humans does *not* support efficacy claims, but more research is needed. (Research that is negative and has only been performed in vitro is so designated in the column.)

NR — Not enough human research has been done yet, or the research quality is poor.

For much more updated information—and more warnings—about many of these and other dietary supplements, refer to the ODS website: ods.od.nih.gov/Health_Information/Information_About_Individual_Dietary_Supplements.aspx.

Other Supplements	Media or Marketing Claims	Effectiveness	Also Be Aware . . . Caution: *Dietary supplements can pose significant and serious health risks,* related to dosage, length of use, health status, age, and interactions with drugs and nutrients. *Before taking them, always* talk to your health-care provider about their safety, risks, and interactions *(not fully listed below),* especially when treating or managing health conditions.
Acidophilus/ lactobacillus acidophilus (LA)	• Reduces lactose intolerance	NR	• No reports of serious adverse effects in human studies
	• Helps control rotaviral diarrhea (LA GG)	↑	• Some products may contain little or no LA; some may contain other strains of lactobacilli or contaminants
	• Prevents antibiotic-associated diarrhea and traveler's diarrhea	↔	• Potential concern for those with weakened immunity, for supplements with live bacteria
	• Prevents or reduces length of vaginal yeast infections	↔ (LA yogurt) NR (LA supplements)	
	• Controls irritable bowel symptoms	↓	
	• Prevents or reduces severity of atopic disease (allergies, eczema, etc.)	NR	
	• Reduces cholesterol	↔	
	• Prevents cancer	NR	
Bee pollen	• Enhances energy, athletic performance	NR	• Evidence supports safe use of 1 teaspoon/day for up to 30 days
	• Reduces symptoms of PMS	NR	• Anaphylactic reaction in some sensitive individuals
	• Prevents gastrointestinal upset	NR	• Not advised for people with asthma or allergies to honey or bee stings
	• Reduces symptoms of chronic prostatitis (inflamed prostate)	NR	• Avoid if you have: liver disease
	• Enhances well-being; "nature's perfect food"	↓	• Avoid during pregnancy due to potential uterine stimulatory effects
Branched chain amino acids (BCAAs)	• Builds muscle; reduces abdominal fat	NR	• Doses higher than 20 g may cause gastrointestinal distress and may impair performance and induce fatigue
	• Improves athletic performance	↓	• May stimulate insulin release and affect medications used to treat high blood glucose
	• Improves appetite in elderly	NR	• Avoid if you have: ALS
	• Helps mental function in people with liver disease	↔	
Carnitine (L-carnitine)	• Improves heart health	↑?	• No serious adverse effects reported with doses ranging from 0.5 to 6 grams a day
	• Improves athletic performance	↓	• Larger doses associated with nausea and diarrhea
	• Increases energy in people with chronic fatigue syndrome or cancer	NR	• Avoid if you have: hypothyroidism, which may inhibit thyroid hormone activity
	• Improves mental function in Alzheimer's disease	NR	• May increase seizure frequency or severity if you have a history of seizures

Other Supplements	Media or Marketing Claims	Effectiveness	Also Be Aware ...
Carnitine (continued)	• Improves thyroid function • Reduces male infertility • Improves immune function • Assists weight reduction	NR ↔ NR NR	
Chondroitin sulfate	• Relieves osteoarthritis pain • Protects joints and tendons from sports injury	↑? NR	• May cause epigastric pain, nausea, diarrhea, constipation • May worsen asthma symptoms • Avoid if you have: (men) prostate cancer or higher prostate cancer risk
Coenzyme Q10 (ubiquinone)	• Improves health of people with heart disease and hypertension • Improves exercise performance • Reduces cancer risk • Improves immune function in individuals with HIV • Helps with neurological disorders • Prevents migraine headache	↑? ↓ NR NR NR NR	• No serious adverse effects reported for 200 mg CoQ$_{10}$ daily for 1 year and 100 mg daily for up to 6 years • May cause mild gastrointestinal distress including nausea, vomiting, diarrhea, appetite suppression, and heartburn • Note: coenzyme Q10 is produced in the body and aids in energy production • May reduce effectiveness of some drugs (e.g., warfarin)
Conjugated linoleic acid (CLA)	• Helps control weight • Stimulates immune function • Prevents cancer • Reduces risk for heart disease • Improves glucose tolerance	↓? ↓ NR ↓ ↓	• No serious adverse effects found in short-term studies. • Most common side effect: gastrointestinal upset (diarrhea, nausea, loose stools, and dyspepsia); fatigue also possible • Some forms may increase insulin resistance in individuals with abdominal obesity or diabetes.
Creatine	• Increases muscle strength and mass • Delays fatigue in athletes • Increases strength in elderly • Increases strength in muscular disease • Increases strength in heart disease	↑? NR NR ↑? NR	• Avoid exceeding a dose of 2 to 5 g/day • May cause weight gain/water retention, gastrointestinal pain, nausea, or diarrhea. • Avoid if you have: renal disease or insufficiency
DHEA (dehydro-epiandosterone)	• Slows aging; improves age-related memory loss • Improves immune function • Improves heart health • Helps prevent cancer • Reduces symptoms of lupus • Improves health of individuals with AIDS • Assists weight reduction • Reduces menopausal symptoms	NR ↔ ↔ NR ↔ NR ↔ NR	• May increase breast, endometrial, or prostate cancer risks • For women, may promote masculine characteristics • With chronic use, can alter hormone levels: unknown adverse effects. • May decrease HDL cholesterol levels • Avoid if you have: breast, uterine, ovarian cancers; hormone-sensitive conditions; polycystic ovary syndrome; liver problems • Banned by the National Collegiate Athletic Association and the International Olympic Committee
Fish oil, contains omega-3s (DHA, EPA)	• Reduces serum triglyceride levels • Reduces risk for athero-sclerosis/heart disease • Improves glucose levels in people with diabetes • Improves lipid levels in people with diabetes • Reduces blood pressure • Reduces inflammation and pain of arthritis • Improves cognition in individuals with Alzheimer's disease	↑ ↑? NR ↑? - (triglycerides) ↓? (LDL or HDL cholesterol) ↔ ↑? NR	• May prolong bleeding time • Should be monitored if you take anticoagulant medications or have blood clotting disorders • Avoid before surgery • During pregnancy avoid fish oil supplements high in vitamin A (halibut and shark liver oils due to vitamin A's teratogenic effects) • May cause belching, halitosis, heartburn, or gastrointestinal upset • Up to 3 g/day considered safe; > 3 g/day may suppress immune function and may increase risk of hemorrhagic stroke • May cause an adverse reaction in those allergic to seafood • May reduce vitamin E levels

(continued)

OTHER SUPPLEMENTS	MEDIA OR MARKETING CLAIMS	EFFECTIVENESS	ALSO BE AWARE . . .
Fish oil *(continued)*	• Reduces bowel inflammation in colitis or inflammatory bowel disease	↑?	
	• Helps reduce severity of symptoms of psoriasis	↓?	
	• Helps treat depression	NR	
	• Helps treat attention deficit/ hyperactivity disorder	NR	
	• Prevents continued weight loss in people with cancer wasting	NR	
	• Reduces risk of cancer	↓?	
Flaxseed	• Improves blood lipids	↔	• Doses more than 45 g flaxseed powder linked to loose bowels
	• Reduces risk for heart disease and stroke	NR	• Can result in allergic and anaphylactic reactions
	• Reduces risk of estrogen-related and other cancers	NR	• Not advised before surgery or for individuals with clotting disorders
	• Reduces inflammation in individuals with arthritis	NR	• Drink water when consuming whole or cracked flaxseed to prevent intestinal blockage
	• Improves symptoms of lupus, eczema, and other inflammatory diseases	NR	• Fiber in ground flaxseed can interfere with the absorption of other nutrients and some medications affected by fiber
	• Relieves constipation	↑	• May effect antidiabetes drugs; monitor blood glucose
			• No specific safe intake levels for women with breast, uterine, or ovarian cancers, endometriosis, or uterine fibroids
Gamma-linolenic acid (evening primrose oil, black currant oil, borage seed oil)	• Reduces PMS symptoms	↔	• Not to be used with tricyclic antidepressants or anticonvulsants
	• Reduces inflammation in rheumatoid arthritis	↔	• Borage seed shouldn't be taken if drugs with potential liver-related side effects are being taken, too.
	• Reduces atopic dermatitis	↔	• Potential side effects include belching, bloating, nausea, vomiting, flatulence, soft stools, and diarrhea
	• Reduces acne	NR	• Avoid at least 2 weeks before surgery
	• Improves diabetic neuropathy	NR	• Should be monitored by a physician if taking anticoagulant drugs or supplements
	• Reduces cardiovascular disease risk NR	NR	
	• Reduces breast cancer risk; improves response of anti-estrogen breast cancer medications	↔	
Glucosamine	• Relieves osteoarthritis pain in knee, hip, etc.	↔	• Derived from shellfish; possible reaction with shellfish allergy
			• In three-year studies, no serious adverse effects
			• Some controversy regarding glucosamine and blood glucose control. To be safe, people with diabetes should have glucose levels monitored.
Lecithin/ choline	• Improves exercise endurance	↓	• UL: 3.5 g choline/day for adults age 19 years and older
	• Improves dementia in Alzheimer's disease	↓?	• Mild side effects are linked to high doses (20 g): gastro-intestinal symptoms, urinary incontinence, and diarrhea
	• Improves memory, concentration	↓?	• Excess choline (> 20 g) may cause a fishy odor
	• Improves liver health	↓?	• Ongoing use may affect the nervous system
Lutein	• Treats age-related macular degeneration	↑?	• Not likely to have adverse effects, even with long-term use
	• Treats age-related cataracts	NR	
	• Treats retinitis pigmentosa	NR	
	• Prevents cancer	NR	
Lycopene	• Decreases prostate cancer risk	↔	• No scientific studies specifically evaluating the safety of lycopene supplementation. Trials with supplements indicate safety at typical levels, usually at or below 30 mg/day over several weeks
	• Prevents other cancers	NR	• Avoid if diagnosed with prostate cancer
	• Reduces symptoms of exercise-induced asthma	NR	
	• Prevents atherosclerosis	NR	

Other Supplements	Media or Marketing Claims	Effectiveness	Also Be Aware . . .
Melatonin	• Regulates sleep-awake cycles • Reduces jet lag • Reduces cancer risk; eases side effects of cancer treatment • Prevents and treats migraines • Enhances sex drive	↔ ↑? NR NR NR	• Long-term effects and safety have not been studied. No harmful effects reported from short-term use • Driving or using machinery for several hours after taking melatonin not advised • Morning use may affect alertness and reflexes • Do not take if using other sleep aids • Discuss with oncologist if undergoing chemotherapy • Melatonin from animal pineal gland should be avoided due to potential toxin contamination • Avoid if taking blood pressure medication
Noni juice (morinda)	• Prevents cancer • Improves immunity • Reduces blood pressure • Improves cholesterol levels • Acts as a natural pain reliever	NR NR NR NR NR	• Approximately the same amount of potassium as orange juice • May reduce effectiveness of warfarin • High potassium content can cause hyperkalemia in people with kidney disease • Potential liver toxicity for those with compromised liver function
Royal jelly	• Improves immunity • Contributes to a healthy heart • Improves stamina; reduces fatigue • Reduces PMS • Improves mental health, cognition	NR NR NR NR NR	• Not advised for people with asthma or a genetic predisposition to allergies • *Note:* Royal jelly—exotic and expensive—isn't jelly, but instead a substance produced by worker bees to nourish future queen bees
S-adenosyl-methionine (SAM-e)	• Reduces arthritis symptoms • Reduces symptoms of fibromyalgia • Reduces depression symptoms • Improves liver health • Promotes a healthy gallbladder	↑? NR ↑? ↑? NR	• Mild gastrointestinal distress may occur at the beginning of use • Safety well demonstrated for use as long as 2 years • Can interfere with surgery
Soy protein and isoflavones	• Reduces cholesterol levels in individuals with hyper-cholesterolemia • Reduces risk of cancer • Reduces menopausal symptoms • Reduces risk of osteoporosis • Improves kidney function in people with both diabetes and renal impairment	↑? ↔ ↔ ↔ NR	• Avoid if you are: (women) diagnosed with breast cancer or at risk for breast cancer • May reduce the absorption of thyroid medications • Could interfere with estrogen replacement therapy • Avoid if you have a soy allergy or asthma
Shark cartilage	• Cures cancer • Stops cancer spread (in blood supply) • Prevents blood clotting • Treats psoriasis	NR NR NR NR	• No reported adverse interactions • May raise calcium levels—a problem for those taking high dosages of calcium supplements
Spirulina/blue-green algae	• Improves immunity • Reduces cholesterol • Reduces cancer risk • Improves intestinal health • Aids weight loss	NR NR NR NR NR	• Vegans should not rely on spirulina as their sole source of vitamin B_{12} • No long-term studies have evaluated the safety; has been consumed for centuries with few reports of adverse effects • May be contaminated with microbes or heavy metals • Patients with phenylketonuria should avoid consuming spirulina due to potential phenylalanine content
Whey protein	• Builds muscle and improves exercise performance • Improves immunity in individuals with HIV • Acts as an anticancer agent	↔ NR NR	• No long-term human studies • Should be avoided by those diagnosed with allergies or severe sensitivities to milk or milk proteins • For those with lactose intolerance, whey protein concentrate contains lactose. Whey protein isolate has insignificant quantities of lactose • Excess amounts of protein can be harmful for those with kidney disease

Adapted from Allison Sarubin Fragakis, *The Health Professional's Guide to Popular Dietary Supplements,* Third edition online, http://hpgps.adapocketguide.com/index.cfm. Accessed January 1, 2012.

research exists for the safety and effectiveness of one active ingredient, it may not exist for all ingredients, and usually not for the combination. Typically the potency of active ingredients in combination products is less than the amount used in single ingredient studies. More unknowns: There's not enough scientific evidence to know how much of a supplement or its bioactive substitutes offer benefits, how much may be harmful, the health effects of dosages beyond the label dosage, or any interaction with food or with medication.

Good news! When published, sound research data on supplements become available from the National Institutes of Health, including the Office of Dietary Supplements (ODS) and the National Center for Complementary Medicine and Alternative Medicine. Until then, the best advice: a healthy skepticism.

See chapter 24 for more about judging nutrition information, scientific reports, and nutrition quackery.

If You Take a Supplement . . .

Before you head down your store's supplement aisle, order online, or pick up a product at your fitness center, get supplement savvy. Buy and use dietary supplements with the same consumer wisdom you use when you buy a car or make any major investment.

Be aware: For the same supplement in the same dosage, people may react differently.

Warning: Supplement Interactions!

- *Dealing with cancer, diabetes, heart disease, immune problems, kidney problems, thyroid problems, ulcers, or other health problems?* Talk with your doctor before using dietary supplements, and about the potential for harmful interactions.

- *Taking prescription or over-the-counter medication?* Supplements—when combined with medications or other treatments—may interfere with or boost their action, even be harmful or life-threatening. *See "Food and Medicine" in chapter 22.* For example:

  - Folic acid can interact with anticonvulsant medications.

  - Vitamin E, garlic, and ginkgo biloba may thin blood—dangerous when taken with blood-thinning medication such as Coumadin and aspirin.

  - Ginkgo can interact with some psychiatric drugs and some drugs that affect blood glucose levels.

  - Garlic supplements may interact with drugs used in HIV therapy such as saquinavir, which is a protease inhibitor.

  - The combination of foxglove (the source of digitalis, or digoxin) and cardiac medication is dangerous for those with heart disease.

  - St. John's wort may reduce the effect of heart drugs, antidepressants, antiseizure drugs, anti-cancer drugs, birth control drugs, certain HIV drugs, and anti-transplant-rejection drugs.

  - Ginseng can lower blood glucose levels, perhaps interfering with diabetes medication. It can also increase caffeine's effects as a stimulant.

  - Calcium can interact with heart medication (such as Digoxin), thiazide diuretics (Thiazide), and antacids with aluminum and magnesium.

  - Magnesium can interact with thiazide, and loop diuretics (for example, Lasix), some cancer drugs, and antacids with magnesium.

  - Vitamin K and blood thinner (for example, Coumadin)

This isn't a complete list. For more interactions between medications and specific supplements, refer to the ODS website: ods.od.nih.gov/Health_Information/Information_About_Individual_Dietary_Supplements.aspx. *For some nutrient-nutrient interactions, check earlier in this chapter.*

- *Planning for any surgery?* Avoid *all* supplements two to three weeks ahead, according to the American Society of Anesthesiologists. Although herbal supplements may seem "innocent," their use can cause complications such as bleeding, heart instability, low blood glucose level, blood pressure changes, and other interactions. Among those linked to surgical complications: ephedra, garlic, ginkgo, ginseng, kava, St. John's wort, and valerian.

Supplements: If You Have an Adverse Reaction . . .

● Immediately inform your healthcare provider if you think you have suffered a serious harmful effect or illness from a dietary supplement.

● Report any serious problems to the FDA's Med-Watch hotline: (1-800-FDA-1088), fax (1-800-FDA-0178), or online (www.fda.gov/medwatch/how.htm). You and your healthcare provider should do this. Be prepared to identify the suspected product.

● For a general concern or complaint about any supplement, contact your nearest FDA District Office. Find the phone number on the www.cfsan.fda.gov/~dms/district.html website.

Guidelines for Supplement Use

Keeping up with the explosion of supplements and supplement claims can be overwhelming! If you take supplements, ask for expert guidance from a health-care professional.

For All Supplements . . .

Before you decide to take a dietary supplement, go with the tried-and-true. Do you really need a supplement for fitness? Plenty of scientific evidence supports the benefits of physical activity, healthful eating, getting enough sleep, and a healthful lifestyle. If you take a supplement—any supplement—remember:

● Give up the notion that dietary supplements are simple, immediate solutions to your health problems. Even supplements, such as fish oil and calcium, that offer benefits take time and ongoing use to make a difference.

● Skip the lure of this myth: "Even if a supplement won't help me, at least it won't hurt me." High dosages, taken long enough or combined with other supplements, can be harmful.

● Avoid using supplements to replace healthful eating or conventional health care, or to replace a doctor's visit for a health problem. Never self-diagnose a health condition.

● *Best practice:* Talk to your doctor *before* you take any supplement! That's especially important if you're under age eighteen, pregnant or breast-feeding, chronically ill, elderly, or taking prescription or over-the-counter medicines, or planning to have surgery. *See "Warning: Supplement Interactions!" in this chapter.*

● If you're taking a dietary supplement, tell your doctor to make sure it's safe and appropriate for you and your health status. Some interfere with medications. Prepare to discuss:

● Supplement name, type, and daily or weekly dose. (Bring the container if you can.) If it's a dietary supplement, it will have Supplement Facts on the package.

● How long you have taken it and plan to take it, and why—and if you really need it!

● How long you've had symptoms you're treating with supplements; if your symptoms improved.

● Your typical day's food choices. Include fortified foods, such as some cereals and drinks. The combined intake from all supplements and fortified foods needs consideration since excess intakes of some supplements may cause health problems.

● The dosage taken and how often. Keep a daily supplement journal to help remember: what supplement, how often, how much, and why.

● Other medications, supplements (over-the-counter and prescription) you're taking, and other alternative health practices.

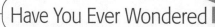 Have You Ever Wondered

. . . if supplements are safe if you have allergies? Remember that herbal and other botanical supplements are made from the bark, flowers, leaves, and seeds of plants. Chitosan, promoted for weight loss (with limited effectiveness), is a fiber from the shells of shellfish—a problem if you have shellfish allergies. If you're prone to allergic reactions, check with your healthcare professional. *See chapter 21 for more about allergies.*

. . . about the difference between vitamin D_2 and D_3 in supplements? Either form increases vitamin D in the blood. However, the D_3 (cholecalciferol) form may do it better and keep levels raised longer. Today many supplements provide vitamin D_3 instead of D_2 (ergocalciferol).

- Any health problems or illnesses:
  - Whether you're pregnant or breast-feeding
  - Whether you drink alcohol or smoke; if so, how often and how much
  - If you have allergies
  - If you're on a special eating plan (self-prescribed or medically prescribed)
- Known side effects (appetite loss, headaches, nausea).
- Cautions or warnings, including amount and upper limit.

For more about talking to your healthcare provider about your nutrition and health needs, see chapter 24.

- If you're pregnant, planning for pregnancy, or breast-feeding, talk to your healthcare provider about supplements! You're at greater risk for side effects.

- Unless your pediatrician prescribes them, avoid giving supplements, including herbals, to your child or teen! *See "What about Nutrient Supplements?" in chapter 17 and "Caution: Herbals Not for Kids!" in this chapter.*

- Look for published research studies on a supplement for the health condition that interests you. The ODS is an excellent science-based resource on specific dietary supplements: ods.od.nih.gov.

- Look for products labeled with the voluntary USP Verified Mark or NF letters, *as described earlier in this chapter.* Although some reputable companies choose

Caution: Herbals Not for Kids!

Even though supplement companies aggressively target kids and parents, herbal and other botanical supplements may not be as safe or effective for your child or teen as you may think! Some are useless; others, potentially harmful. As noted in this chapter, little evidence exists on the safety and effectiveness of botanical supplements for adults. Their use among children and teens is virtually untested. In other words, the short- or long-term benefits, and, more importantly, the risks are mostly unknown.

Warning: Despite the FDA ban against ephedra for anyone—including for those under age eighteen—medications with a form of ephedra may be available to teens. *See "Herbal Ingredients: Hazardous to Health!" in this chapter.*

to pay for independent certification, others don't. Often national brands from larger companies have stricter quality controls. Certification marks represent differing criteria; most important, they indicate whether a label matches the supplement contents, not its safety or effectiveness. The FDA has found contaminants in some products marketed as "natural."

- Remember, "natural" doesn't mean safe or milder. For example, peppermint leaf tea is thought safe; concentrated peppermint oil from leaves can be toxic. Having a "mark" is not necessarily an indicator of quality.

- Stick with the label dosage; heed warnings. The dosage is set by the manufacturer—not by FDA regulations. Boosting the dosage without medical supervision can be dangerous, even for an insignificant substance.

- Follow label directions. Some supplements are more effective taken with food; others, on an empty stomach. Ask your healthcare provider or pharmacist for a list of foods and drinks to avoid consuming with the supplement. Usually water is the best drink.

- Keep dietary supplements in a safe place—away from places where children may reach them! Adult iron supplements are the most common cause of poisoning deaths among children in the United States.

- Keep supplements in a cool, dry place—preferably away from the stove and not in the bathroom. Heat and moisture affect their quality and effectiveness. Keep them in their original containers (label still on).

- Check the expiration date. Supplements lose some potency as they get closer to their expiration date.

- On the same note, skip the urge to "prescribe" a supplement for someone else. Even if it works for you, it may not be safe or effective for someone else.

- Want to know about a supplement's contents? Contact the manufacturer. The FDA doesn't have the resources to analyze supplements. Companies that provide scientific information about their products are more likely to be reliable resources; still, be wary and careful. Supplements aren't standardized by regulation. So even if the label says "standardized" or "certified," the supplement may have more or less than the label says. In addition, manufacturing and storage methods may affect the contents.

● Ask a registered dietitian, pharmacist, or your healthcare provider about the effectiveness of specific supplements—and research behind claims. Show the supplement container; share your information.

● Stay skeptical of supplement marketing—and label or advertising claims. Besides being ineffective, the supplement may be costly and harmful. *See "Play 'Ten Questions'" and "Spotting a Fraud" in chapter 24 to help you evaluate their claims.*

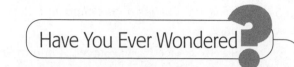

Have You Ever Wondered

. . . if the same supplement can be sold by several names? Yes; that adds to consumer confusion. However, the ingredient list must list the common name.

Botanical supplements may have a common name and a botanical name—for example, St. John's wort, often promoted to treat mild to moderate depression, also is known as *Hypericum perforatum.*

The common name also may refer to a category. Ginseng may refer to *Panax ginseng* or *Panax japonicus* (Asian ginsengs) or to *Panax quinquefolius L.* (American ginseng), each with different effects. Siberian ginseng *(E. senticosus)* isn't botanically related to either!

. . . what "high potency" on a dietary supplement label means? According to government regulations, "high potency" means that a nutrient in a food or a dietary supplement, provides 100 percent or more of the Daily Value (DV) for that vitamin or mineral. The term also can refer to a product with several ingredients if two-thirds of its nutrients contribute more than 100 percent of the DVs. *See chapter 12 for more about DVs.*

. . . if chelated mineral supplements are any better? Chelation binds minerals to other substances, supposedly making minerals easier for the body to absorb. While that may be true, many minerals found naturally in food aren't very bioavailable; that's considered when their Dietary Reference Intakes are established. In the overall picture, chelation isn't important—if you're meeting your day's mineral recommendation.

. . . if dietary supplements contain solid fats (saturated and trans fats)? Some may. Energy and nutrition bars are often classified as supplements. If they have 0.5 grams or more of *trans* or saturated fats, these fats must be on the Supplement Facts.

Caution: Taking dietary supplements for potential health benefits is not uncommon for people diagnosed with cancer, AIDS, or other life-threatening health problems. They may put their hopes and healthcare dollars in supplements and other alternative treatments. Yet, supplements may offer a false sense of security—and a serious problem if well-proven approaches to health care or medical treatment are delayed. If you have a health problem, seek medical attention and proven treatment first. Even if you're healthy now, don't rely on the "security" of supplements to keep you fit!

For Vitamin/Mineral Supplements . . .

● Remember, for most people: food before pills. If you're healthy and self-prescribe a supplement, ask yourself: Do I really need it? Consider your everyday food choices and the nutrients they provide. If you follow a USDA Food Pattern or the DASH Eating Plan, you likely get all the nutrients you need already. *See chapter 10 for more about healthful eating patterns and MyPlate, a visual tool for healthy eating.*

● Use supplements as supplements—not meal replacements. No supplement provides the full complement of vitamins, minerals, and other important nutrients found in food. Supplements only have what's listed on the label. By relying on them, you miss out on the full variety of nutrients, as well as fiber and phytonutrients, that food supplies.

● If your healthcare provider recommends a supplement—either a vitamin-mineral combination or a single nutrient such as calcium—follow his or her professional guidance. *That includes the general guidelines in "For All Supplements . . ." earlier in this chapter.*

● For a vitamin-mineral combination, limit the potency to 100 percent of the Daily Values (DV) for your age for most nutrients; use the label's Supplement Facts to judge the product. A supplement with close to 100 percent DV for most nutrients is likely more than enough, especially if your diet is healthful. Avoid large doses!

● Choose a supplement for your unique needs. Consider your age, gender, and medical status. *Note:* If you're under stress, don't count on a stress vitamin pill to help. Stress doesn't increase nutrient needs.

● For economy, consider the generic brand. Paying

more for the branded product generally offers no additional benefits. Synthetic rather than natural vitamins may cost less. For the most part, their chemical makeup is the same. One exception is "natural" vitamin E (d-alpha-tocopherol on the ingredient list), which is more potent than the synthetic form (dl-tocopherol). In most cases, however, your body won't know the difference between synthetic and natural. "Natural" products likely cost more.

Don't be lured by extra ingredients: inositol, lecithin, PABA, herbs, and enzymes. They add to the cost but offer no proven nutritional benefits.

● Check the expiration date on the label. Over time, nutrient supplements lose some potency.

● Take only the recommended dosage. Instead of double-dosing on days when you've missed a meal, make up for foods you missed with your food choices on the next day.

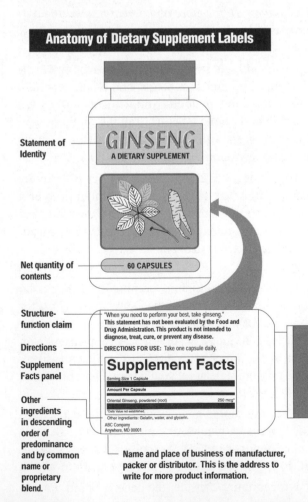

Anatomy of Dietary Supplement Labels

Statement of Identity

GINSENG
A DIETARY SUPPLEMENT

Net quantity of contents — **60 CAPSULES**

Structure-function claim — "When you need to perform your best, take ginseng."
This statement has not been evaluated by the Food and Drug Administration. This product is not intended to diagnose, treat, cure, or prevent any disease.

Directions — DIRECTIONS FOR USE: Take one capsule daily.

Supplement Facts panel —
Supplement Facts
Serving Size 1 Capsule

Amount Per Capsule

Oriental Ginseng, powdered (root) .... 250 mcg*

*Daily Value not established.
Other ingredients: Gelatin, water, and glycerin.
ABC Company
Anywhere, MD 00001

Other ingredients in descending order of predominance and by common name or proprietary blend.

Name and place of business of manufacturer, packer or distributor. This is the address to write for more product information.

● Be cautious about doubling up. If you already take a multivitamin/mineral supplement, taking a single vitamin or mineral supplement, or a food fortified with that nutrient on a regular basis as well may be too much! Read the label.

For Herbal and Other Botanical Supplements . . .

Helpful or harmful? Even though herbal and other botanicals are sold over the counter, use them with caution and discretion. *Besides the guidelines in "For All Supplements . . ." earlier in this chapter,* follow these guidelines:

● Seek unbiased, science-based sources of information about herbals. Relying on product claims may not be a good idea. The poorly defined term "natural" doesn't mean safe or healthful. Ask a registered dietitian or other qualified nutrition expert.

● Find out about the risks and potential side effects. Then decide with your doctor if it's safe and appropriate for you—or if other known health strategies would yield safe, effective results instead.

● Always consult a qualified health professional—preferably one properly trained in herbal medicine. The National Center for Complementary and Alternative Medicine, National Institutes of Health advises that's especially important when taking herbs as part of medical care, including traditional Chinese medicine or Ayurvedic medicine. Be very cautious of those who call themselves a "herbalist," "herb doctor," "health counselor," or "master herbalist." These job titles aren't regulated.

● For serious illness, avoid self-medicating with herbal or other botanical supplements. That may delay known treatment that can help you.

● Talk to your healthcare provider about herbal remedies if you take medication—either prescription or over-the-counter medications. The combination could make your medication ineffective, or create a harmful side effect. *See "Warning: Supplement Interactions" in this chapter*.

● If you get a doctor's okay, use herbal products only as directed. Because herbal supplements can have druglike effects, too much taken at one time can be dangerous.

Take single-herb products, not herbal mixtures, unless recommended by a qualified practitioner with expertise in herbal therapies. If you have an adverse effect, you can identify the source more easily if you're taking single-herb products.

● If a herbal product seems to cause any negative side effects, stop taking it, and contact your doctor right away. Your doctor should contact the FDA's MedWatch hotline, which monitors adverse reactions to food and dietary supplements. *See "Supplements: If You Have an Adverse Reaction . . ." in this chapter.*

See "Pour an 'Herbal' Tea?" in chapter 8.

The Supplement Label

A supplement label looks somewhat like a food label. Required by the Dietary Supplement Health and Education Act, the label must provide specific information you can use to make informed decisions:

● *Statement of identity.* Look for the product name, perhaps "ginseng." The term "dietary supplement" or a descriptive phrase, such as "vitamin and mineral supplement," also must appear. If the product is a botanical, the plant part must be identified.

● *Net quantity of the ingredients.* That might be the number of capsules, perhaps "sixty capsules," in the package or container, or the weight.

● *Disclaimer with any structure/function claim. See "Claim Check!" in this chapter.*

● *Supplement Facts.* This gives the serving (dosage), the amount, the % Daily Values (DVs) per serving if appropriate, and the active ingredient.

● *Directions for use.* This might indicate how often to take the supplement, perhaps "Take one capsule daily"; whether the supplement is best taken with or without food; safety tips; or storage guidelines. Suggested dosage is meaningless when little is known about the benefits and risks of many supplements.

● *Ingredients.* The list must be in descending order by common name or proprietary blend. *See "Ingredients Labeling, Too" in this chapter.*

● *Name and address of the manufacturer, packager, or distributor.* Use this contact information to get more product information.

Need more strategies for appropriate supplement use? Check here for "how-tos":

● Find out about *safe* supplement use for children—see chapter 17.

● Get savvy about ergogenic supplements for athletic performance—see chapter 20.

● Sort through misleading information about supplements—see chapter 24.

● Talk to a qualified nutrition expert about safe and appropriate supplements for you and your family—see chapter 24.

As an option, supplement labels may carry product claims: nutrient content, health, or structure/function claims. Another option, *but not required:* a cautionary statement if adverse effects are linked to the product. In other words, it may or may not carry a warning!

Check the Supplement Facts

How do you know about the nutrition in a dietary supplement? Check the Supplement Facts panel, which must appear on *all* supplements. Its format is similar to the familiar Nutrition Facts you see on food products. To use the Supplement Facts panel:

● Check the serving size, or an appropriate unit, such as a capsule, packet, or teaspoonful. That's what the facts are based on. Unlike Nutrition Facts for foods, serving size isn't standardized for supplements; neither is the potency, or nutrient amount, per serving. Manufacturers make that decision.

● Check the quantity and the % Daily Values (DVs) for any of fourteen nutrients, including sodium, vitamin A, vitamin C, calcium, and iron, if the levels are significant. Other vitamins or minerals must be listed, too, if they are added or referred to with a nutrient content claim on the label.

On the Supplement Facts, you probably won't find a nutrient if it isn't present. For example, cod liver oil lists fat on the panel, but a calcium supplement won't because it doesn't contain fat.

For a substance with no Daily Value, the quantity per serving must be listed—for example, "15 mg omega-3 fatty acids."

Claim Check!

Confused about marketing claims for supplements? Not surprising! Some nutrient content claims and health claims are backed by scientific consensus, yet many (structure/function claims) aren't, at least not yet. One exception: "Calcium helps build strong bones." Loose supplement regulations, including many product claims that push "over the edge" of credibility, leave many consumers misguided, bewildered, or both.

Some product claims are clearly illegal—for example, "cures cancer," "treats arthritis," " prevents impotence." According to FDA regulation, no dietary supplement can legally state or imply that it can help diagnose, lessen, treat, cure, or prevent disease.

Here's what marketers can claim about supplements—and how the claims are regulated—on package labels. *Since claims for food and for dietary supplements are similar, see chapter 12 for more information.*

Nutrient content claims. "High in calcium." "Excellent source of folate." "Iron-free." Like food labels, dietary supplement labels can carry nutrient content claims if they contain a specific level of a nutrient in a serving. The claims, regulated by the FDA, are similar to nutrient content claims for food. For example, any product with at least 20 percent of the Daily Value per serving can be labeled as "high" or "excellent source" of that nutrient.

What does a nutrient content claim tell you? It's just a clue for the relative amount. You need to read the Supplement Facts to know the specific nutrient content of one dose, or "serving."

Why would a supplement be "iron-free"? It's for the age fifty-plus market, when women's iron needs drop. Most men's supplements are also iron-free.

Health claims. "Calcium may reduce the risk of osteoporosis." "Folic acid may reduce the risk of some neural tube defects." Health claims that describe the link between nutrients or food substances and health can be used on supplements. These FDA-regulated statements are based on scientific consensus—you can trust these claims. *For approved health claims for food and supplement labeling, see the appendices.* Some

qualified health claims have been approved for supplements but not for food products: for example, B vitamins (folic acid, vitamin B_6, and vitamin B_{12}) and reduced risk for vascular disease.

Structure/function claims. Echinacea: "boosts the immune system." Zinc: "helps maintain good immunity." Garlic: "helps maintain cardiovascular health." Lutein: "helps maintain healthy eyes."

Structure/function claims may appear on dietary supplements, as on food labels. They describe what the ingredient is intended to do in the body or to promote health. But they can't mention a specific disease. Research to support these claims may be limited, with little or no scientific consensus.

By regulation, the manufacturer, not the FDA, must substantiate that structure-function statements are truthful and not misleading. Because the FDA does not approve them, supplement labels also must carry a disclaimer: "This statement has not been evaluated by the Food and Drug Administration. This product is not intended to diagnose, treat, cure, or prevent any disease."

Ingredients Labeling, Too

The label shows ingredients, with their common name or proprietary blend, in descending order by weight. If an ingredient isn't in the Supplement Facts, it must be in the ingredients statement—for example, rose hips as the vitamin C source. Besides active ingredients, other substances—fillers, colorings or flavors, sweeteners—must be listed.

For herbal and other botanical supplements, potency often differs when different parts of a plant are used. The label must identify what part of the plant it comes from—for example, ginseng may come from a root. The ingredient source may appear on an ingredients statement or near the statement of identity. If the dietary ingredient is the exclusive blend of a manufacturer, both the total weight of the blend and its components must be listed in descending order by weight. Non-dietary ingredients such as fillers, artificial colors, sweeteners, flavors, or binders must be listed, too, in descending order by weight and by common name or proprietary blend.

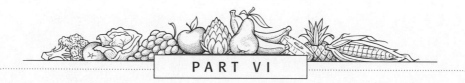

PART VI

Resources

More about Healthful Eating

CHAPTER 24

Well Informed?

Are you well informed . . . or often confused about conflicting nutrition information? Can you easily find reliable nutrition information . . . or do you feel frustrated sorting through a maze of scientific news about healthful eating? For that matter, how do you stay up-to-date?

Popular media—television; print or online magazines, newspapers, and books; and the Internet—are likely part of your health education "mix," alerting you to up-to-date food and nutrition issues, concerns, and popular advice. In fact, many people rely on popular media more than in-person contact with health professionals. Today technology is used for food, nutrition, and health information through computers, handheld/mobile devices, and more. For your own good health, you're wise to find credible sources and learn to judge the value of nutrition advice from any source before using it to make your eating, lifestyle, and health decisions.

Where do teens and children learn about healthful eating? First and foremost, from parents, perhaps you. So being well informed yourself ultimately teaches them. As kids get older, they learn from school, friends, and media, too. Your challenge as a parent, caregiver, or teacher? Knowing enough to direct those in your care to sources of trustworthy eating and lifestyle guidance!

Need Nutrition Advice?

When do you need smart eating advice? Every day! Sometimes you may need to know a little more . . .

- If you're pregnant—or trying to get pregnant
- If you need guidance *and confidence* for breast-feeding
- If you're dealing with the "ups and downs" of infant or child feeding
- If you're trying to steer your teen toward healthier eating
- If you want peak performance for sports
- If you're struggling with your weight—or trying to gain or lose a few pounds
- If you need to change your eating habits to prevent or manage a health problem—yours, or a family member's
- If you're caring for an aging parent or friend
- If you simply want to eat smarter to stay fit

For nutrition advice, ask a qualified expert. Your health—and that of your family—depend on it!

The Real Expert . . . Please Stand Up

Just who is a qualified nutrition expert? Sometimes it's hard to tell. Qualified nutrition experts, with specific academic and training credentials, know the science of nutrition. Their degrees in nutrition, dietetics, public health, or related fields (such as biochemistry, physiology, medicine, or a nutrition specialty in family and consumer sciences) come from well-respected, accredited colleges, universities, or medical schools. The title "dietitian" or "nutritionist" often describes what they do. An "accredited" institution generally is

Who Is a Registered Dietitian?

The initials RD after someone's name mean "registered dietitian." A registered dietitian is a food and nutrition authority who has met academic and training requirements to earn the RD credential—and so provide science-based nutrition guidance to the public.

As an important member of the healthcare team, an RD may have specialized expertise, perhaps in pediatric, maternal, or sports nutrition; oncology, cardiovascular, or renal nutrition; weight counseling; or diabetes education. Besides being in healthcare, education, and research, registered dietitians also provide nutrition and food expertise in business (corporate wellness, consumer affairs, product development, marketing, sales), government (public policy, government programs), food service (restaurant, institutions) management, fitness (education, training), communications (media, public relations, writing), culinary jobs (test kitchen), community services, in private practice counseling and consulting, and more.

To earn the RD credential, an individual must complete a minimum of a bachelor's degree in nutrition or a related field from a U.S. regionally accredited college or university program and coursework approved by the Commission on Accreditation for Dietetics Education (CADE) of the Academy of Nutrition and Dietetics (formerly the American Dietetic Association). He or she must complete a CADE-accredited supervised practice program at a healthcare facility, community agency, or a food-service corporation, which may be combined with undergraduate or graduate studies. Typically, a practice program runs six to twelve months. Many dietetics professionals earn graduate degrees, as well.

To become registered, candidates must pass an extensive examination, administered by the Commission on Dietetic Registration, the credentialing agency of the Academy. All RDs are required to stay current with ongoing continuing education. Only dietitians who have passed the exam and maintain their continuing education are considered "registered."

Some registered dietitians also have specialized credentials, such as Board Certified Specialists in Pediatric Nutrition (CSP) or in Renal Nutrition (CSR), or as Certified Diabetes Educators (CDE).

certified by an agency recognized by the U.S. Department of Education. Check the reference department of your local library for an institution's accreditation.

Letters after a name don't necessarily qualify someone to provide nutrition services. Even when that person holds other academic degrees, nutrition may not be his or her specialty. Probe further.

The initials RD for "registered dietitian" or DTR for "dietetic technician, registered" mean the person has met specific educational requirements in nutrition and health. *See "Who Is a Registered Dietitian?" above and "Who Is a Dietetic Technician, Registered?" on page 659.* Most states have licensing for qualified nutrition experts to help ensure credible nutrition guidance and quality healthcare. The credential may be designated as LD (licensed dietitian), although states differ. Qualifications for licensing typically reflect the same education and training required to become an RD. Many qualified nutrition experts also have advanced degrees, such as M.S., M.Ed., Sc.D., M.D., or Ph.D.

Being qualified in nutrition, dietetics, or any health field doesn't end when a degree is conferred, but continues with lifelong education. A qualified healthcare provider should be able to address current nutrition research and guidance, or help you find a reliable source.

What about job titles such "nutritionist" or "diet counselor"? In many states these titles aren't regulated, so terms like these may be used by those not properly qualified to give accurate nutrition information or sound advice, perhaps with just a little nutrition training or with only mail-order credentials. Mail-order, diploma-mill credentials may appear impressive—but don't be fooled. The U.S. Department of Education defines a "diploma mill" as an organization awarding degrees without requiring its students to meet the established educational standards followed by reputable accredited institutions.

How to Find Nutrition Help . . .

Need personal nutrition counseling? Food assistance for a friend or a family member? Answers to nutrition questions? Check with health, education, and social service organizations in your community, as well as registered dietitians in private practice for direct services.

To Find a Qualified Nutrition Expert

Start with these sources:

- Your doctor, health maintenance organization (HMO), or local hospital for a referral

Who Is a Dietetic Technician, Registered?

The initials DTR after a person's name stand for "dietetic technician, registered." DTRs are trained for support roles in food and nutrition and are an integral part of the healthcare or food service management teams. DTRs often are considered partners in practice with registered dietitians. Job responsibilities may include teaching nutrition classes, offering diet counseling, performing diet histories, assessing a person's nutritional status, or managing aspects of a food-service operation. DTRs typically work in hospitals, day care, or extended care facilities; many also work in food companies, government agencies, education, retail sales and marketing, academic institutions, or fitness centers.

Currently there are two ways to attain the DTR credential. First is by completing requirements for an associate degree from a U.S. regionally accredited college or university and a CADE-accredited dietetic technician program. Second is by completing a baccalaureate degree, a didactic program in dietetics at a CADE (Commission on Accreditation for Dietetics Education)-accredited/approved college or university, and 450 hours of supervised field experience in healthcare facilities, food-service operations, or community nutrition programs through a CADE-accredited DT program. Many DTRs earn additional degrees that complement their food and nutrition background. DTRs also must successfully complete a comprehensive registration exam administered by the Commission on Dietetic Registration, the credentialing agency of the Academy of Nutrition and Dietetics.

Once they earn their credential, DTRs must stay current with ongoing continuing education. Only individuals who pass the exam and maintain their status through continuing education are considered *registered*. In addition, individuals with dietetics education and experience who are not DTRs may have job titles that include "dietetic technician," "diet tech," or "diet clerk."

- Your local dietetic association, public health department, Cooperative Extension Service, or the nutrition department of an area college or university

- The Academy of Nutrition and Dietetics at www.eatright.org (go to "Find a Registered Dietitian"). Or call 800-877-1600, ext. 5000, for a referral to a registered dietitian in your area.

See "The Real Expert . . . Please Stand Up" in this chapter to help you choose a qualified nutrition expert.

To Find Food and Nutrition Services

Agencies, institutions, and businesses—often staffed with qualified nutrition experts—provide direct food or nutrition services. Whether for you or for someone else who might benefit, consider the following:

Child Nutrition Programs. Schools, as well as early childhood centers, after-school programs, and summer camps, may provide nutritious breakfasts, lunches, milk, and snacks for children. Often local programs get support partly through the USDA's Food and Nutrition Service. By regulation, school meals and snacks must meet strict nutrition guidelines. The program also supports nutrition education. *See "For Kids Only—Today's School Meals" in chapter 17.*

Cooperative Extension Service. Each state's Cooperative Extension program provides consumer information on various topics, including food, nutrition, and food safety. State land-grant universities employ nutrition experts through the Extension staff. Look for Extension's food and nutrition information online or perhaps in your local newspaper provided by your grant university.

Click Here! Other Websites to Know . . .

- Academy of Nutrition and Dietetics, www.eatright.org/Public
- Food and Nutrition Service/USDA, fnic.nal.usda.gov/consumer
- International Food Information Council Foundation, www.foodinsight.org
- AND Evidence Analysis Library, www.andevidencelibrary.com or www.eal.org
- QuackWatch, www.quackwatch.com

See "Resources You Can Use" for more websites.

Supplemental Nutrition Assistance Program (SNAP). Formerly the Food Stamp Program, it's administered by state agencies and funded by the U.S. Department of Agriculture (USDA). SNAP provides food assistance to needy families and individuals. Low-income households receive an electronic benefits card to use like cash in most grocery stores and some farmers' markets. For the nearest SNAP (food stamp) office, check your county public health department or the government pages of your phone book.

Health Organizations. For help with specific health issues, check health organizations such as the American Heart Association, the American Diabetes Association, and the Food Allergy and Anaphylaxis Network—as well as the Academy of Nutrition and Dietetics. *Also check "Resources You Can Use" at the end of this book.* Their websites offer a wealth of information, and perhaps a gateway to other credible food, nutrition, and health websites.

Home-Delivered Meals. People who can't leave their homes or who can't prepare food independently may seek services for home-delivered meals. For those who qualify, government or community agencies provide meals at low cost. Check with a social worker, religious group, or state or area Agency on Aging.

Senior Citizens' Meal Programs. Community agencies may offer low-cost meals and social contact for senior citizens. To find services, check with a social worker, health department, religious group, or area Agency on Aging. USDA's Senior Farmers' Market Nutrition Program offers assistance with fresh fruits and vegetables.

Soup Kitchens and Food Pantries. For those who are homeless or have limited resources for food, private and faith-based groups may provide food at no cost. Social workers, social agencies, and religious groups offer referrals.

Women, Infants, and Children (WIC) Program. This federal government program, which also has a Farmers' Market Nutrition Program, offers food assistance and nutrition education to pregnant women, infants, and preschoolers. Again, the county or other local public health department can help, or check the government pages in your phone book or check online.

Child and Adult Care Feeding. For many low-income families, this government program provides nutritious, affordable meals and snacks daily, as part of day care and preschool for children and adult day care for the elderly.

For other government and nonprofit food assistance programs, as well as food assistance for disaster relief, talk with your healthcare provider, Extension office, or local public health department.

For More about Food Products

Food companies and food industry groups provide information about the nutrients and ingredients in their products. Many offer healthful eating and lifestyle information and recipes on their websites, e-newsletters, package labels, and print materials or through their toll-free phone numbers (often printed on food packages). They may provide interactive information through social media, phone apps, and online tutorials. Through their consumer response services—staffed by registered dietitians or other qualified food and nutrition professionals—find answers to your questions, perhaps through their online community.

When You Consult an Expert . . .

Whether you seek nutrition counseling on your own or followup from a doctor's referral, here's how you can make the most of your time with a qualified nutrition professional. For an office visit:

● *Have a medical checkup first.* A qualified nutrition professional needs to know your health status before providing dietary guidance. Your healthcare provider can share your blood pressure and information from blood tests, such as blood cholesterol, triglycerides, blood glucose (sugar), hemoglobin, and hematocrit levels, among other tests.

Some health problems are managed in part or completely by diet and perhaps physical activity. If so, your doctor may refer you to a registered dietitian for appropriate diet therapy. In many states, private health insurance and managed care plans cover nutrition counseling (also known as medical nutrition therapy) with a registered dietitian for some health conditions, such as diabetes. Ask for a referral if you qualify.

● *Share your goals.* If you seek nutrition advice on your own, know what you want to accomplish. Do you want to lose weight? Gain weight? Have more stamina for sports? Improve your blood cholesterol levels? Live a healthier lifestyle? Think about your goals ahead . . . and make them realistic.

● *Forget miracles and magic bullets.* A qualified nutrition professional will focus on changes in your lifestyle and food choices, not on quick results, miracle cures, or costly and unneeded dietary supplements.

● *Tell about dietary supplements you're taking.* That includes herbal remedies and botanicals. Some supplements interact with medications (even over-the-counter types), rendering them ineffective or causing harmful side effects. *See "Food and Medicine" in chapter 22.* Dietary supplements taken in very large doses also may cause adverse health reactions. *See chapter 23, "Dietary Supplements: Use and Misuse."*

● *Keep an ongoing personal health record* to share and aid decisions about your nutrition and healthcare. As technology moves forward, some of this information may be kept for you as part of your electronic health record.

● *Be prepared to answer questions.* Expect to talk about your eating habits, adverse reactions to food, dietary supplements, weight history, food preferences, general medical history, family history of health problems, medications, special diets, any nutrition instruction you've had, and lifestyle habits. With those insights, a dietitian can help you customize food and nutrition advice for your lifestyle and health.

● *For weight or sports nutrition counseling, expect to have your weight and body composition checked*— usually height, weight, and a skinfold measurement in several spots on your body (or other techniques to measure body composition).

● *Ask for clarification.* If you don't understand the terms used in the counseling session, ask! Terms such as "blood glucose level," "HDLs," "triglycerides," "anaphylactic reaction," and "*trans* fatty acids" are nutrition-related lingo. Know what they mean.

● *Be specific with your questions.* You're the most important person on your healthcare team. You can only comply with dietary recommendations if you have a clear understanding of the advice offered.

● *Be open to professional health advice.* For example, if your healthcare provider talks about your weight, it's for your own health benefit.

● *Keep careful eating records*—if you're asked. Record everything you eat and drink, including snacks, perhaps for several days. Record the amounts (in cups, ounces, tablespoons, or the like) and how the foods were prepared, such as "fried" or "baked." If you suspect a food sensitivity, write down any reactions you think may be associated with the food or beverage. *For other tips, see "Dear Journal . . ." in chapter 2.*

● *Involve your family.* If you take a nutrition class or meet with a nutrition professional, bring your family and friends along. Support helps ensure success.

● *Follow up, as advised,* so your progress can be monitored and your questions answered. Follow-up visits are great moral support, too!

● *Stick with it!* A positive change in body weight, blood pressure, blood cholesterol levels, and other physical conditions may take time. With your healthcare provider and support team, plan for gradual results.

Be Your Own Judge!

Do you rely on popular media—magazines, newspapers, TV, radio, blogs, tweeter chat, or information on the Internet—for healthful eating advice and nutrition updates? Fortunately, there's plenty of reliable, consumer-friendly nutrition information available. Many well-qualified food, nutrition, and health experts share trustworthy information through every kind of popular medium, from print to digital! Yet, the airwaves, print, and the web are also full of nutrition hype, misleading reports, and quackery. How can you be a savvy media consumer—and sort fact from fiction?

You Can't Judge a Book by Its Cover

Being a best-seller or highly visible doesn't make advice reliable. Despite threads of truth, the messages may be laced with misinformation or offer advice in a context that doesn't apply to you. Give what you read or hear a reliability check—no matter what the media!

Who Wrote It?

Check the author's qualifications. A reputable nutrition author usually is educated in the field of nutrition, medicine, or a related specialty, with a degree or degrees from an accredited college or university. He or she usually is a credentialed member of a credible

Have You Ever Wondered ?

. . . how to access credible scientific journals? University, medical school, and large urban libraries have them. With Internet access you can check online through the National Library of Medicine, a division of the U.S. National Institutes of Health. Loansome Doc (www.nlm.nih.gov/loansomedoc/loansome_home.html) allows users to order full-text copies of articles from a medical library (local fees and delivery methods vary). Some journals have their own online presence, often available free.

. . . how to master a culinary skill, estimate portion sizes, or learn other food and nutrition how-tos? All kinds of reliable blogs, websites, and phone apps have online tutorials and interactive tools to help you learn, including government and food industry sites. Just use a search engine to find them, *then apply the evaluation criteria in "Nutrition in Cyberspace" in this chapter.*

nutrition organization—for example, an RD or a DTR. *See "The Real Expert . . . Please Stand Up" in this chapter.*

Why Was It Published?

For healthful eating advice, find resources with a balanced nutrition message meant to inform, not advertise. Try to analyze what's being said or implied. If it's not clear, ask a qualified nutrition expert.

Is the Nutrition Advice Credible?

Check the sources cited. Reliable advice is backed up with credible sources such as:

● *Government entities.* For example, the National Academy of Sciences/Institute of Medicine, the U.S. Department of Health and Human Services (DHHS), the U.S. Department of Agriculture (USDA), and Centers for Disease Control and Prevention (CDC) base healthful eating and lifestyle guidelines on the most current research and consensus from scientific experts. Among the guidelines often cited: Dietary Reference Intakes, Dietary Guidelines for Americans, 2010, the DASH Eating Plan, and the CDC's body mass index and Physical Activity Guidelines for Americans.

● *Credible professional nutrition and health organizations.* They base their advice on sound scientific evidence and government guidelines.

● *Peer-reviewed scientific journals.* Research reported in peer-reviewed journals goes through the scrutiny of experts before it can be printed, so in medical news stories, look for the journal citation. If you choose, you can read the original research. Among the many journals: *New England Journal of Medicine, Lancet, Journal of the American Medical Association,* and *Journal of the Academy of Nutrition and Dietetics* (formerly *Journal of the American Dietetic Association*).

Credible nutrition experts don't claim to have all the answers. If scientific evidence isn't conclusive or if the issues are controversial, they say so.

Check "Resources You Can Use" at the back of this book for many—but not all—government and health agencies, professional organizations, and food industry groups that provide credible information.

What Do Credible Experts Say?

Look for reviews by credible experts. For a book, start inside or on the cover itself, where you may find a list of reviewers. Like those of the author, reviewers' credentials or affiliations help you judge the reliability of nutrition information.

For an expert judgment, contact a registered dietitian or other qualified nutritionist connected with a local college, university, hospital, Extension program, public health department, or in private practice.

Read between the Headlines

Every day, nutrition and health news make headlines. In this age of instant communication, research often hits the media before nutrition experts can review and interpret the findings. Today's report may appear to contradict what you heard last week. Adding to the challenge, reporters assigned to medical stories usually need to report complex medical news quickly, in a short, simple way. The result? Confusion.

Legitimate scientists aren't out to mislead you. Responsible journalists aren't, either. Uncovering the mysteries of nutrition and the human body is a complex process. As new findings emerge, research may seem to contradict itself. But differences in two or more reports reflect how scientists continue to learn—sharing research results and questioning each step along the way. Scientific debate leads to more studies. Eventually—perhaps after years of study—recommendations based on sound science (repeated, conclusive evidence) can be shared with the public. In today's popular media, you can listen to the debate.

As science unravels more about the links among nutrition, health, and chronic disease, today's reports will eventually prove to be both true and false. You can't dissect every research report. But you can use caution and common sense before jumping to conclusions and changing your food and lifestyle choices.

● *Go beyond headlines.* An attention-grabbing headline or a short sound bite may leave a different impression than the full newspaper article or news brief itself. Read or listen to the whole story or the full context. Often response from other experts or "bottom line" advice appears at the story's end.

● *Remember—once isn't enough!* Results from one study aren't enough to change food choices. They're just one piece of a bigger scientific puzzle. True nutrition breakthroughs take years of study and the support of repeated findings from many scientific studies. That's why health organizations, government agencies, and health experts may appear conservative; their guidance reflects consistent, well-researched findings.

● *Check the report.* Do other studies support the evidence? And does it build on what scientists know already? Responsible scientists and careful journalists report research within the context of other studies. And one study rarely changes their nutrition advice.

● *Recognize preliminary findings and unpublished data for what they are—preliminary!* Read them with interest. But wait for more evidence before making major changes.

● *Look for the human dimension.* Animal studies may be among the first steps in researching a hypothesis. But the results don't always apply to humans.

● *Learn to be research savvy.* Read more about the study itself before applying its conclusions to you. Ask yourself: Are the people studied like you—perhaps in age, gender, health, ethnicity, geographic location, and lifestyle? Did the study include a large group of people? Was the study long-range? Longer studies, with more people, more likely produce valid results. Even by asking these questions, it's hard for consumers to assess research methods. *See "Scientific Studies: Coming to Terms" in this chapter.*

Words to the Wise

"may," "can"	Does not mean "will"
"contributes to," "is linked to," or "is associated with"	Does not mean "causes"
"proves"	Scientific studies gather evidence in a systematic way, but one study, taken alone, seldom proves anything.
"breakthrough"	This happens only now and then—for example, the discovery of penicillin or polio vaccine. But today this word is so overworked as to be meaningless.
"doubles the risk," "triples the risk," "risky"	May or may not be meaningful. Do you know what the risk was in the first place? If the risk was one in a million, and you double it, that's still only 1 in 500,000. If the risk was 1 in 100 and doubles, that's a big increase.
"significant"	A result is "statistically significant" when the association between two factors has been found to be greater than what might occur at random (this is worked out by a mathematical formula). But people often take "significant" to mean "major" or "important."

Adapted from: © Health Letter Associates, 1996, www.WellnessLetter.com.

● *Consider its context in the real world of healthful eating.* Does the study tell how the findings relate to overall food choices, lifestyle, and other research? A responsible report tells how research fits within the broader context of what is already known.

● *Know what the words mean.* Credible nutrition reports are careful with what they say so they won't mislead you. Research results may "suggest," but that isn't the same as "prove." And "linked to" doesn't mean "causes." *Don't jump to conclusions—get to know "Words to the Wise" on this page.*

● *Check the source.* Ask a qualified nutrition expert. Credible research comes from credible institutions and scientists, and it's reported in credible, peer-reviewed scientific and professional journals. Before nutrition research is published in reputable journals, it must meet well-established standards of nutrition research. If research is attributed simply to "they" or to some elusive source, be wary of its results.

● *Watch for follow-up reports.* Breaking scientific news is often followed by review and advice from nutrition experts. For example, registered dietitians often appear in media, helping to interpret news reports on nutrition issues.

Even when research has been well conducted, scientists may view the results differently. It may take time for nutrition experts to study the research methods and findings. So don't always expect an immediate response. For the best health news, look for a full perspective, not reports of one study.

● *Keep a healthy skepticism.* Every study has strengths and weaknesses. Make nutrition and health decisions based on sound and consensus science. *See "Case against Health Fraud" in this chapter.*

● *Watch out for absolutes!* Responsible scientists don't claim "proof" or "cause" until repeated studies show that the findings are conclusive.

● *Seek a qualified opinion.* Take the article with you! Before you change your eating style, consult a registered dietitian, other qualified nutrition expert, or doctor who can weigh the scientific evidence. Even promising research may not apply to you. For example, a report may suggest that red wine is heart healthy, but if you take an MAO inhibitor (an antidepressant), the combination may raise your blood pressure. Emerging science about wine may not benefit you—and drinking wine may be harmful in your case!

● *Put reports into your own reality.* For any advice, weigh the benefits and risks, as they apply to you, as an individual. And recognize that there's no such thing as "zero risk" for practically anything!

News stories about alternative therapies—supplements, herbal remedies, and holistic therapies—must stand up to the same scrutiny as any scientific research study, and the study itself needs the same rigor and precision. Testimonials and anecdotes aren't enough!

To explore the scientific evidence about a nutrition headline or topic, you can check an evidence-based library. Some are free; others require a subscription. *Check "Resources You Can Use" at the back of this book.*

Nutrition in Cyberspace

Get nutrition tips from a tweet, a phone app, or a blog? Food and nutrition information proliferates in cyberspace. Websites, blogs, discussion forums (chat rooms), list-servs, e-newsletters, video, podcasts, online communities, and other forms of social media can instantaneously spread all kinds of information: breaking news and advice, research findings and sound dietary guidance, healthful recipes and quick food prep tips, food safety recalls and food product information, food scares, and nutrition myths.

Like other media, online information is littered with nutrition misinformation. Science-based content can coexist with questionable, inaccurate, or alarming information, perhaps promoted by those holding unscientific views.

All too often this information goes viral, spreading faster than qualified experts can respond with a credible perspective. Two government agencies—the Federal Trade Commission (FTC) and the Food and Drug Administration (FDA)—are responsible for helping to protect consumers from false or misleading health claims on the Internet. Before you take action or spread the word, read on.

Clearing Up the Web of Confusion

How do you determine if a website, blog, or other social media provides information you can trust, or instead, if credible sources are quoted to "spin" a sense of legitimacy into unreliable sources? Use the same healthy skepticism with online information that you use to evaluate other nutrition information. Also ask yourself: *Does it . . .*

● *Clearly identify its purpose?* Look for a link to information about the site, often called "About This Site," to help you judge its trustworthiness.

● *Identify who runs the site?* That's your clue to the site's perspective, its potential bias, and its intent. The three-letter suffix on a website address is your first clue. Those that end in *.edu* (educational institutions), *.gov* (government agencies), and perhaps *.org* (organizations, often nonprofit) tend to be the most credible. Those ending in *.com* are commercial sites, and those ending in *.net* are networks, Internet service providers, or organizations. Many *.com* sites have responsible consumer information, some written by registered dietitians; just be a savvy consumer.

Scientific Studies: Coming to Terms

You've read news reports of nutrition studies. But what do all the terms mean?

Bias. Problems in the study design that affect the reliability of the results; perhaps the subjects weren't chosen correctly.

Blind (single or double) study. Study (*single blind*) where the subjects don't know if they're in the experimental or placebo group until after the study's over; study (*double blind*) where the researchers don't know either, so they can't influence the outcome.

Clinical trial. Studies done to directly show the effectiveness and the safety of a supplement, medication, or treatment with a selected group of people. The variables are controlled so the study can show cause and effect.

Confounding variable. A "hidden" and related variable (perhaps an unknown phytonutrient) that the researcher attributes to something different.

Control group. The study group that doesn't have the treatment. A control group is used to know if a treatment has an effect.

Correlation. An association between two research variables, such as eating lycopene and reduced risk for prostate cancer. A correlation does not prove cause and effect, but may suggest further study.

Epidemiological study. Study of the incidence and prevalence of a health condition among a specific group of people, such as neural tube defects among newborns.

Generalizability. Describes how much research results apply to the general population of people who are like the studies' subjects.

Incidence. How many new cases of a disease or health condition are reported as of a specific date, for a defined population.

In vitro study. Laboratory study with cells or tissue samples, usually done before an *in vivo* study.

In vivo study. Study with living subjects, either animal or human research.

Meta-analysis. A way to pool quantitative data from many studies to see what overall conclusions can be drawn, such as the pooling of more than forty studies on oats and more than twenty-five studies on soy protein to show their links to cholesterol-lowering.

Morbidity. Number of deaths in relation to a population.

Mortality. Number of people with an illness in relation to a population.

Observational study. Study that identifies a link between a health condition and behavior, such as over-weight and TV-watching, but doesn't prove cause and effect. All the variables aren't controlled; other factors may be responsible for the results. Although the study can't prove or disprove results, it can help develop the hypothesis.

Placebo. A "fake" treatment, perhaps a sugar pill, that appears to be the same as the treatment under study. It's used to remove bias when study subjects don't know which treatment they have.

Placebo effect. Positive results among subjects who think they're getting the real treatment.

Prevalence. How many *existing cases* of a disease or a health condition as of a specific date, for a defined population.

Prospective study. Study that poses the research questions, then follows groups of people, often for decades.

Random sample. A way to choose study subjects whereby anyone from a target population has an equal chance to be picked. In that way the results can be generalized more easily to a larger group.

Reliability. Describes research that is carefully controlled so the data can be reproduced. In other words, the researcher would get the same result with the same study subject several times.

Retrospective study. Study that uses recorded data or recall of the past. Because the study relies on memory or some variables that can't be easily controlled, this type of research has limitations.

Risk. The probability that something (perhaps a heart attack, stroke, cancer, diabetes, osteoporosis) will happen. "Risk" doesn't necessarily mean something will happen.

Risk factor. A factor that's statistically linked to the incidence of disease, such as a high BMI as a risk factor for heart disease. Again, it doesn't necessarily mean cause and effect.

Validity. The accuracy or truthfulness of the study's conclusion, and if the study measured what it meant to study.

Variable. A factor such as age, gender, or food choices in a study that differs among the people being studied. An *independent variable* is the one being studied; a *dependent variable,* perhaps lower blood glucose level or LDL cholesterol level, happens as a result of the treatment.

Adapted from source: Reprinted with permission of the International Food Information Council Foundation, Washington, D.C.

● *Name the writers or perhaps the editorial reviewers or board, with their credentials and perhaps an affiliation?* No matter what the media, credible information comes from qualified nutrition experts. Look for a contact address or phone number.

Today many registered dietitians who work in consulting or private practice have websites or blogs. You can verify their RD credential by contacting the Commission on Dietetic Registration of the Academy of Nutrition and Dietetics. *See "Resources You Can Use" at the back of this book for contact information.*

● *Provide facts with cited sources, not just opinions?* Look for information supported by established scientific findings. Any opinion or advice should be presented as such. And anything posted from other websites or sources should be cited clearly.

● *Link to credible online sites?* Be aware that an unreputable site may hyperlink to a credible site—perhaps a government nutrition site—for a trustworthy perception. Reliable online health sites generally hyperlink only to those sites that meet certain criteria, or their policy may not allow links.

● *Tell how any information you provide will—and will not—be used?* Decide if you want to share the information requested. Read and understand any privacy policy; don't sign up if you don't fully understand its use. Your data may be used for unexpected marketing purposes. Also know that websites routinely track the path users take through their sites to determine what pages are being used.

● *Have an educational purpose, or only a hidden guise of sound nutrition advice? Is it free of advertising, including pop-up ads?* If it's promotional, the information is likely biased or reframed for marketing and sales. Assess information within the context of total nutrition.

● *Indicate regular updates and postings?* Credible websites are updated often to offer the most current advice. Being current is crucial for health information! The most recent date for the update or review should be posted. *Caution:* Being current doesn't necessarily make it accurate. If the links don't work, it's likely old.

● *Pass other credibility tests? See "Read between the Headlines" in this chapter.* Anyone can launch a site. Like any media report, being on the Internet doesn't ensure reliability.

Have You Ever Wondered

. . . how can you judge information from e-mail? E-mail is often used to advertise or bring people to websites; health information may be biased toward that goal. To judge it, consider the origin of the message and its purpose.

. . . how to judge food scares that circulate through e-mail? Being 100 percent sure about these food scares takes research. What appears unsolicited in your e-mail is likely a hoax (1) if it wasn't written by the e-mail sender, (2) if you're asked to forward the e-mail, (3) if it claims not to be a hoax or an urban legend, (4) if it appeals to your emotions, and (5) if it doesn't cite a legitimate source or a credible website. Read critically for obvious false claims, poor logic, and lack of common sense. If you're still not sure, you might want to check websites such as www.quackwatch.com or www.urbanlegends.com that debunk common food myths.

● *Have a qualified nutrition expert host forums and chatrooms?* Many unsponsored bulletin boards bring interested people together, with chat from undisclosed sources who often aren't experts. Be wary! The site should provide the terms of using the service. Before you join in, follow the discussion, then decide.

● *Can you contact the online site's owners with problems, feedback, and questions?*

"Well"-Connected Links

Search engines list legitimate and less reliable websites side-by-side; you need skills to sort them out. Tap health-related resources that indicate high standards:

● To speed your search use gateway sites that link to responsible organizations—for example, the U.S. government's site (www.nutrition.gov). The U.S. Department of Health and Human Services' Healthfinder (www.healthfinder.gov) hyperlinks to hundreds of responsible sites, as does the gateway in the Academy of Nutrition and Dietetics' website (www.eatright.org).

● Review more than one website on the same nutrition topic. With information often presented in "sound bites," usually one site isn't complete enough.

● Look for sites with the HONcode symbol, showing they adhere to the HONcode (Health On the Net Foundation) principles. An example: the WebMD website provides online, consumer-focused health information (www.webmd.com). These sites voluntarily comply with a code of conduct for health and medical websites. HON is an honor symbol and system, so still be a careful online consumer.

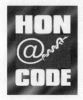

A symbol identifying a URAC-accredited health website is another clue to its reliability; URAC sets high standards for health care.

● Ask a nutrition expert, such as an RD or a DTR, who can see nuances of website bias and inaccuracy. If you find news of interest on the Internet, such as about a phytonutrient link to health, or a dietary supplement, print the information with the name and address of the website or blog; take it to your health-care provider or a nutrition expert for a perspective.

To find reliable nutrition and health websites, see "Resources You Can Use" at the back of this book.

E-Nutrition Advice: Just for You

With a few clicks on your computer or handheld mobile device, you can calculate your BMI, assess your food choices, add to your grocery list, even tie in to online weight-control counseling. But consider this:

● If you wish, use quick, online assessments and counseling on your food choices, physical activity, and health issues, but don't replace your healthcare provider. For a reliable diagnosis and prescribed eating plan, work with a qualified healthcare provider in person, who can review your medical history. Many registered dietitians offer online counseling.

For interactive online tools refer to the USDA's fnic.nal.usda.gov consumer website or check MyPlate, www.ChooseMyPlate.gov. You'll also find a kids' section for food and nutrition games, video clips, and other interactive, fun activities.

● For the same reasons, get advice or a prescription for a dietary supplement from your doctor. As an aside, buying supplements online may, or may not, cost less, and the quality is uneven.

● Even on trustworthy healthcare sites that do online nutrition assessments and counseling, there's a wrinkle: *privacy.* To protect the privacy of your records and avoid a Pandora's box of e-marketing, provide personal data on encrypted, or secured, sites only. If a "closed padlock" appears on the web page, the data you provide are encrypted and secure. And pay attention to "alarms" on the site that warn that you're moving from secure to insecure parts of the website.

As you surf the Internet, keep track of your path. You may be unaware when you pass from a reliable to an unreliable source of information.

Case against Health Fraud

Can you "lose weight while you sleep"? Can a dietary supplement assure "no more arthritic pain" or "cure AIDS"? Can a device guarantee "a bigger bustline" or "spot reduction"?

Americans spend billions of dollars annually on products and services that make such claims. Health quackery is the most common type of fraud aimed at the elderly and others. Easy remedies are hard to resist! Yet many are simply useless; others, potentially harmful. Either way, it's health fraud.

Nutrition quackery thrives among people who are uninformed or already misinformed, desperate for help, overconfident about possible risks, or alienated from traditional healthcare. Quacks can manipulate more easily those who are already leaning in their direction, perhaps with ploys that seem reasonable: "We really care about you." "What have you got to lose?" "Science doesn't have all the answers." "We treat medicine's failures."

Health fraud means promoting, for financial gain, a health remedy that doesn't work—or hasn't yet been proven to work or isn't supported by science. The remedy may be a device, treatment, service, plan, special foods, or other product. Rampant health fraud is often linked to nutrition—perhaps to a dietary supplement, a herbal product, a weight-loss device, or a new diet program.

So what is quackery? The term comes from the term "quacksalver," referring to medieval peddlers of salves who sounded like quacking ducks when talking to promote their wares.

So-called quacks promote health fraud. Their motivation may be strictly financial gain. But often, quacks sincerely believe in the value of their product, treatment, or service but lack both scientific understanding and expertise backed by credentials.

Play "Ten Questions"

Sound too good to be true? To avoid the lure, arm yourself with these questions—even when you aren't suspicious! Ask: Does the promotion of a nutrition product, regimen, service, treatment, or device . . .

YES   NO

☐   ☐   **1.** Try to lure you with scare tactics, emotional appeals, or perhaps a "money-back guarantee" ?

☐   ☐   **2.** Promise to "revitalize," "detoxify," or "balance your body with nature"? Claim to increase your stamina, stimulate your body's healing power, or boost your energy level?

☐   ☐   **3.** Use personal anecdotes or testimonials as "proof" rather than sound science?

☐   ☐   **4.** Advise supplements as "insurance" for everyone? Recommend very large doses of nutrients? "Very large" is significantly more than 100 percent of the Daily Values. *See the appendices.*

☐   ☐   **5.** Claim it can "treat," "cure," or "prevent" diverse health problems . . . from arthritis to cancer to sexual impotence?

☐   ☐   **6.** Make unrealistic claims: "reverse the aging process," "cure disease," or "quick, easy approach"?

☐   ☐   **7.** Blame the food supply as the source of health or behavior problems? Belittle government regulations? Or discredit the advice of recognized medical authorities?

☐   ☐   **8.** Claim that its "natural" benefits surpass those of "synthetic" products?

☐   ☐   **9.** Mention a "secret formula"? Fail to list ingredients on its label or to state possible side effects?

☐   ☐   **10.** Come from a "nutrition expert" without accepted credentials? Does he or she also sell the product?

Now score yourself:

In this game of "Ten Questions," you might spot quackery with just one "yes" answer! Here's why.

1. *Fact:* Playing on emotion, misinformation, or even fear is common among nonscientific pseudo-experts. Emotional words used to promote a product can be an instant tip-off to quackery: "guaranteed," "breakthrough," and "miraculous." So are false claims that foods or additives are "deadly poisons."

2. *Fact:* Pseudo-medical jargon such as "detoxify" or "balance your body chemistry" suggests misinformation. These terms have no meaning in physiology. A supplement can't increase your strength, immunity, stamina, or energy level, either. *For more about supplements promoted to athletes, see "Ergogenic Aids: No Substitute for Training" in chapter 20.*

3. *Fact:* Nutrition is a science, based on fact not emotion or belief. Be skeptical of case histories and testimonials from satisfied users—if that's the only proof that a product works. Instead look for science-based evidence from a reputable institution or a qualified health expert. Without scientific evidence, a reported "cure" actually may be a placebo effect; its benefit may be psychological, not physical. The person may have been misdiagnosed in the first place. Even chronic ailments don't always have symptoms all the time.

4. *Fact:* Everyone does *not* need a vitamin supplement! So ignore the hype! On the contrary, taking too much may be harmful. *See chapter 23, "Dietary Supplements: Use and Misuse."* Most healthy people can get enough nutrients with a varied, balanced eating plan. Quacks rarely say who does *not* need a supplement. *See chapter 10 for more about healthful eating.*

5. *Fact:* No nutrition regimen, device, or product can treat all that ails you. And they can't cure many health conditions, including arthritis, cancer, and sexual impotence. Even when they're part of credible treatment or prevention strategies, nutrition factors are typically just one part of an overall healthcare plan.

6. *Fact:* Claims that sound too good to be true probably are. They say what people want to hear: simple cures and magic ways to change what's imperfect. There's no such thing as a quick fix or a magic bullet.

7. *Fact:* Misleading tactics often belittle the food supply, government regulation, and the established medical community. They may claim that the traditional health community is suppressing their work. Instead they may call for "freedom of choice". . . and describe

Play "Ten Questions" *(continued)*

unproved methods as alternatives to current, proven methods. By discrediting traditional approaches, quacks attempt to funnel healthcare dollars toward their own financial gain.

8. *Fact:* There's nothing magical about supplements promoted as "natural." Even substances found in nature can have natural toxins, with potent, druglike effects.

9. *Fact:* By law, a medication must carry product information on its packaging. That includes the product's ingredients, use, dosage, warnings, precautions, and what to do if adverse reactions occur. However, products or regimens sold through quackery may not report all this information.

10. *Fact:* Be wary when someone tries to assess your health status, then offers to sell you a remedy, such as a routine dietary supplement. Invalid tests may be hard to distinguish from legitimate clinical assessments. Those often used by quacks include hair analysis, iridology, and herbal crystallization analysis, among others. Computerized questionnaires can't supply enough information either to determine your need for a supplement. Get an opinion from a qualified health professional instead.

Quackery underlies many weight loss or gain regimens, too. *To judge their effectiveness and safety, see "Questions to Ask . . . about Weight Loss Programs" in chapter 2.*

Health fraud and misleading tactics have grown dramatically in recent decades. Why? Among the reasons, an unprecedented interest in personal healthcare. In general, people today take more personal responsibility for staying healthy. That interest has created a huge demand for products and services that promote health; while legitimate business uses this opportunity to provide products, treatments, and services that do have scientifically proven benefits, this same wave of interest also has spawned a fanfare of health fraud and quackery, leaving people more vulnerable than ever.

Another common reason for growing health fraud: hope for a quick or easy "health fix." Some people may count on fraudulent products to undo the results of an unhealthful lifestyle. It's not that simple—even if misleading tactics lead you to believe otherwise. With looser government regulation, the misuse of dietary supplements—and hype surrounding them—have grown dramatically. Today supplement manufacturers need to prove harm, not safety. That allows claims for supplements to appear more credible than they really are. *For more about the use and misuse of supplements, see chapter 23.*

Registered dietitians must follow the Academy of Nutrition and Dietetics' Code of Ethics guidelines if they sell supplements.

What Are the Consequences?

Nutrition quackery exploits consumers, and it carries significant health and economic risks along the way:

- *False hopes.* Dream on! Quacks may promise—but unsound nutrition advice, products, or services won't prevent or cure disease or replace unhealthful living.
- *A substitute for reliable healthcare.* False hopes, created through quackery, may delay or replace proper health promotion, medical care, or follow-up treatment. If you follow quackery, you may lose something you can't retrieve: time for effective treatment!
- *Interference with sound eating and lifestyle habits.* That happens when misinformation replaces science-based guidance.
- *Unneeded expense.* In the best case, some products and services touted by quacks simply don't work—yet cause no harm. Why waste hard-earned money on devices, products, and services that have no effect?
- *Potential harm.* Nutrition quackery also can put your health at risk. Taking very large doses of some vitamins and minerals, in the form of dietary supplements, can have toxic side effects. For example, excessive amounts of vitamin A during pregnancy increase the chances of birth defects. Inappropriate supplement

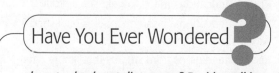

Have You Ever Wondered

. . . how to check out diet scams? Besides talking with a nutrition expert, check the Federal Trade Commission (www.ftc.gov), which may list diet scams it's prosecuted.

use can lead to harmful drug-nutrient interactions. For example, taking vitamin K can be risky if you take blood-thinning drugs. *For more about specific vitamins and minerals, see chapter 6.*

Over-the-counter herbal products, marketed as dietary supplements, are sources of potent drugs. Yet, unlike medications, herbal products aren't well regulated. *See "Herbals and Other Botanicals: Help or Harm?" in chapter 23.*

Quackery: What You Can Do

No one has to be the victim of nutrition fraud. To protect yourself, know how to identify fraud and quackery, and where to find science-based nutrition information.

● Retain a healthy skepticism as your best defense. Take time to be well informed before you invest in a nutrition product, treatment, or service. *Give it the "Ten Questions" test in this chapter.*

● Seek advice from reliable sources. If you're suspicious about a statement, product, or service, contact a credible nutrition source—a registered dietitian,

Spotting a Fraud

Does it sound too good to be true? Then it probably is! The Federal Trade Commission (FTC) advises: Be wary of healthcare products described with claims such as these:

● "Natural" or "non-toxic," suggesting safe or no side effects
● "Scientific breakthrough," "miraculous cure," "secret ingredient," "ancient remedy," "proven science"
● "Money-back" guarantee
● Testimonials with "amazing results" (Testimonials, often undocumented, are no substitute for true scientific evidence.)
● Effective cure for a wide range of ailments
● Impressive-sounding medical terms
● Available from only one source; payment required in advance
● Websites with no company name, physical address, phone number, or other contact information

Ten Red Flags of Junk Science

A new health or nutrition report? Before you jump to conclusions, check it out. Any combination of these signs should send up a red flag of suspicion.

1. Recommendations that promise a quick fix
2. Dire warnings of danger from a single product or regimen
3. Claims that sound too good to be true
4. Simplistic conclusions drawn from a complex study
5. Recommendations based on a single study
6. Dramatic statements that are refuted by reputable scientific organizations
7. Lists of "good" and "bad" foods
8. Recommendations made to help sell a product
9. Recommendations based on studies published without peer review
10. Recommendations from studies that ignore differences among individuals or groups

Source: Developed by the Food and Nutrition Science Alliance (FANSA).

your public health department, the medical or nutrition department of a nearby college or university, or your county Extension office. *See "Need Nutrition Advice?" in this chapter.*

● Report nutrition fraud. If you suspect that a statement, product, or service is fraudulent or false, inquire with the appropriate government agency or file a complaint.

● *To the Postal Service.* Contact your postmaster or someone else in the Postal Service if you've been the victim—or target—of nutrition fraud through the mail. It's illegal to use the Postal Service to make false claims about or to sell fraudulent products or services.

● *To the FDA.* Make inquiries or file complaints about false claims for dietary supplements with the U.S. Food and Drug Administration. That includes concerns about inadequate information on package labels.

● *To the FTC.* For questions or concerns about false or misleading claims in advertising, contact the Federal Trade Commission.

Resources You Can Use

Looking for sound nutrition information? You have many reliable resources: professional associations, health agencies, government agencies, and credible nutrition newsletters. Besides brochures, booklets, and consumer hotlines, many provide reliable online food- and nutrition-information websites, apps, blogs, forums, e-newsletters, RSS feeds, podcasts, videos, and more. Your local hospital, public health, Extension service, and many food industry groups are other reliable resources you might tap.

General Nutrition

Academy of Nutrition and Dietetics
120 South Riverside Plaza, Suite 2000
Chicago, IL 60606-6995
www.eatright.org
800-877-1600

Find a Registered Dietitian
www.eatright.org/iframe/ FindRD.aspx

Center for Nutrition Policy and Promotion
U.S. Department of Agriculture
3101 Park Center Drive, 10th Floor
Alexandria, VA 22302-1594
703/305-7600
www.cnpp.usda.gov

Cooperative Extension Service
(Contact your state's land-grant university.)

Dietitians of Canada
480 University Avenue, Suite 604
Toronto, Ontario Canada
M5G1V2
416/596-0857
www.dietitians.ca

Food and Nutrition Information Center
National Agricultural Library
U.S. Department of Agriculture, Room 105
10301 Baltimore Avenue
Beltsville, MD 20705-2351
301/504-5714
www.fnic.nal.usda.gov

USDA National Nutrient Database for Standard Reference (food composition)
www.ars.usda.gov/ba/bhnrc/ndl

Food and Nutrition Service
U.S. Department of Agriculture
3101 Park Center Drive
Alexandria, VA 22302
www.fns.usda.gov/fns

Supplemental Nutrition Assistance Program (SNAP)
www.fns.usda.gov/snap/

Women, Infants, and Children (WIC) Program
www.fns.usda.gov/wic

International Food Information Council Foundation (IFIC)
1100 Connecticut Avenue, NW, Suite 430
Washington, DC 20036
202/296-6540
www.foodinsight.org

National Academy of Sciences/Health and Medicine
500 Fifth Avenue, NW
Washington, DC 20001
202/334-2000
www.nationalacademies.org/ health

Society for Nutrition Education and Behavior
9100 Purdue Road, Suite 200
Indianapolis, IN 46268
800/235-6690
www.sneb.org

Tufts University Hirsh Health Sciences Library (gateway site)
www.library.tufts.edu/hsl/ subjectguides/nutrition.html

U.S. Department of Agriculture
1400 Independence Avenue, SW
Washington, DC 20250
www.usda.gov

U.S. Government (gateway to health and nutrition sites)
www.nutrition.gov
www.healthfinder.gov
www.kids.gov
www.health.gov

Evidence Based Libraries

Academy of Nutrition and Dietetics (subscription)
www.andevidencelibrary.com or *www.eal.org*

U.S. National Library of Medicine, National Institutes of Health, USHHS
www.nlm.nih.gov/bsd/ pmresources.html

US Department of Agriculture
www.nutritionevidencelibrary .gov

Dietary Supplements

National Center for Alternative and Complementary Medicine
9000 Rockville Pike
Bethesda, MD 20892
888/644-6226
www.nccam.nih.gov

NIH/Office of Dietary Supplements
6100 Executive Blvd.
Bethesda, MD 20892
301/435-2920
www.ods.od.nih.gov

Dietary Supplement Ingredient Database
dietarysupplementdatabase .usda.nih.gov

U.S. Food and Drug Administration
www.cfsan.fda.gov/~dms/ supplmnt.html

U.S. Pharmacopeia
12601 Twinbrook Parkway
Rockville, MD 20852-1790
800/227-8772
www.usp.org

Food Safety, Labeling, and Advertising

American Association of Poision Control Centers
National hotline to local centers: 800/222-1222
www.aapcc.org

Academy of Nutrition and Dietetics/Con Agra
www.homefoodsafety.org

Centers for Disease Control and Prevention
1600 Clifton Rd. Atlanta, GA 30333
800/CDC-INFO (800/232-4636)
www.cdc.gov/foodsafety

Center for Food Safety and Applied Nutrition
Outreach and Information Center
5100 Paint Branch Parkway
HFS-555
College Park, MD 20740-3835
888/723-3366 or 888/SAFE-FOOD
www.fda.gov/food

Federal Trade Commission (FTC)
600 Pennsylvania Avenue, NW, Washington, DC 20580
877/FTC-HELP (877/328-4357)
(Or contact your regional FTC office.)
www.ftc.gov

U.S. Food and Drug Administration (FDA)
10903 New Hampshire Avenue
Silver Spring, MD 20993-0002
888/INFO-FDA
(888/463-6332)
(Or contact your regional FDA office.)
www.fda.gov/food/foodsafety

Food Safety and Inspection Service
U.S. Department of Agriculture
1400 Independence Avenue, SW
Washington, D.C. 20250
888/MPHotline (888/674-6854)
www.fsis.usda.gov
www.befoodsafe.gov

USDA Meat and Poultry Hotline
888/674-6854 or 800/256-7072
www.fsis.usda.gov/mph

National Lead Information Center
1200 Pennsylvania Avenue, NW
Mail Code 7404T
Washington, DC 20460
800/424-LEAD (800/424-5323)
www.epa.gov/lead

The Partnership for Food Safety Education, Fight Bac
www.fightbac.org

U.S. Environmental Protection Agency
Areil Rios Building
1200 Pennsylvania Avenue, NW
Washington, DC 20490

www.water.epa.gov/drink
Safe Drinking Water Hotline
800/426-4791

U.S. Government (gateway to food safety sites)
www.foodsafety.gov

Water Quality Association
International Headquarters & Laboratory
4151 Naperville Road
Lisle, IL 60532-1088
630/505-0160
www.wqa.org

Food Sensitivities

American Academy of Allergy, Asthma, & Immunology
555 East Wells Street, Suite 1100
Milwaukee, WI 53202
414/272-3823
www.aaaai.org

Celiac Disease Foundation
13251 Ventura Blvd., Suite 1
Studio City, CA 91604
818/990-2354
www.celiac.org

Celiac Sprue Association
P.O. Box 31700
Omaha, NE 68131-0700
402/558-0600 or
877/CSA-4CSA
www.csaceliacs.org

Children's P.K.U. Network
3970 Via de la Valle, Suite 120
Del Mar, CA 92014
800/377-6677
www.pkunetwork.org

Food Allergy & Anaphylaxis Network
11781 Lee Jackson Hwy., Suite 160
Fairfax, VA 22033-3309
800/929-4040
www.foodallergy.org

Gluten Intolerance Group
31214 124th Avenue SE
Auburn, WA 98092-3667
253/833-6655
www.gluten.net

National Digestive Diseases Information Clearinghouse (NDDIC)
2 Information Way
Bethesda, MD 20892-3570

800/891-5389
www.digestive.niddk.nih.gov

Maternal, Infant, Child, and Adolescent Nutrition

American Academy of Pediatrics
141 Northwest Point Boulevard
Elk Grove Village, IL 60007-1098
847/434-4000
www.aap.org

The American Congress of Obstetricians and Gynecologists
409 12th Street, SW
PO Box 96920
Washington, DC 20090-6920
202/638-5577
www.acog.org/publications /patient_education

La Leche League International
957 Plum Grove Road
Schaumburg, IL 60173-4808
800/LALECHE
(800/525-3243)
www.lalecheleague.org

March of Dimes
1275 Mamaroneck Avenue
White Plains, NY 10605
914/997-4488
www.marchofdimes.com

National Healthy Mothers, Healthy Babies Coalition
2000 N. Beauregard Street, 6th Floor
Alexandria, VA 22311
703/837-4792
www.hmhb.org

Nemours Center for Children's Health Media
Nemours Foundation
www.kidshealth.org

School Nutrition Association
120 Waterfront Street, Suite 300
National Harbor, MD 20745
301/686-3100
www.asfsa.org

Shaping America's Youth, Academic Network, LLC
120 NW 9th Avenue, Suite 216
Portland, OR 97209-3326

800/SAY-9221
www.shapingamericasyouth.org

Office on Women's Health, U.S. Department of Health and Human Services
200 Independence Avenue, SW
Washington, DC 20201
800/994-9662
www.womenshealth.gov

Nutrition and Aging

American Association of Retired Persons
601 E Street, NW
Washington, DC 20049
888/OUR-AARP
(888/687-2277)
www.aarp.org

Elder Care Locator
800/677-1116
www.eldercare.gov

Meals on Wheels Association of America
203 S. Union Street
Alexandria, VA 22314
703/548-5558
www.mowaa.org

National Association of Area Agencies on Aging
1730 Rhode Island Avenue NW, Suite 1200
Washington, DC 20036
202/872-0888
www.n4a.org

National Association of Nutrition and Aging Services Programs
1612 K Street, NW, Suite 400
Washington, DC 20006
202/682-6899
www.nanasp.org

National Institute on Aging
Building 31, Room 5C-27
31 Center Drive, MSC 2292
Bethesda, MD 20892
301/496-1752
www.nia.nih.gov

General Health and Disease Prevention/ Treatment

General
American Academy of Family Physicians
11400 Tomahawk Creek Parkway

Leawood, KS 66211-2672
800/274-2237 or
    913/906-6000
www.aafp.org

**American Medical
    Association**
515 North State Street
Chicago, IL 60654
800/621-8335
www.ama-assn.org

**American Public Health
    Association**
800 I Street, NW
Washington, DC 20001
202/777-2742
www.apha.org

**Centers for Disease Control
    and Prevention**
1600 Clifton Road Northeast
Atlanta, GA 30333
800/232-4636
www.cdc.gov

**Medline Plus/U.S. National
    Library of Medicine**
8600 Rockville Pike
Bethesda, MD 20894
www.nlm.nih.gov/medlineplus

**National Center for Health
    Statistics**
Centers for Disease Control
    and Protection
3311 Toledo Road
Hyattsville, MD 20782
800/232-4636
cdc.gov/nchs

National Health Council
1730 M Street, NW, Suite 500
Washington, DC 20036
202/785-3910
www.nhcouncil.org

**National Health
    Information Center**
www.health.gov/nhic

**National Institutes of
    Health**
9000 Rockville Pike
Bethesda, MD 20892
301/496-4000
www.nih.gov

**National Wellness Institute,
    Inc.**
P.O. Box 827
Stevens Point, WI 54481-0827
715/342-2969
www.nationalwellness.org

**Office of Disease Prevention
    and Health Promotion**
P.O. Box 1133
Washington, DC 20013-1133
800/336-4797
odphp.osophs.dhhs.gov

Healthy People 2020
www.healthypeople.gov

**Office of Minority Health
    Resource Center**
U.S. Department of Health and
    Human Services
P.O. Box 37337
Washington, DC 20013-7337
800/444-6472
www.minorityhealth.hhs.gov

**U.S. Department of Health
    and Human Services**
200 Independence Avenue, SW
Washington, DC 20201
202/619-0257
www.hhs.gov
www.healthfinder.gov

Alcoholism

**National Institute on Alcohol
    Abuse and Alcoholism**
5635 Fishers Lane, MSC 9304
Bethesda, MD 20892-9304
301/443-3860
www.niaaa.nih.gov

**National Council on
    Alcoholism and Drug
    Dependence, Inc.**
244 East 58th Street, 4th Floor
New York, NY 10022
212/269-7797 or
    800/NCA-CALL
www.ncadd.org

Cancer

American Cancer Society
1599 Clifton Road, NE
Atlanta, GA 30329-4251
800/227-2345
www.cancer.org

**American Institute for
    Cancer Research**
1759 R Street, NW
Washington, DC 20009
202/328-7744
www.aicr.org

National Cancer Institute
NCI Office of Communications
    and Education, Public
    Inquiries Office

6116 Executive Boulevard,
    Suite 300
Bethesda, MD 20892-8322
800/4-CANCER (800/422-
    6237) or 301/435-3848
www.cancer.gov

Cardiovascular (Heart)
Disease

**American Heart
    Association**
7272 Greenville Avenue
Dallas, TX 75231-4596
800/AHA-USA1
    (800/242-8721)
www.heart.org

**National Heart, Lung, and
    Blood Institute/NIH**
P.O. Box 30105
Bethesda, MD 20824-0105
301/592-8573
www.nhlbi.nih.gov

Diabetes

**American Diabetes
    Association**
Attn.: National Call Center
1701 North Beauregard Street
Alexandria, VA 22311
800/342-2383
www.diabetes.org

Joslin Diabetes Center
One Joslin Place
Boston, MA 02215
617/732-2400
www.joslin.org

**Juvenile Diabetes
    Foundation International**
26 Broadway,14th Floor
New York, NY 10004
800/JDF-CURE
    (800/533-2873)
www.jdf.org

**National Diabetes Informa-
    tion Clearinghouse**
1 Information Way
Bethesda, MD 20892-3560
800/860-8747
www. diabetes.niddk.nih.gov

Digestive Disease

**Digestive Disease National
    Coalition**
507 Capitol Court NE, Suite
    200
Washington, DC 20002

202/544-7497
www.ddnc.org

**National Digestive
    Diseases Information
    Clearinghouse/NIH**
2 Information Way
Bethesda, MD 20892-3570
800/891-5389
www.digestive.niddk.nih.gov

Eating Disorders

**National Association of
    Anorexia Nervosa and
    Associated Disorders**
P.O. Box 640
Naperville, IL 60566
630/577-1333
www.anad.org

**National Eating Disorders
    Organization**
165 West 46th Street
New York, NY 10036
212/575-6200
*www.nationaleatingdisorders
    .org*

Oral Health

American Dental Association
211 East Chicago Avenue
Chicago, IL 60611-2678
312/440-2500
www.ada.org

Osteoporosis

**National Osteoporosis
    Foundation**
1150 17th Street, NW,
    Suite 850
Washington, DC 20036
800/231-4222
www.nof.org

Weight

Healthy Weight Network
402 South 14th Street
Hettinger, ND 58639
701/567-2646
www.healthyweightnetwork.com

Overeaters Anonymous
P.O. Box 44020
Rio Rancho, NM 87174
505/891-2664
www.oa.org

Shape Up America!
P.O. Box 149
Clyde Park, MT 59018
www.shapeup.org

**Weight-control Information
Network**
1 WIN Way
Bethesda, MD 20892–3665
877/946–4627
win.niddk.nih.gov/index.htm

Sports Nutrition and Physical Activity

**American Alliance for
Health, Physical
Education, Recreation,
and Dance**
1900 Association Drive
Reston, VA 20191-1598
800/213-7193
www.aahperd.org

**American College of Sports
Medicine**
401 West Michigan Street
Indianapolis, IN 46202-3233
317/637-9200
www.acsm.org

**American Council for Fitness
and Nutrition**
1350 I Street, Suite 300
Washington, DC 20005
800/953-1700
www.acfn.org

**American Council on
Exercise**
4851 Paramount Drive
San Diego, CA 92123
800/825-3626
www.acefitness.org

**America on the Move
Foundation**
www.americaonthemove.org

**American Running
Association**
4405 East-West Highway,
Suite 405
Bethesda, MD 20814
800/776-2732
www.americanrunning.org

**Centers for Disease Control
and Prevention**
*www.cdc.gov/nccdphp/dnpa/ph
ysical/index.htm*

**International Society of
Sports Nutrition**
600 Pembrook Drive
Woodland Park, CO 80863
866/740-4776
www.sportsnutritionsociety.org

**National Physical Activity
Plan**
921 Assembly Street,
Suite 212
Columbia, SC 29208
866/365-5122
www.physicalactivityplan.org

**President's Council on
Physical Fitness Sports &
Nutrition**
1101 Wootton Parkway,
Suite 560
Rockville, MD 20852
240/276-9567
www.fitness.gov
www.presidentschallenge.org
www.fitness.gov

**Women's Sports
Foundation**
Eisenhower Park
East Meadow, NY 11554
800/227-3988
*www.womenssportsfoundation
.org*

YMCA of the USA
101 North Wacker Drive
Chicago, IL 60606
800/USA-YMCA
 (800/872-9622)
www.ymca.net

Vegetarian Eating

**North American Vegetarian
Society**
P.O. Box 72
Dolgeville, NY 13329
518/568-7970
www.navs-online.org

**The Vegetarian Resource
Group**
P.O. Box 1463
Baltimore, MD 21203
410/366-VEGE (8343)
www.vrg.org

Agriculture and Food Technology

**Agricultural Research
Library/USDA**
*www.ars.usda.gov/Services/
docs.htm?docid=1274*

**Alliance to Feed the
Future**
1100 Connecticut Avenue NW,
Suite 430
Washington, DC 20036
*www.alliancetofeedthefuture
.org*

**Biotechnology Industry
Organization**
1201 Maryland Avenue, SW,
Suite 900
Washington, DC 20024
202/962-9200
www.bio.org

**Council for Biotechnology
Information**
1201 Maryland Avenue, SW,
Suite 900
Washington, DC 20024
202/962-9200
www.whybiotech.com

**Institute of Food
Technologists**
525 W. Van Buren,
Suite 1000
Chicago, IL 60607
312/782-8424
www.ift.org

**International Food Additives
Council**
5775 Peachtree-Dunwoody
Road, Suite 500-G
Atlanta, GA 30342
404/252-3663
www.foodadditives.org

**National Institute of Food
and Agriculture/United
States Department of
Agriculture (formerly
CSREES)**
1400 Independence Avenue
SW, Stop 2201
Washington, DC 20250-2201
202-720-4423
www.nifa.usda.gov

Organic Trade Association
28 Vernon Street, Suite 413
Brattleboro, VT 05301
802/275-3800
www.ota.com

**Sustainable Agriculture
Research & Education/
National Institute of Food
and Agriculture, USDA**
1122 Patapsco Building
University of Maryland
College Park, MD 20742-6715
www.sare.org

Health Fraud

**American Council on Science
and Health**
1995 Broadway, Suite 202
New York, NY 10023-5882
866/905-2694
www.acsh.org

**National Council against
Health Fraud**
119 Foster Street
Peabody, MA 01960
978/532-9383
www.ncahf.org

Quackwatch, Inc.
www.quackwatch.org

Food Service, Food Marketing

Food Marketing Institute
2345 Crystal Drive,
Suite 800
Arlington, VA 22202
202/452-8444
www.fmi.org

**Grocery Manufacturers of
America**
1350 I (Eye) Street,
Suite 300
Washington, DC 20005
202/639-590
www.gmaonline.org

**National Food Service
Management Association**
The University of Mississippi
6 Jeanette Phillips Drive
P.O. Drawer 188
University, MS 38677-0188
662/915-7658 or
 800/321-3054
www.nfsmi.org

**National Restaurant
Association**
1200 17th Street, NW
Washington, DC 20036
202/331-5900
www.restaurant.org

Healthy Dining Finder
healthydiningfinder.com

**USDA Agricultural
Marketing Service,
Farmers Market
Search**
*apps.ams.usda.gov/Farmers
Markets/*

Food Industry Associations

Alaska Seafood Marketing Institute
www.alaskaseafood.org

Almond Board of California
www.almondboard.com

American Beverage Association
www.ameribev.org

American Egg Board
www.aeb.org

American Lamb Board
www.americanlamb.com

American Meat Institute
www.meatami.com

The California Avocado Commission
www.avocado.org

California Dried Plum Board
www.californiadriedplums.org

California Fig Advisory Board
californiafigs.com

California Olive Committee
calolive.org

California Olive Oil Council
www.cooc.com

California Raisin Marketing Board
www.calraisins.org

California Strawberry Commission
www.calstrawberry.com

California Walnut Board and Commission
www.walnuts.org

Calorie Control Council
www.caloriecontrol.org

Canned Food Alliance
www.mealtime.org

Canola Council of Canada
www.canolainfo.org

Cherry Marketing Institute
www.choosecherries.com

Corn Refiners Association
www.corn.org

The Cranberry Institute
www.cranberryinstitute.org

Distilled Spirits Council of the United States
www.discus.org

Egg Nutrition Center
www.eggnutritioncenter.org

Georgia Pecan Commission
www.georgiapecans.org

Grain Foods Foundation
www.gowiththegrain.org

The Glutamate Association
www.msgfacts.com

Hazelnut Marketing Board
oregonhazelnuts.org

International Formula Council
www.infantformula.org

International Bottled Water Association
www.bottledwater.org

The International Tree Nut Council
www.nuthealth.org

The McCormick Science Institute (herbs and spices)
www.mccormicksscienceinstitute.com

Mushroom Council
www.mushroomcouncil.org

National Cattlemen's Beef Association Beef Checkoff
www.beefnutrition.org

National Chicken Council
www.eatchicken.com

National Coffee Association of USA
www.ncausa.org

National Dairy Council (Dairy Management, Inc.)
www.dairyinfo.com
www.nationaldairycouncil.org

National Fisheries Institute
www.aboutseafood.com

National Frozen and Refrigerated Foods Association
www.nfraweb.org

National Pasta Association
www.ilovepasta.org

National Peanut Board
www.nationalpeanutboard.org

National Pork Board
www.porkbeinspired.com

National Turkey Federation
www.eatturkey.com

National Watermelon Promotion Board
www.watermelon.org

North Carolina SweetPotato Commission
www.ncsweetpotatoes.com

The Peanut Institute
www.peanut-institute.org

Pistachio Health
www.pistachiohealth.com

Produce for Better Health Foundation
www.fruitsandveggiesmore matters.org

Produce Marketing Association
www.pma.com

Salt Institute
www.saltinstitute.org

Snack Food Association
www.sfa.org

Salmon of the Americas
www.salmonoftheamericas.com

The Soyfoods Council
thesoyfoodscouncil.com

The Sugar Association
www.sugar.org

The Tea Association of the U.S.A.
www.teausa.org

Tuna Council
www.healthytuna.com

United Fresh Fruit & Vegetable Association
www.unitedfresh.org

United Soybean Board
www.soyconnection.org

United States Potato Board
www.healthypotato.com

USA Pears
www.usapears.com

USA Rice Federation
www.usarice.com

US Dry Bean Council
www.beansforhealth.org

US Dry Pea & Lentil Council
www.pea-lentil.com

US Highbush Blueberry Council
www.blueberry.org

Walnut Marketing Board
www.walnuts.org

Wheat Foods Council
www.wheatfoods.org

Whole Grains Council
www.wholegrainscouncil.org

Nutrition Newsletters/ Websites/Blogs

Consumer Reports on Health
www.consumerreports.org

Environmental Nutrition
www.environmentalnutrition .com

Women's Nutrition Connection
Weill Medical College of Cornell University
www.womensnutritionconnec tion.com

Mayo Clinic Health Letter
www.healthletter.mayoclinic .com

Nutrition Blog Network: Powered by Dietitians (aggregate site)
nutritionblognetwork.com

RDs Weigh In/Academy of Nutrition and Dietetics
www.eatright.org/rdsweighin

Supermarket Savvy
www.supermarketsavvy.com

Tufts University Health and Nutrition Letter
www.tuftshealthletter.com

University of California, Berkeley Wellness Letter
www.wellnessletter.com

WebMD
www.webmd.com

Appendices

Dietary Guidelines for Americans, 2010, Key Recommendations

Balance Calories to Manage Weight

● Prevent and/or reduce overweight and obesity through improved eating and physical activity behaviors.

● Control total calorie intake to manage body weight. For people who are overweight or obese, this means consuming fewer calories from foods and beverages.

● Increase physical activity and reduce time spent in sedentary behaviors.

● Maintain appropriate calorie balance during each stage of life—childhood, adolescence, adulthood, pregnancy and breastfeeding, and older age.

Foods and Food Components to Reduce

● Reduce daily sodium intake to less than 2,300 milligrams (mg) and further reduce intake to 1,500 mg among persons who are 51 and older and those of any age who are African American or have hypertension, diabetes, or chronic kidney disease. The 1,500 mg recommendation applies to about half of the U.S. population, including children, and the majority of adults.

● Consume less than 10 percent of calories from saturated fatty acids by replacing them with monounsaturated and polyunsaturated fatty acids.

● Consume less than 300 mg per day of dietary cholesterol.

● Keep *trans* fatty acid consumption as low as possible by limiting foods that contain synthetic sources of *trans* fats, such as partially hydrogenated oils, and by limiting other solid fats.

● Reduce the intake of calories from solid fats and added sugars.

● Limit the consumption of foods that contain refined grains, especially refined grain foods that contain solid fats, added sugars, and sodium.

● If alcohol is consumed, it should be consumed in moderation—up to one drink per day for women and two drinks per day for men—and only by adults of legal drinking age.[1]

Foods and Nutrients to Increase

Individuals should meet the following recommendations as part of a healthy eating pattern while staying within their calorie needs.

● Increase vegetable and fruit intake.

● Eat a variety of vegetables, especially dark-green and red and orange vegetables and beans and peas.

● Consume at least half of all grains as whole grains. Increase whole-grain intake by replacing refined grains with whole grains.

● Increase intake of fat-free or low-fat milk and milk products, such as milk, yogurt, cheese, or fortified soy beverages.[2]

● Choose a variety of protein foods, which include seafood, lean meat and poultry, eggs, beans and peas, soy products, and unsalted nuts and seeds.

● Increase the amount and variety of seafood consumed by choosing seafood in place of some meat and poultry.

[1] The Dietary Guidelines for Americans, 2010, provide additional recommendations on alcohol consumption and specific population groups. There are many circumstances when people should not drink alcohol. *These are discussed in chapter 8 of this book.*
[2] Fortified soy beverages have been marketed as "soymilk," a product name consumers could see in supermarkets and consumer materials. However, FDA's regulations do not contain provisions for the use of the term soymilk. Therefore, in this document, the term "fortified soy beverage" includes products that may be marketed as soymilk.

- Replace protein foods that are high in solid fats with choices that are lower in solid fats and calories and/or are sources of oils.

- Use oils to replace solid fats where possible.

- Choose foods that provide more potassium, dietary fiber, calcium, and vitamin D, which are nutrients of concern in American diets. These foods include vegetables, fruits, whole grains, and milk and milk products.

Build Healthy Eating Patterns

- Select an eating pattern that meets nutrient needs over time at an appropriate calorie level.

- Account for all foods and beverages consumed and assess how they fit within a total healthy eating pattern.

- Follow food safety recommendations when preparing and eating foods to reduce the risk of foodborne illnesses.

Recommendations for specific population groups

Women capable of becoming pregnant[3]

- Choose foods that supply heme iron, which is more readily absorbed by the body; additional iron sources;

and enhancers of iron absorption such as vitamin C-rich foods.

- Consume 400 micrograms (mcg) per day of synthetic folic acid (from fortified foods and/or supplements) in addition to food forms of folate from a varied diet.[4]

Women who are pregnant or breastfeeding

- Consume 8 to 12 ounces of seafood per week from a variety of seafood types.

- Due to their high methyl mercury content, limit white (albacore) tuna to 6 ounces per week and do not eat the following four types of fish: tilefish, shark, swordfish, and king mackerel.

- If pregnant, take an iron supplement, as recommended by an obstetrician or other health care provider.

Individuals ages 50 year and older

- Consume foods fortified with vitamin B_{12}, such as fortified cereals, or dietary supplements.

[3] Includes adolescent girls
[4] Folic acid is the synthetic form of the nutrients, whereas folate is the form found naturally in foods.
Source: Dietary Guidelines for Americans, 2010. For the full document, refer to www.cnpp.usda.gov/DGAs2010-PolicyDocument.htm?.

2008 PHYSICAL ACTIVITY GUIDELINES FOR AMERICANS

AGE GROUP / GUIDELINES

6–17 years

Children and adolescents should do 60 minutes (1 hour) or more of physical activity daily.

- Aerobic: Most of the 60 or more minutes a day should be either moderate[a]- or vigorous[b]-intensity aerobic physical activity, and should include vigorous-intensity physical activity at least 3 days a week.

- Muscle-strengthening[c]: As part of their 60 or more

minutes of daily physical activity children, and adolescents should include muscle-strengthening physical activity on at least 3 days of the week.

- Bone strengthening[d]: As part of their 60 or more minutes of daily physical activity, children and adolescents should include bone-strengthening physical activity on at least 3 days of the week.

- It is important to encourage young people to participate in physical activities that are appropriate for their age, that are enjoyable, and that offer variety.

[a] Moderate-intensity physical activity: Aerobic activity that increases a person's heart rate and breathing to some extent. On a scale relative to a person's capacity, moderate-intensity activity is usually a 5 to 6 on a 1-to-10 scale. Brisk walking, dancing, swimming, or bicycling on a level terrain are examples.

[b] Vigorous-intensity physical activity: Aerobic activity that greatly increases a person's heart rate and breathing. On a scale relative to a person's capacity, vigorous-intensity activity is usually a 7 to 8 on a 1-to-10 scale. Jogging, singles tennis, swimming continuous laps, or bicycling uphill are examples.

[c] Muscle-strengthening activity: Physical activity, including exercise, that increases skeletal muscle strength, power, endurance, and mass. It includes strength training, resistance training, and muscular strength and endurance exercises.

[d] Bone-strengthening activity: Physical activity that produces an impact or tension force on bones, which promotes bone growth and strength. Running, jumping rope, and lifting weights are examples.

Source: Adapted for the Dietary Guidelines for Americans, 2010, from the *2008 Physical Activity Guidelines for Americans*, U.S. Department of Health and Human Services.

(continued)

2008 PHYSICAL ACTIVITY GUIDELINES FOR AMERICANS *(continued)*

18–64 years

● All adults should avoid inactivity. Some physical activity is better than none, and adults who participate in any amount of physical activity at all gain some health benefits.

● For substantial health benefits, adults should do at least 150 minutes (2 hours and 30 minutes) a week of moderate-intensity, or 75 minutes (1 hours and 15 minutes) a week of vigorous-intensity aerobic physical activity, or an equivalent combination of moderate- and vigorous-intensity aerobic activity. Aerobic activity should be performed in episodes of at least 10 minutes, and preferably, it should be spread throughout the week.

● For additional and more extensive health benefits, adults should increase their aerobic physical activity to 300 minutes (5 hours) a week of moderate-intensity, or 150 minutes a week of vigorous-intensity aerobic physical activity, or an equivalent combination of mod-

erate- and vigorous-intensity activity. Additional health benefits are gained by engaging in physical activity beyond this amount.

● Adults should also include muscle-strengthening activities that involve all major muscle groups on 2 or more days a week.

65 years and older

● Older adults should follow the adult guidelines. When older adults cannot meet the adult guidelines, they should be as physically active as their abilities and conditions allow.

● Older adults should do exercises that maintain or improve balance if they are at risk of falling.

● Older adults should determine their level of effort for physical activity relative to their level of fitness.

● Older adults with chronic conditions should understand whether and how their conditions affect their ability to do regular physical activity safely.

USDA FOOD PATTERNS

For each food group or subgroup,[a] recommended average daily intake amounts[b] at all calorie levels. Recommended intakes from vegetable and protein foods subgroups are per week. For more information and tools to use this, go to www.ChooseMyPlate.gov. (For the Lacto-Ovo Vegetarian and Vegan Adaptations of the USDA Food Patterns, refer to the website: www.cnpp.usda.gov/dietaryguidelines.htm.)

CALORIE LEVEL OF PATTERN[c]	1,000	1,200	1,400	1,600	1,800	2,000	2,200	2,400	2,600	2,800	3,000	3,200
Fruits	1 c	1 c	1½ c	1½ c	1½ c	2 c	2 c	2 c	2 c	2½ c	2½ c	2½ c
Vegetables[d]	1 c	1½ c	1½ c	2 c	2½ c	2½ c	3 c	3 c	3½ c	3½ c	4 c	4 c
Dark-green vegetables	½ c/wk	1 c/wk	1 c/wk	1½ c/wk	1½ c/wk	1½ c/wk	2 c/wk	2 c/wk	2½ c/wk	2½ c/wk	2½ c/wk	2½ c/wk
Red and orange vegetables	2½ c/wk	3 c/wk	3 c/wk	4 c/wk	5½ c/wk	5½ c/wk	6 c/wk	6 c/wk	7 c/wk	7 c/wk	7½ c/wk	7½ c/wk
Beans and peas (legumes)	½ c/wk	½ c/wk	½ c/wk	1 c/wk	1½ c/wk	1½ c/wk	2 c/wk	2 c/wk	2½ c/wk	2½ c/wk	3 c/wk	3 c/wk
Starchy vegetables	2 c/wk	3½ c/wk	3½ c/wk	4 c/wk	5 c/wk	5 c/wk	6 c/wk	6 c/wk	7 c/wk	7 c/wk	8 c/wk	8 c/wk
Other vegetables	1½ c/wk	2½ c/wk	2½ c/wk	3½ c/wk	4 c/wk	4 c/wk	5 c/wk	5 c/wk	5½ c/wk	5½ c/wk	7 c/wk	7 c/wk
Grains[e]	3 oz-eq	4 oz-eq	5 oz-eq	5 oz-eq	6 oz-eq	6 oz-eq	7 oz-eq	8 oz-eq	9 oz-eq	10 oz-eq	10 oz-eq	10 oz-eq
Whole grains	1½ oz-eq	2 oz-eq	2½ oz-eq	3 oz-eq	3 oz-eq	3 oz-eq	3½ oz-eq	4 oz-eq	4½ oz-eq	5 oz-eq	5 oz-eq	5 oz-eq
Enriched grains	1½ oz-eq	2 oz-eq	2½ oz-eq	2 oz-eq	3 oz-eq	3 oz-eq	3½ oz-eq	4 oz-eq	4½ oz-eq	5 oz-eq	5 oz eq	5 oz-eq
Protein foods[d]	2 oz-eq	3 oz-eq	4 oz-eq	5 oz-eq	5 oz-eq	5½ oz-eq	6 oz-eq	6½ oz-eq	6½ oz-eq	7 oz-eq	7 oz-eq	7 oz-eq
Seafood	3 oz-eq	5 oz/wk	6 oz-eq	8 oz-wk	8 oz-wk	8 oz-wk	9 oz-wk	10 oz-wk	10 oz-wk	11 oz-eq	11 oz/wk	11 oz/wk
Meat, poultry, eggs	10 oz/wk	14 oz/wk	19 oz/wk	24 oz/wk	24 oz/wk	26 oz/wk	29 oz/wk	31 oz/wk	31 oz/wk	34 oz/wk	34 oz/wk	34 oz/wk
Nuts, seeds, soy products	1 oz/wk	2 oz/wk	3 oz/wk	4 oz/wk	4 oz/wk	4 oz/wk	4 oz/wk	5 oz/wk	5 oz/wk	5 oz/wk	5 oz/wk	5 oz/wk

CALORIE LEVEL OF PATTERN[c]	1,000	1,200	1,400	1,600	1,800	2,000	2,200	2,400	2,600	2,800	3,000	3,200
Dairy[f]	2 c	2½ c	2½ c	3 c	3 c	3 c	3 c	3 c	3 c	3 c	3 c	3 c
Oils[g]	15 g	17 g	17 g	22 g	24 g	27 g	29 g	31 g	34 g	36 g	44 g	51 g
Maximum SoFAS[h] limit, calories (% of calories)	137 (14%)	121 (10%)	121 (9%)	121 (8%)	161 (9%)	258 (13%)	266 (12%)	330 (14%)	362 (14%)	395 (14%)	459 (15%)	596 (19%)

Notes for USDA Food Patterns:

[a] All foods are assumed to be in nutrient-dense forms, lean or low-fat, and prepared without added fats, sugars, or salt. Solid fats and added sugars may be included up to the daily maximum limit identified on the table. Food items in each group and subgroup are:

Fruits All fresh, frozen, canned, and dried fruits, and fruit juices, for example, oranges and orange juice, apples and apple juice, bananas, grapes, melons, berries, and raisins.

Vegetables

- *Dark-green vegetables* All fresh, frozen, and canned dark-green leafy vegetables and broccoli, cooked or raw: for example, broccoli; spinach; romaine; collard, turnip and mustard greens.

- *Red and orange vegetables* All fresh, frozen, and canned red and orange vegetables, cooked or raw: for example, tomatoes, red peppers, carrots, sweet potatoes, winter squash, and pumpkin.

- *Beans and peas (legumes)* All cooked beans and peas: for example, kidney beans, lentils, chickpeas, and pinto beans. Does not include green beans or green peas. (See additional comment under protein foods group.)

- *Starchy vegetables* All fresh, frozen, and canned starchy vegetables: for example, white potatoes, corn, and green peas.
- *Other vegetables* All fresh, frozen, and canned other vegetables, cooked or raw: for example, iceberg lettuce, green beans, and onions.

Grains

- *Whole grains* All whole-grain products and whole grains used as ingredients: for example, whole-wheat bread, whole-grain cereals and crackers, oatmeal, and brown rice.

- *Enriched grains* All enriched refined-grain products and enriched refined grains used as ingredients: for example, white breads, enriched-grain cereals and crackers, enriched pasta, and white rice.

Protein Foods

All meat, poultry, seafood, eggs, nuts, seeds, and processed soy products. Meat and poultry should be lean or low-fat and nuts should be unsalted. Beans and peas are considered part of this group as well as the vegetable group, but should be counted in one group only.

Dairy

All milks, including lactose-free and lactose-reduced products and fortified soy beverages, yogurts, frozen yogurts, dairy desserts, and cheeses. Most choices should be fat-free or low-fat. Cream, sour cream, and cream cheese are not included due to their low calcium content.

[b] Food group amounts are shown in cup (cup) or ounce-equivalents (oz-eq). Oils are shown in grams (g). Quantity equivalents for each food are:

- Grains, l-ounce equivalent is: 1 one-ounce slice bread; l ounce uncooked pasta or rice; ½ cup cooked rice, pasta, or cereal; 1 tortilla (6 diameter): 1 pancake (5 diameter); 1 ounce ready-to-eat cereal (about 1 cup cereal flakes).

- Vegetables and fruits, 1 cup equivalent is: 1 cup raw or cooked vegetable or fruit; ½ cup dried vegetable or fruit; 1 cup vegetable or fruit juice; 2 cups leafy salad greens.

- Protein foods, 1-ounce equivalent is: 1 ounce meat, poultry, seafood; 1 egg; 1 Tbsp. peanut butter; ½ ounce nuts or seeds. Also, ½ cup cooked beans or peas may be counted as a 1-ounce equivalent.

- Dairy, 1 cup equivalent is: 1 cup milk, fortified soy beverage, or yogurt, 1½ ounces natural cheese (e.g., cheddar), 2 ounces of processed cheese (e.g., American).

[c] Food intake patterns at 1,000, 1,200, and 1,400 calories meet the nutritional needs of children ages 2 to 8 years. Patterns from 1,600 to 3,200 calories meet the nutritional needs of children ages 9 years and older and adults. If a child ages 4 to 8 years needs more calories, and, therefore, is following a pattern at 1,600 calories or more, the recommended amount from the dairy group can be 2½ cups per day. Children ages 9 years and older and adults should not use the 1,000, 1,200, or 1,400 calorie patterns.

[d] Vegetable and protein foods subgroup amounts are shown in this table as weekly amounts because it would be difficult for consumers to select foods from all subgroups daily.

[e] Whole-grain subgroup amounts shown in the table are minimums. More whole grains up to all of the grains recommended may be selected, with offsetting decreases in the amount of enriched refined grains.

[f] The amount of dairy foods in the 1,200 and 1,400 calorie patterns have increased to reflect new RDAs for calcium that are higher than previous recommendations for children ages 4 to 8 years.

[g] Oils and soft margarines include vegetables, nut, and fish oils and soft vegetable oil table spreads that have no *trans* fats.

[h] SoFAS are calories from solid fats and added sugars. The limit for SoFAS is the remaining amount of calories in each food pattern after selecting the specified amounts in each food group in nutrient-dense forms (forms that are fat-free or low-fat and with no added sugars). The number of SoFAS is lower in the 1,200, 1,400, and 1,600 calorie patterns than in the 1,000 calorie pattern. The nutrient goals for the 1,200 to 1,600 calorie patterns are higher and require that more calories be used for nutrient-dense foods from the food groups.

Source: Dietary Guidelines for Americans, 2010.

ESTIMATED CALORIE NEEDS PER DAY BY AGE, GENDER, AND PHYSICAL ACTIVITY LEVEL

Estimated amounts of calories[a] needed to maintain calorie balance for various gender and age groups at three different levels of physical activity. The estimates are rounded to the nearest 200 calories. An individual's calorie needs may be higher or lower than these average estimates.

	MALES				FEMALES		
ACTIVITY LEVEL AGE	Sedentary*	Mod. active*	Active*	ACTIVITY LEVEL AGE	Sedentary*	Mod. active*	Active*
2	1000	1000	1000	2	1000	1000	1000
3	1200	1400	1400	3	1000	1200	1400
4	1200	1400	1600	4	1200	1400	1400
5	1200	1400	1600	5	1200	1400	1600
6	1400	1600	1800	6	1200	1400	1600
7	1400	1600	1800	7	1200	1600	1800
8	1400	1600	2000	8	1400	1600	1800
9	1600	1800	2000	9	1400	1600	1800
10	1600	1800	2200	10	1400	1800	2000
11	1800	2000	2200	11	1600	1800	2000
12	1800	2200	2400	12	1600	2000	2200
13	2000	2200	2600	13	1600	2000	2200
14	2000	2400	2800	14	1800	2000	2400
15	2200	2600	3000	15	1800	2000	2400
16	2400	2800	3200	16	1800	2000	2400
17	2400	2800	3200	17	1800	2000	2400
18	2400	2800	3200	18	1800	2000	2400
19-20	2600	2800	3000	19-20	2000	2200	2400
21-25	2400	2800	3000	21-25	2000	2200	2400
26-30	2400	2600	3000	26-30	1800	2000	2400
31-35	2400	2600	3000	31-35	1800	2000	2200
36-40	2400	2600	2800	36-40	1800	2000	2200
41-45	2200	2600	2800	41-45	1800	2000	2200
46-50	2200	2400	2800	46-50	1800	2000	2200
51-55	2200	2400	2800	51-55	1600	1800	2200
56-60	2200	2400	2600	56-60	1600	1800	2200
61-65	2000	2400	2600	61-65	1600	1800	2000
66-70	2000	2200	2600	66-70	1600	1800	2000
71-75	2000	2200	2600	71-75	1600	1800	2000
76 and up	2000	2200	2400	76 and up	1600	1800	2000

*Calorie levels are based on the Estimated Energy Requirements (EER) and activity levels from the Institute of Medicine Dietary Reference Intakes Macronutrients Report, 2002.

Activity levels are based on light physical activity associated with typical day-to-day life:

● "Sedentary" means only the above.

● "Moderately active" means the above plus physical activity equivalent to walking about 1½ to 3 miles a day at 3 to 4 miles per hour.

● "Active" means the above plus physical activity equivalent to walking more than 3 miles per day at 3 to 4 mile per hour.

Estimates for females do not include women who are pregnant or breastfeeding.

Source: Adapted from Dietary Guidelines for Americans, 2010; Britten, Marcoe, Yamini, and Davis. Development of food intake patterns for the MyPyramid Food Guidance System. *J Nutr Educ Behav* 2006:38(6 Suppl): S78-S92.

Sample Menus for a 2000-Calorie Food Pattern

These 7-day menus are motivational tools to help put a healthy eating pattern into practice and to identify creative ideas for healthy meals. Averaged over a week, these menus provide the recommended amounts of key nutrients and foods from each food group. The menus feature many different foods to inspire ideas for adding variety to food choices. They are not intended to be followed day to day as a specific prescription for what to eat. Spices and herbs can be added for flavor.

Day 1

Breakfast

Creamy oatmeal (cooked in milk)
- ½ cup uncooked oatmeal
- 1 cup fat-free milk
- 2 Tbsp. raisins
- 2 tsp. brown sugar

Beverage: 1 cup orange juice

Lunch

Taco salad:
- 2 ounces tortilla chips
- 2 ounces cooked ground turkey
- 2 tsp. corn/ canola oil (to cook turkey)
- ¼ cup kidney beans *
- ½ ounce low-fat cheddar cheese
- ½ cup chopped lettuce
- ½ cup avocado
- 1 tsp. lime juice (on avocado)
- 2 Tbsp. salsa

Beverage: 1 cup water, coffee, or tea**

Dinner

Spinach lasagna roll-ups:
- 1 cup lasagna noodles (2 oz. dry)
- ½ cup cooked spinach
- ½ cup ricotta cheese
- 1 ounce part-skim mozzarella cheese
- ½ cup tomato sauce*
1 ounce whole-wheat roll
- 1 tsp. tub margarine

Beverage: 1 cup fat-free milk

Snacks

2 Tbsp. raisins
1 ounce unsalted almonds

Day 2

Breakfast

Breakfast burrito:
- 1 flour tortilla (8" diameter)
- 1 scrambled egg
- ⅓ cup black beans*
- 1 Tbsp. salsa
½ large grapefruit

Beverage: 1 cup water, coffee, or tea**

Lunch

Roast beef sandwich:
- 1 small whole grain hoagie bun
- 2 ounces lean roast beef
- 1 slice part-skim mozzarella cheese
- 2 slices tomato
- ¼ cup mushrooms
- 1 tsp. corn/canola oil (to cook mushrooms)
- 1 tsp. mustard
Baked potato wedges:
- 1 cup potato wedges
- 1 tsp. corn/canola oil (to cook potato)
- 1 Tbsp. ketchup

Beverage: 1 cup fat-free milk

Dinner

Baked salmon on beet greens:
- 4 ounce salmon filet
- 1 tsp. olive oil
- 2 tsp. lemon juice
- ⅓ cup cooked beet greens (sautéed in 2 tsp. corn/canola oil)
Quinoa with almonds:
- ½ cup quinoa
- ½ ounce slivered almonds

Beverage: 1 cup fat-free milk

Snacks

1 cup cantaloupe balls

Day 3

Breakfast

Cold cereal:
- 1 cup ready-to-eat oat cereal
- 1 medium banana
- ½ cup fat-free milk
1 slice whole-wheat toast
- 1 tsp. tub margarine

Beverage: 1 cup prune juice

Lunch

Tuna salad sandwich:
- 2 slices rye bread
- 2 ounces tuna
- 1 Tbsp. mayonnaise
- 1 Tbsp. chopped celery
- ½ cup shredded lettuce
- 1 tsp. corn/canola oil (to cook mushrooms)
1 medium peach

Beverage: 1 cup fat-free milk

Dinner

Roasted chicken
- 3 ounces cooked chicken breast
1 large sweet potato, roasted
½ cup succotash (limas and corn)
- 1 tsp. tub margarine
1 ounce whole-wheat roll
- 1 tsp. tub margarine

Beverage: 1 cup water, coffee, or tea**

Snacks

¼ cup dried apricots
1 cup flavored yogurt (chocolate)

Day 4

Breakfast

1 whole-wheat English muffin
- 1 Tbsp. all-fruit preserves
1 hard-cooked egg

Beverage: 1 cup water, coffee, or tea**

Lunch

White bean-vegetable soup:
- 1¼ cup chunky vegetable soup with pasta
- ½ cup white beans*
6 saltine crackers*
½ cup celery sticks

Beverage: 1 cup fat-free milk

Dinner

Rigatoni with meat sauce:
- 1 cup rigatoni pasta (2 oz. dry)
- 2 ounces cooked ground beef (95% lean)
- 2 tsp. corn/canola oil (to cook beef)
- ½ cup tomato sauce*
- 3 Tbsp. grated parmesan cheese
Spinach salad:
- 1 cup raw spinach leaves
- ½ cup tangerine sections
- ½ ounce chopped walnuts
- 2 tsp. oil and vinegar dressing

Beverage: 1 cup water, coffee, or tea**

Snacks

1 cup nonfat fruit yogurt

Day 5

Breakfast

Cold cereal:
- 1 cup shredded wheat
- ½ cup sliced banana
- ½ cup fat-free milk
1 slice whole-wheat toast
- 2 tsp. all-fruit preserves

Beverage: 1 cup fat-free chocolate milk

Lunch

Turkey sandwich:
- 1 whole-wheat pita bread (2 oz.)
- 3 ounces roasted turkey, sliced
- 2 slices tomato
- ¼ cup shredded lettuce
- 1 tsp. mustard
- 1 Tbsp. mayonnaise
¼ cup grapes

Beverage: 1 cup tomato juice*

Dinner

Steak and potatoes:
- 4 ounces broiled beef steak
- ⅔ cup mashed potatoes made with milk and 2 tsp. tub margarine
½ cup cooked green beans
- 1 tsp. tub margarine
- 1 tsp. honey
1 ounce whole-wheat roll
- 1 tsp. tub margarine
Frozen yogurt and berries:
- ½ cup frozen yogurt (chocolate)
- ¼ cup sliced strawberries

Beverage: 1 cup fat-free milk

Snacks

1 cup frozen yogurt (chocolate)

Day 6

Breakfast

French toast:
- 2 slices whole-wheat bread
- 3 Tbsp. fat-free milk and
- ⅔ egg (in French toast)
- 2 tsp. tub margarine
- 1 Tbsp. pancake syrup
½ large grapefruit

Beverage: 1 cup fat-free milk

Lunch

3-bean vegetarian chili on baked potato:
- ¼ cup each cooked kidney beans,* navy beans,* and black beans*
- ½ cup tomato sauce*
- ¼ cup chopped onion
- 2 Tbsp. chopped jalapeno peppers
- 1 tsp. corn/canola oil (to cook onion and peppers)
- ¼ cup cheese sauce
- 1 large baked potato
½ cup cantaloupe

Beverage: 1 cup water, coffee, or tea**

Dinner

Hawaiian pizza
- 2 slices cheese pizza, thin crust
- 1 ounce lean ham
- ¼ cup pineapple
- ¼ cup mushrooms
- 1 tsp. safflower oil (to cook mushrooms)
Green salad:
- 1 cup mixed salad greens
- 4 tsp. oil and vinegar dressing

Beverage: 1 cup fat-free milk

Snacks

3 Tbsp. hummus
5 whole-wheat crackers*

Day 7

Breakfast

Buckwheat pancakes with berries:
- 2 large (7") pancakes
- 1 Tbsp. pancake syrup
- ¼ cup sliced strawberries

Beverage: 1 cup orange juice

Lunch

New England clam chowder:
- 3 ounces canned clams
- ½ small potato
- 2 Tbsp. chopped onion
- 2 Tbsp. chopped celery
- 6 Tbsp. evaporated milk
- ¼ cup fat-free milk
- 1 slice bacon
- 1 Tbsp. white flour
10 whole-wheat crackers*
1 medium orange

Beverage: 1 cup fat-free milk

Dinner

Tofu-vegetable stir-fry:
- 4 ounces firm tofu
- ½ cup chopped Chinese cabbage
- ¼ cup sliced bamboo shoots
- 1 Tbsp. chopped sweet red peppers
- 2 Tbsp. chopped green peppers
- 1 Tbsp. corn/canola oil (to cook stir-fry)
- 1 cup cooked brown rice (2 ounces raw)
Honeydew yogurt cup:
- ¾ cup honeydew melon
- ½ cup plain fat-free yogurt

Beverage: 1 cup water, coffee, or tea**

Snacks

1 large banana spread with 2 Tbsp. peanut butter*
1 cup nonfat fruit yogurt

---

* Foods that are reduced sodium, low sodium, or no-salt added products. These foods can also be prepared from scratch with no added salt. All other foods are regular commercial products, which contain variable levels of sodium. Average sodium level of the 7-day menu assumes that no salt is added in cooking or at the table.

** Unless indicated, all beverages are unsweetened and without added cream or whitener.

Italicized foods are part of the dish or food that precedes it.

Source: www.ChooseMyPlate.gov .

DASH Eating Plan at Various Calorie Levels

The number of daily servings in a food group varies depending on calorie needs. DASH Eating Patterns from 1,200 to 1,800 calories meet the nutritional needs of children 4 to 8 years old. Patterns from 1,600 to 3,000 calories meet the nutritional needs of children 9 years and older and adults.

FOOD GROUP	1,600 CALORIES	2,000 CALORIES	2,600 CALORIES	1,600 CALORIES	2,000 CALORIES	2,600 CALORIES	3,100 CALORIES	SERVING SIZES
	NUMBER OF DAILY SERVINGS							
Grains*	4 to 5	5 to 6	6	6	6 to 8	10 to 11	12 to 13	1 slice bread 1 oz. dry cereal ½ cup cooked rice, pasta, or cereal**
Vegetables	3 to 4	3 to 4	3 to 4	4 to 5	4 to 5	5 to 6	6	1 cup raw leafy vegetable ½ cup cut-up raw or cooked vegetable ½ cup vegetable juice
Fruits	3 to 4	4	4	4 to 5	4 to 5	5 to 6	6	1 medium fruit ¼ cup dried fruit ½ cup fresh, frozen, or canned fruit ½ cup fruit juice
Fat-fat or low-fat milk and milk products	2 to 3	2 to 3	2 to 3	2 to 3	2 to 3	3	3 to 4	1 cup milk or yogurt 1½ oz. cheese
Lean meats, poultry, and fish	3 or less	3 to 4 or less	3 to 4 or less	6 or less	6 or less	6 or less	6 to 9	1 oz. cooked meat, poultry, or fish 1 egg
Nuts, seeds, and legumes	3 per week	3 per week	3 to 4 per week	4 per week	4 to 5 per week	1	1	⅓ cup or 1½ oz. nuts 2 Tbsp. or ½ oz. seeds 2 Tbsp. peanut butter 2 Tbsp. or ½ oz. seeds ½ cup cooked dry beans or peas (legumes)
Fat and oils	1	1	2	2 to 3	2 to 3	3	4	1 tsp. soft margarine 1 tsp. vegetable oil 1 Tbsp. mayonnaise 1 Tbsp. salad dressing***
Sweets and added sugars	3 or less per weel	3 or less per week	3 or less per week	5 or less per week	5 or less per week	<2	<2	1 Tbsp. sugar 1 Tbsp. jelly or jam ½ cup sorbet, gelatin dessert 1 cup lemonade
Maximum sodium limit****	2,300 mg/day	2,300 mg/day	2,300 mg/day	2,300 mg/day	2,300 mg/day	2,300 mg/day	2,300 mg/day	

* Whole grains are recommended for most grain servings.

** Serving sizes vary between ½ to 1¼ cups depending on cereal type. Check the Nutrition Facts label.

*** Fat content changes serving counts for fats and oil: For example 1 Tbsp. of regular salad dressing equals 1 serving; 1 Tbsp of low-fat dressing equals ½ serving; 1 Tbsp. of fat-free dressing equals 0 servings.

**** The DASH Eating Plan consists of patterns with a sodium limit of 2,300 mg and 1,500 mg per day.

Source: Adapted from Dietary Guidelines for Americans, 2010.

Dietary Reference Intakes (DRIs): Acceptable Macronutrient Distribution Ranges
Food and Nutrition Board, Institute of Medicine, National Academies

Macronutrient	Range (percent of energy)		
	Children, 1–3 y	Children, 4–18 y	Adults
Fat	30–40	25–35	20–35
n-6 polyunsaturated fatty acids[a] (linoleic acid)	5–10	5–10	5–10
n-3 polyunsaturated fatty acids[a] (α-linolenic acid)	0.6–1.2	0.6–1.2	0.6–1.2
Carbohydrate	45–65	45–65	45–65
Protein	5–20	10–30	10–35

[a] Approximately 10% of the total can come from longer-chain *n*-3 or *n*-6 fatty acids.

Source: Dietary Reference Intakes for Energy, Carbohydrate, Fiber, Fat, Fatty Acids, Cholesterol, Protein, and Amino Acids (2002/2005). This report may be accessed via www.nap.edu. Dietary Reference Intakes reprinted with permission of the National Academy of Sciences, courtesy of the National Academies Press, Washington, D.C.

Dietary Reference Intakes (DRIs): Acceptable Macronutrient Distribution ranges
Food and Nutrition Board, Institute of Medicine, National Academies

Macronutrient	Recommendation
Dietary cholesterol	As low as possible while consuming a nutritionally adequate diet
Trans fatty acids	As low as possible while consuming a nutritionally adequate diet
Saturated fatty acids	As low as possible while consuming a nutritionally adequate diet
Added sugars[a]	Limit to no more than 25% of total energy

[a] Not a recommended intake. A daily intake of added sugars that individuals should aim for to achieve a healthful diet was not set.

Source: Dietary Reference Intakes for Energy, Carbohydrate, Fiber, Fat, Fatty Acids, Cholesterol, Protein, and Amino Acids (2002/2005). This report may be accessed via www.nap.edu. Dietary Reference Intakes reprinted with permission of the National Academy of Sciences, courtesy of the National Academies Press, Washington, D.C.

Dietary Reference Intakes (DRIs): Recommended Dietary Allowances and Adequate Intakes, Total Water and Macronutrients

Food and Nutrition Board, Institute of Medicine, National Academies

Life Stage Group	Total Water[a] (L/d)	Carbohydrate (g/d)	Total Fiber (g/d)	Fat (g/d)	Linoleic Acid (g/d)	α-Linolenic Acid (g/d)	Protein[b] (g/d)
Infants							
0 to 6 mo	0.7*	60*	ND	31*	4.4*	0.5*	9.1*
6 to 12 mo	0.8*	95*	ND	30*	4.6*	0.5*	**11.0**
Children							
1–3 y	1.3*	**130**	19*	ND[c]	7*	0.7*	**13**
4–8 y	1.7*	**130**	25*	ND	10*	0.9*	**19**
Males							
9–13 y	2.4*	**130**	31*	ND	12*	1.2*	**34**
14–18 y	3.3*	**130**	38*	ND	16*	1.6*	**52**
19–30 y	3.7*	**130**	38*	ND	17*	1.6*	**56**
31–50 y	3.7*	**130**	38*	ND	17*	1.6*	**56**
51–70 y	3.7*	**130**	30*	ND	14*	1.6*	**56**
> 70 y	3.7*	**130**	30*	ND	14*	1.6*	**56**
Females							
9–13 y	2.1*	**130**	26*	ND	10*	1.0*	**34**
14–18 y	2.3*	**130**	26*	ND	11*	1.1*	**46**
19–30 y	2.7*	**130**	25*	ND	12*	1.1*	**46**
31–50 y	2.7*	**130**	25*	ND	12*	1.1*	**46**
51–70 y	2.7*	**130**	21*	ND	11*	1.1*	**46**
> 70 y	2.7*	**130**	21*	ND	11*	1.1*	**46**
Pregnancy							
14–18 y	3.0*	**175**	28*	ND	13*	1.4*	**71**
19–30 y	3.0*	**175**	28*	ND	13*	1.4*	**71**
31–50 y	3.0*	**175**	28*	ND	13*	1.4*	**71**
Lactation							
14–18	3.8*	**210**	29*	ND	13*	1.3*	**71**
19–30 y	3.8*	**210**	29*	ND	13*	1.3*	**71**
31–50 y	3.8*	**210**	29*	ND	13*	1.3*	**71**

NOTE: This table (take from the DRI reports, see www.nap.edu) presents Recommended Dietary Allowances (RDA) in **bold type** and Adequate Intakes (AI) in ordinary type followed by an asterisk (*). An RDA is the average daily dietary intake level; sufficient to meet the nutrient requirements of nearly all (97-98 percent) healthy individuals in a group. It is calculated from an Estimated Average Requirement (EAR). If sufficient scientific evidence is not available to establish an EAR, and thus calculate an RDA, an AI is usually developed. For healthy breastfed infants, an AI is the mean intake. The AI for other life stage and gender groups is believed to cover the needs of all healthy individuals in the groups, but lack of data or uncertainty in the data prevent being able to specify with confidence the percentage of individuals covered by this intake.

[a] *Total* water includes all water contained in food, beverages, and drinking water.

[b] Based on g protein per kg of body weight for the reference body weight, e.g., for adults 0.8 g/kg body weight for the reference body weight.

[c]Not determined.

Sources: Dietary Reference Intakes for Energy, Carbohydrate, Fiber, Fat, Fatty Acids, Cholesterol, Protein, and Amino Acids (2002/2005) and *Dietary Reference Intakes for Water, Potassium, Sodium, Chloride and Sulfate* (2005). These reports may be accessed via www.nap.edu. Dietary Reference Intakes reprinted with permission of the National Academy of Sciences, courtesy of the National Academies Press, Washington, D.C.

Dietary Reference Intakes (DRIs): Recommended Dietary Allowances and Adequate Intakes, Vitamins

Food and Nutrition Board, Institute of Medicine, National Academies

Life Stage Group	Vitamin A (µg/d)[a]	Vitamin C (mg/d)	Vitamin D (µg/d)[b,c]	Vitamin E (mg/d)[d]	Vitamin K (µg/d)	Thiamin (mg/d)	Riboflavin (mg/d)	Niacin (mg/d)[e]	Vitamin B6 (mg/d)	Folate (µg/d)[f]	Vitamin B12 (µg/d)	Pantothenic Acid (mg/d)	Biotin (µg/d)	Choline (mg/d)[g]
Infants														
0 to 6 mo	400*	40*	10	4*	2.0*	0.2*	0.3*	2*	0.1*	65*	0.4*	1.7*	5*	125*
6 to 12 mo	500*	50*	10	5*	2.5*	0.3*	0.4*	4*	0.3*	80*	0.5*	1.8*	6*	150*
Children														
1–3 y	**300**	**15**	**15**	**6**	30*	**0.5**	**0.5**	**6**	**0.5**	**150**	**0.9**	2*	8*	200*
4–8 y	**400**	**25**	**15**	**7**	55*	**0.6**	**0.6**	**8**	**0.6**	**200**	**1.2**	3*	12*	250*
Males														
9–13 y	**600**	**45**	**15**	**11**	60*	**0.9**	**0.9**	**12**	**1.0**	**300**	**1.8**	4*	20*	375*
14–18 y	**900**	**75**	**15**	**15**	75*	**1.2**	**1.3**	**16**	**1.3**	**400**	**2.4**	5*	25*	550*
19–30 y	**900**	**90**	**15**	**15**	120*	**1.2**	**1.3**	**16**	**1.3**	**400**	**2.4**	5*	30*	550*
31–50 y	**900**	**90**	**15**	**15**	120*	**1.2**	**1.3**	**16**	**1.3**	**400**	**2.4**	5*	30*	550*
51–70 y	**900**	**90**	**15**	**15**	120*	**1.2**	**1.3**	**16**	**1.7**	**400**	**2.4**[h]	5*	30*	550*
>70 y	**900**	**90**	**20**	**15**	120*	**1.2**	**1.3**	**16**	**1.7**	**400**	**2.4**[h]	5*	30*	550*
Females														
9–13 y	**600**	**45**	**15**	**11**	60*	**0.9**	**0.9**	**12**	**1.0**	**300**	**1.8**	4*	20*	375*
14–18 y	**700**	**65**	**15**	**15**	75*	**1.0**	**1.0**	**14**	**1.2**	**400**[i]	**2.4**	5*	25*	400*
19–30 y	**700**	**75**	**15**	**15**	90*	**1.1**	**1.1**	**14**	**1.3**	**400**[i]	**2.4**	5*	30*	425*
31–50 y	**700**	**75**	**15**	**15**	90*	**1.1**	**1.1**	**14**	**1.3**	**400**[i]	**2.4**	5*	30*	425*
51–70 y	**700**	**75**	**15**	**15**	90*	**1.1**	**1.1**	**14**	**1.5**	**400**	**2.4**[h]	5*	30*	425*
>70 y	**700**	**75**	**20**	**15**	90*	**1.1**	**1.1**	**14**	**1.5**	**400**	**2.4**[h]	5*	30*	425*
Pregnancy														
14–18 y	**750**	**80**	**15**	**15**	75*	**1.4**	**1.4**	**18**	**1.9**	**600**[j]	**2.6**	6*	30*	450*
19–30 y	**770**	**85**	**15**	**15**	90*	**1.4**	**1.4**	**18**	**1.9**	**600**[j]	**2.6**	6*	30*	450*
31–50 y	**770**	**85**	**15**	**15**	90*	**1.4**	**1.4**	**18**	**1.9**	**600**[j]	**2.6**	6*	30*	450*
Lactation														
14–18 y	**1,200**	**115**	**15**	**19**	75*	**1.4**	**1.6**	**17**	**2.0**	**500**	**2.8**	7*	35*	550*
19–30 y	**1,300**	**120**	**15**	**19**	90*	**1.4**	**1.6**	**17**	**2.0**	**500**	**2.8**	7*	35*	550*
31–50 y	**1,300**	**120**	**15**	**19**	90*	**1.4**	**1.6**	**17**	**2.0**	**500**	**2.8**	7*	35*	550*

NOTE: This table (taken from the DRI reports, see www.nap.edu) presents Recommended Dietary Allowances (RDAs) in **bold type** and Adequate Intakes (AIs) in ordinary type followed by an asterisk (*). An RDA is the average daily dietary intake level; sufficient to meet the nutrient requirements of nearly all (97-98 percent) healthy individuals in a group. It is calculated from an Estimated Average Requirement (EAR). If sufficient scientific evidence is not available to establish an EAR, and thus calculate an RDA, an AI is usually developed. For healthy breastfed infants, an AI is the mean intake. The AI for other life stage and gender groups is believed to cover the needs of all healthy individuals in the groups, but lack of data or uncertainty in the data prevent being able to specify with confidence the percentage of individuals covered by this intake.

[a] As retinol activity equivalents (RAEs). 1 RAE = 1 µg retinol, 12 µg β-carotene, 24 µg α-carotene, or 24 µg β-cryptoxanthin. The RAE for dietary provitamin A carotenoids is two-fold greater than retinol equivalents (RE), whereas the RAE for preformed vitamin A is the same as RE.

[b] As cholecalciferol. 1 µg cholecalciferol = 40 IU vitamin D.

[c] Under the assumption of minimal sunlight.

[d] As α-tocopherol. α-Tocopherol includes RRR-α-tocopherol, the only form of α-tocopherol that occurs naturally in foods, and the 2R-stereoisomeric forms of α-tocopherol (RRR-, RSR-, RRS-, and RSS-α-tocopherol) that occur in fortified foods and supplements. It does not include the 2S-stereoisomeric forms of α-tocopherol (SRR-, SSR-, SRS-, and SSS-α-tocopherol), also found in fortified foods and supplements.

[e] As niacin equivalents (NE). 1 mg of niacin = 60 mg of tryptophan; 0–6 months = preformed niacin (not NE).

[f] As dietary folate equivalents (DFE). 1 DFE = 1 µg food folate = 0.6 µg of folic acid from fortified food or as a supplement consumed with food = 0.5 µg of a supplement taken on an empty stomach.

[g] Although AIs have been set for choline, there are few data to assess whether a dietary supply of choline is needed at all stages of the life cycle, and it may be that the choline requirement can be met by endogenous synthesis at some of these stages.

[h] Because 10 to 30 percent of older people may malabsorb food-bound B12, it is advisable for those older than 50 years to meet their RDA mainly by consuming foods fortified with B12 or a supplement containing B12.

[i] In view of evidence linking folate intake with neural tube defects in the fetus, it is recommended that all women capable of becoming pregnant consume 400 µg from supplements or fortified foods in addition to intake of food folate from a varied diet.

[j] It is assumed that women will continue consuming 400 µg from supplements or fortified food until their pregnancy is confirmed and they enter prenatal care, which ordinarily occurs after the end of the periconceptional period—the critical time for formation of the neural tube.

Sources: Dietary Reference Intakes for Calcium, Phosphorous, Magnesium, Vitamin D, and Fluoride (1997); Dietary Reference Intakes for Thiamin, Riboflavin, Niacin, Vitamin B6, Folate, Vitamin B12, Pantothenic Acid, Biotin, and Choline (1998); Dietary Reference Intakes for Vitamin C, Vitamin E, Selenium, and Carotenoids (2000); Dietary Reference Intakes for Vitamin A, Vitamin K, Arsenic, Boron, Chromium, Copper, Iodine, Iron, Manganese, Molybdenum, Nickel, Silicon, Vanadium, and Zinc (2001); Dietary Reference Intakes for Water, Potassium, Sodium, Chloride, and Sulfate (2005); and Dietary Reference Intakes for Calcium and Vitamin D (2011). These reports may be accessed via www.nap.edu. Dietary Reference Intakes reprinted with permission of the National Academy of Sciences, courtesy of the National Academies Press, Washington, D.C.

Dietary Reference Intakes (DRIs): Recommended Dietary Allowances and Adequate Intakes, Elements

Food and Nutrition Board, Institute of Medicine, National Academies

Life Stage Group	Calcium (mg/d)	Chromium (µg/d)	Copper (µg/d)	Fluoride (mg/d)	Iodine (µg/d)	Iron (mg/d)	Magnesium (mg/d)	Manganese (mg/d)	Molybdenum (µg/d)	Phosphorus (mg/d)	Selenium (µg/d)	Zinc (mg/d)	Potassium (g/d)	Sodium (g/d)	Chloride (g/d)
Infants															
0 to 6 mo	200*	0.2*	200*	0.01*	110*	0.27*	30*	0.003*	2*	100*	15*	2*	0.4*	0.12*	0.18*
6 to 12 mo	260*	5.5*	220*	0.5*	130*	11	75*	0.6*	3*	275*	20*	3	0.7*	0.37*	0.57*
Children															
1–3 y	700	11*	340	0.7*	90	7	80	1.2*	17	460	20	3	3.0*	1.0*	1.5*
4–8 y	1,000	15*	440	1*	90	10	130	1.5*	22	500	30	5	3.8*	1.2*	1.9*
Males															
9–13 y	1,300	25*	700	2*	120	8	240	1.9*	34	1,250	40	8	4.5*	1.5*	2.3*
14–18 y	1,300	35*	890	3*	150	11	410	2.2*	43	1,250	55	11	4.7*	1.5*	2.3*
19–30 y	1,000	35*	900	4*	150	8	400	2.3*	45	700	55	11	4.7*	1.5*	2.3*
31–50 y	1,000	35*	900	4*	150	8	420	2.3*	45	700	55	11	4.7*	1.5*	2.3*
51–70 y	1,000	30*	900	4*	150	8	420	2.3*	45	700	55	11	4.7*	1.3*	2.0*
>70 y	1,200	30*	900	4*	150	8	420	2.3*	45	700	55	11	4.7*	1.2*	1.8*
Females															
9–13 y	1,300	21*	700	2*	120	8	240	1.6*	34	1,250	40	8	4.5*	1.5*	2.3*
14–18 y	1,300	24*	890	3*	150	15	360	1.6*	43	1,250	55	9	4.7*	1.5*	2.3*
19–30 y	1,000	25*	900	3*	150	18	310	1.8*	45	700	55	8	4.7*	1.5*	2.3*
31–50 y	1,000	25*	900	3*	150	18	320	1.8*	45	700	55	8	4.7*	1.5*	2.3*
51–70 y	1,200	20*	900	3*	150	8	320	1.8*	45	700	55	8	4.7*	1.3*	2.0*
>70 y	1,200	20*	900	3*	150	8	320	1.8*	45	700	55	8	4.7*	1.2*	1.8*
Pregnancy															
14–18 y	1,300	29*	1,000	3*	220	27	400	2.0*	50	1,250	60	12	4.7*	1.5*	2.3*
19–30 y	1,000	30*	1,000	3*	220	27	350	2.0*	50	700	60	11	4.7*	1.5*	2.3*
31–50 y	1,000	30*	1,000	3*	220	27	360	2.0*	50	700	60	11	4.7*	1.5*	2.3*
Lactation															
14–18 y	1,300	44*	1,300	3*	290	10	360	2.6*	50	1,250	70	13	5.1*	1.5*	2.3*
19–30 y	1,000	45*	1,300	3*	290	9	310	2.6*	50	700	70	12	5.1*	1.5*	2.3*
31–50 y	1,000	45*	1,300	3*	290	9	320	2.6*	50	700	70	12	5.1*	1.5*	2.3*

NOTE: This table (taken from the DRI reports, see www.nap.edu) presents Recommended Dietary Allowances (RDAs) in **bold type** and Adequate Intakes (AIs) in ordinary type followed by an asterisk (*). An RDA is the average daily dietary intake level; sufficient to meet the nutrient requirements of nearly all (97–98 percent) healthy individuals in a group. It is calculated from an Estimated Average Requirement (EAR). If sufficient scientific evidence is not available to establish an EAR, and thus calculate an RDA, an AI is usually developed. For healthy breastfed infants, an AI is the mean intake. The AI for other life stage and gender groups is believed to cover the needs of all healthy individuals in the groups, but lack of data or uncertainty in the data prevent being able to specify with confidence the percentage of individuals covered by this intake.

Sources: Dietary Reference Intakes for Calcium, Phosphorous, Magnesium, Vitamin D, and Fluoride (1997); *Dietary Reference Intakes for Thiamin, Riboflavin, Niacin, Vitamin B₆, Folate, Vitamin B₁₂, Pantothenic Acid, Biotin, and Choline* (1998); *Dietary Reference Intakes for Vitamin C, Vitamin E, Selenium, and Carotenoids* (2000); *Dietary Reference Intakes for Vitamin A, Vitamin K, Arsenic, Boron, Chromium, Copper, Iodine, Iron, Manganese, Molybdenum, Nickel, Silicon, Vanadium, and Zinc* (2001); *Dietary Reference Intakes for Water, Potassium, Sodium, Chloride, and Sulfate* (2005); and *Dietary Reference Intakes for Calcium and Vitamin D* (2011). These reports may be accessed via www.nap.edu. Dietary Reference Intakes reprinted with permission of the National Academy of Sciences, courtesy of the National Academies Press, Washington, D.C.

Dietary Reference Intakes (DRIs): Tolerable Upper Intake Levels, Vitamins
Food and Nutrition Board, Institute of Medicine, National Academies

Life Stage Group	Vitamin A (µg/d)[a]	Vitamin C (mg/d)	Vitamin D (µg/d)	Vitamin E (mg/d)[b,c]	Vitamin K	Thiamin	Riboflavin	Niacin (mg/d)[c]	Vitamin B_6 (mg/d)	Folate (µg/d)[c]	Vitamin B_{12}	Pantothenic Acid	Biotin	Choline (g/d)	Carotenoids[d]
Infants															
0 to 6 mo	600	ND[e]	25	ND	ND	ND	ND	ND	ND	ND	ND	ND	ND	ND	ND
6 to 12 mo	600	ND	38	ND	ND	ND	ND	ND	ND	ND	ND	ND	ND	ND	ND
Children															
1–3 y	600	400	63	200	ND	ND	ND	10	30	300	ND	ND	ND	1.0	ND
4–8 y	900	650	75	300	ND	ND	ND	15	40	400	ND	ND	ND	1.0	ND
Males															
9–13 y	1,700	1,200	100	600	ND	ND	ND	20	60	600	ND	ND	ND	2.0	ND
14–18 y	2,800	1,800	100	800	ND	ND	ND	30	80	800	ND	ND	ND	3.0	ND
19–30 y	3,000	2,000	100	1,000	ND	ND	ND	35	100	1,000	ND	ND	ND	3.5	ND
31–50 y	3,000	2,000	100	1,000	ND	ND	ND	35	100	1,000	ND	ND	ND	3.5	ND
51–70 y	3,000	2,000	100	1,000	ND	ND	ND	35	100	1,000	ND	ND	ND	3.5	ND
>70 y	3,000	2,000	100	1,000	ND	ND	ND	35	100	1,000	ND	ND	ND	3.5	ND
Females															
9–13 y	1,700	1,200	100	600	ND	ND	ND	20	60	600	ND	ND	ND	2.0	ND
14–18 y	2,800	1,800	100	800	ND	ND	ND	30	80	800	ND	ND	ND	3.0	ND
19–30 y	3,000	2,000	100	1,000	ND	ND	ND	35	100	1,000	ND	ND	ND	3.5	ND
31–50 y	3,000	2,000	100	1,000	ND	ND	ND	35	100	1,000	ND	ND	ND	3.5	ND
51–70 y	3,000	2,000	100	1,000	ND	ND	ND	35	100	1,000	ND	ND	ND	3.5	ND
>70 y	3,000	2,000	100	1,000	ND	ND	ND	35	100	1,000	ND	ND	ND	3.5	ND
Pregnancy															
14–18 y	2,800	1,800	100	800	ND	ND	ND	30	80	800	ND	ND	ND	3.0	ND
19–30 y	3,000	2,000	100	1,000	ND	ND	ND	35	100	1,000	ND	ND	ND	3.5	ND
31–50 y	3,000	2,000	100	1,000	ND	ND	ND	35	100	1,000	ND	ND	ND	3.5	ND
Lactation															
14–18 y	2,800	1,800	100	800	ND	ND	ND	30	80	800	ND	ND	ND	3.0	ND
19–30 y	3,000	2,000	100	1,000	ND	ND	ND	35	100	1,000	ND	ND	ND	3.5	ND
31–50 y	3,000	2,000	100	1,000	ND	ND	ND	35	100	1,000	ND	ND	ND	3.5	ND

NOTE: A Tolerable Upper Intake Level (UL) is the highest level of daily nutrient intake that is likely to pose no risk of adverse health effects to almost all individuals in the general population. Unless otherwise specified, the UL represents total intake from food, water, and supplements. Due to a lack of suitable data, ULs could not be established for vitamin K, thiamin, riboflavin, vitamin B_{12}, pantothenic acid, biotin, and carotenoids. In the absence of a UL, extra caution may be warranted in consuming levels above recommended intakes. Members of the general population should be advised not to routinely exceed the UL. The UL is not meant to apply to individuals who are treated with the nutrient under medical supervision or to individuals with predisposing conditions that modify their sensitivity to the nutrient.

[a] As preformed vitamin A only.

[b] As α-tocopherol; applies to any form of supplemental α-tocopherol.

[c] The ULs for vitamin E, niacin, and folate apply to synthetic forms obtained from supplements, fortified foods, or a combination of the two.

[d] β-Carotene supplements are advised only to serve as a provitamin A source for individuals at risk of vitamin A deficiency.

[e] ND = Not determinable due to lack of data of adverse effects in this age group and concern with regard to lack of ability to handle excess amounts. Source of intake should be from food only to prevent high levels of intake.

Sources: *Dietary Reference Intakes for Calcium, Phosphorous, Magnesium, Vitamin D, and Fluoride* (1997); *Dietary Reference Intakes for Thiamin, Riboflavin, Niacin, Vitamin B_6, Folate, Vitamin B_{12}, Pantothenic Acid, Biotin, and Choline* (1998); *Dietary Reference Intakes for Vitamin C, Vitamin E, Selenium, and Carotenoids* (2000); *Dietary Reference Intakes for Vitamin A, Vitamin K, Arsenic, Boron, Chromium, Copper, Iodine, Iron, Manganese, Molybdenum, Nickel, Silicon, Vanadium, and Zinc* (2001); and *Dietary Reference Intakes for Calcium and Vitamin D* (2011). These reports may be accessed via www.nap.edu. Dietary Reference Intakes reprinted with permission of the National Academy of Sciences, courtesy of the National Academies Press, Washington, D.C.

Dietary Reference Intakes (DRIs): Tolerable Upper Intake Levels, Elements
Food and Nutrition Board, Institute of Medicine, National Academies

Life Stage Group	Arsenic[a]	Boron (mg/d)	Calcium (mg/d)	Chromium	Copper (μg/d)	Fluoride (mg/d)	Iodine (μg/d)	Iron (mg/d)	Magnesium (mg/d)[b]	Manganese (mg/d)	Molybdenum (μg/d)	Nickel (mg/d)	Phosphorus (g/d)	Selenium (μg/d)	Silicon[c]	Vanadium (mg/d)[d]	Zinc (mg/d)	Sodium (g/d)	Chloride (g/d)
Infants																			
0 to 6 mo	ND[e]	ND	1,000	ND	ND	0.7	ND	40	ND	ND	ND	ND	ND	45	ND	ND	4	ND	ND
6 to 12 mo	ND	ND	1,500	ND	ND	0.9	ND	40	ND	ND	ND	ND	ND	60	ND	ND	5	ND	ND
Children																			
1–3 y	ND	3	2,500	ND	1,000	1.3	200	40	65	2	300	0.2	3	90	ND	ND	7	1.5	2.3
4–8 y	ND	6	2,500	ND	3,000	2.2	300	40	110	3	600	0.3	3	150	ND	ND	12	1.9	2.9
Males																			
9–13 y	ND	11	3,000	ND	5,000	10	600	40	350	6	1,100	0.6	4	280	ND	ND	23	2.2	3.4
14–18 y	ND	17	3,000	ND	8,000	10	900	45	350	9	1,700	1.0	4	400	ND	ND	34	2.3	3.6
19–30 y	ND	20	2,500	ND	10,000	10	1,100	45	350	11	2,000	1.0	4	400	ND	1.8	40	2.3	3.6
31–50 y	ND	20	2,500	ND	10,000	10	1,100	45	350	11	2,000	1.0	4	400	ND	1.8	40	2.3	3.6
51–70 y	ND	20	2,000	ND	10,000	10	1,100	45	350	11	2,000	1.0	4	400	ND	1.8	40	2.3	3.6
>70 y	ND	20	2,000	ND	10,000	10	1,100	45	350	11	2,000	1.0	3	400	ND	1.8	40	2.3	3.6
Females																			
9–13 y	ND	11	3,000	ND	5,000	10	600	40	350	6	1,100	0.6	4	280	ND	ND	23	2.2	3.4
14–18 y	ND	17	3,000	ND	8,000	10	900	45	350	9	1,700	1.0	4	400	ND	ND	34	2.3	3.6
19–30 y	ND	20	2,500	ND	10,000	10	1,100	45	350	11	2,000	1.0	4	400	ND	1.8	40	2.3	3.6
31–50 y	ND	20	2,500	ND	10,000	10	1,100	45	350	11	2,000	1.0	4	400	ND	1.8	40	2.3	3.6
51–70 y	ND	20	2,000	ND	10,000	10	1,100	45	350	11	2,000	1.0	4	400	ND	1.8	40	2.3	3.6
>70 y	ND	20	2,000	ND	10,000	10	1,100	45	350	11	2,000	1.0	3	400	ND	1.8	40	2.3	3.6
Pregnancy																			
14–18 y	ND	17	3,000	ND	8,000	10	900	45	350	9	1,700	1.0	3.5	400	ND	ND	34	2.3	3.6
19–30 y	ND	20	2,500	ND	10,000	10	1,100	45	350	11	2,000	1.0	3.5	400	ND	ND	40	2.3	3.6
31–50 y	ND	20	2,500	ND	10,000	10	1,100	45	350	11	2,000	1.0	3.5	400	ND	ND	40	2.3	3.6
Lactation																			
14–18 y	ND	17	3,000	ND	8,000	10	900	45	350	9	1,700	1.0	4	400	ND	ND	34	2.3	3.6
19–30 y	ND	20	2,500	ND	10,000	10	1,100	45	350	11	2,000	1.0	4	400	ND	ND	40	2.3	3.6
31–50 y	ND	20	2,500	ND	10,000	10	1,100	45	350	11	2,000	1.0	4	400	ND	ND	40	2.3	3.6

NOTE: A Tolerable Upper Intake Level (UL) is the highest level of daily nutrient intake that is likely to pose no risk of adverse health effects to almost all individuals in the general population. Unless otherwise specified, the UL represents total intake from food, water, and supplements. Due to a lack of suitable data, ULs could not be established for vitamin K, thiamin, riboflavin, vitamin B$_{12}$, pantothenic acid, biotin, and carotenoids. In the absence of a UL, extra caution may be warranted in consuming levels above recommended intakes. Members of the general population should be advised not to routinely exceed the UL. The UL is not meant to apply to individuals who are treated with the nutrient under medical supervision or to individuals with predisposing conditions that modify their sensitivity to the nutrient.

[a] Although the UL was not determined for arsenic, there is no justification for adding arsenic to food or supplements.

[b] The ULs for magnesium represent intake from a pharmacological agent only and do not include intake from food and water.

[c] Although silicon has not been shown to cause adverse effects in humans, there is no justification for adding silicon to supplements.

[d] Although vanadium in food has not been shown to cause adverse effects in humans, there is no justification for adding vanadium to food and vanadium supplements should be used with caution. The UL is based on adverse effects in laboratory animals and this data could be used to set a UL for adults but not children and adolescents.

[e] ND = Not determinable due to lack of data of adverse effects in this age group and concern with regard to lack of ability to handle excess amounts. Source of intake should be from food only to prevent high levels of intake.

Sources: Dietary Reference Intakes for Calcium, Phosphorous, Magnesium, Vitamin D, and Fluoride (1997); Dietary Reference Intakes for Thiamin, Riboflavin, Niacin, Vitamin B$_6$, Folate, Vitamin B$_{12}$, Pantothenic Acid, Biotin, and Choline (1998); Dietary Reference Intakes for Vitamin C, Vitamin E, Selenium, and Carotenoids (2000); Dietary Reference Intakes for Vitamin A, Vitamin K, Arsenic, Boron, Chromium, Copper, Iodine, Iron, Manganese, Molybdenum, Nickel, Silicon, Vanadium, and Zinc (2001); Dietary Reference Intakes for Water, Potassium, Sodium, Chloride, and Sulfate (2005); and Dietary Reference Intakes for Calcium and Vitamin D (2011). These reports may be accessed via www.nap.edu. Dietary Reference Intakes reprinted with permission of the National Academy of Sciences, courtesy of the National Academies Press, Washington, D.C.

BMI: What Does It Mean?

Body mass index (BMI) is a useful tool that can be used to estimate an individual's body weight status in relation to health risk. *See chapter 2 for an explanation of BMI and to find your adult BMI.*

The terms "overweight" and "obese" describe weight ranges that are greater that what is considered healthy for a given height, while "underweight" describes a weight that is lower than what is considered healthy for a given height. These categories are a guide, and some people at a healthy weight also may have weight-responsive health conditions. Those with higher BMIs may have a higher composition of muscle, which accounts for added weight. Adult BMI can be calculated at www.nhlbisupport.com/bmi.

Body mass index (BMI) charts for adults are *not* meant for children and teens. For that reason, growth charts, using BMIs *and* percentiles, were developed by the Centers for Disease Control and Prevention for girls and boys ages two to twenty, to track their growth based on BMI.

BMI/growth charts *are not* meant to diagnose a child's or a teen's weight status. BMI is, however, a reliable indicator of body fatness for most children and teens; it does not measure body fat. Because children and adolescents are growing, their BMI is plotted on growth charts for their gender and age. Their weight changes as they grow, even month by month. The percentile indicates the relative position of the child's BMI among children of the same gender and age. (A child and adolescent BMI calculator is available at apps.nccd.cdc.gov/dnpabmi). Healthcare professionals use these charts to track a child's or a teen's growth over time; your healthcare professional should determine if your child has a weight problem and what action to take, if any, by considering many factors, not just BMI.

Category	Children and Adolescents (BMI for age percentile range)	Adults (BMI)
Underweight	Less than the 5th percentile	Less than 18.5 kg/m²
Healthy weight	5th percentile to less than the 85th percentile	18.5 to 24.9 kg/m²
Overweight	85th percentile to less than the 95th percentile	25.0 to 29.9 kg/m²
Obese	Equal to or greater than the 95th percentile	30.0 kg/m² or greater

Source: Dietary Guidelines for Americans, 2010.

CDC Growth Charts

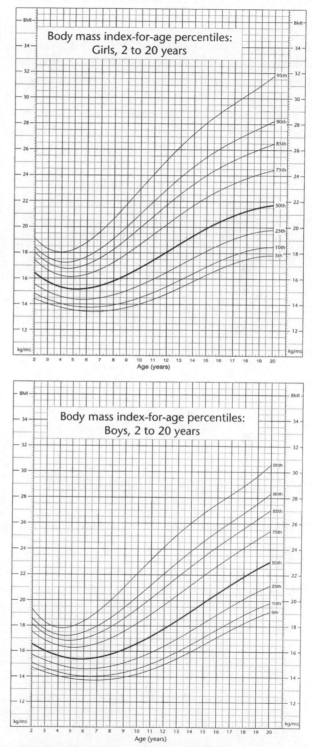

Source: Centers for Disease Control and Prevention, National Center for Health Statistics, CDC 2000 Growth Charts: United States. www.cdc.gov/growthcharts. Accessed June 16, 2011.

% Daily Values: What Are They Based On?

The % Daily Values (% DV) on food and supplement labels are considered average nutrient levels, not necessarily your specific nutrient needs. You may need more or less.

For daily nutrient recommendations specific to your age and gender, see the Dietary Reference Intakes (DRIs)—*shown elsewhere in the appendices and explained in chapter 1.*

The following values are for adults and children ages four and older. Protein levels are different for infants under a year (14 grams); children one to four years (16 grams); pregnant women (60 grams); and nursing mothers (65 grams).

NUTRIENT/FOOD COMPONENT	100% DV IS EQUAL TO THIS AMOUNT
Total fat	65 g*
Saturated fat	20 g*
Cholesterol	300 mg
Sodium	2,400 mg
Potassium	3,500 mg
Total carbohydrate	300 g*

NUTRIENT/FOOD COMPONENT	100% DV IS EQUAL TO THIS AMOUNT
Dietary fiber	25 g†
Protein	50 g*
Vitamin A	5,000 IU
Vitamin C	60 mg
Calcium	1,000 mg
Iron	18 mg
Thiamin	1.5 mg
Riboflavin	1.7 mg
Niacin	20 mg
Vitamin D	400 IU
Vitamin E	30 IU
Vitamin B_6	2 mg
Folate	400 mcg
Vitamin B_{12}	6 mcg
Biotin	300 mcg
Pantothenic acid	10 mg
Phosphorus	1,000 mg
Iodine	150 mcg
Magnesium	400 mg
Zinc	15 mg
Copper	2 mg

*Based on a 2,000-calorie reference diet.
†Based on 11.5 grams per 1,100 calories.

Health Claims on Food Labels

HEALTH CLAIMS ON FOOD LABELS	HOW IT MIGHT APPEAR ON THE LABEL
Calcium and osteoporosis	Adequate calcium as part of a healthful diet, along with physical activity, may reduce the risk of osteoporosis in later life.
Calcium, vitamin D, and osteoporosis	Adequate calcium and vitamin D throughout life, as part of a well-balanced diet, may reduce the risk of osteoporosis.
Sodium and hypertension	Diets low in sodium may reduce the risk of high blood pressure, a disease associated with many factors.
Dietary fat and cancer	Development of cancer depends on many factors. A diet low in total fat may reduce the risk of some cancers.
Saturated fat and cholesterol and the risk of coronary heart disease	While many factors affect heart disease, diets low in saturated fat and cholesterol may reduce the risk of this disease.
Fiber-containing grain products, fruits, and vegetables, and cancer	Low-fat diets rich in fiber-containing grain products, fruits, and vegetables may reduce the risk of some types of cancer, a disease associated with many factors.

HEALTH CLAIMS ON FOOD LABELS *(continued)*

HEALTH CLAIMS ON FOOD LABELS	HOW IT MIGHT APPEAR ON THE LABEL
Fruits, vegetables, and grain products that contain fiber, particularly soluble fiber, and their risk of coronary heart disease	Diets low in saturated fat and cholesterol and rich in fruits, vegetables, and grain products that contain some types of dietary fiber, particularly soluble fiber, may reduce the risk of heart disease, a disease associated with many factors.
Fruits and vegetables and cancer	Low-fat diets rich in fruits and vegetables (foods that are low in fat and may contain dietary fiber, vitamin A, or vitamin C) may reduce the risk of some types of cancer, a disease associated with many factors. Broccoli is high in vitamins A and C, and it is a good source of dietary fiber.
Folate and neural tube defects	Healthful diets with adequate folate may reduce a woman's risk of having a child with a brain or spinal cord defect.
Sugar alcohol and dental caries	*Full claim:* Frequent between-meal consumption of foods high in sugars and starches promotes tooth decay. The sugar alcohols in [name of food] do not promote tooth decay. *Shortened claim* (on small packages): Does not promote tooth decay.
Soluble fiber from certain foods and the risk of coronary heart disease	Soluble fiber from foods such as [name of soluble fiber source], as part of a diet low in saturated fat and cholesterol, may reduce the risk of heart disease. A serving of [food name] supplies _____ grams of the [necessary daily dietary intake for the benefit] soluble fiber from [name of soluble-fiber source] necessary per day to have this effect.
Soy protein and risk of coronary heart disease	1. 25 grams of soy protein a day, as part of a diet low in saturated fat and cholesterol, may reduce the risk of heart disease. A serving of [food name] supplies _____ grams of soy protein. 2. Diets low in saturated fat and cholesterol that include 25 grams of soy protein a day may reduce the risk of heart disease. One serving of [food name] provides _____ grams of soy protein.
Plant sterol/stanol esters and risk of coronary heart disease (interim health claim)	1. Foods containing at least 0.65 gram per serving of vegetable oil sterol esters, eaten twice a day with meals for a daily total intake of at least 1.3 grams, as part of a diet low in saturated fat and cholesterol, may reduce the risk of heart disease. A serving of [food name] supplies _____ grams of vegetable oil sterol esters. 2. Diets low in saturated fat and cholesterol that include two servings of foods that provide a daily total of at least 3.4 grams of plant stanol esters in two meals may reduce the risk of heart disease. A serving of [food name] supplies _____ grams of plant stanol esters.
Whole-grain foods and risk of heart disease and certain cancers	*Required wording:* Diets rich in whole grain foods and other plant foods and low in total fat, saturated fat, and cholesterol may reduce the risk of heart disease and some cancers.
Potassium and the risk of high blood pressure and stroke	*Required wording:* Diets containing foods that are a good source of potassium and that are low in sodium may reduce the risk of high blood pressure and stroke.
Fluoridated water and reduced risk of dental caries	*Required wording:* Drinking fluoridated water may reduce the risk of [dental caries or tooth decay].
Saturated fat, cholesterol, and *trans* fat, and reduced risk of heart disease	*Required wording:* Diets low in saturated fat and cholesterol, and as low as possible in *trans* fat, may reduce the risk of heart disease.

For definitions of terms such as "low," "rich," and "high," see "Label Lingo" in chapters 2, 3, 4, 5, 6, 7, and 12.

Source: Guidance for Industry: A Food Labeling Guide, Appendix C Health Claims (Washington, D.C., Office of Nutritional Products, Labeling, and Dietary Supplements, Center for Food Safety and Applied Nutrition, U.S. Food and Drug Administration). FDA-approved qualified health claims appear in Appendix D Qualified Health Claims. Accessed November 2011.

Index